Review of PHARMACOLOGY

Review of PHARMACOLOGY

Sixteenth Edition

Gobind Rai Garg MBBS MD (Gold Medalist)
Director
Ayush Institute of Medical Sciences
New Delhi, India
Pioneer in Development of Mobile Application
'Pharmacology' by 'Dr Gobind Rai Garg'

Sparsh Gupta MBBS MD (Gold Medalist)
Associate Professor (Pharmacology)
VMMC and Safdarjung Hospital, New Delhi, India
Topper of UPSC (Teaching Specialist, Pharmacology)

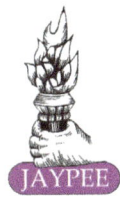

JAYPEE BROTHERS MEDICAL PUBLISHERS
The Health Sciences Publisher
New Delhi | London

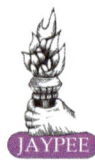 **Jaypee Brothers Medical Publishers (P) Ltd**

Headquarters
Jaypee Brothers Medical Publishers (P) Ltd
EMCA House, 23/23-B
Ansari Road, Daryaganj
New Delhi 110 002, India
Landline: +91-11-23272143, +91-11-23272703
+91-11-23282021, +91-11-23245672
Email: jaypee@jaypeebrothers.com

Corporate Office
Jaypee Brothers Medical Publishers (P) Ltd
4838/24, Ansari Road, Daryaganj
New Delhi 110 002, India
Phone: +91-11-43574357
Fax: +91-11-43574314
Email: jaypee@jaypeebrothers.com

Overseas Office
J.P. Medical Ltd
83 Victoria Street, London
SW1H 0HW (UK)
Phone: +44 20 3170 8910
Fax: +44 (0)20 3008 6180
Email: info@jpmedpub.com

Website: www.jaypeebrothers.com
Website: www.jaypeedigital.com

© 2022, Gobind Rai Garg and Sparsh Gupta

The views and opinions expressed in this book are solely those of the original contributor(s)/author(s) and do not necessarily represent those of editor(s) or publisher of the book.

All rights reserved. No part of this publication may be reproduced, stored or transmitted in any form or by any means, electronic, mechanical, photocopying, recording or otherwise, without the prior permission in writing of the publishers.

All brand names and product names used in this book are trade names, service marks, trademarks or registered trademarks of their respective owners. The publisher is not associated with any product or vendor mentioned in this book.

Medical knowledge and practice change constantly. This book is designed to provide accurate, authoritative information about the subject matter in question. However, readers are advised to check the most current information available on procedures included and check information from the manufacturer of each product to be administered, to verify the recommended dose, formula, method and duration of administration, adverse effects and contraindications. It is the responsibility of the practitioner to take all appropriate safety precautions. Neither the publisher nor the author(s)/editor(s) assume any liability for any injury and/or damage to persons or property arising from or related to use of material in this book.

This book is sold on the understanding that the publisher is not engaged in providing professional medical services. If such advice or services are required, the services of a competent medical professional should be sought.

Every effort has been made where necessary to contact holders of copyright to obtain permission to reproduce copyright material. If any have been inadvertently overlooked, the publisher will be pleased to make the necessary arrangements at the first opportunity. The **CD/DVD-ROM** (if any) provided in the sealed envelope with this book is complimentary and free of cost. **Not meant for sale.**

Inquiries for bulk sales may be solicited at: jaypee@jaypeebrothers.com

Review of Pharmacology

Ninth Edition: 2015,	Tenth Edition: 2016	Eleventh Edition: 2017	Twelfth Edition: 2018
Thirteenth Edition: 2019	Fourteenth Edition: 2020	Fifteenth Edition: 2021	

Sixteenth Edition: 2022

ISBN: 978-93-5465-877-8

Dedicated to

My parents, wife Praveen and sweetheart kids Ayush and Samaira

—Gobind Rai Garg

My family members and my teachers (Shri SK Suri and Ms V Gopalan)

—Sparsh Gupta

GRATITUDE

Life seemed oblivious and dark
Full of dreadful pills
Bombastic names
Giving jitters and chills.

When everything seemed hazy
Someone wiped my glasses
And suggested me to join
Dr GRG's classes.

Had heard about him a lot
Still had apprehensions in mind
But on meeting him personally
Found him very humble and kind

He masters his subject
And teaches with a flair
His wonderful mnemonics
Leave you amazed to stare.

He's hardworking, he's laborious
An entrepreneur in Pharmacology
Always upgrading and improving
With the pace of technology.

Students are his priority
He's an epitome of amiability
Always approachable
To the best of his capabilities.

I feel a dearth of words
To express my gratitude
Indebted to him deeply
In great great magnitude.

My best wishes to you Sir
May you succeed all the way
And reach the heights of glory
Is all that I can say.

Kanav Khanna
MAMC

दूर अन्धकार कर चलो

गिरो, पड़ो, सम्भलो, फिर तेज रफ़्तार कर चलो।
मुट्ठी का विस्तार कर मुट्ठी में संसार कर चलो।।

रब ने बनाया है तुम्हें तुम दुनिया में खास हो।
खुद को संवारकर खुद से अनंत प्यार कर चलो।।

कायरता, घबराहट, कपट, हार का डर क्यों।
आत्मबल से अपनी कमियों पर प्रहार कर चलो।।

तुम ही जीतोगे बेफिक्र होकर कूद पड़ो मैदान में।
वक्त के हमलों के लिए खुद को तैयार कर चलो।।

नयी सुबह, नया सूरज, नयी किरणें होंगे 'पीयूष'
फ़िलहाल दीप बनकर जल उठो दूर अन्धकार कर चलो...

Piyush Shukla

Preface to the Sixteenth Edition

We want to thank all the readers for the overwhelming response and great appreciation of the earlier editions of this book. To meet the expectations of students, we have tried to further improve this new edition.

To meet the constant demand of the students, Dr Gobind Rai Garg has launched his mobile Application 'Pharmacology by Dr Gobind Rai Garg' which is available on both Play store and Apple store. Video lectures of entire Pharmacology are provided in this App along with many other features.

Cracking the 'National Eligibility-cum-Entrance Test (NEET)' and other important PG entrance examinations require a thorough knowledge and understanding of the subject. *Readers of this book have got an edge over others* because of strong theory and conceptual questions. This along with the key points given under the headings of various boxes in the chapters has helped many students to get extremely good ranks in various PG external examinations. We have added golden points at the end of theory of each chapter. Apart from this, **'high yield points' are given separately as boxes in the text.** Boxes are labeled as Key Points for key points, 𝑛 for new drugs and ⚠ Mnemonic for mnemonics. However, we will recommend students to read the theory of each topic thoroughly, which is must. The questions have been asked as one-liners in last year which may not be the case next year and further in AIIMS and PGI exams you need to be well-versed with the theory. Therefore, we will re-emphasize that there is no substitution of knowledge. If you know the subject thoroughly, you can answer any type of question.

In our constant endeavour to improvise the book, we have fully colored the book and added large number of images to make the learning easier and interesting. There has been incorporation of important additions in almost all chapters. For quick revision, we have added 'Golden points' and 'Drug of Choice' sections in every chapter. **Annexures** have been added on 'History of Pharmacology', 'Teratogenic Drugs' 'Drug of Choice' and Special INI-CET Pattern Questions.

In this new edition, we have added a lot of mnemonics, diagrams and flowcharts to make learning interesting and easier. The question bank of every chapter has been divided into subtopics. It will help students to solve MCQs after reading the theory of a particular topic of a chapter. The section of Image Based Questions has been greatly enhanced to incorporate around 100 such questions. These images have been added chapter-wise to retain concepts for longer period.

Recently, in several entrance exams, numerical questions are being asked. To help students to prepare thoroughly for such type of questions, several numerical questions with explanations have been incorporated in the chapter of General Pharmacology.

New topics like 'COVID-19' and 'Anti-smoking Drugs' have been included as per the requirement.

Questions from latest entrance examinations of INI-CET and NEET pattern have been added.

To make the contents of the book more authentic, we have provided appropriate *references* to all the explanations.

In some topics, there are contradictions between different books. In such a situation, we have quoted the text from Harrison's Principles of Internal Medicine, 21st edition.

To help the students understand the Pharmacology in an easy and interesting way, Dr Gobind Rai Garg has started his own institute named 'Ayush Institute of Medical Sciences'. It is the only institute which is meant for teaching Pharmacology only. Dr Gobind Rai Garg himself conducts separate classes for MBBS students and those preparing for PG entrance examinations at Delhi and Hyderabad. For details, you can contact on the www.drgobindraigarg.com/classes.

We must admit hereby that despite keeping an eagle's eye for any inaccuracy regarding factual information or typographical errors, some mistakes must have crept in inadvertently. You are requested to communicate these errors and send your valuable suggestions for the improvement of this book. Your suggestions, appreciation and criticism are most welcome.

Gobind Rai Garg
Sparsh Gupta
E-mail: *gobind_garg@yahoo.co.in*
healing_sparsh@yahoo.co.in

Preface to the First Edition

Pharmacology is one of the most difficult and at the same time most important subject in various postgraduate entrance examinations.

As we experienced it ourselves, most of the students preparing for postgraduate entrance examinations are in a dilemma, whether to study antegrade or retrograde. Antegrade study takes a lot of time and due to bulky textbooks, some important questions are likely to be missed. In a retrograde study, the students are likely to answer the frequently asked MCQs but new questions are not covered. We have tried to overcome the shortcomings of both of the methods while keeping the advantages intact.

In this book, we have given a concise and enriched text in each chapter followed by MCQs from various postgraduate entrance examinations and other important questions likely to come. The text provides the advantage of antegrade study in a short span of time.

After going through the book, it will be easier for the student to solve the questions of most recent examinations, which are given at the end of the book.

More and more questions about new drugs are being asked in the entrance examinations nowadays. These NEW DRUGS have been covered along with the text and a separate chapter has been added at the end. Salient features of the new drugs along with the reference in the text have been included in this chapter.

Recently, the questions are being asked from SOME EMERGING TOPICS like anti-obesity drugs, anti-smoking drugs, drugs for erectile dysfunction and nitric oxide. All these topics have been discussed in a separate chapter.

Large number of questions about first choice drugs is being incorporated in the entrance examinations. To cover these questions, a separate chapter entitled "DRUGS OF CHOICE" has been added.

Important ADVERSE EFFECTS caused by drugs have also been included.

It is very difficult and at times very confusing to remember large number of drugs and adverse effects. To make learning easy, several easy to grasp MNEMONICS have been given throughout the text.

Despite our best efforts, some mistakes might have crept in, which we request all our readers to kindly bring to our notice. Your suggestions, appreciation and criticism are most welcome.

Gobind Rai Garg
Sparsh Gupta
E-mail: *gobind_garg@yahoo.co.in*
healing_sparsh@yahoo.co.in

Acknowledgments

When emotions are profound, words sometimes are not sufficient to express our thanks and gratitude. With these few words, we would like to thank our teachers at University College of Medical Sciences and Guru Teg Bahadur Hospital, Delhi, for the foundation they helped to lay in shaping our careers.

We are especially thankful to **Dr KK Sharma,** Ex-Professor and Head, Department of Pharmacology, UCMS, who is a father figure to whole of the department.

We would also like to acknowledge the encouragement and guidance of **Dr CD Tripathi (Ex-Director-Professor and Head, VMMC), Dr Veena Verma (Director Professor and HOD, VMMC), Dr SK Bhattacharya (Professor and Head, NDMC Medical College and Hindu Rao Hospital), Dr Uma Tekur (Director-Professor, MAMC), Col Dr AG Mathur (Professor and Head, ACMS), Dr Vandana Roy (Director-Professor and Head, MAMC) and Dr Shalini Chawla (Professor, MAMC),** all in the department of Pharmacology, in the completion of this book.

We feel immense pleasure in conveying our sincere thanks to all the residents of department of Pharmacology at MAMC and UCMS for their indispensable help and support.

No words can describe the immense contribution of our family members, Ms Praveen Garg, Ms Ruhee, Ms Anju, Mr Rohit Singla, Mrs Komal Singla, Mr Nitin Misra and Ms Dhwani Gupta, without whose support this book could not have seen the light of the day.

Although it is impossible to acknowledge the contribution of all individuals, we extend our heartfelt thanks to:

- Kanav Khanna (MAMC)
- Mili Rohilla (MAMC)
- Alfa Saifi (MAMC)
- Dr Sapna Pradhan, Associate Professor (Pharmacology), ACMS, Delhi
- Cheshta Sachdeva (VMMC)
- Sukirat Singh Bhatia (VMMC)
- Govinda Bhagat (MAMC)
- Dr Bhupinder Singh Kalra, Associate Professor (Pharmacology), MAMC, Delhi
- Lt Col (Dr) Sushil Sharma, Associate Professor (Pharmacology), AFMC, Pune
- Lt Col (Dr) Dick BS Brashier, Associate Professor (Pharmacology), AFMC, Pune
- Dr Nitin Jain, DCH, DNB (Pediatrics), Delhi
- Dr Sushant Verma, MS (General Surgery), MAMC, Delhi
- Dr Kapil Dev Mehta, MD (Pharmacology), UCMS, Delhi
- Dr Saurabh Arya, MD (Pharmacology), UCMS, Delhi
- Dr Deepak Marwah, MD (Pediatrics), MAMC, Delhi
- Dr Puneet Dwivedi (DA), Hindu Rao Hospital, Delhi
- Dr Sandeep Agnihotri, DVD, Safdarjang Hospital, Delhi
- Dr Harsh Vardhan Gupta MD, Pediatrics, Patiala
- Mr Tarsem Garg, LLB, DM, SBOP
- Ram Gopal Garg (IAS, CBI, Delhi)
- Taral Garg (MBBS, Baba Farid University, Faridkot)
- Dr Pardeep Bansal, MD (Radiodiagnosis), UCMS, Delhi
- Dr Pankaj Bansal, MS (Orthopedics), RML Hospital, Delhi
- Dr Pradeep Goyal, MD (Radiodiagnosis), LHMC, Delhi
- Dr Rakesh Mittal, MS (Surgery), Safdarjung Hospital, Delhi
- Dr Amit Miglani, DM (Gastroenterology), PGI, Chandigarh
- Dr Sachin Gupta DA, DMC (Ludhiana)
- Dr Reenu Gupta DGO BMC (Bengaluru)
- Dr Shiv Narayan Goel, MCh (Urology), KEM, Mumbai

- Dr Anurag Aggarwal (DA, MD Anesthesia, MAMC)
- Dr Kamal Jindal, MD (Physiology), LHMC, Delhi
- Dr Gaurav Jindal, MD (Radiodiagnosis), Resident, Boston, USA
- Dr Saket Kant, MD (Medicine, UCMS), DM (Endocrinology, BHU)
- Dr Mukesh Kr Joon, DM (Cardiology), Udaipur, Rajasthan
- Dr Sonal Pruthi, UCMS, Delhi
- Dr DJ Mohanty, Lecturer, MS (Surgery), UCMS, Delhi
- Dr Amit Garg, MD (Psychiatry), GB Pant Hospital, Delhi
- Dr Ravi Gupta, MD (Psychiatry), GTB Hospital, Delhi
- Dr Shashank Mohanty, MD (Medicine), Udaipur, Rajasthan
- Dr Amit Shersia, MS (Orthopedics), MAMC, Delhi
- Dr Mohit Gupta, DCP, DNB (Pathology), Delhi
- Dr Mayank Dhamija, DCH, DNB (Pediatrics), DNB (Hemato-oncology), Delhi
- Dr Nitin Kumar, NDMC Medical College and Hindu Rao Hospital, Delhi

Last but not least, we would like to thank Shri Jitendar P Vij (Group Chairman), Mr Ankit Vij (Managing Director) Ms Chetna Malhotra (Senior Director – Professional Publishing, Marketing and Business Development) of M/s Jaypee Brothers Medical Publishers (P) Ltd, New Delhi, India, publishers of this book and the entire PGMEE team for their keen interest, innovative suggestions and hardwork in bringing out this edition.

Gobind Rai Garg
Sparsh Gupta

From the Publisher's Desk
We request all the readers to provide us their valuable suggestions/errors (if any)
at: jppgmee@gmail.com
so as to help us in further improvement of this book in the subsequent edition.

References

- **Harrison's** Principles of Internal Medicine, 21st edition
- **Goodman and Gilman's** The Pharmacological Basis of Therapeutics, 13th edition
- **Katzung's** Basic and Clinical Pharmacology, 13th edition
- **HL Sharma and KK Sharma's** Principles of Pharmacology, 2nd edition
- **KD Tripathi's** Essentials of Medical Pharmacology, 8th edition
- **Current Medical Diagnosis and Treatment 2019.**

SYMBOLS USED IN BOXES ON 'HIGH YIELD POINTS'

- Key Points — Key points
- Mnemonic — Mnemonic
- n — New drug
- Controversial question

Unique Features of this Edition

- Fully colored edition
- Special AIIMS pattern questions added
- Plenty of eye-catching images to help aid visual memory
- A separate chapter on Numerical questions with explanations
- New NBE-based pattern (wider coverage and concept development)
- Large NUMBER OF IMAGE BASED QUESTIONS WITH EXPLANATIONS
- Solved MCQs including all recent questions (2022 to 2010)
- Golden points in every chapter
- Recent developments given in every chapter
- Separate annexure of 'New FDA approved drugs
- Mnemonics to remember high yield points regarding new drugs.
- Annexure of 'Drug of Choice' for different conditions
- Chapter-wise concise yet complete text
- Advantage of both antegrade as well as retrograde study
- Doubt solving via telegram group https://t.me/joinchat/CrZcgUJhyP6SJkkPA04Z0A
- Large number of easy to grasp mnemonics
- Authentic and complete question base of various years with latest reframes and explanations of AIIMS, PGI, DNB and NEET pattern examinations.

How to Use this Book

1. **FOR SECOND PROF STUDENTS:**
   It is preferable to begin reading this book during your second year MBBS to build your basics right from the beginning.

   Read the theory of a chapter from this book and then read the textbook. You will be able to easily understand the textbook now.

   Now read the theory of that chapter once again.

   Now solve the MCQs from the book.

   Follow this with another reading from the textbook.
   - This completes your chapter with one reading and revision.
   - While reading the book, either make notes or mark in the book itself for quick revision. Mark the difficult and important MCQ for further revision.
   - Do this for all the chapters.
   - After completing the syllabus, start revising.
   - Remember minimum 4-5 readings are required as Pharmacology is a volatile subject.

2. **FOR STUDENTS WHO HAVE PASSED SECOND PROF (FINAL YEAR STUDENTS, INTERNS AND POST-INTERNS):**
   - We do not recommend studying textbook now due to paucity of time. However, textbook should be kept as a reference material.
   - Do not confuse yourself by studying many books.
   - No other study material is required for entrance exams apart from this book.
   - You should spend 10-15 days for Pharmacology for first reading.

   Read the theory of a chapter and solve MCQs of that chapter. While solving MCQs, solve minimum 50-100 questions at a stretch and only after this compare the answers.

   Re-read the theory of this chapter and now mark the important points for revision. Remember, you should mark only that much so that the next reading of book can be finished in one third of the time. Similarly, encircle or mark the important MCQ for revision.

   Do same for all the chapters.

   During revision, study only marked portion with encircled MCQ only. Second reading should be finished in 4-5 days.

   Similarly third and fourth revision should be completed in 3 days each.

   Give one last revision just before exams in a day or two.
   - Remember, Pharmacology is a very important subject. You can answer nearly 35-40 questions in NEET from this book as it covers not only Pharmacology but many related subjects.

Best wishes

Contents

1. **General Pharmacology** ★★★ 1
   Chapter Review 1
   Golden Points 15
   Image Based Questions 16
   Explanations 20
   Multiple Choice Questions 21
   Explanations 31
   Numerical Questions 41
   Answers 43

2. **Autonomic Nervous System** ★★ 46
   Chapter Review 46
   Golden Points 60
   Drug of Choice 61
   Image Based Questions 62
   Explanations 65
   Multiple Choice Questions 67
   Explanations 77

3. **Autacoids** ★★ 86
   Chapter Review 86
   Golden Points 95
   Drug of Choice 96
   Image Based Questions 97
   Explanations 98
   Multiple Choice Questions 99
   Explanations 104

4. **Cardiovascular System** ★★★ 108
   Chapter Review 108
   Golden Points 129
   Drug of Choice 131
   Image Based Questions 132
   Explanations 137
   Multiple Choice Questions 138
   Explanations 147

5. **Kidney** ★ 153
   Chapter Review 153
   Golden Points 158
   Drug of Choice 159
   Image Based Questions 160
   Explanations 160
   Multiple Choice Questions 161
   Explanations 164

6. **Endocrinology** ★★★ 166
   Chapter Review 166
   Golden Points 186
   Drug of Choice 187
   Image Based Questions 188
   Explanations 192
   Multiple Choice Questions 193
   Explanations 204

7. **Central Nervous System**★★★ 212
    Chapter Review 212
    Golden Points 232
    Drug of Choice 233
    Image Based Questions 234
    Explanations 235
    Multiple Choice Questions 236
    Explanations 249

8. **Anaesthesia**★★ 258
    Chapter Review 258
    Golden Points 268
    Drug of Choice 269
    Image Based Questions 270
    Explanations 272
    Multiple Choice Questions 273
    Explanations 278

9. **Hematology**★★★ 283
    Chapter Review 283
    Golden Points 292
    Drug of Choice 293
    Image Based Questions 294
    Explanations 295
    Multiple Choice Questions 296
    Explanations 302

10. **Respiratory System**★ 306
    Chapter Review 306
    Golden Points 311
    Drug of Choice 312
    Image Based Questions 313
    Explanations 314
    Multiple Choice Questions 315
    Explanations 318

11. **Gastrointestinal Tract**★ 320
    Chapter Review 320
    Golden Points 327
    Drug of Choice 328
    Image Based Questions 329
    Explanations 329
    Multiple Choice Questions 330
    Explanations 334

12. **Chemotherapy A: General Considerations and Non-specific Antimicrobial Agents**★★ 337
    Chapter Review 337
    Golden Points 355
    Image Based Questions 356
    Explanations 358
    Multiple Choice Questions 359
    Explanations 370

13. **Chemotherapy B: Antimicrobials for Specific Conditions**★★★ 379
    Chapter Review 379
    Golden Points 397
    Drug of Choice 398
    Image Based Questions 400
    Explanations 401
    Multiple Choice Questions 402
    Explanations 414

Contents

14. Chemotherapy C: Antineoplastic Drugs ★★ 423
    Chapter Review 423
    Golden Points 437
    Image Based Questions 438
    Explanations 439
    Multiple Choice Questions 440
    Explanations 445

15. Immunomodulators ★★ 449
    Chapter Review 449
    Drug of Choice 455
    Image Based Question 456
    Explanation 456
    Multiple Choice Questions 457
    Explanations 460

16. Miscellaneous Topics ★ 462
    Chapter Review 462
    Multiple Choice Questions 468
    Explanations 471

17. New Drugs with Mnemonics ★ 475

Latest Papers ★★★ 494
    INI CET May, 2022 494
    Explanations 497
    INI CET November, 2021 500
    Explanations 502
    INI CET July, 2021 505
    Explanations 507
    NEET PG May, 2022 510
    Explanations 512
    NEET PG 2021 515
    Explanations 517

Annexures 519
    Annexure I: History of Pharmacology 521
    Annexure II: Drugs of Choice 523
    Annexure III: Important Human Teratogenic Drugs 527
    Annexure IV: Special INI-CET Pattern Questions 528

Most Important ★★★
Very Important ★★
Important ★

CHAPTER 1

General Pharmacology

Pharmacology (Greek pharmakon; means drug) is a science dealing with the drugs. It is divided into several branches like *pharmacokinetics, pharmacodynamics, pharmacotherapeutics, chemotherapy and toxicology* etc.

When a drug is administered to a person, it will exert some effect on the patient (*Pharmacodynamics*) and the patient's body will have some effect on the drug (*Pharmacokinetics*). These are the two major branches of pharmacology. Before discussing about these branches, we will summarize, the various routes by which drugs can be administered to a patient.

ROUTES OF DRUG ADMINISTRATION

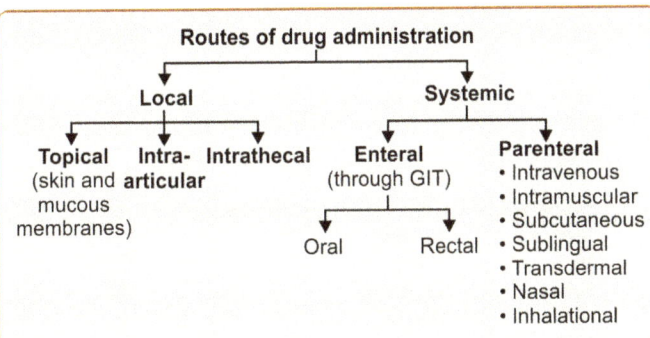

Local Routes include topical application on the skin and mucous membranes as well as the routes like intra-articular (e.g. hydrocortisone) and intrathecal (e.g. amphotericin B).

Absorption of a drug from topical route depends upon thickness of skin. It is generally inversaly proportional to thickness. The sequence of extent of absorption is

Posterior auricular > Scrotal > Scalp > Dorsum of hand > Plantar area

Systemic Routes may be divided into enteral and parenteral routes.

Enteral routes: These include oral and rectal routes:
- **Oral route** is safer and economical but several drugs are not effective by this route because of *high first pass metabolism* in the liver and intestinal wall (e.g. *nitrates, lignocaine, propranolol, pethidine*).
- **Rectal route** avoids first pass metabolism to 50% extent. *Diazepam* is given by this route in children for febrile seizures.

Parenteral routes: These may be injectable or non-injectable.
- **Injectable routes** include intravenous, intramuscular, subcutaneous and intradermal. Angles at which injection should be administered for these routes is shown in the **Figure 1.1**.

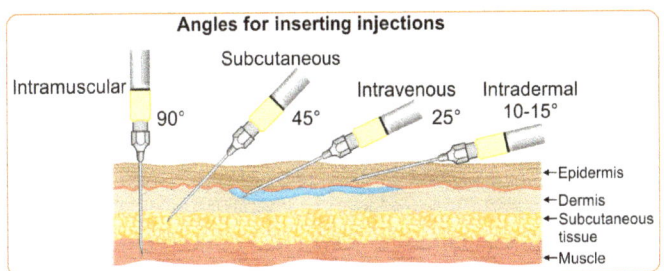

FIG. 1.1: Angles for inserting injections by different routes

  - **Intravenous route** has 100% bio-availability and is useful in emergencies.
  - **Intramuscular** injection is given deep into the muscles, e.g. streptomycin
  - **Subcutaneous route** has the advantage of self administration. Insulin is given by this route.
  - **Intradermal route** is given at an angle of 10–15°C to skin and a bleb must be formed. BCG vaccination and drug testing for allergy is done by this route.
- **Non-injectable** parenteral routes include transdermal, nasal, inhalational and sublingual routes.
  - **Transdermal route** is used only for the drugs which are *highly lipid soluble* and can be absorbed through intact skin. By this route, there is a constant release of the drug (rate of drug delivery to skin is *less than the absorptive capacity of the skin* so that absorption does not become the limiting factor and there is a constant level of the drug in the blood) and it may be administered less frequently. *Nitroglycerine, nicotine, fentanyl and hyoscine* are administered through transdermal patch.
  - Drugs administered by nasal route are **nafarelin** (GnRH agonist), *calcitonin and desmopressin*.
  - **Inhalational route** is the route by which the rate of drug *delivery can be controlled like IV infusion*. The drugs administered by this route include drugs for asthma (*e.g., salbutamol, ipratropium, cromoglycate and inhalational steroids*) and inhalational anaesthetic agents like *nitrous oxide*.
  - **Sublingual route** *avoids first pass metabolism, can be used in emergencies*, can be self-administered and also after getting the desired action, rest of the drug can be spitted. Drugs like **nitroglycerine, isosorbide dinitrate, clonidine, nifedipine** etc. can be administered by sublingual route.

PHARMACOKINETICS

It is the effect of body on the drug i.e. movement of the drug in, through and out of the body. Pharmacokinetics is also called **ADME** study as it deals with Absorption, Distribution, Metabolism and Excretion of a drug.

1. Absorption

It depends on several factors. Only lipid soluble drugs can cross the biological membranes. So, if a drug is administered by oral route, it has to cross the membranes of GIT and blood vessels to reach the blood. Therefore, it should be in lipid soluble form. If a drug is a weak electrolyte, it is the unionized form which is lipid soluble and the ionized form is water soluble.

> **When medium is same, drugs can cross the membrane**

From this statement, we can find that *acidic drugs can cross the membranes in acidic medium* i.e. acidic drugs are lipid soluble in acidic medium (for this acidic drugs must be mainly in the un-ionized form in acidic medium). Opposite is also true for basic drugs. As gastric pH is acidic, therefore acidic drugs are more likely to be absorbed from the stomach, because these will be in unionized (lipid soluble) form here. Thus, aspirin is more likely to be absorbed in the stomach than morphine or atropine (basic drugs).

Weak Acids	Weak Bases
• Barbiturates e.g. phenobarbitone	• Morphine
• NSAIDs e.g. aspirin, diclofenac	• Atropine
• Methotrexate	• Amphetamines
• Sulfonamides	• Quinine
• Penicillins	• Hyoscine

Note
There is never 100% lipid solubility or water solubility, because ionization of a drug is never 100% or 0%. As we have already discussed, when medium is same the drug is lipid soluble. Suppose, we are talking about an acidic drug having pKa of 5.0 (i.e. at pH = 5.0, it will be 50% ionized and 50% unionized). If it is present in a medium with pH = 4.0, it is lipid soluble. But, if the pH of the medium changes to 3.0, what will happen? Obviously, it will become more lipid soluble because more of the drug become un-ionized. We need to remember few concepts:

- If pH of the medium is equal to pKa, then drug is 50% ionized and 50% un-ionized.
- If the pH of the medium is more than pKa (medium becomes alkaline).
  - For acidic drugs, ionized form increases and non-ionized form decreases.
  - For basic drugs, un-ionized form increases and ionized form decreases
- If the pH of the medium is less than pKa, opposite happens, i.e. acidic drugs will be in more un-ionized form and basic drugs be more ionized.
- This ionized or unionized fraction depends on difference (d) between pH and pKa
- When pH = pKa (d = 0) Ionization is 50% and unionized fraction is also 50%.
- When pH – pKa = 1 (d = 1) one form is 90% and other form is 10%
- When d = 2, one form is 99% and other is 1%
- When d = 3, one form is 99.9% and other is 0.1%

	Example for a drug with pKa = 5.0			
pH of Medium	Nature of drug	(pH-pKa)	Ionized form	Non-ionized form
3.0	Acidic	2	1%	99%
4.0	Acidic	1	10%	90%
5.0	Acidic	0	50%	50%
6.0	Acidic	1	90%	10%
7.0	Acidic	2	99%	1%
8.0	Acidic	3	99.9%	0.1%
3.0	Basic	2	99%	1%
4.0	Basic	1	90%	10%
5.0	Basic	0	50%	50%
6.0	Basic	1	10%	90%
7.0	Basic	2	1%	99%
8.0	Basic	3	0.1%	99.9%

Note
It is simplified form of Henderson-Hasselbach equation:
$$pH = pKa + \log \frac{[\text{Protonated form}]}{[\text{Unprotonated form}]}$$

Bioavailability

- It is the fraction of administered drug that reaches the systemic circulation in the unchanged form.
- When we administer a drug orally, first it is absorbed into the portal circulation and reaches the liver. Here, some of the drug may be metabolized (*first pass metabolism or pre-systemic metabolism*) and rest of the drug reaches the systemic circulation. Thus, absorption and first pass metabolism are two important determinants of bioavailability.

Drugs with High First pass Metabolism	
Nitrates	- Nitrates
Have	- Hydrocortisone
Large	- Lignocaine
Pre	- Propranolol
Systemic	- Salbutamol
Metabolism	- Morphine

- By *IV route*, bioavailability is *100%*.
- Bioavailability can be *calculated by comparing the AUC* (area under plasma concentration time curve) for IV route and for that particular route **(Fig. 1.2)**. It can also be calculated by comparing the excretion in the urine.

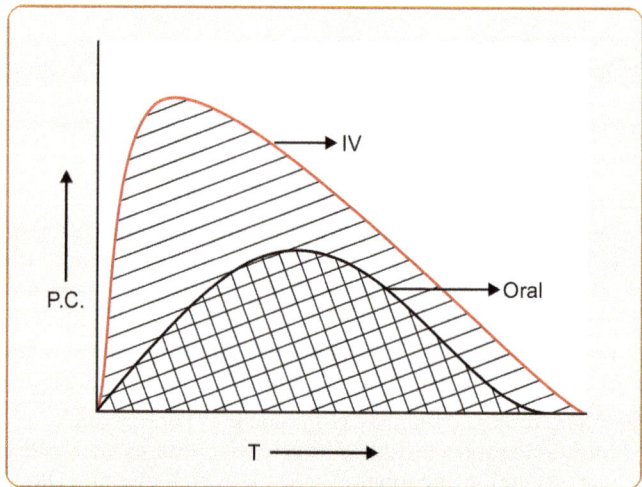

FIG. 1.2: Graph to calculate bioavailability

- AUC tells about the **extent of absorption** of the drug.
- T_{max} tells about the time to reach maximum concentration, i.e. **rate of absorption**
- C_{max} is the **maximum concentration** of a drug that can be obtained (Fig. 1.3)

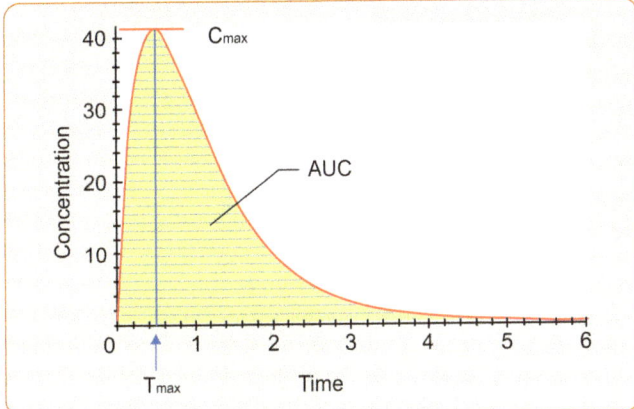

FIG. 1.3: Plot between plasma concentration and time to calculate bioavailability

Bioequivalence

Many different pharmaceutical companies can manufacture same compound (with same dose as well as dosage form) e.g. phenytoin is available as tab. Dilantin as well as Tab. Eptoin. *If the difference in the bioavailability of these two preparations (same drugs, same dose, same dosage forms) is less than 20%, these are known to be bioequivalent.* As the term implies, these are biologically equal i.e. will produce similar plasma concentrations.

2. Distribution

After the drug reaches the blood, it may be distributed to various tissues. This is determined by a hypothetical parameter, **Volume of distribution** (V_d). It is the volume that would be required to contain the administered dose if that dose was evenly distributed at the concentration measured in plasma. If more amount of drug is entering the tissues, it has a higher volume of distribution and vice-a-versa. It depends on several factors like lipid solubility and plasma protein binding.

- Drugs which are **lipid soluble** are more likely to cross the blood vessel wall and thus have **high volume of distribution**.
- If a drug is highly **bound to plasma proteins**, (*e.g.,* warfarin, benzodiazepines, furosemide, calcium channel blockers, digitoxin etc.) it will behave like a large molecule and more likely to stay in the plasma. Therefore, less will go to tissues resulting in **reduced volume of distribution.**

Key Points

Drugs with high plasma protein binding
- Benzodiazepines
  - *Diazepam*
  - *Chlordiazepoxide*
  - *Midazolam*
- Chlorpropamide
- Tolbutamide
- Cyclosporine
- Fluoxetine
- Imipramine
- Verapamil
- Warfarin

- It is the free form (which is not bound to plasma proteins of a drug that is responsible for the action as well as the metabolism of a drug. Therefore **plasma protein binding** *makes a drug long acting* by reducing its metabolism.
- This property can also expose the drug to several drug interactions due to displacement from the binding site by other drugs.
- The drugs which have low Vd are restricted to the vascular compartment and thus their poisoning can be benefited by dialysis. *Dialysis in not effective in the poisoning due to amphetamines, antidepressants, antipsychotics, benzodiazepines, digoxin, opioids, β-blockers, calcium channel blockers and quinidine.*

Clinical Importance of Plasma Protein Binding

- **D**uration of action: Drugs with high PPB are usually long acting
- **D**istribution: High PPB drugs stay in plasma, thus have low V_d.
- **D**isplacement: Highly PPB drug can be displaced by another highly bound drug
- **D**ialysis: It is not effective for drugs having high PPB

Dialysis in Drug Poisoning

Certain drugs can be removed by dialysis. However,
- Dialysis does not filter proteins. Therefore, *drugs having high plasma protein binding* (e.g. diazepam) *cannot be removed by dialysis*
- Dialysis removes only those drugs which are present in sufficient free concentration in plasma. Thus, *drugs having high volume of distribution* [More in tissues but less in Plasma] *are difficult to be removed by dialysis* e.g. digoxin, propranolol etc.
- Thus, drugs having low V_d and low PPB are good candidates of dialysis e.g. salicylates.

MNEMONIC

Dialysis is not effective in poisoning of
A	- Amphetamines
V	- Verapamil
O	- Organophosphates
	- Opioids
I	- Imipramine
D	- Digitalis
Dialysis	- Diazepam

Volume of Distribution

It can be calculated by dividing the plasma concentration attained to the dose of a drug administered IV Initial plasma concentration (Co) is calculated by extrapolating the graph of plasma concentration vs time to y-axis.

$$V_d = \frac{\text{Dose administrated (IV)}}{\text{Plasma concentration } (C_o)}$$

It is a measure of the distribution of a drug. If V_d is more, it means more amount of drug is in the tissues and less is in the plasma. Thus, higher dose has to be administered to attain the same plasma concentration for drugs having high V_d than those having low V_d. This high dose is called **loading dose**. Thus, **V_d is the main determinant of loading dose**. **Chloroquine** is the drug with **highest V_d** (1300 L/Kg).

3. Metabolism

The primary site of metabolism is liver. Most of the drugs are inactivated by metabolism but some may be activated from the inactive compounds (**Prodrugs**) and others may give rise to active metabolites from the active compound (e.g. diazepam, propranolol).

> **MNEMONIC**
>
> **PRODRUGS**
> All   - ACE inhibitors (except captopril and lisinopril)
> Prefer   - Prednisone
>   - Proton pump inhibitors
>   - Proguanil
> Doing   - Dipivefrine
> M   - Mercaptopurine
>   - Methyldopa
>   - Minoxidil
> D   - Levo-dopa
> In   - Irinotecan
> Clinical - Cyclophosphamide
>   - Clopidogrel
>   - Carbimazole
> Subjects - Sulfasalazine

- Metabolism may occur with the help of **microsomal** (*present in smooth endoplasmic reticulum*) or **non-microsomal** enzymes. Microsomal enzymes (*monooxygenases, cytochrome P450 and glucuronyl transferase*) may be **induced** or **inhibited** by other drugs whereas non-microsomal enzymes are not subjected to these interactions.

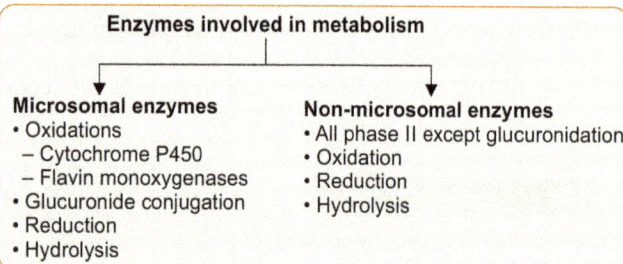

- The drug which is metabolized by a microsomal enzyme is known as substrate and the chemical increasing or decreasing the number of enzymes is known as inducer or inhibitor respectively.

- **Enzyme inducers** will increase the metabolism of other drugs and thus their effect will decrease. Therefore dose of such drugs (which are metabolized by microsomal enzymes) should be increased when administered along with microsomal enzyme inducers. Potent inducers of microsomal enzymes include **rifampicin, phenobarbitone, phenytoin, griseofulvin, phenylbutazone and chloral hydrate**.

> **MNEMONIC**
>
> **Enzyme Inducers**
> G   - Griseofulvin
> P   - Phenytoin
> R   - Rifampicin
> S   - Smoking
> Cell - Carbamazepine
> Phone - Phenobarbitone

- Further, **rate-limiting** enzyme of porphyrin synthesis i.e. δ-ALA synthase is a microsomal enzyme. Enzyme inducers like phenytoin and phenobarbitone induce it and increase porphyrin synthesis. Thus, these drugs are contra-indicated in acute intermittent porphyria.
- **Enzyme inhibitors** will decrease the metabolism of drugs metabolized by microsomal enzymes, thus predisposes to the toxicity by such agents. Inhibitors include **ketoconazole, cimetidine, erythromycin and metronidazole**.

> **MNEMONIC**
>
> **Enzyme Inhibitors**
> Vitamin   - Valproate
> K   - Ketoconzole
> Cannot   - Cimetidine
> Cause   - Ciprofloxacin
> Enzyme   - Erythromycin
> Inhibition - INH

Phases of Metabolic Reactions

Metabolic reactions may be classified into phase I (non-synthetic) and phase II (synthetic) reactions. Function of **phase I reactions** is to attach a **functional group** to the drug molecule whereas **phase II reactions** serve to **attach a conjugate** to the drug molecule. After phase I reaction, drug may be water soluble or lipid soluble whereas **after phase II reaction, all drugs become water soluble** (lipid insoluble). Phase I reactions include oxidation, reduction, hydrolysis, cyclization and decyclization etc. whereas phase II reactio1ns include glucuronidation, acetylation, methylation, sulfation and glycine conjugation etc.

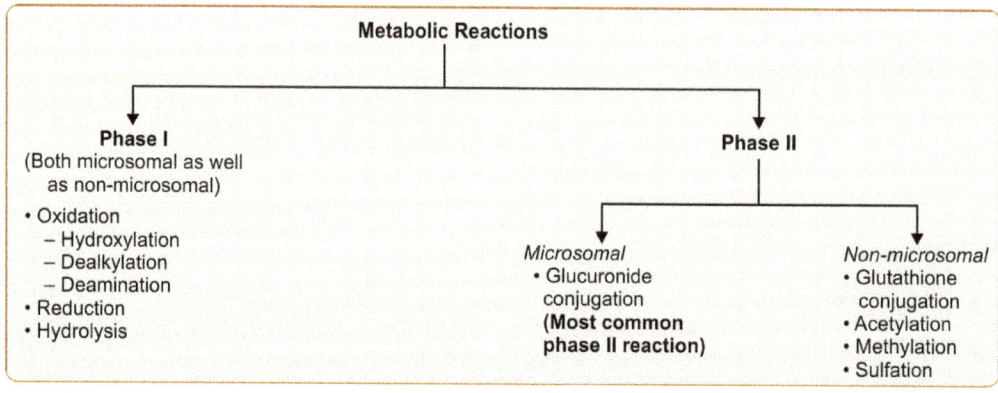

Cytochrome P450 Enzymes

These are **one group of microsomal enzymes** and are commonly abbreviated as CYP enzymes. In P450, **P** stands for **pigment** that has maximum light absorption at **wavelength 450 nm**. Several families of CYP enzymes are involved in metabolism of xenobiotics. These are named as CYP followed by a number (denotes family), then alphabet (subfamily) and again a number (specific isoform of the enzyme) e.g. in CYP 3A4; 3 is family, A is subfamily and 4 is specific isoform.

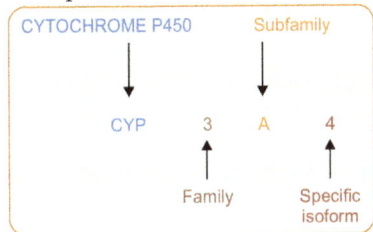

CYP 3A4 forms the maximum hepatic content (26%) of CYP enzymes and is also involved in metabolism of maximum percentage of drugs (33%). On the other hand, CYP 2D6 is involved in metabolism of 23% of drugs although it constitutes only 2% of hepatic CYP content.

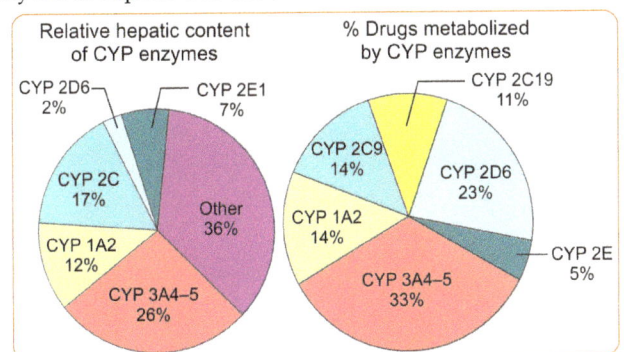

FIG. 1.4: Relative hepatic content and percentage drugs metabolized by different CYP enzymes.

CYP	Substrate	Inducer	Inhibitor

3A4	C–Cyclosporine
	   Calcium channel
	   blockers
	T–Tacrolimus
	S–Statins
	C–CAT drugs
	   – Cisapride
	   – Astemizole
	   – Terfenadine
	A–Amiodarone
	N–Navirs (Protease
	   inhibitors)
		Barbiturates
		Rifampicin
		Phenytion
		Carbamazepine
		St. John's wort
			Erythromycin
			Ketoconazole
			Fluconazole
			Grapefruit juice
			Ritonavir

2D6	• Most antidepressants
	   – TCA
	   – SSRI
	   – MAO inhibitors
	• Most beta blockers
	• Most antiarrhythmics
		No known inducer	Quinidine
			Paroxetine

2C19	• Omeprazole • Clopidogrel	Rifampicin Barbiturates	Fluconazole
2C9	• Phenytion • Tolbutamide • Warfarin	Rifampicin Barbiturates	Erythromycin Cimetidine
1A2	• Theophylline warfarin	Smoking Rifampicin	Ciprofloxacin
2E1	• Acetaminophen • Enflurane • Halothane	Ethanol	Disulfiram

4. Excretion

The major route of excretion is kidney. Excretion through kidneys occurs by glomerular filtration, tubular reabsorption and tubular secretion.

Glomerular filtration depends on the *plasma protein binding and renal blood flow*. It **does not depend on the lipid solubility** because all substances (whether water soluble or lipid soluble) can cross the fenestrated glomerular membrane.

Tubular reabsorption depends on the *lipid solubility*. If a drug is lipid soluble, more of it will be reabsorbed and less will be excreted. Opposite is true for lipid insoluble drugs. As lipid solubility depends on ionization, the ionized drug will be excreted by the kidney. Thus, in acidic drug poisoning (*salicylate, barbiturates, chlorpropamide, methotrexate etc.*) urine should be *alkalinized* with sodium bicarbonate because weak acids are in ionized form in alkaline urine and thus are easily excreted. Similarly for basic drug poisoning (e.g. *morphine, amphetamine* etc.), urine should be *acidified* using ammonium chloride.

Tubular secretion does not depend on lipid solubility or plasma protein binding. In the nephron, separate pumps are present for acidic and basic drugs. Drugs utilizing the same transporter may show drug interactions e.g. *probenecid decreases the excretion of penicillin* and increases the excretion of uric acid. Remember, exogenous substances e.g. penicillins are removed whereas endogenous substances like uric acid are retained by these pumps.

> **Key Points**
>
> Lithium, KI and rifampicin are secreted in saliva

KINETICS OF ELIMINATION

Rate of Elimination is the *amount of drug eliminated per unit time*. If we want to calculate the rate of elimination (R) of a particular organ (e.g. liver), it will be

> R = Amount of drug entering the organ per unit time –
> Amount of drug leaving the organ per unit time
> = $Q.C_A - Q.C_V$

Where Q is Rate of blood flow to that organ
C_A is Concentration of drug in arteries entering that organ
C_V is Concentration of drug in veins leaving that organ
Thus, $R = Q.(C_A - C_V)$

> **Clearance** is the amount of plasma completely cleared off a drug per unit time. It is calculated as:
>
> $$CL = \frac{\text{Rate of Elimination}}{\text{Plasma concentration}}$$
>
> If we calculate clearance by a particular organ, it will be
>
> $$CL = \frac{R}{PC} = Q.\left(\frac{C_A - C_V}{C_A}\right) = Q. \text{Extraction Ratio.}$$
>
> Thus, clearance is calculated from rate of blood flow and extraction ratio of an organ.

Order of Kinetics

Drugs may follow zero order or first order kinetics. It depends on the following formula:

Rate of Elimination ∝ {Plasma Concentration}^{order}

- Thus, if a drug follows zero order kinetics, {Plasma Concentration}^{0} is equal to one, in other words rate of elimination is independent of plasma concentration or rate of elimination is constant.
- From the above formula, rate of elimination is proportional to plasma concentration for the drugs following first order kinetics.

First Order Kinetics (Linear kinetics)	Zero Order Kinetics (Non linear Kinetics)
1. Constant fraction of drug is eliminated per unit time.	1. Constant amount of the drug is eliminated per unit time.
2. Rate of elimination is proportional to plasma concentration.	2. Rate of elimination is independent of plasma concentration.
3. Clearance remains constant.	3. Clearance is more at low concentrations and less at high concentrations.
4. Half life remains constant.	4. Half life is less at low concentrations and more at high concentrations.
5. Most of the drugs follow first order kinetics.	5. Very few drugs follow pure zero order kinetics e.g. alcohol
	6. Any drug at high concentration (when metabolic or elimination pathway is saturated) may show zero order kinetics.

Drugs Showing Zero/Pseudo Zero Order Kinetics

MNEMONIC

Zero	Zero order kinetics shown by
W	Warfarin and Heparin
A	Alcohol and Aspirin
T	Theophylline
T	Tolbutamide
Power	Phenytoin

Half Life ($t_{1/2}$)

It is the time required to reduce the plasma concentration to half (50%) of the original value. If metabolism is more, half life is less and vice-versa. It is a *secondary pharmacokinetic parameter derived from two primary parameter; V_d and CL. It determines the dosing interval and time required to reach the steady state* (It does not affect the dose of the drug). Drugs having short half lives are administered more frequently than those having longer half life. It takes 4 to 5 half lives for a drug to reach its steady state.

$$t_{1/2} = \frac{0.693 \times V_d}{CL}$$

If a drug follows **first order kinetics**, its **half life is constant**. This is *true both for rising as well as falling plasma concentrations*. When a drug is given by constant IV infusion, initially the plasma level rises, it reaches a steady state and when infusion is stopped this level starts declining. Elimination of the drug from plasma is 50% in one half life, 75% (50 + 25) in two half lives, 87.5% (50 + 25 + 12.5) in three half lives and so on. The same is true for rising plasma concentration also i.e. with constant IV infusion, in one half life the plasma concentration is half of steady state and in two half lives, it is 75% and so on.

Steady State (Fig. 1.5)

If fixed dose of a drug is administered after regular intervals, its plasma concentration starts increasing. However, as plasma concentration rises, rate of elimination also starts increasing. When rate of administration becomes equal to rate of elimination, plasma concentration stabilizes. This is called steady state.

1. Time to reach steady state depends on $t_{1/2}$. It takes approximately 5 half lives.
2. Steady state plasma concentration achieved depends on dose rate.
3. Variation between peak and trough concentration at steady state depends on dosing interval. However, average steady state plasma concentration remains same irrespective of dosing interval provided dose rate remains same.

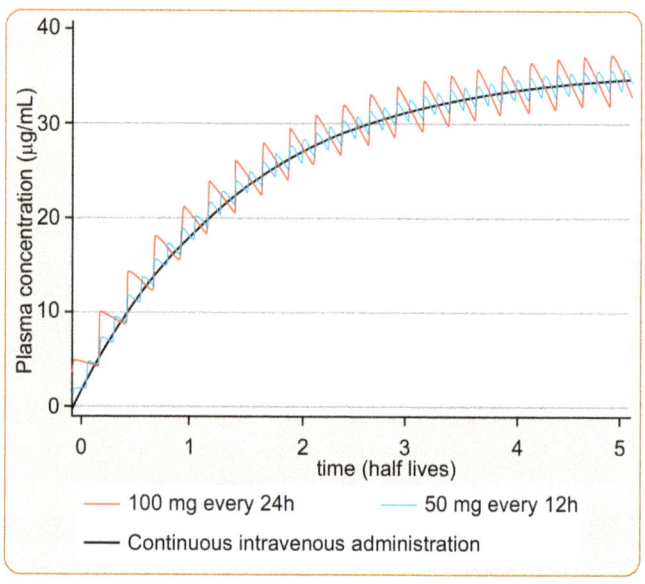

FIG. 1.5: Concept of steady state plasma concentration

Two Dose Strategy

The drugs having high volume of distribution are given by this strategy. First a large dose (loading dose) is administered to attain the steady state quickly and later on, to maintain the plasma concentration smaller dose is given (maintenance dose).

Loading dose: It is mainly used for drugs having long $t_{1/2}$ and large volume of distribution. It is given to load (saturate) the tissue stores. So it is mainly dependent on V_d.

Loading dose = V_d × Target plasma concentration

Maintenance dose: It is mainly dependent on CL.

Maintenance dose = CL × Target plasma concentration

Therapeutic Drug Monitoring (TDM)

- TDM is a process by which the dose of a drug is adjusted according to its plasma concentration.
- It is done for drugs having *known correlation between serum level and drug response or toxicity.*
- It is done for drugs having *wide variation in pharmacokinetics* (absorption, metabolism or excretion), both intra- as well as inter- individual.

General Pharmacology

- It is done for drugs having *low therapeutic index* like digitalis, aminoglycosides, tricyclic antidepressants, theophylline, lithium, antiepileptics, immuno-modulators and antiarrhythmics etc.
- TDM is done for those drugs whose *effect cannot be easily measured* (like effect of antihypertensive drugs can be easily measured by monitoring BP, so TDM is not used). Due to same reason, TDM is not indicated for anticoagulants (e.g. warfarin) or antidiabetics (e.g. metformin).
- TDM is **not done for** the drugs which are *activated in the body* or produce active metabolites.

Key Points

TDM is required for
- **A** — **A**minoglycosides (e.g. gentamicin)
- **D**rug — **D**igitalis
- **P**ossessing — **P**henytoin (anti-epileptics)
- **L**ow — **L**ithium
- **T**herapeutic — **T**ricyclic antidepressants
- **I**ndex — **I**mmunomodulators (e.g. cyclosporine)

PHARMACODYNAMICS

This is the study dealing with the effect of drugs on the body. It includes actions of drugs as well as their mechanism.

Drugs may act by *physical mechanism* (e.g. osmotic diuretics), *chemical action* (e.g. antacids), stimulation or inhibition of *enzymes* (competitive and non-competitive inhibition) or via *receptors*.

Enzyme Inhibition

Drugs may act by inhibiting the enzymes competitively, non-competitively or un-competitively.

Competitive Inhibition (Fig. 1.6)

Important points about this type of enzyme inhibition (e.g. sulfonamides) are:

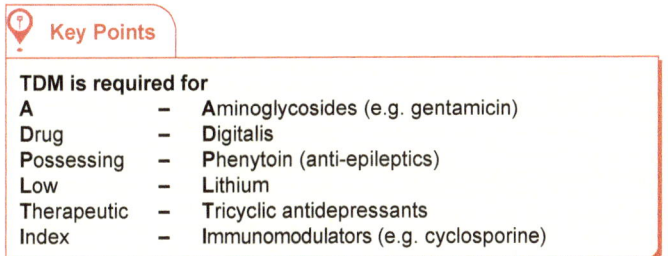

FIG. 1.6: Competitive inhibition

- It **binds only to enzyme** and not to enzyme-substrate complex (ES)
- Drug should have *similar structure* as that of substrate of the enzyme.
- Inhibitor *binds to the active site* of the enzyme.
- This type of inhibition is mostly *surmountable*, i.e. inhibition can be overcome by increasing the dose of the substrate.
- K_m is Michaelis Menton's constant and is calculated as amount of substrate required to produce half of the maximal velocity whereas V_{max} is maximum reaction velocity.
- It results in increase in K_m but does not affect the V_{max}
- If the drug binds very strongly to the active site, so that it cannot be displaced even by large concentration of substrate, it can result in **irreversible competitive inhibition**. In this type of inhibition, K_m rises and V_{max} decreases. **Organophosphates are irreversible competitive inhibitors.**

⚠ MNEMONIC

K_m looks like kilometers, In competition one need to run more kilometers i.e. K_m increases.

Noncompetitive Inhibition (Fig. 1.7)

Important points about this type of enzyme inhibition (e.g. cyanide) are:

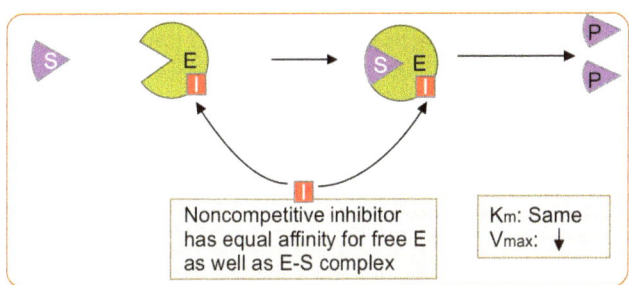

FIG. 1.7: Noncompetitive inhibition

- It **binds to both enzyme as well as ES** with equal affinity
- Drug *need not have similar structure* as that of substrate of the enzyme.
- It *binds to* a different site of the enzyme, known as *allosteric site*.
- This type of inhibition is *insurmountable*, i.e. inhibition cannot be overcome by increasing the dose of the substrate.
- It result in decrease in V_{max} but does not affect the K_m.
- Mostly non-competitive inhibitors are irreversible but **carbonic anhydrase inhibitors are reversible non-competitive inhibitors**.

Uncompetitive Inhibition (Fig. 1.8)

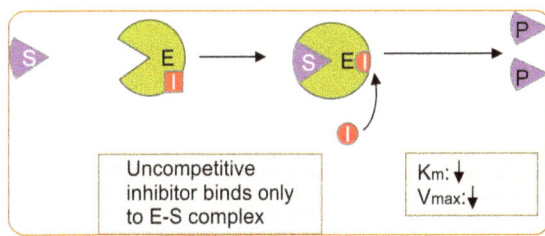

FIG. 1.8: Uncompetitive inhibition

- It has **affinity for only ES** and is not able to bind to enzyme.
- It decreases the activity of enzyme-substrate complex, so V_{max} **decreases**.
- As ES is removed, the binding of substrate to enzyme increases (affinity increases). resulting in **decrease in Km**.
- It is rare type of enzyme inhibition.

Inhibition	Binds to	Km	V_{max}	Example
Competitive	E only	↑	No change	Physostigmine Neostigmine
Non-competitive	Both E and ES complex	No change	↓	Cyanide
Un-competitive	ES complex only	↓	↓	Lithium

Receptors

These are the binding sites of the drug with funtional correlate. Two important terms related to the receptors are affinity and intrinsic activity (IA).

Affinity is the *ability of a drug to combine with the receptor*. If a drug has no affinity, it will not bind to the receptor. So, all type of drugs acting via receptors (agonist, antagonist, inverse agonist and partial agonist) possess some affinity for the receptors. Drugs with high affinity can be used in low concentrations.

After binding to the receptor, the *ability to activate the receptor* is called its **intrinsic activity**. It *varies from –1 through zero to +1*.

Drugs may be divided into four types *based on their intrinsic activities*.

- **Agonist:** It will bind to the receptor and *activate it maximally*. i.e. **IA is +1**
- **Antagonist:** Binds to the receptor but produces **no effect (IA is 0)**. But now agonist is not able to bind to the receptor because these are already occupied by the antagonist. Thus, it decreases the action of the agonist but itself has no effect.
- **Partial agonist:** It activates the receptor submaximally (**IA between 0 and +1**). It will produce the similar effect in the absence of agonist but it will decrease the effect of a pure agonist. e.g. pindolol has partial agonistic activity at β_1 receptors. In the presence of agonists like adrenaline and nor-adrenaline it will produce antagonistic effect i.e. decrease in heart rate but even in high doses it does not result in severe bradycardia due to some agonistic action.
- **Inverse agonist:** These type of drugs bind to the receptor and produce opposite effect (**IA is negative**) e.g. β carboline is an inverse agonist at BZD receptors.

Types of Antagonism

These may be physical, chemical, physiological or pharmacological.

- **Physical antagonist** binds to the drug and prevents its absorption like charcoal binds to the alkaloids and prevents their absorption.
- **Chemical antagonist** combines with a substance chemically like chelating agents bind with the metals.
- **Physiological antagonist** produces an action opposite to a substance but *by binding to the different receptors* e.g. adrenaline is a physiological antagonist of histamine because adrenaline causes bronchodilation by binding to β_2 receptors, which is opposite to bronchoconstriction caused by histamine through H_1 receptors.
- **Pharmacological antagonists** produce opposite actions by *binding to the same receptor* e.g. beta blockers.

Classification of Receptors

The receptors are classified into four types based on the signal transduction mechanisms.

G-Protein Coupled Receptors (Fig. 1.10)

These are also called metabotropic receptors or heptahelical (serpentine) receptors i.e. have seven transmembrane spanning segments. Drugs bind to the receptor which in turn activates a G-protein (GTP activated protein). G-proteins consist of three subunits; α, β and γ. When all three are joined together (along with GDP), G-protein is inactive. When GTP replaces GDP, α-subunit seperates from β-γ subunit and become activated. Activated α-subunit may result in one of the 3 actions:

1. **Activation (by Gs) or inhibition (by Gi) of enzyme adenyl cyclase:** It changes the concentration of cAMP that acts by activating protein kinases (e.g. protein kinase A). Latter produce action by phosphorylation of their substrates. Examples include β-receptors (increase cAMP) and somatostatin (works by decreasing cAMP).
2. **Activation of phospholipase C (by Gq):** This enzyme converts PIP_2 to IP_3 and DAG. Final result is increase in intracellular calcium and thus action e.g. α-receptors, vasopressin V_1 receptors.
3. **Stimulation or inhibition of ion channels** e.g. M_2 receptors of ACh.

Cyclic AMP, IP_3 and DAG act as second messengers whereas Ca^{2+} is both a second as well as **third messenger**.

After the action, the intrinsic GTPase activity of alpha subunit result in joining it with β-γ subunits and thus G-protein is available for action again.

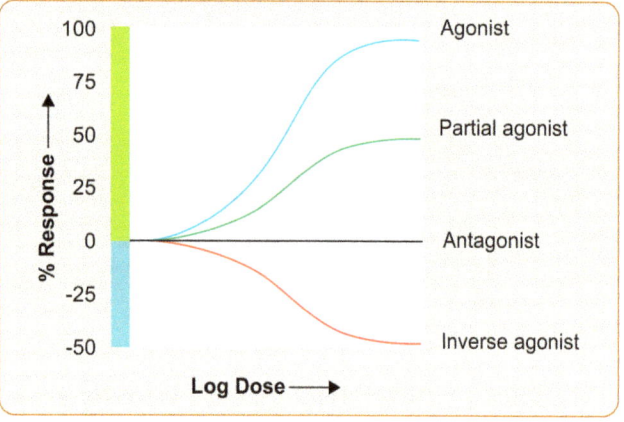

FIG. 1.9: Log DRC with different types of drugs

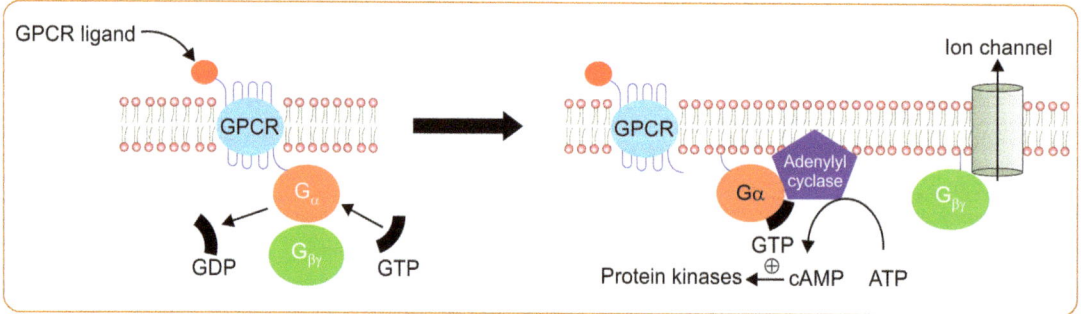

FIG. 1.10: G-protein coupled receptors

General Pharmacology

Ionotropic Receptors (Fig. 1.11)

The drug binds directly to the receptor located on an ion channel without mediation by G proteins. These are the **fastest acting receptors**. It includes **GABA$_A$, N$_M$, N$_N$, NMDA** (receptors of glutamate) and **5-HT$_3$** receptors.

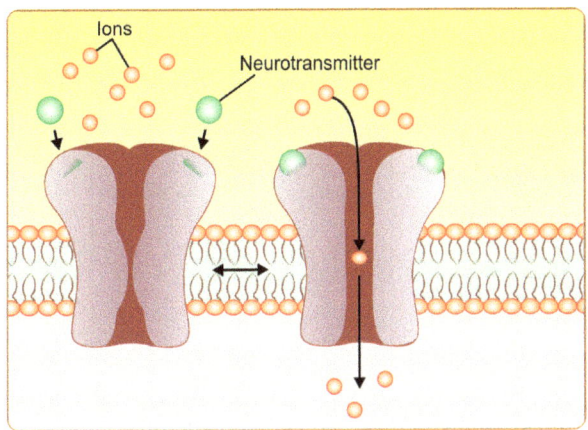

FIG. 1.11: Ionotropic receptors

Enzymatic Receptors (Fig. 1.12)

This type of receptor has two sites, the drug binds on the extracellular site and the intracellular site has enzymatic activity (mostly *tyrosine kinase*). This enzyme can be activated via JAK-STAT pathway. Cytokines, prolactin, insulin and growth hormone acts via these receptors.

⚠ MNEMONIC

Enzymatic receptors
- P – Prolactin
- I – Insulin
- G – Growth hormone

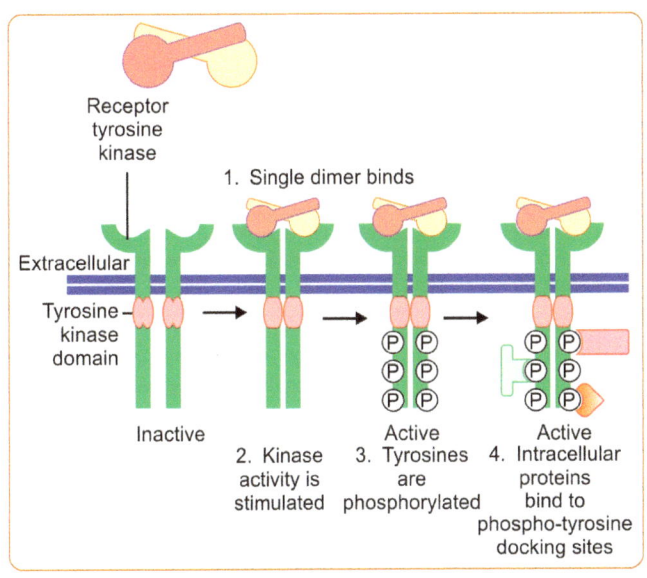

FIG. 1.12: Enzymatic receptors

Intracellular Receptors (Fig. 1.13)

These types of receptors are **slowest acting**. These may be present in the **cytoplasm (glucocorticoids, mineralocorticoids, and vitamin D)** or in the **nucleus (T$_3$, T$_4$, Retinoic acid, PPAR, estrogen, progesterone and testosterone)**. *Both type of receptors finally act by nuclear mechanisms (i.e. by affecting transcription).* All the intracellular receptors are considered a part of '**Nuclear Receptor Superfamily**'.

⚠ MNEMONIC

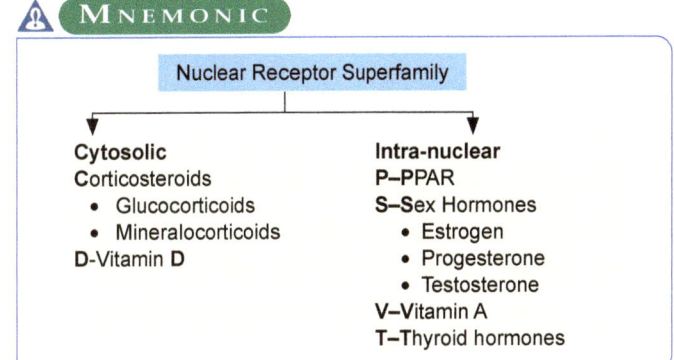

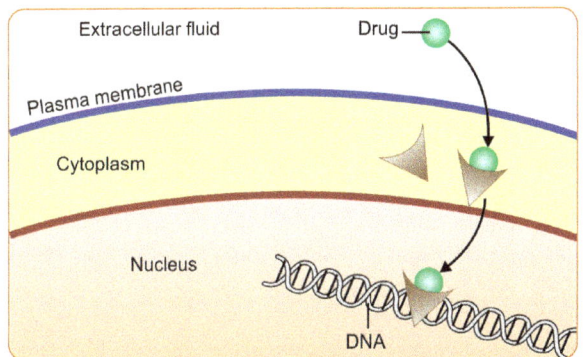

FIG. 1.13: Intracellular receptors

> **Note**
> Progesterone and testosterone receptors are present in both nucleus as well as cytoplasm.

Dose Response Curve (DRC)

It is a graph between the dose of a drug administered (on X-axis) and the effect produced by the drug (on Y-axis). It consists of two components; *dose-plasma concentration curve and plasma concentration-response curve*. As plasma concentration is more closely related to response, the graph between plasma concentration and response is usually called **DRC**. Two types of DRC can be described: *Quantal and graded*.

Quantal DRC

Variation in sensitivity of response to increasing doses of the drug in different individuals can be obtained from quantal DRC. When the response is an *'all or none'* phenomenon (e.g. antiemetic drug stopping the vomiting or not), the y-axis (response axis) shows the number of person responding and X-axis shows the plasma concentration. It is used to calculate ED$_{50}$ and LD$_{50}$.

- **Median Effective Dose (ED$_{50}$):** It is the *dose that will produce the desired response in half of the (50%) recepients*. More is ED$_{50}$, lower is the potency and vice a versa.
- **Median Lethal Dose (LD$_{50}$):** It is the dose that will result in death of 50% of the animals receiving the drug. *More is LD$_{50}$, safer is the drug.*
- **Therapeutic Index (T.I.):** It is a *measure of the safety* of a drug. It is calculated as a ratio of LD$_{50}$ to ED$_{50}$. Drugs having high T.I. are safer whereas those having low T.I. are more likely to be toxic.

$$T.I = \frac{LD_{50}}{ED_{50}}$$

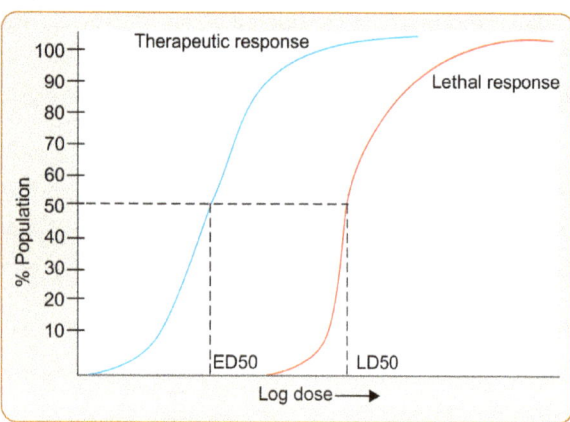

FIG. 1.14: Quantal DRC showing ED50 and LD50

Graded DRC

When the response can be graded (e.g. reduction in BP), the *y*-axis shows the magnitude of response.

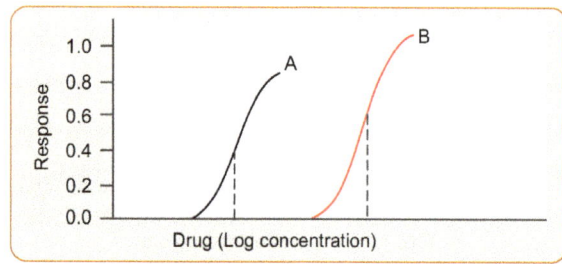

FIG. 1.15: Log DRC of two drugs A and B

DRC is **usually hyperbola** in shape. As curved lines cannot give good mathematical comparisons, so usually the dose is converted to log dose to form **log DRC**, which gives a **sigmoid shaped curve (Fig. 1.15)**. The middle portion (which is of therapeutic importance) is straight line in the log DRC. Another advantage of converting it into logarithmic form is that large variation in doses can be plotted on the same curve. **Three important parameters** (*potency, efficacy and slope of curve*) can be determined from DRC.

Potency

It is the measure of the amount of a drug needed to produce the response. *Drugs producing the same response at lower dose are more potent* whereas those requiring large dose are less potent. *In DRC, more a drug is on left side* of the graph, *higher is its potency* and vice a versa. In **Figure 1.15**, drug A is more potent than drug B.

Efficacy

It is the *maximum effect produced by a drug. More the peak of the curve greater is the efficacy*. It is *clinically* more important than potency. In **Figure 1.15**, drug B is more efficacious than drug A.

Slope

If the DRC is steeper, that means the response will increase dramatically with slight increase in dose. Thus, *drugs having steeper DRC have narrow therapeutic index* (like barbiturates) than those having less steep curves (e.g. benzodiazepines).

DRC can also be utilized to know whether a drug is competitive or non-competitive inhibitor **(Fig. 1.16)**.

- **In case of competitive inhibitor, curve will shift to right**, i.e. now the same agonist will have less potency in the presence of antagonist. It does not affect the efficacy.
- In case of **noncompetitive inhibitor**, there will be **flattening of DRC**, i.e. efficacy decreases. It usually does not affect potency. If the antagonist is **irreversible competitive**, then there will be *decrease in potency as well as efficacy*.

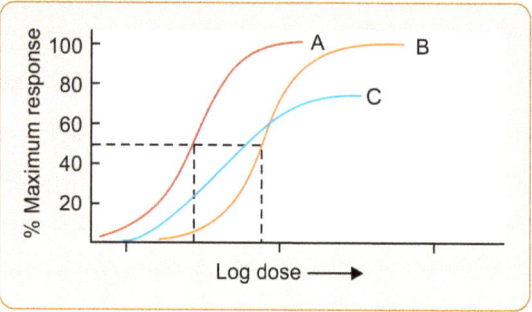

FIG. 1.16: Effect of different drugs on Log DRC. A: Drug alone; B: Drug with competitive antagonist (potency decreases; parallel shift to right; C: Drug with noncompetitive antagonist (Efficacy decreases)

Pharmacogenetic Conditions

Due to different genetic make up, some drugs have different effects in different individuals, so these drugs may show either toxicity or lack of effect in certain individuals, if used in conventional dosage. These conditions include:

1. **Acetylator Polymorphism:** Some individuals are *slow acetylators* and some are *fast acetylators*. The drugs metabolized by this route may be ineffective in fast acetylators and may show toxicity in slow acetylators.
   Important drugs metabolized by acetylation include (remembered as **SHIP**)

   - **S**ulfonamides including dapsone and PAS
   - **H**ydralazine
   - **I**soniazid
   - **P**rocainamide

   > **Note**
   > - All SHIP drugs can also cause lupus erythematosis.
   > - Other drugs metabolized by acetylation include acebutolol, amantadine, amrinone, benzocaine, clonazepam, nitrazepam and phenelzine etc.

2. **Glucose-6-phosphate Dehydrogenase (G-6-PD) Deficiency:** Oxidant drugs may produce *hemolysis* in the patient with deficiency of this enzyme. The important drugs are:

   - Primaquine
   - Chloroquine
   - Menadione
   - Sulfonamides including dapsone
   - Nitrofurantoin
   - Isoniazid
   - Quinine
   - Nalidixic acid

3. **Atypical Pseudocholinesterase and Succinylcholine:** Succinylcholine is a very short acting drug due to metabolism by pseudocholinesterase. In some individuals, this enzyme is not functioning well (atypical). In such individuals this drug may produce *prolonged apnea*.
4. **Inability to Hydroxylate Phenytoin**
5. **Resistance to Coumarin Anticoagulants**
6. **Malignant Hyperthermia by Halothane.**

General Pharmacology

NEW DRUG DEVELOPMENT

Drug development process is broadly divided into:
- Drug discovery phase
- Preclinical studies
- Clinical trials

Drug Discovery Phase

Most new drugs are discovered through random screening, compound oriented approach, target oriented approach or rational drug designing.

These all approaches result in selection of several compounds (process called **lead finding**). These are then subjected to various procedures to identify one or two drug candidates (now called **lead compounds**) suitable for further investigations. (This process is called **lead optimization**). These lead compounds are then evaluated in preclinical phase.

For a molecule to be developed as a drug, certain properties should be present. These properties determine the molecule to be drug-like and are called **Lipinski's Rule of Five**. According to this rule, the molecule should have

- < 5 hydrogen bond donors
- < 500 dalton molecular weight
- < 5 Partition coefficient log P (measure of lipid solubility)
- < 10 Hydrogen bond acceptors.

Pre-clinical Studies

The lead compounds are tested on animals to know the whole pharmacological profile. Tests are first performed on small animals (mice, rat, guinea pig etc. and then on large animal (like cat, dog, monkey etc). All studies like pharmacokinetics, pharmacodynamics, toxicology, therapeutic index etc. are performed and promising compounds are selected that can be evaluated in humans.

Clinical Trials

Before a new drug comes to the market, it is extensively tested in animals and in vitro studies for safety and efficacy. If the drug is found to be promising in these studies, an application called **IND (Investigational New Drug)** is filed with the United States Food and Drug Administration (main regulatory authority). If the permission is granted, then drug is tested in humans. This testing is called clinical trials. These are divided into four phases.

Phase 1: Here, the drug is tested in **normal human volunteers** (extremes of ages; elderly and children are excluded). As the drug is not tested in the patients, so we **cannot determine efficacy** in this phase. This is mainly for **toxicity** and **pharmacokinetic studies**. This is *first in human study*. The idea of testing the new drug in normal humans is based on the fact that healthy persons are more likely to tolerate the adverse effects of the drug than diseased persons. Because anti-cancer drugs can produce unacceptable toxicity and we cannot expose healthy humans to such a toxicity, the *phase-1 trials for anticancer drugs are done in the patients*.

Phase 2: The drug in this phase is tested in *small number of (20-200) patients*. We can determine *both efficacy and safety* in this phase. This is **first in patient** study.

Phase 3: Here the drug is tested in *large number* of patients *at several centers* to include patient with different genetic makeup. This is done to generalize the results of the study to variable genetic and ethnic groups.

If the drug is found to be safe and effective in these trials, then another application is filed with FDA (**New Drug Application or NDA**) to market the drug. If approval is granted, the drug is marketed.

Phase 4: This is **post marketing surveillance** of a drug to know the rare adverse effects or those occurring with prolonged use of the drug. In this phase **ethical clearance is not required**.

Phase 0: These are also called **microdosing studies**. Here, a very low dose 1/100th of human dose; maximum 100 µg) of the drug is administered to **healthy volunteers**. As the dose is sub-therapeutic, so *safety and efficacy cannot be known* in phase 0. However, the drug is radiolabelled and thus **movement of drug in the body can** be known. This could avoid costly phase I studies for candidate drugs with unsuitable pharmacokinetics.

All phases of clinical trials must follow the ICH-GCP (Good clinical practice guidelines given by International Conference for Harmonization, so that the data generated is credible and interest of the patients/volunteers can be safeguarded.

SUMMARY OF CLINICAL TRIALS

Phase	Name	Conducted on	Blinding and control	Purpose
I	Human Pharmacology and safety	**Healthy** volunteers (20 – 100)	**OPEN LABEL** (No blinding)	• To know maximum tolerable dose (MTD) • Safety and tolerability
II	Therapeutic exploratory	100 – 150 **Patients (homogenous** population)	**Single blind** controlled	• To establish therapeutic efficacy • Dose ranging and ceiling effect
III	Therapeutic confirmatory	Up to 5000 patients from several centres (**heterogenous** population)	**Double blind** Randomized Controlled	• To confirm therapeutic efficacy • To establish the value of drug in relation to existing therapy
IV	Post marketing surveillance	Large number of patients being treated by practicing physicians	—	• To know rare **and long-term adverse effects** • Special groups like children, pregnancy etc. can be tested
0 (Zero)	**Microdosing** studies	**Healthy** volunteers (small number)	—	• To **know pharmacokinetics**. • Could avoid costly phase I studies for candidate drugs with unsuitable pharmacokinetics.

THE PHARMACOVIGILANCE PROGRAM OF INDIA (PVPI)

Pharmacovigilance is the science of detection, assessment, understanding and prevention of adverse effects or any other possible drug-related problems

The **Central Drugs Standard Control Organization (CDSCO)**, New Delhi, under the aegis of Ministry of Health and Family Welfare (MOHFW) has initiated the PvPI in July 2010. Initially **National coordinating centre (NCC)** was AIIMS, New Delhi but it was shifted to **Indian Pharmacopoeia commission (IPC)**, Ghaziabad (UP) in April 2011. The vision of PvPI is to improve patient safety in Indian population by monitoring drug safety and there by reducing the risks associated with the use of medicines.

Adverse drug reaction Monitoring Centres (AMCs) play a vital role in PvPI. These AMCs include MCI approved medical colleges and hospitals, autonomous institutes and even corporate hospitals. AMCs are responsible for collecting the ADR (adverse drug reaction) reports from patients and sending it to NCC via entry in a software called **Vigiflow**. NCC then assesses the ICSR (individual case safety reports) by various methods of causality assessment like **Naranjo scale**, and if found valid will commit to **Uppsala Monitoring centre (UMC) in Sweden**.

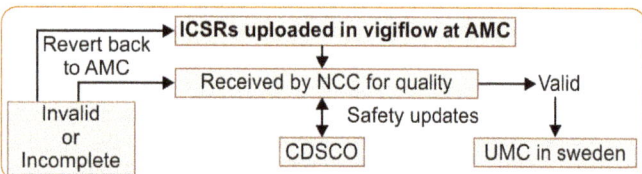

DRUG CATEGORIES WITH PECULIAR NAMES

Some category of drugs have been given names like spurious drugs, misbranded drugs, contaminated drugs, me-too drugs, orphan drugs and essential drugs etc.

Spurious Drugs

A drug shall be deemed to be spurious if
- It is manufactured under a name which belongs to another drug or
- It is an imitation of another drug or
- It has been substituted partly or wholly by another drug or
- It wrongly claims to be product of another manufacturer.
- Contaminated and misbranded drugs.

Misbranded Drugs

A drug shall be deemed to be misbranded:
- If it is so colored, coated, powdered or polished that damage is concealed or if it is made to appear of better or greater therapeutic value than it really is; or
- If it is not labelled in the prescribed manner; or
- If its label or container or anything accompanying the drug bears any statement, design or device which makes any false claim for the drug or which is false or misleading in any particulars.

Adulterated Drugs

For the purposes of this chapter, a drug shall be deemed to be adulterated:
- If it consists in whole or in part, of any filthy, putrid or decomposed substance; or
- If it has been prepared, packed or stored under insanitary conditions whereby it may have been contaminated with filth or whereby it may have been rendered injurious to health; or
- If its container is composed, in whole or in part, of any poisonous or deleterious substance which may render the contents injurious to health; or
- If it bears or contains, for purposes of coloring only, a color other than one which is prescribed; or
- If it contains any harmful or toxic substance which may render it injurious to health; or
- If any substance has been mixed therewith so as to reduce its quality or strength.

Me-Too Drugs

A drug that is structurally very similar to already known drugs with only minor differences is called me-too drug. These drugs have **similar mechanism of action** and mostly similar indications and adverse effects. These mainly differ in pharmacokinetic parameters like V_d, $t\frac{1}{2}$, etc. Enalapril, ramipril, perindopril, captopril etc. are me-too drugs.

Orphan Drugs

Orphan drugs are defined as the medicines which are **unlikely to be developed by pharmaceutical industry due to economic reasons** but which respond to public health needs. An **orphan drug** is mostly a pharmaceutical agent that has been developed specifically to treat a rare medical condition (*affecting fewer than 200,000 people*), the condition itself being referred to as an orphan disease. Examples include *deferipirone* to treat iron overload in thalasemia patients, *N-acetylcysteine* to treat paracetamol poisoning etc. The term orphan drug is **also used for medicines for some common diseases in third world countries** and also to some products formed by research process that cannot be patented. Since the pharmaceutical companies will not like to develop such a drug due to lack of financial benefits, a separate law known as '*The Orphan Drug Act*' was passed in 1983. The intent of the Orphan Drug Act is to stimulate the research, development, and approval of products that treat rare diseases.

Essential Drugs

- These are the drugs **that satisfy the priority healthcare needs of a population.** These are selected with regard to
  - Incidence and pravelence of disease (public health relevance)
  - Evidence on safety and efficacy
  - Comparative cost-effectiveness
  - Assurance of quality
- Most essential drugs are formulated as **single compounds**
- WHO brought first essential drug list in 1977. It is updated every 2 years. The current version is 18th WHO essential medicines list and 4th WHO essential medicines list for children updated in April 2013.
- The first national essential medicine list of India was prepared in 1996. It was revised in 2003, 2011 and in 2013. The latest list contains 406 drugs.

Golden Points

1. Two drugs having opposite response via action on different receptors are called physiological antagonists, e.g. adernaline (causes bronchodilation by actiion on $β_2$ receptors) is physiological antagonist of histamine (cause bronchoconstriction by acting on H_1 receptors).

2. Two drugs having opposite response via action on same receptors are called **pharmacological antagonists,** e.g. propranolol (causing bradycardia by acting on $β_1$ receptors) is pharmacological antagonist of adrenaline (cause tachycardia by acting on $β_1$ receptors)

3. Alpha 1 ($α_1$) receptors act by increasing Ca^{2+} whereas $β_1$ increase cAMP in the cell.

4. Apparent volume of distribution is more than total body fluids (very high), if the drug is sequestered by tissues.

5. Essential medicines are the drugs that cater to priority health-care needs of a population. Most of these are formulated as single compounds.

6. Important drugs causing hemolysis in a patient with G-6-PD deficiency are primaquine, sulfonamides, dapsone and methylene blue.

7.
Clinical Trial	Other Name
Phase 0	Microdosing studies
Phase I	Human pharmacology and safety
Phase II	Therapeutic exploratory
Phase III	Therapeutic confirmatory
Phase IV	Post marketing surveillance

8. **Grapefruit juice** acts as inhibitor of CYP3A4 due to its content of **furanocumarins** and narigin.

9. Therapeutic index is a measure of safety of a drug. It is calculated as LD50/ED50.

10. **Schedule H** of drugs and cosmetics act deal with **drugs that must be sold by retail only when a prescription by registered medical practitioner is produced**. Most drugs fall under this schedule.

11. Efficacy refers to maximum response a drug can produce regardless of its dose.

12. Phocomelia is defect in development of long bones. It is caused by thalidomide when given to pregnant females.

13. Drugs metabolized by acetylation and causing SLE like syndrome are:
    - Sulfonamides (including dapsone)
    - Hydralazine
    - Isoniazid
    - Procainamide

14. Rifampicin can result in failure of oral contraceptives due to its enzyme inducing property.

15. Pharmacogenetics refers to study dealing with how variations in human genome affect the response to drugs.

16. Drugs following zero-order kinetics are warfarin, alcohol, high dose aspirin, theophylline, tolbutamide and phenytoin.

17. Most accurate method of calculating drug dosage in children is body surface area.

18. Therapeutic drug monitoring is not required for antihypertensive (e.g. ACE inhibitors), antidiabetic (e.g. metformin) and anticoagulant (e.g. warfarin) drugs.

19. Important microsomal enzyme inhibitors are valproate, ketoconazole, cimetidine, macrolides (except azithromycin), ciprofloxacin and protease inhibitors.

20. Gastric lavage is contra-indicated in corrosive [strong acid or strong base] and kerosene poisoning.

21. Forced alkaline diuresis is effective for management of acidic drug poisoning like phenobarbitone, aspirin and methotrexate, etc.

Image Based Questions

1. In the given pharmacodynamic curve, point A corresponds to:

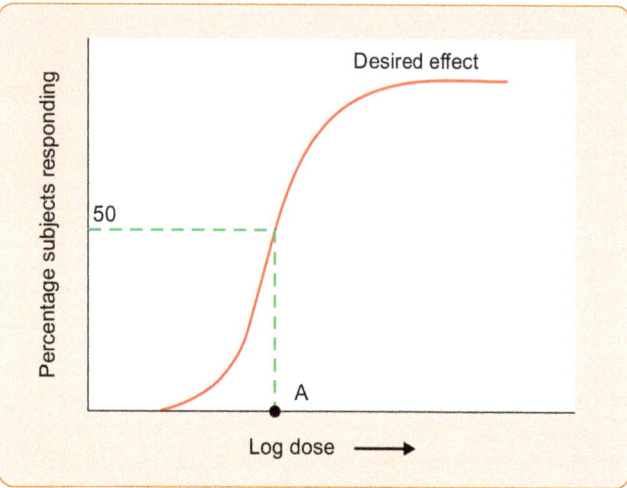

   (a) Potency
   (b) Efficacy
   (c) ED_{50}
   (d) LD_{50}

2. The image shows the Log DRC of four drugs A, B, C and D. Which of the following statements about these drugs is true?

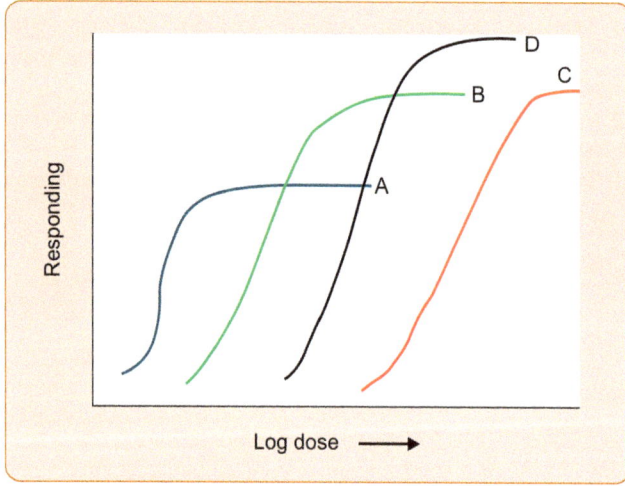

   (a) Drug A is most efficacious
   (b) Drug B and drug C are equipotent
   (c) Drug D is most effective
   (d) Drug B is less potent but more efficacious than drug A

3. Given image shows the Log DRC of a drug alone (A) and in the presence of antagonists (B and C). Identify the type of antagonism shown in the curve B and curve C:

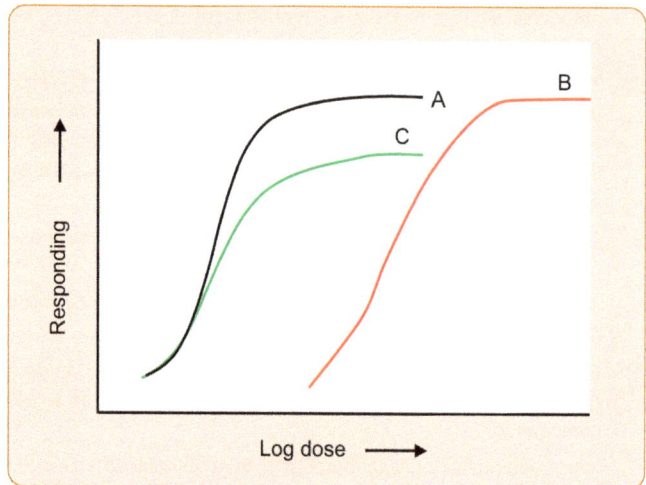

   (a) B is competitive and C is noncompetitive antagonism
   (b) B is noncompetitive an C is competitive antagonism
   (c) Both are competitive antagonists
   (d) Both are noncompetitive antagonists

4. A drug having half life of 12 hours is administered orally twice a day. A graph is plotted between plasma drug concentration and time which is shown in the graph. How much time will be taken for the plasma concentration to reach at point A?

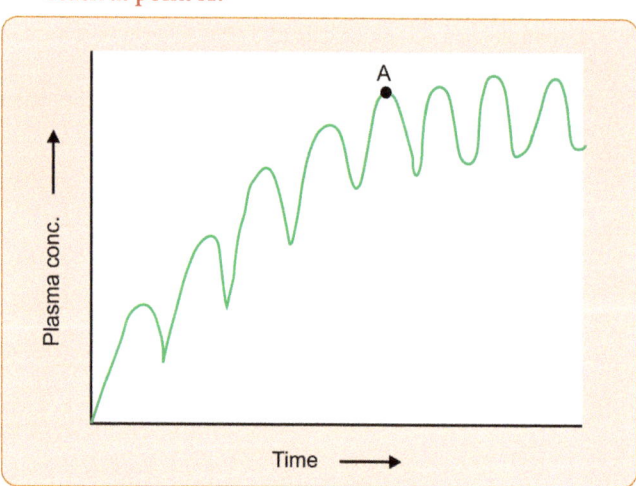

   (a) 12 hours
   (b) 24 hours
   (c) 36 hours
   (d) 60 hours

5. Which of the following drug is likely to act by signal transduction mechanism shown in the image below?

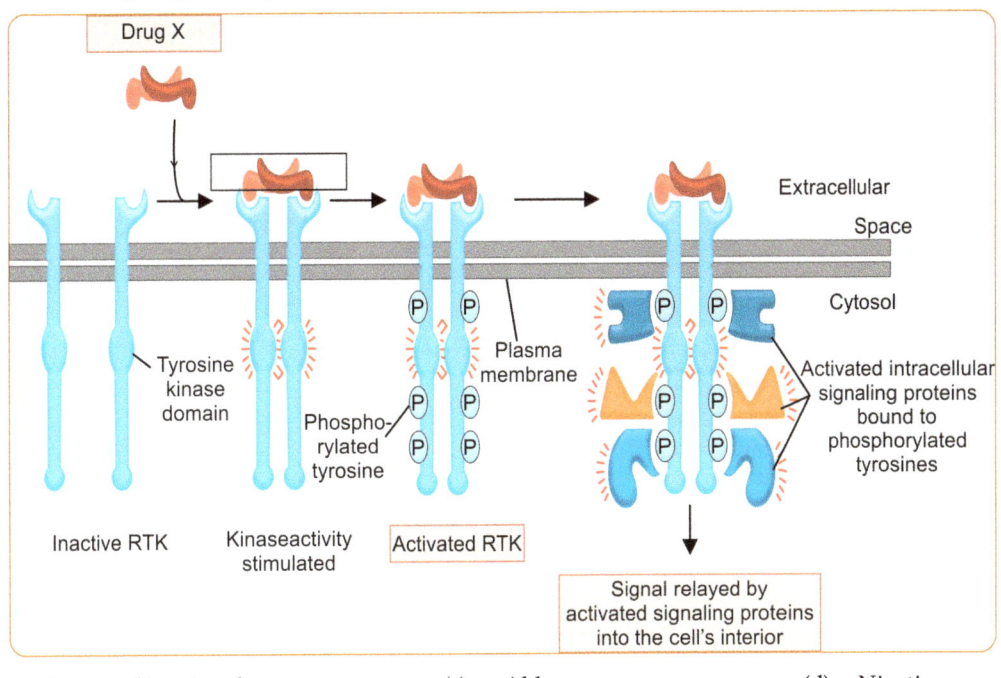

   (a) Salbutamol (b) Insulin (c) Aldosterone (d) Nicotine

6. Till what date the drug salbutamol can be used in the image of the asthalin strip shown in the Figure below?

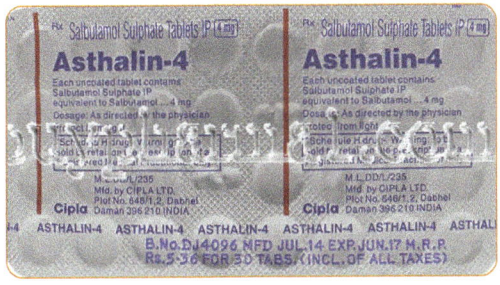

   (a) 14 July 2017 (b) 31 July 2017
   (c) 17 June 2014 (d) 30 June 2017

7. Shelf life of salbutamol in this preparation (shown in the above figure in question 6) is:
   (a) 3 years (b) 14 years
   (c) 5 years
   (d) Cannot be known from the information

8. Expiry date shown in the strip of the tablet (shown in the above figure in question 6) means:
   (a) If this preparation is used after July 2017, it will lose its potency
   (b) If this preparation is used after July 2017, it will become toxic
   (c) Quality of this medicine is not assured after July 2017
   (d) Both a and b

9. What does IP in the above image (in question 6) stand for?
   (a) Drug is meant for Intra Pulmonary use
   (b) Intellectual Property right of the CIPLA
   (c) The standards according to Indian Pharmacopeia
   (d) It is an Instant release Preparation

10. Which of the following route of administration is shown in the given diagram?

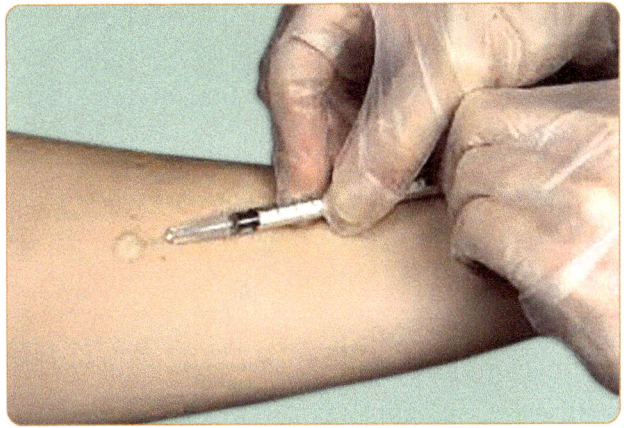

   (a) Intradermal
   (b) Subcutaneous
   (c) Intramuscular
   (d) Intravenous

11. Identify for the route of drug administration shown in the given image:

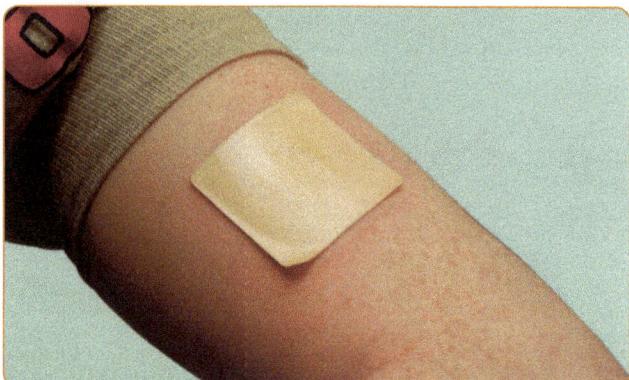

(a) Local
(b) Transdermal
(c) Subcutaneous
(d) Intradermal

12. Calculate the therapeutic index of the drug from given DRC.

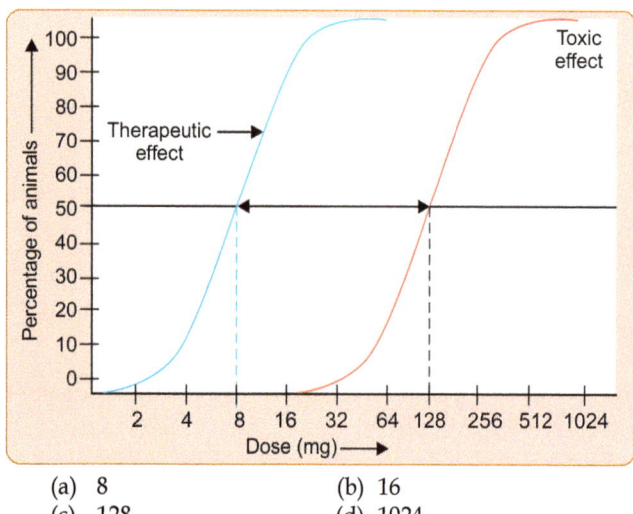

(a) 8
(b) 16
(c) 128
(d) 1024

13. Identify the type of unknown drug Y by looking at the given log DRC.

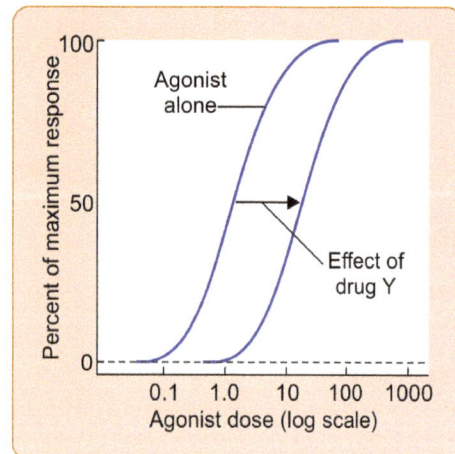

(a) Agonist
(b) Competitive antagonist
(c) Non-competitive antagonist
(d) None of these

14. Identify the type of unknown drug X, by looking at the given log DRC:

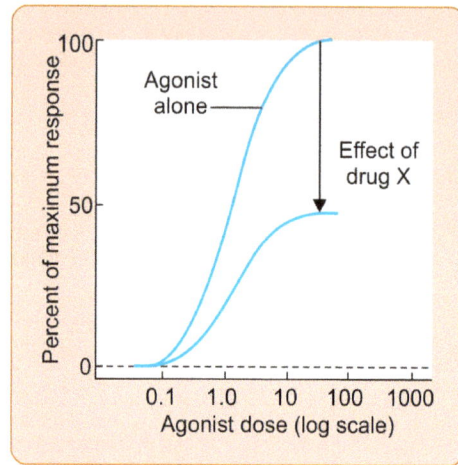

(a) Agonist
(b) Competitive antagonist
(c) Non-competitive antagonist
(d) None of these

15. Which of the following statements about the given plasma concentration vs time graph is correct?

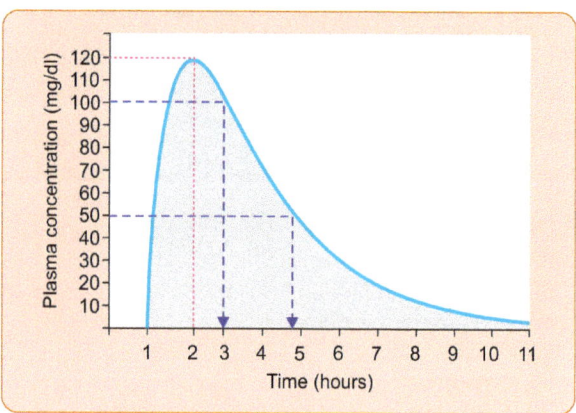

(a) T_{max} of the drug is 3 hours
(b) C_{max} of the drug in this graph is 100 mg/dl
(c) Elimination half life of the drug is approximately 2 hours
(d) The graph can be used to calculate ED_{50}.

16. A new drug X is given orally to a healthy volunteer in a dose of 100 mg. Plasma concentration of the drug is measured at hourly interval and a graph is plotted between plasma concentration and time as shown in below figure.

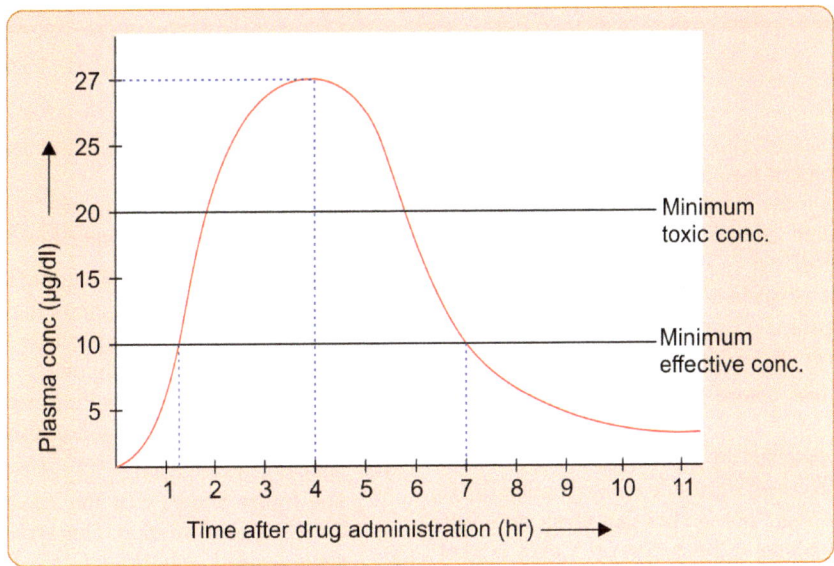

Which of the following statements about drug X is TRUE?
(a) Its C_{max}. Is 20 μg/dL.
(b) AUC from the above graph reflects rate of absorption
(c) Tmax for drug X is 7 hours.
(d) Instead of 100 mg drug X should be given in divided doses.

Explanations

1. **Ans. (c) ED_{50}**
   Quantal DRC is employed for conditions where there is all or none response. It is used to calculate median effective dose (ED_{50}) and median lethal dose (LD_{50}). ED_{50} is the dose at which 50 percent of the recipient gets the desired (or undesired) action. It is calculated from the quantal DRC as shown in the figure. The same point in graded DRC corresponds to potency of the drug.

2. **Ans. (d) Drug B is less potent but more efficacious than drug A**
   In DRC, potency is assessed by looking at the location of curve on X axis i.e. curves on right side are less potent drugs and those on left are more potent. On the other hand, efficacy is assessed by looking at the curves on Y axis. Higher curves are of more efficacious drugs and lower for less efficacious ones. However, read the statement carefully, we cannot assess effectiveness from the DRC.
   Therefore in the given image:
   - A is most potent, not most efficacious
   - B and C are equally efficacious, not equipotent
   - D is most efficacious, not most effective
   - B is less potent than drug A but has more efficacy than it

3. **Ans. (a) B is competitive and C is noncompetitive antagonist**
   In competitive antagonism, the DRC shifts towards right i.e. potency decreases but efficacy remains same. On the other hand, in case of non-competitive antagonism, the curve becomes flat i.e. potency remains same but efficacy decreases

4. **Ans. (d) 60 hours**
   The point A refers to steady state. The time taken to reach steady state plasma concentration is 4 to 5 half lives. As half life of the drug is 12 hours in the question, so it will take 48-60 hours to reach the steady state.

5. **Ans. (b) Insulin**
   The given figure shows that the signal transduction mechanism of the receptor is through tyrosine kinase. The enzymatic receptors are present for
   - Cytokines
   - Prolactin
   - Insulin
   - Growth Hormone

6. **Ans. (d) 30th June 2017**
   The given strip shows the information that MFD (means manufacturing date) is July 2014 whereas expiry date is June 2017. The drug can be used till last date of month of expiry date. Therefore this product can be used up to 30th June 2014

7. **Ans. (a) 3 years**
   The shelf life is time in which drug can be used ie from manufacturing date to expiry date. In this figure, drug can be used from July 2014 till June 2017, so shelf life is 3 years.

8. **Ans. (c) Quality of this medicine is not assured after July 2017**
   The expiry date means the time till that the product should remain within specified limits if properly stored.

9. **Ans. (c) The standards according to Indian Pharmacopoeia**
   The abbreviations written on the drug label
   - IP: Indian Pharmacopoeia
   - BP: British Pharmacopoeia
   - USP: United Nations Pharmacopoeia
   - BNF: British National Formulary

10. **Ans. (a) Intradermal**
    The figure shows that the needle is at 10-15° angle and there is bleb formation. This is characteristic of intradermal route.

11. **Ans. (b). Transdermal**
    Transdermal route is applied by placing a patch on the skin.

12. **Ans. (b) 16**
    Therapeutic index is calculated as:
    $TI = LD_{50}/ED_{50}$
    = 128 mg/8 mg
    = 16

13. **Ans. (b) Competitive antagonist**
    Competitive antagonist shift the DRC to right (parallel shift). It decreases potency without affecting the efficacy

14. **Ans (c) Noncompetitive antagonist**
    Noncompetitive antagonist shifts the curve down. It decreases the efficacy.

15. **Ans. (c) Elimination half life of the drug is approximately 2 hours.**
    - C_{max} is the maximum concentration obtained with a particular dose. It is 120 mg/dl in this graph
    - T_{max} is the time required to attain C_{max}. It is 2 hours in this graph
    - Half life is the time required for plasma concentration to become 50%. At 3 hours, it was 100 and at 5 hours, it becomes 50 mg/dl. So, 2 hours is the half life.
    - ED_{50} and LD_{50} are calculated from quantal DRC, not from graded DRC.

16. **Ans. (d) Instead of 100 mg, drug X should be given in divided doses.** *(Ref: Goodman Gilman 12/e p35)*
    C_{max} is the maximum plasma concentration obtained. In this question, C_{max} is 27 µg/dl.
    T_{max} is the time to reach C_{max}. It tells about rate of absorption. From the given graph, T_{max} is 4 hours.
    AUC reflects extent of absorption and not the rate of absorption.
    This drug, when given as 100 mg, produce a C_{max} which is higher than the minimum toxic concentration (20 µg/dl.). Thus to avoid the toxic effects, C_{max} must be lower and to produce a lower C_{max}, the dose has to be reduced.

General Pharmacology

Multiple Choice Questions

PHARMACOKINETICS (ADME)

1. Aspirin and phenobarbitone are acidic drugs whereas diazepam is a basic drug. Mention the true/false statements about these drugs. *(AIIMS May 2019)*
   (a) Aspirin is present mainly in non-ionized form in stomach, hence can be easily absorbed
   (b) Diazepam is mostly absorbed form intestine
   (c) Phenobarbitone can be absorbed from stomach but most of the absorption occurs in small intestine due to its large surface area
   (d) No drug is absorbed in large intestine due to its very low surface area
   (e) Diseases decreasing the transit time of drugs like diarrhea will increase the drug absorption in small intestine

2. Low apparent volume of distribution of a drug indicates that: *(AIIMS Nov. 2018)*
   (a) Drug has low half life
   (b) Drug has low bioavailability
   (c) Drug has low efficacy
   (d) Drug is not extensively distributed to tissues

3. Major determinant of loading dose of a drug is: *(AIIMS Nov. 2018)*
   (a) Half life
   (b) Clearance
   (c) Volume of distribution
   (d) Bioavailability

4. From which of the following routes, bioavailability of the drug is likely to be 100 percent? *(AIIMS May 2018)*
   (a) Intravenous   (b) Subcutaneous
   (c) Intramuscular (d) Intradermal

5. Hepatic First pass metabolism will be encountered by which of the following routes of drug administration? *(AIIMS May 2018)*
   (a) Oral   (b) Intravenous
   (c) Sublingual   (d) Subcutaneous

6. Loading dose of a drug depends upon: *(AIIMS May 2018)*
   (a) Volume of distribution
   (b) Clearance
   (c) Half life
   (d) Duration of action

7. High plasma protein binding of a drug result in: *(NEET Pattern Question 2019)*
   (a) Increase in Vd
   (b) Decrease in glomerular filtration
   (c) Increase in tubular secretion
   (d) Decreased drug interactions

8. pKa is the pH at which? *(NEET Pattern question 2018)*
   (a) There is 50% drug in active form
   (b) There is 50% ionized and 50% non-ionized fraction of the drug
   (c) All the drug is in non-ionized form
   (d) All the drug is in ionized form

9. Drug Transport across the cell membrane is mainly by: *(NEET Pattern question 2017)*
   (a) Simple diffusion   (b) Active transport
   (c) Failitated diffusion (d) Pinocytosis

10. Which of the following is not an example of Phase II drug metabolic reaction? *(NEET Pattern Question 2017)*
    (a) Glucuronidation   (b) Decyclization
    (c) Methylation   (d) Acetylation

11. Initial feature of storage of drug in the tissues is suggested by: *(AIIMS Nov 2017)*
    (a) Small apparent volume of distribution
    (b) Large apparent volume of distribution
    (c) Less excretion in urine
    (d) High excretion in saliva

12. Which of the following is a P glycoproteins inducer? *(AIIMS Nov 2017)*
    (a) Ketoconazole   (b) Rifampicin
    (c) Erythromycin   (d) Itraconazole

13. If a drug is absorbed through skin, what is the order of maximum percutaneous absorption of the drug from the given routes? *(AIIMS Nov 2016)*
    (a) Posterior auricular > Scrotum > Scalp > Dorsum of hand > Plantar area
    (b) Scalp > Scrotum > Posterior auricular > Dorsum of hand > Plantar area
    (c) Plantar area > Dorsum of hand > Scalp > Scrotum > Posterior auricular
    (d) Scrotum > Scalp > Posterior auricular > Dorsum of hand > Plantar area

14. Low V_d means: *(AIIMS Nov 2015)*
    (a) The drug has low half life
    (b) The drug does not accumulate in tissues
    (c) The drug has low bioavailability
    (d) The drug has weak plasma protein binding

15. Nitroglycerine is effective when administered sublingually because it is: *(AIIMS May 2015)*
    (a) Non ionized and lipid soluble
    (b) Ionized and lipid soluble
    (c) Non ionized and Water insoluble
    (d) Ionized and water insoluble

16. What is the rationale behind xenobiotic metabolism by CYP enzymes? *(AIIMS May 2015)*
    (a) Increase in water solubility
    (b) Increase in lipid solubility
    (c) Conversion to an active metabolite
    (d) Makes it suitable to evaporate through skin surface

17. Alkaline diuresis is done for treatment of poisoning due to: (AI 2012)
    (a) Morphine (b) Amphetamine
    (c) Phenobarbitone (d) Atropine

18. The mitochondrial enzyme involved in the metabolism of clopidorgel and proton pump inhibitors is: (AI 2012)
    (a) CYP 2A (b) CYP 2B
    (c) CYP 2C19 (d) CYP 2D6

19. Identify the wrong statement:
    (NEET Pattern NEET Pattern Question)
    (a) Acidic drugs bind to albumin in plasma
    (b) Basic drugs bind to alpha-1 acid glycoprotein in plasma
    (c) Drugs having higher affinity for a plasma protein can displace the other drug from the same protein
    (d) Sex steroid hormones do not bind to any protein in plasma

20. The extent to which ionization of a drug takes place is dependent upon pKa of the drug and the pH of the solution in which the drug is dissolved. Which of the following statements is NOT correct? (AIIMS Nov 2010)
    (a) pKa of a drug is the pH at which the drug is 50% ionized
    (b) Small changes of pH near the pKa of a weak acidic drug will not affect its degree of ionization.
    (c) Knowledge of pKa of a drug is useful in predicting its behaviour in various body fluids.
    (d) Phenobarbitone with a pKa of 7.2 is largely unionized at acid pH and will be about 40% nonionized in plasma.

21. All of the following statements regarding bioavailability of a drug are true except: (NEET Pattern Question)
    (a) It is a fraction of administered drug that reaches the systemic circulation in unchanged form
    (b) Bioavailability of an orally administered drug can be calculated by comparing the Area Under Curve after oral and intravenous administration
    (c) Low oral bioavailability always and necessarily means poor absorption
    (d) Bioavailability can be determined from plasma concentration or urinary excretion data.

22. Drugs with high plasma protein binding have:
    (a) Short duration of action (NEET Pattern Question)
    (b) Less drug interactions
    (c) Lower volumes of distribution
    (d) All of the above

23. Which does not induce microsomal enzymes?
    (NEET Pattern Question)
    (a) Cimetidine (b) Griseofulvin
    (c) Rifampicin (d) Phenobarbitone

24. Which of the following is a prodrug?
    (NEET Pattern Question)
    (a) Ampicillin (b) Captopril
    (c) Levodopa (d) Phenytoin

25. Which one of the following drugs does not have active metabolite? (NEET Pattern Question)
    (a) Diazepam (b) Propranolol
    (c) Allopurinol (d) Lisinopril

26. Apparent volume of distribution (Vd) of a drug exceeds total body fluid volume, if a drug is:
    (a) Sequestrated in body tissues
    (b) Slowly eliminated from body
    (c) Poorly soluble in plasma (NEET Pattern Question)
    (d) Highly bound to plasma proteins

27. Which of the following drug acts as microsomal enzyme inhibitor? (NEET Pattern Question)
    (a) Rifampicin (b) Cimetidine
    (c) Phenobarbitone (d) Phenytoin

28. Which of the following is an inducer of microsomal enzymes? (NEET Pattern Question)
    (a) Phenobarbitone (b) Paracetamol
    (c) Digoxin (d) Penicillin

29. Removal of acidic drugs from body is done by using:
    (NEET Pattern Question)
    (a) Ammonium chloride (b) Sodium bicarbonate
    (c) Hydrochloric acid (d) Citric acid

30. Very high first pass metabolism is seen in:
    (NEET Pattern Question)
    (a) Digoxin (b) Dicumarol
    (c) Propranolol (d) Practalol

31. 'Bioavailability' is defined as: (NEET Pattern Question)
    (a) The volume of plasma completely cleared of a specific compound per unit time and measured as a test of kidney function
    (b) The percentage of drug that is detected in the systemic circulation after its administration
    (c) Both (d) None

32. Volume of distribution of drug is given by:
    (NEET Pattern Question)
    (a) $V_d = \dfrac{\text{Dose administrated IV}}{\text{Plasma concentration}}$
    (b) $V_d = \dfrac{\text{Maximum tolerated dose}}{\text{Dose administered IV}}$
    (c) $V_d = \dfrac{\text{Dose administered IV}}{\text{Total lipid solubility}}$
    (d) $V_d = \dfrac{t_{1/2}}{\text{Dose administered IV}}$

33. Redistribution phenomenon is seen in:
    (NEET Pattern Question)
    (a) Halothane (b) Ether
    (c) Thiopentone (d) All

34. Sulphonamide is conjugated with: (NEET Pattern Question)
    (a) Acetylation (b) Methylation
    (c) Hydroxylation (d) None

35. Which of the following statements is correct?
    (NEET Pattern Question)
    (a) Most drugs are absorbed in ionized form
    (b) Basic drugs are generally bound to plasma albumin
    (c) Microsomal enzymes are located in the mitochondria of hepatic cells
    (d) Blood brain barrier is deficient at the chemoreceptor trigger zone

36. Nonsynthetic phase I reaction for drug detoxification is:
    (NEET Pattern Question)
    (a) Glucuronidation (b) Acetylation
    (c) Methylation (d) Oxidation

General Pharmacology

37. Which of the following is NOT a prodrug?
    (NEET Pattern Question)
    (a) Enalapril (b) Imipramine
    (c) Sulphasalazine (d) Cyclophosphamide

38. Loading dose of a drug is given: *(NEET Pattern Question)*
    (a) To achieve steady state concentration in short time
    (b) For drugs with short t½
    (c) To reduce complications
    (d) All of these

39. Alkalinization of urine is done for:
    (NEET Pattern Question)
    (a) Weak acid drugs (b) Weak basics drugs
    (c) Strong acidic drugs (d) Strong basic drugs

40. Loading dose depends on the following factors *except*:
    (NEET Pattern Question)
    (a) Drug concentration to be achieved
    (b) Volume of distribution
    (c) Clearance of the drug
    (d) Bioavailability of drug

41. Which of the following is a Phase I metabolic reaction?
    (NEET Pattern Question)
    (a) Hydroxylation (b) Conjugation
    (c) Glucuronidation (d) Sulfation

42. In drug metabolism, hepatic cytochrome P-450 system is responsible for: *(NEET Pattern Question)*
    (a) Phase I reactions (hydrolysis, oxidation, reduction etc.) only
    (b) Phase II reactions (conjugation, synthesis etc.) only
    (c) Both phase I and II reactions
    (d) Converting hydrophilic metabolites to lipophilic metabolites

43. Time for peak plasma concentration (T max) indicates:
    (NEET Pattern Question)
    (a) The rate of elimination
    (b) The rate of absorption
    (c) The duration of effect
    (d) The intensity of effect

44. One of the potential microsomal enzymes inhibitor drug is: *(NEET Pattern Question)*
    (a) Phenobarbitone (b) Griseofulvin
    (c) Sodium valproate (d) Phenytoin

45. Alkalinization of urine is required to treat toxicity of all *except*: *(NEET Pattern Question)*
    (a) Methotrexate (b) Amphetamine
    (c) Salicylates (d) Barbiturates

46. Cytochrome P450 enzyme most commonly involved in drug metabolism is: *(NEET Pattern Question)*
    (a) CYP 3A4 (b) CYP 1AI
    (c) CYP 2E1 (d) CYP 2D6

47. Which of the following drugs binds to albumin?
    (NEET Pattern Question)
    (a) Penicillin (b) Lidocaine
    (c) Propranolol (d) Verapamil

48. Which of the following is an enzyme inhibitor?
    (NEET Pattern Question)
    (a) Ketoconazole (b) Rifampicin
    (c) Tolbutamide (d) Phenobarbitone

49. All of the following antiepileptics are microsomal enzyme inducers *except*: *(NEET Pattern Question)*
    (a) Valproate (b) Phenobarbitone
    (c) Phenytoin (d) Rifampicin

50. Which of the following is an effect of grapefruit juice on drug metabolism? *(NEET Pattern Question)*
    (a) Enzyme inducer
    (b) Enzyme inhibitor
    (c) Inhibits tubular secretion
    (d) Inhibits tubular reabsorption

51. Which of the following can result in oral contraceptive failure? *(NEET Pattern Question)*
    (a) Valproate (b) Rifampicin
    (c) NSAIDs (d) Ethambutol

52. The drug which may inhibit P450 for warfarin is which one of the following? *(NEET Pattern Question)*
    (a) Cimetidine (b) Ethanol
    (c) Rifampicin (d) Procainamide

53. Forced alkaline diuresis is effective in management of poisoning by which of the following agents?
    (NEET Pattern Question)
    (a) Phenobarbitone (b) Lead
    (c) Iron (d) Organophosphates

54. Which route of drug administration avoids first pass hepatic metabolism and is used with drug preparation that slowly releases drugs for periods as long as seven days? *(NEET Pattern Question)*
    (a) Topical (b) Transdermal
    (c) Sublingual (d) Oral

55. Hemodialysis is useful in all of the following *except*:
    (NEET Pattern Question)
    (a) Barbiturate poisoning (b) Methanol poisoning
    (c) Salicylate poisoning (d) Digoxin poisoning

56. The bioavailability of the drug depends upon:
    (a) First pass metabolism *(NEET Pattern Question)*
    (b) Second pass metabolism
    (c) Volume of distribution
    (d) Excretion

57. Bioavailability is: *(NEET Pattern Question)*
    (a) Amount of drug that reach the systemic circulation
    (b) Drug metabolized in liver before the drug reaches the systemic circulation
    (c) Drug metabolized in liver after the drug reaches the systemic circulation
    (d) Maximum by rectal route

58. About biotransformation untrue is:
    (NEET Pattern Question)
    (a) Inactive metabolites are formed
    (b) Active metabolites are formed
    (c) More fat soluble metabolites are formed
    (d) More water soluble metabolites are formed

59. Which of the following is not a pro-drug?
    (NEET Pattern Question)
    (a) Levodopa (b) Enalapril
    (c) Dipivefrine (d) Amoxicillin

60. Which of the following is a prodrug?
    (NEET Pattern Question)
    (a) Lisinopril (b) Enalapril
    (c) Chlorpromazine (d) Dopamine

61. False regarding Cytochrome P 450 enzymes is:
    (NEET Pattern Question)
    (a) They are involved in the production of steroids.
    (b) They absorb maximum light at 450 nm wavelength
    (c) They are present in endoplasmic reticulum of liver cells
    (d) They are non heme proteins

62. A drug has 40% absorption and hepatic extraction ratio of 0.6. What is the bioavailability of the drug?
    (NEET Pattern Question)
    (a) 16% (b) 24%
    (c) 20% (d) 28%

63. Most variable absorption is seen with which route?
    (NEET Pattern Question)
    (a) Oral (b) Intramuscular
    (c) Intravenous (d) Per rectal

64. Branch of Pharmacology that deals with medicinal drugs obtained from plants and other natural resources is known as:
    (NEET Pattern Question)
    (a) Pharmacognosy (b) Pharmacogenetics
    (c) Pharmacogenomics (d) Pharmacopoeia

PHARMACOKINETICS (CALCULATIONS)

65. Which of the following parameter is used to assess the rate of drug absorption?
    (AIIMS May 2018)
    (a) T_{max}
    (b) C_{max}
    (c) Half life
    (d) Area under the curve

66. A patient require ceftriaxone 180 mg. You have a 2 mL syringe with 10 divisions per mL. The vial contains 100 mg/5 mL of ceftriaxone. How many divisions in the 2 mL syringe will you fill to give 180 mg ceftriaxone?
    (a) 18 (b) 1.8 *(AIIMS Nov 2017)*
    (c) 20 (d) 2

67. A drug X was administered by continuous IV infusion at the rate of 1.6 mg/min. Clearance of drug X is 640 mL/min. If the half-life of the drug is 1.8 h, what would be the concentration of drug after achieving steady state?
    (AIIMS May 2017)
    (a) 0.0025 mg/mL (b) 0.004 mg/mL
    (c) 3.25 mg/mL (d) 1.22 mg/mL

68. A patient was administered 200 mg of a drug. 75 mg of the drug is eliminated from the body in 90 minutes. If the drug follows first order kinetics, how much drug will remain after 6 hrs?
    (AIIMS May 2017)
    (a) 30.5 mg (b) 12.5 mg
    (c) 25 mg (d) 50 mg

69. Digoxin has a half-life of 40 hours. It helps to determine:
    (a) Regimen for smooth discontinuation *(AIIMS Nov 2016)*
    (b) Need for loading dose in order to get immediate effect
    (c) Regimen for maintenance dose
    (d) Single dose will work for 40 hours

70. Which of the following parameters signifies the effective drug removal from the body?
    (AIIMS Nov 2013)
    (a) Clearance (b) Bioavailability
    (c) Safety (d) Volume of distribution

71. True statement about first order kinetics is:
    (AIIMS May 2012)
    (a) A constant amount of a drug is eliminated in unit time
    (b) The half-life increases with an increase in dose
    (c) The rate of elimination is constant
    (d) The rate of elimination is proportional to the plasma concentration

72. Loading dose of a drug primarily depends on:
    (a) Volume of distribution *(NEET Pattern Question)*
    (b) Clearance
    (c) Rate of administration
    (d) Half life

73. True statement regarding first order kinetics is:
    (NEET Pattern Question)
    (a) Rate of elimination is independent of plasma concentration
    (b) A constant proportion of plasma concentration is eliminated per unit time
    (c) Half life increases with dose
    (d) Clearance decreases with dose

74. Zero order kinetics is followed by all of the following drugs *except*: *(NEET Pattern Question)*
    (a) Phenytoin (b) Barbiturates
    (c) Alcohol (d) Theophylline

75. At toxic doses, zero order kinetics is seen in:
    (NEET Pattern Question)
    (a) Penicillin (b) Phenytoin
    (c) Valproate (d) Carbamazepine

76. Inter dose interval depends on: *(NEET Pattern Question)*
    (a) Half life of drug (b) Dose of drug
    (c) Age of patient (d) Bioavailability of drug

77. Time required to reach the steady state after a dosage regimen depends on: *(NEET Pattern Question)*
    (a) Route of administration
    (b) Half life of a drug
    (c) Dosage interval
    (d) Dose of drug

78. Zero order kinetic is shown by all *except*:
    (NEET Pattern Question)
    (a) High dose salicylates (b) Phenytoin
    (c) Ethanol (d) Methotrexate

79. The elimination of alcohol follows:
    (NEET Pattern Question)
    (a) Zero order kinetics (b) 1st order kinetics
    (c) 2nd orders kinetics (d) 3rd orders kinetics

80. The clearance of drug means: *(NEET Pattern Question)*
    (a) Volume of plasma which is cleared of drug in a unit time
    (b) Amount of drug excreted in urine
    (c) Amount of drug metabolized in unit of time
    (d) All of the above

General Pharmacology

81. Zero order kinetics occur in following drug with high dose: *(NEET Pattern Question)*
    (a) Phenytoin and Theophylline
    (b) Digoxin and Propranol
    (c) Amiloride and Probenecid
    (d) Lithium and Theophylline

82. Zero order kinetics means: *(NEET Pattern Question)*
    (a) A constant amount of drug is eliminated per unit time
    (b) A constant fraction of the drug in the body is eliminated per unit time
    (c) The fraction of the administered dose that reaches the systemic circulation
    (d) The effect that can be increased by giving a second agent that boosts the effect ot the liver's enzyme system

83. About first order kinetics true statement is:
    (a) Clearance remains constant *(NEET Pattern Question)*
    (b) Fixed amount of the drug is eliminated
    (c) Half life increase with dose
    (d) Decreased clearance with increasing dose

84. Zero order kinetics occur in following drug with high dose: *(NEET Pattern Question)*
    (a) Phenytoin and propranolol
    (b) Digoxin and propranolol
    (c) Amiloride and prebenecid
    (d) Alcohol and theophylline

85. Elimination after 3 half lives in first order kinetics is: *(NEET Pattern Question)*
    (a) 12.5%   (b) 75%
    (c) 87.5%   (d) 94%

86. Drug remaining in the body after 3 half lives is: *(NEET Pattern Question)*
    (a) 12.5%   (b) 75%
    (c) 87.5%   (d) 94%

PHARMACODYNAMICS AND PHARMACOGENETICS

87. Drug acting via tyrosine kinase receptors is: *(NEET Pattern Question 2020)*
    (a) TRH   (b) TSH
    (c) Insulin   (d) MSH

88. Which of the following drugs shown in the graph below has highest potency? *(NEET Pattern Question 2020)*

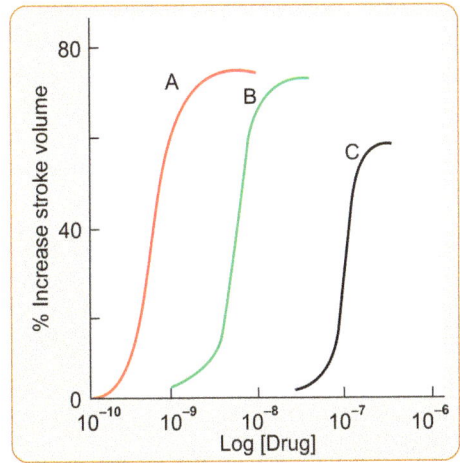

    (a) Drug A   (b) Drug B
    (c) Drug C   (d) Both Drugs A and B

89. True about non-competitive enzyme inhibition is: *(NEET Pattern Question 2020)*
    (a) Km remains same, Vmax decreases
    (b) Km increases, Vmax remains same
    (c) Km decreases, Vmax increases
    (d) Km increases, Vmax increases

90. G-protein coupled receptor that does not act through opening of potassium channels is: *(NEET Pattern Question 2020)*
    (a) Muscarinic M2 receptor
    (b) Dopamine D2 receptor
    (c) Serotonin 5 HT 1 receptor
    (d) Angiotensin 1 receptor

91. Acetazolamide is given to a patient of angle closure glaucoma. It is a non-competitive inhibitor of carbonic anhydrase enzyme. Which of the following should be the effect of this drug? *(AIIMS Nov. 2018)*
    (a) Decrease in V_{max}
    (b) Decrease in K_m
    (c) Decrease in both K_m and V_{max}
    (d) No change in V_{max}

92. Which of the following is correct regarding the mechanism of action of thyroid hormones T4 and T3 at thyroid hormone receptor? *(AIIMS Nov. 2018)*
    (a) These activate phosphatidylinositol/DAG/calcium cascade
    (b) These act by increasing cyclic AMP
    (c) These activate a tyrosine kinase enzyme
    (d) These activate a nuclear transcription factor

93. Which of the following act through G protein coupled receptors? *(AIIMS May. 2018)*
    (a) Muscarinic receptors (b) Insulin receptors
    (c) Nicotinic receptors   (d) GABA-A receptors

94. Variation in sensitivity of response to increasing doses of the drug in different individuals can be obtained from: *(NEET Pattern Question 2019)*
    (a) Graded DRC   (b) Quantal DRC
    (c) Potency   (d) Efficacy

95. Which of the following statement is correct regarding the given Dose Response Curve? *(AIIMS Nov 2016)*
    (a) A and B are full agonists
    (b) C is a non-competitive antagonist
    (c) B is more potent than A
    (d) A more efficacious than B

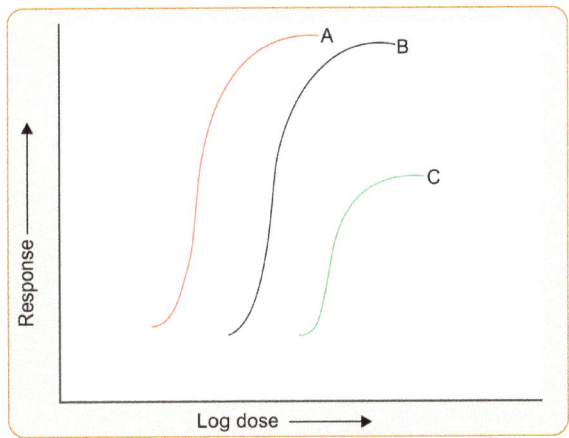

96. All of the following can cause SLE-like syndrome *except*:
 (AIIMS May 2013, 2012)
 (a) Isoniazid (b) Penicillin
 (c) Hydralazine (d) Sulphonamide

97. Which one of the following statements best describes the mechanism of action of insulin on target cells? *(NEET Pattern Question)*
 (a) Insulin binds to cytoplasmic receptor molecule and is transferred as a hormone receptor complex to the nucleus where it acts to modulate gene expression.
 (b) Insulin binds to a receptor molecule on the outer surface of the plasma membrane and the hormone receptor complex activates adenylate cyclase through the Gs protein.
 (c) Insulin binds to a transmembrane receptor at the outer surface of the plasma membrane, which activates the tyrosine kinase that is the cytosolic domain of the receptor.
 (d) Insulin enters the cell and causes the release of calcium ions from intracellular stores.

98. A non-competitive inhibitor of an enzyme:
 (NEET Pattern Question)
 (a) Increase K_m with no or little change in V_{max}
 (b) Decrease K_m
 (c) Decrease V_{max}
 (d) Increase V_{max}

99. All known effects of cyclic AMP in eukaryotic cells results from: *(NEET Pattern Question)*
 (a) Activation of the catalytic unit of adenylate cyclase
 (b) Activation of synthetase
 (c) Activation of protein kinase
 (d) Phosphorylation of G protein

100. All of the following drugs cause hemolysis in patients with G-6-PD deficiency *except*: *(NEET Pattern Question)*
 (a) Primaquine (b) Chloroquine
 (c) Quinine (d) Pyrimethamine

101. All of the following agents act by intracellular receptors *except*: *(NEET Pattern Question)*
 (a) Thyroid hormones (b) Vitamin D
 (c) Insulin (d) Steroids

102. Regarding efficacy and potency of a drug, all are true *except*: *(NEET Pattern Question)*
 (a) In a clinical setup, efficacy is more important than potency
 (b) In the log dose response curve, the height of the curve corresponds with efficacy
 (c) ED_{50} of the drug corresponds to the efficacy
 (d) Drugs that produce a similar pharmacological effect can have different levels of efficacy

103. True statement regarding inverse agonist is:
 (NEET Pattern Question)
 (a) Binds to the receptor and causes intended action
 (b) Binds to the receptor and causes opposite action
 (c) Binds to the receptor and causes no action
 (d) Binds to the receptor and causes submaximal action

104. Which of the following property of the drug will enable it to be used in low concentration? *(NEET Pattern Question)*
 (a) High affinity (b) High specificity
 (c) Low specificity (d) High stability

105. K_m of an enzyme is: *(NEET Pattern Question)*
 (a) Dissociation constant
 (b) The normal physiological substrate concentration
 (c) The substrate concentration at half maximal velocity
 (d) Numerically identical for all isozymes that catalyze a given reaction

106. Which of the following has cytoplasmic receptor?
 (NEET Pattern Question)
 (a) Epinephrine (b) Insulin
 (c) FSH (d) Cortisol

107. Which of the following is true for receptor action of a drug? *(NEET Pattern Question)*
 (a) An antagonist has both intrinsic activity and affinity for receptor
 (b) An antagonist has affinity but no intrinsic activity for receptor
 (c) A partial agonist has no intrinsic activity or affinity for receptor
 (d) Intrinsic activity and affinity are not important for drug action

108. All of the following cross plasma membrane *except*:
 (NEET Pattern Question)
 (a) Epinephrine (b) Thyroxine
 (c) Testosterone (d) Estrogen

109. G-coupled protein receptor is: *(NEET Pattern Question)*
 (a) Metabotropic receptors
 (b) Ionic receptors
 (c) Kinase-linked receptors
 (d) Nuclear receptors

110. Antagonism between acetylcholine and atropine:
 (a) Competitive antagonism *(NEET Pattern Question)*
 (b) Physiological antagonism
 (c) Noncompetitive antagonism
 (d) None

111. When two different chemicals act on two different receptors and their response is opposite to each other on the same cell, this is called as:
 (NEET Pattern Question)
 (a) Physiological antagonism
 (b) Chemical antagonism
 (c) Reversible antagonism
 (d) Competitive antagonism

112. Agonist has: *(NEET Pattern Question)*
 (a) Affinity with intrinsic activity is 1
 (b) Affinity with intrinsic activity is 0
 (c) Affinity with intrinsic activity is -1
 (d) None

113. All of the following drugs can cause SLE like syndrome *except*: *(NEET Pattern Question)*
 (a) Isoniazid (b) Penicillin
 (c) Hydralazine (d) Sulphonamide

114. Two drugs having opposite action on different receptors is which type of antagonism? *(NEET Pattern Question)*
 (a) Physical antagonism
 (b) Competitive antagonism
 (c) Non competitive antagonism
 (d) Physiological antagonism

115. Increase in cAMP is caused by: *(NEET Pattern Question)*
    (a) Somatostatin
    (b) β (Beta) receptor
    (c) α (Alpha) receptor
    (d) Acetylcholine

116. Drug which does not cause hemolysis in G6PD deficiency is: *(NEET Pattern Question)*
    (a) Primaquine
    (b) Dapsone
    (c) Corticosteroids
    (d) Methylene Blue

117. Which of the following is an example of physiological antagonism? *(NEET Pattern Question)*
    (a) Heparin-Protamine
    (b) Prostacycline-Thromboxane
    (c) Adrenaline-Phenoxybenzamine
    (d) Physostigmine-Acetylcholine

118. All the following drugs act on ionic channels *except*: *(NEET Pattern Question)*
    (a) Nicotine
    (b) Insulin
    (c) Glibenclamide
    (d) Diazepam

119. Efficacy of a drug refers to: *(NEET Pattern Question)*
    (a) Affinity of drug to bind to receptors
    (b) Affinity of drug that binds to receptors and activates it
    (c) Dose that requires to produce response
    (d) Maximum response a drug can produce

120. SLE like reaction is caused by: *(NEET Pattern Question)*
    (a) Hydralazine
    (b) Rifampicin
    (c) Paracetamol
    (d) Furosemide

121. When a drug binds to the receptor and causes action opposite to that of agonist this is called as: *(NEET Pattern Question)*
    (a) Complete Agonist
    (b) Partial Agonist
    (c) Inverse agonist
    (d) Neutral antagonist

122. The study of how variation in the human genome affect the response to medications is known as: *(NEET Pattern Question)*
    (a) Pharmacogenomics
    (b) Pharmacokinetics
    (c) Pharmacotherapeutics
    (d) Pharmacovigilance

123. Which ONE of the following is TRUE about a competitive antagonism? *(NEET Pattern Question)*
    (a) Antagonism cannot be completely reversed by increased dose of the agonist
    (b) An agonist cannot displace an antagonists from the receptor
    (c) Agonists and antagonists bind to the same receptor
    (d) Dose-response curve of an agonists shifts to the left in the presence of an antagonist

124. A drug that compete for active binding site is called: *(NEET Pattern Question)*
    (a) Competitive inhibitor
    (b) Non-competitive inhibitor
    (c) Covalent inhibitor
    (d) Any of these

125. Partial agonist possess: *(NEET Pattern Question)*
    (a) Max. intrinsic activity and low affinity
    (b) High intrinsic activity and no affinity
    (c) Low intrinsic activity and high affinity
    (d) Low intrinsic activity and low affinity

126. Pharmacodynamics includes: *(NEET Pattern Question)*
    (a) Drug elimination
    (b) Drug excretion
    (c) Drug absorption
    (d) Mechanism of action

127. Calcitriol acts on: *(NEET Pattern Question)*
    (a) G-protein coupled receptors
    (b) Cytosolic receptors
    (c) Intranuclear receptors
    (d) Enzymatic receptors

128. After giving an enzyme inhibitor, if V_{max} decrease to 60% and Km is same as before. Which type of inhibition is this? *(NEET Pattern Question)*
    (a) Competitive equilibrium type
    (b) Non-competitive
    (c) Competitive non-equilibrium type
    (d) Un-competitive

129. U shaped dose response curve is seen in: *(NEET Pattern Question)*
    (a) Vitamins
    (b) Anti cancer drugs
    (c) Steroids
    (d) Chelators

THERAPEUTIC INDEX AND TDM

130. Therapeutic index is measure of: *(NEET Pattern Question 2020)*
    (a) Safety
    (b) Efficacy
    (c) Potency
    (d) Selectivity

131. Therapeutic monitoring of plasma level of drug is done when using all of the following drugs *except*: *(AI 2012)*
    (a) Warfarin
    (b) Gentamicin
    (c) Cyclosporine
    (d) Phenytoin

132. Therapeutic Drug Monitoring (TDM) involves measurement of plasma concentrations of drugs to find whether the drug levels are within the therapeutic range or not. For TDM to be clinically useful the following criteria should be fulfilled: *(NEET Pattern Question)*
    (a) There should be good relationship between plasma concentration and drug dosage
    (b) The relationship between plasma drug concentration and therapeutic response and/or toxicity should be poor
    (c) When pharmacodynamic tolerance is suspected
    (d) When the clinical response cannot be easily monitored

133. Which of the following drug needs serum level monitoring? *(NEET Pattern Question)*
    (a) Lorazepam
    (b) Lithium
    (c) Amitryptylline
    (d) Haloperidol

134. Which one of the following drugs has narrow therapeutic range? *(NEET Pattern Question)*
    (a) Propranolol
    (b) Phenytoin
    (c) Piroxicam
    (d) Prazosin

135. Therapeutic index is an assessment of: *(NEET Pattern Question)*
    (a) Potency of a drug
    (b) Onset of action
    (c) Duration of action
    (d) Margin of safety

136. Therapeutic Index is: *(NEET Pattern Question)*
    (a) $\dfrac{ED_{50}}{LD_{50}}$
    (b) $\dfrac{LD_{50}}{ED_{50}}$
    (c) $ED_{50} - LD_{50}$
    (d) $ED_{50} \times LD_{50}$

137. ED$_{50}$ is used for determining: *(NEET Pattern Question)*
    (a) Potency (b) Efficacy
    (c) Safety   (d) Toxicity

CLINICAL PHARMACOLOGY

138. Major aim of phase 1 clinical trials is to know the:
    (a) Safety *(AIIMS Nov. 2018)*
    (b) Efficacy
    (c) Maximum tolerable dose
    (d) Pharmacokinetics

139. Which of the following is an example of placebo?
    (a) Herbal medication with no known effect
    (b) Physiotherapy *(AIIMS Nov 2017)*
    (c) Sham surgery
    (d) Cognitive behavioral therapy

140. Which phase of clinical trials is done after the drug enters the market? *(AIIMS May 2016)*
    (a) Phase I   (b) Phase II
    (c) Phase III (d) Phase IV

141. Phase 1 clinical trials are mainly done for assessing: *(AIIMS Nov 2015)*
    a. Safety   b. Efficacy
    c. Pharmacodynamics d. Dosing

142. Design of the study aimed to assess the maximum tolerable dose of a new drug is best described as:
    (a) Case control study *(AIIMS May 2013)*
    (b) Phase II Randomized control trial (RCT)
    (c) Phase I trial
    (d) Phase III Randomized control trial (RCT)

143. Comparison of efficacy of a new drug B with an existing drug A is done in which phase of clinical trials? *(AI 2012)*
    (a) Phase I   (b) Phase II
    (c) Phase III (d) Phase IV

144. True about orphan drug is: *(AIIMS May 2013)*
    (a) Developed for orphans
    (b) Drugs used very rarely
    (c) Drugs used for rare diseases
    (d) Rare drug for common diseases

145. True statement about phase 2 clinical trials is: *(AIIMS 2012)*
    (a) Large number of healthy volunteers are studied
    (b) Used to determine maximum tolerated dose
    (c) Used to determine efficacy
    (d) Used to determine toxicity

146. Good clinical practice (GCP) is not required in: *(AIIMS Nov. 2007)*
    (a) Preclinical phase
    (b) Phase I trial
    (c) Phase II studies
    (d) Phase IV studies

147. In which of the following phases of clinical trials, healthy normal human volunteers participate? *(NEET Pattern Question)*
    (a) Phase-I   (b) Phase-II
    (c) Phase-III (d) Phase-IV

148. There are some undesirable but unavoidable pharmacodynamic effects of a drug, which are known as: *(NEET Pattern Question)*
    (a) Toxic effects (b) Idiosyncrasy
    (c) Side effects (d) Intolerance

149. The aim of post-marketing studies is:
    (a) Efficacy of the drug *(NEET Pattern Question)*
    (b) Dosage of the drug
    (c) Deals with alteration of the drug includes absorption, distribution, binding/storage
    (d) To know rare adverse effects of the drug

150. In which phase of clinical trials, post-marketing surveillance of a drug is carried out? *(NEET Pattern Question)*
    (a) Phase I   (b) Phase II
    (c) Phase III (d) Phase IV

151. Phase 4 clinical trial also called as: *(NEET Pattern Question)*
    (a) Human pharmacology and safety
    (b) Post marketing surveillance
    (c) Therapeutic exploration and dose ranging
    (d) Therapeutic confirmation

152. Phase 4 of clinical trials collect information specially about: *(NEET Pattern Question)*
    (a) Drug efficacy (b) Drug potency
    (c) Drug toxicity
    (d) Pharmacokinetics of the drug

153. Phase 4 clinical trial is carried out: *(NEET Pattern Question)*
    (a) Before the marketing approval of a drug
    (b) After a drug is marketed
    (c) For drugs used in rare diseases
    (d) For drugs used in pediatric patients

MISCELLANEOUS

154. Which of the following is a schedule X-drug?
    (a) Thalidomide *(AIIMS Nov. 2019)*
    (b) Colistin
    (c) Ketamine
    (d) Halothane

155. Which of the following drug must be sold by retail only production of a prescription by a registered medical practitioner? *(AIIMS Nov. 2018)*
    (a) Schedule H (b) Schedule G
    (c) Schedule X (d) Schedule M

156. 'Store in a cool place' is written on a drug label. It means drug should be stored at a temperature of:
    (a) -2 degree Celsius *(AIIMS Nov. 2018)*
    (b) 0 degree Celsius
    (c) 2–8 degree Celsius
    (d) 8–15 degree Celsius

157. Manufacturer of a drug company labels the drug contains 500 mg paracetamol. On govt. analysis, it was found to contain only 200 mg of drug. Which type of drug it is known as? *(AIIMS May 2018)*
    (a) Fake drug
    (b) Spurious drug
    (c) Adulterant drug
    (d) Misbranded drug

General Pharmacology

158. Which of the following statements about fixed dose combination of drugs is true? *(NEET Pattern 2018)*
    (a) Adverse effect of one drug may be neutralized by the other
    (b) In hepatic dysfunction, metabolism of both drugs is altered
    (c) Dose of one drug can be altered as per requirement
    (d) Adverse effect can be ascribed to a single drug

159. Which of the following statements about clinical trials is true? *(NEET Pattern 2019)*
    (a) Phase 1 is done to determine efficacy and dose in patients
    (b) Healthy volunteers are recruited for the first time in phase 2
    (c) Randomized controlled trial in patients is done in phase 3
    (d) Phase 4 is a Pharmacokinetics study in animals

160. Which of the following instructions should be given to a lactating mother regarding drug usage? *(AIIMS Nov 2017)*
    (a) No advice is required as most of the drugs are secreted negligibly in the milk
    (b) Take drugs with longer half-life
    (c) Tell her to feed the baby just before next dose
    (d) Do not feed the baby if you are consuming any drug

161. Which of the following is not necessary to be mentioned on drug advertisement literature? *(AIIMS Nov. 2016)*
    (a) Expiry date of the drug
    (b) References of the information
    (c) Rare but life-threatening adverse effects
    (d) Common but insignificant adverse effects

162. The meaning of 'Store in a cool place' written over a strip of medicine is that it should be kept between temperature of: *(AIIMS Nov. 2015)*
    (a) 2 to 8 °C
    (b) 8 to 15 °C
    (c) Temperature below freezing point of water
    (d) 0 °C

163. Absorption of which of the following drugs is increased when given with a fatty meal? *(AIIMS Nov. 2015)*
    (a) Amphotericin B   (b) Griseofulvin
    (c) Ampicillin   (d) Aspirin

164. For which of the following drugs a warning is written 'To be sold by retail on the prescription of a Registered Medical Practitioner only' *(AIIMS Nov. 2015)*
    (a) Schedule H   (b) Schedule X
    (c) Schedule Y   (d) Schedule J

165. Type A (augmented) adverse drug reactions are characterized by all *except*: *(NEET Pattern Question)*
    (a) Qualitatively abnormal responses to the drug
    (b) Predictable from the drug's known pharmacological or toxicological effects
    (c) Generally dose-dependent
    (d) Usually common

166. In pregnancy, all of the following drugs are contraindicated *except*: *(AIIMS May 2011)*
    (a) ACE Inhibitors
    (b) Angiotensin Receptor Blockers
    (c) Propylthiouracil
    (d) Thalidomide

167. Which of the following is excreted in saliva? *(NEET Pattern Question)*
    (a) Tetracyclines   (b) Ampicillin
    (c) Lithium   (d) Chloramphenicol

168. The pharmacokinetics change occurring in geriatric patients is decline in: *(NEET Pattern Question)*
    (a) Gastric absorption   (b) Liver metabolism
    (c) Renal clearance   (d) Hypersensitivity

169. Drugs used for rare disease are known as: *(NEET Pattern Question)*
    (a) Orphan drugs   (b) Rare drugs
    (c) Over the counter drugs   (d) Emergency drugs

170. Type B adverse drug reaction is: *(NEET Pattern Question)*
    (a) Augmented effect of the drug
    (b) Allergic effect of the drug
    (c) Effect seen on chronic use of the drug
    (d) Delayed effect of the drug

171. Which of the following drug is contraindicated in pregnancy? *(NEET Pattern Question)*
    (a) Enalapril   (b) Amlodipine
    (c) β–blockers   (d) Propylthiouracil

172. Most essential medicines should be formulated as: *(NEET Pattern Question)*
    (a) No compound
    (b) Single compound
    (c) Multiple compounds
    (d) Fixed dose combinations

173. Which is not an alkaloid? *(NEET Pattern Question)*
    (a) Morphine   (b) Neostigmine
    (c) Emetine   (d) Atropine

174. As per "Drugs and cosmetic act" prescription drugs are included in: *(NEET Pattern Question)*
    (a) Schedule C   (b) Schedule H
    (c) Schedule P   (d) Schedule X

175. All the following drugs are teratogenic *except*: *(NEET Pattern Question)*
    (a) Alcohol   (b) Phenytoin
    (c) Warfarin   (d) Metoclopramide

176. Phocomelia is best described as: *(NEET Pattern Question)*
    (a) Defect in development of long bones
    (b) Defect in development of flat bones
    (c) Defect in intramembranous ossification
    (d) Defect in cartilage replacement by bones

177. Which of the following is the most accurate method for calculating drug dosage in children? *(NEET Pattern Question)*
    (a) Weight of the child
    (b) Weight of the child and adult dose
    (c) Age of the child
    (d) Body surface area

178. In which type of poisonings is gastric lavage contraindicated? *(NEET Pattern Question)*
    (a) Organophosphorus poisoning
    (b) Sedative drug poisoning
    (c) Corrosive acid poisoning
    (d) Barium carbonate poisoning

179. All of the following are examples of time dependent late adverse drug reactions *except*: *(NEET Pattern Question)*
    (a) Glucocorticoid induced osteoporosis
    (b) Nitrate induced headache
    (c) Chloroquine induced retinopathy
    (d) Amiodarone induced tissue phospholipid deposition

180. Which of the following drugs can be given safety in pregnancy? *(NEET Pattern Question)*
    (a) Propylthiouracil   (b) Sodium valproate
    (c) Warfarin   (d) Tetracycline

181. Essential medicines are those medicines: *(NEET Pattern Question)*
    (a) That are needed to treat emergency conditions
    (b) That are needed to treat serious diseases
    (c) That satisfy the priority health care needs of the population
    (d) That are introduced recently into the market

182. Counterfeit drug is: *(NEET Pattern Question)*
    (a) Fake medicine
    (b) Contains the wrong ingredient
    (c) They have active ingredient in wrong dose
    (d) All of the above

183. Which of the following statements about clinical trials is true? *(NEET Pattern Question 2019)*
    (a) Phase 1 is done to determine efficacy and dose in patients
    (b) Healthy volunteers are recruited for the first time in phase 2
    (c) Randomized controlled trial in patients is done in phase 3
    (d) Phase 4 is a Pharmacokinetics study in animals

184. Variation in sensitivity of response to increasing doses of the drug in different individuals can be obtained from: *(NEET Pattern Question 2019)*
    (a) Graded DRC   (b) Quantal DRC
    (c) Potency   (d) Efficacy

185. In competitive inhibition, true is: *(NEET Pattern Question 2017)*
    (a) V_{max} increases, km unchanged
    (b) Km unchanged
    (c) Both Km and V_{max} increase
    (d) Km increased, V_{max} unchanged

186. Effect on V_{max} and Km in non-competitive inhibition is: *(NEET Pattern Question 2017)*
    (a) V_{max} increases, Km remains same
    (b) V_{max} decreases, Km remains same
    (c) V_{max} remains same, Km decreases
    (d) V_{max} increases, Km decreases

187. Which of the following drug is contraindicated in acute intermittent porphyria? *(NEET Pattern Question 2017)*
    (a) Lithium   (b) Ampicillin
    (c) Propofol   (d) Barbiturates

188. Drug efficacy is defined as: *(NEET Pattern Question 2017)*
    (a) Ability of a drug to produce maximum effect by acting on target
    (b) Therapeutic maximum response with dose change
    (c) Minimum amount of drug needed to produce a certain response
    (d) Amount of drug which reaches in circulation unchanged

189. Which of the following drug does not act by cAMP pathway? *(NEET Pattern Question 2017)*
    (a) Estrogen   (b) Somatostatin
    (c) Glucagon   (d) ACTH

190. Which of the following statement is true about first order kinetics? *(NEET Pattern Question 2017)*
    (a) Alcohol is eliminated from body by 1st order kinetic
    (b) Constant concentration of drug eliminated in unit time
    (c) Constant fraction of drug eliminated in unit time
    (d) Half-life is dependent on plasma concentration

191. Saftey and efficacy of a drug are best established in which phase of clinical trial? *(NEET Pattern Question 2017)*
    (a) Phase I   (b) Phase II
    (c) Phase III   (d) Phase IV

192. Phase IV clinical trial is: *(NEET Pattern Question 2017)*
    (a) Post marketing trial
    (b) Most important for microdosing of drug
    (c) Not helpful in measuring side effects
    (d) Minimum year of this trial is 10 years

193. Which of the following adverse effect of a drug is explored in the treatment of another disease? *(NEET Pattern Question 2017)*
    (a) Propranolol in migraine
    (b) Nifedipine in migraine
    (c) Metoclopramide in lactation failure
    (d) Minoxidil in alopecia areata

Explanations

1. **Ans. (a) T, (b) T, (c) T, (d) F, (e) F** *(Ref: KDT 8th/e p20-21)*
   Explanation:
   Absorption across any membrane depends on lipid solubility. Non-ionized form of drugs is lipid soluble and can easily cross the membranes.

Drug	Medium	State	Solubility	Permeability
Acidic	Acidic	Non-ionized	Lipid soluble	Yes
Basic	Basic	Non-ionized	Lipid soluble	Yes
Acidic	Basic	Ionized	Water soluble	No
Basic	Acidic	Ionized	Water soluble	No

   So, basic drugs like diazepam are absorbed maximally from intestine (option b).

   Acidic drugs although are mainly non-ionized in stomach but are absorbed very less because the gastric emptying time is very small. So, these are quickly transferred to intestine. These become ionized in intestine due to alkaline medium. However, due to their longer time of stay in intestine and very large surface area as compared to stomach even the small amount of their non-ionised form contributes to significant absorption. So, practically every drug (whether acidic or basic) are absorbed more in intestine as compared to stomach.
   - **Aspirin (acidic drug):** It is non-ionized in stomach and hence easily absorbed.
   - **Diazepam (basic drug):** It is non-ionized in intestine, hence easily absorbed.
   - **Phenobarbitone (acidic drug):** Any drug is maximally absorbed in intestine due to large surface area of intestine.
   - Surface area of large intestine is large, so statement (d) is wrong.
   - Diarrhea decreases the transit time of drug, hence decreases the absorption as the time available for absorption decreases.

2. **Ans. (d) Drug is not extensively distributed to tissues** *(Ref: KDT 8th/e p23)*

   Volume of distribution (Vd) signifies the distribution of drug in the tissues. Low Vd mean less drug is distributed to tissues whereas high value of Vd means drug is being stored in some tissue.

   Volume of distribution is the hypothetical volume of plasma that would be required to contain the administered dose if that dose was evenly distributed at the concentration measured in plasma. If more amount of drug is entering the tissues, it has a higher volume of distribution and vice-a-versa. It depends on several factors like lipid solubility and plasma protein binding.

   - Drugs which are **lipid soluble** are more likely to cross the blood vessel wall and thus have **high volume of distribution**.
   - If a drug is highly **bound to plasma proteins** (e.g. warfarin, benzodiazepines, furosemide, calcium channel blockers, digitoxin, etc.) it will behave like a large molecule and more likely to stay in the plasma. Therefore, less will go to tissues resulting in **reduced volume of distribution**.
   - The drugs which have low Vd are restricted to the vascular compartment and thus their poisoning can be benefited by dialysis. *Dialysis in not effective in the poisoning due to amphetamines, antidepressants, antipsychotics, benzodiazepines, digoxin, opioids, β-blockers, calcium channel blockers and quinidine.*
   - Vd is the main determinant of loading dose of a drug.

3. **Ans. (c). Volume of distribution** *(Ref: KDT 8th/e p41)*
   - *Loading dose is given to saturate the tissue stores so it is mainly dependent on volume of distribution;* Whereas maintenance dose depends on the clearance. Loading dose is used for drugs having very long $t_{1/2}$ (or high Vd). It is calculated as LD = Vd × Target PC
   - Volume of distribution and clearance are primary pharmacokinetic parameters. All other parameters (e.g. half-life) can be calculated from these.

4. **Ans. (a) Intravenous** *(Ref: KDT 8th/e p22)*
   Bioavailability
   - It is the fraction of administered drug that reaches the systemic circulation in the unchanged form.
   - When we administer a drug orally, first it is absorbed into the portal circulation and reaches the liver. Here, some of the drug may be metabolized (*first pass metabolism or pre-systemic metabolism*) and rest of the drug reaches the systemic circulation. Thus, absorption and first pass metabolism are two important determinants of bioavailability.
   - By *IV route*, bioavailability is *100%*.

5. **Ans. (a) Oral** *(Ref: KDT 8th/e p21)*
   - When we administer a drug orally, first it is absorbed into the portal circulation and reaches the liver. Here, some of the drugs may be metabolized (*first pass metabolism or pre-systemic metabolism*) and rest of the drug reaches the systemic circulation.
   - Absorption and first pass metabolism are two important determinants of bioavailability.
   - First pass hepatic metabolism is highest with oral route. It is also noted to some extent with rectal route.

   - **Drugs with High First pass Metabolism**
     - Nitrates - Nitrates
     - Have - Hydrocortisone
     - Large - Lignocaine
     - Pre - Propranolol
     - Systemic - Salbutamol
     - Metabolism - Morphine

6. **Ans. (a) Volume of distribution** *(Ref: KDT 8th/e p41)*
   - **Loading dose:** It is mainly used for drugs having long t½ and large volume of distribution. It is given to load (saturate) the tissue stores. So it is mainly dependent on Vd.
     Loading dose = VD × Target plasma concentration
   - **Maintenance dose:** It is mainly dependent on CL.
     Maintenance dose = CL × Target plasma concentration

7. **Ans. (b) Decrease in glomerular filtration**
   (Ref: Goodman and Gilman 13th/e p18)
   Clinical Importance of Plasma Protein Binding
   1. **Duration of action:** Drugs with high PPB are usually long acting
   2. **Distribution:** High PPB drugs stay in plasma, thus have low Vd.
   3. **Displacement:** Highly PPB drug can be displaced by another highly bound drug
   4. **Dialysis:** It is not effective for drugs having high PPB
   5. As proteins cannot be filtered by glomerulus, so if a drug has high binding to plasma proteins, it tends to have less glomerular filtration.

8. **Ans. (b) There is 50% ionized and 50% non-ionized fraction of the drug** *(Ref: KDT 8th/e p16, 17)*

9. **Ans. (a) Simple diffusion** *(Ref: KDT's 8th/e p16)*

10. **Ans. (b) Decyclization** *(Ref: KDT's 8th/e p31)*

11. **Ans. (b) Large apparent volume of distribution**
    (Ref: KDT 7th/e p21)
    Volume of distribution tells that how much drug is getting distributed in the tissues. A large Vd reflects the storage of drug in tissues.

12. **Ans. (b) Rifampicin** *(Ref: Katzung 13th/e p70)*
    Rifampicin is a powerful inducer of microsomal enzymes as well as P glycoprotein.

13. **Ans. (a) Posterior auricular > Scrotum > Scalp > Dorsum of arm > Plantar area** *(Ref: Katzung 13th/e p.1045)*
    Percutaneous absorption depends upon thickness of the skin. Higher the thickness lesser is absorption. Therefore order of percutaneous absorption of drug applied topically is posterior auricular > Scrotum > Vulva > Forehead > Scalp > Fore arm > Plantar surface

14. **Ans. (b) The drug does not accumulate in tissues**
    (Ref: KDT 8th/e p23, 24)
    Vd means volume of distribution. It signifies the distribution of drug in the tissues. Low Vd mean less drug is distributed to tissues whereas high value of Vd means drug is being stored in some tissue.

15. **Ans. (a) Non ionized and lipid soluble** *(Ref: KDT 8th/e p28)*
    *Nitroglycerin is effective when retained sublingually because it is **non-ionized** and has **very high lipid solubility**. Thus, the drug is **absorbed very rapidly**.*

16. **Ans. (a) Increase in water solubility**
    (Ref: Goodman Gillman KDT 8th/e p28)
    The aim of xenobiotics metabolism is to increase water solubility so that these compounds can be excreted in urine.

17. **Ans. (c) Phenobarbitone** *(Ref: KDT 8th/e p37)*
    Phenobarbitone is a barbiturate which is a derivative of barbituric acid (weakly acidic drug) and its excretion can be enhanced by making the urine alkaline. Morphine, atropine and amphetamines are basic drugs.

18. **Ans. (c) CYP2C19** *(Ref: Katzung 13th/e p80)*
    Clopidogrel and proton pump inhibitors are metabolized mainly by CYP2C19 and by CYP3A4. Due to this reason there is potential of interaction between these two drugs

19. **Ans. (d) Sex steroid hormones do not bind to any protein in plasma** *(Ref: KDT 8th/e p26-27)*
    - Acidic drugs mainly bind to albumin and basic drugs to alpha-1 acid glycoprotein. Drugs having high PPB like sulfonamides can displace other drugs bound to same site and may result in toxicity.
    - Sex steroids bind to steroid hormone binding globulin as well as albumin.

20. **Ans. (b) Small changes of pH near the pKa of a weak acidic drug will not affect its degree of ionization**
    (Ref: Katzung 13th/e p9)
    - pKa is the pH at which half of the drug is in the ionized form. There is maximum variation in the ionization of a drug at pH near its pKa value.
    - Phenobarbitone is an acidic drug having pKa of 7.2. Therefore, at pH = 7.2, 50% of drug is ionized and 50% un-ionized. In acidic medium, more of it will be unionized (because it is acidic in nature). In plasma (pH = 7.4), more will be ionized (60%) and less (40%) un-ionized.

21. **Ans. (c) Low oral bioavailability always and necessarily mean poor absorption** *(Ref: KDT 8th/e p22)*
    - Low oral bioavailability can also be due to high first pass metabolism. *For detail see text.*

22. **Ans. (c) Lower volumes of distribution** *(Ref: KDT 8th/e p26)*
    - The clinically significant implications of plasma protein binding are:
    1. Plasma protein binding causes restriction of drugs in the vascular compartment and thus *lower volume of distribution.*
    2. *Longer duration of action* – as the protein-bound fraction is not available for metabolism or excretion.
    3. Plasma protein bound drugs tend to have *more drug interactions* due to displacement of a drug with lower affinity by a drug with higher affinity for plasma proteins.
    4. Hypoalbuminemia can lead to high concentration of free drug and thus drug toxicity.

23. **Ans. (a) Cimetidine**
    (Ref: KDT 8th/e p30; Goodman and Gilman 13th/e p1098)

24. **Ans. (c) Levodopa** *(Ref: KDT 8th/e p29)*

25. **Ans. (d) Lisinopril** *(Ref: KDT 8th/e p29)*
    - Captopril and lisinopril are ACE inhibitors that are not prodrugs.
    - Diazepam produce many active metabolites like oxazepam.
    - Propranolol can produce 4-hydroxypropranolol which has β-antagonist activity.
    - Allopurinol gives rise to oxypurinol which can inhibit xanthine oxidase.

General Pharmacology

26. **Ans. (a) Sequestered in body tissues** *(Ref: KDT 8th/e p24)*
    - Apparent volume of distribution (V_d) is more for drugs sequestered in tissues.
    - *Lipid insoluble drugs do not enter cells, Vd approximates ECF volume.*

27. **Ans. (b) Cimetidine** *(Ref: KDT 8th/e p33)*
28. **Ans. (a) Phenobarbitone** *(Ref: KDT 8th/e p30)*
29. **Ans. (b) Sodium bicarbonate** *(Ref: KDT 8th/e p37)*
30. **Ans. (c) Propranolol** *(Ref: KDT 8th/e p35)*
31. **Ans. (b) The percentage of drug that is detected in the systemic circulation after its administration** *(Ref: KDT 8th/e p22)*
32. **Ans. (a)** $V_d = \dfrac{\text{Dose administrated by IV route}}{\text{Plasma concentration}}$
    (Ref: KDT 8th/e p23)
33. **Ans. (c) Thiopentone** *(Ref: KDT 8th/e p24)*
34. **Ans. (a) Acetylation** *(Ref: KDT 8th/e p31)*
35. **Ans. (d) Blood brain barrier is deficient at the chemoreceptor trigger zone** *(Ref: KDT 8th/e p24)*
36. **Ans. (d) Oxidation** *(Ref: KDT 8th/e p29)*
37. **Ans. (b) Imipramine** *(Ref: KDT 8th/e p29)*
38. **Ans. (a) To achieve Steady State concentration in short time** *(Ref: KDT 8th/e p41)*
39. **Ans. (a) Weak acid drugs** *(Ref: KDT 8th/e p37)*
40. **Ans. (c) Clearance of the drug** *(Ref: KDT 8th/e p41)*
41. **Ans. (a) Hydroxylation** *(Ref: Katzung 13th/e p60)*
42. **Ans. (a) Phase I reactions (hydrolysis, oxidation, reduction etc.) only** *(Ref: Katzung 13th/e p60; KDT 8th/e p32)*
    Cytochrome P450 enzymes are responsible for phase I reactions only whereas microsomal enzymes can be involved in phase II also (glucuronide conjugation)
43. **Ans. (b) The rate of absorption** *(Ref: Katzung 11/e p44)*
44. **Ans. (c) Sodium valproate** *(Ref: Goodman and Gilman 13th/e p320)*
45. **Ans. (b) Amphetamine** *(Ref: KDT 8th/e p37)*
46. **Ans. (a) CYP 3A4** *(Ref: KDT 8th/e p29)*
47. **Ans. (a) Penicillin** *(Ref: KDT 8th/e p26)*
    - Acidic drugs bind to albumin whereas basic drugs bind to α_1 acid glycoprotein.
    - Penicillin is an acidic drug, so it binds to albumin.
48. **Ans. (a) Ketoconazole** *(Ref: KDT 8th/e p33)*
49. **Ans. (a) Valproate** *(Ref: KDT 8th/e p30)*
50. **Ans. (b) Enzyme inhibitor** *(Ref: KDT 8th/e p30)*
    - Grapefruit juice contains furano cumarins and naringin that are CYP 3A4 inhibitors.
51. **Ans. (b) Rifampicin** *(Ref: KDT 8th/e p352)*
52. **Ans. (a) Cimetidine** *(Ref: KDT 8th/e p670)*
53. **Ans. (a) Phenobarbitone** *(Ref: KDT 8th/e p37)*
54. **Ans. (b) Transdermal** *(Ref: KDT 8th/e p12)*
55. **Ans. (d) Digoxin poisoning** *(Ref: KDT 8th/e p24)*
56. **Ans. (a) First pass metabolism** *(Ref: KDT 8th/e p22, 23)*
57. **Ans. (a) Amount of drug that reach the systemic circulation** *(Ref: KDT 8th/e p22)*
58. **Ans. (c) More fat soluble metabolites are formed** *(Ref: KDT 8th/e p28)*
59. **Ans. (d) Amoxicillin** *(Ref: KDT 8th/e p29)*
60. **Ans. (b) Enalapril** *(Ref: KDT 8th/e p29)*
61. **Ans. (d) They are non heme proteins** *(Ref: Goodman and Gilman 13th/e p88)*
    - Cytochrome P 450 enzymes are microsomal i.e. these are present in endoplasmic reticulum of hepatocytes and other cells.
    - They contain cytochrome which is a heme protein.
    - The pigment has maximum light absorption at a wavelength of 450 nm.
    - These are involved in the synthesis of steroids and bile acids apart from metabolism of xenobiotics.
62. **Ans. (a) 16%** *(Ref: Goodman and Gilman 13th/e p22)*
    If we administer 100 molecules of the drug.
    - Amount absorbed = 40 molecules (40% absorption)
    - Amount removed by liver = 40 × 0.6 (Hepatic extraction ratio) = 24 molecules
    - Drug available to produce action = 40 − 24 = 16 molecules
    - So, Bioavailability = 16 percent
63. **Ans. (a) Oral** *(Ref: KDT 8th/e p10)*
    Oral route has maximum variability in absorption
64. **Ans. (a) Pharmacognosy** *(Ref: K K sharma 2nd/e p4)*
65. **Ans. (a) T_{max}** *(Ref: KK Sharma 3rd/e p31)*
    - AUC tells about the **extent of absorption** of the drug.
    - T_{max} tells about the time to reach maximum concentration, i.e. **rate of absorption**
    - C_{max} is the **maximum concentration** of a drug that can be obtained after giving a particular dose.
66. **Ans. (a) 18** *(Ref: See below)*
    Volume the syringe can contain = 2 mL
    Total number of divisions = 10 (divisions per mL) × 2 = 20
    Concentration of ceftriaxone = 100 mg/mL
    Ceftriaxone in 1 mL = 100 mg
    Ceftriaxone in 2 mL = 100 × 2 = 200 mg
    200 mg ceftriaxone in how many divisions = 20
    180 mg ceftriaxone in how many divisions = 20/200 × 180 = 18
67. **Ans. (a) 0.0025 mg/mL** *(Ref: See below)*
    Maintenance dose rate = Clearance × Target steady state plasma concentration
    1.6 mg/min = 640 mL/min × Steady state plasma concentration
    Steady state plasma conc. = 1.6/640 = 0.0025 mg/mL
68. **Ans. (a) 30.5 mg** *(Ref: See below)*
    In first order kinetics percentage of drug eliminated per unit time is constant
    Here amount eliminated is 75 mg (from 200 mg) in 1.5 hours (90 minutes)
    So, percentage eliminated is 75/200 = 37.5% in 1.5 hours

- **Method 1:** So, every 1.5 hours 37.5% will be eliminated
- After 3 hours remaining will be 125 − [125 × 37.5/100] = 78.125
- After 4.5 hours remaining will be 78.125 − [78.125 × 37.5/100] = 48.82
- After 6 hours remaining will be 48.82 − [48.82 × 37.5/100] = 30.5

Method 2: Every 1.5 hours 100 − 37.5 = 62.5% will remain
After 3 hours = 125 × 62.5/100
After 4.5 hours = 125 × 62.5/100 × 62.5/100
After 6 hours = 125 × 62.5/100 × 62.5/100 × 62.5/100 = 30.5

69. **Ans. (b) Need for loading dose in order to get immediate effect** *(Ref: KDT 8th/e p41)*
    Loading dose of a drug is required for

    - Drugs with high volume of distribution like chloroquine
    - Drugs with long half-life but action is required quickly like digoxin

    Steady state reaches in 5 half lives. In this example, it will take 200 hours (40 × 5) for digoxin to reach steady state plasma concentration. As we require it to produce action quickly and we cannot wait so long, so a loading dose is given to achieve steady state quickly.

70. **Ans. (a) Clearance** *(Ref: KDT 8th/e p38)*
    Clearance of a drug is the theoretical volume of plasma from which the drug is completely removed in unit time.

71. **Ans. (d) The rate of elimination is proportional to the plasma concentration** *(Ref: KDT 8th/e p38-39)*
    Drugs may follow zero order or first order kinetics. It depends on the following formula:
    Rate of Elimination α {Plasma Concentration}^{order}
    - Thus, if a drug follows zero order kinetics, {Plasma Concentration}^{0} is equal to one, in other words rate of elimination is independent of plasma concentration or rate of elimination is constant.
    - From the above formula, rate of elimination is proportional to plasma concentration for the drugs following first order kinetics.

72. **Ans. (a) Volume of distribution** *(Ref: KDT 8th/e p41)*

    - *Loading dose is given to saturate the tissue stores so it is mainly dependent on volume of distribution; Whereas maintenance dose depends on the clearance. Loading dose is used for drugs having very long $t\frac{1}{2}$ (or high V_d). It is calculated as LD = V_d × Target PC*
    - **Volume of distribution and clearance are primary pharmacokinetic parameters. All other parameters (e.g. half-life) can be calculated from these.**

73. **Ans. (b) A constant proportion of plasma concentration is eliminated per unit time** *(Ref: KDT 8th/e p38-39)*

    In first order kinetics, rate of elimination is proportional to plasma concentration of the drug. Half life and clearance are constant in first order kinetics.

74. **Ans. (b) Barbiturates** *(Ref: KDT 8th/e p38, 246, 440)*
75. **Ans. (b) Phenytoin** *(Ref: KDT 8th/e p440)*
76. **Ans. (a) Half life of drug** *(Ref: KDT 8th/e p39)*
77. **Ans. (b) Half life of a drug** *(Ref: KDT 8th/e p40-41)*
    - After a dosage regimen, concentration of the drug to reach the steady state (when the elimination balances the input) is called **steady state plasma concentration Cpss.**
    - Cpss is reached in about 4-5 half lives.
    - The amplitude of fluctuations in Cpss depends on the dose interval relative to $t_{1/2}$.

78. **Ans. (d) Methotrexate** *(Ref: KDT 8th/e p38, 214, 440)*
79. **Ans. (a) Zero order kinetics** *(Ref: KDT 8th/e p38)*
80. **Ans. (a) Volume of plasma which is cleared of drug in unit of time** *(Ref: KDT 8th/e p38)*
81. **Ans. (a) Phenytoin and Theophylline** *(Ref: KDT 8th/e p246, 440)*
82. **Ans. (a) A constant amount of drug is eliminated per unit time** *(Ref: KDT 8th/e p38-39)*
83. **Ans. (a) Clearance remains constant** *(Ref: KDT 8th/e p38-39)*
84. **Ans. (d) Alcohol and theophylline** *(Ref: KDT 8th/e p38, 246)*
85. **Ans. (c) 87.5%** *(Ref: KDT 8th/e p39)*
86. **Ans. (a) 12.5%** *(Ref: KDT 8th/e p39)*
87. **Ans. (c) insulin** *(Ref: KDT 8th/e p248)*
    Explanation:
    - Drugs acting via tyrosine kinase receptors— Cytokines, prolactin, insulin and growth hormone
    - TRH, TSH and MSH acts through GPCR receptors

88. **Ans. (a) Drug A** *(Ref: KDT 8th/e p63-64)*
    Explanation:
    - Potency determines the affinity of a drug for its receptor.
    - In Log DRC, more the curve is on left side, more potent is the drug. In the given figure, the order of potency is A>B>C.
    - Efficacy is maximum response of a drug regardless of dose. In DRC, it is determined by highest point of the curve. In the given graph, efficacy of drug A and B is same but higher than drug C.

89. **Ans. (a) Km remains same, Vmax decreases** *(Ref: KDT 8th/e p47)*

    Explanation:
    Km remains same whereas Vmax decreases in non-competitive inhibition

	Km	Vmax
Competitive	↑	No effect
Noncompetitive	No effect	↓
Uncompetitive	↓	↓

90. **Ans. (d) Angiotensin 1 receptor** *(Ref: KDT 8th/e p56)*
    Explanation:
    - GPCR that acts through opening of K$^+$ channels can result in hyper-polarisation, thus leading to

inhibition. So, receptor which causes stimulation cannot act through opening of K⁺ channels.
- Muscarinic M2 receptor, Dopamine D2 receptor and serotonin 5HT1 receptor act through opening of K⁺ channels.
- Whereas Angiotensin 1 receptor act by increasing Ca^{2+}.

91. **Ans (a) Decrease in V_{max}** *(Ref: KDT 8th/e p47)*
   - In competitive inhibition, there is increase in K_m and V_{max} remains same.
   - In Non-competitive inhibition, V_{max} decreases but K_m remains same.
   - In un-competitive inhibition, both K_m as well as V_{max} decrease.

Inhibition	Binds to	K_m	V_{max}
Competitive	E only	↑	No change
Non-competitive	Both E and ES complex	No change	↓
Un-competitive	ES complex only	↓	↓

92. **Ans (d) These activate a nuclear transcription factor** *(Ref: KDT 8th/e p60-61)*

Thyroid hormones act through intracellular receptors which activate a nuclear transcription factor.
   - Intracellular receptors (Nuclear receptor superfamily) are **slowest acting**.
   - These may be present in the

   - **Cytoplasm**
     - Glucocorticoids
     - Mineralocorticoids
     - Vitamin D
   - **Nucleus**
     - Thyroid hormones (T3, T4)
     - Retinoic acid
     - PPAR
     - Sex hormones like estrogen

   - *Both types of receptors finally act by nuclear mechanisms* (i.e. by affecting transcription).
   - All the intracellular receptors are considered a part of '**Nuclear Receptor Superfamily**'.

93. **Ans. (a) Muscarinic receptors** *(Ref: KDT 8th/e p55)*
The receptors are classified into four types based on the signal transduction mechanisms.
G Protein Coupled Receptors
These are also called metabotropic receptors or **heptahelical (serpentine) receptors** i.e. have seven transmembrane spanning segments.
   - **Activation (by Gs) or inhibition (by Gi) of enzyme adenyl cyclase:**
     a. Beta adrenergic receptors (increase cAMP)
     b. Histamine H2 receptors (increase cAMP)
     c. Somatostatin (works by decreasing cAMP).
   - **Activation of phospholipase C (by Gq):**
     a. Alpha adrenergic receptors
     b. Vasopressin V1 receptors
     c. Histamine H_1 receptors
   - **Stimulation or inhibition of ion channels**
     a. M2 muscarinic receptors of ACh
     b. GABA-B receptors

94. **Ans. (b) Quantal DRC** *(Ref: KDT 8th/e p65)*

Quantal DRC
When the response is an 'all or none' phenomenon (e.g. antiemetic drug stopping the vomiting or not), the y-axis (response axis) shows the number of person responding and X-axis shows the plasma concentration. It thus shows that how many people respond to a particular dose of the drug. It is used to calculate ED50 and LD50.

- **Median Effective Dose (ED50):** It is the *dose that will produce the desired response in half of the (50%) recipients.* More is ED50, lower is the potency and vice a versa.
- **Median Lethal Dose (LD50):** It is the dose that will result in death of 50% of the animals receiving the drug. *More is LD50, safer is the drug.*
- **Therapeutic Index (T.I.):** It is a *measure of the safety* of a drug. It is calculated as a ratio of LD50 to ED50. Drugs having high T.I. are safer whereas those having low T.I. are more likely to be toxic.

95. **Ans. (a) A and B are full agonists** *(Ref: KDT 8th/e p64)*
The graph given in the question depicts that
   - A and B have equal efficacy whereas C has lower efficacy than both.
   - A is most potent followed by B and C is least potent.
   - As the curve is shifting downwards in case of drug C (means efficacy decreases), it cannot be competitive antagonist. Decrease in efficacy is feature of non-competitive antagonism. In case of competitive antagonism, curve shifts towards right only.
   - A and B have equal efficacy, although we cannot generalize but these are likely to be full agonists.

96. **Ans. (b) Penicillin** *(Ref: Harrison 18/e p2735)*
Important drugs causing SLE like syndrome include:

S	Sulfonamides
H	Hydralazine
I	Isoniazid
P	Procainamide

97. **Ans. (c) Insulin binds to a transmembrane receptor at the outer surface of the plasma membrane, which activates the tyrosine kinase that is the cytosolic domain of the receptor.** *(KDT 8th/e p58)*
Enzymatic Receptors have two sites, the drug binds on the extracellular site and the intracellular site has enzymatic activity (mostly tyrosine kinase). This enzyme can be activated via JAK-STAT pathway. Insulin, growth hormone, prolactin and cytokines act via enzymatic receptors.

98. **Ans. (c) Decreases V_{max}** *(Ref: KDT 8th/e p47)*
   - Competitive inhibitors increase K_m value whereas non-competitive inhibitors decreases V_{max} of an enzyme

99. **Ans. (c) Activation of protein kinase** *(Ref: KDT 8th/e p55)*
   - Cyclic AMP exerts most of its effects by stimulating cAMP-dependent protein kinases. These phosphorylate enzymes resulting in their activation or inhibition.

100. **Ans. (d) Pyrimethamine** *(Ref: KDT 8th/e p76)*
   - Important drugs causing hemolysis in G-6-PD deficiency are

– Primaquine	– Dapsone	– Sulfonamides
– Nitrofurantoin	– Aspirin	– Menadione
– Chloroquine	– Quinine	– Nalidixic acid

- Sulfonamides can cause hemolysis in patients with G-6-PD deficiency and not pyrimethamine.

101. **Ans. (c) Insulin** *(Ref: KDT 8th/e p60)*
    - Insulin acts through enzymatic receptors
    - Thyroid hormones, sex hormones, steroids, vitamin D and vitamin A act through intracellular receptors.

102. **Ans. (c) ED_{50} of the drug corresponds to the efficacy**
    (Ref: Katzung 13th/e p35)
    ED_{50} corresponds to potency of a drug, not its efficacy. All other statements are true.

103. **Ans. (b) Binds to the receptor and causes opposite action** *(Ref: KDT 8th/e p50)*

104. **Ans. (a) High affinity** *(Ref: KDT 8th/e p50)*

105. **Ans. (c) The substrate concentration at half maximal velocity** *(Ref: KDT 8th/e p47)*
    K_m of an enzyme is similar to potency of a drug. It is the *substrate concentration at which the velocity reaches half of the maximum* known as V_{max} (similar to efficacy of a drug). Higher is the Km, lesser is the speed of the reaction.

106. **Ans. (d) Cortisol** *(Ref: KDT 8th/e p60)*

107. **Ans. (b) An antagonist has affinity but no intrinsic activity for receptor** *(Ref: KDT 8th/e p50)*

108. **Ans. (a) Epinephrine** *(Ref: KDT 8th/e p60)*

109. **Ans. (a) Metabotropic receptors** *(Ref: Katzung 13th/e p358)*

110. **Ans. (a) Competitive antagonism** *(Ref: Katzung 13th/e p122)*

111. **Ans. (a) Physiological antagonism**
    (Ref Katzung KDT 13th/e p25)

112. **Ans. (a) Affinity with intrinsic activity is 1**
    (Ref: KDT 8th/e p50)

113. **Ans. (b) Penicillin** *(Ref: KDT 8th/e p76)*

114. **Ans. (d) Physiological antagonism** *(Ref: KDT 8th/e p68)*

115. **Ans. (b) β (Beta) receptor** *(Ref: KDT 8th/e p55)*

116. **Ans. (c) Corticosteroids** *(Ref: KDT 8th/e p76)*

117. **Ans. (b) Prostacycline-Thromboxane** *(Ref: KDT 8th/e p68)*

118. **Ans. (b) Insulin** *(Ref: KDT 8th/e p58)*
    - Nicotine acts on N_M and N_N receptors which are ionotropic receptors.
    - Diazepam acts on GABA-BZD-CL channel complex that mediates entry of chloride.
    - Glibenclamide is a sulfonylurea that acts on ACh sensitive K^+ channels.
    - Insulin acts on enzymatic receptors.

119. **Ans. (d) Maximum response a drug can produce**
    (Ref: KDT 8th/e p64)

120. **Ans. (a) Hydralazine** *(Ref: KDT 8th/e p76)*

121. **Ans. (c) Inverse agonist** *(Ref: KDT 8th/e p50)*

122. **Ans. (a) Pharmacogenomics** *(Ref: KDT 8th/e p75)*

123. **Ans. (c) Agonists and antagonists bind to the same receptor** *(Ref: KDT 8th/e p50)*

124. **Ans. (a) Competitive inhibitor** *(Ref: KDT 8th/e p47)*

125. **Ans. (c) Low intrinsic activity and high affinity**
    (Ref: KDT 8th/e p50)

126. **Ans. (d) Mechanism of action** *(Ref: KDT 8th/e p1)*

127. **Ans. (b) Cytosolic receptors**
    (Ref: KDT 8th/e p367; Goodman Gilman 13th/e p893)

Cytosolic Receptors	Intranuclear Receptors
• Vitamin D	• Sex Hormone receptors
• Mineralocorticoids	• Vitamin A
• Glucocorticoids	• Thyroid Hormones
	• PPAR

128. **Ans. (b) Non-competitive** *(Ref: KDT 8th/e p47)*

	Km	V_{max}
Competitive	Increases	No change
Noncompetitive	No change	Decreases
Uncompetitive	Decreases	Decreases

129. **Ans. (a) Vitamins** *(Ref: Goodman Gilman 13th/e p55)*
    - Normal log DRC is sigmoid in shape
    - Non-monotonic DRC may be of following shapes:
      - **Vitamins and essential** metals show **U-shaped DRC**
      - Formaldehyde exhibit J-shaped (Hockey stick shaped) DRC.
      - Estrogen may show inverted U-shaped DRC.

130. **Ans. (a) Safety** *(Ref: KDT 8th/e p65)*
    Therapeutic Index (TI)
    - It is a *measure of the safety* of a drug.
    - It is calculated as a ratio of LD50 to ED50.
    - Drugs having high TI are safer whereas those having low TI are more likely to be toxic.

131. **Ans. (a) Warfarin** *(Ref: KDT 8th/e p42)*
    Therapeutic drug monitoring is not required for oral anticoagulants like warfarin. The effect of warfarin is monitored by measuring prothrombin time or INR (International Normalized Ratio).

132. **Ans. (d) When the clinical response cannot be easily monitored.** *(Ref: KDT 8th/e p42)*
    - TDM is a process by which the dose of a drug is adjusted according to its plasma concentration.
    - For performing TDM, there should be good relation between drug concentration and response. Note that there may not be good relation between dose and plasma concentration.
    - TDM is done for those drugs whose effect cannot be easily measured (like effect of antihypertensive drugs can be easily measured by monitoring BP, so TDM is not used).
    - TDM is **not done for** the drugs which are activated in the body or produce active metabolites, when pharmacological tolerance is suspected and when there is poor relation between drug concentration and effect.

133. **Ans. (b) Lithium** *(Ref: KDT 8th/e p42)*

134. **Ans. (b) Phenytoin** *(Ref: KDT 8th/e p65)*

135. **Ans. (d) Margin of safety** *(Ref: KDT 8th/e p65)*

136. **Ans. (b) $\dfrac{LD_{50}}{ED_{50}}$** *(Ref: KDT 8th/e p65)*

137. **Ans. (a) Potency** *(Ref: KDT 8th/e p64)*

138. **Ans. (c) Maximum tolerable dose** *(Ref: KDT 8th/e p90)*

Phase I trial is designed as a dose-escalation study to determine the maximum tolerable dosage (MTD), that is, the maximum dose associated with an acceptable level of dose-limiting toxicity.

139. **Ans. (c) Sham surgery** *(Ref: KK Sharma 2/e p103)*
Placebo is used as a control to compare the active treatment with something with all similarities except the active treatment. Mostly inactive substances are used as placebo but rarely sham surgery can be used as placebo in surgical cases.

140. **Ans. (d) Phase IV** *(Ref: KDT 8th/e p91)*

Clinical Trial	Other Name
Phase 0	Microdosing studies
Phase I	Human pharmacology and safety
Phase II	Therapeutic exploratory
Phase III	Therapeutic confirmatory
Phase IV	Post marketing surveillance

141. **Ans. (d) Dosing** *(Ref: KDT 8th/e p90)*
Phase 1 trails are done to assess the maximum tolerable dose of a new chemical entity. Thus pharmacokinetic parameters are assessed in these trials. These are mostly done in healthy volunteers. These are exposed to the drug one by one, starting with the lowest estimated dose and increasing stepwise to reach the maximum tolerable dose. Although the emphasis is on safety, tolerability and to detect any potentially dangerous effects on vital functions, however these are assessed in terms of dose. So among the safety and dosing, the better answer seems to be dosing.
Aim of phase I trials should be answered in the following sequence.
MTD > Dosing > Pharmacokinetics > Safety

142. **Ans. (c) Phase I trial** *(Ref: KDT 8th/e p90)*
Phase I trial is designed as a dose-escalation study to determine the maximum tolerable dosage (MTD), that is, the maximum dose associated with an acceptable level of dose-limiting toxicity.

143. **Ans. (c) Phase III** *(Ref: KDT 8th/e p91)*
"The purpose of phase III trials is to obtain adequate data about the efficacy and safety of drugs in a larger number of patients of either sex in multiple centres usually in comparison with the standard drug."

144. **Ans. (c) Drugs used for rare diseases** *(Ref: KDT 8th/e p7)*
Orphan drugs are the drugs that are used for the treatment of rare diseases. e.g. N-acetylcysteine for paracetamol poisoning. Other examples include fomepizole, sodium nitrite, digibind etc.

145. **Ans. (c) Used to determine efficacy** *(Ref: KDT 8th/e p91)*
For details, see text.

146. **Ans. (a) Preclinical Phase** *(Ref: KDT 8th/e p90)*
    - GCP guidelines are made to safeguard the interest of subjects in clinical trials. These have to be adhered to in all phases of clinical trials.
    - Preclinical trials are performed in animals for which different regulations are given by CPCSEA (Committee for the Purpose of Control and Supervision of Experiments on Animals).

147. **Ans. (a) Phase-I** *(Ref: KDT 8th/e p90)*

148. **Ans. (c) Side effects** *(Ref: KDT 8th/e p94)*
"**Side effects** are unwanted but often-unavoidable pharmacodynamic effects that occur at therapeutic dose" (less than toxic dose)
Intolerance is the appearance of characteristic toxic effects of a drug in an individual at therapeutic doses.
Toxic effects are the result of excess pharmacological action of the drug due to overdose or prolonged use. Effects are predictable and dose related.

149. **Ans. (d) To know rare adverse effects of the drug** *(Ref: KDT 8th/e p91)*

150. **Ans. (d) Phase IV** *(Ref KDT 8th/e p91)*

151. **Ans. (b) Post marketing surveillance** *(Ref: KDT 8th/e p91)*

152. **Ans. (c) Drug toxicity** *(Ref: KDT 8th/e p91)*

153. **Ans. (b) After a drug is marketed** *(Ref: KDT 8th/e p91)*

154. **Ans. (c) Ketamine** *(Ref: Drugs and Cosmetics Act 1945)*
Explanation:
    - Schedule X is for the psychotropic drugs i.e. addictive drugs.
    - Among given options, drug that comes under schedule X is KETAMINE.

Important drug schedules
    - Schedule G: Deals with details of drugs to be labeled 'Caution: It is dangerous to take this medicine except under medical supervision'.
    - Schedule H: Deals with drugs and medicine to be sold on prescription-only.
    - Schedule R: Deals with standards for contraceptives.
    - Schedule X: Deals with psychotropic drugs which require special license for manufacturing and sale.

Note: Category X is pregnancy category of drugs. It means highly teratogenic drugs. Do not get confused between schedule X and category X drugs.

155. **Ans. (a) Schedule H** *(Ref: KK Sharma 2nd/e p6)*
Drugs are broadly of 2 types:
    1. **Schedule H drugs:** Must be sold by retail only when a prescription by registered medical practitioner is produced.
    2. **OTC:** These are over the counter drugs, which may be sold without prescription.

156. **Ans. (d) 8–15 degree Celsius** *(Ref: Park 22nd/e p100)*
    - **Storage condition of drugs (according to IP)**
        - Store frozen:–2 °C
        - Do not freeze or Keep Cold: 2-8 °C
        - Keep cool: 8–15 °C

157. **Ans. (d) Misbranded drug** *(Ref: Drugs and Cosmetics Act)*
The Drugs and Cosmetics (amendment) Act, 2008 provides deterrent penalties for offences relating to manufacture of spurious or adulterated drugs which have serious implications on public health.
Spurious drugs: These products are manufactured concealing the true identity of the product and made to resemble another drug, especially some popular brand, to deceive the buyer and cash on the popularity of original

product. The product may or may not contain the active ingredients. Spurious drugs are usually manufactured by unlicensed anti-social elements but sometimes licensed manufacturers may also be involved.

Adulterated drugs: These are those drugs which are found to contain an adulterant/substituted product or contaminated with filth rendering it injurious to health

Misbranded drugs: A drug shall be deemed to be misbranded,
a. If it is so colored, coated, powdered or polished that damage is concealed or if it is made to appear of better or greater therapeutic value than it really is; or
b. If it is not labeled in the prescribed manner; or
c. If its label or container or anything accompanying the drug bears any statement, design or device which makes any false claim for the drug or which is false or Misleading in any particulars.

158. **Ans. (a) Adverse effect of one drug may be neutralized by the other** *(Ref: KDT 8th/e p72)*

Fixed dose combination (FDC) refers to a combination of two or more therapeutically active entities in a fixed ratio of doses. The term is used generically to mean a particular combination of drugs irrespective of the formulation or brand.

Criteria for choosing FDCs
- The FDCs must be based on convincing therapeutic rationalization and be carefully justified and clinically relevant.
- FDCs must be shown to be safe and effective for the claimed indications and it cannot be assumed that benefits of the FDC outweigh its risks.
- As for any new medicine, the risks and benefits must be defined and compared. Specifically, attention should be drawn to the doses of each active substance in the FDC.

Advantages of using FDC
- Increased compliance
- Reduced incidence of adverse effects as side effects of one may be counteracted by the other; example loop diuretic with a potassium sparing diuretic
- Increased efficacy as some drugs act synergistically e.g. levodopa + carbidopa/ benserazide
- May help to lower the cost of therapy as well
- Reduced development of resistance in case of antibiotics. This is particularly relevant for the treatment of TB, HIV

Disadvantages of using FDC
- Either the doses of the components, and/or the ratio of doses may differ from patient to patient (inter-patient variability)
- The patients may be taking different doses at different stages of treatment (as in initial treatment compared with long-term treatment; intra-patient variability)
- When the dose adjustment is required; becomes particularly significant when one or more of the actives has a narrow therapeutic index.
- Difficult of establishing causality of a newly reported adverse drug reaction.
- Presence of allergic reaction to any component of the FDC precludes its use as a whole.
- There is a higher incidence or greater severity of adverse reactions to the combination than with any of the ingredients given alone, or there are adverse reactions not seen in response to treatment with any of the individual ingredients.
- There are unfavorable pharmacokinetic interactions between the ingredients, for example when one drug alters the absorption, distribution, metabolism or excretion of another.
- Dose adjustment is required necessarily in special populations, such as in people with renal or hepatic impairment, or the elderly.
- The product (tablets or capsules), is so large that patients find it difficult to swallow.

159. **Ans. (c) Randomized controlled trial in patients is done in phase 3** *(Ref: KDT 8th/e p90-91)*

SUMMARY OF CLINICAL TRIALS

Phase	Name	Conducted on	Blinding and control	Purpose
I	Human Pharmacology and safety	**Healthy** volunteers (20–100)	**OPEN LABEL** (No blinding)	• **To know maximum tolerable dose (MTD)** • Safety and tolerability
II	Therapeutic exploratory	100–150 **Patients (homogenous** population)	**Single blind** controlled	• **To establish therapeutic efficacy** • Dose ranging and ceiling effect
III	Therapeutic confirmatory	Up to 5000 patients from several centres (**heterogeneous** population)	**Double blind** randomized controlled	• **To confirm therapeutic efficacy** • To establish the value of drug in relation to existing therapy
IV	Post marketing surveillance	Large number of patients being treated by practicing physicians	—	• To know rare **and long-term adverse effects** • Special groups like children, pregnancy etc can be tested
O (Zero)	**Microdosing** studies	**Healthy** volunteers (small number)	—	• To **know pharmacokinetics** • Could avoid costly phase I studies for candidate drugs with unsuitable pharmacokinetics.

160. **Ans. (c) Tell her to feed the baby just before next dose** *(Ref: Katzung 13/e p1020)*

161. **Ans. (a) Expiry date of the drug** *(Ref: WHO criteria for drug advertisement, Practical Manual of Pharmacology by Dinesh Badyal 1st/e p211-212)*

According to WHO criteria and OPPI (Organization of Pharmaceutical Producers of India) code of Pharmaceuti-

General Pharmacology

cal practices 2012, the printed drug promotional literature (DPL) must contain

- Name of the drug: Brand name should be available with the active ingredient (generic name). The ratio of size of brand name to generic name should not be more than 3:1
- Indications: Approved therapeutic indications must be present on the DPL.
- Dosage: Content of active ingredient(s) per dosage form and whole regiment should be written on the DPL
- Precautions and warnings
- Contraindications
- Adverse effects: All serious adverse effects and common non-serious adverse effects should be mentioned on the DPL
- Major interactions
- Price: Price of the drug as well as whole regimen should be present on DPL.
- Information of manufacturer: The name and address of the pharmaceutical company or its agent responsible for marketing the product must be present on DPL
- **Reference to scientific literature:** Appropriate references should be available regarding the claims made by the DPL.

162. **Ans. (b) 8 to 15° C** *(Ref: Park 22nd/e p100)*
- Storage condition of drugs (according to IP)

Store frozen:–20ºC

Do not freeze or Keep Cold: 2-8ºC

Keep cool: 8-25ºC

Store at room temperature: Dry, clean, well ventilated area at temp 15-25ºC or upto 30ºC depending on climatic conditions

Protect from moisture: To be stored in normal humidity at room temperature (relative humidity less than 60%)

Protect from light: Store in a light resistant cupboard/drawer

163. **Ans. (b) Griseofulvin** *(Ref: KDT 8th/e p842)*
Important drugs whose absorption is increased by food
- Vitamin a analogs like acitretin and isotretinoin
- Carbamazepine
- Griseofulvin
- Halofantrine
- Mefloquine
- Protease inhibitors like saquinavir
- Statins
- Tyrosine kinase inhibitors like imatinib

164. **Ans. (a) Schedule H** *(Ref: KK Sharma 2nd/e p6)*
Drugs are broadly of 2 types:
Schedule H drugs: Must be sold by retail only when a prescription by registered medical practitioner is produced.
OTC: These are over the counter drugs, which may be sold without prescription.

165. **Ans. (a) Qualitatively abnormal responses to the drug**
(Ref: Principles of Pharmacology by HL Sharma and KK Sharma, 1st/e p71; KDT 8th/e p92)

Adverse Drug Reactions are noxious or unintended effects produced by drugs. These may be classified as

- **Type A:** Augmented pharmacologic effects - Dose dependent and predictable e.g. hypoglycemia caused by anti-hyperglycemic drugs like sulfonylureas
- **Type B:** Bizarre effects (or idiosyncratic) - Dose independent and unpredictable e.g. allergic reactions caused by penicllins
- **Type C:** Chronic effects e.g. peptic ulcer caused by chronic use of NSAIDs
- **Type D:** Delayed effects e.g. teratogenicity caused by thalidomide
- **Type E:** End-of-treatment effects e.g. withdrawal response to morphine
- **Type F:** Failure of therapy

166. **Ans. (c) Propylthiouracil** *(Ref: KDT 7th/e p964)*
- Among the given options, the best answer seems to be propylthiouracil. Although, the latter can cause hepatotoxicity in mother.

167. **Ans. (c) Lithium** *(Ref: KDT 8th/e p476)*
168. **Ans. (c) Renal clearance** *(Ref: Katzung 11th/e p1039)*
169. **Ans. (a) Orphan drugs** *(Ref: KDT 8th/e p7)*
170. **Ans. (b) Allergic effect of the drug** *(Ref: KDT 8th/e p92)*
171. **Ans. (a) Enalapril** *(Ref: KDT 8th/e p531)*
172. **Ans. (b) Single compound** *(Ref: KDT 8th/e p6)*
173. **Ans. (b) Neostigmine** *(Ref: KDT 8th/e p116)*
174. **Ans. (b) Schedule H** *(Ref: KDT 8th/e p7)*

Schedule of Drugs
'Drugs and cosmetics act 1940' along with 'Drugs and cosmetic rules 1945' and its amendments describe various schedule of drugs. Important schedules are:

Schedule	Deals with
C and C1	Biological and special products
F and F1	Bacterial vaccines
G	Drugs to be labelled with the word "Caution"-It is dangerous to take this preparation except under medical supervision
H	Drugs that must be sold by retail only when a prescription by RMP is produced
M	Good manufacturing practices (GMP)
P	Expiry period of drug formulations
W	Drugs that shall be marketed under generic names only
X	Psychotropic drugs requiring special licence for manufacture and sale
Y	Requirements and guidelines on clinical trials, import and manufacture of new drugs

175. **Ans. (d) Metoclopramide** *(Ref: KDT 8th/e p100)*
176. **Ans. (a) Defect in development of long bones** *(Ref: KDT 8th/e p100)*
177. **Ans. (d) Body surface area** *(Ref: KDT 8th/e p73)*
178. **Ans. (c) Corrosive acid poisoning** *(Ref: KDT 8th/e p95)*
179. **Ans. (b) Nitrate induced headache** *(Ref: KDT 8th/e p96)*
180. **Ans. (a) Propylthiouracil** *(Ref: KDT 8th/e p100)*
181. **Ans. (c) That satisfy the priority health care needs of the population** *(Ref: KDT 8th/e p6)*

182. **Ans. (d) All of the above** *(Ref: Satoskar 24th/e p54)*
    Counterfeit Drugs
    It is a fake medicine. These are illegal drugs and
    - May be contaminated
    - May contain wrong active ingredient
    - May contain no active ingredient
    - May have right active ingredient but in wrong dose
183. **Ans (c) Randomized controlled trial in patients is done in phase 3** *(Ref: KDT 8th/e p90-91)*
184. **Ans. (b) Quantal DRC** *(Ref: KDT 8th/e p65)*
    Quantal DRC
    When the response is an *'all or none' phenomenon* (e.g. antiemetic drug stopping the vomiting or not), the y-axis (response axis) shows the number of person responding and X-axis shows the plasma concentration. It thus shows that how many people respond to a particular dose of the drug. It is used to calculate ED50 and LD50.

185. **Ans. (d) Km increased, V_{max} unchanged** *(Ref: KDT 8th/e p47)*
186. **Ans. (b) V_{max} decreases, Km remains same** *(Ref: KDT's 8th/e p47)*
187. **Ans. (d) Barbiturates** *(Ref: KDT's 8th/e p427)*
188. **Ans. (a) Ability of a drug to produce maximum effect by acting on target** *(Ref: KDT 8th/e p64)*
189. **Ans. (a) Estrogen** *(Ref: KDT's 8th/e p55)*
190. **Ans. (c) Constant fraction of drug eliminated in unit time** *(Ref: KDT's 8th/e p38)*
191. **Ans. (c) Phase III** *(Ref: KDT 8th/e p91)*
192. **Ans. (a) Post marketing trial** *(Ref: KDT 8th/e p91)*
193. **Ans. (d) Minoxidil in alopecia areata** *(Ref: KDT's 8th/e p613)*

Numerical Questions

1. Half-Life of propranolol in a 60 kg patient is 7 hours and V_d is 6 L/kg. Determine:
   (a) Total clearance of propranolol
   (b) What will be renal clearance if fraction excreted unchanged in urine is 0.3
   (c) If drug is eliminated only by hepatic and renal routes, what will be hepatic extraction ratio if blood flow to liver is 90 L/hour
   (d) If blood flow to liver is reduced to 45 L/hour in a CHF patient, what will be new
      i. Renal clearance
      ii. Hepatic clearance
      iii. Total clearance

2. Lignocaine was administered at a dose of 100 mg intravenously to a 60 kg man. The concentration of lignocaine in arteries entering the liver is 10 µg/L whereas it is 2 µg/L in veins leaving the liver. If hepatic blood flow is 1.5 L/hour, find the hepatic clearance of lignocaine.

3. A new drug X is being evaluated for its hypnotic action. From the information provided in the figure below, find the therapeutic index of the drug X

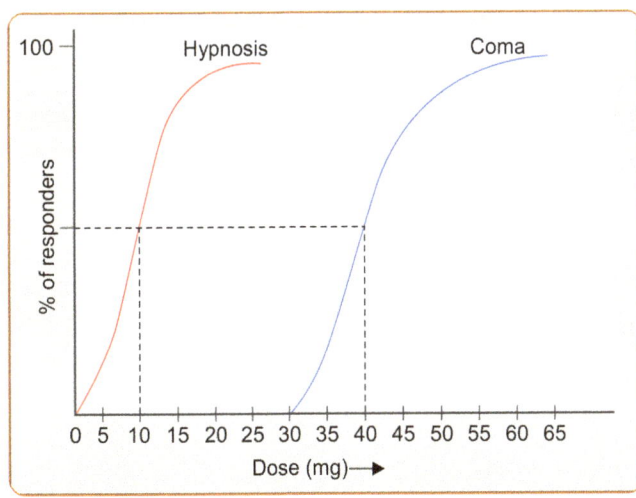

4. Cimetidine is a weak base with pKa of 7.0. How much percentage of cimetidine can be absorbed from stomach (pH = 3.0)?

5. A patient suffering from UTI was prescribed 500 mg norfloxacin by oral route. Fractional oral bioavailability of norfloxacin is 0.8 and $t_{1/2}$ is 6 hours. If initial plasma concentration (Co) obtained is 80 µg/mL, what is volume of distribution of norfloxacin?

6. A graph is plotted between log plasma concentration vs time after administration of 100 mg drug Y to a person. Calculate half-life, V_d and total clearance of the drug Y.

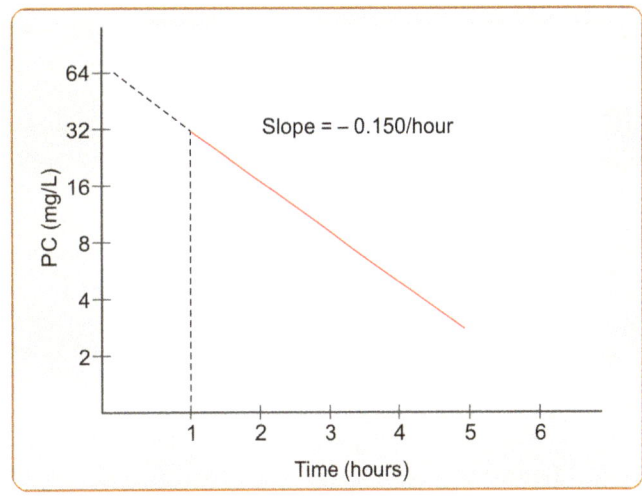

7. Initial plasma concentration of a drug given IV at 8 AM is 200 mg/L. If half-life of drug is 4 hours and it follows first order kinetics, what will be its plasma concentration at 8 PM same day?

8. A new drug A is administered at 9 am at a dose of 1000 mg intravenously. When plasma concentration was measured at 11 am, 300 mg drug was eliminated from body. Calculate the remaining drug in the body at 3 pm same day, if
   i. It follows first order kinetics throughout
   ii. It follows zero order kinetics throughout.

9. A drug X was administered by continuous IV infusion at the rate of 1.6 mg/min. Clearance of drug X is 640 mL/min. If the $t_{1/2}$ of the drug is 1.8 hours, what would be the concentration of drug after achieving steady state?

10. A patient was administered 200 mg of a drug. 75 mg of the drug is eliminated from the body in 90 minutes. If the drug follows first order kinetics, how much drug will remain after 6 hrs?

11. An 80 kg patient is brought in the causality in shock. Dopamine needs to be started at 10 micrograms/kg/min rate. A 5 mL vial contains 200 mg of dopamine. Two vials are diluted to a solution of 250 mL with the help of normal saline. Calculate drops per minute required to be administered if 1 mL = 16 drops.

12. Amount of a drug X administered to a patient is 4.0 g and its plasma concentration is found to be 50 µg/mL, what will be the volume of distribution of drug X?

13. Rate of elimination of a new drug is 20 mg/hr at a steady state plasma concentration of 10 mg/L. Find its clearance.

14. A drug following first order kinetics is being administered by constant IV infusion at a rate of 10 mg/min. Its steady state plasma concentration is 2 mg/min. If the dose rate is increased to 20 mg/dL, what will be the new steady state plasma concentration?

15. Ram Prashad is admitted to Guru Teg Bahadur Hospital with respiratory infection for which antibiotic tobramycin is ordered. The clearance and Vd of tobramycin in him are 160 mL/min and 40 L, respectively. If you wish to give Ram Prashad an intravenous loading dose to achieve the therapeutic plasma concentration of 4 mg/L rapidly, how much should be given?

16. A 30-year-old patient on digoxin therapy has developed digitalis toxicity. The plasma digoxin level is 4 ng/mL. Renal function is normal and the plasma $t_{1/2}$ for digoxin in this patient is 1.6 days. How long should you withhold digoxin in order to reach a safer yet probably therapeutic level of 1 ng/mL?

17. A young male Kallu is brought to the hospital with severe asthma. The pharmacokinetics of theophylline include the following parameters: Vd = 35 L; CL = 48 mL/min; half-life is 8 hrs. If an intravenous infusion of theophylline is started at a rate of 0.48 mg/min, how long will it take the plasma concentration to reach 93.75% of the final steady state?

18. A patient requires an infusion of procainamide. Its half-life is 2 hrs. The infusion is begun at 9 am. At 1 pm on the same day, the blood concentration is found to be 3 mg/L. What is the probable steady state concentration after 2 days of infusion?

19. A volunteer Ram will receive a new drug in a phase I clinical trial. The clearance and the volume of distribution of the drug in Ram are 1.386 L/hr and 80 L respectively. Calculate the approximate half-life of the drug in him.

20. Drug X is normally administered to patients at a rate of 50 mg/hour. Elimination of the drug X from body takes place as:
    - Hepatic Metabolism 10%
    - Biliary Secretion 10%
    - Renal Excretion 80%

    This drug has to be administered to a 65 years old patient Uttaam Singh, with a GFR of 60 mL/min. (assuming normal GFR is 120 mL/min). Liver and biliary functions are normal in this patient. What should be the dose rate of drug X in this patient?

Answers

1. **(a) Total clearance (CL)**

   $t_{1/2} = \dfrac{0.693 \times V_d}{CL}$, So, $CL = \dfrac{0.693 \times V_d}{t_{1/2}}$

   So, $CL = \dfrac{0.693 \times 6 \text{ L/kg}}{7 \text{ hours}} = \dfrac{0.693 \times 6 \times 60}{7}$

   = App. 36 L/hour

   (b) Renal Clearance (CL_R)

   Total Clearance (CL) = $CL_R + CL_H + CL_{other\ organs}$

   Here, kidney contributes 0.3 fraction,

   So, $CL_R = 0.3 \times CL = 0.3 \times 36 = 10.8$ L/hour

   and $CL_H = 36 - 10.8 = 25.2$ L/hour

   (If only by liver and kidney)

   (c) Hepatic Extraction Ratio (HER)

   $CL_H = Q \times HER$ [Q is Rate of blood blow to liver]

   $HER = \dfrac{CL_H}{Q} = \dfrac{25.2}{90} = 0.28$

   (d) If Q' is 45 L/hour

   (i) New $CL_R = 10.8$ L/hour   (Same as early)

   (ii) New $CL_H = HER \times Q = 0.28 \times 45 = 12.6$ L/hour

   (iii) New $CL = CL_R + CL_H = 10.8 + 12.6 = 23.4$ L/hour

2. Hepatic Extraction Ratio = $\dfrac{C_A - C_V}{C_A}$

   C_A = Conc. of drug in artery

   C_V = Conc. of drug in veins

   $= \dfrac{10 - 2}{10} = 0.8$

   $H_{CL} = Q \times HER = 0.8 \times 1.5$ L/hour = 1.2 L/hour

3. Therapeutic Index = $\dfrac{LD_{50}}{ED_{50}} = \dfrac{40}{10} = 4$

4. **Nature of drug = Basic**

   pKa = 7.0

   pH = 3.0

   Drugs cross in same medium

   Here, Drug is basic but medium is acidic, so less will be able to cross the membrane.

pH	Drug Crossing
7	50%
6	10%
5	1%
4	0.1%
3	0.01%

5. $V_d = \dfrac{\text{Amount given}}{\text{Initial plasma concentration}} \times \text{Fraction Bioavailability}$

   $= \dfrac{500 \text{ mg}}{80 \text{ μg/mL}} \times 0.8$

   $= \dfrac{500 \text{ mg}}{80 \text{ mg/L}} \times 0.8 = 5$ L

6. Slope = $-\dfrac{k}{2.303}$ where k = Elimination rate constant

   so, $k = 2.303 \times 0.150 = 0.345$ hr^{-1}

   Now, $t_{1/2} = \dfrac{0.693}{K} = \dfrac{0.693}{0.345} = 2$ hours

   Further, from the graph (by extrapolation);

   $C_O = 64$

   so, $V_d = \dfrac{\text{Amount given}}{PC(C_O)} = \dfrac{100}{64} = 1.56$ L

   and $t_{1/2} = 0.693 \times \dfrac{V_d}{CL}$

   so, $CL = \dfrac{0.693 \times V_d}{t_{1/2}} = \dfrac{0.693 \times 1.56}{2} = 0.54$ L/hour

7. **Initial concentration = 200 mg/L**

   $t_{1/2}$ = 4 hours

   Number of $t_{1/2}$ in 12 hours (8 am to 8 pm) = 3

   Remaining plasma concentration =

   200
   ↓ 1 $t_{1/2}$
   100
   ↓ 2 $t_{1/2}$
   50
   ↓ 3 $t_{1/2}$
   25

   Ans is 25 mg/L

8. **(i) In first order kinetics, fraction of drug eliminated per unit time is constant.**

   Here, fraction is $\dfrac{300}{1000} \times 100 = 30\%$ in 2 hours (9 to 11 am)

   So, every 2 hours, 30% will be eliminated. Means every 2 hours, 70% will remain.

   Therefore,

   Remaining drug: At 11 am = 70% of 1000

   $= \dfrac{1000 \times 70}{100} = 700$ mg

   At 1 pm = 70% of 700

   $= \dfrac{70 \times 700}{100} = 490$ mg

   At 3 pm = 70% of 490

   $= \dfrac{490 \times 70}{100} = 343$ mg

   So, remaining at 3 pm is 343 mg

   (ii) In zero order kinetics, same amount is eliminated per unit time

   Here, 300 mg is eliminated in 2 hours

   So, remaining at 11 am : 1000 − 300 = 700 mg

   So, remaining at 1 pm : 700 − 300 = 400 mg

   So, remaining at 3 pm : 400 − 300 = 100 mg

9. Maintenance dose rate = Clearance × Target steady state plasma concentration

   1.6 mg/min = 640 mL/min × Steady state plasma concentration

   Steady state plasma conc. = 1.6/640 = 0.0025 mg/mL

10. Applying the formula

    $\log[C_0] - \log[C_t] = kt$

    Where C_0 is initial drug concentration

    C_t is concentration of drug at time t

    k is Elimination constant

    To solve this

    We can use 2 properties of logarithms

    1. $\log A - \log B = \log A/B$
    2. $Z \times \log A = \log A^z$

    Step 1: Calculation of k

    C_0 = 200 mg

    C 1.5 hour = 200–75 = 125 mg

    t = 1.5 hour

    $\log[200] - \log[125] = k \times 1.5$

    $\log[200/125] = 1.5\, k$

    $k = \dfrac{\log[200/125]}{1.5}$

    Step 2: Calculation of remaining drug

    Now t = 6 hours

    C_t = ?

    $\log C_0 - \log C_t = kt$

    $\log[C_0/C_t] = kt$

    $\log[200/C_t] = 6 \times \dfrac{\log[200/125]}{1.5}$

    $\log[200/C_t] = 4 \log[200/125]$

    $\log[200/C_t] = \log[200/125]^4$

    $200/C_t = [200/125]^4$

    $200/C_t = [8/5]^4$

    $C_t/200 = [5/8]^4$

    $C_t = 200 \times 5 \times 5 \times 5 \times 5/8 \times 8 \times 8 \times 8 = 30.5$

    Simpler method to calculate

    In first order kinetics percentage of drug eliminated per unit time is constant

    Here amount eliminated is 75 mg (from 200 mg) in 1.5 hours

    So percentage eliminated is 75/200 = 37.5% in 1.5 hours

    Method 1:

    So every 1.5 hours 37.5% will be eliminated

    After 3 hours remaining will be 125 – [125 × 37.5/100] = 78.125

    After 4.5 hours remaining will be 78.125 – [78.125 × 37.5/100] = 48.82

    After 6 hours remaining will be 48.82 – [48.82 × 37.5/100] = 30.5

    Method 2:

    Every 1.5 hours 100–37.5 = 62.5% will remain

    After 3 hours = 125 × 62.5/100

    After 4.5 hours = 125 × 62.5/100 × 62.5/100

    After 6 hours = 125 × 62.5/100 × 62.5/100 × 62.5/100 = 30.5

11. Amount of dopamine required to be infused (@10 mcg/kg/min) = 80 × 10

    = 800 micro g/min = 0.8 mg/min

    Amount of dopamine in 250 mL of solution

    = 200 mg × 2 = 400 mg

    Amount of dopamine in 1 mL solution

    = 400/250 mg = 1.6 mg

    Or

    1.6 mg dopamine present in = 1 mL solution

    0.8 mg dopamine present in = 0.5 mL solution

    So, solution should be infused @ 0.5 mL per min.

    As 1 mL = 16 drops

    So, infusion should be started at 8 drops per min.

12. Vd = Amount administered/Plasma concentration

    = 4 g/50 mcg/mL = 80 L

13. Clearance = Rate of elimination/plasma concentration

    $= \dfrac{20\ \text{mg/hour}}{10\ \text{mg/L}} = 2\ \text{L/hour}$

14. Dose Rate = Clearance × Steady state plasma concentration

    This means plasma concentration at steady state is a direct function of the dose rate, if clearance is constant. In first order kinetics (clearance is constant), plasma concentration attained is directly proportional to the dose rate. Thus, doubling of dose rate from 10 to 20 mg/min, will double the steady state plasma concentration (from 2 to 4 mg/dL).

15. Loading dose = Vd × target plasma concentration

    = 40 L × 4 mg/L = 160 mg

    Clearance plays no role in the determination of loading dose. It is given just to confuse you.

16. We want to decrease the plasma concentration of digoxin from 4 ng/mL to 1 ng/mL. It will take two half lives. Thus time required will be 2 × $t_{1/2}$ i.e. 2 × 1.6 = 3.2 days.

17. For a drug following first order kinetics, rise in plasma concentration as well as fall in plasma concentration is similar. When the steady state is attained and the drug administration is stopped, it will be eliminated from the body. 50% will be eliminated in one half-life, 75% in 2 $t_{1/2}$, 87.5% (50 + 25 + 12.5%) in 3 $t_{1/2}$ and 93.75% (50 + 25 + 12.5 + 6.25%) in four half lives.

- When constant IV infusion is administered, plasma concentration increases in the same manner. In one half-life, it is 50% of the steady state and to reach 93.75% of steady state, 4 half-lives will be required.
- As half-life of this drug is 8 hours, approximately 32 hours (4 × 8) will be taken.

18. Half-life of this drug is 2 hours and its plasma concentration is 3 mg/L after 4 hours (9 am to 1 pm).
    - This means, after 2 half lives (4 hours) plasma concentration is 3 mg/L. We know, by constant IV infusion, plasma concentration attained is 75% of the steady state in 2 half-lives.

    Thus,

    75% of steady state plasma concentration = 3 mg/L

    Steady state plasma concentration $= \dfrac{3}{75} \times 100$ mg/L
    $= 4$ mg/L

19. **Half life = 0.693 × V_d/CL**
    = 0.693 × 80/1.386 = 40 hours

20. In this question 80% of drug is eliminated by renal route and 20% by non-renal routes (10% by hepatic metabolism and 10% by biliary secretion).

    This patient has 50% renal function (60 mL/min of GFR instead of 120 mL/min). Thus, the drug that can be eliminated in this person is 20% (Non-renal route) + 40% (Renal route; 50% of 80%) = 60%

    Thus, the dose rate should be 60% of the original. i.e. 50 mg/hr × 60% = 30 mg/hr.

CHAPTER 2

Autonomic Nervous System

Autonomic Nervous System (ANS) is involuntary in nature and the activities of this system are maintained autonomically. In contrast to somatic nervous system, organs supplied by ANS *do not atrophy* even after the section of an autonomic nerve (rather, denervation supersensitivity of receptors occur). ANS is divided into **three main divisions**.

- *Sympathetic*
- *Parasympathetic*
- *Enteric nervous system.*

Division of ANS into sympathetic and parasympathetic system is *anatomical* in origin. Fibres of sympathetic system originates from thoracic and lumbar spinal cord (*thoracolumbar outflow*) whereas parasympathetic system originates from cranial nerves (III, VII, IX and X) and sacral ($S_{2,3,4}$) spinal cord (*craniosacral outflow*). All autonomic fibres form a synapse in the ganglion before supplying the organ and thus can be divided into pre and post-ganglionic fibres. In *sympathetic* system, *postganglionic fibres are either equal to or longer* than preganglionic fibres whereas in *parasympathetic system preganglionic fibres are much longer* than postganglionic fibres (ganglia are closer to the organs).

- **Acetylcholine (ACh)** is the principal neurotransmitter (NT) at neuromuscular junction (NMJ) as well at *all preganglionic* fibres.

- In *parasympathetic* system, NT released at *postganglionic* fibres is also ACh.
- In *sympathetic* system, at most of the postganglionic fibres, NT secreted is *nor-adrenaline* (NA) but it can be *dopamine* (renal and mesenteric vasculature), ACh (sweat glands; sympathetic cholinergic) or *adrenaline* (adrenal medulla).

Impulse is conducted along the axon till it reaches the cell body forming the synapse. Cell body releases the NT that acts on the receptors present on the post-synaptic membrane (post-synaptic receptors) as well as on the pre-synaptic membrane (pre-synaptic receptors). Pre-synaptic receptors increase (**nicotinic, β**) or decrease (**muscarinic, α_2**) the release of neurotransmitter from their own neuron (autoreceptors) or from adjoining neurons (heteroreceptors).

Most of the actions of sympathetic and parasympathetic systems are opposite. To remember major actions, we can assume that sympathy is related to heart, so sympathetic system stimulates it (i.e. tachycardia, positive inotropic action etc.). On the other hand, parasympathetic system has opposite action, so depress heart. At most other parts action is reverse i.e. sympathetic system inhibits and parasympathetic system stimulates.

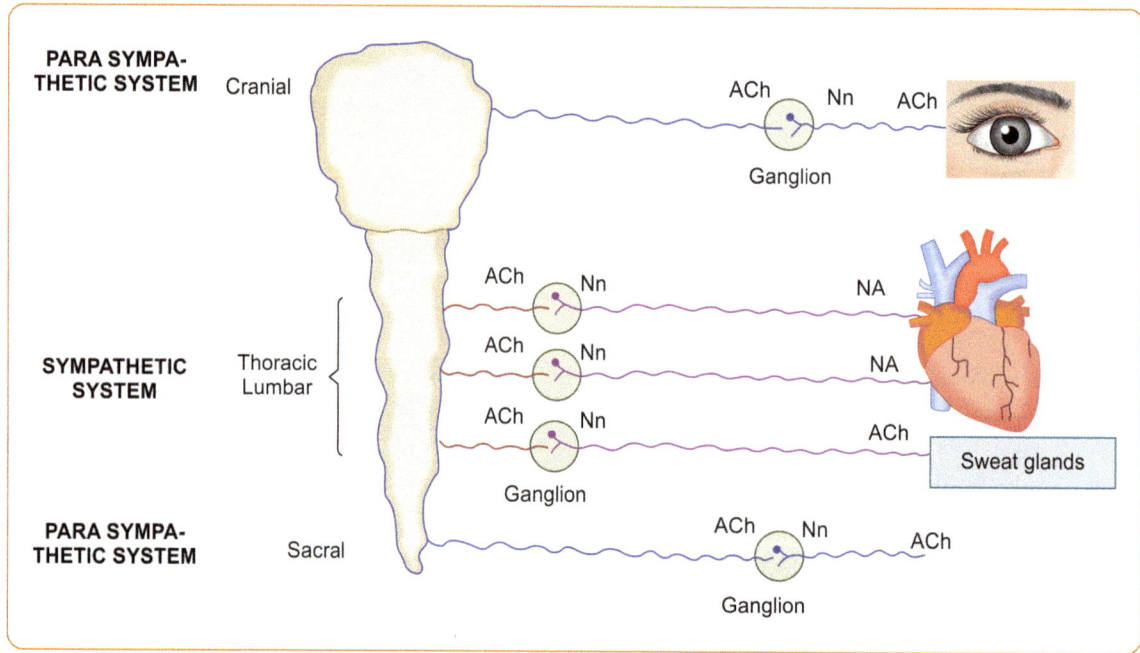

FIG. 2.1: Divisions of autonomic nervous system

Autonomic Nervous System

Site	Sympathetic Action	Parasympathetic Action
Heart	Stimulate	Depress
Bronchus	Dilation	Contraction
GI motility	Decrease	Increase
Urine outflow	Decrease	Increase
Pupil	Mydriasis	Miosis
Secretions	Decrease (except sweating)	Increase

PARASYMPATHETIC NERVOUS SYSTEM

In parasympathetic system, **acetylcholine is the principal NT** secreted by preganglionic as well as postganglionic fibres. Therefore, it is also known as cholinergic nervous system. ACh is synthesized (from acetyl Co-A and choline) and stored within the cholinergic neurons.

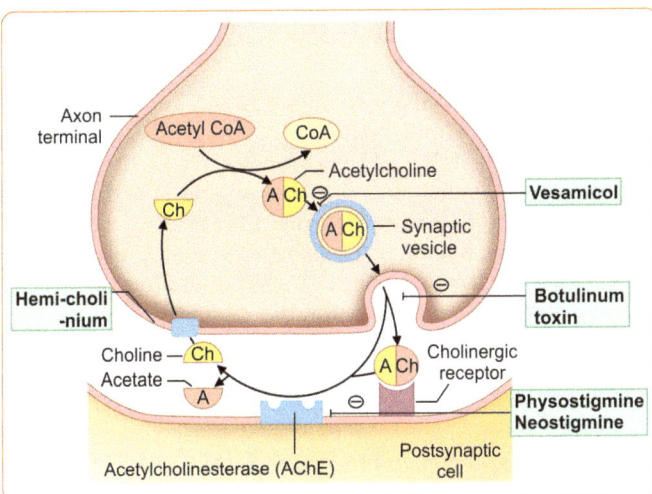

FIG. 2.2: Drugs acting at cholinergic neurons

Uptake of choline by the neurons is the *rate limiting step* in the biosynthesis of this NT. After its synthesis, ACh is stored in the vesicles. It is released in the synaptic cleft (by exocytosis) when nerve impulse stimulates the neuron. Here, it stimulates post-ganglionic as well as pre-ganglionic cholinergic receptors and produces the response.

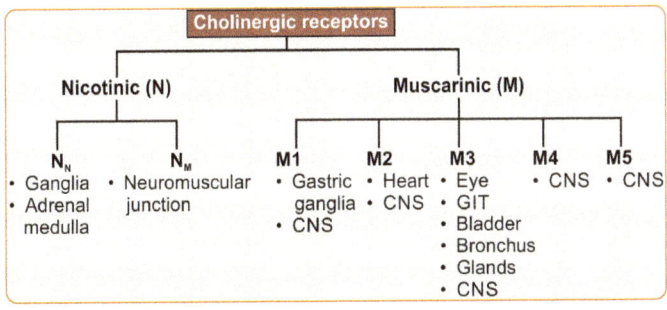

⚠ MNEMONIC

To remember location of cholinergic receptors, read in Hindi
—Pehle khao, Phir dil lagao, Baki kaam bad mein
i.e. M_1 in stomach, M_2 in heart and M_3 at all other places.

Functions of Cholinergic System

Sympathetic and parasympathetic systems have opposite actions on most of the organs. At almost all organs except heart, cholinergic system has excitatory activity and adrenergic system has relaxing properties.

Muscarinic Actions

- **Heart:** Parasympathetic system has *inhibitory effect on the heart (M_2)* and is responsible for the negative chronotropic (decreased heart rate) and dromotropic (decreased conduction) effects. Bradycardia occurs due in decrease in slope of phase 4 of action potential (delay in spontaneous diastolic depolarization) whereas decrease in conduction occcurs due to delay in AV node. Anticholinergic drugs stimulate the heart by decreasing the inhibitory effect of ACh on heart.
- **Blood vessels:** *No direct cholinergic supply is present in blood vessels but cholinergic receptors (M_3) are present on endothelium of blood vessels.* Stimulation of these receptors causes *release of NO* from endothelium *resulting in vasodilation.* Additional mechanism of vasodilation is inhibitory action of ACh on nor-adrenaline release from tonically active vasoconstrictor nerve endings. However, if endothelium is damaged, ACh can stimulate M_3 receptors in the vascular smooth muscle leading to vasoconstriction.
- **Eye:** Cholinergic system stimulates sphincter pupillae (circular muscle of eye) and thus results in *miosis (M_3)*. ACh also causes contraction of ciliary muscle of the eye and thus accommodation is possible. Anticholinergic drugs result in mydriasis and loss of accommodation (blurred vision).
- **Glands:** Cholinergic system stimulates the secretion of glands and results in the *increased salivation, lacrimation as well as sweating (M_3).* On the other hand anticholinergic drugs will result in dry mouth, dry eyes and difficulty in swallowing (due to decreased saliva).
- **Urinary bladder:** Cholinergic drugs *stimulate detrusor and relax the trigone* (sphincter) of urinary bladder resulting in increased micturition (M_3). Anticholinergic drugs may result in urinary retention.
- **Gastrointestinal tract:** Hydrochloric acid secretion in the stomach (M_1 and M_3) is stimulated by parasympathetic system and thus increases the *risk of peptic ulcer disease.* Peristalsis of GIT is increased and sphincters are relaxed by the cholinergic drugs. Anticholinergic drugs can be used as spasmolytic agents for intestinal colic.
- **Bronchus:** Cholinergic system causes *bronchoconstriction (M_3)* and anticholinergic drugs may lead to bronchodilation.
- **Male sex organs:** Due to vasodilation, cholinergic system is responsible for *erection of the male organ.*

Nicotinic Actions

- **Autonomic ganglia:** Both sympathetic and parasympathetic ganglia are stimulated by ACh through the stimulation of N_N receptors.
- **Neuromuscular junction:** ACh stimulates skeletal *muscle contraction* by its action on NMJ (N_M receptors).

PARASYMPATHOMIMETIC DRUGS

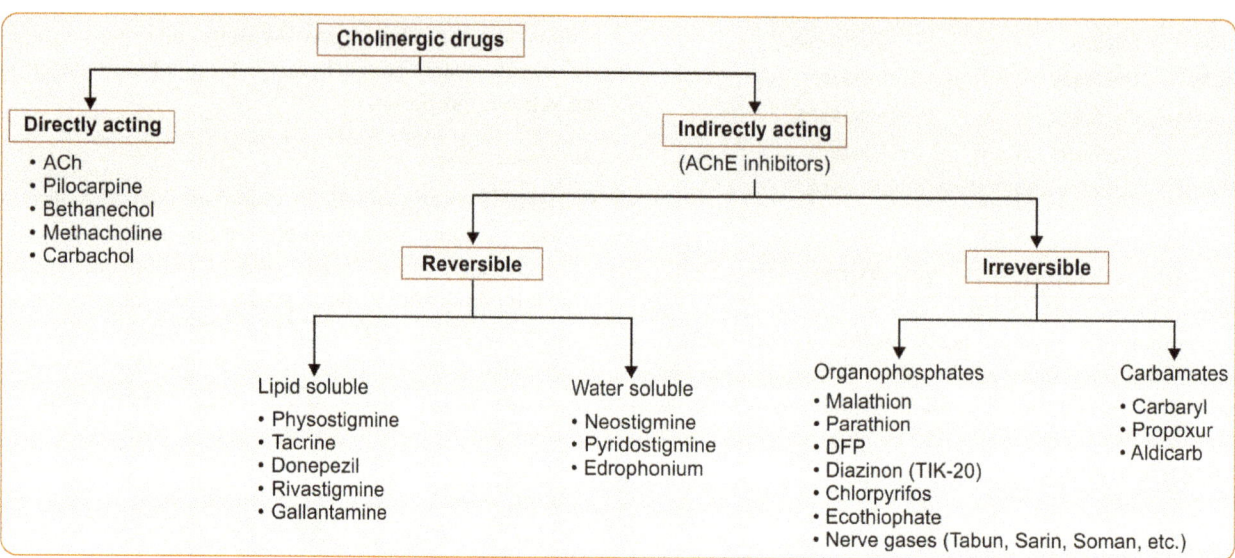

These drugs may directly activate the muscarinic receptors (directly acting) or may act by increasing the availability of ACh at the synaptic cleft (indirectly acting).

Directly Acting Drugs

These are the esters of choline and may be **natural alkaloids** (*ACh, muscarine, nicotine, pilocarpine and arecoline*) or **synthetic derivatives** (*methacholine, carbachol and bethanechol*).

- *Acetylcholine* is not used clinically because it is *metabolized very quickly* by cholinesterases in the plasma and is not effective even by i.v. route.
- **Methacholine** has maximum action on **m**yocardium. It can be given inhalationally for the diagnosis of bronchial hyperreactivity in patients who do not have clinically apparent asthma **methacholine challenge test**.
- **Bethanechol** is mainly used for its action on urinary **b**ladder and has no nicotinic activity.
- **Pilocarpine** is used in glaucoma due to its **p**upillary constrictor (miotic) action. However because of its *very short duration of action*, intraocular tension may increase even if one or two doses are missed.
- **Carbachol** has **c**ommon activity on nicotinic and muscarinic receptors.
- Pilocarpine and Cevimeline are used to treat dry mouth associated with Sjogren syndrome and that caused by radiation damage of salivary glands.

Indirectly Acting Drugs

These drugs act by *inhibiting the enzyme acetylcholinesterase*, thus increasing the availability and prolonging the action of ACh. These drugs are also known as anticholinesterases. Cholinesterase inhibitors may be reversible or irreversible.

Reversible Anticholinesterases

Physostigmine, neostigmine, pyridostigmine, edrophonium, tacrine, donepezil, galantamine and rivastigmine are the important drugs in this group. These drugs inhibit the enzyme AChE reversibly and prolong the duration of action of ACh.

- **Physostigmine** is naturally occurring *tertiary amine* and is *lipid soluble*. Tacrine, donepezil, rivastigmine and galantamine are also lipid soluble drugs. **All other** reversible anti-cholinesterases are synthetic *quaternary* compounds and are *lipid insoluble*. Due to high lipid solubility, physostigmine can be administered orally and it can cross blood brain barrier and corneal membrane. Lipid insoluble compounds are ineffective orally and do not enter CNS or eye.
- *Physostigmine* is *used in glaucoma* as a miotic drug *and in belladona (atropine) poisoning* as a specific antidote.
- **Neostigmine** is preferred for the treatment of *myasthenia gravis*. It does not produce adverse effects in the CNS (does not cross BBB) and it also has *direct NM receptor agonistic action*. It can also be used for the *treatment of cobra bite* (cobra venom contain the compounds that cause skeletal muscle paralysis), *postoperative paralytic ileus, atony of urinary bladder and the reversal of competitive skeletal muscle relaxants*.
- **Pyridostigmine** is *longer acting* than neostigmine and can be used for all these indications. Atropine is added to neostigmine therapy when action is required on N_M receptors [to avoid adverse effects due to muscarinic receptor stimulation] as in case of myasthenia gravis and cobra bite.

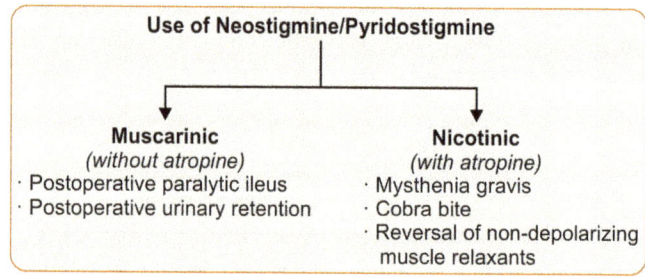

- **Edrophonium** is a short acting synthetic anticholinesterase and is useful in the *diagnosis of myasthenia gravis*. 1-2 mg i.v. dose of edrophonium improves skeletal muscle activity if the weakness is due to myasthenia whereas it will worsen the condition if it is due to cholinergic crisis. (**Tensilon test**)
- **Tacrine** was the drug of choice for Alzheimer's disease but due to several limitations (*frequent dosing requirement, hepatotoxicity, diarrhea*), other drugs like donepezil, rivastigmine and galantamine are now the preferred agent.
- **Rivastigmine** has been approved for the treatment of dementia in Alzheimer's as well as Parkinson's disease.

Autonomic Nervous System

Irreversible Anticholinesterases

This group includes **organophosphates** (*malathion, parathion, ecothiophate, chlorpyrifos, nerve gases like tabun, sarin, soman, etc. and diflos*) and **carbamates** (*carbaryl and propoxur*).

- Except ecothiophate these are *not used therapeutically. Ecothiophate is useful in glaucoma.*
- Other drugs are used as insecticides and are important due to their potential to cause poisoning.
- **Symptoms of anti-cholinesterase poisoning** are simply the extension of the pharmacological actions of ACh and are manifested as *pin-point pupil, salivation, lacrimation, sweating, bronchoconstriction, diarrhea, urination, bradycardia, hypotension and coma*. Blood pressure and heart rate may increase rarely due to stimulation of nicotinic receptors.
- **Atropine** is an *antidote of choice for both organophosphate and carbamate poisoning.*
- **Enzyme reactivators** like *pralidoxime, obidoxime and diacetylmonoxime* can be used to regenerate AChE in the organophosphate poisoning but are *contra-indicated in the carbamate poisoning. Principle indications* of oximes are **muscle weakness and respiratory depression.** The site on which oximes bind and reactivate the enzyme (anionic site) is occupied by carbamates whereas it is free in the organophosphate poisoning. (organophosphates binds to esteritic site only whereas carbamates bind to both esteritic as well as anionic sites) Further *oximes themselves possess weak AChE inhibitory action.* Due to these two reasons, oximes should not be given in carbamate poisoning.
- *Diacetylmonoxime can cross BBB* and regenerate AChE in the brain whereas pralidoxime and obidoxime cannot cross BBB.
- Chronic exposure to certain organophosphates e.g. triorthocresyl phosphate (additive in lubricating oils) may cause:
  - *Delayed neuropathy* (appear 1-2 weeks after exposure) associated with demyelination of axons. It is not caused by cholinesterase inhibition but rather by NTE (neuropathy target esterase) inhibition.
  - *Intermediate syndrome* (occurs after 1-4 days) caused by cholinesterase inhibition.

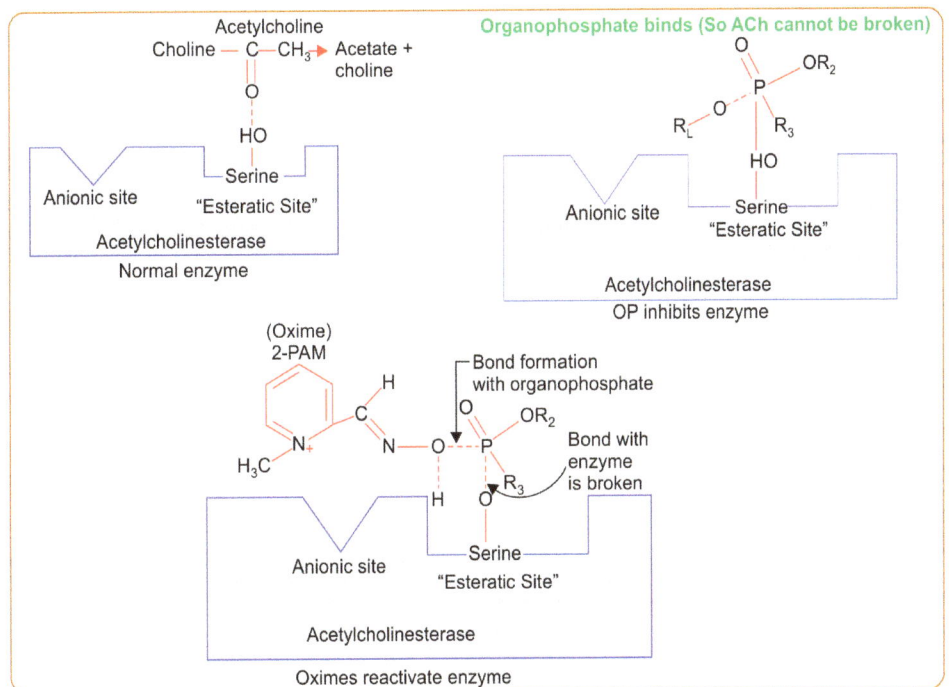

FIG. 2.3: Inhibition and reactivation of acetylcholinesterase

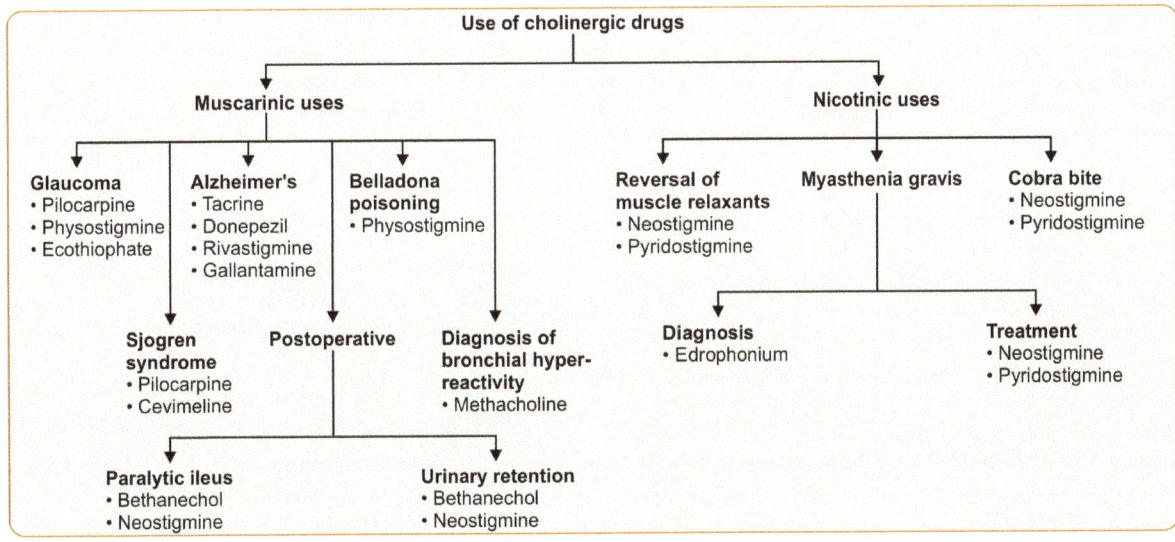

ANTICHOLINERGIC DRUGS

These drugs act by blocking muscarinic (*antimuscarinic*) or nicotinic receptors. Drugs blocking N_M receptors are called *neuromuscular blocking* agents and those blocking N_N receptors are called *ganglion blockers*.

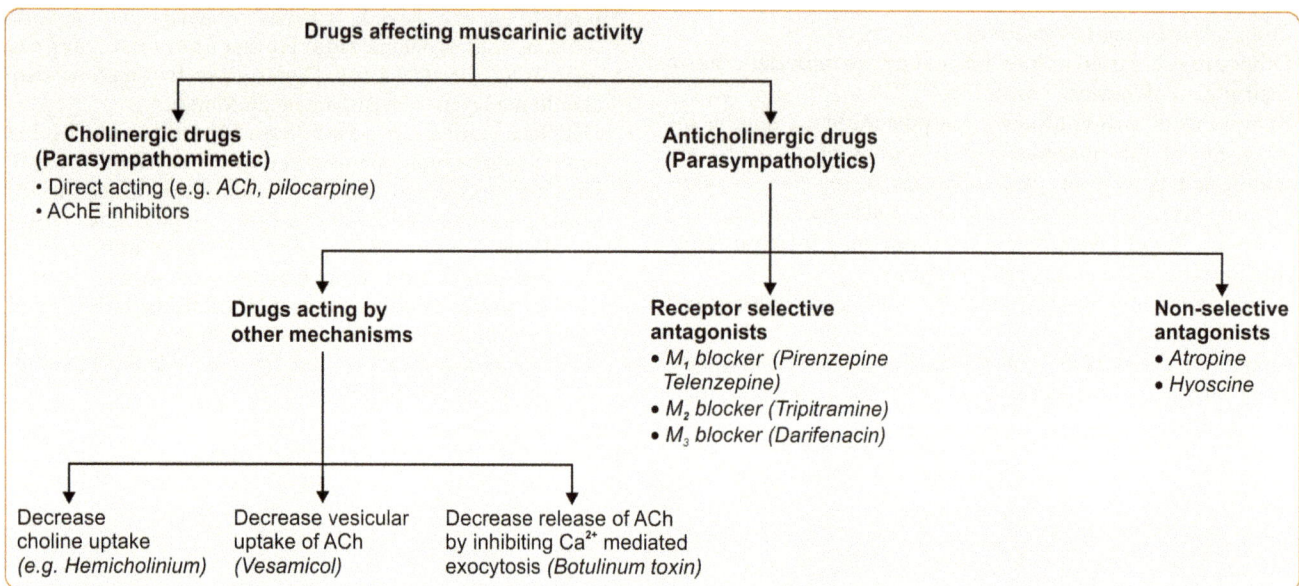

Atropine (obtained from *Atropa belladonna*) and scopolamine (l-hyoscine) are natural alkaloids that act as non-selective antagonists at all muscarinic receptors.

Actions of Antimuscarinic Agents

Central Nervous System

- Atropine is a CNS stimulant whereas scopolamine causes CNS depression.
  - Due to its amnesic and CNS depressant action, hyoscine induces "twilight sleep" and has been used as a *lie detector or truth serum* in suspects.
  - *Transdermal patch* of scopolamine (applied behind the pinna) is used for prevention of *motion sickness*. (Please note: Drug of choice for prophylaxis of mountain sickness is acetazolamide).
  - Central anticholinergic agents like *trihexiphenidyl* (benzhexol), *benztropine* and *biperidin* are drugs of choice for the treatment and prevention of *drug induced Parkinsonism*.

Onabotulinum toxin A has recently been approved to prevent headaches in adult patients with chronic migraine.

Eye

- Anticholinergic drugs cause mydriasis and cycloplegia.
  - *Atropine, homatropine, cyclopentolate and tropicamide* are used as *mydriatic* and cycloplegic agents. Mydriatic action is useful in fundus examination [maximum part of retina can be visualized] whereas cycloplegic action allows correct assessment of refractive error [due to loss of error resulting from accomodation]. Further, pain in iridocyclitis occur due to spasm of ciliary muscle which can be relieved due to cycloplegic action. *Atropine has very long duration of action* (3-5 days) in the eye (therefore avoided in adults) whereas it has shorter action in other organs. Hyoscine possess *similiar cycloplegic* action and *more potent mydriatic action as compared to atropine*. Its duration of action is also quite long (but less than atropine).
  - *Tropicamide is the shortest acting mydriatic.*
  - Anticholinergic agents are *contra-indicated in glaucoma*.

Cardiovascular System

- Atropine causes *bradycardia initially* due to inhibition of presynaptic muscarinic receptors (M_2) but further increase in dose causes *tachycardia* due to inhibition of post-synaptic M_2 receptors. Atropine is useful in the treatment of arrhythmias like AV block and digitalis induced bradycardia. It has negligible effect on BP and cardiac contractility.

Respiratory System

- Anticholinergic drugs *reverse the bronchoconstriction* caused by stimulation of M_3 receptors. **Ipratropium and tiotropium** are muscarinic receptor antagonists useful in the *treatment of COPD* and bronchial asthma. *Ipratropium has non-selective action* on all muscarinic receptors whereas tiotropium is somewhat selective blocker of M_1 and M_3 receptors. **Glycopyrolate** is used as a *pre-anaesthetic medication* to decrease the secretions and reflex bronchospasm during general anaesthesia.

Gastrointestinal Tract

- Anticholinergic drugs decrease the motility, tone and secretions in the gastrointestinal tract.
  - *Pirenzepine and telenzepine* are selective M_1 blockers useful in peptic ulcer disease.
  - *Hyoscine, dicyclomine, propantheline, oxyphenonium and clidinium* are useful as *anti-spasmodic* agents for the treatment of intestinal colic.
  - *Darifenacin and solefenacin* are selective M_3 blockers useful for irritable bowel syndrome and overactive bladder.

Genitourinary Tract

- Anticholinergic drugs decrease the motility of urinary tract and thus may *result in urinary retention* (therefore contra-indicated in BPH).
  - *Dicyclomine, flavoxate and oxybutynin* are useful for the treatment of *urinary incontinence* [detrusor instability] and renal colic.
  - *Tolterodine, fesoterodine (a prodrug of tolterodine), darifenacin and solefenacin* (selective M_3 antagonist) are also useful for urinary incontinence.

> ⚠️ **MNEMONIC**
>
> S – Solefenacin
> O – Oxybutynin
> F – Flavoxate, Fesoterodine
> T – Tolterodine, Trospium
>   blad DAR - DARifenacin
>
> Soft bladder means bladder is relaxed, so these can be used for overactive bladder.

- **Oxybutynin** has maximum risk of **dry mouth** and other anticholinergic adverse effects.
- **Trospium** has **minimum CNS penetration** because of quarternary amine structure. It has thus *lesser risk of causing impairment of cognition* and is safe in elderly also. It is the only drug from this group that **can be used with AChE inhibitors**.
- **Tolterodine, solefenacin and darifenacin** are vesicoselective M_3 antagonists and thus are less likely to block M_1 muscarinic receptors present in CNS. These also can be used in elderly and cognitive impaired person.
- **Trospium** is the only drug in this group that is *not metabolized by liver*. Thus, it is safe to be used with CYP inhibitors.
- **Oxybutynin** is *shortest acting* and **solefenacin** is *longest acting* drug from this **group**.
- **Mirabegron** and **Vibegron** are newer drugs approved for overactive bladder. These *act by stimulating β_3 receptors*.
- In refractory cases, intrabladder injection of botulinum toxin A can be done.
- *Behavioural therapy* (bladder training, pelvic floor exercises, fluid management) *is first line of treatment for overactive bladder* whereas antimuscarinic drugs are second line treatment.
- Any antimuscarinic drug may be used because these have similar efficacy. If both extended release (ER) and immediate release (IR) preparations are available, ER is preferred.

Glands

- Anticholinergic drugs decrease the secretions and *cause dry mouth*, reduced sweating, salivation and lacrimation. **Atropine is contra-indicated in children due to the risk of hyperthermia** (due to decreased sweating).

Other Uses

- **Botulinum toxin type A** has been approved for *treatment of strabismus, blepharospasm, cervical dystonia and glabellar lines* whereas botulinum toxin **type B** has been approved for the treatment of *cervical dystonia*.
- *Onabotulinum toxin A has recently been approved to prevent headaches in adult patients with chronic migraine (given every 12 weeks as multiple injections).*
- **Prabotulinum toxin-A** also inhibit release of acetylcholine. It is given intramuscularly for temporary improvement of glabellar lines.
- **Rimabotulinum toxin B** inhibits release of ACh. It is injected into salivary glands for treatment of chronic sialorrhea.

Atropine is the drug of choice for early mushroom poisoning due to Inocybe species. (It is contra-indicated in poisoning due to Amanita muscaria). Thiotic acid is useful for late mushroom poisoning due to Amanita phalloides.

- It is also the drug of choice for *organophosphate and carbamate poisoning*.
- It is used along *with neostigmine* (to decrease its muscarinic side effects) for the treatment of Myasthenia gravis and cobra bite.
- It is also added to diphenoxylate (anti-motility drug) to reduce its addictive potential.

Adverse Effects

These include *dry mouth, blurred vision* (due to mydriasis and cycloplegia), *urinary retention, constipation, hyperthermia, confusion, delirium and restlessness* etc. Anticholinergic drugs are **contraindicated in glaucoma and BHP**.

SYMPATHETIC NERVOUS SYSTEM

In this part of ANS, *nor-adrenaline is the neurotransmitter at most of the sites*. Circulating tyrosine is transported into the neuronal cytoplasm where it is hydroxylated to form l-dopa (**di** hydr**o**xy **p**henyl**a**lanine). This *rate limiting step is catalysed by an enzyme, tyrosine hydroxylase* that is amenable to inhibition by **metyrosine**. Latter can be used to control the discharge of catecholamines during surgical removal of the tumor in patients with pheochromocytoma. L-dopa is converted to dopamine by the action of a *non specific decarboxylase* (that also decarboxylates 5-hydroxytryptophan to serotonin), which can be *inhibited by carbidopa and benserazide*. Dopamine is transported to the storage vesicles (inhibited by **reserpine, tetrabenazine, deutetrabenazine and valbenazine**), where it is converted to nor-adrenaline by dopamine β hydroxylase. This enzyme is inhibited by disulfiram. Action of NA is terminated mainly by reuptake in the vesicles (inhibited by cocaine and TCA) and partly by the metabolism through MAO and COMT. Further conversion of NA to adrenaline (A) is carried out in the adrenal medulla. This methylation step occurs in the cytoplasm with the help of phenyl ethanolamine-N-methyl transferase. Sympathetic neurons lack this enzyme; therefore catecholamine synthesis is stopped at NA level.

NA remains stored in the vesicles. Stimulation of this neuron by the action potential increases the influx of Ca^{2+} and results in exocytosis of NA in the synaptic cleft. *Exocytosis is inhibited by bretylium and guanethidine*. NA released in the synapse acts on post-synaptic receptors (to produce various effects) as well as presynaptic receptors (to modulate its own release).

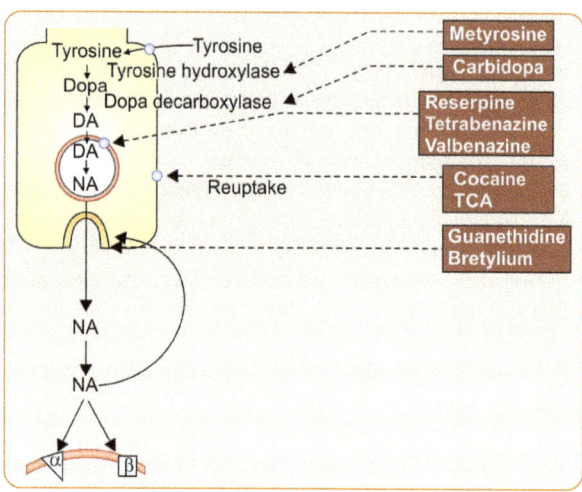

FIG. 2.4: Drugs acting at adrenergic neurons

Actions of Sympathetic System

- **Heart:** Positive chronotropic, inotropic and dromotropic effects are seen due to stimulation of β_1 receptors.
- **Blood vessels:** Stimulation of α_1 receptors causes *vasoconstriction* whereas β_2 stimulation leads to *dilation of blood vessels*. Effect of sympathetic system depends on the predominant type of receptor (α_1 or β_2) present in a particular vascular bed. Skin, mucosal and splanchnic blood vessels are constricted due to predominance of α_1 receptors whereas skeletal muscular blood vessels and coronaries are dilated because of the presence of β_2 receptors in excess. Renal vessels contain both α_1 (vasoconstriction) and D_1 (vasodilator) receptors and sympathetic stimulation cause less increase in vascular resistance here than in other vascular beds.
- **GIT:** Smooth muscles of GIT are relaxed by direct action of β_2 receptors and indirect action of α_2 receptors. Latter are present presynaptically on the cholinergic neurons (heteroreceptors) and results in decreased release of ACh.
- **Urinary system:** Urinary retention can occur due to *relaxation of detrusor by β_2 action* and *contraction of trigone (sphincter) by α_1 action*.
- **Genital system:** Pregnant *uterus is relaxed by β_2 stimulation*. Activation of α_1 receptors in vas deferens, seminal vesicle and prostate *facilitates ejaculation*.
- **Bronchus:** Bronchial smooth muscle contains β_2 *receptors but no sympathetic supply*. Exogenous drugs can cause *bronchodilation* by stimulation of β_2 receptors. Mucosal vasoconstriction (by action on α_1 receptors) further increases the luminal diameter of bronchus.
- **Eye:** Stimulation of α_1 *receptors* present on the dilator pupillary muscle causes *mydriasis*. Ciliary vasodilation by stimulation of β_2 receptors *increases the formation of aqueous humor* whereas α receptor stimulation decreases the secretion. Thus β blockers and α agonists are useful in the treatment of glaucoma.
- **Glands:** Secretion of salivary glands becomes thick. *Sweating is stimulated by sympathetic cholinergic receptors (M_3 action)*.
- **Metabolic effects:** Stimulation of β_3 receptors causes breakdown of triglycerides to free fatty acids. Hyperglycemia is caused by promotion of *glycogenolysis and gluconeogenesis on β_2 stimulation*. Initially it causes efflux of K^+ from liver (hyperkalemia) that is *followed by hypokalemia (due to uptake by skeletal muscles)*. α_2 stimulation also contributes to hyperglycemia by *reducing the release of insulin* from β cells. Minor β_2 mediated increase in glucagon secretion also is responsible for the elevation in blood glucose.
- **Other effects:** Stimulation of β_1 receptors in the JG cells of kidney is responsible for renin release. β_2 stimulation can cause tremors.

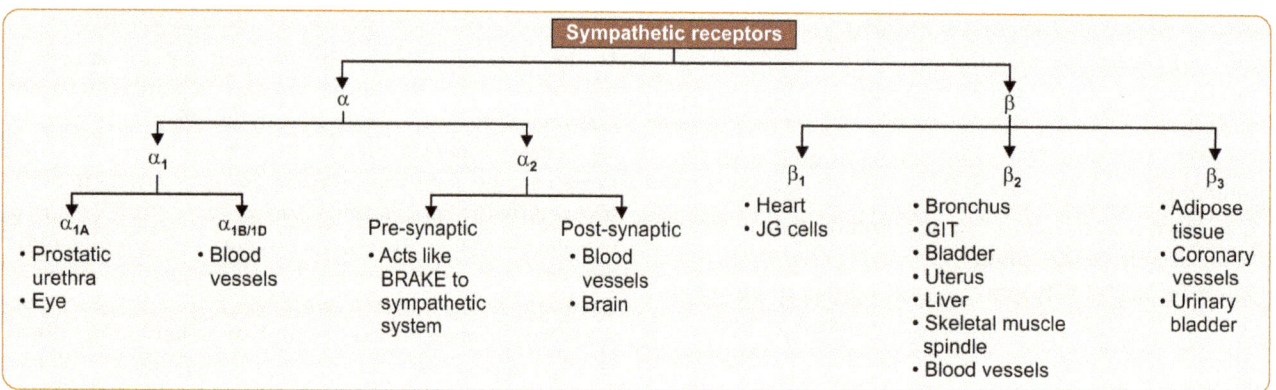

⚠ MNEMONIC

1. We have one heart and two lungs i.e. β_1 is in heart and β_2 is in lungs (bronchus).
2. Sympathetic system stimulates heart and inhibits at other places. In heart, we have β_1 receptor, so its function is to stimulate (i.e. tachycardia etc.) whereas at other places, we have β_2, so it relaxes (i.e. bronchodilation, tocolytic action, relaxation of GIT and bladder).
3. In emergencies, we require sympathy. Thus, the tremors occuring during fear are due to β_2 receptor stimulation.
4. Blood vessels contain α_1 receptors (causing vasoconstriction) and β_2 receptor (causing vasodilation). To remember, we have ABCD.
   A (Alpha 1) → C (Constriction)
   B (Beta 2) → D (Dilation)
5. When sympathetic system is stimulated, both α_1 and β_2 receptors are stimulated, so what will happen to blood vessels? It depends upon the relative number of receptors. If a blood vessel contain more α_1 receptors, it contracts whereas those having more β_2 receptors will dilate. To remember this, When we see a lion, we require sympathy, so sympathetic system is activated. We need to run now, so muscles require more blood. They get this because blood vessels of skeletal muscle contain more β_2 receptors. At this time of emergency, blood requirement in skin and internal organs is minimal, so vasoconstriction occur here due to more α_1 receptors.
6. Hypoglycemia is an emergency. Sympathetic system protect from it by:
   – Causing warning symptoms (tachycardia, palpitations via β_1 stimulation) and tremors by β_2 activation.
   – Beta-2 receptor in liver reverse hypoglycemia by increasing the formation (stimulate gluconeogenesis and glycogenolysis) of glucose.

Autonomic Nervous System

SYMPATHOMIMETIC DRUGS

These drugs increase the activity of adrenergic system and may be divided into directly acting, indirectly acting and mixed action sympathomimetics. Directly acting drugs stimulates alpha and beta receptors directly whereas indirectly acting drugs increase the amount of NA in the synapse. Mixed action sympathomimetics possess both of these actions.

Directly Acting Sympathomimetics

These drugs may be catecholamines (containing di hydroxy benzene nucleus) or non-catecholamines. A, NA and dopamine (DA) are the *endogenous catecholamines* whereas *isoprenaline, dobutamine, dopexamine and fenoldopam are synthetic catecholamines*. Non-catecholamines may act as selective agonists of α_1, α_2, β_1 and β_2 receptors.

Catecholamines

A, NA and DA are high potency compounds with short half life (due to rapid inactivation by MAO and COMT). Being polar, these drugs have poor penetration in the CNS. Metabolism in intestine (by MAO and COMT) and liver (by MAO) precludes their oral use.

Adrenaline acts on α_1, α_2, β_1 and β_2 receptors whereas NA has poor β_2 activity (i.e. α_1, α_2 and β_1) **and isoprenaline possess little α activity** (β_1 and β_2 only). Effect of these drugs on the heart rate and blood pressure are given below:

Systolic blood pressure (SBP) is *determined by cardiac output* (β_1 *action*) *whereas diastolic BP (DBP) depends on the state of blood vessels*. Stimulation of α_1 increases DBP by causing vasoconstriction whereas β_2 activation results in reduction of DBP due to vasodilation. *Increased DBP stimulates* baroreceptor mediated release of ACh (reflex action) that decreases heart rate via activation of M_2 receptors. Reduction in DBP increases central sympathetic outflow and thereby increases heart rate. NA normally decreases heart rate but if given after a dose of atropine, increase in heart rate will be seen (reflex action is abolished).

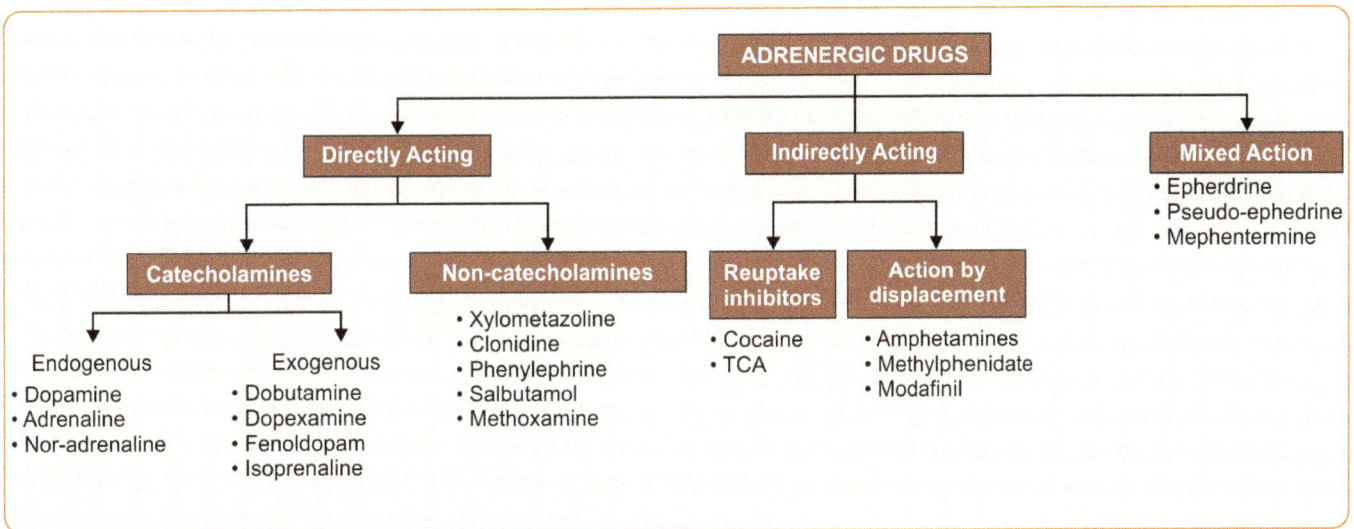

	SBP (β_1)	DBP (β_2 and α)	Heart Rate		
			Direct action (β_1)	Reflex action (M_2)	Net effect
A	↑↑	Nil	↑	Nil	↑
NA	↑↑	↑↑	↑	↓↓	↓
Iso	↑↑	↓↓	↑	↑	↑↑

- **Adrenaline** is the *drug of choice for anaphylactic shock*. It is given as 0.5 mL of 1:1000 solution (i.e. 0.5 mg) IM/SC injection. **Intramuscular route** (on Lateral thigh) **is preferred** because of variability in absorption from SC sites. Intravenous route is avoided but can be used rarely in much lower concentration (1:10,000).
- Adrenaline is also used to *prolong the duration of action and decrease the systemic toxicity of local anaesthetics*.
- Adrenaline is also used in patients with cardiac arrest. The preferred route is i.v. followed by intra-osseus and endotracheal.
- **Dopamine** is the *drug of choice for cardiogenic shock with oliguric renal failure*. It acts on D_1 (at a dose of 1-2 µg/kg/min.), β_1 (at 2-10 µg/kg/min.) and α_1 (at > 10 µg/kg/min.) receptors. It causes renal vasodilation by acting on D_1 receptors and maintains renal perfusion and GFR. Other inotropic agents like NA cause renal vasoconstriction and thus worsen renal failure.
- **Ibopamine** has similar properties as DA.
- **Dobutamine** is *relatively selective β_1 agonist with no action on DA receptors. It increases cardiac output with little action on heart rate*.
- **Dopexamine** *combines β_2 and D_1 agonistic activity with NA reuptake inhibitory action*.
- **Fenoldopam** *is D_1 agonist useful in hypertensive emergencies*.

Non-Catecholamines

α_1 **agonists:** These drugs can be used as nasal decongestants like *naphazoline, oxymetazoline and xylometazoline*. When effect of these drugs subside, after-congestion is seen. If used for prolonged periods, these can result in **atrophic rhinitis** (*Rhinitis medicamentosa*). **Phenylephrine** can also be used as a mydriatic (*does not cause cycloplegia*). Methoxamine and mephentermine can be used to inrease BP in hypotensive states. **Midodrine** is a prodrug (active metabolite is *desglymidodrine*) used for the treatment of orthostatic hypotension.

- Phenylpropanolamine was banned due to risk of hemorrhagic stroke

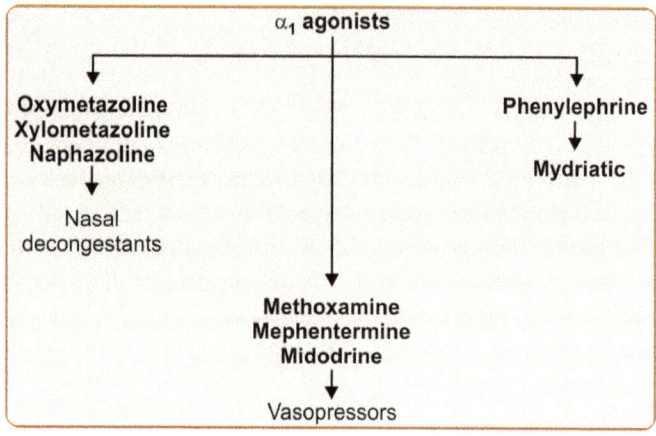

α_2 **agonists:** *Clonidine* and *α methyldopa* (a prodrug) are α_2 agonists that can be **used for the treatment** of hypertension. Other uses of clonidine include:

- To control *diarrhea in diabetic patients* with autonomic neuropathy.
- *Prophylaxis of migraine.*
- *Management of withdrawal symptoms* of alcohol, nicotine and opioids.
- Epidurally, in combination with opioids for relief of pain.
- For treatment of ADHD [as monotherapy or adjunctive to other drugs]
- Tourette syndrome

Apraclonidine and brimonidine are selective α_2 agonists used *topically for the treatment of glaucoma*. **Dexmeditomidine** (central α_2 agonist) is used for *pre-anaesthetic medication*. It is also indicated for sedation of initially intubated and mechanically ventilated patients during treatment in ICU. **Lofexidine** is a new α_2 agonist recently approved to decrease opioid withdrawal symptoms. Guanfacine and guanabenz are α_2 agonists similar to clonidine and are rarely used now. Tizanidine is used as a muscle relaxant.

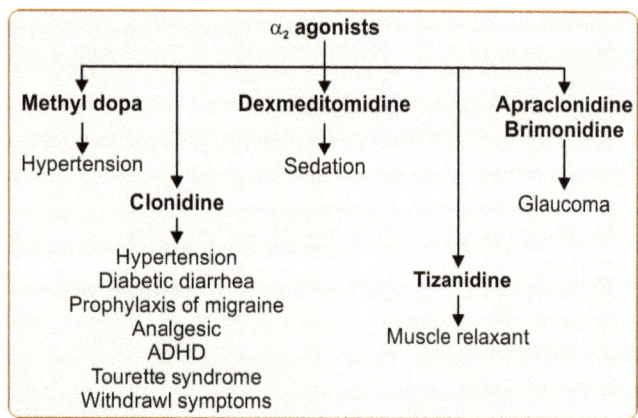

β_1 **agonists:** *Prenalterol* is the only non-catecholamine β_1 selective agent. It has been promoted recently for the reversal of β blockade.

β_2 **agonists:** *Salbutamol* (albuterol), levalbuterol, bitolterol, fenoterol, *metaproterenol, terbutaline, pirbuterol, salmeterol, formoterol, arformoterol, carmoterol and indacterol* are selective β_2 agonists useful in bronchial asthma. *Ritodrine and isoxsuprine* are agonists useful as tocolytic (uterine relaxant) agents.

β_3 **agonists:** *Mirabegron* is a new drug that acts by stimulating β_3 receptors in urinary bladder. It is indicated for treatment of overactive bladder.

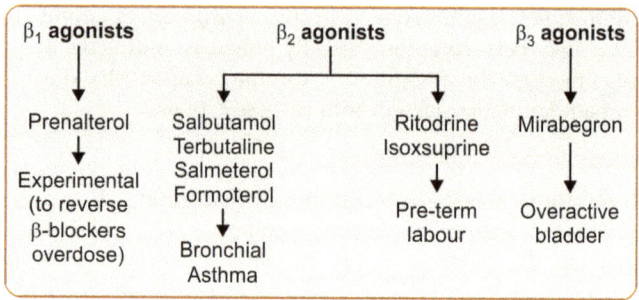

Indirectly Acting Sympathomimetics

These drugs act by increasing the release of NA in the synaptic cleft or by inhibiting the reuptake of NA. These agents *enter the neuronal cytoplasm by the same transporter that is responsible for the reuptake of NA*. From the cytoplasm, these drugs enter the storage vesicles and displace and release the stored NA (because each vesicle has fixed storage capacity). Released NA activates adrenergic receptors. On repeated dosing at short intervals, *tachyphylaxis* (rapid development of tolerance) is seen with these drugs.

- *Tyramine* is normally present in certain foods and can lead to *cheese reaction* in patients taking MAO inhibitors
- *Methylphenidate* is the preferred drug for the treatment of *attention deficit hyperkinetic disorder* (ADHD). **Dexmethylphenidate** is d-isomer of methylphenidate and **serdexmethylphenidate** is a prodrug of dexmethylphenidate. Both of these have recently been approved for ADHD. **Viloxazine** is a new drug that acts by inhibiting reuptake of 5HT and noradrenaline. It is also approved for treatment of ADHD. Other drugs used for this indication are *amphetamines, atomoxetine and pemoline*. **Pemoline** has been withdrawn due to life threatening **hepatotoxicity**.
- *Amphetamines* are addictive substances and can result in tolerance and dependence. As these are basic drugs, *urinary acidification* (with NH_4Cl) is employed *for the treatment of their toxicity*. On the other hand, amphetamine addicts use sodium bicarbonate to obtain the "kick".
- **Modafinil** is approved for treatment of *narcolepsy, in shift workers, to relieve fatigue in multiple sclerosis and as an adjunct in obstrutive sleep apnea.*
- **Solriamfetol** is a new drug approved for treatment of excessive daytime sleepiness in obstructive sleep apnea and narcolepsy. It acts by inhibiting reuptake of dopamine and noradrenaline.

Mixed Action Sympathomimetics

These drugs enhance the release of NA (like indirectly acting drugs) apart from activating α and β receptors directly. Ephedrine and pseudoephedrine are present in the cold remedies for nasal decongestant and bronchodilator action. **Ephedrine** can also be used for the treatment of bronchial asthma. It is the *vasopressor of choice in pregnancy* because due to β_2 mediated vasodilatory action, it does not interfere with placental circulation [methoxamine, mephentermine and other selective α_1 agonists can cause placental vasoconstriction and compromise fetal circulation].

SYMPATHOLYTIC DRUGS

These drugs may act by blocking α and/or β-adrenergic receptors.

Alpha Blockers

Nonselective α-Blockers

Phenoxybenzamine is an *irreversible antagonist* whereas *phentolamine and tolazoline* are *reversible* blockers of α_1 and α_2 receptors. These agents result in *vasodilation and postural hypotension* (due to antagonism of vasoconstrictor α_1 receptors). Reflex increase in sympathetic discharge and increased sympathetic outflow (due to blockade of α_2 receptors) are responsible for *marked tachycardia* seen with the use of these agents. Use of these drugs before adrenaline results in **vasomotor reversal of Dale**. Intravenous injection of adrenaline normally causes increase in blood pressure (α effect) followed by prolonged fall (β_2 effect). If it is administered after giving α blockers, only fall in BP is seen *(vasomotor reversal of Dale)*.

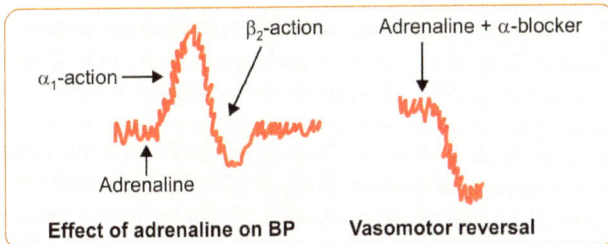

FIG. 2.5: Vasomotor reversal of Dale

- *Phenoxybenzamine* is used to prevent hypertensive episodes during operative manipulation of tumor in *pheochromocytoma*.
- *Phentolamine and tolazoline* are preferred agents for the treatment of hypertensive crisis in *clonidine withdrawal and cheese reaction*.

Selective α₁-Blockers

These drugs (*prazosin, terazosin, doxazosin and alfuzosin*) cause decrease in blood pressure with lesser tachycardia than non selective blockers (due to lack of α_2 blocking action, sympathetic outflow is not increased).

- Selective α_1 blockers have **favorable effect on lipid profile** (increase HDL and decrease LDL and TG)
- Due to relaxation of smooth muscle in the neck of urinary bladder and prostatic urethra, urinary flow is improved by these drugs. Therefore, selective α_1 blockers are *drugs of choice for patients with hypertension and benign hyperplasia of prostate* (BHP).
- Alpha receptors play a vital role in pathogenesis of heart failure and pulmonary edema due to scorpion sting. **Prazosin** (and other α_1 blockers) are useful for the treatment of **scorpion sting.**
- **Major adverse effect** of these drugs is *postural hypotension*. It is seen with first few doses or on dose escalation (*First dose effect*). If used continuously, tolerance develops to this adverse effect. **Inhibition of ejaculation** is another side effect of these agents.
- **Tamsulosin** and **Silodosin** *selectively inhibits subtype of α_1 receptors present in the prostate (α_{1A}) without affecting those present in the blood vessels. These are therefore preferred for the treatment of BHP because of their reduced propensity to cause postural hypotension. These has been found to cause intra-operative* **'floppy iris syndrome'** *during cataract surgery.*
- **Indoramin** and **urapadil** are occasionally used for *hypertensive emergencies.*

Selective α₂-Blockers

Yohimbine and idazoxan are blockers of α_2 receptors having no established clinical role.

Beta Blockers

Nonselective β-Blockers [First generation β-blockers)

Drugs in this category are *propranolol, timolol, nadolol, pindolol, alprenolol and oxprenolol.*

Important effects of these drugs are:

- Myocardial oxygen demand is decreased due to blockade of β_1 receptors in the heart (*useful in classical angina*) but coronary vasoconstriction can occur due to blockade of vasodilatory β_2 receptors (*contraindicated in variant angina*).
- *Decrease in blood pressure* (mainly due to β_1 blockade).
- *Bronchoconstriction* may occur due to blockade of β_2 receptors (*contraindicated in asthmatics*).

Limitations of Non-selective β-Blockers

- Contraindicated in bronchial asthma due to their *bronchoconstrictor action.*
- Hypoglycemia is commonly observed in diabetic patients receiving insulin and oral hypoglycemic drugs. Symptoms of hypoglycemia (like tachycardia, sweating and tremors) are due to sympathetic stimulation that act as warning signs for the patient. Beta blockers mask these symptoms (**except sweating** because *it is mediated by sympathetic cholinergic system*) and patient can go directly into coma. Further, these agents *delay the recovery* from hypoglycemia due to inhibition of β_2 mediated hyperglycemia. These drugs are therefore *contraindicated in diabetic patients.*
- On long-term use non-selective β blockers can *adversely affect serum lipid profile and can cause glucose intolerance.*
- By causing vasoconstriction (β_2 is vasodilatory), these drugs can *worsen peripheral vascular disease* (contraindicated in Raynaud's disease).
- These drugs can *impair exercise capacity* due to blockade of skeletal vascular β_2 receptors.

> **MNEMONIC**
>
> **Contraindications of non-selective β-blockers**
> A – **A**sthma
> B – **B**lock (AV)
> C – **C**HF
> D – **D**iabetes

Cardioselective (Selective β1) β-Blockers [Also known as Second-Generation β-blockers)

- These agents are *preferred in patients with diabetes mellitus, bronchial asthma, peripheral vascular disease or hyperlipidemia.* The drugs in this group are:

New	– Nebivolol (**Most cardioselective**)
Beta	– Betaxolol
Blockers	– Bisoprolol
Acting	– Acebutolol
Exclusively	– Esmolol
At	– Atenolol
Myo	– Metoprolol
Cardium	– Celiprolol

> **Key Points**
>
> **Advantages of cardioselective β-blockers:**
> - Safe in asthma
> - Safe in diabetes
> - Safe in PVD
> - Less likely to impair exercise capacity
> - Less risk of hyperglycemia
> - Less risk of dyslipidemia

Beta-Blockers with Intrinsic Sympathomimetic Activity (ISA)

These drugs are partial agonists at $β_1$ receptors (apart from having β blocking property). These are preferred in the *patients prone to develop severe bradycardia with β blocker therapy.* However, these drugs are less useful in angina (because of stimulation of heart by $β_1$ receptors). The drugs can be remembered as:

- **CO**ntain — Celiprolol, Oxprenolol
- **Partial** — Pindolol, Penbutolol
- **Agonistic** — Alprenolol
- **Activity** — Acebutolol

Beta-Blockers with Membrane-Stabilizing Activity

These drugs possess Na^+ channel blocking (local anaesthetic) activity. It can contribute to *antiarrhythmic action.* These drugs should be *avoided in glaucoma* due to the risk of corneal anaesthesia. The drugs are:

- **Possess** — Propranolol (*maximum*)
- **Membrane stabilizing or** — Metoprolol
- **Local** — Labetalol
- **Anaesthetic** — Acebutolol
- **Property** — Pindolol

Lipid-Insoluble β-Blockers

These agents are mainly *excreted by kidney* and are therefore *contraindicated in renal failure.* Most of these have *long duration of action.*

- **Not** — Nadolol (*longest acting β blocker*)
- **Soluble** — Sotalol
- **A** — Atenolol
  — Acebutolol
- **B** — Betaxolol
  — Bisoprolol
- **C** — Celiprolol

Other β blockers are metabolized mainly by liver and are short acting (**shortest acting β blocker is esmolol**).

> **Note**
> Acebutolol possesses all activities i.e. cardioselectivity, ISA, membrane stabilizing action and lipid insolubility.

Third-Generation β-Blockers

These drugs possess *additional vasodilatory property.* It may be due to α blockade (*labetalol, carvedilol*), $β_2$ agonism (*celiprolol, carteolol, bopindolol*), release of NO (*nebivolol, nipradilol*), opening of K^+ channels (*tilisolol*) or inhibition of Ca^{2+} channels (*carvedilol, bevantolol, betaxolol*).

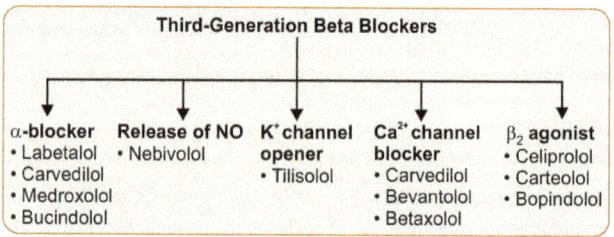

Uses of β-Blockers

Cardiac (Due to $β_1$ blockade)	Extra cardiac (Due to $β_2$ blockade)
Hypertension	Pheochromocytoma (after α blockade)
Classical angina	Hyperthyroidism
Myocardial infarction	Performance anxiety
Supraventricular arrhythmias	Tremors
Chronic CHF	Akathisia
Hypertrophic obstructive cardiomyopathy (DOC)	Prophylaxis of migraine
Emergency management of symptoms of TOF	Glaucoma (*timolol and betaxolol*)
Mitral valve prolapse	Alcohol and opioid withdrawal
	Prophylaxis of bleeding in portal hypertension

Combined Alpha and Beta Blockers

Labetalol and *carvedilol* are the important drugs in this group. These are useful for the control of hypertensive episodes in *pheochromocytoma*. **Carvedilol** is the *most commonly used beta blocker in chronic CHF* due to its **antioxidant and antimitogenic properties.** Other drugs having both α and β blocking activity are *medroxalol* and *bucindolol*.

> **Note**
> Carvedilol has maximum plasma protein binding (98%) whereas celiprolol has minimum (< 5%).

GLAUCOMA

- Glaucoma is characterized by progressive damage to optic nerve associated with raised intraocular pressure (> 21 mm Hg). Rise in intraocular tension is either due to excessive production or due to less drainage of aqueous humor. So, the drugs used for glaucoma act by either **decreasing the secretion** (*β-blockers, $α_2$ agonists and carbonic anhydrase inhibitors*) or by **increasing the outflow** (*miotics, dipivefrine and prostaglandins*) of aqueous humor.

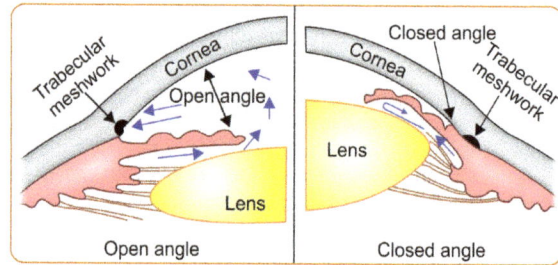

FIG. 2.6: Pathogenesis of open and closed angle glaucoma

- Various drugs useful in **primary open angle glaucoma (POAG)** are:
  - **β-blockers:** These are among the first line drugs for POAG. Ciliary processes contain $β_2$ (vasodilatory) and $α_2$ (vasoconstrictor) receptors. Whenever vasodilation occurs, amount of blood reaching in the ciliary body

Autonomic Nervous System

increases resulting in excessive secretion of aqueous humor. Therefore, β-blockers and α agonists can decrease the secretion of aqueous. **Timolol, betaxolol, levobetaxolol, levobunolol, carteolol and metipranolol** have been approved for use in glaucoma. *Levobunolol is longest acting* whereas betaxolol is cardioselective (therefore less efficacious but safe in asthmatics) β-blocker.

Beta blockers
Blepharoconjunctivitis

- **Prostaglandin analogs:** $PGF_{2\alpha}$ increases uveoscleral outflow. **Latanoprost, bimatoprost and unoprostone** are $PGF_{2\alpha}$ derivatives useful in glaucoma. These are **now the drug of choice for POAG.** These *cause growth of eyelashes as an adverse effect which can be utilized for treatment of hypotrichosis.* All $PGF_{2\alpha}$ analogs can cause **cystoid macular edema** especially in aphakic patients.

Pigmentation of iris
Growth of eyelashes
Fluid in macula (macular edema)
P G $F_{2\alpha}$ analogs

- **α-Agonists: Dipivefrine** (prodrug of adrenaline) and adrenaline act by increasing trabecular outflow (main action), reducing aqueous secretion and increasing uveoscleral outflow. **Epinephrine** can cause **black pigmentation on conjunctiva** due to its oxidation to a product, **adrenochrome. Apraclonidine and brimonidine** (selective α_2 agonists) act by decreasing aqueous secretion. *Apraclonidine can cause lid retraction whereas brimonidine is associated with CNS depression.*

apracLonIDine
L ID retraction

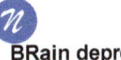

BRain depression
Iridocyclitis
BRI monidine

- **Carbonic anhydrase inhibitors:** Acetazolamide (oral), brinzolamide and dorzolamide (both topical) act by decreasing the secretion of aqueous humor.
- **Miotics: Pilocarpine** (directly acting cholinomimetic) and **physostigmine** (indirectly acting cholinomimetic) increase aqueous outflow by causing miosis. *Pilocarpine is short acting*, therefore requires frequent daily dosing. **Demacarium and ecothiophate** (both are long acting cholinomimetics) are rarely used because they *accelerate cataract development.*

miotiCS
Stenosis (Punctal)
Cataract

- **Netarsudil** is a Rho kinase inhibitor. It can be used for treatment of open angle glaucoma in combination with latanoprost as topical therapy.
- For closed-angle glaucoma, definitive treatment is surgery (Laser peripheral iridotomy or surgical peripheral iridectomy). The only drugs used to control intra-ocular tension preceeding surgery are cholinomimetics (miotics), acetazolamide and osmotic diuretics (e.g. mannitol). The onset of other agents is too slow in this situation. Initial treatment of choice in acute cases is **intravenous acetazolamide**.

> **Note**
> All patients with primary acute angle-closure glaucoma should undergo prophylactic laser peripheral iridotomy to the unaffected eye.

Drugs used in Glaucoma

Group	Drugs	Mechanism	Adverse effects	Special points
1. MIOTICS – Directly acting muscarinic agonist – AChE inhibitor	Pilocarpine Physostigmine Echothiophate	Increase trabecular outflow	• Blurred vision due to induced myopia • Headache and brow pain • AChE inhibitors can lead to cataract formation	• Pilocarpine is short acting and can result in fluctuations in IOP • Miotics increase the risk of retinal tears in susceptible individuals • Can cause **punctal stenosis of nasolacrimal system**
2. BETA BLOCKERS – Non-selective ($\beta_1+\beta_2$) blockers – Cardioselective (β_1) blockers	Timolol Levobunolol Carteolol Metipranolol Betaxolol	↓ Formation of aqueous humor	• Allergic blepharo-conjunctivitis • Precipitates asthma • Transient stinging and burning in eye	• Should be avoided in: – Asthma – Bradycardia – CHF – Diabetes • Betaxolol is less likely to precipitate asthma but is less efficacious
3. $PGF_{2\alpha}$ ANALOGS	Latanoprost Bimatoprost Travoprost Tafluprost Unoprostone	↑ Uveoscleral outflow	**Iris pigmentation** **Growth of eyelashes** **Macular edema** in aphakics (Latanoprost) **Reactivation of uveitis** (Latanoprost)	• **Drug of choice** for POAG

Contd...

Contd...

Group	Drugs	Mechanism	Adverse effects	Special points
4. α_2 AGONISTS	Apraclonidine Brimonidine	↓ Aqueous formation	• **Lid retraction** • Dry Mouth • Ocular burning and allergic conjunctivitis	• Brimonidine is less likely to cause ocular allergy • These can cause **CNS depression and apnea in neonates** and are contra-indicated in children < 2 years
5. NON-SELECTIVE ADRENERGIC DRUGS	Dipivefrine Adrenaline	↑ Trabecular outflow ↑ Uveoscleral outflow ↓ Secretion	• Conjunctival hyperemia (Red Eye) • Ocular allergy	
6. CARBONIC ANHYDRASE INHIBITORS	Dorzolamide Brinzolamide Acetazolamide	↓ Aqueous formation	• Ocular allergy • Corneal edema • Bitter taste	• These can **increase retinal blood flow**

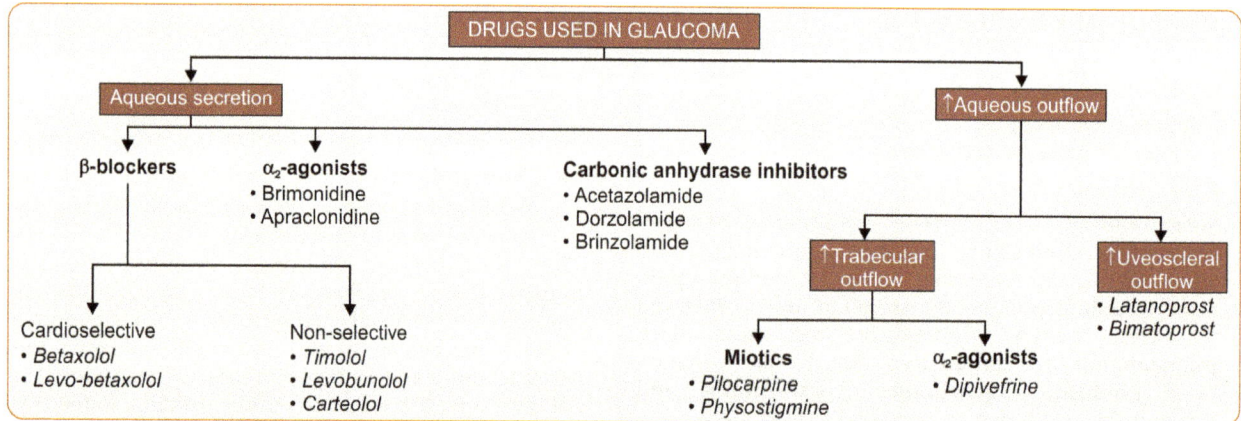

EFFECT OF DRUGS ON RABIT EYE EXPERIMENT

Rabbit (scientific name; **Oryctalagus cuniculus**) is commonly used animal in pharmacological studies. Average weight of rabbit is 1.5–2.5 kg. Effects of drugs on rabbit eye are as follows:

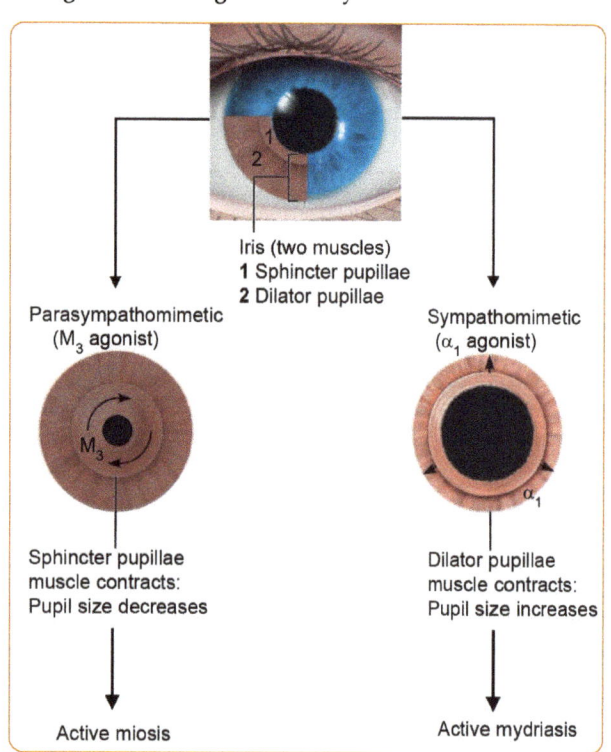

FIG. 2.7: Active miosis and mydriasis

- **Sympathomimetic** drugs cause contraction of dilator pupillae and thus result in *active mydriasis* whereas **parasympathomimetic** drugs contract sphincter pupillae leading to *active miosis*.
- **Parasympatholytic** drugs like atropine stop the action of ACh on sphincter pupillae resulting in *passive mydriasis*.
- In addition parasympatholytic drugs can result in loss of light reflex.
- **Local anesthetics** cause *loss of corneal reflex*.

Drug group	Example	Pupil	Light reflex	Corneal reflex
Sympathomimetics	Adrenaline	Mydriasis	Present	Present
Parasympatho-mimetics	Physostigmine Pilocarpine	Miosis	Present	Present
Parasympatholytics	Atropine	Mydriasis	Absent	Present
Local Anaesthetics	Lignocaine	No change	Present	Absent

EFFECT OF DRUGS ON RABBIT ILEUM EXPERIMENT

Parasympathetic drugs like ACh stimulate rabbit ileum (increase tone and frequency) that is blocked on pretreatment with atropine. Similarly, sympathomimetics inhibit rabbit ileum contractions which is abolished by pre-treatment with beta-blockers

Drug	Effect on ileum	Effect of atropine	Effect of beta-blocker
Acetylcholine	Stimulate	Block the effect	No effect
Adrenaline	Inhibit	No effect	Block the effect
Papaverine	Inhibit	No effect	No effect
$CaCl_2$	Stimulate	No effect	No effect

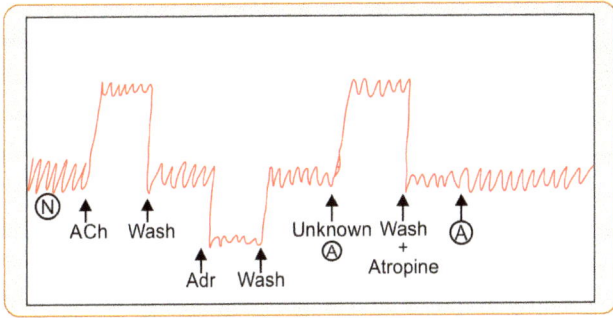

FIG. 2.8: Drug A is parasympathetic (like ACh). It stimulates ileum and its effect is abolished by atropine

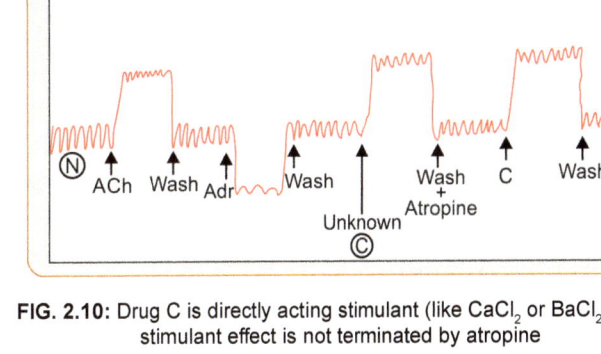

FIG. 2.10: Drug C is directly acting stimulant (like $CaCl_2$ or $BaCl_2$) as its stimulant effect is not terminated by atropine

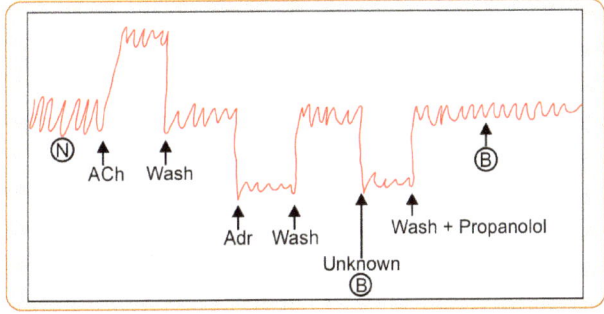

FIG. 2.9: Drug B is sympathomimetic (like adrenaline). It relaxes ileum and this depressant effect is abolished by beta-blockers

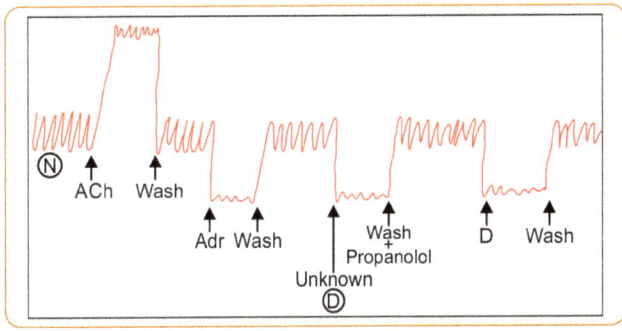

FIG. 2.11: Drug D is directly acting relaxant (like papaverine) as its depressant effect is not abolished by beta-blockers

To identify the unknown drug,

First see, whether the drug increases the tone (stimulant) or decreases (depressant).

If it is **stimulant**, it is likely to be *acetylcholine or barium chloride*. Then see, whether the effect can be abolished by atropine or not. If stimulant effect is absent after atropine, the drug is acetylcholine but if it is still present, then it is directly acting drug like barium or calcium chloride.

If it is **depressant**, it is likely to be *adrenaline or papaverine*. Then see, whether the effect can be abolished by beta blocker or not. If depressant effect is absent or reduced after giving beta blocker (completely abolished by alpha plus beta blocker), the drug is adrenaline but if it is still present, then it is directly acting drug like papaverine.

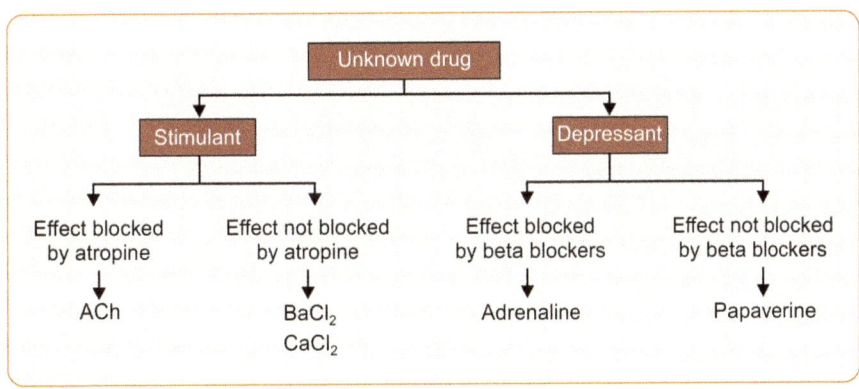

Golden Points

1. Acetylcholine (ACh) is the principal neurotransmitter at neuromuscular junction as well at all preganglionic fibres.

2. Uptake of choline by the neurons is the rate limiting step in the biosynthesis of acetylcholine.

3. No direct cholinergic supply is present in blood vessels but cholinergic receptors (M_3) are present on endothelium of blood vessels.

4. Atropine is an antidote of choice for both organophosphate and carbamate poisoning.

5. Oximes should not be given in carbamate poisoning.

6. Triopicamide is the shortest acting mydriatic.

7. Atropine is longest acting mydriatic.

8. Trospium has minimum CNS penetration among drugs used in overactive bladder.

9. Solefancin is longest acting and oxybutynin is shortest acting drug among this group.

10. Rate-limiting enzyme in catecholamine biosynthesis is tyrosine hydroxylase.

11. Adrenaline is the drug of choice for anaphylactic shock.

12. Dopamine is the drug of choice for cardiogenic shock with oliguric renal failure.

13. **Mirabegron** is a new drug approved for overactive bladder. It acts by stimulating $β_3$ receptors

14. Ephedrine is the vasopressor of choice in pregnancy.

15. **Selective $α_1$ blockers have favorable effect on lipid profile** (increase HDL and decrease LDL and TG).

16. **Tamsulosin and Silodosin** are **selective $α_{1A}$ blockers** and are preferred for the treatment of BHP because of reduced propensity to cause postural hypotension.

17. **Tamsulosin and silodisin have** been found to cause intra-operative '**floppy iris syndrome**' during cataract surgery.

18. **Latanoprost** causes **growth of eyelashes** as an adverse effect which can be utilized for treatment of hypotrichosis.

19. **Apraclonidine** can cause **lid retraction** whereas brimonidine is associated with CNS depression.

20. $PGF_{2α}$ analogs can cause cystoid macular edema in aphakics.

21. **Beta blockers contraindicated in renal failure:**
    A – Atenolol
    N – Nadolol
    S – Sotalol

Drug of Choice

Condition	Drug of Choice
Mushroom poisoning	
– Early (Inocybe sp.)	Atropine
– Delayed (Amanita sp.)	Thioctic acid
Glaucoma	
– Open angle	Latanoprost
– Angle closure	Acetazolamide
Myasthenia gravis	
– Diagnosis	Edrophonium
– Treatment	Neostigmine/pyridostigmine
Belladonna poisoning	Physostigmine
Atropine poisoning	Physostigmine
Datura poisoning	Physostigmine
Alzheimer's dementia	Donepezil/Rivastigmine/Galantamine
Cobra bite	Anti-venom
Anticholinesterase poisoning	
– Organophosphate	Atropine
– Carbamate	Atropine
Colicky pain	Anticholinergics like hyoscine/dicyclomine
Bronchial asthma	Salbutamol
Refraction testing	
– In adults	Tropicamide
– In children	Atropine
Fundoscopy	Phenylephrine
Uveitis	
– Iridocyclitis	Atropine + steroids
– Posterior uveitis	Steroids
– Panuveitis	Steroids
Bradycardia	Atropine
Atrioventricular block	Atropine
Drug induced Parkinsonism	Anticholinergics like benzhexol

Condition	Drug of Choice
Shock	
– Cardiogenic	Nor-adrenaline or dopamine
– With oliguria	Dopamine
– Anaphylactic	Adrenaline
– Distributive	Noradrenaline or phenylephrine
– Septic	Broad spectrum antimicrobials
– Shock due to adrenal insufficiency	Corticosteroids
– Hypovolemic	Fluids (crystalloids)
– Secondary	Prazosin (α-blockers)
Postural hypotension	Fludrocortisone
Attention deficit hyperkinetic disorder	Methylphenidate
Narcolepsy	Modafinil or armodafinil
Pheochromocytoma	
– Before surgery	Phenoxybenzamine
– Long term	Calcium channel blockers like nifedipine or nicardipine extended release
Cheese reaction	Phentolamine or tolazoline
Rebound hypertension due to clonidine withdrawal	Phentolamine or tolazoline
Raynaud's phenomenon	Calcium channel blockers like nifedipine ER or amlodipine
Essential tremors	Propranolol
Akathisia	Propranolol
Hypertrophic obstructive cardiomyopathy	Propranolol
Beta blocker poisoning	Glucagon
Benign hyperplasia of prostate	Tamsulosin
– Without hypertension	Prazosin or doxazosin
– With hypertension	
Performance anxiety	Propranolol

Image Based Questions

1. The unknown drug is likely to be:

   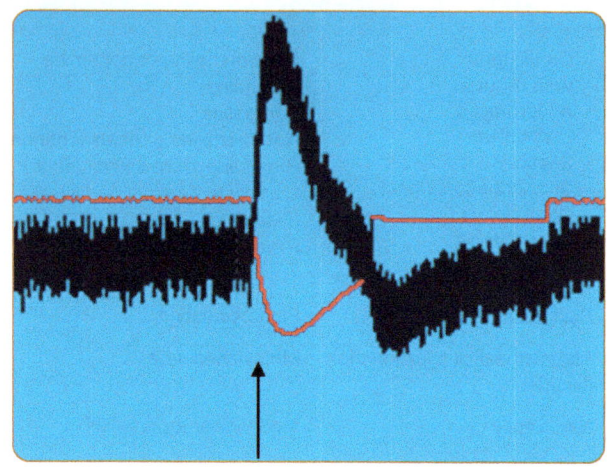

   (a) Low dose adrenaline (b) High dose adrenaline
   (c) Nor-adrenaline   (d) Isoprenaline

2. What is this effect known as?

   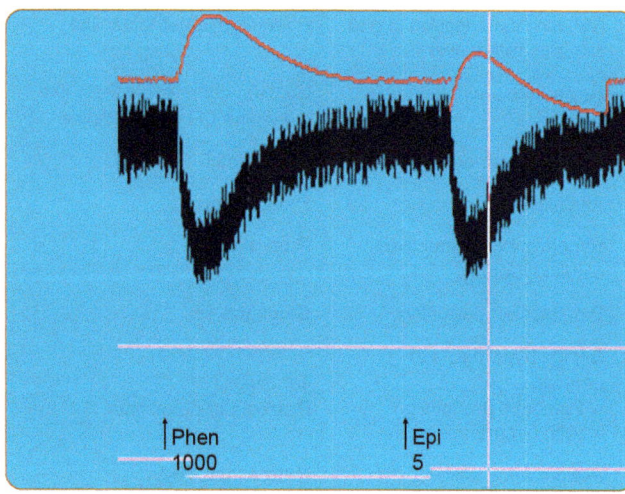

   (a) Tachyphylaxis
   (b) Nicotinic actions of ACh
   (c) Biphasic response of Adr
   (d) Vasomotor reversal of Dale

3. What is this effect known as?

   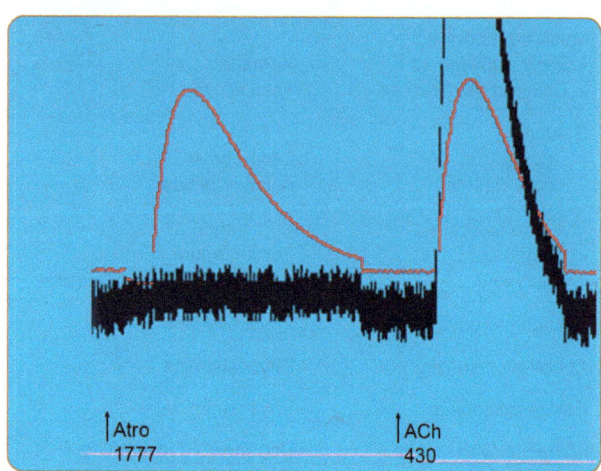

   (a) Tachyphylaxis
   (b) Nicotinic actions of ACh
   (c) Biphasic response of Adr
   (d) Vasomotor reversal of Dale

4. What is this phenomenon known as?

   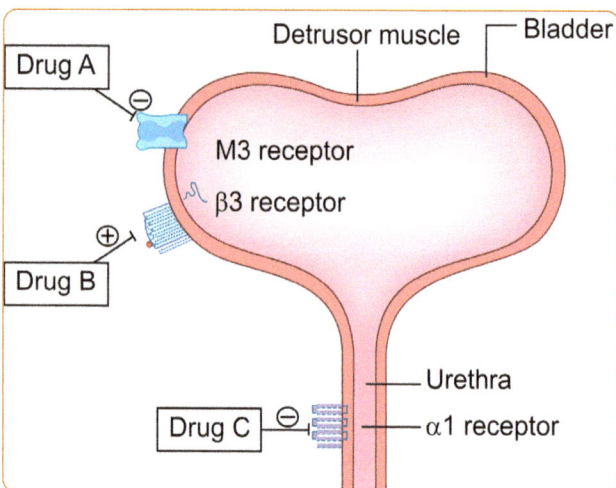

   (a) Tachyphylaxis
   (b) Nicotinic actions of ACh
   (c) Biphasic response of Adr
   (d) Vasomotor reversal of Dale

Autonomic Nervous System

5. Apart from the effects shown in the image, the light and corneal reflex were present. Drug A is likely to be:

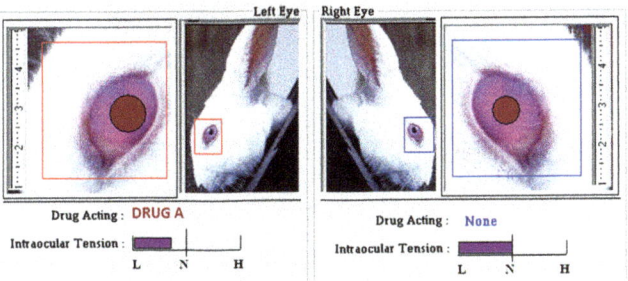

   (a) Parasympathomimetic   (b) Sympathomimetic
   (c) Parasympatholytic   (d) Sympatholytic

6. Apart from the effects shown in the image, the light and corneal reflex were present. Drug B is likely to be:

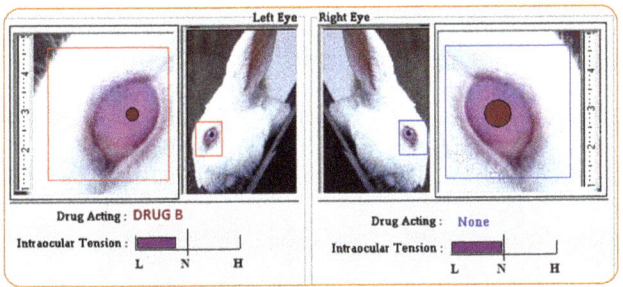

   (a) Parasympathomimetic   (b) Sympathomimetic
   (c) Parasympatholytic   (d) Local anaesthetic

7. Identify the unknown drug by its action on rabbit ileum:

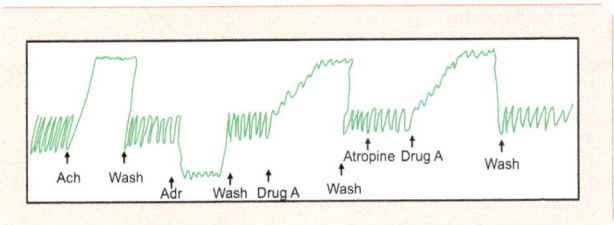

   (a) Acetylcholine   (b) Adrenaline
   (c) Barium chloride   (d) Papaverine

8. Identify the unknown drug by its action on rabbit ileum:

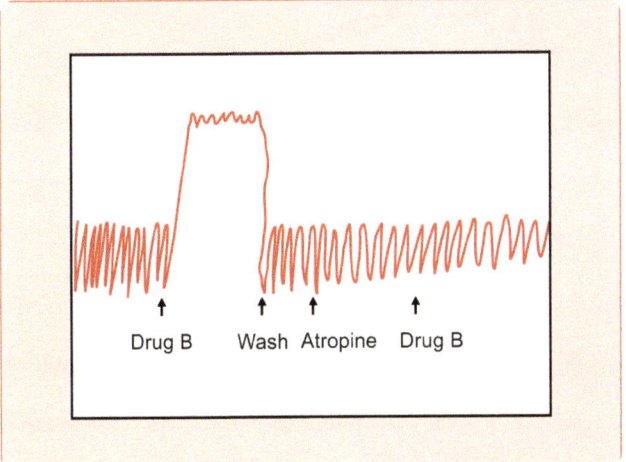

   (a) Acetylcholine   (b) Adrenaline
   (c) Barium chloride   (d) Papaverine

9. Identify the unknown drug by its action on rabbit ileum:

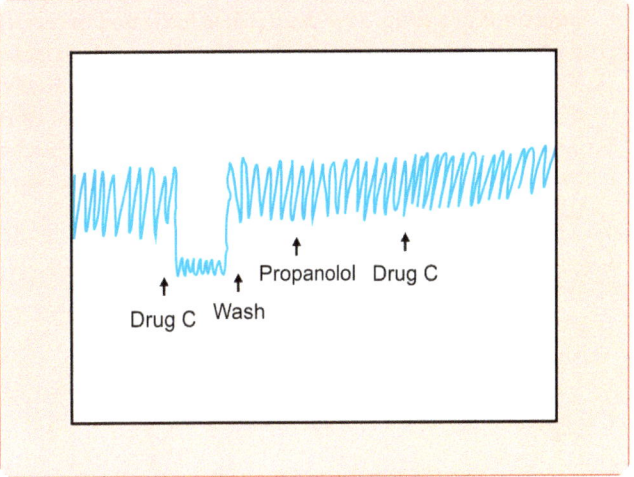

   (a) Acetylcholine   (b) Adrenaline
   (c) Barium chloride   (d) Papaverine

10. Identify the unknown drug by its action on rabbit ileum:

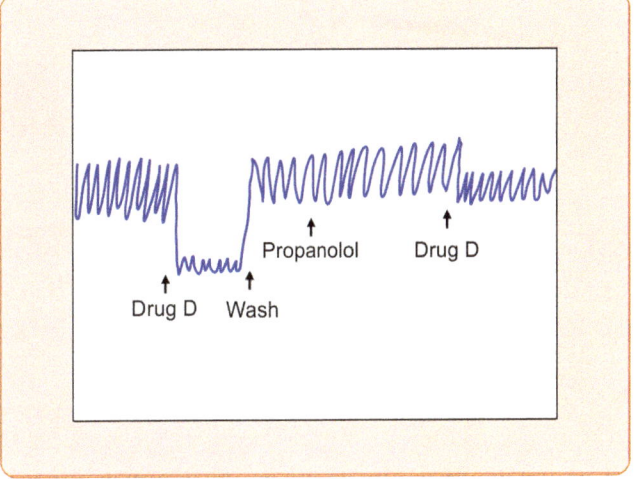

   (a) Acetylcholine   (b) Adrenaline
   (c) Barium chloride   (d) Papaverine

11. Identify the unknown drug by its action on rabbit ileum:

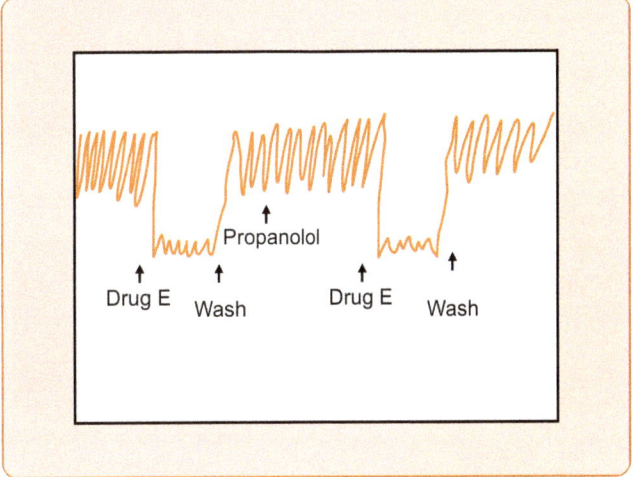

   (a) Acetylcholine   (b) Adrenaline
   (c) Barium chloride   (d) Papaverine

12. A 30-year-old theatre actress developed few wrinkles on the face. The treating physician advised her to have local injections of a drug. This drug is also indicated in cervical dystonia and other spastic disorders like cerebral palsy. Very recently, it has also been approved for prophylaxis of migraine. The physician warned of the drug to cause dry mouth and blurring of vision. The actress searched the compound on internet and found the site of action of the drug as shown in the Figure below.

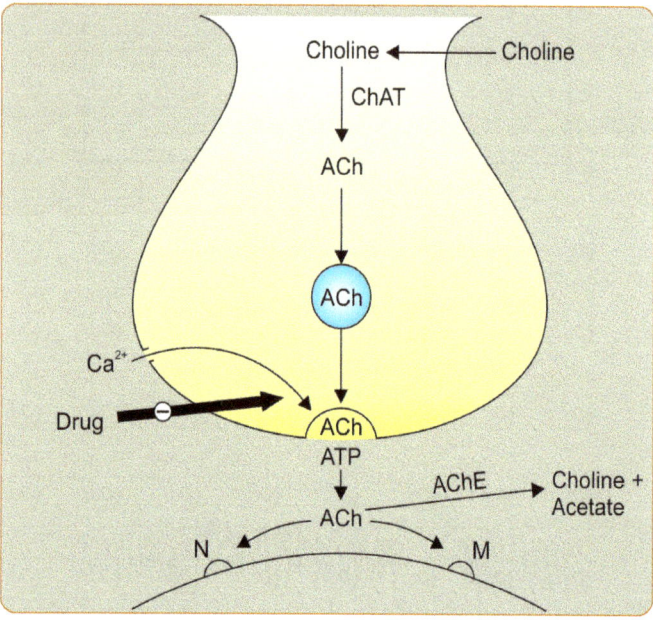

Which of the following drug is being talked about?

(a) Hemicholinium
(b) Vesamicol
(c) Botulinum toxin
(d) Physostigmine

13. A patient was given topical antiglaucoma drug for several months. He presents with the features shown in the image. Likely drug responsible for the adverse effect is

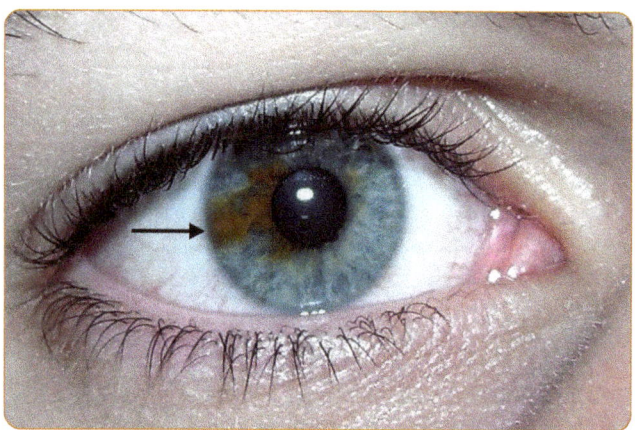

(a) Timolol
(b) Brimonidine
(c) Brinzolamide
(d) Latanoprost

14. Which of the following antiglaucoma drugs can result in this adverse effect?

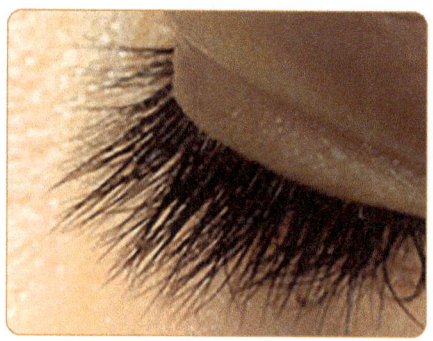

(a) Apraclonidine   (b) Latanoprost
(c) Pilocarpine   (d) Dipivefrine

15. A patient presents with the increase in the drooping of the eyelid (as shown in image) as the day progresses which drug can be used to differentiate between myasthenia gravia and cholinergic crisis?

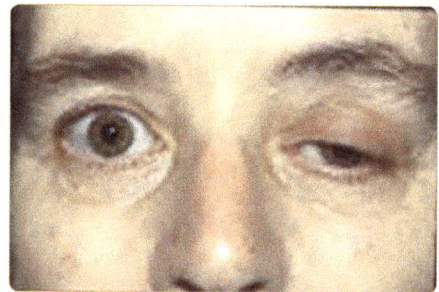

(a) Edrophonium   (b) Neostigmine
(c) Atropine   (d) Pilocarpine

16. Mechanism of action of 3 drugs used in urology is shown in the figure. Which of the following statements regarding these drugs is false?

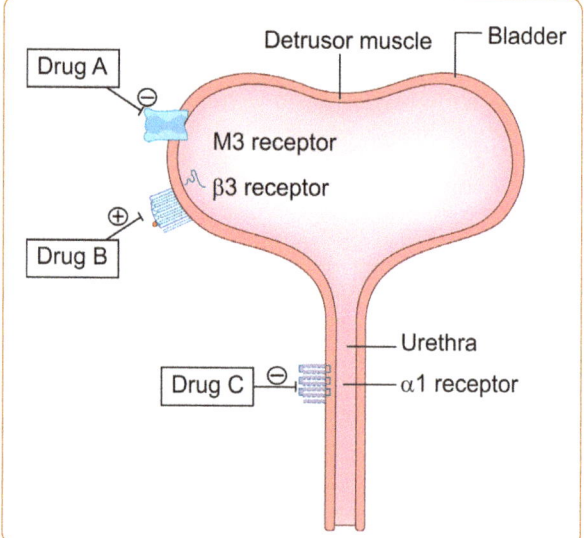

(a) Drug A may be oxybutynin and is used for treatment of overactive bladder
(b) Drug B may be mirabegron and is used for treatment of atonic bladder
(c) Drug C may be tamsulosin and is used to relieve urinary symptoms of BHP
(d) All the statements are correct

Explanations

1. **Ans. (b) High dose adrenaline**
   Given figure shows that after giving a drug, blood pressure first increases and then decreases. It is known as biphasic response which is characteristic of high dose adrenaline. At low doses, adrenaline stimulates only beta 2 receptors and thus cause only fall in BP. But at high doses, It stimulates both alpha and beta receptors and initially cause rise in BP due to alpha receptor stimulation, however as plasma concentration falls, it lead to decrease in BP due to stimulation of only beta 2 receptors. This is known as biphasic response

2. **Ans. (d) Vasomotor reversal of Dale**
   Adrenaline normally produce biphasic response at high doses as explained in the question above. However, if alpha blocker (Phentolamine in the given figure) is given before giving adrenaline, this biphasic response is not seen. Only fall in BP is noted. This is called vasomotor reversal of Dale.

3. **Ans. (b) Nicotinic actions of acetylcholine**
   Acetylcholine normally produces fall in BP due to its effect on muscarinic receptors to cause vasodilation. However, when given in very high doses, it can stimulate nicotinic receptors present on the ganglia that can result in increase in blood pressure. However, to demonstrate this effect, muscarinic receptors should be blocked by giving high dose atropine.

4. **Ans. (a) Tachyphylaxis**
   When repeated doses of a drug produce lesser response than original, it is called tachyphylaxis. It is shown by indirectly acting sympathomimetic drugs like tyramine and ephedrine

5. **Ans. (b) Sympathomimetic**
   The drug is causing mydriasis with decrease in IOP whereas both light reflex and corneal reflex are present. These are changes of sympathomimetic drugs like adrenaline.
   We can identify the nature of some drugs by their action on rabbit eye.

Drug	Pupil size	Light reflex	Corneal reflex	Intraocular tension
Sympathomimetic like adrenaline	Mydriasis	Present	Present	Decreases
Parasympathomimetics like pilocarpine	Miosis	Present	Present	Decreases
Parasympatholytics like atropine	Mydriasis	Absent	Present	No effect or increase
Local anaesthetic like lignocaine	No change	Present	Absent	No effect
Cocaine	Mydriasis	Present	Absent	Decreases

6. **Ans. (a) Parasympathomimetics**
   As explained in the question above, the drug is causing miosis with decrease in IOP whereas both light reflex and corneal reflex are present. These are changes of parasympathomimetic drugs like pilocarpine.

7. **Ans. (c) Barium chloride**
   The given figure shows that the drug is stimulant at rabbit ileum and its stimulatory effects are not blocked by atropine. So, it seems to be a directly acting stimulant like Barium chloride or calcium chloride.
   We can identify the nature of some drugs by their effect on rabbit ileum

Drug	Effect on rabbit intestine	Acts through	Effect stopped by
Acetylcholine	Stimulant	Muscarinic receptors	Atropine
Barium chloride	Stimulant	Directly	None
Adrenaline	Depressant	Alpha and Beta receptors	Alpha plus beta blocker
Papaverine	Depressant	Directly	None

To identify the unknown drug,
First see whether the drug increases the tone (stimulant) or decreases (depressant).
If it is **stimulant**, it is likely to be *acetylcholine or barium chloride*. Then see, whether the effect can be abolished by atropine or not. If stimulant effect is absent after atropine, the drug is acetylcholine but if it is still present, then it is directly acting drug like barium or calcium chloride.
If it is **depressant**, it is likely to be *adrenaline or papaverine*. Then see, whether the effect can be abolished by beta-blocker or not. If depressant effect is absent or reduced after giving beta blocker (completely abolished by alpha plus beta blocker), the drug is adrenaline but if it is still present, then it is directly acting drug like papaverine or KCl.

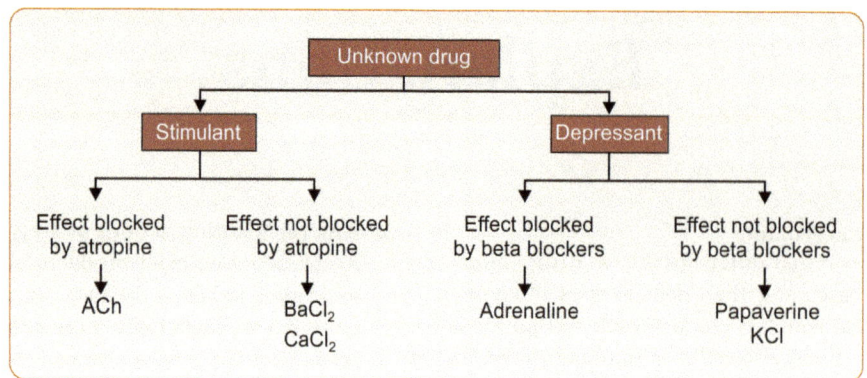

8. **Ans. (a) Acetylcholine**
 The drug is stimulant whose effect is abolished after giving atropine
9. **Ans. (b) Adrenaline**
 The given drug is depressant whose effect is abolished after beta blocker
10. **Ans. (b) Adrenaline**
 The given drug is depressant whose effect is significantly reduced by beta blocker. So the drug is working through beta receptors but as some effect is still present means the drug is acting on alpha receptors also. The likely drug is adrenaline
11. **Ans. (d) Papaverine**
 The given drug is a depressant whose effects are not abolished by beta blocker. So the drug is directly acting depressant like papaverine or KCl.
12. **Ans. (c) Botulinum toxin**   *(Ref: KK Sharma 2/e p211)*
 As shown in the diagram, the drug is inhibiting the exocytosis of ACh. Botulinum toxin act by this mechanism. Other features pointing towards botulinum toxin are:
 • Anticholinergic adverse effects (dry mouth, blurring of vision)
 • Use in wrinkles, spastic disorders, prophylaxis of migraine.

13. **Ans. (d) Latanoprost**
 The given image is of pigmentation of iris known as heterochromia iridis. It is caused by $PFG_{2\alpha}$ analogs like latanoprost.
14. **Ans. (b) Latanoprost**
 The image shows overgrowth of eyelashes, It is also known as hyper trichosis. It is an adverse effect of $PGF_{2\alpha}$ analogs like latanoprost.
15. **Ans (a) Edrophonium**
 Edrophonium is a short-acting AChE inhibitor. It is used to differentiate between myasthenia gravis and cholinergic crisis.
16. **Ans. (b) Drug B may be mirabegron and is used for treatment of atonic bladder**

Drug	Example	Mechanism	Use
A	Oxybutynin Tolterodine	M_3 antagonist	Overactive bladder
B	Mirabegron	β_3 agonist	Overactive bladder
C	Tamsulosin Prazosin	α_1 antagonist	BHP

Autonomic Nervous System

Multiple Choice Questions

PARASYMPATHOMIMETICS AND GLAUCOMA

1. A patient of diabetes mellitus developed postoperative urinary retention. Which of the following drugs can be used for short term treatment to relieve the symptoms of this person? *(NEET Pattern 2020)*
   - (a) Bethanechol
   - (b) Methacholine
   - (c) Terazosin
   - (d) Tamsulosin

2. Anti-glaucoma drug that acts by increasing uveoscleral outlfow is: *(NEET Pattern 2020)*
   - (a) Latanoprost
   - (b) Timolol
   - (c) Pilocarpine
   - (d) Dorzolamide

3. A patient presented to emergency with overdose of some drug. There was increased salivation and increased bronchial secretions. On examination, blood pressure was 88/60 mm Hg. RBC esterase level is 50. What should be the treatment of this person? *(NEET Pattern 2020)*
   - (a) Neostigmine
   - (b) Atropine
   - (c) Flumazenil
   - (d) Physostigmine

4. All of the following can be used to decreased intraocular pressure in glaucoma *except*: *(AIIMS Nov. 2019)*
   - (a) Mannitol
   - (b) Methazolamide
   - (c) Clonidine
   - (d) Dexamethasone

5. Acetylcholine decrease heart rate by which of the following mechanisms? *(AIIMS Nov. 2018)*
   - (a) By decreasing the rate of diastolic depolarization of SA node
   - (b) By causing delay through AV node
   - (c) By blocking calcium channels and prolonging the plateau phase
   - (d) By reducing the rate of ventricular repolarization

6. Which drug used for differentiating myasthenia gravis from cholinergic crisis? *(NEET Pattern 2019)*
   - (a) Edrophonium
   - (b) Neostigmine
   - (c) Atropine
   - (d) Acetylcholine

7. Drug causing ocular hypotension with apnea in an infant is: *(NEET Pattern 2019)*
   - (a) Latanoprost
   - (b) Brimonidine
   - (c) Timolol
   - (d) Acetazolamide

8. Which drug used for differentiating myasthenia gravis from cholinergic crisis? *(NEET Pattern Question 2019)*
   - (a) Edrophonium
   - (b) Neostigmine
   - (c) Atropine
   - (d) Acetylcholine

9. Drug causing ocular hypotension with apnea in an infant is: *(NEET Pattern Question 2019)*
   - (a) Latanoprost
   - (b) Brimonidine
   - (c) Timolol
   - (d) Acetazolamide

10. Which of the following are post-ganglionic receptors? *(AIIMS May 2017)*
    - (a) Dopaminergic
    - (b) Cholinergic
    - (c) Adrenergic
    - (d) Serotonergic

11. Methacholine has maximum agonist action at which of the following cholinergic receptors? *(AIIMS May 2015)*
    - (a) M1
    - (b) M2
    - (c) M3
    - (d) M4

12. Organophosphates act by inhibiting the enzyme acetylcholinesterase. Which type of enzyme inhibitors are they? *(AIIMS May 2015)*
    - (a) Competitive and reversible
    - (b) Non-competitive and irreversible
    - (c) Uncompetitive and reversible
    - (d) Competitive and irreversible

13. Cholinomimetics are useful in all of the following conditions *except*: *(AIIMS Nov 2013, 14)*
    - (a) Glaucoma
    - (b) Myasthenia gravis
    - (c) Post operative atony of bladder
    - (d) Partial heart block

14. Which of the following drugs acts on trabecular meshwork and affects the aqueous outflow? *(AIIMS May 2014)*
    - (a) Timolol
    - (b) Pilocarpine
    - (c) Brimonidine
    - (d) Brinzolamide

15. Correct match of drug and mechanism of action is: *(AIIMS May 2013)*
    - (a) Brimonidine: Decreases aqueous production
    - (b) Latanoprost: Carbonic anhydrase inhibitor
    - (c) Pilocarpine: Increases uveoscleral outflow
    - (d) Betaxolol: Increases trabecular outflow

16. Cholinomimetic drugs can be used for the treatment of all the following conditions *except*: *(AIIMS Nov 2012)*
    - (a) Closed angle Glaucoma
    - (b) Bradycardia
    - (c) Cobra bite
    - (d) Myasthenia gravis

17. A patient presents to emergency with pinpoint pupil, salivation, lacrimation, tremors and red tears. Plasma cholinesterase level was 30% of normal. Most probable Diagnosis is: *(AIIMS May 2012)*
    - (a) Organophosphate poisoning
    - (b) Datura poisoning
    - (c) Opioid poisoning
    - (d) Pontine hemorrhage

18. Synaptic transmission in the autonomic ganglion is usually: *(Recent NEET Pattern Question)*
    - (a) Adrenergic
    - (b) Peptidergic
    - (c) Cholinergic
    - (d) Mediated by substance P

19. Which of the following cranial nerve does not contain parasympathetic motor (GVE) fibers? *(Recent NEET Pattern Question)*
    - (a) III
    - (b) VI
    - (c) IX
    - (d) X

20. Major neurotransmitter released at end organ effectors of the sympathetic division of the autonomic nervous system is: *(Recent NEET Pattern Question)*
    (a) Adrenaline (b) Noradrenaline
    (c) Dopamine (d) Acetylcholine

21. All of the following agents are used in glaucoma treatment, *except*: *(Recent NEET Pattern Question)*
    (a) Apraclonidine (b) Timolol
    (c) Pilocarpine (d) Metoprolol

22. Which of the following antiglaucoma medication is UNSAFE in infants? *(Recent NEET Pattern Question)*
    (a) Timolol (b) Brimonidine
    (c) Latanoprost (d) Dorzolamide

23. A patient complains of muscle weakness. It was reversed on administration of neostigmine, because: *(Recent NEET Pattern Question)*
    (a) It blocks action of acetylcholine
    (b) It interferes with the action of mono amine oxidase
    (c) It interferes with the action of carbonic anhydrase
    (d) It interferes with the action of acetyl cholinesterase.

24. How would a drug that competes with ACh for receptors at the motor end plate affect skeletal muscle? It would: *(Recent NEET Pattern Question)*
    (a) Produce uncontrolled muscle spasms
    (b) Cause the muscles to contract and be unable to relax
    (c) Cause muscles to relax and be unable to contract
    (d) Make the muscles more excitable

25. All are cholinergic agents *except*: *(Recent NEET Pattern Question)*
    (a) Galantamine (b) Donepezil
    (c) Tacrine (d) Memantine

26. Neostigmine is not able to cross blood brain barrier because of its: *(Recent NEET Pattern Question)*
    (a) Primary structure (b) Secondary structrure
    (c) Tertiary structure (d) Quaternary structure

27. True statement about pralidoxime is: *(Recent NEET Pattern Question)*
    (a) Signs of atropinization occur more slowly when pralidoxime is used as compared to the use of atropine alone
    (b) It can be used for chlorinated pesticides
    (c) It should not used for nerve gases used in chemical warfare
    (d) Therapy with pralidoxime should ideally be monitored by measuring blood cholinesterase concentration

28. Which drug is not used now in Alzheimer's disease? *(Recent NEET Pattern Question)*
    (a) Tacrine (b) Galantamine
    (c) Donepezil (d) Rivastigmine

29. Organophosphates bind to: *(Recent NEET Pattern Question)*
    (a) Anionic site of AChEs (b) Esteratic site of AChEs
    (c) ACh (d) None

30. Drug used in ameliorative test for myasthenia gravis is: *(Recent NEET Pattern Question)*
    (a) Physostigmine (b) Edrophonium
    (c) Tacrine (d) Pyridostigmine

31. Atropine is useful in organophosphate poisoning because it: *(Recent NEET Pattern Question)*
    (a) Reactivates acetylcholinesterase
    (b) Competes with acetylcholine release
    (c) Binds with both nicotinic and muscarinic acetylcholine receptors
    (d) Is a competitive antagonist of acetylcholine

32. 2-PAM (Pralidoxime) is useful in treatment of: *(Recent NEET Pattern Question)*
    (a) Paracetamol overdose (b) DDT Poisoning
    (c) Malathion Poisoning (d) Lead Poisoning

33. Pin-point pupil suggests poisoning with: *(Recent NEET Pattern Question)*
    (a) DDT (b) Opiates
    (c) Belladonna (d) Barbiturates

34. Drug of choice in treatment of myasthenia gravis is: *(Recent NEET Pattern Question)*
    (a) d-Tubocurarine (b) Hexamethonium
    (c) Neostigmine (d) Gallamine

35. Which of the following does not cross the blood brain barrier? *(Recent NEET Pattern Question)*
    (a) Pralidoxime (b) Obidoxime
    (c) Diacetyl-monoxime (d) Physostigmine

36. Anti-cholinesterases are ineffective against: *(Recent NEET Pattern Question)*
    (a) Belladona poisoning (b) Carbamate poisoning
    (c) Postoperative ileus (d) Cobra bite

37. Acetylcholine is not used commercially because: *(Recent NEET Pattern Question)*
    (a) Long duration of action
    (b) Costly
    (c) Rapidly destroyed in the body
    (d) Crosses blood brain barrier

38. Which one of the following acts commonly both on parasympathetic and sympathetic division?
    (a) Atropine *(Recent NEET Pattern Question)*
    (b) Pilocarpine
    (c) Acetylcholine
    (d) Adrenaline

39. The short acting anticholinesterase drug is: *(Recent NEET Pattern Question)*
    (a) Edrophonium (b) Demecarium
    (c) Dyflos (d) Ectothiophate

40. Anticholinesterase with effect on CNS is: *(Recent NEET Pattern Question)*
    (a) Neostigmine (b) Pyridostigmine
    (c) Physostigmine (d) Edrophonium

41. Which of the following anticholinesterase is derived from natural source? *(Recent NEET Pattern Question)*
    (a) Physostigmine (b) Neostigmine
    (c) Pyridostigmine (d) Tacrine

42. The α_2 agonist used in glaucoma is: *(Recent NEET Pattern Question)*
    (a) Guanacare (b) Guanabenz
    (c) Brimonidine (d) Tizanidine

Autonomic Nervous System

43. Which antiglaucoma drug can be used in an asthmatic patient? *(Recent NEET Pattern Question)*
    (a) Timolol (b) Betaxolol
    (c) Propranolol (d) All

44. Cholinesterase activators are useful for treatment of which poisoning? *(Recent NEET Pattern Question)*
    (a) Paraquat (b) Parathion
    (c) Carbamates (d) Organochlorocompounds

45. Neostigmine used in treatment of myasthenia gravis acts by: *(Recent NEET Pattern Question)*
    (a) Increasing the number of receptors for acetylcholine
    (b) Increasing synthesis of acetylcholine
    (c) Decreasing breakdown of acetylcholine
    (d) Increasing actylcholine degradation

46. Which of the following is not a carbamate? *(Recent NEET Pattern Question)*
    (a) Physostigmine (b) Neostigmine
    (c) Edrophonium (d) Pyridostigmine

47. Which among the following is contraindicated in a myasthenic patient? *(Recent NEET Pattern Question)*
    (a) Aminoglycosides (b) Sulphonamides
    (c) Penicillin (d) All

48. A patient requires mild cholinomimetic stimulation following surgery. Physostigmine and bethanechol in small doses have significantly different effects on which of the following? *(Recent NEET Pattern Question)*
    (a) Gastric secretion (b) Neuromuscular junction
    (c) Sweat glands (d) Ureteral tone

49. In oral poisoning with carbamate insecticides .... may be hazardous: *(Recent NEET Pattern Question)*
    (a) Pralidoxime
    (b) Atropine
    (c) Magnesium sulfate purgative
    (d) Gastric lavage with activated charcoal

50. Pralidoxime is ineffective in case of which poisoning? *(Recent NEET Pattern Question)*
    (a) Organophosphorous (b) Carbaryl
    (c) Both (d) None

51. Which of the following is the most reliable clinical end-point to indicate adequate atropinisation in organophosphate poisoning? *(Recent NEET Pattern Question)*
    (a) Pupillary dilatation
    (b) Control of diarrhea
    (c) Heart rate more than or equal to 100 beats/min
    (d) Absence of pulmonary secretions

52. Regarding neostigmine, all of the following are correct except: *(Recent NEET Pattern Question)*
    (a) A quaternary ammonium compound
    (b) Shorter acting than edrophonium
    (c) Poorly absorbed orally
    (d) Used in myasthenia gravis

53. Nicotinic receptor sites include all of the following except:
    (a) Bronchial smooth muscle
    (b) Adrenal medulla *(Recent NEET Pattern Question)*
    (c) Skeletal muscle
    (d) Sympathetic ganglia

54. All of the following are used in organophosphorus poisoning except: *(Recent NEET Pattern Question)*
    (a) Pralidoxime (b) Atropine
    (c) Activated charcoal (d) Naltrexone

55. A 35-year-old man was found unconscious. Examination revealed bilateral constricted pupils, bradycardia, excessive sweating and secretion. Most likely cause is:
    (a) Opium poisoning *(Recent NEET Pattern Question)*
    (b) Acute alcohol intoxication
    (c) Organophosphate poisoning
    (d) Pontine hemorrhage

56. A 24-year-old farm worker is rushed to a nearby emergency department after an accidental exposure to parathion. Which of the following drugs can be given to increase the activity of his acetyl cholinesterase? *(Recent NEET Pattern Question)*
    (a) Atropine (b) Dimercaprol
    (c) Physostigmine (d) Pralidoxime

57. Pilocarpine reduce the intraocular pressure in persons with closed angle glaucoma by: *(Recent NEET Pattern Question)*
    (a) Reducing aqueous humor secretion
    (b) Contracting iris sphincter muscle
    (c) Increasing aqueous humor outflow
    (d) Relaxing ciliary muscle

58. Sweating as a result of exertion is mediated through:
    (a) Adrenal hormones *(Recent NEET Pattern Question)*
    (b) Sympathetic adrenergic
    (c) Parasympathetic cholinergic
    (d) Sympathetic cholinergic

59. All are cholinergic actions except: *(Recent NEET Pattern Question)*
    (a) Bronchoconstriction (b) Tachycardia
    (c) Salivation (d) Miosis

60. Edrophonium test is used in the diagnosis of:
    (a) Marcus gunn jaw winking ptosis
    (b) Horner's syndrome *(Recent NEET Pattern Question)*
    (c) Blepharophimosis syndrome
    (d) Myasthenic ptosis

61. Which of the following anti-glaucoma drugs can cause heterochromia iridis? *(AIIMS May 2015)*
    (a) Timolol (b) Latanoprost
    (c) Apraclonidine (d) Acetazolamide

PARASYMPATHOLYTICS

62. All of the following can cause miosis except: *(NEET Pattern 2020)*
    (a) Organophosphates (b) Belladona
    (c) Morphine (d) Pilocarpine

63. A 3-year-old child was undergoing squint surgery. Initial heart rate was 140 beats per min. After anaesthesia and start of surgery heart rate dropped to 40 beats/min. What should be the next step? *(NEET Pattern 2018)*
    (a) Stop surgery
    (b) Decrease plane of anaesthesia
    (c) Inj glycopyrrolate
    (d) Inj atropine

64. Atropine is indicated in all the following poisonings except: (AIIMS Nov 2017)
    (a) Baygon (b) Tik 20
    (c) Parathion (d) Endrin

65. Which of the following is NOT a tertiary amine? (Recent NEET Pattern Question)
    (a) Atropine (b) Hyoscine
    (c) Glycopyrrolate (d) Physostigmine

66. Which of the following drugs does not cross blood placental barrier? (AI 2012)
    (a) Atropine
    (b) Glycopyrrolate
    (c) Physostigmime
    (d) Hyoscine hydro bromide

67. Botulinum toxin blocks neuromuscular transmission by which of the following mechanism? (Recent NEET Pattern Question)
    (a) Closure of Ca^{++} channels at presynaptic membrane
    (b) Closure of Na$^+$ channels at the postsynaptic membrane
    (c) Opening of K$^+$ channels at the presynaptic membrane
    (d) Opening of Cl$^-$ channels at the postsynaptic membrane

68. Which is the shortest acting mydriatic? (Recent NEET Pattern Question)
    (a) Atropine (b) Tropicamide
    (c) Cyclopentolate (d) Homatropine

69. Oxybutynin acts by: (Recent NEET Pattern Question)
    (a) Nicotine receptor stimulation
    (b) Muscarinic receptor stimulation
    (c) Muscarinic receptor inhibition
    (d) α receptor inhibition

70. Atropine does not cause: (Recent NEET Pattern Question)
    (a) Increase bowel sound
    (b) Decrease bowel sound
    (c) Dryness
    (d) Tachycardia

71. Atropine poisoning causes all, except: (Recent NEET Pattern Question)
    (a) Dilated pupil
    (b) Excitement
    (c) Excessive salivation
    (d) Hot skin

72. Which of the following drugs is useful in prophylaxis of motion sickness? (Recent NEET Pattern Question)
    (a) Hyoscine (b) Metoclopramide
    (c) Prochlorperazine (d) Ondansetron

73. Clinical signs of atropine intoxication are as follows, except: (Recent NEET Pattern Question)
    (a) Decreased bowel sounds
    (b) Dry skin
    (c) Scarlet flushing of face
    (d) Increased bowel sounds

74. Atropine is substituted by phenylephrine to facilitate fundus examination when: (Recent NEET Pattern Question)
    (a) Mydriasis is required without cycloplegia
    (b) Cycloplegia is required
    (c) Mydriasis and cycloplegia both are required
    (d) Cycloplegia and Mydriasis both are not required

75. The following drug is a selective blocker (antagonist) of M1 muscarinic receptors: (Recent NEET Pattern Question)
    (a) Methacholine
    (b) Bethanechol
    (c) Methoctramine
    (d) Pirenzepine

76. Which of the following drugs has no cycloplegic action? (Recent NEET Pattern Question)
    (a) Atropine (b) Cyclopentolate
    (c) Tropicamide (d) Phenylepherine

77. The main mechanism of hyperpyrexia induced by atropine includes: (Recent NEET Pattern Question)
    (a) Vasodilation
    (b) Inhibition of sweating
    (c) Through central actions
    (d) Increase in basal metabolic rate

78. Pirenzepine acts on which receptor? (Recent NEET Pattern Question)
    (a) Muscarinic (b) Nicotinic
    (c) Alfa (d) Beta

79. Which one of the following drugs increases gastro-intestinal motility? (Recent NEET Pattern Question)
    (a) Glycopyrrolate (b) Atropine
    (c) Neostigmine (d) Fentanyl

80. Retinoscopy in 5-year-old is best done with: (Recent NEET Pattern Question)
    (a) Atropine (b) Homatropine
    (c) Cyclopentolate (d) Tropicamide

81. Atropine is most sensitive to:
    (a) Mucous and pharyngeal secretions
    (b) Heart (Recent NEET Pattern Question)
    (c) Pupil
    (d) GI tract motility

82. Which is not an effect of atropine? (Recent NEET Pattern Question)
    (a) Rise of body temperature
    (b) Decreased salivary secretion
    (c) Bradycardia
    (d) Increased A-V conduction

83. Atropine is used in all except:
    (a) Glaucoma (Recent NEET Pattern Question)
    (b) As a mydriatic
    (c) As a cyclopegic
    (d) Preanaesthetic medication

84. Atropine is added to commercial preparations containing diphenoxylate to: (Recent NEET Pattern Question)
    (a) Potentiate us anti-spasmodic effect
    (b) To reduce excretion of salt and water
    (c) To prevent overdosage and discourage opioid dependence
    (d) To prolong its duration of action

Autonomic Nervous System

85. Blockade of neuromuscular transmission by botulinum toxin is an example of: *(Recent NEET Pattern Question)*
    (a) Depolarizing blockade
    (b) Competitive blockade
    (c) Presynaptic blockade
    (d) Postsynaptic blockade

86. Atropine when used as a pre-medication causes all of the following symptoms *except*: *(Recent NEET Pattern Question)*
    (a) Skin flush
    (b) Bronchoconstriction
    (c) Prevents bradycardia
    (d) Dryness of mouth

87. Which of the following drug is not used in treatment of iridocyclitis: *(Recent NEET Pattern Question)*
    (a) Atropine eye ointment
    (b) Pilocarpine eye drops
    (c) Timolol eye drops
    (d) Steroid eye drops

88. All of the following are the feature of atropine poisoning *except*: *(Recent NEET Pattern Question)*
    (a) Mydriasis
    (b) Hallucinations
    (c) Hypothermia
    (d) Coma

89. The drug that is contraindicated in angle closure glaucoma is: *(Recent NEET Pattern Question)*
    (a) Pilocarpine
    (b) Atropine
    (c) Dorzolamide
    (d) Timolol

90. Atropine is contraindicated in: *(Recent NEET Pattern Question)*
    (a) Early mushroom poisoning
    (b) Myasthenia gravis
    (c) Organophosphate poisoning
    (d) Glaucoma

91. Antidote for nicotine poisoning is: *(Recent NEET Pattern Question)*
    (a) Neostigmine
    (b) Atropine sulphate
    (c) Phentolamine
    (d) Trimethaphan

ADRENERGIC DRUGS

92. A patient was given ampicillin 2 g intravenously. After that, the person developed rash on skin, hypotension and difficulty in breathing. The patient should be managed by: *(NEET Pattern 2018)*
    (a) 0.5 mL of 1:1000 adrenaline by intramuscular route
    (b) 0.5 mL of 1:1000 adrenaline by intravenous route
    (c) 0.5 mL of 1:10000 adrenaline by intramuscular route
    (d) 0.5 mL of 1:10000 adrenaline by intravenous route

93. Alternative drug to epinephrine for pulseless cardiac arrest in ACLS is: *(NEET Pattern Question 2017-2018)*
    (a) Low dose dopamine
    (b) Conivaptan
    (c) Vasopressin
    (d) Atropine

94. Stimulation of Alpha adrenoreceptor causes: *(NEET Pattern Question 2016-17)*
    (a) Increased gut motility
    (b) Decreased gland secretion
    (c) Vasodilatation
    (d) Vasoconstriction

95. The drug recently approved to be used along with phentermine in the management of obesity is: *(NEET Pattern Question 2016-17)*
    (a) Lorcaserin
    (b) Orlistat
    (c) Topiramate
    (d) Sibutramine

96. All of the following drugs are useful in treatment of obesity *except*: *(NEET Pattern Question 2016-17)*
    (a) Orlistat
    (b) Chlorpropamide
    (c) Metformin
    (d) Lorcaserin

97. Most appropriate route for adrenaline use in cardiac arrest is: *(NEET Pattern Question 2016-17)*
    (a) Intraosseus
    (b) Intratracheal
    (c) Intravenous
    (d) Intrascardiac

98. An unknown drug is being tested in experimental set-up. The results obtained are given in the table. From these actions, new drug is likely to be: *(AIIMS Nov 2017)*

Parameter	Placebo treated	New drug treated
Heart rate	72	86
Systolic BP	110	150
Diastolic BP	80	68
Tremors	Absent	Present

    (a) Beta 1 and Beta 2 agonist
    (b) Alpha 1 antagonist and Beta 2 agonist
    (c) M2 and M3 agonist
    (d) Alpha 1 and Beta 1 agonist

99. Treatment of choice for anaphylactic shock is: *(AIIMS Nov 2017)*
    (a) Adrenaline 0.5 mL of 1:1000 solution by intramuscular route
    (b) Adrenaline 1 mL of 1:10000 by intravenous route
    (c) Atropine 3 mg intravenously
    (d) Adenosine 12 mg intravenously

100. In animal models, how will you demonstrate vasomotor reversal of Dale? *(AIIMS Nov 2017)*
    (a) Low dose adrenaline and then beta 1 blockade
    (b) Beta 1 stimulation by nor-adrenaline and then alpha 1 stimulation
    (c) High dose adrenaline followed by alpha 1 block
    (d) Alpha 1 stimulation followed by beta 1 stimulation

101. Which of the following statements is correct regarding the graph given below? *(AIIMS Nov 2016)*

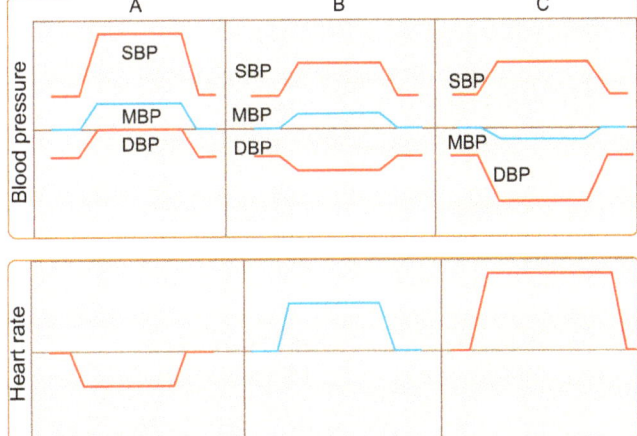

    (a) Drug A in the graph is epinephrine
    (b) The effect on heart rate in graph A can be prevented by anti-muscarinic agents
    (c) Drug acting on graph B is isoprenaline
    (d) Drug acting in the graph C is nor-epinephrine

102. An 80 kg patient is brought in the causality in shock. Dopamine needs to be started at 10 micro/kg/min rate. A 5 mL vial contains 200 mg of dopamine. Two vials are diluted to a solution of 250 mL with the help of normal saline. Calculate drops per minute required to be administered if 1 mL = 16 drops. *(AIIMS Nov 2016)*
    (a) 8 (b) 16
    (c) 24 (d) 32

103. Action of adrenaline on which of the following receptor is not required in treatment of anaphylactic shock?
    (AIIMS May 2016)
    (a) Alpha 1
    (b) Presynaptic alpha 2 receptors
    (c) Beta 1
    (d) Beta 2

104. Which of the following combinations will show vasomotor reversal of Dale? *(AIIMS May 2016)*
    (a) Phentolamine followed by adrenaline
    (b) Propranolol followed by adrenaline
    (c) Phentolamine followed by nor-adrenaline
    (d) Propranolol followed by nor-adrenaline

105. Dopamine given in acute CHF DOES NOT act on which of the following receptors? *(AIIMS May 2016)*
    (a) Receptors present on renal blood vessels
    (b) D1 receptors
    (c) Beta 1 receptors
    (d) Alpha 1 receptors

106. Action of dopamine in 1-2 mcg/kg/min dose is:
    (a) Vasoconstriction *(AIIMS Nov 2015)*
    (b) Increases renal blood flow
    (c) Increases cardiac contractility
    (d) Increases blood pressure

107. Adrenergic beta-receptors having lipolysis property in fat cells is: *(AIIMS May 2015)*
    (a) Alpha-1 (b) Alpha-2
    (c) Beta-1 (d) Beta-3

108. Dexmedetomidine is a: *(AIIMS Nov 2014)*
    (a) Centrally acting α_2 agonist
    (b) Peripherally acting α_2 agonist
    (c) Centrally acting α_2 antagonist
    (d) Peripherally acting α_2 antagonist

109. Alpha 2 agonists cause all of the following *except*:
    (AIIMS May 2014)
    (a) Analgesia (b) Hyperalgesia
    (c) Sedation (d) Anxiolysis

110. Which of the following is a mixed alpha and beta agonist?
    (AIIMS May 2014)
    (a) Dobutamine (b) Fenoldopam
    (c) Epinephrine (d) Phenylephrine

111. Which of the following agent is not used in erectile dysfunction? *(AIIMS Nov. 2012)*
    (a) PGE$_2$ (b) Vardenafil
    (c) Phenylephrine (d) Alprostadil

112. Which of the following concentrations of epinephrine does not correspond to the respective route of administration? *(Recent NEET Pattern Question)*
    (a) 1 : 10000 for intravenous route
    (b) 1 : 1000 for inhalational route
    (c) 1 : 1000 for intramuscular route
    (d) 1 : 1000 for *subcutaneous route*

113. One of the following activities is not mediated through β_2 adrenergic receptors: *(Recent NEET Pattern Question)*
    (a) Stimulation of lipolysis
    (b) Increased hepatic gluconeogenesis
    (c) Increased muscle glycogenolysis
    (d) Smooth muscle relaxation

114. Fenoldopam is used in the management of:
    (Recent NEET Pattern Question)
    (a) Hypertensive emergencies
    (b) Congestive heart failure
    (c) Migraine prophylaxis
    (d) Tachyarrhythmia

115. The rate limiting step for norepinephrine synthesis is:
    (Recent NEET Pattern Question)
    (a) Conversion of phenylalanine to tyrosine
    (b) Conversion of tyrosine to DOPA
    (c) Conversion of DOPA to dopamine
    (d) Conversion of dopamine to norepinephrine

116. Dopamine is preferred in treatment of shock because of:
    (Recent NEET Pattern Question)
    (a) Renal vasodilatory effect
    (b) Increased cardiac output
    (c) Peripheral vasoconstriction
    (d) Prolonged action

117. Which of the following increases systolic and diastolic BP for prolonged period? *(Recent NEET Pattern Question)*
    (a) Epinephrine (b) Dopamine
    (c) Ephedrine (d) All of these

118. TRUE statement regarding use of adrenaline in anaphylactic shock is: *(Recent NEET Pattern Question)*
    (a) The usual dose is 0.5-1 mg by IM route
    (b) Cerebral hemorrhage never occurs as an adverse effect to epinephrine when used in treatment of anaphylactic shock
    (c) It is repeated after every 2-4 hours
    (d) Same solution can be given for SC as well as IV route

119. Renal dose of dopamine is: *(Recent NEET Pattern Question)*
    (a) 2.5 µg/kg/min
    (b) 5-10 µg/kg/min
    (c) 10-20 µg/kg/min
    (d) 1-2 µg/kg/min

120. Half life of Dobutamine is:
    (Recent NEET Pattern Question)
    (a) 120 seconds (b) 200 seconds
    (c) 20 seconds (d) 20 minutes

121. All are side effects of salbutamol *except*:
    (Recent NEET Pattern Question)
    (a) Palpitation (b) Muscle tremors
    (c) Sedation (d) Hypokalemia

122. Treatment of choice for anaphylactic shock is:
    (Recent NEET Pattern Question)
    (a) Intravenous hydrocortisone
    (b) Subcutaneous adrenaline
    (c) Intravenous aminophylline
    (d) Subcutaneous antihistaminic

Autonomic Nervous System

123. Norepinephrine action at the synaptic cleft is terminated by: *(Recent NEET Pattern Question)*
(a) Metabolism by COMT
(b) Metabolism by MAO
(c) Reuptake
(d) Metabolism by acetylcholinesterase

124. Epinephrine is most useful in:
(a) Bronchial asthma *(Recent NEET Pattern Question)*
(b) Anaphylactic shock
(c) Peripheral vascular disease
(d) Wide angle glaucoma

125. Exogenous adrenaline is metabolized by: *(Recent NEET Pattern Question)*
(a) AChE (b) COMT
(c) Decarboxylase (d) Acetyl transferase

126. Which of the following is NOT true about adrenergic receptors? *(Recent NEET Pattern Question)*
(a) α_1 receptors are usually presynaptic
(b) β_1 receptors are predominantly found in heart
(c) Noradrenaline stimulates β_1 receptors
(d) α_2 receptor stimulation inhibits transmitter release

127. Drug given in cardiogenic shock is: *(Recent NEET Pattern Question)*
(a) Dopamine (b) Phenylephrine
(c) Atropine (d) Digoxin

128. Which one of the following is a relatively selective α_2 adrenergic blocker with short duration of action? *(Recent NEET Pattern Question)*
(a) Prazosin (b) Yohimbine
(c) Terazosin (d) Doxazosin

129. Biphasic reaction on blood pressure is seen with the administration of: *(Recent NEET Pattern Question)*
(a) Adrenaline (b) Nor adrenaline
(c) Dopamine (d) Dobutamine

130. Methyl dopa acts on which of the following receptor? *(Recent NEET Pattern Question)*
(a) α_2 (b) α_1
(c) β_1 (d) D_1

131. Salbutamol is preferred over adrenaline in an asthmatic due to: *(Recent NEET Pattern Question)*
(a) β_1 selectivity (b) β_2 selectivity
(c) α_1 selectivity (d) None

132. Adrenaline increases all of the following blood pressures significantly *except*: *(Recent NEET Pattern Question)*
(a) Systolic (b) Diastolic
(c) Mean BP (d) Pulse pressure

133. Most common adverse effect of salbutamol is: *(Recent NEET Pattern Question)*
(a) Tremors (b) Hypertension
(c) Rhinorrhoea (d) Headache

134. Methylphenindate is drug of choice for: *(Recent NEET Pattern Question)*
(a) Obsessive compulsive disorder
(b) ADHD (attention deficit hyperkinetic disorder)
(c) Enuresis
(d) Autism

135. Which of the following statement is not true regarding dobutamine? *(Recent NEET Pattern Question)*
(a) Agonist of D_1 and D_2 receptors
(b) Derivative of dopamine
(c) Selective beta-agonistic action
(d) Reduced chances of arrhythmia than adrenaline

136. Epinephrine act through beta 1 receptors by stimulating: *(Recent NEET Pattern Question)*
(a) Adenyl cyclase (b) Phosohodiestarase
(c) Phospholipase (d) None

137. Vasomotor reversal of Dale is due to: *(Recent NEET Pattern Question)*
(a) α blocker (b) β-blocker
(c) α and β-blocker (d) None

138. Depression occurs as a side effect due to the use of: *(Recent NEET Pattern Question)*
(a) Reserpine (b) Propranolol
(c) Morphine (d) Amphetamine

139. Catecholamine action on α-receptors causes: *(Recent NEET Pattern Question)*
(a) Increased atrial contraction
(b) Increased heart rate
(c) Detrusor relaxation
(d) Gastrointestinal sphincter contraction

140. Which is not an endogenous catecholamine? *(Recent NEET Pattern Question)*
(a) Isoprenaline (b) Dopamine
(c) Noradrenaline (d) Adrenaline

141. Clonidine has the following attributes *except*: *(Recent NEET Pattern Question)*
(a) Acts on α_2 adrenergic receptors
(b) Can produce rebound hypertension on abrupt withdrawal
(c) Can produce CNS stimulation
(d) Inhibits salivation

142. Clonidine is used for: *(Recent NEET Pattern Question)*
(a) Migraine
(b) Opioid withdrawal syndrome
(c) Diabetic diarrhea
(d) All of the above

143. Which of the following is a non-catecholamine sympathomimetic drug? *(Recent NEET Pattern Question)*
(a) Ephedrine (b) Dopamine
(c) Isoproterenol (d) Dobutamine

144. Dobutamine increases: *(Recent NEET Pattern Question)*
(a) Heart rate
(b) Cardiac output
(c) Blood pressure
(d) Plasma volume

145. All of the following statements about dopamine are true *except*: *(Recent NEET Pattern Question)*
(a) Causes increase in GI Ischemia
(b) Positive inotropic
(c) Improves renal perfusion
(d) Causes vasoconstriction

146. Most potent cardiac stimulant of the following is: *(Recent NEET Pattern Question)*
(a) Adrenaline (b) Noradrenaline
(c) Ephedrine (d) Salbutamol

147. Mechanism of action of clonidine is mediated by which of the following receptors? *(Recent NEET Pattern Question)*
    (a) Alpha 1
    (b) Alpha 2
    (c) Beta 1
    (d) Beta 2

148. Which of the following drugs is most effective for control of orthostatic hypotension? *(Recent NEET Pattern Question)*
    (a) Clonidine
    (b) Fludrocortisone
    (c) Esmolol
    (d) Phenylephrine

149. In Anaphylactic shock, epinephrine is given by which route? *(Recent NEET Pattern Question)*
    (a) Intravenous route
    (b) Oral
    (c) Subcutaneous
    (d) Intramuscular

150. Catecholamines are synthesized from: *(Recent NEET Pattern Question)*
    (a) Alanine
    (b) Glycine
    (c) Cysteine
    (d) Tyrosine

151. In shock, Dopamine is used at the following dose rate: *(Recent NEET Pattern Question)*
    (a) <1 – 2 µg/kg/min
    (b) 1 – 2 µg/kg/min
    (c) 2 – 10 µg/kg/min
    (d) Greater than 10 µg/kg/min

152. Stimulation of which receptor will release renin? *(Recent NEET Pattern Question)*
    (a) Alpha 1
    (b) Alpha 2
    (c) Beta 1
    (d) Beta 2

153. Selective α_2 agonist is: *(Recent NEET Pattern Question)*
    (a) Clonidine
    (b) Prazosin
    (c) Adrenaline
    (d) Propranolol

154. Tachyphylaxis is seen after use of: *(Recent NEET Pattern Question)*
    (a) Tamoxifen
    (b) Ephedrine
    (c) Morphine
    (d) Chlorpromazine

155. Mydriatic which does not cause cycloplegia is: *(Recent NEET Pattern Question)*
    (a) Tropicamide
    (b) Atropine
    (c) Homatropine
    (d) Phenylephrine

156. Sibutramine is indicated for: *(Recent NEET Pattern Question)*
    (a) Smoking cessation
    (b) Obesity
    (c) Severe weight loss
    (d) Mania

157. Drug of choice for attention deficit hyperactivity disorder is: *(Recent NEET Pattern Question)*
    (a) Fluoxetine
    (b) Haloperidol
    (c) Deriphylline
    (d) Methylphenidate

ADRENERGIC ANTAGONISTS

158. A hypertensive patient was on metoprolol treatment. Verapamil was added to the therapy of this patient. This can result in: *(AIIMS Nov. 2018)*
    (a) Atrial fibrillation
    (b) Bradycardia with AV block
    (c) Torsades' de pointes
    (d) Tachycardia

159. Drug used for hypertension and pulmonary edema due to scorpion sting: *(NEET Pattern Question 2019)*
    (a) Prazosin
    (b) Clonidine
    (c) Furosemide
    (d) Mannitol

160. The approximate weight of the rabbit used in pharmacological studies for assessing the effect of drugs on rabbit eye is: *(AIIMS Nov 2016)*
    (a) 0.5-1 kg
    (b) 1.5-2.5 kg
    (c) 4-5 kg
    (d) 10-12 kg

161. Which of the following anti-glaucoma drugs is likely to cause black pigmentation on conjunctiva? *(AIIMS May 2016)*
    (a) Adrenaline
    (b) Latanoprost
    (c) Beta blockers
    (d) Pilocarpine

162. Which of the following drug produce analogous action on dilator pupillae as is produced by pilocarpine on sphincter pupillae? *(AIIMS May 2015)*
    (a) Epinephrine
    (b) Hydroxyamphetamine
    (c) Cocaine
    (d) Timolol

163. A guinea pig is dissected and a portion of its intestine is fixed in the Dales organ bath to study the effect of some drugs on intestinal contractility. A substance C was infused in the organ bath and the following graph was obtained (as shown in the figure). Substance C most closely resembles which of these substances? *(AIIMS May 2015)*

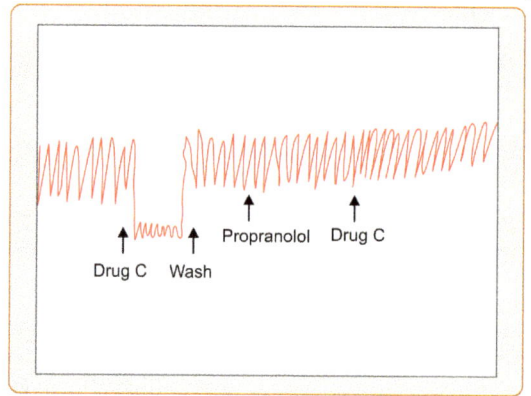

    (a) Adrenaline
    (b) Acetylcholine
    (c) Barium chloride
    (d) Potassium chloride

164. All of the following are therapeutic uses of prazosin, except: *(Recent NEET Pattern Question)*
    (a) Peripheral vascular disease
    (b) Pheochromocytoma
    (c) Lupus erythematosus
    (d) Scorpion sting

165. All of the following are cardioselective beta blockers except: *(Recent NEET Pattern Question)*
    (a) Atenolol
    (b) Esmolol
    (c) Bisoprolol
    (d) Propranolol

166. Beta blocker without local anaesthetic effect is: *(Recent NEET Pattern Question)*
    (a) Metoprolol
    (b) Pindolol
    (c) Propranolol
    (d) Timolol

167. Drug used for treatment of scorpion sting is: *(Recent NEET Pattern Question)*
    (a) Adrenaline
    (b) Morphine
    (c) Captopril
    (d) Prazosin

Autonomic Nervous System

168. Beta blockers are indicated for all of the following conditions *except*: *(Recent NEET Pattern Question)*
    (a) Hypothyroidism
    (b) Alcohol withdrawal
    (c) Portal hypertension
    (d) Performance anxiety

169. Propranolol can be used in all of the following conditions *except*: *(Recent NEET Pattern Question)*
    (a) Thyrotoxicosis
    (b) Variant angina
    (c) Migraine
    (d) Hypertension

170. Propranolol is useful in all *except*: *(Recent NEET Pattern Question)*
    (a) Atrial flutter
    (b) Parkinsonian tremor
    (c) Thyrotoxicosis
    (d) Hypertrophic cardiomyopathy

171. Timolol is contraindicated in: *(Recent NEET Pattern Question)*
    (a) Hypertension
    (b) Glaucoma
    (c) COPD
    (d) Aphakia

172. Atenolol is indicated in all *except*: *(Recent NEET Pattern Question)*
    (a) Hypertension
    (b) Partial heart block
    (c) Hypertrophic obstructive cardiomyopathy
    (d) Classical angina

173. Which of the following is a selective β_2 antagonist? *(Recent NEET Pattern Question)*
    (a) Esmolol
    (b) Betaxolol
    (c) Butoxamine
    (d) Celiprolol

174. Propranolol is contraindicated in diabetes mellitus because it: *(Recent NEET Pattern Question)*
    (a) Causes hyperglycemia
    (b) Causes seizures
    (c) Masks the hypoglycemic symptoms
    (d) Causes hypotension

175. An ultrashort acting β–blocker devoid of partial agonistic or membrane stabilizing action is: *(Recent NEET Pattern Question)*
    (a) Esmolol
    (b) Timolol
    (c) Atenolol
    (d) Pindolol

176. Which of the following alpha-blocker drug is used in the treatment of benign hypertrophy of prostate without producing significant hypotension? *(Recent NEET Pattern Question)*
    (a) Dexazosin
    (b) Phentolamine
    (c) Tamsulosin
    (d) Terazosin

177. Old patient taking beta blockers is prone to develop: *(Recent NEET Pattern Question)*
    (a) Asthma
    (b) CHF
    (c) Bradycardia
    (d) All

178. Beta blocker having both α and β blocking property is: *(Recent NEET Pattern Question)*
    (a) Carvedilol
    (b) Sotalol
    (c) Nadolol
    (d) Pindolol

179. Heart rate is decreased by: *(Recent NEET Pattern Question)*
    (a) Propranolol
    (b) Isoprenaline
    (c) Dopamine
    (d) Dobutamine

180. Which of the following is a false statement? *(Recent NEET Pattern Question)*
    (a) Esmolol is mainly metabolized in liver
    (b) Celiprolol has inherent vasodilatory properly
    (c) Nevibolol releases nitric oxide.
    (d) Metoprolol is used in congestive cardiac failure and prolongs survival

181. Tamsulosin, a competitive αadrenoceptor antagonist has affinity for which of the following receptors? *(Recent NEET Pattern Question)*
    (a) α_{1A}
    (b) α_{1D}
    (c) None of the above
    (d) Both (a) and (b)

182. The beta blocker having intrinsic sympathomimetic activity is: *(Recent NEET Pattern Question)*
    (a) Propranolol
    (b) Atenolol
    (c) Sotalol
    (d) Pindolol

183. Ideal drug employed in the preoperative preparation for surgical excision of pheochromocytoma is: *(Recent NEET Pattern Question)*
    (a) Atenolol
    (b) Phenoxybenzamine
    (c) Reserpine
    (d) Clonidine

184. Short elimination half-life (8-10 min) of esmolol (beta-adrenergic blocker) is due to: *(Recent NEET Pattern Question)*
    (a) Rapid redistribution
    (b) Rapid elimination by kidney
    (c) Hydrolysis by blood esterase
    (d) Rapid protein binding

185. Adverse effects of beta-blockers may include: *(Recent NEET Pattern Question)*
    (a) Congestive heart failure
    (b) Blunting of sympathetic response of oral hypoglycaemic drugs
    (c) Bronchial asthma
    (d) All of above

186. An example of covalent drug receptor interaction is: *(Recent NEET Pattern Question)*
    (a) Noradrenaline binding to β_1 adrenergic receptor
    (b) Acetylcholine binding to muscarinic receptor
    (c) Prazosin binding to α_1 adrenergic receptor
    (d) Phenoxybenzamine binding to alpha adrenergic receptor.

187. All are alpha blockers *except*: *(Recent NEET Pattern Question)*
    (a) Atenolol
    (b) Prazosin
    (c) Indoramine
    (d) Idazoxan

188. Beta blockers are not indicated in: *(Recent NEET Pattern Question)*
    (a) Acute CHF
    (b) Hypertension
    (c) Chronic CHF
    (d) Arrhythmia

189. Which of the following is not a cardioselective β-blocker? *(Recent NEET Pattern Question)*
    (a) Acebutolal
    (b) Atenolol
    (c) Pindolol
    (d) Metoprolol

190. Drug of choice for bradycardia due to beta blocker overdose is: *(Recent NEET Pattern Question)*
    (a) Atropine
    (b) Dopamine
    (c) Adrenaline
    (d) Isoprenaline

191. Which of the following is an selective alpha 2 antagonist? *(Recent NEET Pattern Question)*
    (a) Prazosin
    (b) Labetalol
    (c) Yohimbine
    (d) Butoxamine

192. Alpha 1a (α₁ₐ) adrenergic blocker providing symptomatic relief in BPH is: *(Recent NEET Pattern Question)*
    (a) Tamsulosin   (b) Prazosin
    (c) Doxazosin   (d) Tolazoline

193. Alpha I blocker without any effect on blood pressure is: *(Recent NEET Pattern Question)*
    (a) Tamsulosin   (b) Prazosin
    (c) Doxazosin   (d) Terazosin

194. Beta blockers are contraindicated in: *(Recent NEET Pattern Question)*
    (a) Decompensated CHF   (b) Asthma
    (c) Variant angina   (d) All of the above

195. Which β₁ selective blocker is used in glaucoma? *(Recent NEET Pattern Question)*
    (a) Levobunolol   (b) Timolol
    (c) Betaxolol   (d) Carteolol

196. Propranolol is useful for all of the following *except*: *(Recent NEET Pattern Question)*
    (a) Angina
    (b) Familial tremor
    (c) Hypertension
    (d) Partial AV block

197. Beta-adrenoceptor blocking agent that should be avoided in patients with renal failure is: *(Recent NEET Pattern Question)*
    (a) Atenolol   (b) Metoprolol
    (c) Propranolol   (d) Esmolol

198. Which one of the following drugs does not induce mydriasis? *(Recent NEET Pattern Question)*
    (a) Phentolamine   (b) Ephedrine
    (c) Phenylephrine   (d) Cocaine

199. Patients taking a β-adrenergic receptor blocking drug may experience all of the following *except*: *(Recent NEET Pattern Question)*
    (a) Exacerbation of existing heart block
    (b) Precipitation of heart failure
    (c) Nasal blockage
    (d) Cold extremities

200. Beta blocker with peripheral vasodilator action is: *(Recent NEET Pattern Question)*
    (a) Propranolol   (b) Carvedilol
    (c) Atenolol   (d) Acebutolol

201. A hypertensive patient has heart rate of 50 beats/min and taking tablet atenolol 200 mg/day in divided doses. After anesthesia, heart rate further fell down to 40 beats/min. What will be the appropriate treatment to improve heart rate? *(Recent NEET Pattern Question)*
    (a) IV adrenaline   (b) IV atropine
    (c) IV isoprenaline
    (d) Dobutamine infusion intravenously

202. Which drug is contraindicated in a glaucoma patient suffering from bronchial asthma? *(Recent NEET Pattern Question)*
    (a) Timolol maleate (b) Latanoprost
    (c) Betaxolol   (d) Brimonidine

203. A 33-year-old patient with history of asthma is being treated for symptoms of hypertension. Which of the following beta blocker would be an appropriate therapy for this patient? *(Recent NEET Pattern Question)*
    (a) Isoprenaline   (b) Labetalol
    (c) Metoprolol   (d) Propranolol

204. Propranolol is not used in: *(Recent NEET Pattern Question)*
    (a) A-V block
    (b) Hypertension
    (c) Hypertrophic obstructive cardiomyopathy
    (d) Migraine

Explanations

1. **Ans. (a) Bethanechol** *(Ref: KDT 8th/e p115)*
   Among the given options only bethanechol is used for treatment of post-operative urinary retention.
   - Bethanechol is mainly used for its action on urinary bladder and has no nicotinic activity. Therefore used in post-operative urinary retention. It can cause bronchospasm due to stimulation of M3 receptors on the bronchus. Therefore, it is avoided in patients with respiratory diseases like asthma and COPD
   - Methacholine has maximum action on myocardium. It can be given inhalationally for the diagnosis of bronchial hyper-reactivity in patients who do not have clinically apparent asthma. It is known as methacholine challenge test.
   - Terazosin and Tamsulosin are used in benign prostatic hypertrophy. Tamsulosin is being investigated for prevention of postoperative urinary retention. However, it has no role in treatment of postoperative urinary retention.

2. **Ans. (a) Latanoprost** *(Ref: KDT 8th/e p168)*

Mechanism of action of topical antiglaucoma drugs				
Drug/ class	Example	Aqueous secretion	Trabecular outflow	Uveo-scleral outflow
β- blockers	Timolol	↓	–	–
Sympatho-mimetics	Adrenaline Dipivefrine	↓	↑	↑
Alpha 2 agonists	Apraclonidine Brimonidine	↓	–	↑
Prostaglandins	Latanoprost	–	–	↑
Miotics	Pilocarpine	–	↑	–
Carbonic anhydrase inhibitors	Dorzolamide Brinzolamide	↓	–	–

3. **Ans. (b) Atropine** *(Ref: KDT 8th/e p122)*
   - Low esterase levels are suggestive of overdose of drug inhibiting acetyl choline esterase like organophosphate poisoning.
   - Inhibition of choline esterase results in cholinergic symptoms like salivation, lacrimation, urination, emesis, increased bronchial secretions, and reduction in blood pressure. So treatment of choice is Atropine.
   - **Atropine:** It is highly effective in counter-acting the muscarinic symptoms, but higher doses are required to antagonize the central effects. It does not reverse peripheral muscular paralysis which is a nicotinic action. All cases of anti-ChE (carbamate or organophosphate) poisoning must be promptly treated with atropine 2 mg IV repeated every 10 min till dryness of mouth or other signs of atropinization appear (up to 200 mg has been administered in a day). Continued treatment with maintenance doses may be required for 1-2 weeks.
   - Neostigmine and physostigmine worsens the signs and symptoms as these also act by inhibiting cholinesterase.
   - Physostigmine and flumazenil are respectively used for Atropine and benzodiazepines poisoning.

4. **Ans. (d) Dexamethasone** *(Ref: KDT 8th/e p318, 167, 170)*
   - Dexamethasone is a corticosteroid. Corticosteroids are contraindicated in glaucoma, as they result in further increase in the intraocular pressure.
   - Mannitol is drug of choice for acute congestive glaucoma by intravenous route. Mannitol decongest the eye by its osmotic action.
   - Methazolamide is a carbonic anhydrase inhibitor and clonidine is an alpha 2 agonist. These can also cause decrease in intraocular pressure.

Topical drugs for glaucoma				
β-Adrenergic blockers	α-Adrenergic agonists	Prostaglandin analogues	Carbonic anhydrase inhibitors	Miotics
Timolol	Dipivefrine	Latanoprost	Dorzolamide	Pilocarpine
Betaxolol	Apraclonidine	Travoprost	Brinzolamide	Physostigmine
Levobunolol	Brimonidine	Bimatoprost		Echothiophate
Carteolol				

5. **Ans. (a) By decreasing the rate of diastolic depolarization of SA node** *(Ref: KDT 8th/e p114)*
   - Spontaneous diastolic depolarization (Phase 4 of action potential) of SA node is required for automaticity of SA node.
   - By decreasing the slope of phase 4, acetylcholine decreases the rate of impulse generation and thus decreases heart rate.
   - ACh decreases the AV conduction by increasing the refractory period of AV node and His-Purkinje fibres.

6. **Ans. (a) Edrophonium** *(Ref: KDT 8th/e p120)*
   - Patients with myasthenia gravis may present in the emergency with muscle weakness. This could be because of the aggravation of their primary problem (myasthenic crisis) or due to the overdose of the drugs like neostigmine (cholinergic crisis). The etiology of the two conditions is important to understand because in myasthenic crisis, there is deficiency of acetylcholine whereas in cholinergic crisis, there is excess of acetylcholine.
   - Edrophonium is an inhibitor of the enzyme acetylcholinestrase and thus, increases the concentration of acetylcholine at the neuromuscular junction. The increased availability of ACh causes dramatic improvement in the symptoms of patients with myasthenic crisis.
   - In contrast, the symptoms of patients with cholinergic crisis worsen with edrophonium (because it further increases ACh in cholinergic crisis). The drug, therefore, is useful to clinically differentiate the actual cause of muscle weakness in an emergency situation.
   - The reason for preferring edrophonium over other inhibitors of acetyl cholinesterase is its short duration

of action. This may be *desirable for patients presenting with cholinergic crisis as the the worsening in their condition would be only for a short time.*

7. **Ans. (b) Brimonidine** *(Ref: Goodman and Gilman 13th/e p1259)*

Brimonidine causes CNS depression in newborn babies and can result in apnea, so it is contraindicated in such patients.

Ocular adverse effects of anti-glaucoma drugs

Drug	Adverse Effect
Miotics (Pilocarpine)	Cataract Stenosis of nasolacrimal system
PGF2 analogs (Latanoprost)	Heterochromia iridis Growth of eyelashes Cystoid macular edema
Apraclonidine	Lid retraction
Brimonidine	CNS depression and apnea in newborn
Adrenaline	Conjunctival pigmentation

8. **Ans. (a) Edrophonium** *(Ref: KDT 8th/e p120)*
   - Patients with myasthenia gravis may present in the emergency with muscle weakness. This could be because of the aggravation of their primary problem (myasthenic crisis) or due to the overdose of the drugs like neostigmine (cholinergic crisis). The etiology of the two conditions is important to understand because in myasthenic crisis, there is deficiency of acetylcholine whereas in cholinergic crisis, there is excess of acetylcholine.
   - Edrophonium is an inhibitor of the enzyme acetylcholinestrase and thus, increases the concentration of acetylcholine at the neuromuscular junction. The increased availability of ACh causes dramatic improvement in the symptoms of patients with myasthenic crisis.
   - In contrast, the symptoms of patients with cholinergic crisis worsen with edrophonium (because it further increases ACh in cholinergic crisis). The drug, therefore, is useful to clinically differentiate the actual cause of muscle weakness in an emergency situation.
   - The reason for preferring edrophonium over other inhibitors of acetylcholinesterase is its short duration of action. This may be *desirable for patients presenting with cholinergic crisis as the worsening in their condition would be only for a short time.*

9. **Ans. (b) Brimonidine**
   (Ref: Goodman and Gilman 13th/e p1259)
   Brimonidine causes CNS depression in newborn babies and can result in apnea, so it is contraindicated in such patients.

Ocular adverse effects of anti-glaucoma drugs

Drug	Adverse Effect
Miotics (Pilocarpine)	Cataract Stenosis of nasolacrimal system
PGF2 analogs (Latanoprost)	Heterochromia iridis Growth of eyelashes Cystoid Macular Edema
Apraclonidine	Lid retraction
Brimonidine	CNS depression and apnea in newborn
Adrenaline	Conjunctival pigmentation

10. **Ans. (b) Cholinergic** *(Ref: Katzung 13th/90; KDT 8th/e p112)*
    Postsynaptic receptors on the ganglia are NM receptors which are cholinergic.

    - All preganglionic fibres (Both sympathetic as well as parasympathetic) secrete ACh
    - Post-ganglionic parasympathetic fibres secrete ACh.
    - Post-ganglionic sympathetic fibres secrete mostly nor-adrenaline.

11. **Ans. (b) M2** *(Ref: Goodman Gillman 12th/e p; Katzung 12th/e p100; KDT 8th/e p113)*
    Methacholine is a non-selective muscarinic agonist. It has maximum agonist action on M2 receptors.
    Relatively selective agonist of cholinergic receptors are:
    - M1 selective: Oxotremorine
    - M2 selective: Methacholine
    - M3 selective: Bethanechol

12. **Ans. (d) Competitive and irreversible** *(Ref: Goodman Gillman 12th/e p242; Katzung 12th/e p106; KDT 8th/e p110)*
    Both organophosphates and carbamates cause competitive inhibition of acetylcholineesterase by binding to esteratic site. However organophosphates are irreversible and most carbamates (except carbaryl and propoxur) are reversible inhibitors. Thus, the type of inhibition of acetyl cholinesterase caused by organophosphates is competitive & irreversible.

13. **Ans. (d) Partial heart block** *(Ref: KDT 8th/e p119-122)*
    - Cholinergic drugs decrease the conduction from atrium to ventricle, thus should be avoided in partial heart block
    - Cholinergic drugs like pilocarpine and physostigmine are used in angle closure glaucoma
    - Neostigmine (acetylcholinesterase inhibitor, a cholinergic drug) is used for treatment of myasthenia gravis
    - Neostigmine is also used for post operative paralytic ileus and post operative urinary retention.

14. **Ans. (b) Pilocarpine** *(Ref: Katzung 13/e p161)*
    Miotics-like pilocarpine act by increasing the trabecular outflow.

Drugs for Glaucoma	Mechanism of Action
Brimonidine	Reducing aqueous production and Increasing uveoscleral flow
Latanoprost	Increase the uveoscleral outflow
Pilocarpine	Increases trabecular outflow
Betaxolol	Reduces aqueous secretion by ciliary body

15. **Ans. (a) Brimonidine: Decreases aqueous production** *(Ref: KDT 8th/e p168)*

Drug	Mechanism of action in glaucoma
Apraclonidine/Brimonidine	Decrease aqueous production
Latanoprost	Increase uveoscleral outflow
Miotics (Pilocarpine)	Increase trabecular outflow
Beta blockers (Timolol/betaxolol)	Decrease aqueous production
Carbonic anhydrase inhibitors (acetazolamide)	Decrease aqueous secretion.

16. **Ans. (b) Bradycardia** *(Ref: KDT 8th/e p114)*
    Cholinomimetic drug will cause bradycardia as an adverse effect and thus cannot be used for its treatment.

Autonomic Nervous System

17. Ans. (a) Organophosphate poisoning
(Ref: Katzung 12/e p110)
These are characteristic features of anti-cholinestearse (organophosphate and carbamate) poisoning.
Features of Organophosphate poisoning:
- **Muscarinic symptoms:** Pin point pupil, salivation, lacrimation, urination, defecation, gastrointestinal distress, vomiting, bronchospasm, bradycardia
- **Nicotinic symptoms:** Fasciculations and fibrillations of muscle, tachycardia, tachypnea
- **CNS symptoms:** Temors, giddiness, ataxia, coma
- **Red tears:** Due to accumulation of porphyrin in the lacrimal glands

18. Ans. (c) Cholinergic *(Ref: Katzung 10/e p76; KDT 8th/e p104)*
- Autonomic ganglia (both sympathetic as well as parasympathetic) release ACh that stimulates the N_N nicotinic receptors on the post-ganglionic fibres.

19. Ans. (b) VI *(Ref: Katzung 10/e p75; KDT 8th/e p105)*
- Parasympathetic system is craniosacral in outflow. Cranial part involves III (oculomotor), VII (facial), IX (glossopharyngeal) and X (vagus) nerves whereas sacral portion includes S2 to S4.

20. Ans. (b) Noradrenaline
(Ref: Katzung 10/e p76; KDT 8th/e p104)
- Neurotransmitter secreted at end organ effectors of sympathetic system is mostly nor-adrenaline (except in sweat glands and hair follicle, where it is acetylcholine) whereas it is acetyl-choline at parasympathetic system.

21. Ans. (d) Metoprolol
(Ref: Katzung 10/e p103, 152; KDT 8th/e p162)
- Metoprolol is a beta blocker with local anaesthetic activity. Such beta blockers are not indicated in glaucoma.
- Apraclonidine (alpha 2 agonist), timolol (beta blocker without local anaesthetic activity) and pilocarpine (directly acting miotic) are used in glaucoma.

22. Ans. (b) Brimonidine
(Ref: Goodman & Gilman 12/e p1788; KDT 8th/e p168)
- Apraclonidine and brimonidine can cross blood brain barrier and may result in CNS depression and apnea in neonates. These are therefore contra-indicated in children less than 2 years.

23. Ans. (d) It interferes with the action of acetyl cholinesterase *(Ref: Katzung 11/e p105)*
Neostigmine acts by inhibiting the enzyme acetylcholinesterase. This enzyme is involved in degradation of ACh, consequently neostigmine increases the synaptic level of ACh. Muscle weakness can be improved by stimulation of N_M receptors at muscle end plate due to increased ACh.

24. Ans. (c) Cause muscles to relax and be unable to contract
(Ref: KDT 8th/e p375)
Drugs competing with ACh at neuromuscular junction are competitive or non-depolarizing neuromuscular blockers. These drugs are used as muscle relaxants. In contrast to depolarizing muscle relaxants, these do not cause initial fasciculations.

25. Ans. (d) Memantine *(Ref: KDT 8th/e p518-19)*
- Donepezil, rivastigmine, gallantamine and tacrine are cholinergic (due to inhibition of cholinesterase enzyme) drugs useful for Alzheimer's disease.
- Memantine is an NMDA blocker, used for Alzheimer's disease.

26. Ans. (d) Quaternary structure *(Ref: KDT 8th/e p116)*
Quaternary ammonium compounds are water soluble and thus cannot cross blood brain barrier. Neostigmine is a quaternary derivative whereas physostigmine is a tertiary amine.

27. Ans. (d) Therapy with pralidoxime should ideally be monitored by measuring blood cholinesterase concentration.
(Ref: KDT 6/e p105, Drug facts and comparisons 2010/599)
- Pralidoxime is ACh esterase reactivator used for organophosphate poisoning.
- Blood cholinesterase levels can be used to monitor therapy, however RBC cholinesterase levels better reflect ACh esterase activity than serum or plasma levels because *with chronic exposure to organophosphates, serum levels may return to normal but RBC levels remain depressed.*
- Chlorinated pesticides like DDT are CNS stimulants and their overdose is treated by diazepam like drugs. Pralidoxime has no role in their treatment.
- Nerve gases used in warfare act by inhibiting acetyl cholinesterase. Atropine and oximes are used for their treatment.
- When atropine and pralidoxime are used together, the signs of atropinization may occur earlier than might be expected when atropine is used alone.

28. Ans. (a) Tacrine *(Ref: KDT 8th/e p119, 518)*
Because of hepatotoxicity, and requirement of frequent dosing, tacrine is less often used than other agents.

29. Ans. (b) Esteratic site of AChEs *(Ref: KDT 8th/e p123)*
- The active region of Acetylcholinesterase (AChE) has two sites, i.e. an anionic site and an esteratic site. Anticholinesterase poisoning like Organophosphate compounds binds to esteratic site of AChE.

30. Ans. (b) Edrophonium *(Ref: KDT 8th/e p121)*
- Drug used in ameliorative test (**tensilon test**) for myasthenia gravis is *edrophonium*. It is a cholinergic drug and can be used for diagnosis of myasthenia gravis *because of its short duration of action (10 – 30 min.)*

31. Ans. (d) Is a competitive antagonist of acetylcholine
(Ref: KDT 8th/e p122)
Atropine acts as an antagonist at muscarinic receptors. It has no activity on nicotinic receptors and do not interfere with the release of ACh.

32. Ans. (c) Malathion Poisoning *(Ref: KDT 8th/e p123)*
- Pralidoxime is cholinesterase reactivator useful for organophosphate (malathion, parathion) poisoning.

33. Ans. (b) Opiates *(Ref: KDT 8th/e p120, 501)*
Causes of Pin-Point Pupil

- Opioids Poisoning
- Organophosphate Poisoning
- Carbamate Poisoning
- Carbolic acid Poisoning
- Pontine Hemorrhage

34. Ans. (c) Neostigmine *(Ref: KDT 8th/e p120)*

35. Ans. (a) Pralidoxime *(Ref: Katzung 11/e p121; KDT 8th/e p123)*

36. **Ans. (b) Carbamate poisoning**
    (Ref: Katzung 11/e p106-107; KDT 8th/e p123)
37. **Ans. (c) Rapidly destroyed in the body** *(Ref: Katzung 11/e p97)*
38. **Ans. (c) Acetylcholine** *(Ref: KDT 8th/e p104-105)*
39. **Ans. (a) Edrophonium** *(Ref: KDT 8th/e p119)*
40. **Ans. (c) Physostigmine** *(Ref: KDT 8th/e p119)*
41. **Ans. (a) Physostigmine** *(Ref: KDT 8th/e p120)*
42. **Ans. (c) Brimonidine** *(Ref: KDT 8th/e p168)*
43. **Ans. (b) Betaxolol** *(Ref: KDT 8th/e p168)*
44. **Ans. (b) Parathion** *(Ref: KDT 8th/e p123)*
45. **Ans. (c) Decreasing breakdown of acetylcholine**
    (Ref: KDT 8th/e p101)
46. **Ans. (c) Edrophonium**
    (Ref: KDT 8th/e p116, Katzung 11/e p104)
    Physostigmine, neostigmine and pyridostigmine are carbamates by chemical nature, whereas edrophonium is an alcohol.
47. **Ans. (a) Aminoglycosides** *(Ref: KDT 8th/e p795)*
    Aminoglycosides can result in neuromuscular blockade that can aggravate myasthenia gravis.
48. **Ans. (b) Neuromuscular junction** *(Ref: Katzung 11/e p98)*
    Bethanechol acts on muscarinic receptors only whereas physostigmine increases ACh, thus can stimulate both muscarinic and nicotinic receptors. Neuromuscular junction contains N_M receptors, thus will be affected by physostigmine but not by bethanechol.
49. **Ans. (a) Pralidoxime** *(Ref: KDT 8th/e p123)*
    Oximes are ineffective in carbamate poisoning. Rather, these can worsen the poisoning due to weak anticholinesterase activity of its own.
50. **Ans. (b) Carbaryl** *(Ref: KDT 8th/e p123)*
51. **Ans. (d) Absence of pulmonary secretions**
    (Ref: emedicine.medscape.com)
52. **Ans. (b) Shorter acting than edrophonium**
    (Ref: KDT 8th/e p116-121)
53. **Ans. (a) Bronchial smooth muscle** *(Ref: KDT 8th/e p113)*
54. **Ans. (d) Naltrexone** *(Ref: KDT 8th/e p122-123)*
55. **Ans. (c) Organophosphate poisoning** *(Ref: KDT 8th/e p123)*
56. **Ans. (d) Pralidoxime** *(Ref: KDT 8th/e p123)*
57. **Ans. (c) Increasing aqueous humor outflow**
    (Ref: KDT 8th/e p170)
58. **Ans. (d) Sympathetic cholinergic** *(Ref: KDT 8th/e p104)*
59. **Ans. (b) Tachycardia** *(Ref: KDT 8th/e p114)*
60. **Ans. (d) Myasthenic ptosis** *(Ref: KDT 7/e p110)*
61. **Ans. (b) Latanoprost**
    (Ref: Katzung 12th/e p328; KDT 8th/e p169)
    PGF2a agonists like Latanoprost can cause iris pigmentation (heterochromia iridis) and growth of eyelashes (hypertrichosis) as adverse effects.
62. **Ans. (b) Belladona** *(Ref: KDT 8th/e p115,122,127,499)*
    Miosis or pin point pupil is caused by:
    - Organophosphate poisoning
    - Opioids like morphine
    - Phenol poisoning
    - Pontine hemorrhage
    - Cholinergic drugs like pilocarpine

    Belladona is a plant (Atropa belladona) from which atropine (Anticholinergic drug) is obtained. It causes mydriasis not miosis.

63. **Ans. (d) Inj atropine** *(Ref: KDT 8th/e p131)*
    - We need to immediately reverse the bradycardia by giving atropine.
64. **Ans. (d) Endrin** *(Ref: KDT 7/e p105)*
    Endrin is an organochlorine whereas all other drugs in the options like baygon (contains carbaryl), Tik 20 (contains diazinon) and parathion are acetylcholinesterase inhibitors (organophosphates or carbamates). Atropine is drug of choice for anticholinesterase poisoning. There is no specific antidote for organochlorine poisoning.
65. **Ans. (c) Glycopyrrolate** *(Ref: KDT 8th/e p124)*
    The structure of tertiary and quaternary amines can be depicted as

Tertiary amine	Quarternary amine
R–C–R with R above	R–C–R with R above and R below, with ⊕ charge

    - As seen in the diagram, quarternary amines are ionized and thus water soluble. These drugs are not able to cross the blood brain barrier.
    - Atropine, hyoscine and physostigmine are tertiary amines (thus lipid soluble) and can cross the blood brain barrier whereas glycopyrrolate is quaternary amine and cannot cross blood brain barrier.
66. **Ans. (b) Glycopyrrolate** *(Ref: KDT 8th/e p124)*
    - Glycopyrrolate is a quaternary ammonium compounds and is thus water soluble and unable to penetrate BBB.
67. **Ans. (a) Closure of Ca++ channels at the presynaptic membrane** *(Ref: Katzung 10/e p90; KDT 8th/e p110)*
    Botulinum toxin acts by inhibiting the calcium mediated exocytosis of ACh from the vesicles in the synapse.
68. **Ans. (b) Tropicamide** *(Ref: Katzung 11/e p124)*
    Atropine is longest acting (5-6 days) whereas tropicamide is the shortest acting (15-60 min) mydriatic.
69. **Ans. (c) Muscarinic receptor inhibition**
    (Ref: KDT 8th/e p124)
    - Oxybutynin is a synthetic anticholinergic agent.
70. **Ans. (a) Increase bowel sound** *(Ref: KDT 8th/e p132)*
    - Atropine is an anticholinergic drug. It decreases bowel sounds.
71. **Ans. (c) Excessive salivation** *(Ref: KDT 8th/e p132)*
    Atropine is an *anticholinergic drug*. Its toxicity causes:
    - *Dry mouth* (and not excessive salivation)
    - Hot skin
    - Dilated pupil and photophobia
    - Excitement
    - Flushing of skin
    - Hypotension → cardiovascular collapse
    - Convulsions and coma

Autonomic Nervous System

72. **Ans. (a) Hyoscine** *(Ref: KDT 8th/e p132)*
    Hyoscine is used for the prophylaxisof motion sickness whereas other drugs listed in the question are used for the treatment of vomiting.

73. **Ans. (d) Increased bowel sounds** *(Ref: KDT 8th/e p132)*
    Atropine is an anticholinergic drug. It will decrease GI motility. Atropine flushing is seen in overdose, the exact mechanism of which is not known.

74. **Ans. (a) Mydriasis is required without cycloplegia**
    (Ref: KDT 8th/e p148)

75. **Ans. (d) Pirenzepine** *(Ref: KDT 8th/e p112)*

76. **Ans. (d) Phenylepherine** *(Ref: KDT 8th/e p148)*

77. **Ans. (b) Inhibition of sweating** *(Ref: KDT 8th/e p108)*

78. **Ans. (a) Muscarinic** *(Ref: KDT 6/e p111)*

79. **Ans. (c) Neostigmine** *(Ref: KDT 8th/e p119)*

80. **Ans. (a) Atropine** *(Ref: KDT 8th/e p131)*

81. **Ans. (a) Mucous and pharyngeal secretions**
    (Ref: KDT 8th/e p125, 126)

82. **Ans. (c) Bradycardia** *(Ref: KDT 8th/e p126)*

83. **Ans. (a) Glaucoma** *(Ref: KDT 8th/e p132)*

84. **Ans. (c) To prevent overdosage and discourage opioid dependence** *(Ref: KDT 8th/e p733)*

85. **Ans. (c) Presynaptic blockade** *(Ref: KDT 8th/e p110)*

86. **Ans. (b) Bronchoconstriction** *(Ref: KDT 8th/e p126)*

87. **Ans. (c) Timolol eye drops** *(Ref: CMDT 2014/175)*

88. **Ans. (c) Hypothermia** *(Ref: KDT 8th/e p132)*
    Atropine poisoning is associated with hyperthermia (not hypothermia)

89. **Ans. (b) Atropine** *(Ref: KDT 8th/e p132)*

90. **Ans. (d) Glaucoma** *(Ref: KDT 8th/e p132)*

91. **Ans. (d) Trimethaphan** *(Ref: KDT 8th/e p135)*

92. **Ans. (a) 0.5 mL of 1:1000 adrenaline by intramuscular route** *(Ref: KDT 8th/e p97)*
    Features like rash on skin, hypotension, and difficulty in breathing are suggestive of anaphylactic shock.
    In case of anaphylactic shock the resuscitation council of UK has recommended the following measures:
    - Put the patient in reclining position, administer oxygen at high flow rate and perform cardiopulmonary resuscitation if required.
    - Inject adrenaline 0.5 mg (0.5 mL of 1 in 1000 solution for adult, 0.3 mL for child 6–12 years and 0.15 mL for child up to 6 years) im; repeat every 5–10 min in case patient does not improve or improvement is transient. This is the only life saving measure. Adrenaline should not be injected IV (can itself be fatal) unless shock is immediately life-threatening. If adrenaline is to be injected IV, it should be diluted to 1:10,000 and infused slowly with constant monitoring.
    - Administer a H1 antihistaminic (pheniramine 20–40 mg or chlorpheniramine 10–20 mg) IM/slow IV. It may have adjuvant value.
    - Intravenous glucocorticoid (hydrocortisone sodium succinate 200 mg) should be added in severe/recurrent cases. It acts slowly, but is especially valuable for prolonged reactions and in asthmatics. It may be followed by oral prednisolone for 3 days.

93. **Ans. (c) Vasopressin** *(Ref: Harrison 19th/1769)*

94. **Ans. (d) Vasoconstriction** *(Ref: KDT's 8th/140)*

95. **Ans. (c) Topiramate** *(Ref: FDA New drugs)*

96. **Ans. (b) Chlorpropamide** *(Ref: Harrison's 19th/e pg. 2397)*

97. **Ans. (c) Intravenous** *(Ref: Harrison's 19th/e pg.1769)*

98. **Ans. (a) Beta 1 and Beta 2 agonist** *(Ref: KDT 7th/e p130)*
    The features shown are:
    Tachycardia (due to beta 1 stimulation), increase in systolic BP (due to beta 1 stimulation), decrease in diastolic BP (due to beta 2 stimulation) and tremors (due to beta 2 stimulation). From these features, it seems the drug is beta 1 and beta 2 agonist.

99. **Ans. (a) Adrenaline 0.5 mL of 1:1000 solution by intramuscular route** *(Ref: Harrison 19th/e p2117)*
    - Drug of choice for anaphylactic shock is adrenaline.
    - Route of choice is intramuscular > subcutaneous
    - Concentration of choice is 1:1000
    - If repeated injections by intramuscular route are not effective, then intravenous adrenaline (1:10000) is given

100. **Ans. (c) High dose adrenaline followed by alpha 1 block**
     (Ref: KDT 7th/e p131)
     Vasomotor reversal of Dale is fall in blood pressure noted with high dose of adrenaline when the person is treated with alpha blockers. It is due to un-opposed beta 2 action.

101. **Ans. (b) The effect on heart rate in graph A can be prevented by anti-muscarinic agents**
     (Ref: Goodman and Gilman 12th/283)
     Decoding the graph
     Drug A: It increases systolic as well as diastolic BP and cause bradycardia. These properties suggest that it is nor-epinephrine. Increased BP lead to reflex bradycardia due to vagal stimulation. This reflex decrease in heart rate can be prevented by anti-muscarinic drugs like atropine. After giving atropine, same dose of nor-epinephrine produces tachycardia instead of bradycardia because of its direct action only.
     Drug B: It increases systolic BP, slighltly decreases diastolic BP and cause tachycardia. These features suggest the drug to be epinephrine.
     Drug C: It increases systolic BP, markedely decreases diastolic BP and cause severe tachycardia. These findings suggest drug C to be isoproterenol (isoprenaline).

102. **Ans. (a) 8** *(Ref: See below)*
     Amount of dopamine required to be infused (@10 micro/kg/min) = 80 × 10
     $$= 800 \text{ micro g/min}$$
     $$= 0.8 \text{ mg/min}$$
     Amount of dopamine in 250 mL of solution
     $$= 200 \text{ mg} \times 2$$
     $$= 400 \text{ mg}$$
     Amount of dopamine in 1 mL solution
     $$= 400/250 \text{ mg}$$
     $$= 1.6 \text{ mg}$$

Or
1.6 mg dopamine present in
= 1 mL solution
0.8 mg dopamine present in
= 0.5 mL solution
So, solution should be infused @ 0.5 mL per min.
As 1 mL = 16 drops
So, infusion should be started at 8 drops per min.

103. **Ans. (b) Presynaptic alpha 2 receptors**
(Ref: Katzung 13th/148-149)
Action of adrenaline in anaphylactic shock by different receptors is

Receptor	Action	Use
Alpha 1	Vasoconstriction	Increase in diastolic BP
Beta 1	Cardiac stimulation	Increase systolic BP
Beta 2	Bronchodilation	Reverse bronchoconstriction

104. **Ans. (a) Phentolamine followed by adrenaline**
(Ref: KDT 8th/e p143)
Intravenous injection of adrenaline normally causes increase in blood pressure (α effect) followed by prolonged fall (β_2 effect). If it is administered after giving α blockers (like phentolamine), only fall in BP is seen. This is called *vasomotor reversal of Dale*.

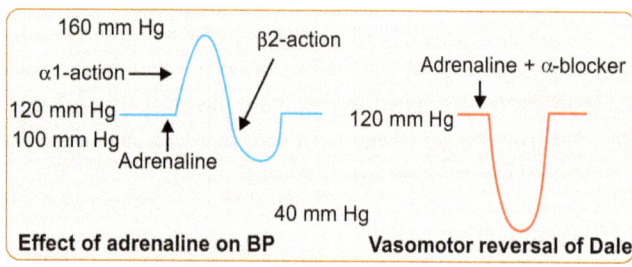

105. **Ans. (d) Alpha 1 receptors** *(Ref: Katzung 13th/142, 144)*
Dopamine is used in CHF for its stimulatory effects on beta 1 receptors. It has dose dependent effects as follows

Receptor stimulated	Action	Dose required
D1	Renal vasodilation	1–2 µg/kg/min
β_1	Cardiac stimulation	2–10 µg/kg/min
α_1	Vasoconstriction	> 10 µg/kg/min

Therefore, in CHF, it is used at a dose of 2-10 mcg/kg/min. Thus, dopamine stimulates D1 and beta 1 receptors but not alpha 1 receptors.

106. **Ans. (b) Increases renal blood flow**
(Ref: Goodman Gilman 12th/e p355; KDT 8th/e p146)
Dopamine has dose dependent actions
Low dose (1-2 mcg/kg/min): It stimulates only D1 receptors leading to renal vasodilation and thus increase in renal blood flow.
Medium dose (2-10 mcg/kg/min): It stimulates both D1 and beta 1 receptors means it will lead to inotropic action also.
High dose (>10 mcg/kg/min): It stimulates D1, beta 1 and alpha 1 receptors resulting in additional vasoconstriction.

107. **Ans. (d) Beta-3** *(Ref: KDT 8th/e p139, 142)*
Beta-3 receptors are present on adipose tissue (cause lipolysis), coronary artery (cause vasodilation) and on urinary bladder (cause relaxation).

108. **Ans. (a) Centrally acting α_2 agonist**
(Ref: KDT 8th/e p412, Katzung 12th/445)
Dexmedetomidine is a highly selective central α_2- adrenergic agonist (like clonidine). It is the active S-enantiomer of medetomidine (used in veterinary medicine).

109. **Ans. (b) Hyperalgesia** *(Ref: Goodman and Gilman 12th/296; Katzung 12th/176; KDT 8th/e p140)*
- Alpha 2 agonists cause analgesia, not the hyperalgesia.
- Clonidine is used for treatment of hypertension. It decreases blood pressure by acting on central alpha-2 adrenergic receptors.
- Dexmedetomidine is another alpha-2 receptor agonist that is used to produce sedation and anxiolytic state by action on alpha 2 receptors in the brain. It can also produce analgesia by acting on alpha-2 receptors in spinal cord.

110. **Ans. (c) Epinephrine**
(Ref: Goodman and Gilman 12th/277; KDT 8th/e p142)
- Epinephrine is having both alpha (1 and 2) and beta (1 and 2) agonist property.
- Dobutamine stimulates only beta 1 whereas phenylephrine acts only on alpha 1 receptors.
- Fenoldopam does not act on alpha or beta receptors, rather it is D1 agonist.

111. **Ans. (c) Phenylephrine** *(Ref: Harrison /18th/e p377-378)*
Alpha blockers are used in erectile dysfunction not alpha agonists (phenyephrine).

Drugs useful in the management of erectile dysfunction (ED)

• Phosphodiesterase inhibitors
  – *Sildenafil*
  – *Vardenafil*
  – *Tadalafil*
  – *Udenafil*
• PGE_1 analog – Alprostadil
• Aviptadil

112. **Ans. (b) 1 : 1000 for inhalational route**
(Ref: Drug Facts and Comparisons, 2010/837)
For inhalational route, adrenaline is used in a concentration of 1:100 for treatment of bronchial asthma by nebulizer.

Concentration of adrenaline for different routes and indications

Route and Indication	Concentration of Adrenaline required
Bronchial asthma, inhalational	1:100
Anaphylactic shock, intramuscular	1:1000
Anaphylactic shock, subcutaneous	1:1000
Anaphylactic shock, intravenous	1:10000
Cardiac arrest, intravenous	1:10000
With Local anaesthetics, subcutaneous	1:200000

Autonomic Nervous System

113. Ans. (a) Stimulation of lipolysis
(Ref: Katzung 10/e p86; KDT 8th/e p139)
Lipolysis is mediated by β_3 receptors whereas other actions are done by stimulation of β_2 receptors.

114. Ans. (a) Hypertensive emergencies
(Ref: Katzung 10/e p133, 174)
- Fenoldopam is a D_1 agonist useful for i.v. treatment of hypertensive emergencies.

115. Ans. (b) Conversion of tyrosine to DOPA
(Ref: Katzung 10/e p78; KDT 8th/e p136)
- Rate limiting enzyme in norepinephrine synthesis is tyrosine hydroxylase that catalyses the conversion of tyrosine to dopa. In ACh synthesis, rate limiting step is uptake of choline by the neurons.

116. Ans. (a) Renal vasodilatory effect *(Ref: Katzung 11/e p137)*
Dopamine acts on D_1, β_1 and α_1 receptors. Stimulation of D_1 receptors cause renal vasodilation, which is useful clinically to improve renal perfusion in shock with oliguria.

117. Ans. (c) Ephedrine *(Ref: KDT 8th/e p147)*
- Ephedrine acts directly as well as indirectly through release of nor-adrenaline. Latter increases systolic (β_1) as well as diastolic (α_1 action) blood pressure. This is due to lack of β_2 mediated vasodilation.
- Adrenaline transiently increase diastolic BP which later on decreases due to its β_2 stimulatory action.

118. Ans. (a) The usual dose is 0.5-1 mg by IM route
(Ref: KDT 8th/e p150)

- Adrenaline 0.5 ml of 1:1000 solution (i.e., 0.5 mg) by i.m. route is drug of choice for anaphylactic shock. It can also be used by s.c. route
- If not responding, it can be repeated after 5 minutes (not 2-4 hours). In desperate circumstances i.v. route can be used but it must be diluted 10 times (i.e., 1:10000 concentration is used), therefore same solution cannot be utilized, However, in rare circumstances, i.v. adrenaline can result in cerebral hemorrhage due to uncontrolled rise in blood pressure.

119. Ans. (d) 1-2 µg/kg/min *(Ref: Harrison 17th/1453)*

Dose of Dopamine	Effects
1-2 micro gm/kg/min	Renal vasodilation (Renal dose)
2-10 micro gm/kg/min	Stimulates β-1 receptors of heart
> 10 µ gm/kg/min	Stimulates peripheral α receptors leading to vasoconstriction

120. Ans. (a) 120 seconds *(Ref: Lawrence 9/e p453)*
Dobutamine is an inotropic drug which has onset of action = 1-2 min.
Peak action = 1-10 min.
Duration of action = < 10 min.
Half life = 2 min.

121. Ans. (c) Sedation *(Ref: KDT 8th/e p243)*
- Side effects of salbutamol:
  1. Palpitation
  2. Muscle tremors
  3. Hypokalemia
  4. Nervousness
  5. Ankle edema

122. Ans. (b) Subcutaneous adrenaline *(Ref: KDT 8th/e p150)*

123. Ans. (c) Reuptake *(Ref: KDT 8th/e p137)*
Endogenous adrenaline action is terminated mainly by reuptake whereas exogenous agent is metabolized by COMT and MAO.

124. Ans. (b) Anaphylactic shock *(Ref: KDT 8th/e p150)*

- Epinephrine is the agent of choice for the treatment of anaphylactic shock. It increases BP by α action and causes bronchodilation by β_2 action.
- For bronchial asthma, selective β_2 agonists like salbutamol are preferred.
- For glaucoma, a prodrug of epinephrine, dipivefrine is useful (as adrenaline cannot cross corneal membrane).
- Treatment for PVD is α blockers.

125. Ans. (b) COMT *(Ref: KDT 8th/e p137)*
Endogenous adrenaline action is terminated mainly by reuptake whereas exogenous agent is metabolized by COMT and MAO.

126. Ans. (a) α_1 receptors are usually presynaptic
(Ref: KDT 8th/e p140)
Presynaptic sympathetic receptors are usually α_2. Other statements are true.

127. Ans. (a) Dopamine *(Ref: KDT 8th/e p146)*
128. Ans. (b) Yohimbine *(Ref: KDT 8th/e p140)*
129. Ans. (a) Adrenaline *(Ref: KDT 8th/e p143)*
130. Ans. (a) α_2 *(Ref: KDT 8th/e p612)*
131. Ans. (b) β_2 selectivity *(Ref: KDT 8th/e p243)*
132. Ans. (b) Diastolic *(Ref: KDT 8th/e p143)*
133. Ans. (a) Tremors *(Ref: KDT 8th/e p242)*
134. Ans. (b) ADHD (attention deficit hyperkinetic disorder)
(Ref: KDT 8th/e p152)
135. Ans. (a) Agonist of D_1 and D_2 receptors
(Ref: KDT 8th/e p147)
136. Ans. (a) Adenyl cyclase *(Ref: KDT 8th/e p55)*
137. Ans. (a) α blocker *(Ref: KDT 8th/e p143)*
138. Ans. (a) Reserpine *(Ref: KDT 8th/e p614)*
139. Ans. (d) Gastrointestinal sphincter contraction
(Ref: KDT 8th/e p140)
140. Ans. (a) Isoprenaline *(Ref: KK Sharma 1/e p172)*
141. Ans. (c) Can produce CNS stimulation *(Ref: KDT 8th/e p611)*
142. Ans. (d) All of the above *(Ref: KDT 8th/e p611-612)*
143. Ans. (a) Ephedrine *(Ref: Katzung 11/e p134)*
144. Ans. (b) Cardiac output *(Ref: KDT 8th/e p147)*
145. Ans. (a) Causes increase in GI Ischemia *(Ref: KDT 7th/134)*
Dopamine causes vasodilation in renal and splanchnic vessels by stimulating D_1 receptors.

146. Ans. (a) Adrenaline *(Ref: KDT 8th/e p143)*
147. Ans. (b) Alpha 2 *(Ref: KDT 8th/e p611)*
148. Ans. (b) Fludrocortisone *(Ref: CMDT 2014/941)*

149. Ans. (d) Intramuscular (Ref: KDT 8th/e p150)
150. Ans. (d) Tyrosine (Ref: KDT 8th/e p140)
151. Ans. (d) Greater than 10 µg/kg/min (Ref: KDT 8th/e p146)
152. Ans. (c) Beta 1 (Ref: KDT 8th/e p142)
153. Ans. (a) Clonidine (Ref: KDT 8th/e p140)
154. Ans. (b) Ephedrine (Ref: KDT 8th/e p147)
155. Ans. (d) Phenylephrine (Ref: KDT 8th/e p148)
156. Ans. (b) Obesity (Ref: KDT 8th/e p149)
157. Ans. (d) Methylphenidate (Ref: KDT 8th/e p152)
158. Ans. (b) Bradycardia with AV block (Ref: KDT 8th/160)
    - Beta blockers like metoprolol depress the heart. They decrease the heart rate, conduction as well as contractility
    - Calcium channel blockers like verapamil and diltiazem also depress the heart.
    - Beta blockers should never be combined with verapamil or diltiazem due to additive cardiac depression leading to severe bradycardia and AV block.
159. Ans. (a) Prazosin (Ref: Harrison 20th/e p3329)
    - Scorpion sting is a dreadful medical emergency.
    - Scorpion stings cause a wide range of symptoms, from severe local reactions to cardiovascular, respiratory and neurological manifestations.
    - Alpha-receptors play vital role in the pathogenesis of cardiac failure and pulmonary edema due to scorpion sting.
    - Prazosin is a selective alpha-1 adrenergic receptor blocker. It dilates veins and arterioles, thereby reducing pre-load and left ventricular impedance without rise in heart rate and renin secretion. It also inhibits sympathetic outflow in central nervous system. It enhances insulin secretion, which is inhibited by venom action. It has also been found useful even in cases with hypotension. Thus, its pharmacological properties can antagonize the hemodynamic, hormonal and metabolic effects of scorpion venom action.
160. Ans. (b) 1.5-2.5 kg (Ref: Practical Manual of Pharmacology by Dinesh Badyal 1st ed/75)

    > Important points regarding rabbits used in pharmacological studies
    > - **Scientific name:** *Oryctalagus cuniculus*
    > - **Adult weight:** 1.5-2.5 Kg
    >   Age suitable for experiment: 5-6 months

161. Ans. (a) Adrenaline
    Adrenaline is oxidized to produce adrenochrome which can cause black pigmentation of conjunctiva. Remember pigmentation of iris is caused by latanoprost
162. Ans. (a) Epinephrine (Ref: KDT 8th/e p114, 144)
    Pilocarpine is a parasympathomimetic drug. It causes contraction of sphincter pupillae and result in miosis. Epinephrine results in contraction of dilator pupillae and result in mydriasis.
163. Ans. (a) Adrenaline (Ref: Goodman Gilman 12th/e p188, 285; Katzung 12th/e p90; KDT 8th/e p144)
    Decrease in tone, amplitude and frequency of intestinal contractions seen in the graph depicts the drug to be a depressant drug. Important depressants drugs on intestinal smooth muscle are sympathomimetics like adrenaline and directly acting drugs like papaverine. As the depressant effect of the drug was abolished by propranolol, it must be mediated by beta receptors. So, the likely drug among the options seem to be adrenaline.
164. Ans. (c) Lupus erythematosus (Ref: KDT 8th/e p156-157)
    Prazosin is a selective α_1 blocker and can be used for treatment of pheochromocytoma, peripheral vascular disease, benign hyperplasia of prostate and hypertension. It is the drug of choice for scorpion sting.
165. Ans. (d) Propranolol (Ref: Goodman & Gilman 11/e p286)
166. Ans. (d) Timolol (Ref: Katzung 11/e p157)
167. Ans. (d) Prazosin (Ref: Harrison 17/e p2752)
    Prazosin is used for treatment of scorpion sting.
168. Ans. (a) Hypothyroidism (Ref: KDT 8th/e p164-165)
    - Beta blockers are used to treat hyperthyroidism (not hypothyroidism).
    - These are the only drugs that offer prophylactic benefits in a patient of varices who has never bled.
169. Ans. (b) Variant angina (Ref: KDT 8th/e p161)
    - **Propranolol worsens variant angina, due to unopposed α receptor mediated coronary constriction.**
    - For indications of β-blockers, refer to text.
170. Ans. (b) Parkinsonian tremor (Ref: KDT 8th/e p164)
    Propranolol is useful in the management of tremor due to overdose of sympathomimetic agents (β_2 mediated). Metoprolol as well as propranolol are effective in *essential or familial tremor* (β_1 *mediated*). β-blockers are ineffective in intention tremor and rest (parkinsonian) tremors.
171. Ans. (c) COPD (Ref: KDT 8th/e p160-161)
    Timolol is a non-selective β-blocker. It can prevent β_2 mediated bronchodilation and thus worsen the condition in patients of bronchial asthma and COPD.
172. Ans. (b) Partial heart block (Ref: KDT 8th/e p160-161)
    β-blockers are contraindicated in partial or complete heart block as they cause bradycardia.
173. Ans. (c) Butoxamine (Ref: Katzung 11/e p160)
174. Ans. (c) Masks the hypoglycemic symptoms
     (Ref: CMDT 2010/402)
175. Ans. (a) Esmolol (Ref: KDT 8th/e p163)
176. Ans. (c) Tamsulosin (Ref: KDT 8th/e p156)
177. Ans. (d) All (Ref: KDT 8th/e p160)
178. Ans. (a) Carvedilol (Ref: KDT 8th/e p165)
179. Ans. (a) Propranolol (Ref: Katzung 11/e p 162)
180. Ans. (a) Esmolol is mainly metabolized in liver
     (Ref: KDT 8th/e p141)
181. Ans. (a) α_{1A} (Ref: KDT 8th/e p156)
182. Ans. (d) Pindolol (Ref: KDT 8th/e p162)
183. Ans. (b) Phenoxybenzamine (Ref: KDT 8th/e p154-155)
184. Ans. (c) Hydrolysis by blood esterase (Ref: KDT 8th/e p141)
185. Ans. (d) All of above (Ref: KDT 8th/e p160-161)

Autonomic Nervous System

186. **Ans. (d) Phenoxybenzamine binding to alpha adrenergic receptor** *(Ref: Katzung 10/e p16; KDT 8th/e p154-155)*
     - Phenoxybenzamine is an irreversible (covalent) antagonist at alpha receptors. All other drugs mentioned are reversibly interacting with their receptors.
187. **Ans. (a) Atenolol** *(Ref: KDT 8th/e p153)*
188. **Ans. (a) Acute CHF** *(Ref: KDT 8th/e p160)*
189. **Ans. (c) Pindolol** *(Ref: KDT 8th/e p158)*
190. **Ans. (a) Atropine** *(Ref: KDT 8th/e p160)*
     - **Dopamine, adrenaline and isoprenaline** act by *stimulating β1 receptors* in heart. As patient has β-blocker overdose, these are likely to be ineffective
     - **Atropine** can increase heart rate in this person by *blocking parasympathetic* action on heart.
191. **Ans. (c) Yohimbine** *(Ref: KDT 8th/e p156)*
192. **Ans. (a) Tamsulosin** *(Ref: KDT 8th/e p156)*
193. **Ans. (a) Tamsulosin** *(Ref: KDT 8th/e p156)*
194. **Ans. (d) All of the above** *(Ref: KDT 8th/e p160-161)*
195. **Ans. (c) Betaxolol** *(Ref: KDT 8th/e p168)*
196. **Ans. (d) Partial AV block** *(Ref: KDT 8th/e p161)*
197. **Ans. (a) Atenolol** *(Ref: KDT 8th/e p162-163)*
198. **Ans. (a) Phentolamine** *(Ref: KDT 8th/e p155)*
199. **Ans. (c) Nasal blockage** *(Ref: KDT 8th/e p160-161)*
200. **Ans. (b) Carvedilol** *(Ref: KDT 8th/e p165)*
201. **Ans. (b) IV atropine** *(Ref: KDT 8th/e p131)*
202. **Ans. (a) Timolol maleate** *(Ref: KDT 8th/e p167)*
203. **Ans. (c) Metoprolol** *(Ref: KDT 8th/e p161)*
204. **Ans. (a) AV block** *(Ref: KDT 8th/e p161)*

Autacoids

CHAPTER 3

These are the substances produced by wide variety of cells that act locally at the site of production. Autacoids are classified as

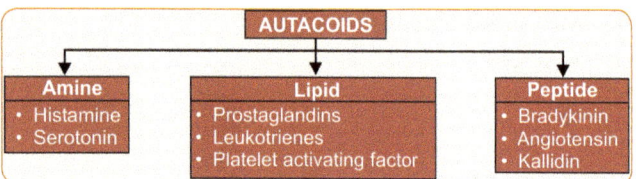

HEREDITARY ANGIONEUROTIC EDEMA (HAE)

It is a condition characterized by recurrent attacks of severe swelling that may affect arms, legs, face, GIT and airway. The pathophysiology mainly involves deficient or dysfunctional C1 inhibitor protein. As the name suggests, C1 inhibitor is involved in inhibition of various proteases in Complement, Coagulation and Contact pathways. Normally, the level of bradykinin remains low because C-1 inhibitor interferes with activity of factor XIIa and plasma kallikrein. Therefore, in patients with C-1-inhibitor deficiency, bradykinin level increases and is responsible for HAE. Various drugs can be used to treat or prevent the attacks of HAE. These include:

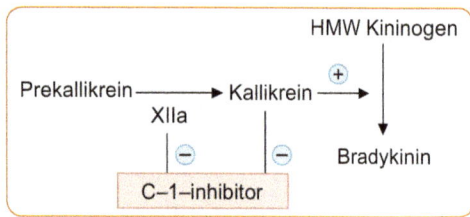

- **C-1 inhibitor replacement:** Various preparations of C-1 inhibitors are available for long-term prophylaxis or for short-term use before surgery or dental procedures. Many plasma derived preparations can be used. Recombinant C-1-inhibitors like **conestat-alpha** and **Ruconest** have been approved for HAE.

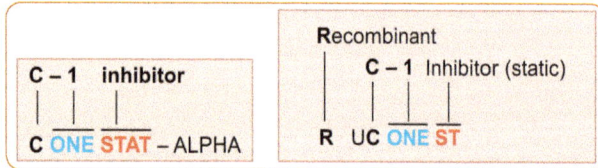

- **Kallikrein inhibitors: Ecallantide, Lanadelumab** and **Berotralstat** are the drugs that decrease bradykinin by inhibiting kallikrein. Ecallantide is approved for treatment of HAE whereas other drugs are used for long-term prophylaxis of HAE.

- **Bradykinin antagonist: Icatibant** is a bradykinin B-2 receptor antagonist and is approved for treatment of HAE.

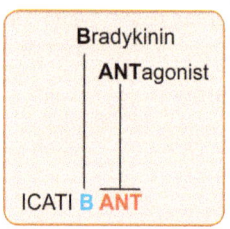

- **Androgens:** Androgens increase the level of C-1-inhibitor. Therefore drugs like **danazol** and **stanozolol** can be used for long-term prophylaxis of HAE.

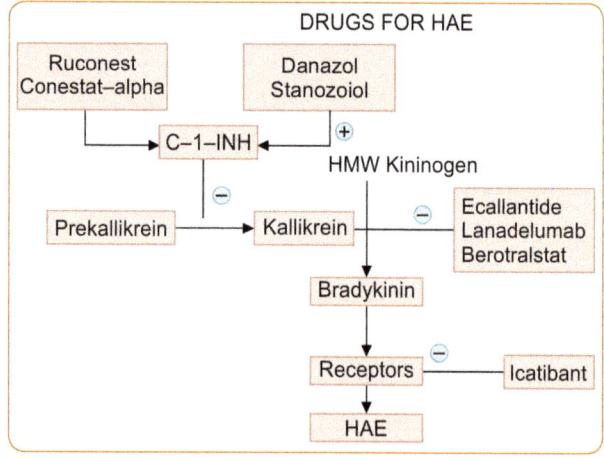

HISTAMINE

Histamine is *synthesized from histidine* and is stored within the storage granules of mast cells. It acts mainly on H_1 and H_2 receptors. Recently H_3 (presynaptic) and H_4 receptors have also been isolated.

Actions

- It causes dilation of small blood vessels and can result in *flushing and hypotension*. Fall in blood pressure is mediated by both H_1 (early; by release of NO) as well as H_2 (delayed and persistent; direct action on smooth muscles of blood vessels) receptors.
- Histamine is a powerful contractor of visceral smooth muscles through H_1 receptors and results in *bronchocons-triction and abdominal cramps*.
- Histamine *increases gastric secretion* by stimulation of H_2 receptors.

- Histamine synthesized within the brain *stimulates reticular activating system and maintains wakefulness* (through H_1 receptors).
- **H_3 receptors** are pre-synaptic in location and inhibit the release of histamine. Inverse agonist or antagonist of these receptors may increase histamine leading to wakefulness. **Pitolisant (tiprolisant)** is such a drug approved for **Narcolepsy**.
- **H_4 receptors** are present in hematopoietic cells like eosinophils, basophils and mast cells. These promote chemotaxis.

Antagonists of these receptors are being developed for allergic conditions.
- Histamine serves as a *mediator of inflammation and immediate type of hypersensitivity reactions*
  - **Betahistine** is an oral histamine analogue used *to control vertigo* in Meniere's disease
  - Some **basic drugs** like *d-tubocurarine, morphine, atropine, vancomycin and polymyxin B etc. may result in histamine release.*

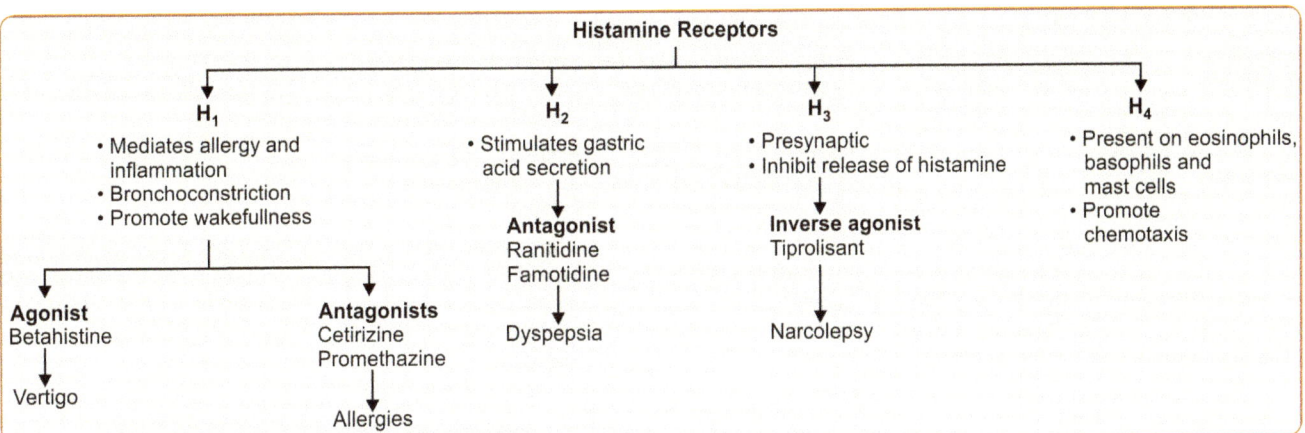

H_1 ANTI-HISTAMINICS

These drugs act as competitive antagonists at H_1 receptors. These may be classified into first generation and second generation compounds on the basis of CNS penetration and anticholinergic properties.

(a) First Generation Anti-histaminics

These drugs *can penetrate blood brain barrier* and thus result in sedation and psychomotor impairment. Therefore, these drugs are *contraindicated in persons requiring constant attention* (like truck drivers, machinery operators and swimmers).

Another property of first generation compounds is the presence of *anticholinergic activity*. This property is responsible for their wide spectrum of uses and more adverse effects than second generation compounds. First generation drugs may be classified as:

Highly sedating	Moderately sedating	Mildly sedating
Diphenhydramine	Pheniramine	Chlorpheniramine
Dimenhydrinate	Cyproheptadine	Mepyramine
Promethazine	Meclizine	Cyclizine
Hydroxyzine	Buclizine	Clemastine
Doxepin	Cinnarizine	

Uses

Based on H_1 blocking action	Based on anticholinergic properties	
1. Allergic conditions like itching, urticaria, hay fever etc.	Possess Anti-dystonia	- Parkinsonism - Acute muscular
2. Insect bite, ivy poisoning and to prevent the adverse effects due to histamine releasers	Cholinergic Properties	- Common cold - Prophylaxis of motion sickness

Adverse Effects

Major adverse effects of first generation agents are *sedation, psychomotor impairment and anticholinergic effects* (dryness of mouth, blurred vision, urinary retention, constipation etc.)

(b) Second Generation Anti-histaminics

These drugs have little CNS penetration (do not cause sedation) and do not possess anticholinergic activity. Some drugs like cetirizine and azelastine possess additional anti-allergic mechanisms. These drugs *lack sedation* (can be used in truck drivers) *and anticholinergic adverse effects* but their use is also restricted to antiallergic effects.

Important Drugs

- **Terfenadine** is the fastest acting antihistaminic drug. In overdose, it blocks cardiac delayed rectifier K^+ channels and may result in polymorphic ventricular tachycardia (torsades de' pointes) manifested as prolongation of QTc interval. Use of this drug with microsomal enzyme inhibitors like ketoconazole, erythromycin, clarithromycin and itraconazole increases the risk of this arrhythmia. Terfenadine is metabolized to an active metabolite **"fexofenadine"** (available as a separate drug) that lacks K^+ channel blocking property.
- **Astemizole** is **slowest and longest** acting agent and possesses arrhythmogenic property similar to terfenadine. Therefore, it should not be administered with ketoconazole, erythromycin, clarithromycin and itraconazole.
- *Loratidine* is another *long acting* second generation antihistaminic and is metabolized to *desloratidine* (available as a separate drug).
- *Cetirizine* is an active metabolite of a first generation antihistaminic drug, hydroxyzine. *All second generation antihistaminics are metabolized to active products except cetirizine and mizolastine.* It possesses additional anti-allergic mechanisms like inhibition of release of cytotoxic mediators from platelets and inhibition of chemotaxis. Some persons acquire sedative effects with cetirizine. *Levocetirizine* is l-isomer of cetirizine that is more potent and less sedative.
- *Azelastine* possesses *maximum topical activity* and can be given by nasal spray for allergic rhinitis.
- *Mizolastine, ebastine, levocabastine, rupatidine, acrivastine* and *olopatadine* are other second generation antihistaminic agents.

- **Olopatadine** is a recently approved topical H_1-antihistaminic used as nasal spray for seasonal allergic rhinitis.
- **Alcaftadine** is approved as ophthalmic solution for allergic conjunctivitis.
- Some authorities describe the term **3rd generation antihistaminics** for the active enantiomer (like levocetirizine) or metabolite (e.g. desloratidine and fexofenadine) of 2nd generation drugs.

SEROTONIN				
5 HT_1		**5 $HT_{2A/2C}$**	**5 HT_3**	**5 HT_4**
5 HT_{1A}	5 $HT_{1B/1D}$			
Presynaptic autoreceptor	Cause constriction of cranial vessels	Responsible for most of the direct actions of serotonin	**Ionotropic receptor** (all others 5 HT receptors are G-protein coupled receptors)	Present in GIT Responsible for the increase in peristalsis
Modulates the release of serotonin		Ketanserin and ritanserin (antagonists) are useful as antihypertensive agents	Mediates most of the reflex and indirect actions of serotonin	
Partial agonist of this receptor *(buspirone, ipsapirone, gepirone)* are useful as **antianxiety drugs**	**Agonists** at this receptor *(sumatriptan, naratriptan)* are useful for the treatment of **acute migraine** attacks	Clozapine and risperidone are atypical antipsychotic agents that act through antagonistic activity at this receptor.	**Antagonists** like *ondansetron, grainsetron and* tropisetron are the agents of choice for **chemotherapy induced vomiting**	**Agonists** (cisapride, mosapride, renzapride, tegaserod) are useful in the treatment of gastroesophageal reflux disease

5-hydroxytryptamine (5HT; serotonin) is synthesized from tryptophan. It acts by activation of several serotonin receptors (5- HT_1 - HT_7 receptors).

RECEPTORS

5HT receptors include $5HT_1$, $5HT_2$, $5HT_3$, $5HT_4$, $5HT_5$, $5HT_6$ and $5HT_7$.

Non-selective Drugs

- **Cyroheptadine**: It blocks 5 HT_{2A}, H_1 and muscarinic receptors. It increases appetite and can be used in children to *promote weight gain*.
- **Methysergide**: It is a 5 $HT_{2A/2C}$ antagonist and a 5 HT_1 agonist. It is indicated for the *prophylaxis of migraine* attacks but prolonged use *can result in pulmonary, endocardial and retroperitoneal fibrosis*.
- **LSD**: It is an ergot derivative and a *powerful hallucinogen*. It acts as an agonist at several serotonin receptors including 5 HT_{1A}, 5 $HT_{2A/2C}$ and 5 HT_{5-7} receptors.
- **Flibanserin** is a new drug approved for hypoactive sexual desire disorder in premenopausal women. It is $5HT_{1A}$ receptor agonist and $5HT_{2A}$ receptor antagonist.
- **Lorcaserin** is $5HT_{2C}$ agonist indicated in obesity.

Ergot Alkaloids

These are derived from a fungus *Claviceps purpurea*. Important compounds are *ergotamine, ergometrine (ergonovine), ergotoxine, bromocriptine, dihydroergotamine and methysergide*. These drugs possess partial agonistic and antagonistic effect at 5HT, α and dopaminergic receptors. **These drugs are only α blockers that can cause vasoconstriction** due to their partial agonistic activity on α and $5HT_2$ receptors (maximum with ergotamine). **Hydrogenation of the compound decreases α agonistic activity but increases the α blocking potential**. Therefore dihydroergotamine has very little vasoconstricting activity. Ergot derivatives *can cause dry gangrene of hand and feet as well as coronary vasospasm*.

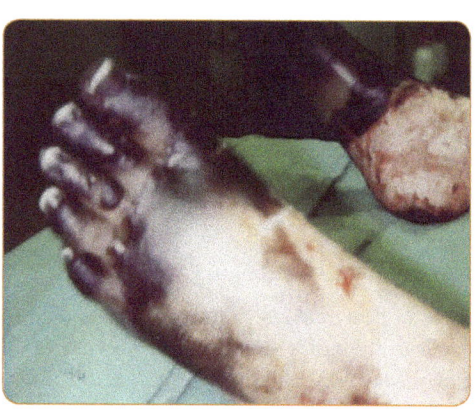

FIG. 3.1: Ergot induced gangrene

- **Ergotamine and dihydroergotamine** are used for the treatment of *acute attack of migraine*. These are *contraindicated in patients with ischemic heart disease* (due to their propensity to cause coronary vasospasm).
- **Dihydroergotoxine** (codergocrine) is useful for the treatment of *dementia*.
- **Bromocriptine** is useful in *Parkinsonism, hyperprolactinemia and acromegaly*.
- **Methysergide** is useful for the *prophylaxis of migraine attacks*.

MIGRAINE

It is unilateral pulsatile headache due to dilation and inflammation of the affected cerebral vessels. **Calcitonin Gene-related Peptide (CGRP)** is assumed to be the principal mediator of neurogenic inflammation of migraine and vasodilation seen in migraine. Mild and moderate attacks of migraine are usually controlled by NSAIDs whereas severe attacks require ergot alkaloids or triptans for termination.

- **Ergotamine** (*oral/sublingual*) or dihydroergotamine (*parenteral*) can be used **to abort acute attack of migraine**. Caffeine *enhances the absorption* of ergotamine and is a *powerful vasoconstrictor*. It is usually combined with ergotamine. These drugs however, *increase the nausea and vomiting during migraine attack*.

- *Sumatriptan (subcutaneous) is the drug of choice for aborting acute attack of migraine.* It acts as a selective agonist at $5HT_{1B/1D}$ receptors. It also suppresses the vomiting of migraine. It is a short acting drug and has low oral bioavailability. *Frovatriptan is the longest acting and rizatriptan is the fastest acting congener.* Other drugs useful are *zolmitriptan, eletriptan, naratriptan and almotriptan*. All of these drugs can cause **coronary vasospasm** and are *contraindicated in ischemic heart disease*. Triptans are also contra-indicated in patients with *hypertension, epilepsy, pregnancy, liver and renal impairment. Triptans and ergotamine should not be administered within 24 hours of each other.*
- **Pharmacokinetic properties** of triptans:

	Maximum	Minimum
Oral bioavailability	Naratriptan	Sumatriptan
Duration of action	Frovatriptan (Longest)	Sumatriptan (Shortest)
Onset of action	Rizatriptan (Fastest)	Frovatriptan (Slowest)
Plasma protein binding	Eletriptan	Sumatriptan
Potency	Naratriptan	Sumatriptan

- For patients with history of CAD, triptans or ergotamine are contra-indicated, therefore opioids like **intranasal butorphanol** should be used for acute severe migraine. If not controlled, these can be treated by droperidol and last resort is propofol.
- **Prophylaxis of migraine** is required if the attacks are frequent (>2-3 per month). The *drugs useful for prophylaxis are:*

> - **Propranolol is the most commonly used drug** for prophylaxis of migraine attacks. Timolol, atenolol, metoprolol and nadolol can also be used but the drugs with ISA (e.g. pindolol) are ineffective.
> - Calcium channel blockers like **flunarizine** (also blocks Na^+ channels) is also effective. Diltiazem, verapamil and nimodipine can also be used.
> - **Methysergide, cyproheptadine and TCAs** like amitriptyline, imipramine and nor-triptyline can also be used.
> - **Clonidine** can be used orally for the prophylaxis of migraine attacks.
> - **Topiramate** (anticonvulsant drug) has recently been approved for prophylaxis of migraine Valproate and gabapentin also possess some prophylactic activity.
> - **Onabotulinum toxin A** has recently been approved for prophylaxis when headaches occur for more than 14 days per month. It is given every 12 weeks as multiple injections around the head and neck to try to dull future headache symptoms.
> - **Candesartan** can also be used for migraine prophylaxis
> *(Ref CMDT 2015 pg 956)*

NEW DRUGS FOR MIGRAINE

Recently three group of drugs have been approved for migraine. These include $5HT_{1F}$ agonists **(ditans)**, CGRP receptor antagonists **(gepants)** and monoclonal antibodies against CGRP receptor.

- **$5HT_{1F}$ agonists: Lasmiditan** is a prototype drug in this group. 'Ditans' act by stimulating $5HT_{1F}$ receptor and thus inhibiting release of CGRP. Unlike 'triptans', these drugs do not cause vasoconstriction directly and therefore are unlikely to cause coronary vasospasm. These are **given orally** for acute attack of migraine.
- **CGRP receptor antagonists:** The drugs in this group are called **gepants** (calcitonin GEne related Peptide ANTagonists). The approved drugs are **rimegepant** and **ubrogepant**. These are **given orally** for acute attack of migraine.
- **Monoclonal antibodies against CGRP receptor:** These are given by **subcutaneous** route for *prophylaxis* of migraine. The drugs in this group include **Erenumab, Galcanezumab, Fremanezumab** and **Eptinezumab** (approved as slow IV infusion also).

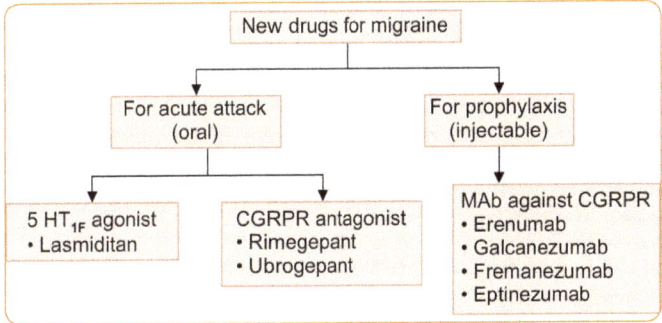

Monoclonal antibodies against CGRP have recently been approved for prophylaxis of migraine. All these are given subcutaneously. The approved drugs in this category are:
- Erenumab
- Galcanezumab
- Fremanezumab
- Eptinezumab

PROSTAGLANDINS

Prostaglandins and thromboxanes are synthesized from arachidonic acid (obtained from membrane phospholipids due to the action of phospholipase A_2; rate limiting enzyme) with the help of enzyme cyclooxygenase (COX).

COX-1	COX-2	COX-3
• Consitutive (Always present in Cells) • Serves house-keeping function e.g. gastro-protection	• Inducible (Synthesis Simulated by endotoxins and other inflammatory mediators) • Participates in inflammation • Constitutive in brain, endothelium and kidney • Pro-carcinogenic due to inhibitory activity on apoptosis, stimulation of cell migration and invasiveness.	• Recently isolated from cerebral cortex • Involved in pain perception and fever • Not involved in inflammation • Paracetamol targets COX-3

COX acts on arachidonic acid to produce cyclic endoperoxides (PGG_2/PGH_2) in all cells. Further fate of these compounds depends on the presence of different enzymes in the cells. *Platelets contain thromboxane synthetase and results in the production of TXA_2 whereas vascular endothelium contains prostacyclin synthase and thus produces PGI_2.* Various cells contain enzyme isomerase and can convert cyclic endoperoxides to PGD_2, PGE_2 and $PGF_{2\alpha}$. **Corticosteroids** inhibit the enzyme phospholipase A_2 by *inducing the production of lipocortins (Now known as annexins).* **NSAIDs** *decrease PG and TX production by inhibiting COX.*

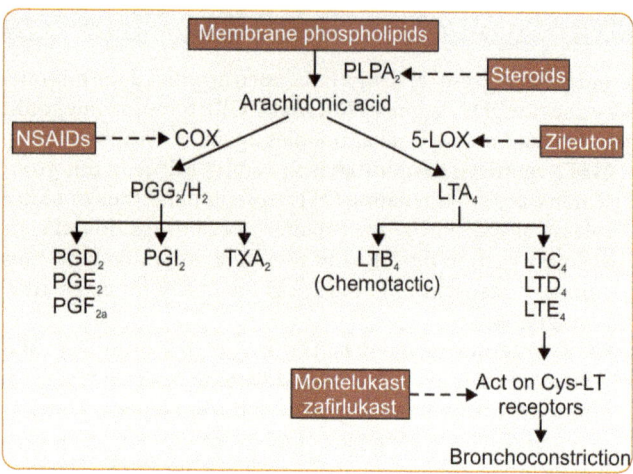

ACTIONS

CNS

PGE₁ and PGE₂ are pyrogenic and cause fever. NSAIDs act as antipyretic agents by inhibiting these PGs.

Peripheral Nerve Endings

PGE₂ and PGI₂ sensitize pain receptors to various mediators. NSAIDs act as analgesics by decreasing the synthesis of PGs.

CVS

- PGE₂ and PGI₂ are vasodilators whereas PGF₂ₐ and TXA₂ are vasoconstrictor agents. *Epoprostenol (PGI₂) and treprostinil (longer acting PGI₂ analogue) can be used for the treatment of pulmonary hypertension.*
- PGE₂ increases capillary permeability.
- PGE₂ and PGI₂ keeps ductus arteriosus patent. In some congenital heart diseases (like transposition of great vessels), it becomes essential **to keep ductus arteriosus patent** before surgery. For this indication, *alprostadil* (PGE₁) *and epoprostenol* (PGI₂) *can be given intravenously.* If ductus arteriosus fails to close (**patent ductus arteriosus**) at birth, *NSAIDs like aspirin and indomethacin are given to close it.*

Platelets

- *PGI₂ inhibits platelet aggregation whereas TXA₂ is a potent aggregator of platelets.* Non-selective COX inhibitors inhibit the generation of both of these compounds. TXA₂ is synthesized in platelets and its synthesis cannot be resumed, once it is inhibited by **NSAIDs** (because platelets lack nuclei) whereas synthesis of PGI₂ resumes after sometime (endothelial cells can synthesize new COX). Net result of this process is inhibition of TXA₂ synthesis and *platelet anti-aggregation.*
- **Low dose aspirin** can be used as an *antiplatelet* drug for the prophylaxis of MI and stroke.
- *Epoprostenol* (PGI₂) can be used as an *anti-aggregatory drug in dialysis and cardiopulmonary bypass.* It can also be used for storage of platelets for transfusion.

⚠ MNEMONIC

PGI₂ Inhibits platelet aggregation whereas TXA₂ is a potent aggregator of platelets.

Uterus

- PGE₂ and PGF₂ₐ are powerful uterine stimulants (contractor). *Dinoprostone (PGE2) intravaginally and carboprost (PGF₂ₐ) intraamniotic injection can be used for inducing mid trimester abortion.* **Misoprostol (PGE₁)** along with methotrexate or mifepristone is used **for induction of abortion in first few weeks of pregnancy.**
- PGE₂ causes softening of cervix (cervical ripening) during labour. *Dinoprostone or misoprostol intravaginally are employed for cervical ripening during labour.*
- *Carboprost (PGF₂ₐ)* can be used to *control post partum hemorrhage* (contraction of uterus leads to compression of blood vessels resulting in decreased bleeding).
- PGs are responsible for pain during menstruation (*dysmenorrhoea*) and NSAIDs like *mefenamic acid* are useful for relieving this pain.
- Use of *misoprostol in pregnancy* is associated with *moebius syndrome* (abnormal development of cranial nerves; most commonly VI and VII).

Bronchus

- PGI₂ and PGE₂ are bronchodilators and TXA₂ and PGF₂ₐ are bronchoconstrictor agents.
- *Aerosolized PGE₂* has been used effectively *to abort acute attacks of asthma.*
- COX inhibitors like aspirin cause more production of LTs (because due to enzyme inhibition arachidonic acid now produces only LTs). *Aspirin can result in precipitation of asthma attacks* because LTs are the main bronchoconstricting mediators in human asthma.

GIT

- PGE₂ and PGI₂ decrease acid secretion and increase mucus production and mucosal blood flow. All these factors decrease the chances of peptic ulcer. NSAIDs on long term use can precipitate PUD due to inhibition of PG synthesis.
- *Misoprostol is the most specific drug for the treatment of peptic ulcer due to chronic NSAID use.* [Remember, the drug of choice is proton pump inhibitors]
- PGE₂ and PGF₂ₐ cause *diarrhea and colicky pain* in the abdomen. These symptoms are important side effects of these drugs.
- PG seems to play some role in colonic cancer. *Regular use of aspirin or celecoxib decreases the risk of colonic polyps and cancers.*

Kidney

- PGE₂ and PGI₂ cause *renal vasodilation, natriuresis* and increased water clearance due to inhibition of the action of ADH. These agents also *facilitate renin release.*
- Loop diuretics act partly by increasing the stimulation of COX; therefore *NSAIDs attenuate the diuretic action* of these drugs.
- **Bartter syndrome** is characterized by *excess PGs* leading to *hyperreninemia, excess aldosterone and the resultant hypokalemia and alkalosis.* **Indomethacin** is used for *treatment of this syndrome.*

Male Reproductive System

PGE₂ and PGI₂ increases sperm motility and enhances penile erection. *Alprostadil can be used to treat erectile dysfunction.*

Eye

$PGF_{2\alpha}$ decreases intraocular pressure **by increasing the uveoscleral outflow.** Latanoprost ($PGF_{2\alpha}$) is being used as eye drops for glaucoma. *Bimatoprost, travaprost and unoprostone are new prostaglandin analogues for this indication.*

LEUKOTRIENES

These are synthesized from arachidonic acid with the help of the enzyme, 5-lipoxygenase. This enzyme must associate with **5-lipoxygenase activating protein (FLAP)** for leukotriene synthesis. First step is the production of LTA_4 that is converted either to LTB_4 or to cysteinyl leukotrienes (LTC_4, D_4 and E_4). LTC_4 *and* LTD_4 are also known as **slow reacting substance of anaphylaxis (SRS-A)** due to their powerful bronchoconstricting action. LTB_4 *is a powerful chemotactic agent* and is an important mediator of all types of inflammation.

Action of LTs can be inhibited by:
- *Corticosteroids* (decrease the production of LTs by inhibiting phospholipase A_2)
- Lipoxygenase inhibitors (*zileuton*)
- LT receptor antagonists (*zafirlukast, montelukast, iralukast*)

NON STEROIDAL ANTI INFLAMMATORY DRUGS (NSAIDS)

NSAIDs act by inhibiting COX enzyme and thus prostaglandin synthesis. These drugs act as antipyretic, analgesic and anti-inflammatory agents. Prostaglandins play a protective role in the stomach and non-selective COX inhibitors can cause GI toxicity (peptic ulcer) on long term use.

CLASSIFICATION

- Non selective COX inhibitors (inhibit both COX 1 and COX 2)
- Preferential COX 2 inhibitors (inhibitory activity on COX 2 is greater than COX 1)
- Selective COX 2 inhibitors

Non-selective COX Inhibitors

(a) Paracetamol (Acetaminophen)

- It **does not possess anti-inflammatory activity** because it is ineffective in the presence of peroxides generated at the site of inflammation. Other explanation offered is **selective COX 3 inhibition** in the brain.
- It is thought that the analgesic action of paracetamol may be attributed to **activation of vanilloid receptors** (TRPV1) by its metabolite.
- It produces **very little GI toxicity** and can be administered in patients intolerant to other NSAIDs.
- It is metabolized to N-acetyl paraaminobenzo quinoneimine (NAPQ) by microsomal enzymes. This metabolite has high affinity for sulfhydryl groups and can combine with the enzymes and other biomolecules resulting in **hepatotoxicity**.
- Normally acetaminophen is a safe drug because glutathione (contain sulfhydryl group due to presence of sulfur containing amino acid, cysteine) produced by the liver combines with NAPQ to detoxify it. However **chronic alcoholics are predisposed to toxicity** because:
  - Glutathione production decreases due to liver disease.
  - Alcohol is a powerful inducer of microsomal enzymes. It increases the production of NAPQ from acetaminophen resulting in toxicity.

Acetaminophen toxicity can be decreased by providing sulfhydryl donors like *N-acetylcysteine* (*antidote of choice*). Gastric lavage (with activated charcoal) should be done to prevent further absorption but it is **ineffective after 4 hours** of ingestion.

(b) Salicylates

Aspirin is the only **irreversible inhibitor** of COX enzyme (other salicylates are reversible inhibitors). Apart from antipyretic, analgesic and anti inflammatory effects, aspirin has several other indications.

- At low doses (40–325 mg), it acts as an *antiplatelet drug* and is useful in the prophylaxis of myocardial infarction and stroke. It acts by inhibiting cyclooxygenase enzyme and thus decreasing the synthesis of TXA_2 (platelet aggregator). However it also inhibits PGI_2 (anti-aggregatory) synthesis. Net effect is to decrease TXA_2 synthesis because:

  - TXA_2 is synthesized by *platelets* and these *are exposed to aspirin in the portal circulation.* Here, it acetylates COX enzyme and irreversibly inhibits the generation of TXA_2. Very little aspirin reaches the systemic circulation to inhibit PGI_2 synthesis.
  - *Platelets lack nuclei* and cannot synthesize new COX enzyme once it is inhibited whereas endothelium can regenerate COX enzyme to produce PGI_2. Net effect is thus inhibition of TXA_2 generation.

- Aspirin and indomethacin are useful for the closure of ductus arteriosus in children with **PDA** (Alprostadil is used to keep it patent).
- Aspirin is used to **inhibit niacin induced flushing** (it is PG mediated).
- It is also useful in *dysmenorrhoea and pre-eclampsia*.
- COX-2 inhibitory action is responsible for *decreased incidence of colorectal carcinoma* in patients on long term aspirin therapy.

Adverse Effects

- Salicylates can cause **dose dependent effects on acid base balance**. Respiratory alkalosis occurs first characterized by *headache, vertigo, tinnitus, vomiting and hyperventilation* (salicylism). Excessive metabolic compensation can result in **metabolic acidosis** manifested as loss of vision, hyperpyrexia, vasomotor collapse, dehydration, convulsions and coma. Chances of metabolic acidosis are **more in infants** because early symptoms like tinnitus and vertigo are frequently missed. *Salicylate poisoning is treated by supportive measures,* gastric lavage, correction of metabolic acidosis and urinary alkalinization to increase the excretion.
- Aspirin can **prolong bleeding time** and should be used cautiously with anticoagulants.
- **At therapeutic doses, it can cause hyperuricemia** by decreasing the excretion of uric acid. It, therefore, should not be used in patients with gout. It also decreases the uricosuric action of probenecid. At high doses (>5 g/d), it increases the excretion of uric acid, but such high doses are not tolerated.
- Aspirin is **contraindicated in children** (<12 yrs old) **due to increased risk of Reye's syndrome.**

(c) Other Non-selective COX Inhibitors

- **Indomethacin** inhibits PLPA$_2$ and possesses immunosuppressive properties apart from its COX inhibitory action. It causes more GI upset than other NSAIDs. It is implicated in causing *headache* (analgesic causing pain) and *sedation*. Treatment with *indomethacin*, combined with *potassium repletion* and *spironolactone* is associated with *improvement* in the symptoms and biochemical derangements of *Bartter's syndrome*.
- **Phenylbutazone** causes agranulocytosis due to bone marrow suppression.
- Propionic acid derivatives include **ibuprofen, ketoprofen and flurbiprofen.** Ketoprofen possesses additional lysosomal stabilizing action and flurbiprofen can be used topically as eye drops. Ibuprofen has been cleared for paediatric patients.
- **Naproxen and oxaprozin** are long acting drugs that also inhibit leucocyte migration.
- **Mefenamic acid** also possesses PG receptor antagonistic and PLPA$_2$ inhibitory activity. It is very useful in dysmenorrhoea.
- **Phenacetin** (prodrug of paracetamol) is implicated in causing analgesic nephropathy
- **Ketorolac** is the only NSAID that can be used i.v apart from paracetamol. It is also available as eye drops. Course longer than 5 days is not recommended.
- **Piroxicam and tenoxicam** are longest acting NSAIDs due to enterohepatic cycling. **Oxaprozin** is another very long acting NSAID.
- **Apazone** possess potent uricosuric activity. It is indicated in conditions, in which other NSAIDs have failed.

Preferential COX-2 Inhibitors

These drugs have more inhibitory action on COX-2 than COX-1. Drugs included in this group are **nimesulide** (*potential of causing hepatotoxicity*), meloxicam, **nabumetone** (*prodrug*), etodolac and diclofenac. *All NSAIDs are acidic in nature except nabumetone.* Relatively less GI toxicity is experienced with the use of these drugs.

Selective COX-2 Inhibitors

These drugs have advantage of **very little GI toxicity**. However renal toxicity is similar and **chances of thrombosis** (acute MI and stroke) are **increased on prolonged use**. *Rofecoxib and valdecoxib were withdrawn due to increased risk of thrombotic disorders like myocardial infarction.*

- Celecoxib, rofecoxib and valdecoxib are sulfonamide derivatives, thus can cause rash and hypersensitivity.
- **Etoricoxib** is *longest acting coxib* and monitoring of hepatic function is must during its use.
- **Lumiracoxib** is a newer COX 2 inhibitor that has *more activity in the acidic medium*
- **Parecoxib** is a prodrug of valdecoxib that can be administered parenterally.

RHEUMATOID ARTHRITIS

Rheumatoid arthritis (RA) is an autoimmune multisystem disease. *NSAIDs are used to provide symptomatic relief but exert no effect on the progression of the disease.* Disease modifying anti rheumatoid drugs (DMARDs) slow the progression of disease but act slowly (takes 6 weeks to 6 months).

Drugs for Treatment of Rheumatoid Arthritis

Corticosteroids
- Used as **bridge therapy** to reduce disease activity till slower acting DMARDs take effect
- Can be used as **adjunctive therapy** for active disease that persists despite treatment with DMARDs

Synthetic DMARDs
- Methotrexate
- Sulfasalazine
- Leflunomide
- Hydroxychloroquine
- Minocycline
- Tofacitinib
- Gold salts
- Penicillamine
- Baricitinib

Biological DMARDs
- **TNF-α inhibitors**
  – Etanercept
  – Infliximab
  – Adalimumab
  – Golimumab
  – Certolizumab
- **Co-stimulation inhibitors**
  – Abatacept
  – Belatacept
- **IL-6 inhibitor**
  – Tocilizumab
  – Sarilumab
- **B-cell depleter**
  – Rituximab
- **IL-IR antagonist**
  – Anakinra

A. Corticosteroids

Low-dose corticosteroids can be used as a bridge therapy (until DMARDs start to work) or as adjunctive therapy (with DMARDs) in rheumatoid arthritis:

B. Synthetic DMARDs

1. Methotrexate

It is **first choice DMARD** and is used at much lower doses (7.5 mg weekly) than required in cancer chemotherapy (30 mg daily). Methotrexate inhibits Amino Imidazole Carboxy Amide Ribonucleotide (AICAR) reductase enzyme. It results in intracellular accumulation of AICAR. Later **increases the local release of adenosine** which acts as anti-inflammatory agent.

Adverse effects of methotrexate

- Gastric irritation and stomatitis (most common)
- Pancytopenia
- **Hepatotoxicity** with fibrosis and cirrhosis **Risk factors are:**

- Chronic hepatitis
- Heavy alcohol consumption
- Diabetes mellitus
- Obesity
- Kidney disease

- Interstitial pneumonitis (Hypersensitivity reaction)
- Teratogenicity
- Increased risk of B-cell lymphomas
- Amoxycillin and probenecid increase risk of methotrexate toxicity

2. Sulfasalazine

It is metabolized to *sulfapyridine and 5-aminosalicylic acid*. Former is the active moiety in RA and latter is useful for ulcerative colitis. It is used in patients when methotrexate is contraindicated.

3. Leflunomide

It is a **prodrug** (converted in the body to an active metabolite) that **inhibits the enzyme dihydro orotate dehydrogenase**. This enzyme is required for pyrimidine synthesis and thus growth of B cells is arrested by leflunomide. *Cholestyramine decreases its toxicity by enhancing its clearance.* It is *faster acting* (action is manifested in 4 weeks as compared to 3 months with other DMARDs) *alternative to methotrexate*.

Teriflunomide is dihydro-orotate dehydrogenase inhibitor (like leflunomide). It is indicated for relapsing-remitting multiple sclerosis.

4. Chloroquine and hydoxychloroquine

These antimalarial drugs are also useful as DMARDs. Hydoxychloroquine is preferred over chloroquine due to less chances of retinal damage by the former.

5. Minocycline

It is reserved for early mild cases and works better during the first year of RA. Mechanism of action is not clear but it has anti-inflammatory property including the ability to inhibit collagenase. Most common adverse effect of minocycline is dizziness.

6. Janus Kinase Inhibitors

Tofacitinib, baricitinib and upadacitinib are inhibitors of Janus kinase 3. These are approved for severe RA refractory to methotrexate. These are effective orally. Like TNF-α inhibitors, screening of patients for latent TB must be done prior to receiving these drugs.

> **Note**
> Tofacitinib is also being tried with remdesivir for COVID-19 patients.

7. Old drugs

Gold and d-penicillamine are highly efficacious DMARDs but are rarely used now due to severe toxic reactions. Gold salts can be used orally (auranofin) as well as intramuscularly (aurothiomalate). *Dermatitis is the most common adverse effect seen with gold salts.* These can also result in kidney and liver damage, peripheral neuropathy, pulmonary fibrosis, encephalopathy and bone marrow depression.

C. Biological DMARDs

1. TNF-α blocking agents

TNF-α plays a major role in the joint destruction in patients with RA. Five drugs **etanercept, adalimumab, infliximab, golimumab** and **certolizumab** act as DMARDs by blocking the action of TNF-α. All of these are given subcutaneously except infliximab which is given I.V. These drugs can cause *activation of latent tuberculosis*. **Infliximab** is *also indicated in Crohn's disease, psoriatic arthritis, Wegener's granulomatosis and sarcoidosis.*

2. Co-stimulation inhibitors

Abtacept and **belatacept** act by inhibiting CD80 and CD86 co-stimulatory molecules on antigen presenting cells. Interaction of these with CD 28 on T-cells is necessary for T-Cell activation. These are indicated for RA resistant to combination of methotrexate and TNF-α inhibitors.

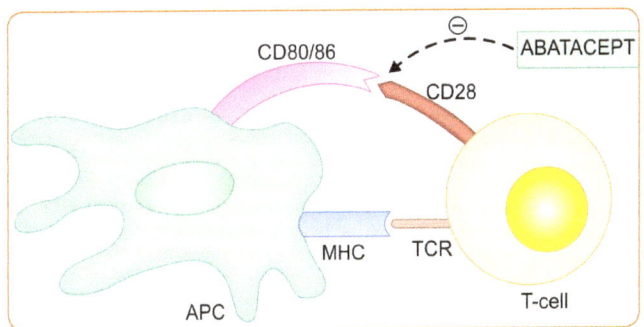

3. IL-6 receptor antagonists

Tocilizumab is a monoclonal antibody against IL-6. It is approved for RA in combination with methotrexate. Tocilizumab is also approved now for *cytokine release syndrome*. **Sarilumab** is a new IL-6R antagonist for RA.

4. Rituximab

It is a monoclonal antibody that depletes B-cells and is used for RA in combination with methotrexate.

5. Anakinra

It is IL-1 receptor antagonist used for RA.

DISEASE MODIFYING ANTI-OSTEOARTHRITIS DRUGS

Osteoarthritis is treated by NSAIDs but these do not arrest the disease progression or joint destruction. Recently two compounds; *Diacerin (IL-1 antagonist) and Licofelone (combined COX-LOX inhibitor)* have been developed to slow the progression of the disease.

GOUT

It is a disease characterized by elevated serum uric acid level. Uric acid has low water solubility and gets precipitated in the joints, kidney and subcutaneous tissues. Secondary hyperuricemia may result due to excessive production (breakdown of proteins and nucleic acids during cancer chemotherapy) or decreased excretion (due to the use of thiazides, loop diuretics, ethambutol, clofibrate etc.) of uric acid.

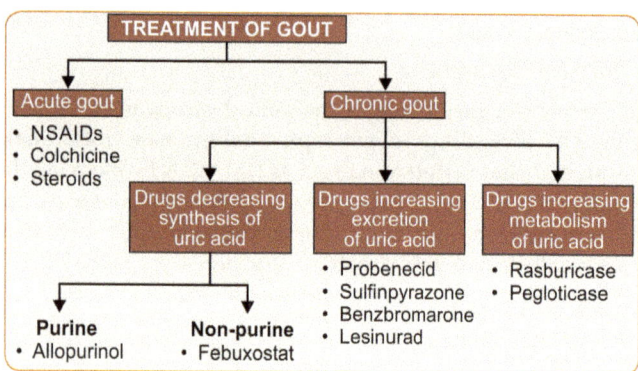

Acute Gout

It is manifested as severe inflammation of joints (due to precipitation of uric acid crystals)

- **NSAIDs** like indomethacin are *drug of choice* due to better tolerability. *Aspirin is not used* as it may cause hyperuricemia. **Tolmetin is not effective.**
- **Colchicine** is *more effective and faster acting* than NSAIDs but *is used rarely* due to its high toxicity. **It acts by inhibiting granulocyte migration** into the inflamed joint. It *causes metaphase arrest* (other drugs causing metaphase arrest are *vinca alkaloids, ixabepilone and taxanes*). Most common and dose limiting toxicity is diarrhea. It can also cause *kidney damage, myopathy and bone marrow depression.*

> **MNEMONIC**
>
> **Uses of Colchicine**
> U – Uric acid raised [Prophylaxis of recurrent attacks of gouty arthritis]
> C – Cirrhosis
> M – Mediterranean fever [Acute]
> S – Sarcoid arthritis

- Intra-articular corticosteroids can be used in the refractory cases.

Chronic Gout

Strategies to decrease uric acid in the serum are to *decrease the synthesis or to increase the excretion and metabolism.*

Drugs Decreasing Synthesis

Allopurinol (hypoxanthine analog) and recently approved drug, **febuxostat** (a non-purine drug) decrease the production of uric acid by *inhibiting the enzyme xanthine oxidase*. Allopurinol is metabolized by the same enzyme to alloxanthine which is a long acting inhibitor of xanthine oxidase. These are indicated as **drug of choice for chronic gout** in the inter-critical period (between two acute attacks) and also with anticancer drugs (to decrease secondary hyperuricemia). 6-Mercaptopurine and *azathioprine are metabolized by xanthine oxidase; therefore dose of these drugs should be decreased* when given with allopurinol. *Allopurinol is also used as an adjuvant to sodium stibogluconate in the treatment of kala azar.* **It is contraindicated in acute gout** because uric acid has inhibitory effect on release of cytokines and allopurinol may aggravate the inflammation by reducing uric acid.

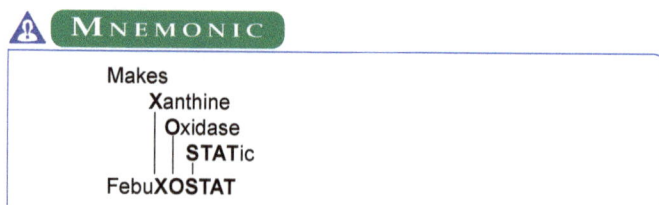

- Most frequent adverse effect with xanthine oxidase inhibitors is precipitation of acute attack of gout.
- There is strong association between HLA–B*5801 and allopurinol hypersensitivity
- Combined use of allopurinol and ampicillin causes a drug rash in 20% of patients.
- Allopurinol requires dose adjustment in renal failure whereas febuxostat can be administered without dose adjustment.
- Febuxostat can result in abnormal liver function tests

Drugs Increasing Excretion

Probenecid, sulfinpyrazone, benzbromarone and **lesinurad** acts as competitive inhibitors of reabsorption of uric acid in proximal tubules. Plenty of fluids and urinary alkalinizers should be given concurrently to prevent precipitation of uric acid crystals in the kidney tubules. These drugs are *ineffective in the presence of renal damage*. Probenecid is also used along *with penicillins to decrease their renal excretion.*

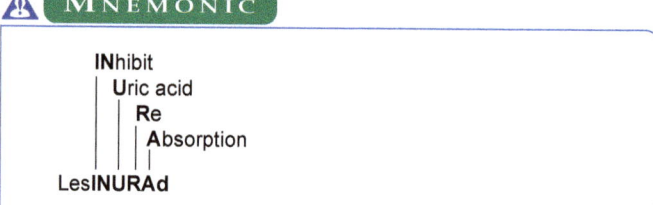

- Uricosuric drugs should not be used if:
  - Creatinine clearance is <50 mL/min.
  - History of nephrolithiasis (uric acid or calcium stones)
  - Evidence of overproduction of uric acid (> 800 mg of uric acid in a 24-hour urine collection)

Drugs Increasing Metabolism

Urate oxidase (uricase) metabolizes insoluble uric acid to soluble allantoin in the birds. This enzyme is absent in humans. *Recombinant urate oxidase is now available as* **rasburicase**. **Pegloticase** is another similiar drug that is pegylated to increase duration of action. Pegloticase and rasburicase are administered by i.v. route and are indicated only in patients with chronic gout refractory to other treatments.

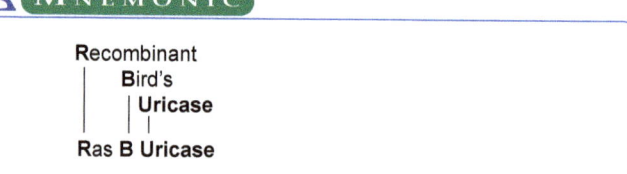

Golden Points

1. Intradermal injection of histamine may result in *triple response* consisting of
   - Red reaction (due to vasodilation).
   - Wheal (exudation of fluid due to increased permeability)
   - Flare (spreading redness *due to axon reflex*).

2. First generation anti-histaminics are *contraindicated in persons requiring constant attention*.

3. First generation anti-histaminics are *contraindicated in persons requiring constant attention*.

4. **Tiprolisant** is H_3 inverse agonist used for **Narcolepsy**

5. Doxepin is a tricyclic antidepressant having most potent H_1 blocking action (800 times more potent than diphenhydramine).

6. **Terfenadine** and **Astemizole** result in polymorphic ventricular tachycardia (**Torsades de' pointes**) manifested as prolongation of QTc interval.

7. Ergot derivatives *can cause dry gangrene of hand and feet and coronary vasospasm*.

8. *Sumatriptan is the drug of choice for aborting acute attack of migraine*.

9. *Frovatriptan is the longest acting and rizatriptan is the fastest acting $5HT_{1B/1D}$ agonist*.

10. Both triptans and ergot alkaloids can cause **coronary vasospasm** and are *contraindicated in ischemic heart disease*.

11. Triptans and ergotamine should not be administered within 24 hours of each other.

12. **Propranolol is the most commonly used drug** for prophylaxis of migraine attacks.

13. Phospholipase A_2 is rate limiting enzyme in synthesis of prostaglandins.

14. **Alprostadil is used to keep ductus arteriosus patent** before surgery whereas NSAIDs like aspirin and indomethacin are used for treatment of **Patent ductus arteriosus**

15. *Misoprostol is the most specific* drug whereas **proton pump inhibitors are drugs of choice** for the treatment of **peptic ulcer due to chronic NSAID use.**

16. Use of *misoprostol in pregnancy* is associated with *Moebius syndrome*

17. Most potent agent known to cause increase in the capillary permeability is platelet activating factor.

18. $PGF_{2\alpha}$ decreases intraocular pressure **by increasing the uveoscleral outflow.**

19. *Licofelone is combined COX-LOX inhibitor* that is being investigated as a *disease modifying anti-osteoarthritis drug* (DMAOAD).

20. Paracetamol acts by inhibiting COX-3 in brain

21. *N-acetylcysteine is antidote of choice* for paracetamol poising.

22. **Paracetamol** *(acetaminophen) has no anti-inflammatory activity* and **Nimesulide and nefopam** *do not act by decreasing PG synthesis*

23. Aspirin is the only **irreversible inhibitor** of COX enzyme

24. **At low doses (40-325 mg),** it acts as an *antiplatelet drug*

25. **Aspirin** is contraindicated in children (<12 yrs old) due to increased risk of **Reye's syndrome.**

26. **Sulindac** and nabumetone are prodrugs.

27. **Piroxicam and tenoxicam** are *longest acting NSAIDS due to enterohepatic cycling.*

28. Methotrexate is first choice DMARD

29. **Hydroxychloroquine** is the safest DMARD in pregnancy.

30. **Tofacitinib** is an inhibitor of Janus kinase 3 and is approved for severe rheumatoid arthritis refractory to methotrexate. It can be given orally.

31. **Abatacept** is a co-stimulation inhibitor indicated for severe refractory rheumatoid arthritis.

32. NSAIDs like indomethacin are drug of choice for acute gout

33. Drugs decreasing uric acid synthesis are contra-indicated in acute gout

34. Plenty of fluids and urinary alkalinizers should be given with probenecid to prevent precipitation of uric acid crystals in the kidney tubules.

35. Dose of 6-Mercaptopurine and *azathioprine should be decreased* when given with allopurinol.

36. **Lesinurad** is a new drug for govt. It acts as uricosuric agent by inhibiting reabsorption of uric acid through URAT-1

Drug of Choice

Drug of choice

Condition	Drug of choice
Migraine	
– Acute-mild to moderate	NSAIDs
– Acute-severe	Sumatriptan
– Prophylaxis	Propranolol
Abortion < 7 weeks	Mifepristone + misoprostol
Induction of labour	Oxytocin
Post-partum hemorrhage	Oxytocin
Cervical priming	Misoprostol
NSAID-induced peptic ulcer	Proton pump inhibitors
Open angle glaucoma	Latanoprost
To maintain patency of ductus arteriosus	Alprostadil
Treatment of patent ductus arteriosus (PDA)	Indomethacin
Bartter syndrome	Indomethacin
Erectile dysfunction	Sildenafil
Rheumatoid arthritis	
– Pain relief	NSAIDs
– Bridge therapy	Corticosteroids
– DMARD	Methotrexate
Flushing due to nicotinic acid	Aspirin
Prophylaxis of MI and stroke	Aspirin
Acetaminophen (Paracetamol) poisoning	N-Acetyl cysteine
Anaphylactic shock	Adrenaline
Acute mediterranean fever	Colchicine
Cancer chemotherapy induced vomiting	$5HT_3$ antagonists like ondansetron
Cisplatin induced vomiting	
– Early	Ondansetron
– Delayed	Aprepitant
Gout	
– Acute	NSAIDs except aspirin
– Refractory acute	Colchicine
– Chronic	Allopurinol
– Chronic (in patient allergic to allopurinol)	Febuxostat
Hyperuricemia secondary to anticancer drugs	Allopurinol

Image Based Questions

1. A patient of rheumatoid arthritis was on DMARDs since 7 years. The fundus examination revealed the features shown in the image. Which of the following is the likely drug responsible for these features?

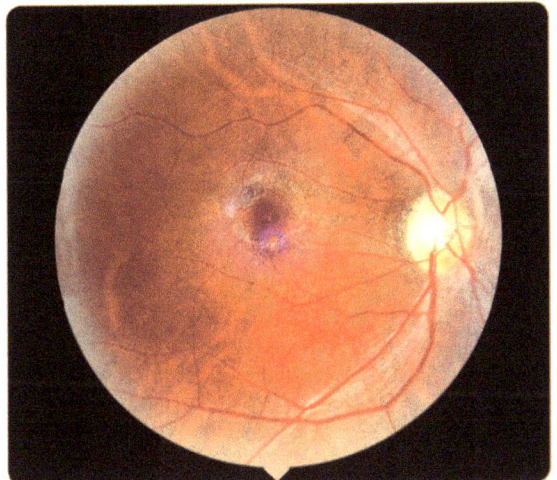

   (a) Methotrexate
   (b) Hydroxychloroquine
   (c) Leflunomide
   (d) Sulfasalazine

2. Erenumab is a new drug recently approved for prophylaxis of migraine. According to the mechanisms shown in the figure, it is likely to be:

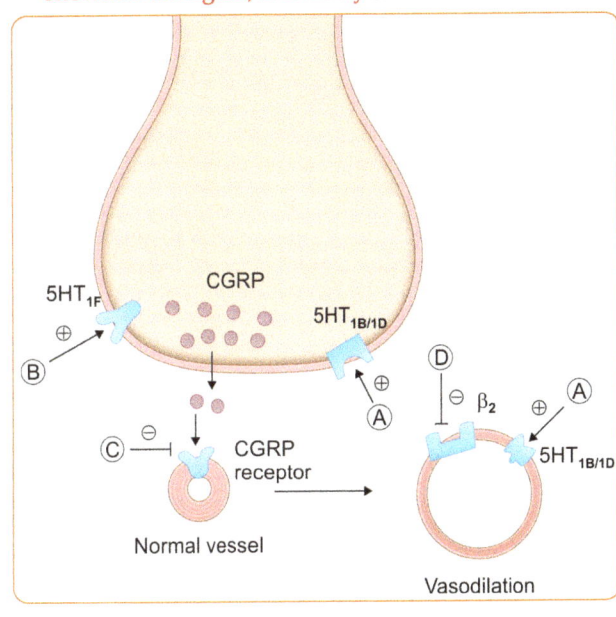

   (a) A
   (b) B
   (c) C
   (d) D

3. Which of the following anti-gout drugs act at the site marked by arrow in the image?

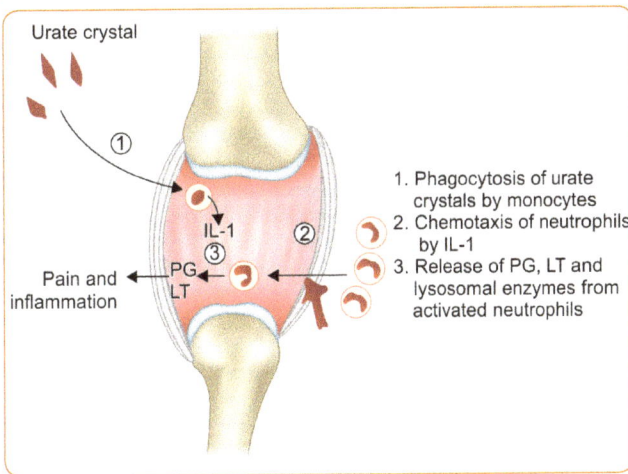

   (a) Indomethacin
   (b) Colchicine
   (c) Allopurinol
   (d) Rasburicase

Explanations

1. **Ans. (b) Hydroxychloroquine**
   The image shows the characteristic Bull's Eye maculopathy. It is caused by chloroquine group of drugs.

2. **Ans. (c) C**
   - Erenumab is a monoclonal antibody against CGRP. It is approved for prophylaxis of migraine
   - Drug B is likely to be a 'ditan' (e.g. lasmiditan). These drugs act by stimulating $5HT_{1F}$ that decreases the release of CGRP.
   - Drug A is $5HT_{1B/1D}$ agonist like sumatriptan
   - Drug D is a beta blocker like propranolol.

3. **Ans. (b) Colchicine**
   Colchicine acts by inhibiting the recruitment of neutrophils.

Autacoids

Multiple Choice Questions

HISTAMINE AND SEROTONIN

1. A boy is planning to travel by bus. Which of the following drug can be used to prevent motion sickness in this person? *(NEET Pattern Question 2020)*
   - (a) Promethazine
   - (b) Cetirizine
   - (c) Loratidine
   - (d) Fexofenadine

2. Buspirone acts on: *(NEET Pattern Question 2019)*
   - (a) 5HT1A
   - (b) 5 HT2
   - (c) 5 HT3
   - (d) 5 HT4

3. Chemical name of serotonin is: *(NEET Pattern Question 2017-2018)*
   - (a) 5 Hydroxytryptamine
   - (b) 5 Hydroxytryptophan
   - (c) 5 Deoxy tryptophan
   - (d) 5 Deoxy tryptamine

4. Which of the following anti-histaminic has very less cholinergic side effects? *(NEET Pattern Question 2016-17)*
   - (a) Promethazine
   - (b) Chlorpheniramine
   - (c) Triprolidine
   - (d) Loratadine

5. A vasodilator is obtained by decarboxylation of: *(NEET Pattern Question 2016-17)*
   - (a) Histidine
   - (b) Arginine
   - (c) Tyrosine
   - (d) Glycine

6. Which is not a 2nd generation anti-histaminic agent? *(AIIMS Nov 2012)*
   - (a) Cetirizine
   - (b) Cyclizine
   - (c) Loratidine
   - (d) Fexofenadine

7. A peptide that causes increased capillary permeability and edema is: *(AI 2012)*
   - (a) Histamine
   - (b) Angiotensin II
   - (c) Bradykinin
   - (d) Renin

8. The non sedative antihistamines are all except one: *(Recent NEET Pattern Question)*
   - (a) Fexofenadine
   - (b) Desloratidine
   - (c) Levocetirizine
   - (d) Cinnarizine

9. Ketanserin is: *(Recent NEET Pattern Question)*
   - (a) $5HT_{1B}$ antagonist
   - (b) $5HT_2$ antagonist
   - (c) $5HT_{1A}$ agonist
   - (d) $5HT_{1D}$ antagonist

10. Which of the following drugs, if given with terfenadine, can cause ventricular arrhythmias? *(Recent NEET Pattern Question)*
    - (a) Ketoconazole
    - (b) Griseofulvin
    - (c) Ampicillin
    - (d) Sparfloxacin

11. One of the following is not a 5-HT receptor antagonist: *(Recent NEET Pattern Question)*
    - (a) Ketanserin
    - (b) Lanreotide
    - (c) Methysergide
    - (d) Tropisetron

12. Antihistaminic used in motion sickness is: *(Recent NEET Pattern Question)*
    - (a) Cetirizine
    - (b) Meclizine
    - (c) Diphenhydramine
    - (d) Fexofenadine

13. Ondansetron is a potent: *(Recent NEET Pattern Question)*
    - (a) Antiemetic
    - (b) Anxiolytic
    - (c) Analgesic
    - (d) Antidepressant

14. Fexofenadine is metabolic product of: *(Recent NEET Pattern Question)*
    - (a) Loratidine
    - (b) Astemizole
    - (c) Cetrizine
    - (d) Terfenadine

15. Histamine blocker in stomach act through: *(Recent NEET Pattern Question)*
    - (a) Decreasing cAMP in stomach
    - (b) Increasing cAMP in stomach
    - (c) Increasing IP_3 in stomach
    - (d) Decreasing IP_3 in stomach

16. $5 HT_1$ agonists are used as: *(Recent NEET Pattern Question)*
    - (a) Anti anxiety drugs
    - (b) Antipsychotic drugs
    - (c) For GERD
    - (d) For chemotherapy induced vomiting

17. Which of the following is a $5HT_3$ antagonist? *(Recent NEET Pattern Question)*
    - (a) Cisapride
    - (b) Ondansetron
    - (c) Clozapine
    - (d) Buspirone

18. H_1 antagonist has all the functions *except*: *(Recent NEET Pattern Question)*
    - (a) Antipruritic
    - (b) Sedation
    - (c) Decrease gastric acid secretion
    - (d) Antivertigo

19. Effects mediated by H_1 histamine receptor include: *(Recent NEET Pattern Question)*
    - (a) Inhibition of gastric acid secretion
    - (b) Induction of hepatic cytochrome P450 enzymes
    - (c) Maintenance of a wakeful state
    - (d) Vasoconstriction of arterioles

20. Which of the following H_1 blocker has high anti-cholinergic activity? *(Recent NEET Pattern Question)*
    - (a) Cetrizine
    - (b) Chlorpheniramine
    - (c) Fexofenadine
    - (d) Astemizole

21. Which one of the following drug and active metabolite combination is incorrect? *(Recent NEET Pattern Question)*
    - (a) Hydroxyzine-Cetirizine
    - (b) Terfenadine-Fexofenadine
    - (c) Chlorpromazine-Promethazine
    - (d) Loratidine-Desloratidine

22. The drug which blocks both H_1 and $5 HT_2$ receptor is: *(Recent NEET Pattern Question)*
    - (a) Phenoxybenzamine
    - (b) Cyproheptadine
    - (c) Ritanserin
    - (d) Ondansetron

23. Serotonin can be synthesized from: *(Recent NEET Pattern Question)*
    - (a) Tryptophan
    - (b) Tyrosine
    - (c) Dopa
    - (d) Epinephrine

ERGOT ALKALOIDS AND MIGRAINE

24. Sumatriptan acts as an agonist at this receptor:
  (NEET Pattern Question 2016-17)
    (a) 5HT-1A (b) 5HT-2A/2C
    (c) 5HT 1B/1D (d) 5HT 2A/2C

25. Sumatriptan should not be given to the patient of:
  (NEET Pattern Question 2016-17)
    (a) Peptic ulcer
    (b) Hypertension
    (c) Ischemic heart disease
    (d) Migraine

26. Antiepileptic drug used for prophylaxis of migraine is:
  (NEET Pattern Question 2016-17)
    (a) Propranolol (b) Sumatriptan
    (c) Topiramate (d) Flunarizine

27. Methysergide which was once used as a drug of choice for prophylaxis of migraine is not used now-a-days because of risk of: *(NEET Pattern Question 2016-17)*
    (a) Peptic ulcer (b) Arrhythmias
    (c) Pulmonary fibrosis (d) Carcinoid

28. After taking some drug for acute attack of migraine, a patient developed nausea and vomiting. He also developed tingling and numbness in the tip of the finger that also turned blue. Which of the following is the most likely drug implicated in causing the above findings? *(AI 2012)*
    (a) Dihydroergotamine (b) Sumatriptan
    (c) Aspirin (d) Butorphanol

29. Drugs used in migraine prophylaxis are all *except*:
  (Recent NEET Pattern Question)
    (a) Flunarizine (b) Propranolol
    (c) Cyproheptadine (d) Sumatriptan

30. Sumatriptan is used in: *(Recent NEET Pattern Question)*
    (a) Mania (b) Depression
    (c) Schizophrenia (d) Migraine

31. Sumatriptan is: *(Recent NEET Pattern Question)*
    (a) $5HT_{1D}$ antagonist (b) $5HT_{1A}$ agonist
    (c) $5HT_{1D}$ agonist (d) $5HT_{1A}$ antagonist

32. Drug of choice in acute severe migraine is:
  (Recent NEET Pattern Question)
    (a) Ergotamine (b) Sumatriptan
    (c) Dihydroergotamine (d) Propranol

33. Methyl ergometrine is used in the prophylaxis of:
    (a) Migraine *(Recent NEET Pattern Question)*
    (b) Postpartum hemorrhage
    (c) PIH
    (d) None of the above

34. Which one of the following is true about sumatriptan?
  (Recent NEET Pattern Question)
    (a) Antagonist of serotonin
    (b) Interacts with alpha and beta adrenergic receptors
    (c) Has antimigraine activity
    (d) Can be used in a patient with ischaemic heart disease

35. Ergometrine is not used for initiation of labour because:
    (a) Slow onset of action *(Recent NEET Pattern Question)*
    (b) Fetal hypoxia
    (c) Increases blood pressure
    (d) Act on D2 receptors to cause vomiting

36. Most commonly used drug for prophylaxis of migraine is: *(Recent NEET Pattern Question)*
    (a) Sumatriptan (b) Propranolol
    (c) Valproate (d) Flunarizine

37. Which of the following drug is useful in prophylaxis of migraine? *(Recent NEET Pattern Question)*
    (a) Propranolol (b) Sumatriptan
    (c) Domperidone (d) Ergotamine

38. Which of the following drug is useful in acute attack of migraine? *(Recent NEET Pattern Question)*
    (a) Bromocriptine (b) Cinnarizine
    (c) Sumatriptan (d) Ondansetron

39. Which one is a contraindication to the use of ergot derivatives? *(Recent NEET Pattern Question)*
    (a) Migraine
    (b) Hyperprolactinemia
    (c) Obstructive vascular disease
    (d) Postpartum hemorrhage

40. Triptans used in migraine headaches are agonists at which receptor? *(Recent NEET Pattern Question)*
    (a) $5HT_{ID/IB}$ (b) $5HT_{1A}$
    (c) $5HT_3$ (d) $5HT_{2A}$

EICOSANOIDS AND NSAIDs

41. All of the following drugs are used for the treatment of post-partum hemorrhage *except*: *(AIIMS May 2019)*
    (a) Misoprostol
    (b) Dinoprostone
    (c) Prostaglandin F2 alpha
    (d) Oxytocin

42. Bimatoprost is used as: *(NEET Pattern Question 2016-17)*
    (a) Topical eye drops in open angle glaucoma
    (b) Systemically to maintain patency of ductus arteriosus
    (c) Cervical gel for ripening of cervix
    (d) Orally for gastric ulcer

43. All are true about alprostadil *except*:
    (a) PGE1 inhibitor *(NEET Pattern Question 2016-17)*
    (b) Penile fibrosis is very rare
    (c) Used to maintain patency of ductus arteriosus
    (d) Gastroprotective in nature

44. The COX-inhibitor which causes increased risk of myocardial infarction is: *(NEET Pattern Question 2016-17)*
    (a) Rofecoxib (b) Meloxicam
    (c) Ketorolac (d) Indomethacin

45. Which of the following statement about NSAIDs is FALSE? *(AIIMS Nov, 2014)*
    (a) They interfere with the antihypertensive effect of diuretics
    (b) NSAIDs are useful in neuropathic pain
    (c) NSAIDs should be avoided in renal disease as they can cause nephrotoxicity
    (d) Many NSAIDs can be used topically

46. The therapeutic efficacy of antihypertensive drugs is blunted by NSAIDs because they:
  (Recent NEET Pattern Question)
    (a) Cause sodium excretion
    (b) Increase the clearance of antihypertensive drugs
    (c) Decrease the absorption of antihypertensive drugs
    (d) Decrease the synthesis of vascular prostacyclin

47. Aspirin should be used with caution in the following groups of patients because of which of the following reason? *(Recent NEET Pattern Question)*
    (a) In diabetics because it can cause hyperglycemia
    (b) In children with viral disease, because of the risk of acute renal failure
    (c) In gout, because it can increase serum uric acid
    (d) In pregnancy, because of high risk of teratogenicity

48. Aspirin inhibits which of the following enzymes? *(Recent NEET Pattern Question)*
    (a) Lipoprotein lipase (b) Lipoxygenase
    (c) Cyclooxygenase (d) Phospholipase D

49. The antidote of choice in paracetamol poisoning is: *(Recent NEET Pattern Question)*
    (a) Flumazenil (b) Sodium bicarbonate
    (c) N-acetylcysteine (d) Methylene Blue

50. Prostaglandin useful for the prevention of duodenal ulcer is: *(Recent NEET Pattern Question)*
    (a) Dinoprost (b) Misoprostol
    (c) Alprostadil (d) Carboprost

51. Prostaglandin inhibiting action of aspirin is useful in the treatment of all of the following conditions, *except*: *(Recent NEET Pattern Question)*
    (a) Analgesia and antipyresis
    (b) Closure of ductus arteriosus
    (c) Uricosuria
    (d) Antiinflammatory and anti platelet aggregation

52. Which of the following drugs inhibit an enzyme in the prostaglandin synthesis? *(Recent NEET Pattern Question)*
    (a) Aminocaproic acid (b) Aspirin
    (c) Aprotinin (d) Alteplase

53. Misoprostol, a prostaglandin analogue is useful as: *(Recent NEET Pattern Question)*
    (a) Uterine relaxant (b) Anti-ulcer
    (c) Bronchodilator (d) Vasodilator

54. Drug commonly causing analgesic nephropathy is: *(Recent NEET Pattern Question)*
    (a) Aspirin (b) Ibuprofen
    (c) Phenacetin (d) Phenylbutazone

55. Which one of the following is aspirin? *(Recent NEET Pattern Question)*
    (a) Methyl salicylate
    (b) Para-aminobenzoic acid
    (c) Para-aminosalicylic acid
    (d) Acetyl salicylic acid

56. True about COX-2 are all *except*: *(Recent NEET Pattern Question)*
    (a) It is constitutionally expressed on some cell surfaces
    (b) Activation of COX-2 leads to ulceroprotective effect on gastric mucosa
    (c) Induced at the site of inflammation
    (d) It is utilized in generation of eicosanoids with a ring structure

57. Which of the following is non opioid analgesic and does not inhibit prostaglandin synthesis? *(Recent NEET Pattern Question)*
    (a) Nefopam (b) Tenoxicam
    (c) Ketorolac (d) Piroxicam

58. All are true about Reye's Syndrome *except*: *(Recent NEET Pattern Question)*
    (a) Hepatic encephalopathy
    (b) Seen with ampicillin therapy
    (c) Fever and rash
    (d) Viral associated

59. Ibuprofen acts on: *(Recent NEET Pattern Question)*
    (a) Lipoxygenase pathway
    (b) Cyclooxygenase pathway
    (c) Kinin system
    (d) Serotonin system

60. Which of the following prostaglandin analogues is used in glaucoma? *(Recent NEET Pattern Question)*
    (a) Misoprostol (b) Latanoprost
    (c) Enprostil (d) Rioprostil

61. Cycloxygenase enzyme is not inhibited by: *(Recent NEET Pattern Question)*
    (a) Aspirin (b) Warfarin
    (c) Phenylbutazone (d) Diclofenac

62. Which prostaglandin helps in cervical ripening? *(Recent NEET Pattern Question)*
    (a) PGI_2 (b) PGF_2
    (c) PGE_2 (d) PGD_2

63. Development of hepatic central lobular necrosis secondary to acetaminophen overdose can be prevented effectively by which of the following if given within a few hours after ingestion? *(Recent NEET Pattern Question)*
    (a) N-acetylcysteine (b) Dimercaprol
    (c) Sodium nitrite (d) Amyl nitrite

64. For pain control in a patient having history of GI bleeding, which of the following is given? *(Recent NEET Pattern Question)*
    (a) Nimesulide (b) Ibuprofen
    (c) Rofecoxib (d) Pentazocin

65. Rofecoxib was withdrawn due to: *(Recent NEET Pattern Question)*
    (a) Ischemic heart disease (b) Renal complication
    (c) Liver adenoma (d) Gastric ulcer

66. Which of the following statements is true of ketorolac? *(Recent NEET Pattern Question)*
    (a) Has potent anti-inflammatory activity
    (b) Its analgesic efficacy is equal to morphine in postoperative pain
    (c) Is used as preanaesthetic analgesic
    (d) It interacts with opioid receptor

67. Use of aspirin in children with viral disease is associated with: *(Recent NEET Pattern Question)*
    (a) Metabolic acidosis (b) Reye's syndrome
    (c) Renal tubular acidosis (d) Fixed drug eruption

68. Which enzyme is irreversibly inhibited by aspirin? *(Recent NEET Pattern Question)*
    (a) Lipooxygenase (b) Cyclooxygenase
    (c) Thromboxane synthase (d) Phospholipase

69. Prostaglandins are used in all of the following conditioins *except*: *(Recent NEET Pattern Question)*
    (a) Cervical ripening
    (b) Post partum haemorrhage
    (c) Erectile dysfunction
    (d) Palliative treatment of patent ductus arteriosus

70. Irreversible inhibition of COX is done by:
    (Recent NEET Pattern Question)
    (a) Aspirin   (b) Nimesulide
    (d) Celecoxib   (d) Naproxen

71. NSAID with least anti-inflammatory action is:
    (Recent NEET Pattern Question)
    (a) Indomethacin (b) Paracetamol
    (c) Ketorolac   (c) Ibuprofen

72. Dinoprost is: *(Recent NEET Pattern Question)*
    (a) PG E_1 (b) PG E_2
    (c) PGF_{2a} (d) PGI_2

73. Prostaglandin derivatives are used in following conditions *except*: *(Recent NEET Pattern Question)*
    (a) Cervical ripening
    (b) As an abortificient
    (c) NSAID induced peptic ulcer
    (d) Patent ductus arteriosus

74. Which of the following NSAID has good tissue penetrability with concentration in synovial fluid?
    (Recent NEET Pattern Question)
    (a) Ketorolac   (b) Diclofenac sodium
    (c) Sulindac   (d) Piroxicam

75. Alprostadil is not used for:
    (a) Erectile dysfunction *(Recent NEET Pattern Question)*
    (b) Pulmonary hypertension
    (c) Patent ductus arteriosus
    (d) Critical limb ischemia

76. NSAID given in once daily dose is:
    (Recent NEET Pattern Question)
    (a) Naproxen   (b) Ketorolac
    (c) Piroxicam   (d) Paracetamol

77. All of the following drugs are reversible inhibitors of cyclo-oxygenase *except*: *(Recent NEET Pattern Question)*
    (a) Diclofenac   (b) Ibuprofen
    (c) Aspirin   (d) Indomethacin

78. Latanoprost (PGF_2 alpha) is used in:
    (Recent NEET Pattern Question)
    (a) Maintenace of ductus arteriosus
    (b) Pulmonary hypertension
    (c) Gastric mucosal protection
    (d) Glaucoma

79. Misoprostol is an analogue of:
    (Recent NEET Pattern Question)
    (a) PGE_1 (b) PGE_2
    (c) PGF_2 (d) PGI_2

80. N-acetylcysteine reduces the severity of hepatic necrosis in toxicity due to: *(Recent NEET Pattern Question)*
    (a) Isoniazid   (b) Acetaminophen
    (c) Halothane   (d) Methyldopa

81. Prostaglandins are synthesized from:
    (Recent NEET Pattern Question)
    (a) Lignoceric acid   (b) Nervonic acid
    (c) Arachidonic acid (d) Butyric acid

82. Which of the following actions are performed by prostacyclin PGI_2? *(Recent NEET Pattern Question)*
    (a) Vasodilation and platelet aggregation
    (b) Vasodilation and inhibition of platelet aggregation
    (c) Vasoconstriction and platelet aggregation
    (d) Vasoconstriction and inhibition of platelet aggregation

83. All of the following are true about prostaglandin E_2 *except*: *(Recent NEET Pattern Question)*
    (a) It is the principal prostaglandin synthesized in the stomach
    (b) Its biosynthesis is inhibited by aspirin
    (c) It stimulates gastric acid secretion
    (d) It causes dilatation of submucosa blood vessels

RHEUMATOID ARTHRITIS AND GOUT

84. Pegloticase is used for treatment of:
    (a) Ankylosing spondylosis *(NEET Pattern Question 2020)*
    (b) CPPD
    (c) Chronic tophaceous gout
    (d) Refractory rheumatoid arthritis

85. A patient diagnosed with rheumatoid arthritis was on medications. After 2 years, he developed blurring of vision and was found to have corneal opacity. Which drug is most likely to cause this?
    (NEET Pattern Question 2020)
    (a) Sulfasalazine   (b) Chloroquine
    (c) Methotrexate   (d) Leflunomide

86. Pegloticase is used in the treatment of: *(AIIMS Nov. 2019)*
    (a) Chronic gout   (b) Paralytic ileus
    (c) Psoriatic arthritis (d) Rheumatoid arthritis

87. Which of the following drugs is not used in Rheumatoid arthritis? *(AIIMS Nov. 2018)*
    (a) Febuxostat   (b) Leflunomide
    (c) Etanercept   (d) Methotrexate

88. Which of the following drugs act by inhibiting granulocyte migration? *(NEET Pattern Question 2019)*
    (a) Colchicine   (b) Montelukast
    (c) Cromoglycate   (d) Allopurinol

89. A patient of RA is taking methotrexate, steroids and NSAIDs since 4 months but activity of disease progression is same. Next step is:
    (NEET Pattern Question 2019)
    (a) Start monotherapy with anti-TNF alpha drugs
    (b) Continue methotrexate and steroids
    (c) Stop oral methotrexate and start parenteral methotrexate
    (d) Add sulfasalazine and hydroxychloroquine

90. Which of the following drugs act by inhibiting granulocyte migration? *(NEET Pattern Question 2019)*
    (a) Colchicine   (b) Montelukast
    (c) Cromoglycate   (d) Allopurinol

91. Mechanism of action of colchicine in acute gout is:
    (NEET Pattern Question 2017-2018)
    (a) Prevention of granulocyte migration
    (b) Inhibition of leukotriene synthesis
    (c) Inhibition of uric acid formation
    (d) Inhibition of purine metabolism

92. Which of the following DMARD acts by increasing adenosine extracellularly? *(AIIMS May 2017)*
    (a) Methotrexate   (b) Sulfasalazine
    (c) Azathioprine   (d) Leflunomide

Autacoids

93. Which of the following DMARDs require liver function testing? *(AIIMS Nov 2016)*
    (a) Methotrexate (b) Infliximab
    (c) Abatacept (d) Cyclophosphamide

94. Etanercept is a biological disease-modifying agent used in the management of rheumatoid arthritis. Its mechanism of action is: *(AIIMS Nov 2015)*
    (a) TNF alpha blockade
    (b) COX-2 inhibition
    (c) IL-6 inhibition
    (d) Stabilization of mast cells

95. Which of the following is a DMARD? *(Recent NEET Pattern Question)*
    (a) Desferrioxamine (b) Penicillamine
    (c) Succimer (d) Dimercaprol

96. Which of the following increases uric acid excretion? *(Recent NEET Pattern Question)*
    (a) Allopurinol (b) Aspirin
    (c) Colchicine (d) Probenecid

97. Which of the following drugs is useful in acute attack of gout? *(Recent NEET Pattern Question)*
    (a) Furosemide (b) Sulfinpyrazone
    (c) Allopurinol (d) Piroxicam

98. Allopurinol potentiates the action of: *(Recent NEET Pattern Question)*
    (a) Corticosteroids (b) Probenecid
    (c) 6-Mercaptopurine (d) Ampicillin

99. Probenecid interacts with: *(Recent NEET Pattern Question)*
    (a) Streptomycin (b) Ampicillin
    (c) Vancomycin (d) Erythromycin

100. Drug useful for gout is: *(Recent NEET Pattern Question)*
    (a) Pyrazinamide (b) Rifampicin
    (c) Allopurinol (d) Naloxone

101. Loading dose of leflunomide in rheumatoid arthritis is: *(Recent NEET Pattern Question)*
    (a) 20 mg (b) 10 mg
    (c) 100 mg (d) 400 mg

102. Allopurinol specifically inhibits: *(Recent NEET Pattern Question)*
    (a) Xanthine oxidase (b) Arginase
    (c) Carbamoyl transferase (d) Urease

103. Leflunomide is used in the treatment of:
    (a) Rheumatoid arthritis *(Recent NEET Pattern Question)*
    (b) Dermatomyositis
    (c) Bony metastasis
    (d) Postmenopausal osteoporosis

104. Which of the following disease modifying anti-rheumatic drugs (DMARDs) is the drug of first choice? *(Recent NEET Pattern Question)*
    (a) Methotrexate (b) Gold compounds
    (c) D-penicillamine (d) Anakinra

105. The most common effect of colchicine which is dose limiting is: *(Recent NEET Pattern Question)*
    (a) Diarrhea (b) Dyspepsia
    (c) Retinal damage (d) Loss of taste sensation

106. Which drug is not included in DMARDs? *(Recent NEET Pattern Question)*
    (a) Chloroquine (b) Vincristine
    (c) Penicillamine (d) Leflunomide

107. Allopurinol is used in the treatment of: *(Recent NEET Pattern Question)*
    (a) Gout (b) Hypothyroidism
    (c) Hypertension (d) Hyperlipidemia

108. Best drug for chronic gout in patient with renal impairment is: *(Recent NEET Pattern Question)*
    (a) Naproxen (b) Probenecid
    (c) Allopurinol (d) Sulfinpyrazone

109. Allopurinol is a competitive inhibitor of: *(Recent NEET Pattern Question)*
    (a) Uricase
    (b) Xanthine oxidase
    (c) Guanase
    (d) Adenosine deaminase

110. Gout is a disorder associated with: *(Recent NEET Pattern Question)*
    (a) Increase in lactic acid
    (b) Increase in uric acid
    (c) Increase in hippuric acid
    (d) Increase in glutamic acid

111. Uricosuric drug among these is: *(Recent NEET Pattern Question)*
    (a) Probenecid (b) Colchicine
    (c) Allopurinol (d) All of these

112. Allopurinol works on the basis of: *(Recent NEET Pattern Question)*
    (a) Decreased excretion of uric acid
    (b) Decreased metabolism of uric acid
    (c) Increased excretion of uric acid
    (d) Decreased synthesis of uric acid

MISCELLANEOUS

113. Most common cause of Mobius syndrome is use of which of the following drug in pregnancy? *(AI 2012)*
    (a) Misoprostol (b) Thalidomide
    (c) Methotrexate (d) Dinoprostone

114. Inhibitor of platelet aggregation includes: *(Recent NEET Pattern Question)*
    (a) TXA_2 (b) PGI_2
    (c) PGG_2 (d) All of the above

115. Bosentan is a/an: *(Recent NEET Pattern Question)*
    (a) Serotonin uptake inhibitor
    (b) Endothelin receptor antagonist
    (c) Leukotriene modifier
    (d) Phosphodiestease inhibitor

116. All of the following are well known ototoxic drugs *except*: *(Recent NEET Pattern Question)*
    (a) Aspirin
    (b) Acetaminophen
    (c) Aminoglycosides
    (d) Loop diuretics

Explanations

1. **Ans. (a) Promethazine** *(Ref: KDT 8th/e p180)*
   Explanation:
   - Promethazine is a first generation anti-histaminic drug. It has strong anti-cholinergic properties and good entry in brain. Therefore, it can be used as an alternative to scopolamine for prophylaxis of motion sickness.
   - Cetirizine, loratidine and fexofenadine are second generation anti-histaminic agents. These have poor CNS penetration and are thus not effective in prophylaxis of motion sickness.

1st Generation	2nd Generation
Cross BBB, cause sedation	Do not cross BBB, no sedation
Anticholinergic action present	No anticholinergic action
Useful for • Motion sickness • Drug induced parkinsonism • Muscular dystonias • Allergy	Useful only for allergy
Promethazine Diphenhydramine Dimenhydrinate Pheniramine Chlorpheniramine Cyclizine Cinnarizine	Terfenadine – not used (due to QT prolongation) Fexofenadine Astemizole–not used (TDP) Loratidine Des loratidine Cetrizine, Levocetrizine Azelastine, Olopatadine – Topical

2. **Ans. (a) 5HT1A** *(Ref: Goodman and Gilman 13th/e p234)*
   Drugs acting on serotonergic receptors
   - 5-hydroxytryptamine (serotonin) is synthesized from tryptophan. It acts by activation of several serotonin receptors (5-HT1 to HT7).
   - 5-HT1A (presynaptic receptor) modulates the release of serotonin. Partial agonists of this receptor (buspirone, ipsapirone, gepirone) are useful as anti anxiety drugs.
   - 5-HT1B/1D (presynaptic receptor) cause constriction of cranial vessels and agonists at this receptor (sumatriptan, naratriptan) are useful for the treatment of acute migraine attacks.
   - 5-HT2A/2C receptor is responsible for most of the direct actions of serotonin. Ketanserin and ritanserin are antagonists at this receptor and are useful as antihypertensive agents. Clozapine and risperidone are *atypical antipsychotic* agents that act through antagonistic activity at this receptor.
   - 5-HT3 receptor is an **ionotropic receptor** (other 5 HT receptors are GPCRs) and mediates most of the reflex and indirect actions of serotonin. Stimulation of this receptor is responsible for vomiting induced by anticancer drugs. *5-HT3 receptor antagonists like ondansetron are the drug of choice for chemotherapy induced vomiting.*
   - 5-HT4 receptor is present in GIT and is responsible for increase in peristalsis. Agonists at his receptor (cisapride, tegaserod) are useful as *prokinetic* agents in the treatment of gastroesophageal reflux disease.

3. **Ans. (a) 5 Hydroxytryptamine** *(Ref: KDT 8th/e p185)*
4. **Ans. (d) Loratadine** *(Ref: KDT's 8th/e p180)*
5. **Ans. (a) Histidine** *(Ref: KDT's 8th/e p174)*
6. **Ans. (b) Cyclizine** *(Ref: Goodman and Gilman 12th/e p921,922)*
   Antihistaminics may be classified into first generation and second generation compounds on the basis of CNS penetration and anticholinergic properties. First Generation Anti-histaminics can penetrate blood brain barrier and possess additional anticholinergic properties which are lacking in second generation drugs. Cyclizine is a first generation whereas cetririzine, loratidine and fexofenadine are second generation drugs.
7. **Ans. (c) Bradykinin** *(Ref: KDT 8th/e p549)*
   Although both histamine as well as bradykinin can cause edema and increase in permeability, histamine is an amine whereas bradykinin is a peptide.
8. **Ans. (d) Cinnarizine** *(Ref: KDT 8th/e p179)*
9. **Ans. (b) 5HT$_2$ antagonist** *(Ref: KDT 8th/e p190)*
10. **Ans. (a) Ketoconazole** *(Ref: KDT 8th/e p844)*
11. **Ans. (b) Lanreotide** *(Ref: KDT 8th/e p189-190)*
    Lanreotide is a somatostatin analog used in acromegaly.
12. **Ans. (c) Diphenhydramine** *(Ref: Katzung 11th/e p278)*
    Diphenhydramine and promethazine have maximum anti-cholinergic activity and maximum ability to cross the blood brain barrier and are thus most effective in motion sickness.
13. **Ans. (a) Antiemetic** *(Ref: KDT 8th/e p190)*
14. **Ans. (d) Terfenadine** *(Ref: KDT 8th/e p181)*
15. **Ans. (d) Decreasing IP$_3$ in stomach** *(Ref: KDT 8th/e p175)*
16. **Ans (a) Anti anxiety drugs** *(Ref: KDT 8th/e p189)*
17. **Ans (b) Ondansetron** *(Ref: KDT 8th/e p190)*
18. **Ans. (c) Decrease gastric acid secretion** *(Ref: KDT 8th/e p182-183)*
19. **Ans. (c) Maintenance of a wakeful state** *(Ref: KDT 8th/e p177)*
20. **Ans. (b) Chlorpheniramine** *(Ref: KDT 8th/e p179)*
21. **Ans. (c) Chlorpromazine-Promethazine** *(Ref: KDT 8th/e p181-182)*
22. **Ans. (b) Cyproheptadine** *(Ref: KDT 8th/e p189)*
23. **Ans. (a) Tryptophan** *(Ref: KDT 8th/e p185)*
24. **Ans. (c) 5HT 1B/1D** *(Ref: KDT 8th/e p193)*
25. **Ans. (c) Ischemic heart disease** *(Ref: KDT's 8th/e p194)*
26. **Ans. (c) Topiramate** *(Ref: KDT's 8th/e p195)*
27. **Ans. (c) Pulmonary fibrosis** *(Ref: KDT's 8th/e p190)*

Autacoids

28. **Ans. (a) Dihydroergotamine** *(Ref: Katzung 11th/e p289)*
    This is a classical sign of ergot induced vasoconstriction. Dihydroergotamine can be used for acute attack of migraine and can result in these symptoms. Due to their vasoconstricing potential, ergot alkaloids are contra-indicated in a patient with peripheral vascular disease. These may also lead to development of gangrene.

29. **Ans. (d) Sumatriptan** *(Ref: Harrison 17th/e p102, CMDT-2010/874)*

30. **Ans. (d) Migraine** *(Ref: KDT 8th/e p193-194)*

31. **Ans. (c) $5HT_{1D}$ agonist** *(Ref: KDT 8th/e p193)*

32. **Ans. (b) Sumatriptan** *(Ref: KDT 8th/e p193)*

33. **Ans. (b) Postpartum hemorrhage** *(Ref: KDT 8th/e p357)*

34. **Ans. (c) Has antimigraine activity** *(Ref: KDT 8th/e p194)*

35. **Ans. (b) Fetal hypoxia** *(Ref: Goodman Gilman 12th/e p349)*

36. **Ans. (b) Propranolol** *(Ref: KDT 8th/e p195)*

37. **Ans. (a) Propranolol** *(Ref: KDT 8th/e p195)*

38. **Ans. (c) Sumatriptan** *(Ref: KDT 8th/e p194)*

39. **Ans. (c) Obstructive vascular disease** *(Ref: KDT 8th/e p191)*

40. **Ans. (a) $5HT_{ID/IB}$** *(Ref: KDT 8th/e p193)*

41. **Ans. (b) Dinoprostone** *(Ref: KDT 8th/e p206)*
    Dinoprostone is a PGE2 analogue whereas misoprostol is PGE1 analogue.
    - Misoprostol, Dinoprostone and Prostaglandin F2 alpha cause contraction of upper segment of uterus, hence can be used in PPH.
    - Oxytocin is drug of choice for treatment as well prophylaxis of post partum hemorrhage.
    - Therefore, all the four drugs given in the options can be used for PPH. However, Dinoprostone is given intravaginally or per rectally and it cannot be given as injection, so it is not a preferred drug.

42. **Ans. (a) Topical eye drops in open angle glaucoma** *(Ref: KDT's 8th/e p169)*

43. **Ans. (a) PGE1 inhibitor**
    (Ref: KDT 8th/e p206, 304; Goodman Gilman 12th/e p665, 666)

44. **Ans. (a) Rofecoxib** *(Ref: KDT's 8th/e p225)*

45. **Ans. (b) NSAIDs are useful in neuropathic pain**
    (Ref: KDT 8th/e p214-217, Katzung 12th/e p637-638)
    - All NSAIDs may cause nephrotoxicity and hepatotoxicity.
    - NSAIDs are ineffective in neuropathic pain.
    - NSAIDs blunt the antihypertensive effects of diuretics and ACE inhibitors.
    - Diclofenac, ibuprofen, piroxicam etc. are available as topical NSAID preparations.

46. **Ans. (d) Decrease the synthesis of vascular prostacyclins** *(Ref: KDT 8th/e p215)*
    - PGE_2 and PGI_2 cause *renal vasodilation, natriuresis* and increased water clearance due to inhibition of the action of ADH.
    - Loop diuretics act partly by increasing the stimulation of COX; therefore *NSAIDs attenuate the diuretic action* of these drugs.

47. **Ans. (c) In gout, because it can increase serum uric acid** *(Ref: KDT 8th/e p214, 215)*

    - At therapeutic doses, Aspirin can cause hyperuricemia by decreasing the excretion of uric acid. It, therefore, should not be used in patients with gout. It also decreases the uricosuric action of probenecid. At high doses (>5 g/d), it increases the excretion of uric acid, but such high doses are not tolerated.
    - Aspirin is contraindicated in children (<12 yrs old) due to increased risk of Reye's syndrome, which is a type of hepatic encephalopathy.
    - It should be avoided in diabetics because of risk of hypoglycemia
    - It should be avoided in pregnancy because it may be responsible for low birth weight babies, however, it does not cause congenital malformations.

48. **Ans. (c) Cyclooxygenase** *(Ref: Katzung 10th/e p554; KDT 8th/e p212)*
    - Aspirin is an NSAID and acts by irreversible inhibition of cyclooxygenase enzyme that decreases the formation of prostaglandins.

49. **Ans. (c) N-acetylcysteine** *(Ref: KDT 8th/e p224)*

50. **Ans. (b) Misoprostol** *(Ref: KDT 8th/e p206)*

51. **Ans. (c) Uricosuria** *(Ref: KDT 8th/e p212, 213)*
    Inhibition of PG synthesis is responsible for analgesic, antipyretic, anti-inflammatory and antiplatelet actions of aspirin. This action is also utilized in the treatment of PDA. High doses of aspirin cause uricosuria whereas therapeutic doses result in hyperuricemia. These effects are unrelated to its action on PG synthesis.

52. **Ans. (b) Aspirin** *(Ref: KDT 8th/e p212)*

53. **Ans. (b) Anti-ulcer** *(Ref: KDT 8th/e p702)*

54. **Ans. (c) Phenacetin** *(Ref: KDT 8th/e p223)*
    It is a prodrug of paracetamol and is commonly implicated in the causation of analgesic nephropathy.

55. **Ans. (d) Acetyl salicylic acid** *(Ref: KDT 8th/e p212)*

56. **Ans. (b) Activation of COX-2 leads to ulceroprotective effect on gastric mucosa**
    (Ref: KDT 8th/e p202-203, Katzung 9th/e p582)

    - COX-2 is constitutively active within kidney, endothelium and brain. Recommended doses of COX-2 inhibitors cause renal toxicities similar to those associated with other NSAIDs.
    - COX-2 inhibitors have been shown to have less gastrointestinal side effects because COX-1 is mainly involved in protection from gastric ulcers.
    - Constitutive COX-1 isoform tend to be house keeping in function while COX-2 is induced during inflammation.
    - COX have role in synthesis of PG's from arachidonic acid, PGs have 20C fatty acids containing cyclopentane ring.
    - Selective COX-2 inhibitors increase the risk of MI.

57. **Ans. (a) Nefopam** *(Ref: KDT 8th/e p224)*

58. **Ans. (b) Seen with ampicillin therapy** *(Ref: KDT 8th/e p214)*

59. Ans. (b) Cyclooxygenase pathway
    (Ref: Katzung 11th/e p626-627)
60. Ans. (b) Latanoprost   *(Ref: Katzung 11th/e p315)*
61. Ans. (b) Warfarin   *(Ref: KDT 8th/e p209)*
62. Ans. (c) PGE_2 *(Ref: KDT 8th/e p206)*
63. Ans. (a) N-acetylcysteine   *(Ref: KDT 8th/e p224)*
64. Ans. (c) Rofecoxib   *(Ref: KDT 8th/e p225)*
65. Ans. (a) Ischemic heart disease   *(Ref: KDT 8th/e p221, 222)*
66. **Ans. (b) Its analgesic efficacy is equal to morphine in postoperative pain**   *(Ref: KDT 8th/e p219)*
    - Ketorolac is an NSAID promoted for systemic use mainly as an analgesic, not as an anti-inflammatory drug (though it has typical NSAID properties).
    - The drug does appear to have significant analgesic efficacy and has been used successfully to replace morphine in some situations involving mild to moderate postsurgical pain.
67. Ans. (b) Reye's syndrome   *(Ref: KDT 8th/e p214)*
68. Ans (b) Cyclooxygenase   *(Ref: KDT 8th/e p212)*
69. Ans (d) Palliative treatment of patent ductus arteriosus   *(Ref: KDT 8th/e p206-207)*
70. Ans (a) Aspirin   *(Ref: KDT 8th/e p212)*
71. Ans (b) Paracetamol   *(Ref: KDT 8th/e p224)*
72. Ans (c) $PGF_{2\alpha}$ *(Ref: KDT 8th/e p206)*
73. Ans. (d) Patent ductus arteriosus   *(Ref: KDT 8th/e p207)*
    In PDA, drugs decreasing PGs are used.
74. Ans. (b) Diclofenac sodium   *(Ref: KDT 8th/e p221)*
75. Ans. (c) Patent ductus arteriosus   *(Ref: Goodman Gilman 12/e p952, CMDT 2014 p1184; KDT 8th/e p207)*
    - Alprostadil is used to keep the ductus open and not for already patent ductus arteriosus.
76. Ans. (c) Piroxicam   *(Ref: KDT 8th/e p218)*
77. Ans. (c) Aspirin   *(Ref: KDT 8th/e p210)*
78. Ans. (d) Glaucoma   *(Ref: KDT 8th/e p206)*
79. Ans. (a) PGE_1 *(Ref: KDT 8th/e p206)*
80. Ans. (b) Acetaminophen   *(Ref: KDT 8th/e p223, 224)*
81. Ans. (c) Arachidonic acid   *(Ref: KDT 8th/e p197)*
82. Ans. (b) Vasodilation and inhibition of platelet aggregation   *(Ref: KDT 8th/e p199-200)*
83. Ans. (c) It stimulates gastric acid secretion
    (Ref: KDT 7th/e p186)
84. **Ans. c. Chronic tophaceous gout**   *(Ref: KDT 8th/e p235)*
    Pegloticase is a recombinant uricase, an enzyme which oxidises uric acid to highly soluble allantoin, that is easily excreted by kidney. Humans lack this enzyme.
    - It is indicated only in rare cases of refractory symptomatic chronic gout because it is immunogenic and carries high risk of infusion reactions, including anaphylaxis.

85. **Ans. (b) Chloroquine**   *(Ref: KDT 8th/e p880)*
    - Prolonged use of high doses of chloroquine (as needed for rheumatoid arthritis, DLE etc.) may cause loss of vision due to retinal damage. Corneal deposits may also occur and affect vision, but are reversible on discontinuation.
    - Sulfasalazine, methotrexate and leflunomide are used in rheumatoid arthritis but do not cause blurring of vision due to corneal opacity.
86. **Ans. (a) Chronic gout**   *(Ref: KDT 8th/e p235)*
    Pegloticase is a recombinant uricase, an enzyme which oxidises uric acid to highly soluble allantoin, that is easily excreted by kidney. Humans lack this enzyme.
    - It is indicated only in rare cases of refractory symptomatic chronic gout because it is immunogenic and carries high risk of infusion reactions, including anaphylaxis.
87. **Ans. (a) Febuxostat**   *(Ref: KDT 8th/e p235)*
    Febuxostat is a xanthine oxidase inhibitor used in chronic gout, it is not used for rheumatoid arthritis.
88. **Ans (a) Colchicine**   *(Ref: Goodman and Gilman 13th/e p702-703)*
    - **Colchicine** is *more effective and faster acting* than NSAIDs *but is used rarely* due to its high toxicity.
    - It *acts by inhibiting granulocyte migration* into the inflamed joint.
    - It *causes metaphase arrest* (other drugs causing metaphase arrest are *vinca alkaloids, ixabepilone and taxanes*).
    - *Most common and dose limiting toxicity is diarrhea.*
    - It can also cause *kidney damage, myopathy and bone marrow depression.*
89. **Ans. (d) Add sulfasalazine and hydroxychloroquine**
    (Ref: Harrison 20th/e p2539)

> **MANAGEMENT OF RHEUMATOID ARTHRITIS**
> - Therapy with disease-modifying antirheumatic drugs (DMARDs) should be started as soon as the diagnosis of RA is made.
> - Treatment should be aimed at reaching a target of sustained remission or low disease activity in every patient.
> - Monitoring should be frequent in active disease (every 1 to 3 months); if there is no improvement by at most 3 months after the start of treatment or the target has not been reached by 6 months, therapy should be adjusted.
> - Methotrexate should be part of the first treatment strategy.
> - In patients with a contraindication to methotrexate (or early intolerance), leflunomide or sulfasalazine should be considered as part of the (first) treatment strategy.
> - Short-term glucocorticoids should be considered when initiating or changing conventional synthetic DMARDs (csDMARDS) in different dose regimens and routes of administration but should be tapered as rapidly as clinically feasible. csDMARDs include hydroxychloroquine, leflunomide and sulfasalazine.

Autacoids

- If the treatment target is not achieved with the first csDMARD strategy, in the absence of poor prognostic factors, other csDMARDs should be considered. Double drug therapy with methotrexate and sulfasalazine and triple therapy with methotrexate, sulfasalazine and hydroxychloroquine can be tried
- If the treatment target is not achieved with csDMARD strategy, when poor prognostic factors are present, addition of a biological DMARD (bDMARD) like TNF alpha inhibitors or IL-6 antagonists etc or a targeted synthetic DMARD (tsDMARD) like tofacitinib should be considered; current practice would be to start a bDMARD.
- If treatment with a bDMARD or tsDMARD has failed, treatment with another bDMARD or tsDMARD should be considered; if one TNF-inhibitor therapy has failed, patients may receive another TNF-inhibitor or an agent with another mode of action.

90. **Ans. (a) Colchicine** *(Ref: Goodman and Gilman 13th/e p702-703)*
    - **Colchicine** is *more effective and faster acting* than NSAIDs but is used rarely due to its high toxicity.
    - It **acts by inhibiting granulocyte migration** into the inflamed joint.
    - It *causes metaphase arrest* (other drugs causing metaphase arrest are *vinca alkaloids, ixabepilone and taxanes*).
    - *Most common and dose limiting toxicity is diarrhea.*
    - It can also cause *kidney damage, myopathy and bone marrow depression.*

91. **Ans. (a) Prevention of granulocyte migration**
    (Ref: KDT 8th/e p231, KK Sharma 2nd/e p382)
    Colchicine is used in acute gout. It acts by two main mechanisms
    1. By binding to tubulin, it inhibits the granulocyte migration into the inflamed joint
    2. It also inhibits the release of glycoprotein from lysosomes which is responsible for inflammatory activity

92. **Ans. (a) Methotrexate** *(Ref: Katzung 13/e p627)*
    Major mechanism of methotrexate at low doses used in rheumatoid arthritis is inhibition of AICAR (Amino-imidazole carboxamide ribonucleotide) transformylase and thymidylate synthase enzymes. This results in accumulation of AICAR in the cells. AICAR is a competitive inhibitor of AMP deaminase resulting in accumulation of AMP. Later is converted to adenosine which is a powerful anti-inflammatory compound.

93. **Ans. (a) Methotrexate** *(Ref: KDT 8th/e p228)*
    Methotrexate is hepatotoxic, so it requires liver function test monitoring for therapy

94. **Ans. (a) TNF alpha blockade** *(Ref: KDT 8th/e p943)*
    TNF alpha blocking drugs are used in rheumatoid arthritis and Crohn disease. These include
    - Adalimumab
    - Certolizumab
    - Etanercept
    - Infliximab
    - Golimumab

95. **Ans. (b) Penicillamine** *(Ref: KDT 8th/e p229)*
96. **Ans. (d) Probenecid** *(Ref: KDT 8th/e p232-233)*
97. **Ans. (d) Piroxicam** *(Ref: KDT 8th/e p218)*

NSAIDs and colchicine are highly effective in acute attack of gout whereas allopurinol and sulfinpyrazone are used for chronic gout. Furosemide causes hyperuricemia and should be avoided in patients with gout.

98. **Ans. (c) 6-Mercaptopurine** *(Ref: KDT 8th/e p234)*
    Allopurinol inhibits xanthine oxidase, which metabolises 6-MP and azathioprine, so dose of 6-MP is reduced to ¼-½ if used along with allopurinol.

99. **Ans. (b) Ampicillin** *(Ref: KDT 8th/e p233)*

Interactions of Probenecid

> - It competitively blocks active transport of organic acids at all sites especially renal tubules. It inhibits excretion of penicillin/ampicillin and increases its blood level.
> - It also inhibits urinary excretion of cephalosporins, sulfonamides, methotrexate and indomethacin.
> - It inhibits tubular secretion of nitrofurantoin.
> - Salicylates, pyrazinamide and ethambutol inhibit uricosuric action of probenecid.
> - It inhibits biliary excretion of rifampicin.

100. **Ans. (c) Allopurinol** *(Ref: KDT 8th/e p233)*
101. **Ans. (c) 100 mg** *(Ref: KDT 8th/e p229)*
102. **Ans. (a) Xanthine oxidase** *(Ref: KDT 8th/e p233)*
103. **Ans. (a) Rheumatoid arthritis** *(Ref: KDT 8th/e p229)*
104. **Ans. (a) Methotrexate** *(Ref: KDT 8th/e p228)*
105. **Ans. (a) Diarrhea** *(Ref: KDT 8th/e p232)*
106. **Ans (b) Vincristine** *(Ref: KDT 7th/e p210)*
107. **Ans (a) Gout** *(Ref: KDT 8th/e p233)*
108. **Ans. (c) Allopurinol** *(Ref: KDT 8th/e p217)*
     - NSAIDs like naproxen have no role in chronic gout
     - Uricosuric drugs like probenecid and sulfinpyrazone are ineffective in the presence of renal insufficiency
     - Allopurinol is drug of choice for most cases of chronic gout.

109. **Ans. (b) Xanthine oxidase** *(Ref: KDT 8th/e p233)*
110. **Ans. (b) Increase in uric acid** *(Ref: KDT 8th/e p230)*
111. **Ans. (a) Probenecid** *(Ref: KDT 8th/e p232)*
112. **Ans. (d) Decreased synthesis of uric acid**
     (Ref: KDT 8th/e p233)
113. **Ans. (a) Misoprostol** *(Ref: Katzung 11/e p1029)*

> Moebius syndrome is extremely rare congenital condition characterized by facial paralysis and inability to move the laterally. It results due to paralysis of sixth and seventh cranial nerves. Important causes of this syndrome are:
> - Birth trauma
> - Use of misoprostol in mother during pregnancy
> - Use of thalidomide in mother during pregnancy
> - Use of cocaine in mother during pregnancy

114. **Ans. (b) PGI_2** *(Ref: KDT 8th/e p200)*
115. **Ans. (b) Endothelin receptor antagonist**
     (Ref: Katzung 11th/e p304)
116. **Ans. (b) Acetaminophen** *(Ref: KDT 8th/e p223)*

Cardiovascular System

CHAPTER 4

CONGESTIVE HEART FAILURE

Fundamental problem in heart failure is inability of the heart to meet the metabolic demands of the body. Heart failure may be **low output failure** in which there is decreased contractility of heart leading to decreased cardiac output or it may be **high output failure** (demands of body are high, which are not met even with increased cardiac output like in cases of **severe anemia**, **thyrotoxicosis** and **thiamine deficiency**).

Acute or decompensated heart failure is the condition in which heart is not able to pump the blood effectively; therefore it is *amenable to treatment with positive inotropic drugs*. Human body also has compensatory mechanisms to maintain the homeostasis. Thus, it leads to increased sympathetic activity that causes increased cardiac output by stimulation of β_1 adrenergic receptors in the heart. This maintains the cardiac output in short run which leads to compensation of heart failure. But, increased sympathetic activity also results in two other effects i.e. vasoconstriction due to α receptor stimulation and increased renin release from the kidney due to β_1 stimulation. Elevated renin stimulates renin angiotensin aldosterone system, thus increasing angiotensin II (causes vasoconstriction) and aldosterone (retains salt and water and is responsible for cardiac remodeling or left ventricular hypertrophy). Vasoconstriction of arterioles increases the after load and that of venules increases the preload, thus leading to increased workload on the heart. Cardiac remodeling is responsible for the increased mortality in CHF.

TREATMENT OF ACUTE HEART FAILURE

It is aimed at *decreasing the congestive symptoms* with diuretics and *increasing the contractility* with positive inotropic agents.

Diuretics

In heart failure, there is accumulation of fluid in the lungs and peripheral organs leading to congestive symptoms. Diuretics help in decreasing these symptoms by mobilizing the edema fluid. **Diuretics of choice are loop diuretics** like furosemide and bumetanide which possess high ceiling diuretic effect. These will decrease the preload and reduce the symptoms. Loop diuretics produce venodilation prior to diuresis and result in immediate relief from dyspnea in pulmonary edema. Same function is achieved by morphine also. Chronic use of these diuretics may lead to development of tolerance that can be overcome by combination with other diuretics like thiazides or spironolactone. Diuretics do not alter the basic pathology; therefore have no effect on mortality except *spironolactone*, which decreases *mortality*.

Inotropic Drugs

Major inotropic drugs used in CHF are dobutamine, dopamine, inodilators and cardiac glycosides. These drugs are used for **short term management of acute CHF** (*except digoxin that can be used orally for maintenance also*).

A. Dobutamine

It is a selective β_1 agonist and has no effect on dopamine receptors. By acting on β_1 receptors, it increases cAMP in the heart that is responsible for increased cardiac contractility and thus increased output. This drug is given by IV infusion. It has *half life of 2 min.*

B. Dopamine

It acts on dopamine, β and α receptors depending on the concentration. At a dose of 1-2 μg/kg/min., it stimulates only dopamine receptors leading to renal vasodilation. Intravenous infusion at the rate of 2-10 μg/kg/min. stimulates heart by the agonistic action at β_1 receptors. At still higher dose (>10 μg/kg/min) there is intense vasoconstriction via stimulation of α receptors.

C. Inodilators

Drugs in this group include **inamrinone** (previously known as amrinone), **milrinone, enoximone** and **vesnarinone**. The name inodilators is obtained from their action as inotropic agents as well as their vasodilatory actions. These drugs inhibit the enzyme phosphodiesterase III and thus increase cAMP in heart and blood vessels. cAMP increases transmembrane influx of Ca^{++} in myocardial cells and thus increases contractility whereas it results in the relaxation of vascular smooth muscle (vasodilation). These drugs are indicated for short term IV use in severe and refractory CHF. **Thrombocytopenia is the major adverse effect of inamrinone** and is rare with milrinone (so, latter is preferred). Both of these drugs can result in arrhythmias. **Levosimendan** is an inodilator that acts by a different mechanism. It **sensitizes the myocardium to Ca^{++}** by binding to troponin C. In addition, it **opens K+ channels** to cause vasodilation.

Nesiritide

BNP is particularly valuable in differentiating cardiac from pulmonary causes of dyspnoea. Nesiritide is a **recombinant BNP** (brain derived natriuretic peptide, normally secreted by ventricles). Like ANP, it also **increases cGMP** and thus **causes vasodilation**. As the name suggests, it *increases the excretion of sodium through the kidney*. It has a *short half life* and has been used IV for acute CHF associated with dyspnoea at rest. The limiting factor is its breakdown by the enzyme, *neutral endopeptidase (NEP)* in the body. Inhibitor of this enzyme, **sacubitril** is approved for CHF in combination with valsartan.

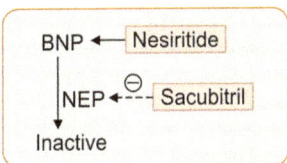

TREATMENT OF COMPENSATED/CHRONIC CHF

Main aim is *to decrease the work of heart* by decreasing the preload and afterload *and to decrease the mortality* by reversing cardiac remodeling **(Fig. 4.1)**. Major drugs used for chronic CHF are vasodilators, ACE inhibitors, ARBs, beta blockers and aldosterone antagonists. Oral inotropic drugs like digoxin can be used in some patients to maintain cardiac output.

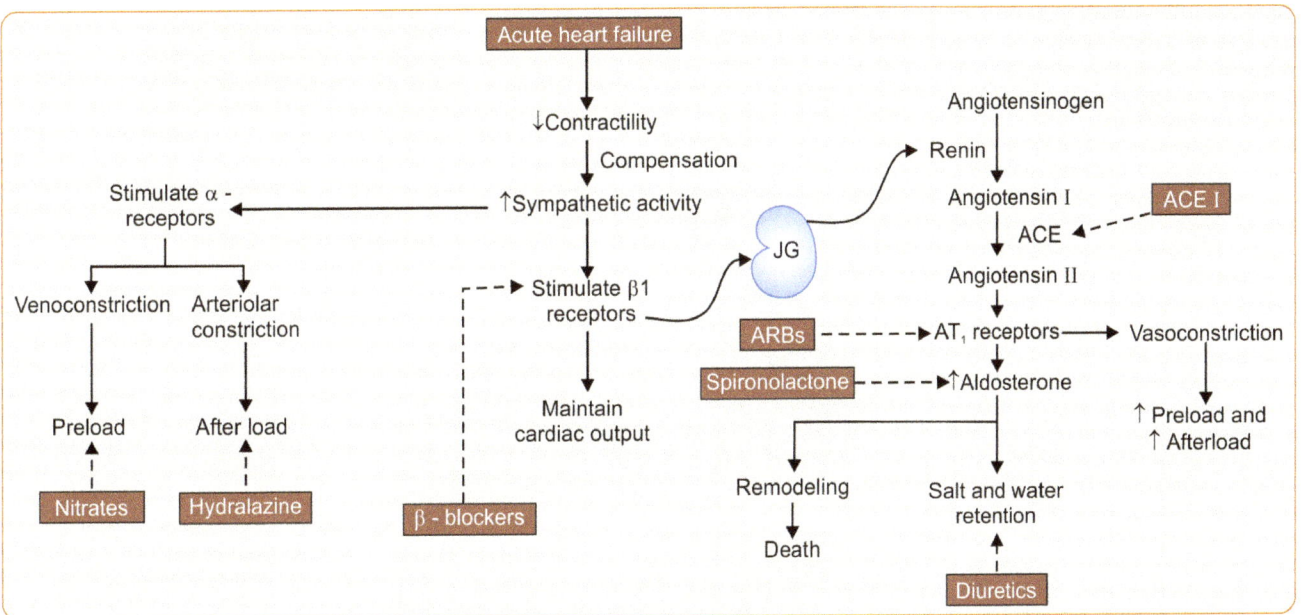

FIG. 4.1: Pathogenesis and drug therapy of chronic CHF

A. Vasodilators

- These drugs may act by reducing preload (*venodilators*), afterload (*arteriolar dilators*) or both (*combined* arteriolar and venodilators).
- **Nitrates preferentially dilate veins** therefore benefit in CHF is due to preload reduction.
- **Hydralazine, minoxidil and calcium channel blockers** like nifedipine are **primarily arteriolar dilators** and cause afterload reduction.
- **Calcium channel blockers should not be used in CHF** because these drugs may increase the mortality in CHF patients (due to reflex sympathetic activation in case of nifedipine and direct cardiodepressant action in case of verapamil and diltiazem).
- Agents reducing both preload and afterload include ACE inhibitors, angiotensin receptor blockers (ARBs), nitroprusside and alpha blockers.
- Combination of **hydralazine and isosorbide dinitrate** has also been shown to **decrease the mortality**. Other vasodilators do not prolong the survival in CHF.

B. ACE Inhibitors and Angiotensin Receptor Blockers

These drugs are indicated in all grade of CHF unless contraindicated. These can decrease mortality in CHF. These decrease the mortality via prevention and reversal of cardiac remodeling due to aldosterone (final mediator of remodeling).

C. Aldosterone Antagonists

Spironolactone and epleronone are the aldosterone antagonists. These are used as potassium sparing diuretics. Their diuretic effect is quite feeble, but in CHF these drugs **reduce the mortality** (at doses lower than diuretic doses) by antagonizing the effect of aldosterone (**reversal of remodeling**). These can also be added to thiazides if tolerance develops.

D. Beta Blockers

Previously beta blockers were considered to be contra-indicated in CHF due to their negative inotropic action but now it has been found that if used carefully, these drugs **can increase the longevity** of CHF patients. Beta-1 causes release of renin which stimulate RAAS and finally increase in aldosterone results. Beta blockers antagonize this pathway resulting in reversal of remodeling. **Most widely used beta blocker is carvedilol** followed by metoprolol and bisoprolol. These are best indicated in mild to moderate heart failure (NYHA class II and III) with dilated cardiomyopathy and are **absolutely contraindicated in decompensated heart failure** (because beta blockers decrease cardiac contractility). These should be *started at very low doses and the dose should be gradually increased* to get the maximum benefit.

E. Cardiac Glycosides

These consist of a sugar (glycone) and a non-sugar moiety (aglycone). These drugs are collectively known as digitalis as they are obtained from a plant *Digitalis purpurea* **(Fig. 4.2)**.

Compounds in this group include **digoxin, digitoxin, strophanthin and ouabain etc**. Cardiac glycosides are positive inotropic drugs but unlike other inotropes, these do not increase heart rate or oxygen consumption (rather heart rate and oxygen consumption are decreased by digitalis). These drugs can be used as acute treatment of CHF as well as for maintenance (digoxin) but these do not alter the basic pathology and thus are unable to decrease the mortality. Cardiac glycosides are also used for treatment of atrial fibrillation, atrial flutter and paroxysmal supraventricular tachycardia (DOC is adenosine). **Digoxin** is the only inotropic drug available that can be **given orally**.

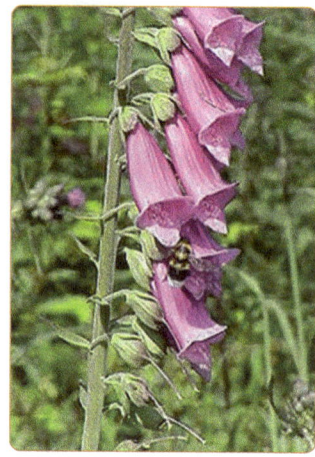

FIG. 4.2: Digitalis purpurea (Foxglove plant)

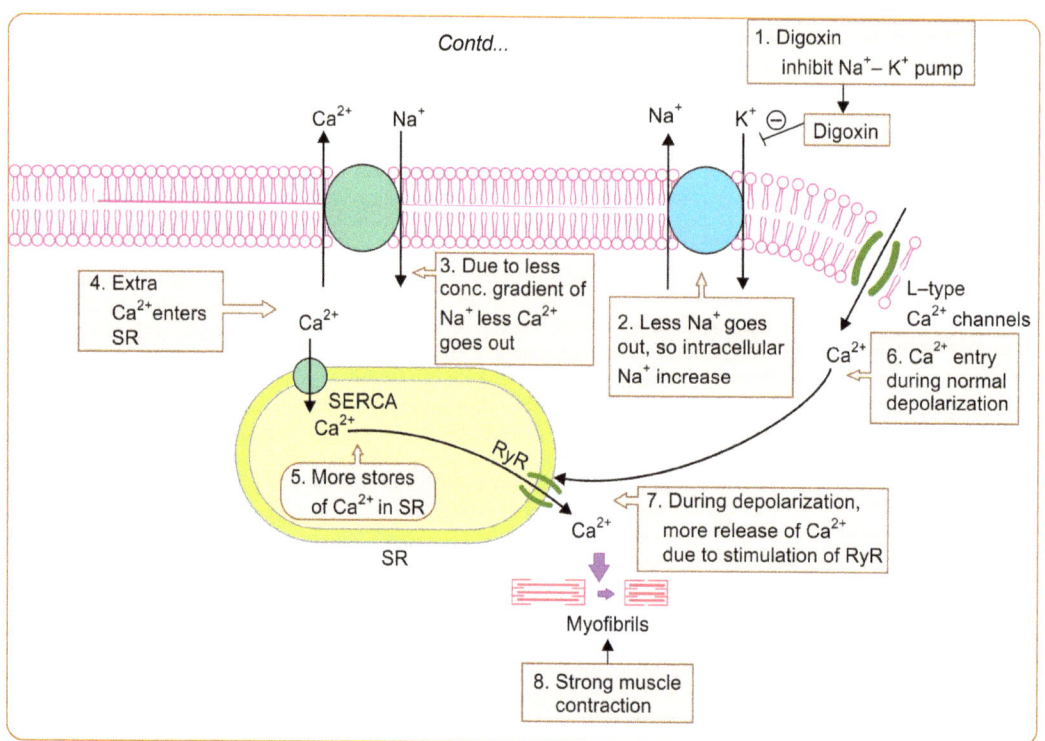

FIG. 4.3: Mechanism of action of digitalis in CHF

Mechanism of Action in CHF (Fig. 4.3)

- These drugs act by inhibiting $Na^+K^+ATPase$ of myocardial fibres by binding to its extracellular face. This result in the accumulation of sodium in the cardiac cell, which in turn results in increased intracellular calcium. Normally Na^+ comes inside the cell in exchange with Ca^{2+} by $Na^+ - Ca^{++}$ exchanger. When intracellular Na^+ is high, more sodium is not required in the cell, so Ca^{++} is not extruded resulting in raised Ca^{++} in the cell. This Ca^{2+} is shifted to sarcoplasmic reticulum with the help of SERCA (sarcoplasmic endoplasmic reticulum calcium ATPase) for storage. Thus, during systole, entry of calcium from membrane Ca^{2+} channels triggers release of high amount of Ca^{++} from the sarcoplasmic reticulum and result in increased contractility.
- *Binding of cardiac glycosides to Na^+K^+ ATPase is slow and also after binding, intracellular Ca^{++} increases gradually. These factors are responsible for the delayed action of digitalis (even on IV injection).*
- *Raised extracellular K^+ decreases the binding of cardiac glycosides to this enzyme* that explains the increased risk of toxicity of these drugs in presence of hypokalemia.

Mechanism of Action in Atrial Fibrillation

- **In atrial fibrillation (AF)**, the mechanism of action of digitalis is to cause *increased refractoriness of AV nodal pathway* (due to vagomimetic action).
- In AF, atrium beats at very high rate (500 beats/minute), and at such high rates the contractions become ineffective.
- This is not of very much disadvantage in case of atrium, because it has to give blood only to the ventricles. But if all the contractions are passed to ventricles, cardiac output will decrease, because ventricular contractions will also become ineffective due to this high rate.
- Thus, *aim of treatment in atrial fibrillation is to maintain ventricular rate at low levels.*

- Digitalis does so by its vagomimetic effect that decreases AV conduction.
- *Vagomimetic effect is also responsible for bradycardia due to digitalis therapy.*
- In atrial flutter, it is difficult to control the ventricular rate. **Digitalis converts atrial flutter to AF**, *in which ventricular rate can be controlled easily.*

Cardiac Effects of Digitalis

- Digitalis **increases the force of contraction sub-bullets and decreases the heart rate.** It also *decreases the AV conduction.*
- The changes in ECG include
    - Inversion of T wave
    - Increased PR interval
    - Shortening of QT interval (duration of systole is shortened)
    - Depression of ST segment

Adverse effects and toxicity

Earliest adverse effect	Nausea, Vomiting
MC adverse effect	Nausea, Vomiting
MC cardiac adverse effect	Arrhythmias
MC arrhythmia	Ventricular bigeminy
Most characteristic arrhythmia	Non-paroxysomal supraventricular tachycardia with variable AV block
Arrhythmia not seen in digoxin toxicity	Atrial flutter Mobitz type 2 heart block
Other adverse effects	Gynaecomastia Yellow vision (xanthopsia)

Treatment of digoxin toxicity

- Mild digitalis toxicity can be decreased with potassium (It decreases binding of the drug to Na$^+$K$^+$ATPase) but *in severe digitalis toxicity, K$^+$ is rather contraindicated* because already there is excess of K$^+$ in the extracellular fluid.
- For ventricular arrhythmias, lignocaine is the drug of choice (phenytoin is an alternative).
- For atrial tachyarrhythmia, beta blockers like propranolol may be administered and for bradyarrhythmias and AV block, atropine is the agent of choice.
- **For very severe toxicity**, digoxin antibody (**digibind**) is preferred.

Istaroxime is an investigational steroid (in Phase II trials) that acts by inhibiting Na$^+$ - K$^+$ - ATPase. But in addition, it also increases the entry of Ca^{2+} in sarcoplasmic reticulum. This action may render the drug less arrhythmogenic than digoxin.

Contraindications and Interactions

 MNEMONIC

Contraindications of digoxin

Contra-indicated	-	Carditis (Myocarditis)
In	-	Increased Ca^{2+} (Hypercalcemia)
Weak	-	WPW Syndrome
H	-	Hypokalemia and Hypomagnesemia
E	-	Elderly
A	-	AV Block (Partial)
R	-	Renal failure (Digoxin)
T	-	Thyroid (hyper or hypothyroidism)

- *Diuretics* like thiazides and furosemide (cause hypokalemia and hypomagnesemia) should be *used cautiously.*
- **Quinidine and calcium channel blockers** (verapamil, diltiazem) decreases the renal clearance and thus *increases the toxicity by pharmacokinetic mechanisms.*
- Antacids, metoclopramide and sulfasalazine decrease the absorption of digitalis from GIT.
- *Digitalis can convert partial AV block to complete block, so should not be used in such patients.*
- It should be used in MI only when it is accompanied by heart failure and atrial fibrillation.
- It is **contraindicated in Wolff-Parkinson-White (WPW) syndrome** because it decreases the conduction through the AV node but not through the aberrant pathway (manifested as widened QRS complex).

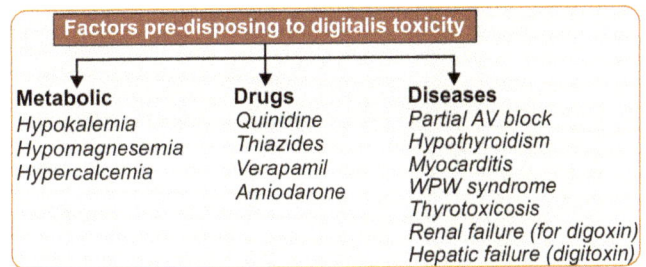

Factors pre-disposing to digitalis toxicity

Metabolic: Hypokalemia, Hypomagnesemia, Hypercalcemia
Drugs: Quinidine, Thiazides, Verapamil, Amiodarone
Diseases: Partial AV block, Hypothyroidism, Myocarditis, WPW syndrome, Thyrotoxicosis, Renal failure (for digoxin), Hepatic failure (digitoxin)

NEW DRUGS FOR CHF

Ivabradine

It is a **funny current blocker** used in angina pectoris. It decreases myocardial oxygen demand by causing bradycardia. European guidelines recommend it for CHF in patients with heart rate >70 bpm with ejection fraction ≤ 35% and symptomatic despite treatment with beta blockers, ACE inhibitors and aldosterone antagonists.

Vasopeptidase Inhibitors

These are the drugs inhibiting two enzymes, ACE and NEP. **Omapatrilat and sampatrilat** are the drugs that can be used orally for the treatment of chronic CHF. These drugs possess all the actions of ACE inhibitors and also result in natriuresis due to increased BNP (decreased metabolism due to inhibition of NEP). Major limiting factor of these drugs is angioedema. Recently, a combination of **valsartan** and **sacubitril** known as **ARNI** (Angiotensin Receptor blocker and Neprilysin Inhibitor) has been approved for CHF.

Vericiguat

It is a soluble guanylate cyclase (sGC) stimulator. Normally nitric oxide (NO) activates to generate cGMP that regulates vascular tone, cardiac contractility and remodelling. In CHF patients, there is impaired synthesis of NO, leading to myocardial vascular dysfunction. Vericiguat can activate sGC in the absence

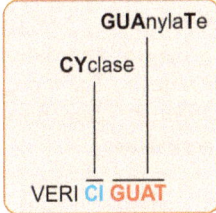

of NO (and synergistically also) resulting in increase in cGMP and smooth muscle relaxation and vasodilation. It is given orally for chronic CHF.

> **Key Points**
>
> **Agents Decreasing Mortality in CHF**
> - ACE inhibitors
> - Angiotensin receptor antagonists
> - Beta blockers
> - Aldosterone antagonists
> - Isosorbide dinitrate plus hydralazine combination

HYPERTENSION

Blood pressure ≥ 140/90 mm Hg is considered hypertension. Four main group of drugs used for controlling hypertension are,

- Diuretics (decrease blood volume and sodium retention)
- Sympathoplegics
- Vasodilators
- Renin-angiotensin aldosterone system (RAAS) inhibitors

1. DIURETICS

Sodium ions contribute to hypertension by increasing the stiffness of blood vessels and thus TPR. Salt restriction and diuretics reverse these effects of sodium. Initially, diuretics cause sodium and water loss that leads to decrease in cardiac output but later on, cardiac output returns to normal while there is net sodium deficit that results in the decrease in TPR. **Thiazides are the first line drugs in hypertension**. Thiazides *should be used at low doses only* because by increasing the dose, antihypertensive effect does not increase but adverse effects tend to increase.

- *Indapamide* is *effective as an antihypertensive at lower doses than those required for the diuretic effect* (due to its direct vasodilatory action). It also produces less metabolic adverse effects (hypokalemia, hyperglycemia, hyperuricemia etc.) and can be used as an antihypertensive in diabetic patients (whereas other thiazides are contra-indicated).
- *Loop diuretics* are not indicated for mild to moderate hypertension because of the brisk diuresis leading to severe reduction in blood volume and electrolyte imbalance. However, these drugs are *indicated in severe hypertension with CHF and renal dysfunction*. **Indacrinone** can be used in patients of gout because it **inhibits reabsorption of uric acid in the nephron** (other loop diuretics and thiazides cause hyperuricemia).
- *Potassium sparing diuretics* (amiloride, triamterene, spironolactone and eplerenone) are used only in combination with thiazides or loop diuretics *to decrease the risk of hypokalemia*.

2. SYMPATHOPLEGICS

This group of drugs is aimed at decreasing the activity of sympathetic system. This task may be accomplished with the use of drugs that decrease central sympathetic outflow, block the autonomic ganglia, deplete the neurotransmitter store or block the adrenergic receptors **(Fig. 4.4)**.

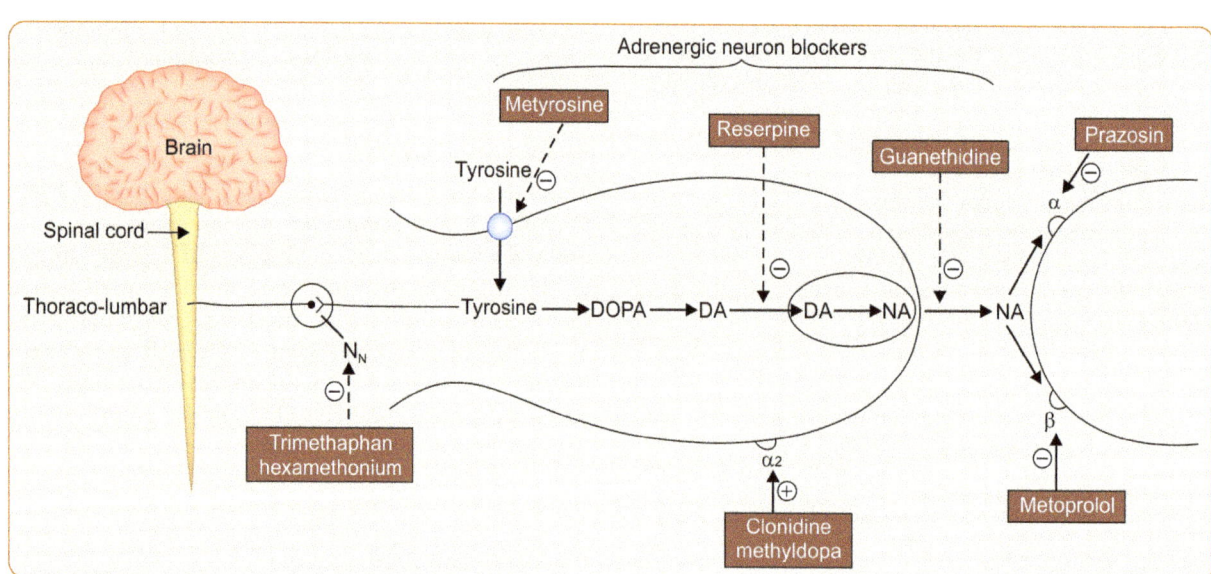

FIG. 4.4: Antihypertensive drugs targeting sympathetic system

A. Drugs Inhibiting Central Sympathetic Outflow

Stimulation of α_2 receptors in CNS leads to decrease in sympathetic outflow whereas stimulation of β receptors in the brain has opposite effects. Therefore, α_2 **agonists** and β_1 **antagonists** can decrease the sympathetic activity and are useful for the treatment of hypertension.

- *Clonidine and α-methyl dopa act as α2 agonists in the brain*. Clonidine acts directly whereas α **methyl dopa is a prodrug**.

Both of these drugs can cause *sedation*. Abrupt discontinuation of clonidine therapy can lead to *rebound hypertension (treated by phentolamine)*; therefore this drug is not suitable for people having travelling job like business executives who are likely to miss the doses. *Methyl dopa can cause hemolytic anemia* as an adverse effect. Both of these drugs are safe *in pregnancy (α methyl dopa is preferred)*. Clonidine, if administered by IV route initially leads to rapid rise in blood pressure followed by prolonged fall. The initial rise is due to the activation of vascular post-synaptic α_2 receptors by high concentration of clonidine. Oral dose is slowly absorbed and such high concentrations are not attained, so orally it results only in antihypertensive effects.

- New drugs like **moxonidine and rilmenidine** are congeners of clonidine with *longer half lives*. These drugs are **selective for imidazoline receptors** *that modulate the central α2 receptor activity*.
- β_1 receptor antagonists like *atenolol, metoprolol and propranolol* etc. can also produce reduction in the central sympathetic outflow. These drugs also act by several other mechanisms (discussed later in the chapter).
- **All of these drugs can result in sodium and water retention on prolonged use due to compensatory mechanisms.** *Diuretics* can be added to these agents to *restore the sensitivity*.

B. Ganglion Blockers

These drugs *inhibit the NN type of nicotinic receptors* that are present on the autonomic ganglia (both sympathetic and parasympathetic). The therapeutic effect (decrease in blood pressure) is due to the decrease in neurotransmission through sympathetic ganglia whereas decreased transmission through parasympathetic ganglia is responsible for the adverse effects like urinary retention and dry mouth. *Hexamethonium and trimethaphan* are the drugs in this group and are used as **antidotes for nicotine poisoning**. *Trimethapan* is used along *with nitroprusside as a slow IV infusion for hypertensive emergencies in aortic dissection*. Mec**amylam**ine is a ganglion blocker used for smoking cessation.

C. Adrenergic Neuron Blockers

Drugs of this group deplete the sympathetic neurotransmitter and thus decrease the sympathetic system activity. **Reserpine, bretylium and guanethidine** are the drugs in this group and are rarely used now.

- **Reserpine** inhibits the vesicular uptake of neurotransmitters causing depletion of adrenaline, dopamine and serotonin in the synaptic vesicles. Due to deficiency of serotonin in the brain, **severe depression** can result with use of reserpine sometimes **leading to suicidal tendencies**.
- **Guanethidine and bretylium** is taken up inside the synaptic vesicles and displaces the stored noradrenaline (which is metabolized), resulting in the decreased neurotransmission. Both of these drugs can be given orally.
- All these drugs can cause *postural hypotension even if used for prolonged periods* (unlike α blockers this is not first dose phenomenon).

D. Adrenergic Receptor Antagonists

Two main types of adrenergic receptors are α and β receptors. Alpha 1 is present on the smooth muscles of blood vessels (cause vasoconstriction) whereas β_1 is present mainly in the myocardium (causing increased heart rate and cardiac output) and juxtaglomerular (JG) cells of the kidney (stimulate renin release).

(i) **Alpha blockers:** Phenoxybenzamine, phentolamine and tolazoline are non-selective alpha blockers (at both α_1 and α_2 receptors). **Phenoxybenzamine** is used for hypertensive crisis in **pheochromocytoma** whereas **phentolamine and tolazoline are drugs of choice for hypertensive emergencies in clonidine withdrawal and cheese reaction**. These drugs cause much *greater tachycardia* than selective α_1 blockers like prazosin due to the inhibition of presynaptic α_2 receptors (α_2 decreases sympathetic outflow) in addition to reflex tachycardia due to vasodilation (caused by both non-selective as well as selective α_1 blockers). *Prazosin, terazosin, and doxazosin* are selective α_1 blockers and cause less tachycardia. These drugs are the **treatment of choice for patient with hypertension and benign hyperplasia of prostate** (BHP). Major adverse effect of alpha blockers is **first dose hypotension** (postural hypotension occurring at the start of treatment or on dose escalation). These drugs do not impair the metabolism, thus *can be safely used in patients with diabetes* (no change in blood glucose), *coronary artery disease* (improves lipid levels) *and gout* (do not affect uric acid).

(ii) **Beta blockers:** Mechanism of action of beta blockers as antihypertensive drugs include:

> - Inhibition of cardiac β_1 receptors leading to decreased cardiac output.
> - Decrease in renin due to inhibition of β_1 receptors in JG cells of the kidney.
> - Inhibition of central and peripheral sympathetic outflow due to the inhibition of presynaptic stimulatory β_1 receptors on adrenergic neurons.
> - Increased vasodilatory prostacyclin synthesis in the vascular beds.

(iii) **Combined α and β blockers:** Labetalol and carvedilol are the drugs having antagonistic activity at both α and β adrenergic receptors. These are used mainly for controlling hypertension in pheochromocytoma. *Carvedilol*, due to its *antioxidant and anti-mitogenic property* is also useful in CHF.

3. VASODILATORS

Drugs may cause vasodilation by opening potassium channels, by releasing nitric oxide, by blocking calcium channels or by acting as agonists of dopamine receptors. **All vasodilators can lead to reflex tachycardia due to vasodilation and sodium and fluid retention due to compensatory mechanisms**; therefore these are *best utilized in combination with diuretics and beta blockers*. Major *adverse effect* of vasodilators is *tachycardia and headache* (due to dilation of cerebral blood vessels).

A. Potassium Channel Openers

> Drugs in this group include *hydralazine, minoxidil and diazoxide*. By opening potassium channels, these drugs cause dilatation of mainly arterioles. These have negligible effect on venules. **Hydralazine in addition acts by releasing nitric oxide (NO) from the endothelium.** Latter action requires the presence of intact endothelium.
> - Minoxidil and hydralazine can be given orally for the treatment of severe hypertension whereas diazoxide is administered in hypertensive emergencies as rapid IV injection.

Contd...

Contd...

- **Hydralazine is metabolized by acetylation** and thus its effect is genetically determined due to the presence of slow and fast acetylators. On prolonged administration it can lead to *drug induced lupus erythematosis*.
- **Minoxidil is a prodrug** and is *activated* in liver to produce minoxidil sulphate (*by phase II reaction*), which opens potassium channels. Its levels are not changed in renal disease, so it is particularly *useful in patients with chronic renal failure*. Minoxidil can cause abnormal hair growth in females (hirsutism) and this adverse effect has been utilized as a *treatment of alopecia in males*.
- **Diazoxide** is a thiazide derivative and can cause hyperuricemia and hyperglycemia (by inhibiting insulin release from beta cells of pancreas). The latter effect has lead to its *use in insulinoma*.

B. Nitric Oxide (NO) Releasers

Sodium nitroprusside *and* **hydralazine** act by releasing nitric oxide from the endothelium, which in turn increases intracellular cGMP by stimulation of guanylyl cyclase leading to vasodilation. **Nitroprusside, in addition can directly stimulate guanylyl cyclase** to cause increase in cGMP. Nitroprusside is a **very short acting drug**; therefore has to be administered by *constant IV infusion* for the treatment of **hypertensive emergencies**. Its solution should be freshly prepared because it is unstable and *sensitive to light*. Prolonged administration of this drug can result in accumulation of *cyanide* leading to *toxicity* particularly in patients with renal disease. It can also result in *hypothyroidism* due to the accumulation of thiocyanate (antithyroid compound). It is *contraindicated in pregnancy*.

 Key Points

Riociguat is a stimulator of soluble guanylate cyclase and is indicated for **Chronic thromboembolic pulmonary hypertension**.

C. Dopamine Agonist

Fenoldopam is dopamine D_1 receptor agonist that causes dilation of peripheral arteries and natriuresis. It can be used IV for short term control of blood pressure in *hypertensive emergencies* particularly in patients with renal dysfunction (because of improved renal perfusion).

D. Calcium Channel Blockers (CCBs)

- These are the drugs that **block L-type of voltage gated calcium channels** present in blood vessels and heart. Three groups of CCBs include **phenylalkylamines** (*verapamil, nor-verapamil*), **benzothiazepines** (*diltiazem*) **dihydropyridines** (*nifedipine, nicardipine, nimodipine, nisoldipine, nitrendipine, isradipine, lacidipine, felodipine and amlodipine*).
- By inhibiting the calcium channels, these agents result in vasodilation and decreased activity of the heart (decrease heart rate, AV conduction and contractility).
- **Dihydropyridine** (DHP) group has little direct cardiac activity and acts mainly on blood vessels, therefore are also called **peripherally acting CCBs**.
- Verapamil and diltiazem have strong direct cardiodepressant (verapamil > diltiazem) activity.
- CCBs tend to cause reflex tachycardia (because of their vasodilatory action), which is nullified by the direct depressant action on the heart (except DHPs).
- **Nicardipine** is **longest** acting parenteral calcium channel blocker and is **drug of choice for hypertensive emergencies** (CMDT 2017/469). It is combined with beta blockers to avoid tachycardia.

 Key Points

DOC for hypertensive emergencies is calcium channel blockers (nicardipine or clevidipine). Nitroprusside is no longer preferred now.

Effect of different CCBs on the heart rate and blood pressure

	Blood vessel	BP	Heart rate		
			Direct effect	Reflex action	Net effect
Verapamil	Vasodilation	↓	↓↓↓	↑	↓↓
Diltiazem	Vasodilation	↓	↓↓	↑	↓
DHP	Vasodilation	↓	No effect	↑	↑

- Reflex tachycardia is more marked in case of drugs with short half lives (nifedipine) whereas in long acting drugs like *amlodipine* (**maximum half life**), effects of reflex activity are hardly discernible. Due to the above reason, *promptly acting nifedipine can increase the risk of angina* (increases cardiac work due to increase in heart rate) whereas sustained release preparation of nifedipine and amlodipine are safer in this regard. Earlier *nifedipine* was used sublingually for hypertensive emergencies but now this practice has been banned due to *increased risk of MI and mortality*. Nifedipine, in addition also possesses *natriuretic* property.
- **Nimodipine** is a relatively cerebro-selective vasodilator, thus used to reverse the compensatory vasoconstriction after **sub-arachnoid hemorrhage**.
- **Verapamil** has maximum depressant action on the heart and it causes vasodilation by causing blockade of calcium channel. It is indicated *for the treatment of angina, PSVT, hypertension and hypertrophic obstructive cardiomyopathy* (HOCM). Diltiazem has lesser effect on the heart than verapamil and is also indicated for these conditions.
- CCBs are especially suitable for *elderly* patients, patients with *low renin* hypertension, patients with diseases like *asthma, migraine or peripheral vascular disease* and in cases of *isolated systolic hypertension*. DHPs are *safe in pregnancy*.
- **CCBs (verapamil and diltiazem) should be avoided in conditions involving decreased conductivity of the heart like sick sinus syndrome, CHF and along with beta blockers** (both cause myocardial depression leading to bradycardia and AV block). **Clevidipine** is an ultrashort acting DHP, recently approved for hypertensive emergencies.

4. DRUGS DECREASING THE ACTION OF RAAS

Angiotensinogen secreted from the liver is converted to angiotensin I with the help of renin (secreted by JG cells of the kidney). JG cells are stimulated either due to less fluid delivery to the macula densa or by β_1 receptors. Angiotensin I is converted to angiotensin II mainly by angiotensin converting enzyme (also known as kininase II). An insignificant amount of angiotensin II is also produced by chymase enzymes (*non- ACE pathway*). This latter pathway assumes importance when ACE is inhibited by the drugs like enalapril, and can result in the decreased effect of these drugs. ACE is also involved in the breakdown of bradykinin, which is a potent vasodilator. **Bradykinin is involved in the causation of dry cough and angioedema.** Angiotensin II acts on AT_1 (main action) and AT_2 (less important) receptors. AT_1 stimulation causes vasoconstriction (by direct action, by release of adrenaline from adrenal medulla and by increasing central sympathetic outflow) and stimulation of aldosterone release. Aldosterone is involved in salt and water retention as well as in the causation of cardiac remodeling. Thus **RAAS results in vasoconstriction as well as salt and water retention leading to increase in blood pressure**. Therefore, drugs that antagonize the action of RAAS can be used for decreasing the blood pressure. This group of drugs is more effective in sodium depleted states (like diuretic use) because activity of RAAS is more in such cases (to compensate for salt loss). *These drugs may cause postural hypotension in diuretic treated patients*, which otherwise is a relatively rare adverse effect. Beta blockers, renin inhibitors, ACE inhibitors, AT_1 antagonists and aldosterone antagonists can act by decreasing the activity of RAAS **(Fig. 4.5)**.

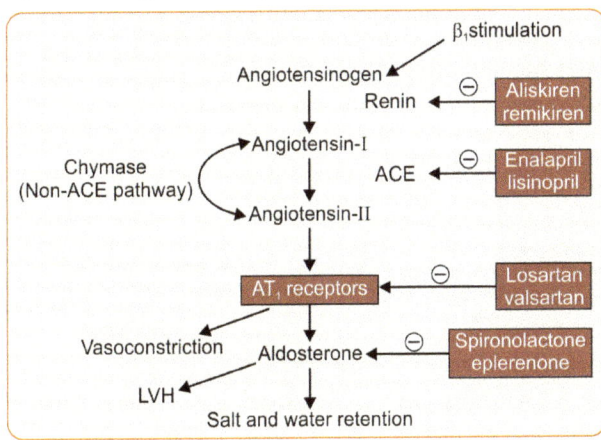

FIG. 4.5: Renin angiotensin aldosterone system and target of drugs

Renin Inhibitors

Aliskiren, remikiren and enalkiren are the drugs that inhibit the enzyme renin. So these drugs decrease the activity of RAAS causing fall in blood pressure. These drugs **can be used orally** for the treatment of chronic hypertension.

Angiotensin Converting Enzyme Inhibitors (ACEI)

This group of drugs inhibits the enzyme kininase II or ACE. So, these drugs decrease the activity of RAAS and also potentiate the vasodilatory action of bradykinin. *Because these prevent the conversion of angiotensin I to angiotensin II, so these can decrease the action of the former but not the latter.*

- *Captopril, enalapril, lisinopril, ramipril, perindopril, trandolapril, fosinopril and moexipril* etc are the compounds in this group.
- Important differences between captopril and other ACEIs is that *captopril is less potent, has fast onset and short duration of action and less absorption in presence of food* in GIT. Because of short and fast action, it *can cause postural hypotension* which is not seen with other ACEI.

- **Perindopril** is *longest acting* whereas **captopril** is *shortest acting* ACE inhibitor.
- **All ACEI are prodrugs except captopril and lisinopril**. Other drugs like enalapril are converted to its active metabolite (enalaprilat) and thus are slow acting.
- **Enalaprilat** is available as a separate drug meant for use in hypertensive emergencies by IV route.
- ACEI are used for the treatment of *hypertension, CHF, evolving MI, diabetic nephropathy, diabetic retinopathy, non-diabetic renal disease and* also in *scleroderma crisis*. These drugs reduce proteinuria in diabetic as well as non-diabetic renal disease and also prevent the manifestations of scleroderma crisis which are mediated by angiotensin II.
- **Most frequent adverse effect associated with these agents is dry cough**. It can be reduced by iron supplements and aspirin. ACEI can also cause **angioedema (Fig. 4.6)**. Both cough and angioedema is *due to elevated levels of bradykinin*.
- These can cause hyperkalemia if used along with other agents causing elevation of serum potassium (like potassium sparing diuretics).
- Other adverse effects include *rashes, dysguesia (altered taste sensation), and acute renal failure (if used in bilateral renal artery stenosis)*. It is important to distinguish between acute renal failure and a normal predictable rise in serum creatinine secondary to ACE inhibitor therapy. An increase in serum creatinine upto 30% within 2-5 days can be expected in most patients started on ACE inhibitors. It stabilizes in 2-3 weeks and is reversible on stopping drug therapy. These drugs are *contra-indicated in pregnancy and when serum creatinine is more than 3.5 mg/dL*.

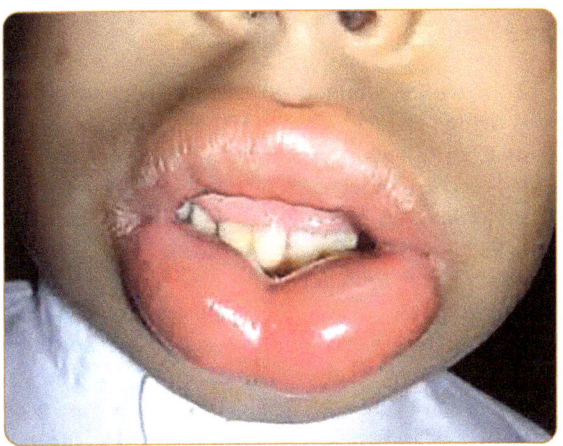

FIG. 4.6: Captopril-induced angioedema

⚠ MNEMONIC

C - **C**ough
A - **A**ngioedema
P - **P**rodrugs (except captopril and Lisinopril)
T - **T**aste disturbances
O - **O**rthostatic hypotension (when combined with diuretics)
P - **P**regnancy (contra- indicated)
R - bilateral **R**enal artery stenosis (contra-indicated)
I - **I**ncreased K⁺ (contra-indicated)
L - **L**ower the formation of Ang II (Mechanism)

Angiotensin Receptor Blockers (ARBs)

- *Losartan, valsartan, irbesartan, candesartan, telmisartan and eprosartan* act by antagonizing the action of angiotensin II at AT_1 receptors.
- These drugs do not increase bradykinin and thus have **less** chances of causing **cough and angioedema**.
- ARB act at a distal site, so these will inhibit the activity of RAAS even when angiotensin II is generated by non-ACE pathway. Due to this reason, ARB can be combined with ACEI for various indications.
- All indications, adverse effects and contra-indications of ACEI also apply to ARB except that incidence of cough and angioedema is less with ARB.

- Special features of **losartan** are:
  - Produce active metabolite
  - Has anti-platelet action due to competitive antagonism of TXA_2.
  - Mild uricosuric effect

- **Telmisartan** has additional PPAR-γ agonistic activity. This activity can help in patients with dysglycemia.
- **Telmisartan** is *longest acting* whereas **eprosartan** is *shortest acting ARB*.

AMERICAN SOCIETY FOR HYPERTENSION GUIDELINES FOR HYPERTENSION 2018

Blood pressure categories in the new guidelines are:

Category	SBP (mm Hg)	DBP (mm Hg)
Normal	<120	<80
Elevated BP	120–129	<80
Stage 1 Hypertension	130–139	80–89
Stage 2 Hypertension	≥ 140	≥ 90

- These guidelines eliminate the category of prehypertension, categorizing patients as having either Elevated (120-129 and less than 80) or Stage I hypertension (130-139 or 80-89).
- While previous guidelines classified 140/90 mm Hg as Stage 1 hypertension, this level is classified as Stage 2 hypertension under the new guidelines.
- In addition, the guidelines stress the importance of using proper technique to measure blood pressure.
- ASH guidelines recommend prescribing medication for Stage I hypertension only if a patient has already had a cardiovascular event such as a heart attack or stroke, or is at high risk of heart attack or stroke based on age, the presence of diabetes mellitus, chronic kidney disease or calculation of atherosclerotic risk.

JOINT NATIONAL COMMITTEE GUIDELINES FOR HYPERTENSION

Classification of hypertension according to JNC-VIII is given in the table. All patients should be advised life style modification (physical exercise, weight reduction, salt restriction etc.) and the patients, who are not controlled with this, should be prescribed thiazides diuretics, if not contra-indicated. Combination of drugs should be considered for the patients not responding to above medication.

Classification of blood pressure according to JNC VIII

Blood pressure classification	SBP (mm Hg)	DBP (mm Hg)
Normal	< 120	and < 80
Prehypertension	120-139	Or 80-89
Stage I Hypertension	140-159	Or 90-99
Stage II Hypertension	≥ 160	Or ≥ 100

SALIENT FEATURES OF JNC-8 GUIDELINES

- Goal BP should be < 140/90 mmHg in all patients < 60 years irrespective of presence or absence of diabetes (DM) or chronic kidney disease (CKD).
- **Goal BP for elderly** (> 60 years) without CKD and DM is relaxed to < 150/90 mmHg
- Goal BP for elderly (> 60 years) with CKD or DM or both is < 140/90 mmHg.
- **Beta blockers are no longer considered as first-line drugs** due to increased mortality.
- First line drugs include thiazides, ACE inhibitors, ARBs and calcium channel blockers (CCBs).
- Rest of the drugs are considered later-line drugs as blood pressure should be controlled by first line drugs alone or in combination.
- ACE inhibitors and ARBs should not be given simultaneously to a person.
- ACE inhibitors or ARBs are first choice drugs in patients with CKD irrespective of ethnic backgrounds.
- For patients with African descent without CKD, CCBs or thiazides should be preferred.

DOC for various conditions

Condition	According to JNC	According to standard books
Hypertension	Thiazides	Thiazides
Hypertensive Emergency	Nitroprusside	CCBs
Gestational Hypertension	Methyldopa	Labetalol (oral)
Hypertensive Emergency in pregnancy	Hydralazine	Labetalol (iv)

SAFE ANTIHYPERTENSIVE DRUGS IN PREGNANCY

Better Mother Care During Hypertensive Pregnancy	Beta blockers (Cardioselective and Labetalol) Methyl dopa (Preferred drug) Clonidine Dihydropyridine CCB (sustained release nifedipine, amlodipine) Hydralazine (DOC for hypertensive emergencies in pregnancy, *according to JNC-VII*) Prazosin (and other alpha blockers)

ANTI-HYPERTENSIVES AND PLASMA RENIN ACTIVITY

Renin is secreted from JG cells, either due to stimulation by β_1 receptor activation or due to decreased fluid delivery to macula densa. Therefore, the drugs that inhibit activation of β_1 receptors (directly by β-blockers and indirectly by sympatholegic drugs) will result in decrease in plasma renin activity whereas other antihypertensive drugs will increase plasma renin activity due to compensatory mechanisms (diuretics, ACEI and ARBs

Cardiovascular System

decrease the fluid volume resulting in reduction of fluid delivery to macula densa and vasodilators increase sympathetic activity and therefore result in activation of β₁ receptors).

  Key Points

The drugs that inhibit activation of β_1 receptors (directly by β-blockers and indirectly by sympatholegic drugs) will result in decrease in plasma renin activity.

TREATMENT OF IDIOPATHIC PULMONARY HYPERTENSION

- If the patient responds to intravenous vasodilators (< 5%), then oral calcium channel blockers (including amlodipine, diltiazem, and nifedipine) are the first-line therapy.
- If these are ineffective or the patient does not respond to vasodilators, then therapy depends on function.
  - If the patient has WHO Class 2 symptoms, then either phosphodiesterase inhibitors (sildenafil or tadalafil) or endothelin receptor blockers (bosentan or ambrisentan) are recommended.
  - If the patient has WHO Class 3 symptoms, then prostacyclin analogs (epoprostenol intravenously, iloprost by inhalation, or beraprost or treprostinal subcutaneously or selexipag orally) should be added to the regimen.
  - For patients with WHO Class 4 symptoms, either epoprostenol or iloprost should be used as the sole agent, though some experts still advocate combination therapies.

DRUGS USEFUL IN PULMONARY HYPERTENSION

Group	Examples	Route of administration
Calcium channel blockers	Amlodipine Diltiazem	Oral
Endothelin receptor antagonists	Bosentan Ambresentan Macicentan	Oral
Phosphodiesterase-5 inhibitors	Sildenafil Tadalafil	Oral
Prostacyclins	Epoprostenol Treprostinil Iloprost	Epoprostenol: iv Treprostinil: iv, sc and inhalational Iloprost: Inhalational
PGI₂ agonist	Selexipag	Oral
Soluble guanylate cyclase activator	Riociguat	Oral

MNEMONIC

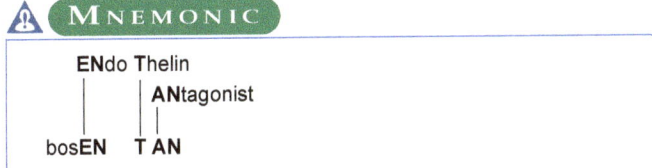

MNEMONIC

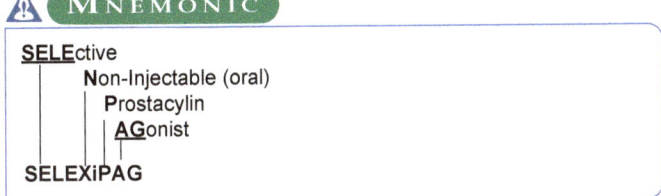

Note

Pulmonary hypertension
- Drug of choice
- MC used drug
- Most effective drug
- Endothelin antagonist
- Warfarin > Bosentan
- PGI_2

ANGINA PECTORIS

Major symptom of angina is the chest pain that occurs due to imbalance between oxygen supply and demand. Coronary arteries are the large conducting arteries that run epicardially and gives collateral vessels to endocardial region. Blood flow to endocardium occurs mainly during diastole. In classical angina, there is a fixed atherosclerotic narrowing of the coronary arteries (Figs. 4.7 and 4.8). At rest, the patient does not develop pain because demand is also less which can be met even with reduced flow. However, during exercise or emotional stimuli, myocardial oxygen requirement increases that result in anginal pain (because blood supply is fixed and cannot be increased). Two major strategies for the treatment and prevention of angina are to decrease the oxygen requirement or to increase the blood supply to the ischemic region.

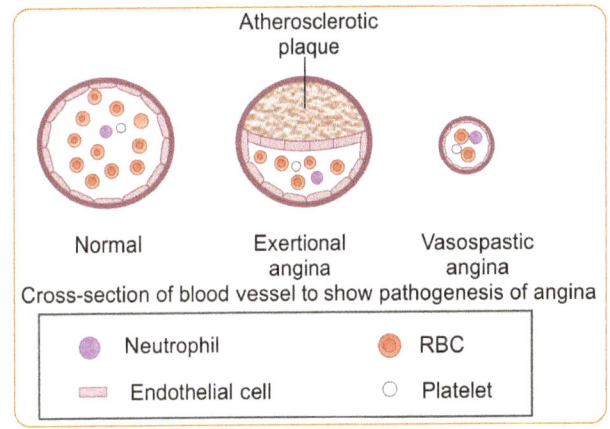

FIG. 4.7: Cross-section of blood vessel to show pathogenesis of angina

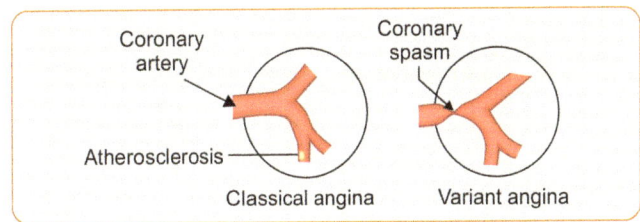

FIG. 4.8: Mechanism of classical and variant angina

Oxygen demand of the heart is increased by increase in heart rate, contractility and heart size. Increase in myocardial fibre tension and ventricular pressure also increases oxygen requirement. Increase in end diastolic pressure (more blood in left ventricle at the end of diastole) increases the duration of systole and heart spends less time in the diastole. This may further increase the chances of anginal attacks because coronary flow occurs mainly during diastole. *Beneficial effect of nitrates in classical angina is through the reduction of preload* that leads to less end diastolic pressure. *Beta blockers and calcium channel blockers act by decreasing the heart rate and contractility.*

In **variant angina** (vasospastic or prinzmetal angina), the major problem is spasm of major coronary arteries (Figs. 4.7 and 4.8). Due to spasm, even normal blood cannot be delivered to heart leading to pain even during rest. All the drugs used in variant angina act by causing dilation of coronary artery. **Recently, a new strategy developed for use in angina is to make efficient utilization of substrates by the heart.**

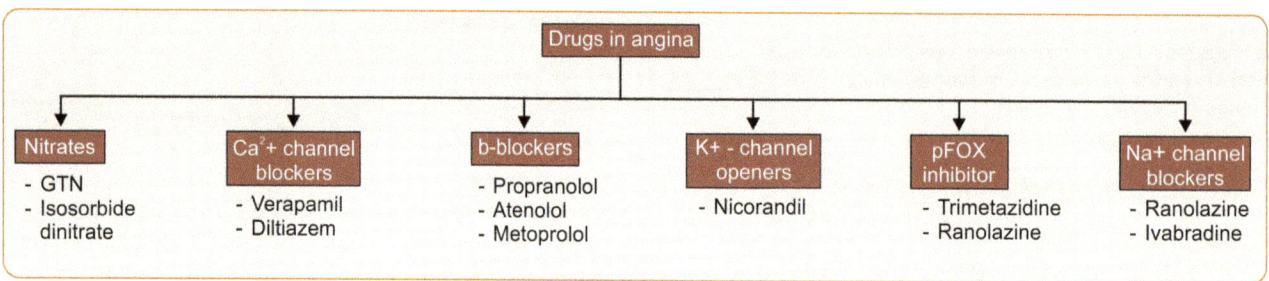

Nitrates

Glyceryl trinitrate (*nitroglycerine*), **isosorbide dinitrate** (IDN), **isosorbide mononitrate** (IMN), **erythrityl trinitrate, pentaerythritol tetranitrate and amyl nitrite** are important compounds in this category. These drugs *act by releasing NO*, which increase cGMP and results in *venodilation*. At high doses arteriolar dilation can also occur. *The enzyme responsible for releasing NO from the nitrates is present mainly in the veins* (therefore selective venodilator action). Venodilation results in peripheral pooling of the blood and consequently decrease in preload and end diastolic pressure. This is the main action of nitrates responsible for relief in classical angina **(Fig. 4.9)**.

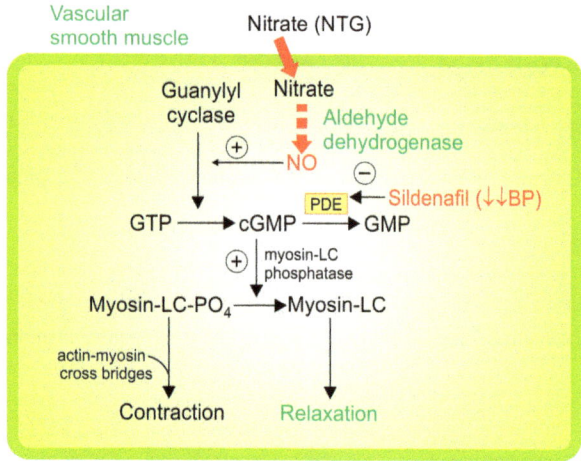

FIG. 4.9: Mechanism of action of nitrates to cause vasodilation

Nitrates *also cause favourable redistribution of blood flow to the ischemic area* (**total coronary flow is not increased**) by dilation of large epicardial coronary arteries. Because small vessels in the ischemic area are already maximal dilated (ischemia is a powerful vasodilator), blood flow to this area is selectively increased on dilation of large vessels and collaterals. **Coronary vasodilatory action is mainly responsible for the therapeutic benefit of nitrates in variant/prinzmetal angina** (vasospasm is the main factor) On the other hand, *dipyridamole* dilates small autoregulatory vessels. Because vessels in the ischemic area cannot be dilated further, blood in diverted away from this area to non-ischemic region (dilation of blood vessels occurs in this area). This phenomenon is known as *coronary steal phenomenon* and is responsible for the therapeutic failure of this drug.

- **Nitroglycerine and isosorbide dinitrate sublingually can be used for aborting the acute attack of angina.**
- Nitroglycerine (by oral or transdermal route) and other *nitrates by oral routes* are used *for prophylaxis* of anginal attacks.
- *Pentaerythritol tetranitrate is the longest acting and amyl nitrite* (by inhalation) *is the shortest acting drug in this group.*
- All nitrates undergo very high first pass metabolism *except IMN (100% bioavailability).*
- Nitroglycerine can also be used for treatment of *acute LVF* by slow intravenous infusion.
- These drugs relax other smooth muscles also, therefore are useful in *biliary colic and oesophageal spasm*.
- Amyl nitrite and sodium nitrite can be used for the treatment of cyanide toxicity. Toxic effects of cyanides are present due to chelation of iron in cytochrome oxidase by this compound. *Nitrites convert hemoglobin to methemoglobin* (which possesses very high affinity for cyanide ions) and forms cyanomethemoglobin. Cytochrome oxidase is freed in this process and the toxicity is abated. Excess cyanomethemoglobin is removed from the body by administration of sodium thiosulphate (forms sodium thiocyanate that can be easily excreted).

As with all vasodilators; *tachycardia, flushing and headache* are the major adverse effects of nitrates. Another problem with nitrate use is the development of **tolerance** on chronic use (not seen with sublingual use) requiring at least 8 hours of drug free period per day. **Molsidomine** is an emerging agent in this category to which *tolerance does not develop*. Phosphodiesterase inhibitors like *sildenafil should never be prescribed with nitrates*. Cyclic GMP is increased by nitrates and its breakdown is prevented by the inhibition of phosphodiesterase, resulting in profound hypotension (due to excess cGMP) and the risk of death.

Calcium Channel Blockers

Verapamil, diltiazem and long acting DHPs can be used in angina. *Short acting DHPs like nifedipine should be avoided* because these can accentuate the symptoms of angina by causing tachycardia. CCBs are effective for the treatment of *both classical as well as variant angina*. **Nifedipine** can cause *hyperglycemia* (by decreasing insulin release) *and voiding difficulty* in elderly (by causing relaxation of urinary bladder). CCBs particularly *verapamil* can also *cause constipation and ankle edema*. These drugs should be *avoided in* *sick sinus syndrome and along with beta blockers. These drugs also increase plasma digoxin concentration by decreasing its excretion.*

Beta Blockers

Major *beneficial effect* of beta blockers in angina pectoris is by *reducing cardiac work*. These drugs do not dilate coronary vessels; rather vasoconstriction may occur (unopposed α mediated vasoconstriction due to blockade of $β_2$ mediated vasodilation). These drugs are therefore, **contraindicated in variant angina**. Abrupt withdrawal may precipitate acute angina and MI (dose *should be gradually tapered*). Beta blockers can be combined with nitrates and DHPs to counteract tachycardia. **Beta blockers are the only anti-anginal drugs that decrease mortality in patients with CAD (Post-MI).**

Potassium Channel Openers

Nicorandil is the agent that causes coronary dilation by activating myocardial ATP sensitive K⁺ channels. *In addition it possesses NO releasing property*; to which tolerance does not develop.

Partial Fatty Acid Oxidation Inhibitors

Trimetazidine is a drug which act in angina by this new strategy. Heart normally utilizes fatty acids as fuel (not very efficient fuel). Heart starts utilizing glucose (very efficient fuel) as a fuel, if oxidation of fatty acids is inhibited by these drugs **(Fig. 4.10)**. Further by inhibiting the lipid peroxidation, these drugs *reduce the generation of free radicals* and protect the myocardium from harmful effects of ischemia. Thus, it can provide beneficial effects in angina via *non-hemodynamic mechanisms*.

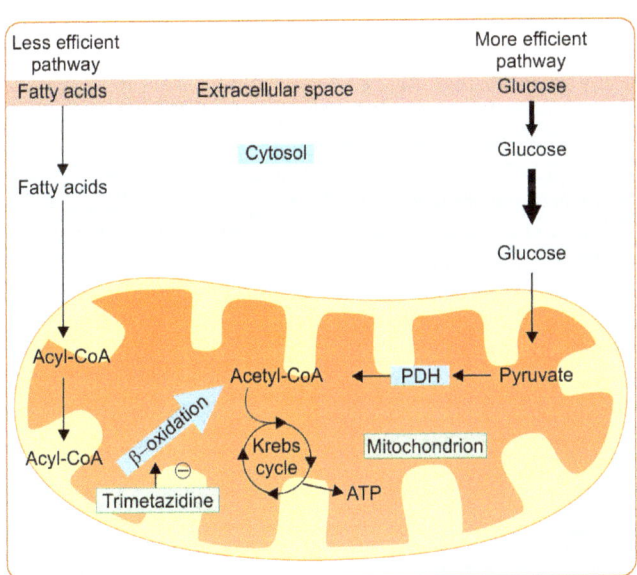

FIG. 4.10: Mechanism of action of metabolic modulators

- **Ranolazine** was initially assigned to this group. However, now it is believed that it acts by blocking a late sodium current that facilitates calcium entry via NCX. Ranolazine is the first new antianginal drug to be approved by the FDA in many years, and it is **approved as first-line agent for chronic angina**. It has **no effect on heart rate and blood pressure,** and it has been shown in clinical trials to prolong exercise duration and time to angina, both as monotherapy and when administered with conventional antianginal therapy.

It is **safe to use with erectile dysfunction drugs like sildenafil** (as compared to nitrates which can result in severe hypotension when used along with phosphodiesterase inhibitors). Because, Ranolazine **can cause QT prolongation,** it is contraindicated in patients with existing QT prolongation; in patients taking QT prolonging drugs, such as class I or III antiarrhythmics (eg, quinidine, dofetilide, sotalol); and in those taking potent and moderate CYP450 3A inhibitors. It also decreases occurrence of atrial fibrillation and results in a **small decrease in HbA1C. It is contraindicated in patients with significant liver and kidney disease. Ranolazine is not to be used for treatment of acute anginal episodes.**

New Drugs

- **Ivabradine** is a new drug for angina. It is known as **bradycardiac agent** (as it decreases heart rate without affecting the conduction or contractility). It acts by blocking a hyperpolarization activated sodium channel (known to carry **funny current;** I_f). Apart from bradycardia, **visual disturbances** is the most important adverse effect of ivabradine

MNEMONIC

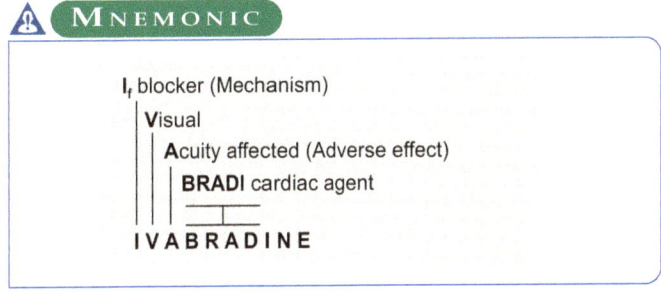

I_f blocker (Mechanism)
Visual
Acuity affected (Adverse effect)
BRADI cardiac agent
I V A B R A D I N E

- **Fasudil** is a selective Rho A/**Rho kinase (ROCK) inhibitor**. ROCK is an enzyme that plays important role in vasoconstriction and cardiac remodeling. By inhibiting this enzyme, fasudil acts as a vasodilator and thus can be used in **angina** and **cerebral vasospasm.**

MYOCARDIAL INFARCTION

For the treatment of acute ST elevation MI, thrombolytic therapy (*streptokinase, urokinase, anistreplase, alteplase, reteplase, tenecteplase etc.*) should be instituted as early as possible, preferably *within first 3 hours*. Ten percent reduction in mortality can still be attained even if these are administered after 12 hours. **Morphine**-like opioid is administered IV **to decrease pain and increased sympathetic activity** (pain in MI results in the increased sympathetic outflow). *Pentazocine and pethidine should not be used* for this indication since these agents cause tachycardia and can worsen the symptoms. *Aspirin* should be started at low doses (40-325 mg) for its antiplatelet action. If aspirin is contra-indicated *clopidogrel* can be used. **Beta blockers** like metoprolol *reduce infarct size, prevents reinfarction and decrease the incidence of arrhythmias*. Oral anticoagulants can be administered to prevent thrombus extension and embolism. Statins can be added to reduce associated dyslipidemia.

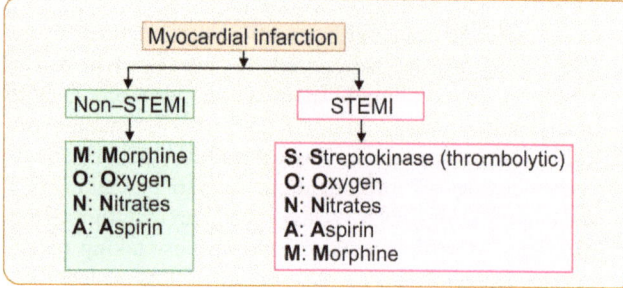

> **Key Points**
>
> Pentazocine and pethidine should not be used for myocardial infarction since these agents cause tachycardia and can worsen the symptoms.

CARDIAC ARRHYTHMIA

Deviation from the normal pattern of cardiac rhythm is known as arrhythmia. Knowledge of the action potential of heart muscle is necessary for understanding the basic pharmacology of anti-arrhythmic drugs.

Cardiac action potential

The cardiac action potential differs significantly in different portions of the heart. At rest, myocardial cell has a negative membrane potential. Stimulation above a threshold value induces the opening of voltage-gated ion channels. Entry of cations (positively charged ions) inside the cell, results in depolarization. There are important physiological differences between nodal cells and ventricular cells that give rise to unique properties to SA node (most importantly, automaticity necessary for pacemaker activity).

Resting membrane potential (RMP)

The resting membrane potential is caused by the difference in the ionic concentration and conductance across the membrane of the cell during phase 4 of the action potential. The normal RMP of ventricles is about –85 to –95 mV. This potential is determined by the selective permeability of the cell membrane to various ions. The membrane is most permeable to K⁺ and is relatively impermeable to other ions. Therefore, **K⁺ is the main cation that determines the RMP of cardiac cells.** K⁺ is the principal cation within the cells whereas Na⁺ and Cl⁻ predominate extracellularly.

Phases of the cardiac action potential (Fig. 4.11)

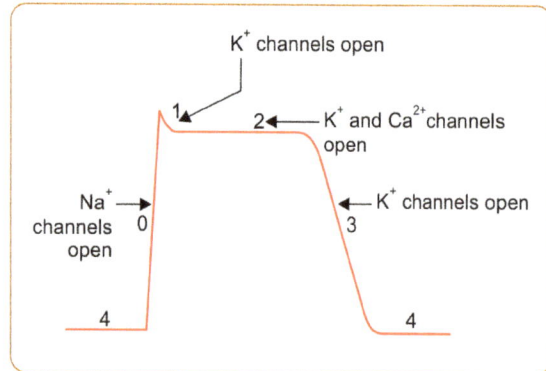

FIG. 4.11: Phases of cardiac action potential

The action potential of a ventricular cell has 5 phases (numbered 0-4).

> **Phase 4:** Phase 4 is the resting membrane potential (when the cell is not being stimulated). This phase is associated with diastole. Certain cells of the heart have the ability to undergo spontaneous depolarization, in which an action potential is generated without any stimulation (automaticity). Spontaneous depolarization is fastest in the SA node of the heart, therefore it is the pacemaker. Electrical activity that originates from the SA node is propagated to the rest of the heart.
>
> **Phase 0:** Phase 0 is the rapid depolarization phase. The slope of phase 0 represents the maximum rate of depolarization of the cell and is known as V_{max}. This phase is due to the opening of the fast Na⁺ channels causing a rapid influx of Na⁺ ions into the cell. **Na⁺ channels exist in three forms;** *open, inactivated and closed.* When cell is stimulated, Na⁺ channels open and result in inward movement of Na⁺ for a brief period. These channels then enter in an inactivated state from which these cannot be stimulated. Slowly Na⁺ channels recover from this inactivated state and enter the closed state (in this stage channels can open on the arrival of a sufficiently strong stimulus). The ability of the cell to open the fast Na⁺ channels during phase 0 is related to the membrane potential at the moment of excitation. If the membrane potential is at its baseline (about -85 mV), all the fast Na⁺ channels are closed, and excitation will open them all, causing a large influx of Na⁺ ions. If, however, the membrane potential is less negative, some of the fast Na⁺ channels will be in the inactivated state (resistant to opening), thus causing a lesser response to excitation of the cell membrane and a lower V_{max}. For this reason, if the resting membrane potential becomes too positive, the cell may not be excitable and conduction through the heart may be delayed. This increases the risk of arrhythmias.
>
> **Phase 1:** Phase 1 of the action potential occurs with the inactivation of the fast Na⁺ channels. The downward deflection of the action potential is due to the movement of K⁺ and Cl⁻.
>
> **Phase 2:** This "plateau" phase of the cardiac action potential is sustained by a balance between the inward movement of Ca²⁺ through L-type calcium channels and outward movement of K⁺ through the slow delayed rectifier potassium channels.
>
> **Phase 3:** During phase 3 of the action potential, Ca²⁺ channels close, while the K⁺ channels are still open. This ensures a net outward current responsible for repolarization. The delayed rectifier K⁺ channels close when the membrane potential is restored to about -80 to -85 mV.

> **Note**
>
> In the SA node and AV node, the upstroke of action potential is due to opening of Ca²⁺ channels rather than Na⁺ channels.

MECHANISM OF ACTION OF ANTI-ARRHYTHMIC DRUGS

Drugs may decrease automatic rhythms by 4 mechanisms:

1. Increase APD (K channel blockers) **(Fig. 4.12)**
2. Increase threshold potential (Na and Ca channel blockers) **(Fig. 4.13)**
3. Make maximum diastolic potential more negative (e.g. Ach and adenosine) **(Fig. 4.14)**
4. Decrease slope of phase 4 (Beta blockers) **(Fig. 4.15)**

Cardiovascular System

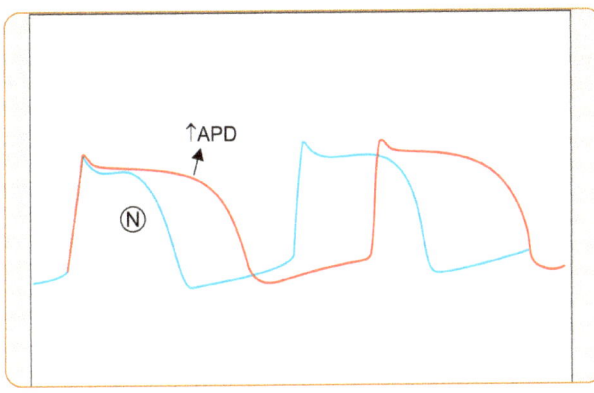

FIG. 4.12: Mechanism of K⁺ channel blockers

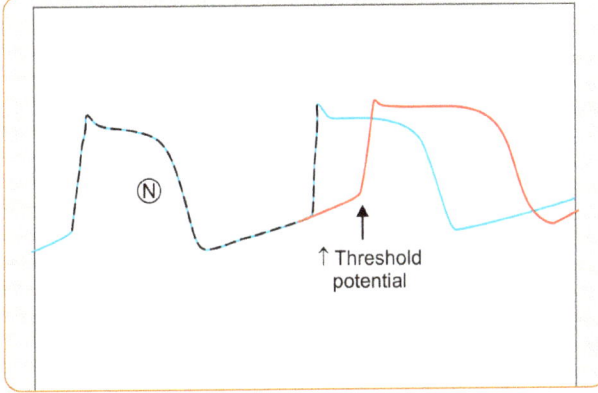

FIG. 4.13: Mechanism of Na⁺ channel blockers and Ca²⁺ channel blockers

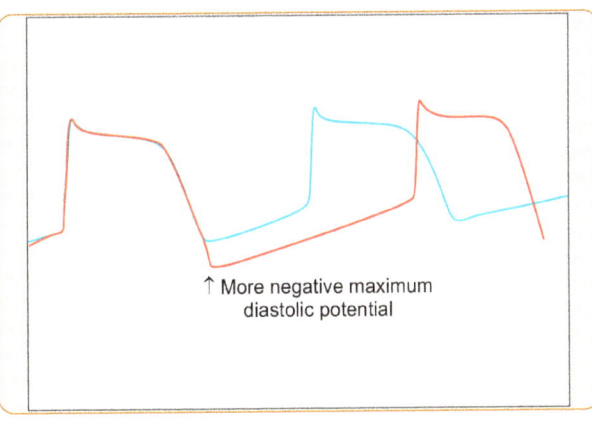

FIG. 4.14: Mechanism of action of adenosine

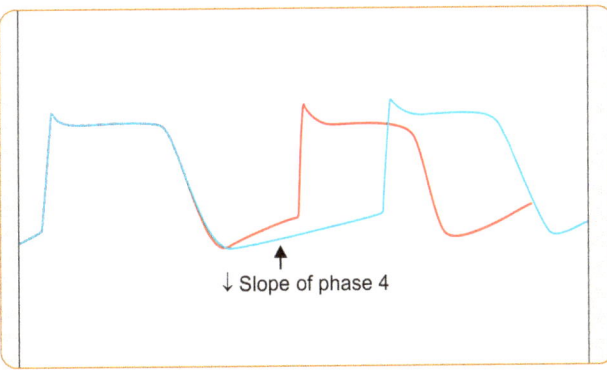

FIG. 4.15: Mechanism of beta blockers

RELATION OF VARIOUS PHASES OF CARDIAC ACTION POTENTIAL WITH ECG

Phase 0 and 1	QRS complex (depolarization)
Phase 2	ST segment (plateau phase)
Phase 3	T wave (repolarization)

SINGH AND VAUGHAN WILLIAM'S CLASSIFICATION OF ANTIARRHYTHMIC DRUGS

This scheme classifies a drug based on its primary mechanism of action. There are five main classes of antiarrhythmic agents.

Class I	Na⁺ channel blockers
Class II	Beta blockers
Class III	K⁺ channel blockers
Class IV	Ca²⁺ channel blockers
Class V	Miscellaneous drugs

CLASS I AGENTS

The class I antiarrhythmic agents *interfere with the activity of Na⁺ channels*. Thus, all of these drugs can decrease the slope of phase 0 (V_{max}). More frequently the sodium channels open, greater will be the blockade by these drugs (*use dependent blockade*). These are further classified according to action of these drugs on K⁺ channels.

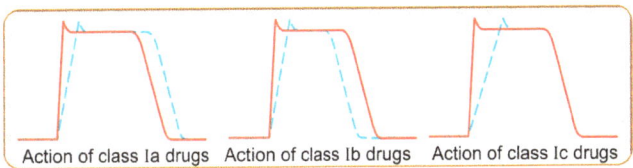

FIG. 4.16: Effect of Class I antiarrhythmic drugs on cardiac action potential. (Bold lines indicate normal action potential and dotted lines indicate the effects of the drug)

Class Ia Agents (Fig. 4.16)

Apart from its action on sodium channels (block Na⁺ channel in **open state**), these drugs *also block cardiac K⁺ channels* (thus delaying repolarization resulting in prolonged action potential duration). Due to prolongation of APD, these drugs *can precipitate torsades de'pointes (prolonged QT interval)*. Agents in this class also cause decreased conductivity and increased refractoriness. These drugs *dissociate from the sodium channels with intermediate kinetics*. Time of recovery of sodium channels (τ) is 1-10 ms. *Quinidine, procainamide, and disopyramide* are the important members of Class Ia.

- **Quinidine** is a derivative of cinchona plant but its antimalarial action is poorer than quinine. In overdose, it can result in **cinchonism** which manifests as *tinnitus, vertigo, deafness, headache, visual disturbances and mental changes*. It decreases renal (digoxin) and biliary (digitoxin) clearance of cardiac glycosides, thus *may precipitate digitalis toxicity*.

- **Procainamide** is an orally active derivative of a local anaesthetic, procaine. It is metabolized in liver by **acetylation** to produce N-acetyl-procainamide that retains the K⁺ channel blocking activity. There are fast and slow acetylators of procainamide similar to isoniazid. Long term therapy with high dose of this drug can result in *drug induced lupus* erythematosis (DLE) particularly in slow acetylators. It is **drug of choice for atrial fibrillation associated with WPW syndrome**.
- While procainamide and quinidine may be used for conversion of atrial fibrillation to normal sinus rhythm, they should only be used in conjunction with an AV node blocking agent (like digoxin, verapamil, or a beta blocker), because these drugs can increase AV nodal conductivity resulting in paradoxical tachycardia.

used for acute treatment of Wolff Parkinson White (WPW) syndrome (Fig. 4.17). [*Treatment of choice for WPW syndrome is radiofrequency ablation of the aberrant pathway*].

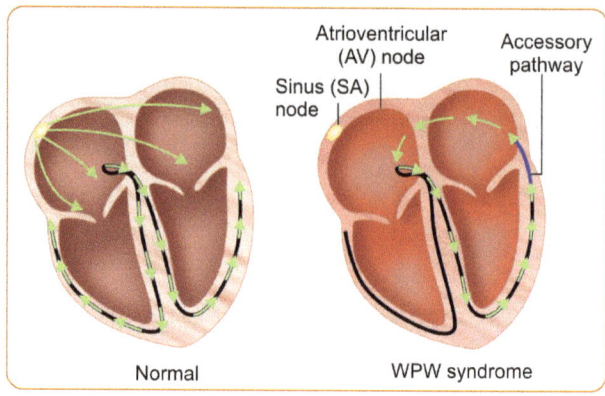

FIG. 4.17: Pathogenesis of WPW syndrome

Class IB Agents (Fig. 4.16)

Class Ib antiarrhythmic agents *(lignocaine, mexiletine, tocainide and phenytoin)* are sodium channel blockers (**block Na channels in inactivated state**) that possess K⁺ channel opening property. Class Ib agents have fast onset and offset kinetics (τ < 1s), meaning that they have little or no effect at slower heart rates, and more effects at faster heart rates. These agents shorten the APD and reduce refractoriness (because of the opening of K⁺ channels). These agents will decrease Vmax in partially depolarized cells with fast response action potential. They do not change the APD in non-depolarized tissues. These drugs are **used only for ventricular arrhythmia.**

- **Lignocaine** is the most commonly used local anaesthetic agent. It has very high first pass metabolism, therefore administered only by IV route. Excessive dose can lead to neurological toxicity (drowsiness, paraesthesia, convulsions and coma) and myocardial depression. It is the **drug of choice** for the treatment of **ventricular arrhythmias due to digitalis toxicity** (ineffective in atrial arrhythmias). It is also the first-line drug for ventricular arrhythmias after myocardial infarction.
- **Mexiletine** is an **orally active** lignocaine derivative with all the properties of lignocaine.
- **Phenytoin** is a popular antiepileptic drug. It can be used as an alternative to lignocaine for digitalis induced ventricular arrhythmias.
- **Tocainide** (group Ib drug having similar name as group Ic drugs like encainide and flecainide) can be given orally but not used widely because of risk of **agranulocytosis**.

Class IC Agents (Fig. 4.16)

These agents have the most potent sodium channel blocking effects with *negligible effect on K+ channels* (therefore no effect on APD). These have slow kinetics (τ > 10s). Drugs in this group include *encainide, moricizine, flecainide and propafenone*. These drugs have *maximum pro-arrhythmic property*, therefore indicated only for the resistant and life-threatening ventricular tachycardia or ventricular fibrillation and for the treatment of refractory supraventricular tachycardia. **Flecainide can be**

CLASS II AGENTS

Class II agents are conventional *beta blockers*. They act by blocking the effects of adrenaline and nor-adrenaline at the β₁ receptors, thereby decreasing the sympathetic activity on the heart. These agents are particularly useful in the treatment of *supraventricular tachycardia*. These drugs *decrease the slope of phase 4 (responsible for automaticity) and conduction* through the AV node. Important β blockers used as antiarrhythmic agents are *esmolol, propranolol, and metoprolol*. Esmolol is the shortest acting beta blocker. It can be used IV for the emergency control of ventricular rate in atrial fibrillation or flutter.

CLASS III AGENTS

Class III agents predominantly *block the potassium channels*, thereby prolonging repolarization (prolongation of APD) (**Fig. 4.18**). These drugs *may precipitate torsades de'pointes* due to prolongation of QT interval.

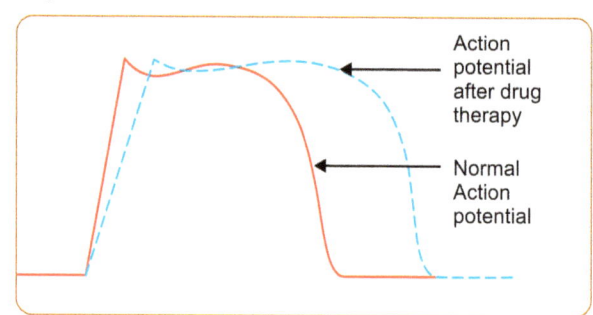

FIG. 4.18: Action of class III anti-arrhythmic agents (shown by dotted line)

Drugs in this group are *amiodarone, bretylium, sotalol, ibutilide and dofetilide*.

> ⚠️ **MNEMONIC**
>
> **Class III Anti-arrhythmic drugs**
> B – Bretylium
> I – Ibutilide
> n
> D – Dofetilide
> A – Amiodarone
> S – Sotalol

- **Amiodarone** is **longest acting** ($t_{1/2}$ = 3-8 weeks) anti-arrhythmic drug. It possesses **action of all classes** of antiarrhythmic drugs (Na^+ channel blockade non-competitive, β blockade, K^+ channel blockade and Ca^{2+} channel blockade). Due to this property, it has the **widest anti-arrhythmic spectrum**. It carries less chances of causing torsades despite prolongation of QT interval. It **contains iodine** (approx. 37.5%) and can result in **hyperthyroidism** (similar drug dronaderone do not contain iodine). It can also cause **hypothyroidism** by inhibiting peripheral conversion of T_4 to T_3. Other adverse effects include **peripheral neuropathy, myocardial depression, pulmonary fibrosis, hepatotoxicity, corneal microdeposits** and **photosensitivity**. Dronedarone is a similar drug but lacks iodine and thus adverse effects on thyroid are not seen. Amiodarone is indicated for the treatment of refractory VT or VF, particularly in the setting of acute ischemia. Amiodarone is also safe to use in individuals with cardiomyopathy and atrial fibrillation, to maintain normal sinus rhythm. It can be used for the prophylaxis of almost all arrhythmias except torsades de'pointes.

⚠️ MNEMONIC

Adverse effects of amiodarone

The	Thyroid (both hypo and hyperthyroidism)
Periphery of	Peripheral neuropathy
My	Myocardial depression
Lung	Lung fibrosis
Liver and	Liver Toxicity [including cirrhosis]
Cornea is	Corneal microdeposits
Photosensitive	Photosensitivity

- **Bretylium** is an adrenergic neuron blocking drug used only parenterally for arrhythmias. Its major adverse effect is postural hypotension. It was considered as a '**pharmacological defibrillator**'.
- **Sotalol** is a non-selective lipid insoluble beta blocker. It has actions of both class II as well as class III antiarrhythmic agents. It is indicated for the treatment of atrial or ventricular tachyarrhythmias, and AV re-entrant arrhythmias.
- **Ibutilide** is a structural analog of sotalol (but no beta blocking property) used for the treatment of atrial fibrillation or atrial flutter by IV route only. **Ibutilide is the only antiarrhythmic agent currently approved by FDA for acute conversion of atrial fibrillation to sinus rhythm** (other drugs used in atrial fibrillation are for controlling ventricular rate).
- **Dronedarone** is non-iodinated compound which has **fewer adverse effects** but also **less efficacy** than amiodarone. It is indicated for atrial fibrillation and atrial flutter. It has lesser incidence of pulmonary fibrosis, peripheral neuropathy and hypothyroidism than amiodarone.
- **Vernakalant** is a multi-ion channel blocker that selectively prolongs atrial refractory period without affecting ventricles. It is indicated for converting atrial fibrillation of short duration (< 7 days) to sinus rhythm. It has little or no pro-arrhythmic action.

CLASS IV AGENTS

Class IV agents are the *blockers of L-type voltage gated calcium channels*. They decrease the rate of phase 4 depolarization in SA and AV nodes. This results in decreased automaticity of SA node and decreased conduction through the AV node. *Verapamil and diltiazem are mainly indicated for PSVT and for control of ventricular rate in atrial fibrillation and flutter*. **Verapamil is drug of choice for the treatment of supraventricular tachycardia (SVT) and for the prophylaxis of PSVT.**

CLASS V AGENTS

Class V agents include *digoxin, adenosine, magnesium, atropine and potassium*.

- **Digoxin** *increases vagal activity* and is used for controlling ventricular rate in atrial fibrillation and flutter.
- **Adenosine** opens the potassium channels and lead to *hyperpolarization of AV node*. It is the *drug of choice for treatment of PSVT*. It is *very short acting* ($t_{1/2}$ = 10 seconds) drug, therefore adverse effects like flushing of face and bronchospasm are also short lived. *Theophylline* being adenosine receptor antagonist *inhibits its action* whereas *dipyridamole potentiates* its action by inhibiting the reuptake of adenosine.
- **Magnesium** is used for treatment of both congenital and acquired **long QT syndrome**.

Drug Treatment of Arrhythmias

Type of arrhythmia	Drugs for acute therapy	Drugs for chronic therapy	Remarks
AF/AFL	Propranolol (Rate control) Ibutilide (to convert to sinus rhythm)	Digoxin Amiodarone Verapamil	Only ibutilide is indicated for conversion to sinus rhythm, other drugs control ventricular rate only
PSVT	**Adenosine**	Verapamil Propranolol Amiodarone	
Ventricular tachycardia	**Lignocaine** Magnesium	Sotalol Amiodarone Quinidine	
Ventricular fibrillation	**Lignocaine** Bretylium	Amiodarone	**Cardioversion** is the treatment of choice
WPW syndrome	Flecainide	Propranolol Amiodarone	**Laser ablation** of aberrant pathway is definitive treatment
Torsades de' pointes	**Magnesium** (for both congenital and acquired)	**Propranolol** (only congenital)	Amiodarone should not be used
Digitalis induced ventricular arrhythmia	**Lignocaine** Phenytoin	Propranolol	For bradyarrhythmias atropine can be used.

> **Note**
> *Amiodarone can be used for chronic treatment of all arrhythmias except torsades de pointes and digitalis induced arrhythmias.*

DYSLIPIDEMIA

Dietary triglycerides (TGs) and cholesterol are transported by chylomicrons whereas VLDL carries endogenous TGs from the liver to blood. TG content of chylomicrons is more than the cholesterol content. In the wall of blood vessels, TGs contained in the chylomicrons are metabolized by lipoprotein lipase (LPL) and the free fatty acids so formed are utilized by various tissues like fat and muscle. Hepatic lipase (HL) present on the surface of liver metabolizes remaining TGs and the chylomicron remnants (with only cholesterol) are taken up by the liver. Net result of this process is transport of dietary cholesterol to the liver and free fatty acids to fat and muscle.

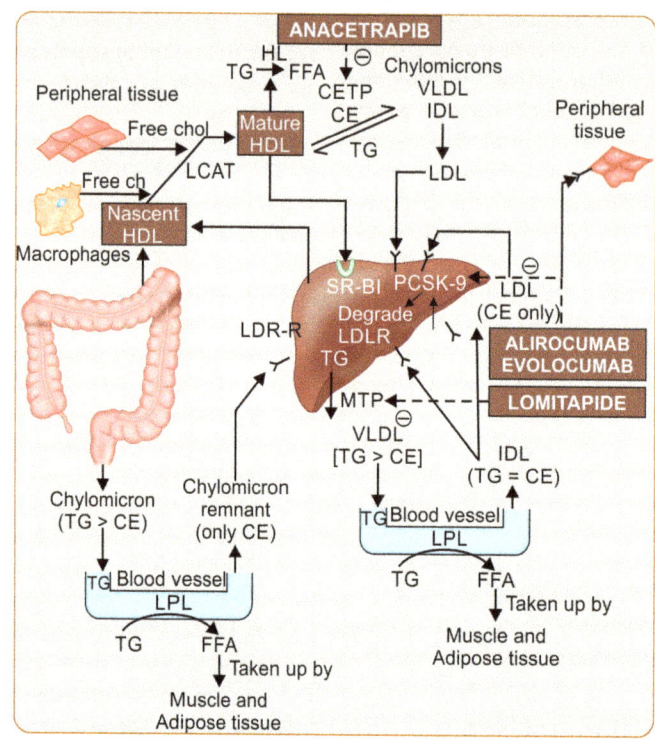

FIG. 4.19: Cholesterol transport and site of action of new anti-dyslipidemic drugs

When TG production in the liver increases, VLDL is formed and is released in the circulation. Microsomal triglyceride transport protein (MTP) helps in packaging of TG and other components to form VLDL. It contains more TG than cholesterol ester (CE). TGs are metabolized by LPL and VLDL is converted to IDL (TG = CE). IDL has two fates; either it is converted to LDL by the metabolism of remaining TGs by HL (LDL contains only CE) or it is taken up in the liver through LDL receptors (LDLR). LDL transports its CE either to various tissues or is taken up in the liver by LDLR. Proprotein convertase subtilisin/kexin type 9 (PCSK 9) is a protein that binds LDL-receptors and target it for degradation. TG and CE transported by LDL-R are sent to lysosome where these are broken down by lysosomal acid lipase (Fig. 4.19).

HDL is formed by taking cholesterol from tissues and helps in the transport of this cholesterol to the liver (reverse cholesterol transport). Thus *HDL is a good cholesterol and LDL, IDL and VLDL are bad cholesterols*. Nascent HDL is secreted by hepatocytes and enterocytes. It takes free cholesterol from peripheral tissues and macrophages. Enzyme lecithin cholesterol acetyl transferace (LCAT) converts the free cholesterol to cholesteryl ester (CE). This mature HDL has 2 fates.

1. It may be taken by liver through scvanger receptor SR-B1.
2. CE are transferred to chylomicrons or VLDL in exchange with TG. This requires enzyme cholesterylester TG transport protein (CETP). This converts VLDL to LDL which is taken by liver through LDL receptor. TG rich HDL is now acted upon by hepatic lipase.

Altered level of these lipoproteins may be secondary to some diseases like diabetes and nephrotic syndrome. Primary hyperlipoproteinemia is familial or genetic in origin. Various types of primary hyperlipoproteinemia are given in the table and important points to remember are:

- TG is elevated in all except type IIa
- Cholesterol is elevated only in type II (IIa, IIb) and type III
- Type II is treated with statins and III and IV with fibrates
- Type I and V do not increase the risk of atherosclerosis and require no treatment.

Type of disorder	LP increased	Lipids elevated		Risk of atherosclerosis	Treatment
		TG	CH		
I	CM	+++	N	No	None
IIa	LDL	N	++	+++	Statins
IIb	VLDL and LDL	++	++	+++	Statins, fibrates, nicotinic acid
III	IDL and CMR	++	++	++	Fibrates
IV	VLDL	++	N	++	Fibrates, nicotinic acid
V	VLDL and CM	++	N	No	None

Cardiovascular System

ANTI-DYSLIPIDEMIC DRUGS

First line drugs include *statins, bile acid binding resins and intestinal cholesterol absorption inhibitors* whereas **second line** drugs include *fibrates and niacin.*

Statins

HMG CoA reductase catalyses the *rate limiting step* in cholesterol biosynthesis (conversion of HMG CoA to mevalonate). *Statins act by inhibiting this enzyme* competitively and result in decreased cholesterol synthesis in the liver. As liver requires cholesterol for synthesis of bile acids and steroid hormones, it responds by increasing the uptake of LDL from the plasma. This is done by *increasing LDL receptors on its surface* **(Fig. 4.20)**. **Statins are most powerful LDL lowering agents.** These drugs also lower TG, IDL and VLDL and increases HDL slightly. However, these drugs have **no effect on lipoprotein (a)**. *Most potent statin is* **pitavastatin followed by rosuvastatin** whereas fluvastatin and lovastatin are least potent compounds in this group. Activity of HMG CoA reductase is maximum at night, so these drugs are administered at night. *Rosuvastatin (t1/2 =19 hours) and atorvastatin (t1/2 = 14 hours) are long acting drugs,* therefore can be administered at any time of the day. In addition to lipid lowering effects, statins also possess **additional antioxidant, anti-inflammatory and anti-proliferative properties**. These are **known as pleotropic effects** of statins and are responsible, in part for lowering the risk of stroke and MI. *Pravastatin also causes decrease in plasma fibrinogen levels.*

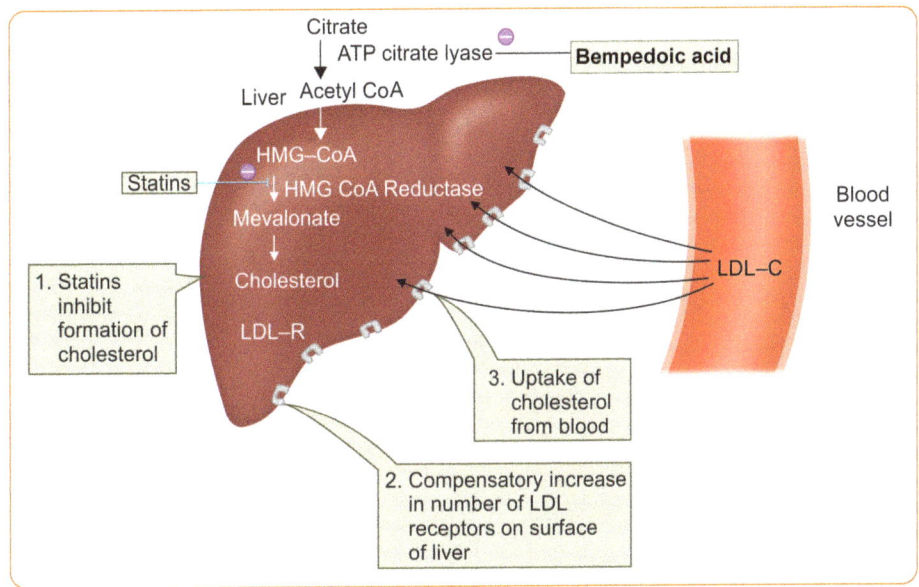

FIG. 4.20: Mechanism of action of stations

> **Key Points**
>
> **Pleotropic Effects of Statins**
> - Antioxidant
> - Anti-inflammatory
> - Anti-proliferative

> **Key Points**
>
> **Risk of statin induced myopathy is increased by**
> - Old age
> - Renal insufficiency
> - Erythromycin
> - Ketoconazole
> - Fibrates
> - Immunosuppressants

- Structurally lovastatin and simvastatin are inactive lactone prodrugs, pravastatin has active lactone ring whereas atorvastatin, fluvastatin and rosuvastatin are fluorine-containing congeners.

- All statins can be **absorbed** orally (*maximum fluvastatin*). **Food increases absorption of all drugs except pravastatin. Lovastatin and simvastatin** undergo extensive first pass metabolism and are administered as **prodrugs**.

- Pravastatin, fluvastatin, atorvastatin and rosuvastatin are administered as active drugs. *All drugs except pravastatin are metabolized extensively by hepatic microsomal enzymes.* Pravastatin is metabolized by sulfation (non-microsomal) and thus has least chances of drug interactions.

- **Rosuvastatin** is *longest acting* whereas **pitavastatin** is *most potent* statin.

- Major adverse effect of these drugs is **myopathy and hepatotoxicity**. Chances of myopathy increases if these are co-administered with fibrates (maximum with gemfibrozil) or niacin. Myopathy can proceed to rhabdomyolysis with resultant renal shutdown. *Pravastatin remains confined to the liver and is safer in this regard.* These agents should be *avoided in pregnancy and lactation.*

- Some **patients taking statins develop diabetes mellitus** but the benefits associated with reduction in cardiovascular events outweigh the risk of diabetes.

- Statins are the **first line drugs for type IIa, type IIb and secondary hyperlipoproteinemia** (in these conditions, cholesterol level is raised more than TG).
- In children with heterozygous familial hypercholesterolemia, pravastatin is approved for children ≥ 8 years whereas other statins are approved for children ≥ 10 years. Pitavastatin has not been studied for this indication.

> ⚠️ **MNEMONIC**
>
> **Pravastatin**
> - **Minimum** drug interactions [metabolized by non-microsomal enzymes]
> - **Minimum** Food interactions [Food increase absorption of all statins except pravastatin]
> - **Minimum** risk of myopathy
> - **Minimum** CNS penetration
> - **Minimize** (Decrease) Fibrinogen Level

Intestinal Cholesterol Absorption Inhibitor

Ezetimibe inhibits a transporter involved in intestinal absorption of cholesterol called NPC1L1. Due to decreased absorption, cholesterol content of the liver decreases and it responds by increasing LDL receptor synthesis. It can be used alone or combined with statins for type IIa and IIb hyperlipoproteinemia. It is effective in reducing LDL-C in patients with **sitosterolemia**

Bile Acid Binding Resins

These drugs *bind to bile acids in the intestinal lumen and decrease its reabsorption* (resulting in more excretion through faeces) (**Fig. 4.21**). Cholesterol pool of liver is depleted because it is utilized for the formation of bile acids. Liver acquires cholesterol from the plasma by increasing LDL receptors. *Bile acids inhibit TG production in the liver* and their deficiency results in **elevation of TGs. Bile acid binding resins are used only for type IIa disorder (TGs are normal in this condition)**. Drugs in this group include *cholestyramine, colestipol and colesevelam*.

Cholestyramine and colestipol are available as sachets. These are mixed with water, kept for some time (to increase the palatability) and then taken with meals. *Colesevelam is available as a tablet and has better patient compliance*. Major adverse effect of these drugs is constipation. **These are cholesterol lowering agent of choice in children, pregnancy and lactation.**

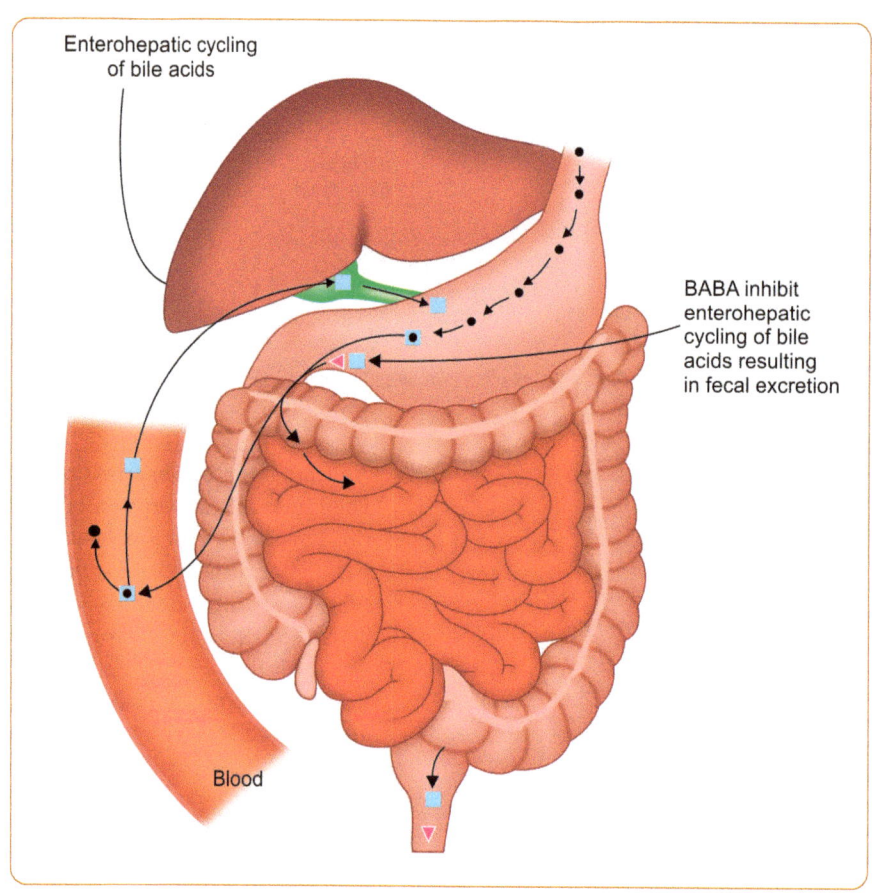

FIG. 4.21: Mechanism of action of bile acid binding agents

Fibric Acid Derivatives

This group of drugs *acts by activating LPL* by activating a nuclear receptor, **PPARα** (peroxisome proliferator activated receptor alpha). Major effect of the fibrates is to *reduce TG* (contained in VLDL) and to increase HDL. Clofibrate is not used now because it resulted in increased mortality (due to malignancies and post cholecystectomy complications) and did not prevent fatal MI. *Gemfibrozil, fenofibrate and bezafibrate are currently* *available*. **Fenofibrate is a prodrug with longest half life. It has maximum LDL cholesterol lowering action.** *Fibrates also reduce plasma fibrinogen level*. Fibrates are the **drugs of choice in hypertriglyceridemia (type III and IV)** and can be used with other drugs in type IIb. **Fenofibrate is uricosuric and can be used in the setting of hyperuricemia.** GI distress and elevation of aminotransferases are important adverse effects of fibric acid derivatives. *Risk of myopathy is increased* if these are used *with statins except bezafibrate*. **Fibrates can potentiate the effects of warfarin and oral hypoglycemic agents.**

Nicotinic Acid

Niacin (not nicotinamide) is an inexpensive drug (vitamin B_3) that produces decrease in LDL cholesterol and VLDL triglycerides along with increase in HDL cholesterol. It **acts by inhibiting lipolysis in the adipose tissue**.

- Among all hypolipidemic drugs, niacin has **maximum HDL increasing property;** therefore it is useful in patients having increased risk of CAD.
- Further, *it can also* **decrease lipoprotein (a) and fibrinogen.** It is *useful for type IIb, III and IV disorders*.
- Main **compliance limiting feature is cutaneous flushing and pruritis.** These symptoms are due to vasodilatory action of niacin through release of PGs and can be **prevented by pretreatment with aspirin**. To minimize the side effects, niacin should be started at low doses.
- Niacin should be **avoided in diabetic patients** because it impairs insulin sensitivity.
- Other important adverse effects are **GI toxicity and hyperuricemia.**
- Niacin can also lead to **hepatotoxicity** which is *manifested by fall in both LDL as well HDL cholesterol*.
- **Acanthosis nigricans** (dark colored skin lesion) and **maculopathy** are infrequent side effects of niacin.

> **Key Points**
>
> | | |
> |---|---|
> | Maximum LDL lowering drugs: | **Statins** |
> | Maximum TG lowering drugs: | **Fibrates** |
> | Maximum HDL increasing drugs: | **Niacin** |

Miscellaneous Drugs

Probucol is useful because of its *antioxidant* action. It inhibits oxidation of LDL and causes reduction in levels of both HDL and LDL cholesterol. **Gugulipid** is the drug developed by Central Drug Research Institute, Lucknow. It causes modest decrease in LDL and slight increase in HDL cholesterol. Diarrhea is the only adverse effect of this drug.

New Drugs

CETP Inhibitors

Cholesteryl Ester Triglyceride transport Protein (CETP) is required for exchange of TG and CE between HDL and apo-B rich lipoproteins. This leads to formation of TG rich HDL which is acted upon by hepatic lipase. Inhibitors of CETP can thus increase HDL cholesterol level. **Torcetrapib, dalcetrapib and evacetrapib failed the clinical trials**. Torcetrapib resulted in excessive deaths whereas other two had lack of efficacy. **Anacetrapib is undergoing clinical trials.**

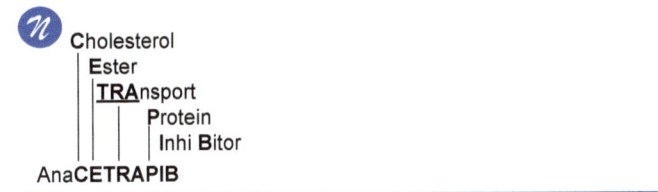

MTP Inhibitors

Lomitapide inhibits microsomal triglyceride transport protein (MTP) which is necessary for VLDL assembly and secretion in liver. It is indicated for familial homozygous hyper cholesterolemia.

> **Key Points**
>
> Niacin can cause hepatotoxicity and hyperuricemia.

Mipomersen

It is an antisense oligonucleotide that targets the mRNA for apo-B. It is FDA-approved for familial homozygous hyper-cholesterolemia. It is administered subcutaneously once a week. FDA-has issued a black box warning of liver disease for this drug.

> **Key Points**
>
> Drugs approved for homozygous familial hypercholesterolemia
> - Mipomersen
> - Lomitapide
> - Evolocumab

PCSK9 Inhibitors

Proprotein convertase subtilisin kexin type 9 (PCSK 9) is a protein that binds LDL-receptors and transport them to lysosomes where these are degraded. Therefore instead of recycling of LDL-R to surface of hepatocytes, they get destroyed. Inhibitors of PCSK 9, therefore prevent destruction of LDL-R resulting in lowering of LDL-cholesterol. **Alirocumab** and **evolocumab** are monoclonal antibodies against PCSK 9 and are approved for familial hypercholesterolemia as an adjunct to diet and maximally tolerated statin therapy.

> **Key Points**
>
> **Alirocumab** and **Evolocumab** are PCSK 9 inhibitors for familial hypercholesterolemia

Avasimibe

It is an *inhibitor of enzyme ACAT-1* (acyl coenzyme A: cholesterol acyl transferase-1) which forms cholesterol ester from cholesterol.

Evinacumab

It is a monoclonal antibody against ANGPTL3 (Angiopoietin-like 3 protein). Normally, ANGPTL3 inhibits lipoprotein lipase (LPL) and endothelial lipase (EL). LPL breaks TG within chylomicrons and VLDL. By inhibiting ANGPTL3, the function of LPL is enhanced and there will be more breakdown of chylomicrons and VLDL resulting in decrease in TG, VLDL as well as LDL-cholesterol (VLDL is required to form LDL). However, function of EL is to break HDL-cholesterol. So, evinacumab result in **decrease in TG, Total cholesterol, LDL, VLDL as well as HDL-cholesterol**. The major advantage of this drug is that, it decreases cholesterol **independent of LDL-receptor levels**. Evinacumab is approved for treatment of familial homozygous hypercholesterolamia by intravenous route.

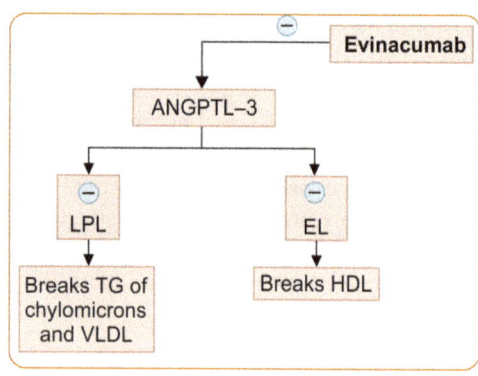

Bempedoic Acid

It inhibits the enzyme ATP-citrate lyase. This enzyme helps in conversion of citrate from TCA cycle to acetyl-CoA which is required for formation of cholesterol. It is used orally for treatment of hypercholesterolemia

Golden Points

1. *Spironolactone is the only diuretic* which decreases *mortality in patients with CHF.*
2. Digoxin is the only inotropic drugs available that can be given orally.
3. *Mechanism of action of digitalis in CHF is inhibition of Na^+-K^+-ATPase* whereas its vagonmimetic action is used for treatment of atrial fibrillation
4. **Digitalis** is **contraindicated in Wolff-Parkinson-White (WPW) syndrome** because it decreases the conduction through the AV node but not through the aberrant pathway.
5. Evaluation of adequate response to digitalis therapy is primarily done by monitoring clinical symptoms.
6. Earliest appearing adverse effect of digitalis is *nausea and vomiting*
7. Digitalis can cause almost any cardiac arrhythmia *except Mobitz type II heart block and Atrial flutter.*
8. **Most characteristic arrhythmia** due to digitalis toxicity is non-paroxysmal supra-ventricular tachycardia with variable atrio-ventricular block whereas most common is ventricular bigeminy.
9. For digitalis-induced ventricular arrhythmias, lignocaine is the drug of choice
10. **Sacubitril** is a neprilysin (NEP) inhibitor recently approved for CHF
11. ACE inhibitors and ARBs are indicated for all grades of CHF unless these are contraindicated.
12. Most widely used beta blocker for CHF is carvedilol followed by metoprolol and bisoprolol.
13. Beta blockers are absolutely contra- indicated in decompensated heart failure
14. In CHF, Beta blockers should be *started at very low doses and the dose should be gradually increased*
15. **Moxonidine and rilmenidine** are congeners of clonidine with *longer half lives*. These drugs are **selective for imidazoline receptors**.
16. Mecamylamine is a ganglion blocker used for smoking cessation.
17. Due to deficiency of serotonin in the brain, **severe depression** can result with use of reserpine sometimes **leading to suicidal tendencies.**
18. Phentolamine and tolazoline are drugs of choice for hypertensive emergencies in clonidine withdrawal and cheese reaction.
19. Diuretics has maximum risk of causing erectile dysfunction whereas ACE inhibitors decrease the risk of erectile dysfunction.
20. Minoxidil can cause abnormal hair growth in females (hirsutism) and this adverse effect has been utilized as a *treatment of alopecia in males.*
21. Prolonged administration of sodium nitroprusside can result in accumulation of *cyanide* leading to *toxicity* particularly in patients with renal disease.
22. Nimodipine is a cerebro-selective CCB, used to reverse the compensatory vasoconstriction after sub-arachnoid hemorrhage.
23. **Clevidipine** is an ultrashort acting DHP, recently approved for hypertensive emergencies.
24. Bradykinin is involved in the causation of dry cough and angioedema due to ACE inhibitors.
25. *ACE inhibitors and ARBs may cause postural hypotension in sodium depleted conditions as in diuretic treated patients.*
26. *Aliskiren, remikiren and enalkiren* are oral renin inhibitors
27. All ACEI are prodrugs except captopril and lisinopril.
28. **ARBs** do not increase bradykinin and thus have **less** chances of causing **cough and angioedema as compared to ACE inhibitors.**
29. **Beta blockers are not considered first line antihypertensives by JNC-VIII guidelines.**
30. **Goal BP for patients > 60 yrs without CKD or DM is < 150/90 mm Hg according to JNC-VIII**
31. **Selexipag** is a new oral PGI_2 receptor agonist indicated for pulmonary artery hypertension
32. Tolerance can develop to nitrates on chronic use (not seen with sublingual use). Thus, for clinical use, at least 8 hours of drug free period per day is required.
33. Phosphodiesterase inhibitors like sildenafil should never be prescribed with nitrates due to risk of profound hypotension
34. Beta blockers are contra-indicated in variant angina.
35. Ranolazine has no effect on heart rate and blood pressure
36. **Ivabradine** is a relatively selective I_f sodium channel blocker (I_f: funny current) that reduce cardiac rate by inhibiting the hyperpolarization-activated sodium channel in SA node.
37. Thrombolytic drugs should be administered within 12 hours for STEMI and within 3 hours of ischemic stroke
38. K^+ is the main cation that determines the RMP of cardiac cells.
39. The class I antiarrhythmic agents *interfere with the activity of Na^+ channels*. Thus, all of these drugs can decrease the slope of phase 0 (V_{max}).
40. In overdose, quinidine can result in **cinchonism** which manifests as *tinnitus, vertigo, deafness, headache, visual disturbances and mental changes.*
41. Class Ib agents are used only for ventricular arrhythmias.
42. Lignocaine is drug of choice for digitals-induced ventricular arrhythmias
43. Procainamide is metabolized in liver by acetylation
44. *Treatment of choice for WPW syndrome is radiofrequency ablation of the aberrant pathway*
45. Amiodarone is **longest acting** whereas adenosine is shortest acting anti-arrhythmic drug.

46. **Vernakalant** is a multi-ion channel blocker recommended for converting recent onset atrial fibrillation to normal sinus rhythm.

47. Adenosine is the drug of *choice for treatment of PSVT.*

48. Bile acid binding agents and ezetimibe are best drugs for sitosterolemia

49. *Bile acids inhibit TG production in the liver* and their deficiency results in elevation of TGs.

50. *Bile acid binding agents are DOC for cholesterol lowering in children, pregnancy and lactation.*

51. **Mipomersen** is an antisense oligonucleotide inhibitor of **mRNA of apo B-100 synthesis**. It is indicated as **once weekly injection** for treatment of **homozygous familial hypercholestrolemia**

52. Fibrates are drugs of choice in hypertriglyceridemia (type III and IV)

53. **Lomitapide** acts by inhibiting microsomal triglyceride transfer protein (MTP). This protein is necessary for VLDL assembly and secretion in liver.

54. *Risk of myopathy is increased* if fibrates are used *with statins except bezafibrate.*

Cardiovascular System

Drug of Choice

Condition	Drug of choice
Diabetic nephropathy	ACE inhibitors or ARBs
Scleroderma hypertensive crisis	Captopril
Congestive heart failure	
– Decompensated	Dobutamine
– Compensated	ACEI/ARB
Hypertrophic obstructive cardiomyopathy	Propranolol
Angina pectoris	
– Acute attack	Sublingual nitroglycerine
– Prophylaxis	Oral/transdermal nitrates
Esophageal spasm	Nitroglycerine
Cyanide poisoning	Hydroxocobalamin/amyl nitrite
Raynaud's phenomenon	Nifedipine ER or amlodipine
Myocardial infarction	
– Pain relief	Sublingual nitroglycerine ↓ Morphine
– Prophylaxis	Aspirin
– Thrombolytic for STEMI	Reteplase or alteplase
Hypertension	Thiazides
– With BHP	Prazosin
– With diabetes mellitus	ACE inhibitors
– With ischemic heart disease (angina)	Beta blockers
– With chronic kidney disease	ACE inhibitors
– In pregnancy	Labetalol
Acute severe digitalis toxicity	Digibind
Hypertensive emergencies	Nicardipine + Esmolol
– In cheese reaction	Phentolamine
– in clonidine withdrawl	Phentolamine
– In aortic dissection	Nitroprusside + esmolol
– In Pregnancy	Labetalol
Hyperlipidemia	
– Type IIa and IIb	Statins
– Type III (hypertriglyceridemia)	Fibrates
– Type IV	Statins
– Secondary to diabetes or nephrotic syndrome	Statins
Supraventricular tachycardia	
– Narrow QRS complex	Verapamil or beta blockers
– Wide complex	Flecainide
– WPW syndrome	Flecainide
Paroxysmal supraventricular tachycardia (PSVT)	
– Acute treatment	Adenosine
– Prophylaxis	Verapamil
Ventricular tachycardia	Lignocaine
– Digitalis induced	Lignocaine
– Post MI	Lignocaine or amiodarone
Long QT syndrome (Torsades' de pointes)	Magnesium
Pulmonary Hypertension	Bosentan

Image Based Questions

1. Mechanism of action of 3 antihypertensive drugs (X, Y and Z) is shown in the given figure. These are likely to be (in sequence):

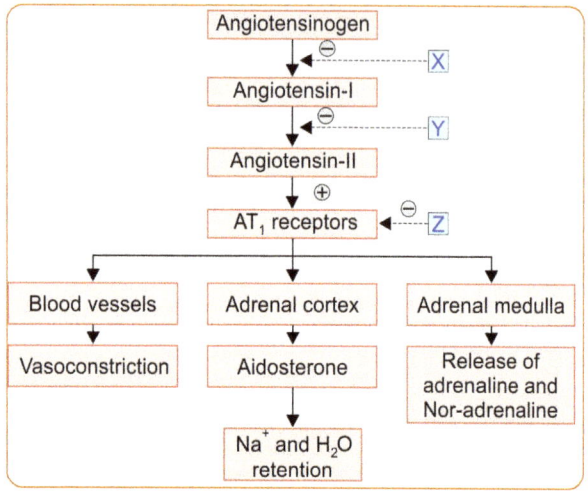

   (a) Enalapril, Enalkerin and Losartan
   (b) Losartan, Enalapril and Enalkerin
   (c) Enalkerin, Enalapril, Losartan
   (d) Enalkerin, Losartan, Enalapril

2. Which of the following drug is likely to produce the effect on action potential as shown in the diagram?

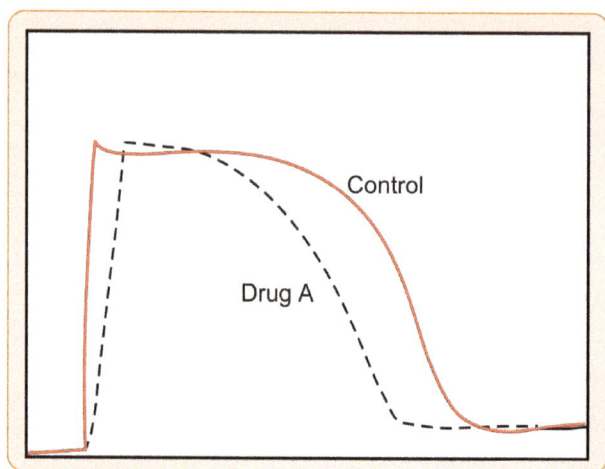

   (a) Quinidine
   (b) Amiodarone
   (c) Lignocaine
   (d) Flecainide

3. Drug which can act at both sites 1 and 2 as shown in the diagram is:

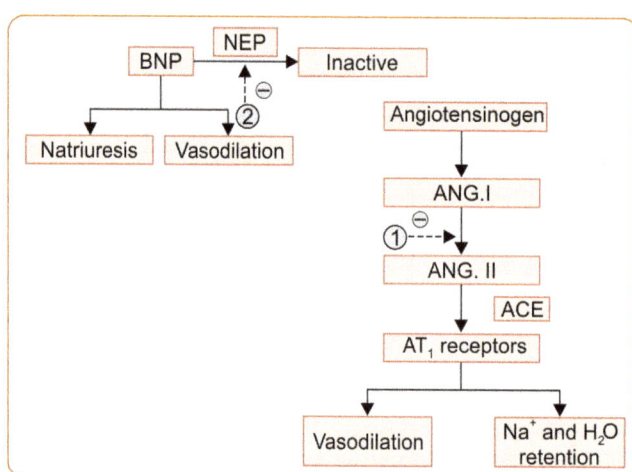

   (a) Sacubitril   (b) Samptrilat
   (c) Losartan   (d) Nesiritide

4. Which of the following is likely to be drug A?

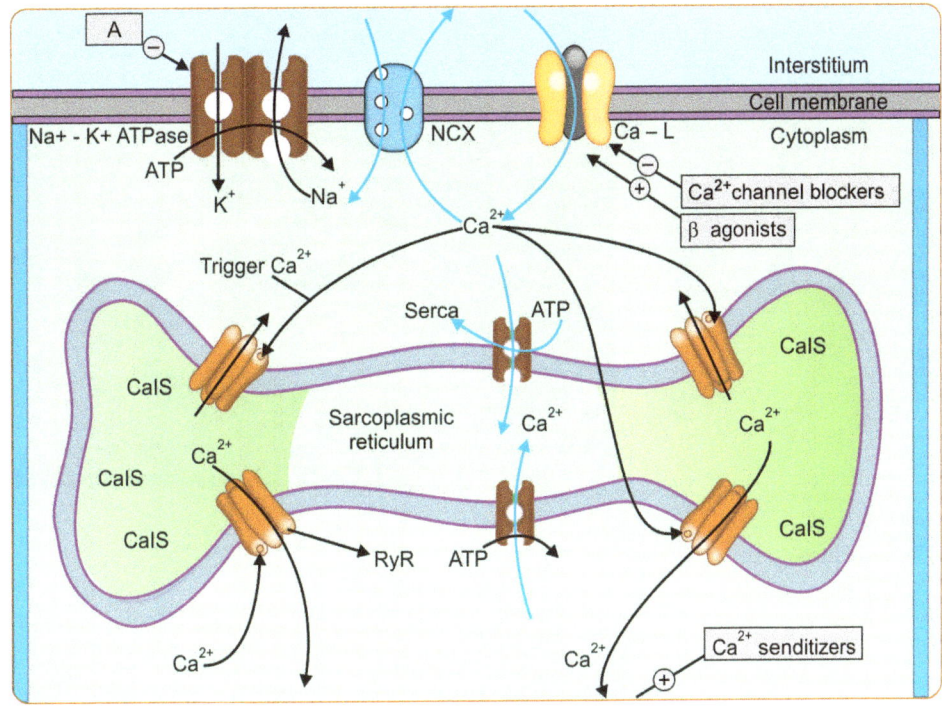

(a) Digoxin
(b) Levosimendan
(c) Amrinone
(d) None of these

5. Which of the following drugs are likely to cause the given change in ECG?

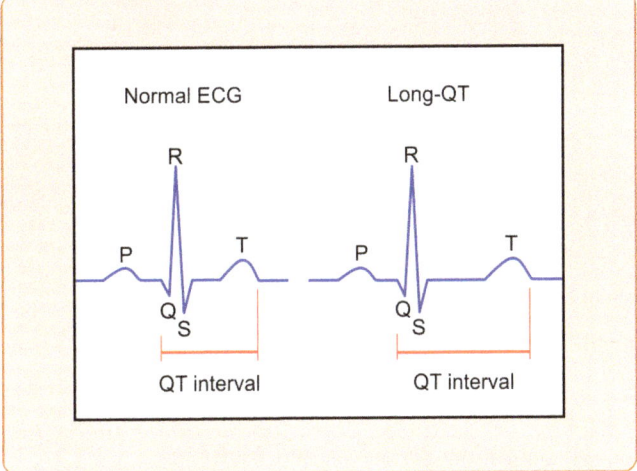

(a) Quinidine
(b) Lignocaine
(c) Verapamil
(d) Propranolol

6. The drug obtained from this plant is used for the treatment of:

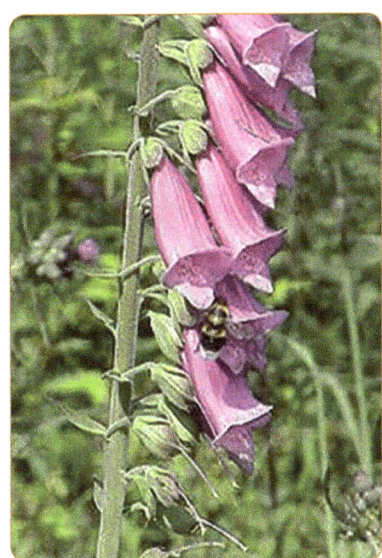

(a) Malaria
(b) Congestive heart failure
(c) Myocardial infarction
(d) Iridocyclitis

7. The drug obtained from the plant is used for the treatment of:

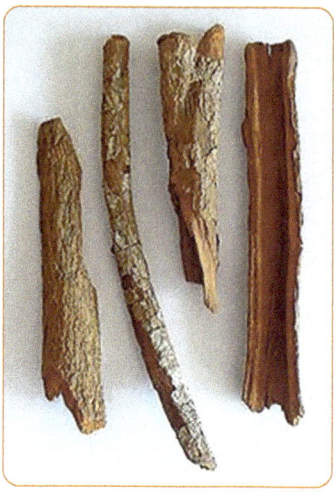 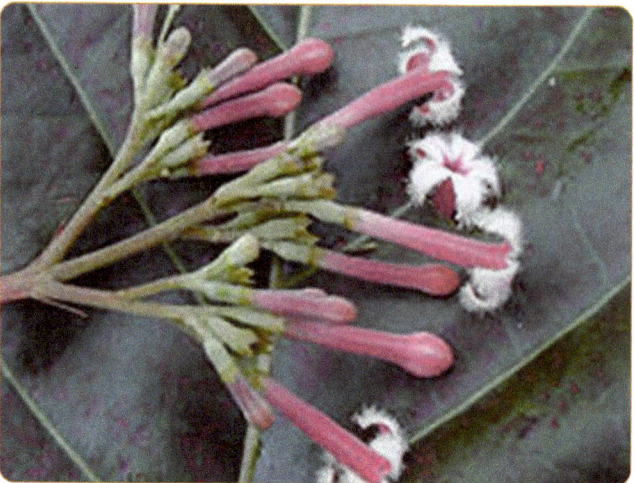

   (a) Malaria
   (b) Congestive heart failure
   (c) Myocardial infarction
   (d) Iridocyclitis

8. The drug obtained from the plant is used for the treatment of:

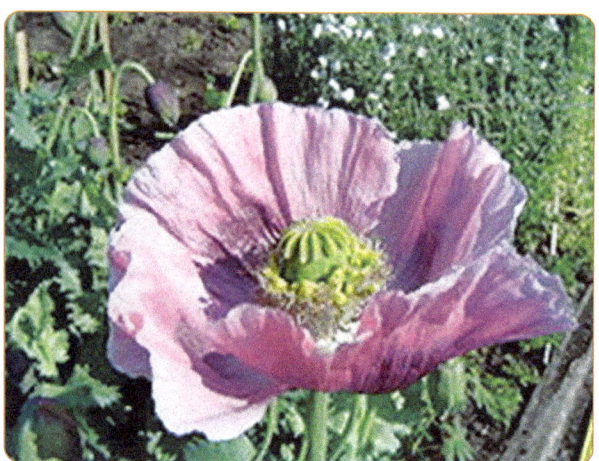

   (a) Malaria
   (b) Congestive heart failure
   (c) Myocardial infarction
   (d) Iridocyclitis

9. The plant shown in the figure is a source of:

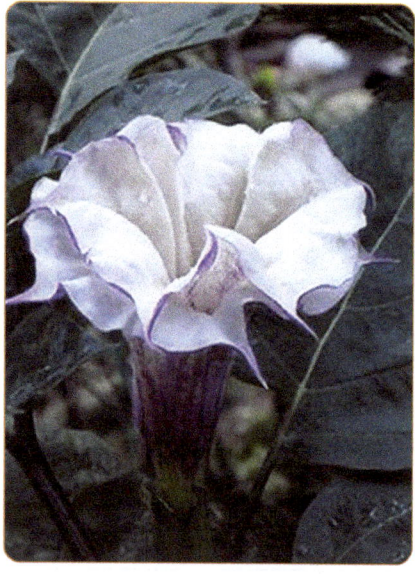

   (a) Atropine   (b) Morphine
   (c) Quinine   (d) Digoxin

10. A 30-year-old female was treated with an antihypertensive drug and presented with following features. The likely drug was:

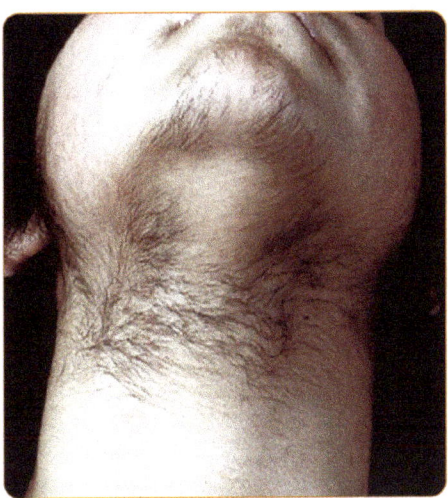

(a) Minoxidil
(b) Fenoldopam
(c) Methyl Dopa
(d) Enalapril

11. A 60-year-old male presents with acute severe chest pain associated with sweating 30 min before. The ECG of the person is shown below. Which of the following drug should be given to this person?

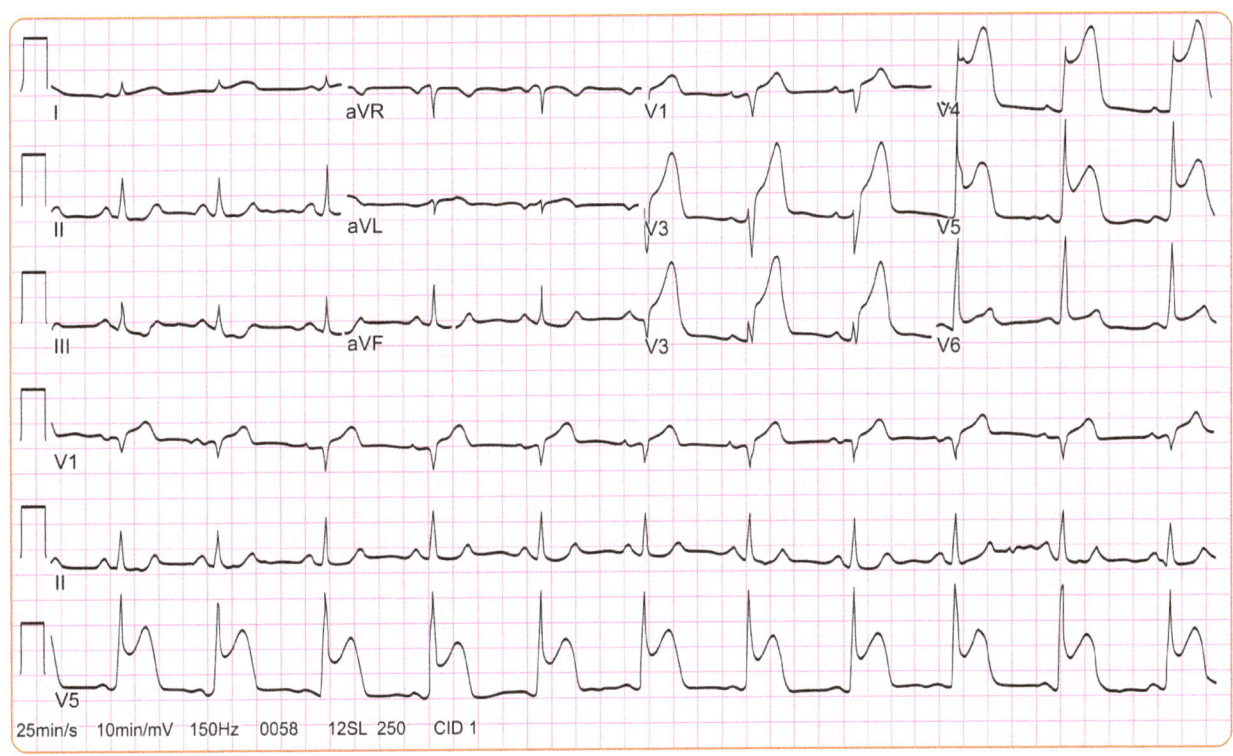

(a) Atropine
(b) Streptokinase
(c) Amiodarone
(d) Adenosine

12. A 30-year-old athlete went for routine examination. He has no symptoms. The ECG is shown below. What advise will you give to him?

    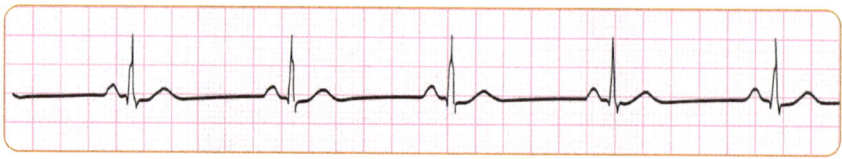

    (a) No treatment is required
    (b) Permanent pacemaker should be placed
    (c) Atropine should be given
    (d) Electrical defibrillation should be done

13. A new antiarrhythmic drug is found to be effective against both atrial and ventricular arrhythmias. Its effect on action potential is shown below. The effect of this new drug is most similar to:

    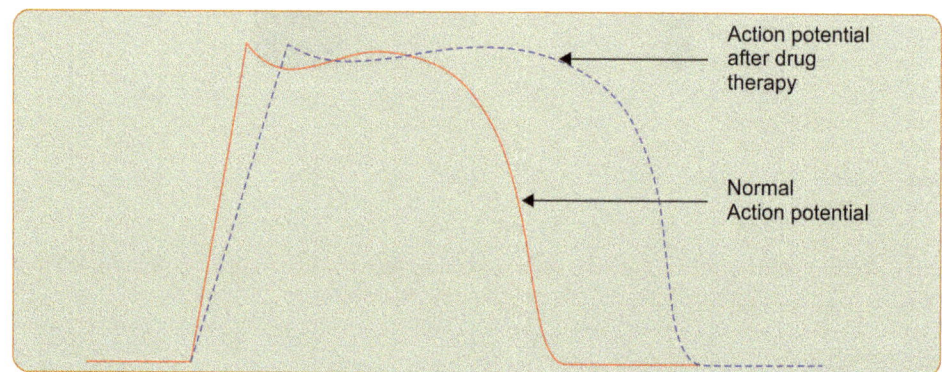

    (a) Lignocaine   (b) Propranolol
    (c) Encainide   (d) Quinidine

14. Which of the following drug is not indicated in a person with the given ECG?

    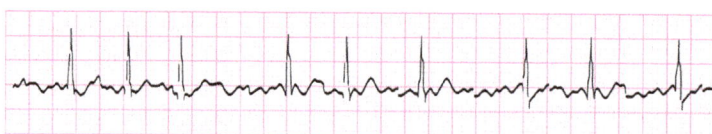

    (a) Amiodarone   (b) Propranolol
    (c) Verapamil   (d) Adenosine

15. A 52-year-old male, Vivek was treated with enalapril for hypertension. It was able to control his blood pressure. Which of the following is the most likely combination of changes in response to this patient's treatment?

	Renin	Angiotensin I	Angiotensin II	Aldosterone	Bradykinin
(a)	↑	↑	↓	↓	↑
(b)	↑	↑	↓	↓	↓
(c)	↑	↓	↓	↓	↓
(d)		↓	↓	↓	No change

Explanations

1. **Ans. (c) Enalkerin, Enalapril, Losartan**
   The figure shows the drugs inhibiting the renin angiotensin pathway
   - Renin inhibitors: Enalkerin, Remikerin, Aliskiren
   - ACE inhibitors: Enalapril, Ramipril, Perindopril
   - ARB: Losartan, Valsartan, Telmisartan

2. **Ans. (c) Lignocaine**
   The figure shows that the drug decreases slope of phase 0 (Na channel blockade) and also it decreases action potential duration (K channel opener). These are the actions of antiarrhythmic drugs belonging to class Ib like lignocaine

3. **Ans. (b) Sampatrilat**
   Sampatrilat and omapatrilat are vasopeptidase inhibitors that inhibit both neutral endopeptidase as well as ACE.

4. **Ans. (a) Digoxin**
   The figure shows the mechanism of action of digitalis ie Na K pump inhibitor drug

5. **Ans. (a) Quinidine**
   Drugs that block K channels in the heart can cause increase in QT interval and predispose to Torsades' de pointes. Antiarrhythmic drugs having K channel blocking property are:
   Class 1a: Quinidne and Procainamide
   Class 3: Amiodarone, Sotalol, Bretylium etc

6. **Ans. (b) Congestive heart failure**
   The figure shows the plant digitalis purpura. It can identified from name itself. The flowers of the plant can be put in fingers (digits). Digoxin is the drug obtained from this plant and is used in CHF

7. **Ans. (a) Malaria**
   The figure shows the bark of cinchona plant. The drugs obtained from this plant are quinine and quinidine. Former is used for malaria whereas latter can be used for arrhythmias

8. **Ans. (c) Myocardial infarction**
   The plant shown in the figure is papaver somniferum. Crud extract of this plant is known as opium which is source of opioids like morphine.

9. **Ans. (a) Atropine**
   The plant shown in the figure is dhatura stramomium which is source of atropine

10. **Ans. (a) Minoxidil**
    The figure shows male pattern hair growth in females known as hirsutism. It is adverse effect of minoxidil. Other important drugs causing hirsutism are cyclosporine and phenytoin apart from androgens.

11. **Ans. (b) Streptokinase**
    The given ECG shows the ST elevation in leads V3 to V6 whereas there is associated ST depression in contiguous leads I, II and aVF. These ECG findings along with clinical features points towards acute ST elevation MI. Thrombolytics like streptokinase are indicated in these patients.

12. **Ans. (a) No treatment is required**
    The given ECG shows the patient in normal sinus rhythm. However, the heart rate is very low (approximately 50 beats per minute). As the patient is asymptomatic and is athlete (heart rate is usually low in these patients), no treatment is required. However this person should not be prescribed any drug that can reduce heart rate further (like beta blockers or calcium channel blockers).
    Also see the ECG findings in different types of heart block.
    First degree block

    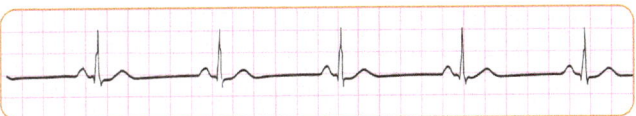

    Second degree type 1

    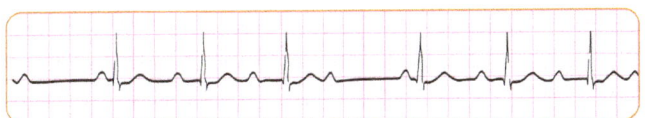

    Second degree type 2

    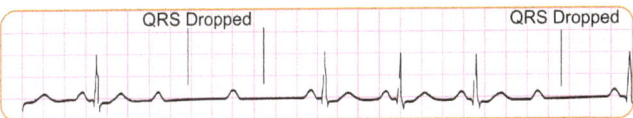

13. **Ans. (d) Quinidine** *(Ref: KK Sharma 2nd/e p301)*
    This drug is decreasing the slope of phase 0 (Na^+ channel blocking property) as well as increasing the action potential duration (K^+ channel blocking property). Thus, it exhibits the properties of class Ia anti-arrhythmic agents like quinidine.

14. **Ans. (d) Adenosine** *(Ref: Harrisons 19th/e p2080)*
    The ECG shows the features of atrial fibrillation as
    Irregularly irregular rhythm
    Absence of P waves
    The drugs used for atrial fibrillation include:
    a. Anticoagulants like warfarin, heparin etc
    b. Drugs to control atrial rate:
       i. Beta blockers: Propranolol, metoprolol etc.
       ii. Calcium channel blockers: Diltiazem and Verapamil
       iii. Digoxin
    c. Drugs to control rhythm:
       i Sodium channel blockers: Flecainide, Propafenone, quinidine
       ii. Pottasium channel blockers: Amiodarone, ibutilide, dofetilide
    Adenosine has very very short half life (less than 10 sec.). It is indicated for treatment of PSVT only.

15. **Ans. (a)** *(Ref: KK Sharma 2nd/e p265)*
    ACE inhibitors decrease angiotenisn II by inhibiting the conversion of Ang I to Ang II and thus aldosterone also decrease. Due to compensatory increase in plasma renin activity, renin and angiotensin I levels increase. By inhibiting the metabolism of bradykinin, the level of these vasoactive peptides also increase.

Multiple Choice Questions

CONGESTIVE HEART FAILURE

1. Which of the following is not used in heart failure?
   (NEET Pattern 2020)
   (a) Metoprolol (b) Trimetazidine
   (c) Sacubitril (d) Nesiritide

2. Mention the true/false statements about digoxin toxicity:
   (AIIMS Nov. 2019)
   (a) Earliest manifestation of digoxin are gastrointestinal symptoms
   (b) Nonspecific vision changes may be noted in digoxin toxicity
   (c) Early toxicity may not correlate with serum levels
   (d) Neurological symptoms may occur without corresponding cardiovascular changes
   (e) Hypokalemia is associated with increased risk of toxicity

3. Active metabolite of sodium nitroprusside acts via activation of: *(AIIMS Nov. 2018)*
   (a) Phospholipase A (b) Phospholipase C
   (c) Guanylate cyclase (d) Protein kinase C

4. Sacubitril is: *(NEET Pattern 2017-2018)*
   (a) Renin inhibitor
   (b) ACE inhibitor
   (c) Angiotensin receptor antagonist
   (d) NEP inhibitor

5. Which of the following is first line drug for acute congestive heart failure? *(NEET Pattern 2016-17)*
   (a) Carbonic anhydrase inhibitor
   (b) Loop diuretic
   (c) Thiazide diuretic
   (d) Morphine

6. Digoxin is contraindicated in:
   (Recent NEET Pattern Question)
   (a) Supraventricular tachycardia
   (b) Atrial fibrillation
   (c) Congestive heart failure
   (d) Hypertrophic obstructive cardiomyopathy

7. Which one of the following provides hemodynamic stability and prolongs survival in congestive heart failure?
   (Recent NEET Pattern Question)
   (a) Lisinopril (b) Furosemide
   (c) Digoxin (d) Milrinone

8. The drug that is NOT useful in congestive heart failure is: *(Recent NEET Pattern Question)*
   (a) Adrenaline (b) Digoxin
   (c) Hydrochlorothiazide (d) Enalapril

9. Which of the following is not a contraindication for use of digitalis? *(Recent NEET Pattern Question)*
   (a) Acute rheumatic carditis
   (b) Thyrotoxicosis
   (c) WPW syndrome
   (d) Hyperkalemia

10. Therapeutic plasma level of digoxin is:
    (Recent NEET Pattern Question)
    (a) 0.1-0.3 ng/mL (b) 0.8-1.5 ng/mL
    (c) 1.2 to 2 ng/mL (d) More than 2.4 ng/mL

11. Digibind is used to: *(Recent NEET Pattern Question)*
    (a) Potentiate the action of digoxin
    (b) Decrease the metabolism of digoxin
    (c) Treat digoxin toxicity
    (d) Rapidly digitalize the patient

12. All are true about digoxin *except*:
    (Recent NEET Pattern Question)
    (a) Causes bradycardia due to increased vagal tone
    (b) Acts by inhibiting Na^+K^+ ATPase in myocardial fibres
    (c) It is 95% plasma protein bound
    (d) Primarily excreted unchanged by glomerular filtration

13. All of the following drugs reduce afterload, *except*:
    (Recent NEET Pattern Question)
    (a) Enalapril (b) Propranolol
    (c) Hydralazine (d) Sodium nitroprusside

14. Sodium-nitroprusside acts by activation of:
    (Recent NEET Pattern Question)
    (a) Guanylate cyclase (b) K^+ channels
    (c) Ca^{++} channels (d) Cyclic AMP

15. Ouabain acts by inhibiting:
    (Recent NEET Pattern Question)
    (a) Adenyl cyclase (b) Ca^{++} channels
    (c) H^+K^+ ATPase (d) Na^+K^+ ATPase

16. Time taken for digitalization is:
    (Recent NEET Pattern Question)
    (a) 36 hours (b) 12 hours
    (c) 5 day (d) 10 day

17. Drug directly acting on blood vessels is:
    (Recent NEET Pattern Question)
    (a) Hydralazine (b) Verapamil
    (c) Propranolol (d) Methyldopa

18. Digitalis toxicity can cause:
    (Recent NEET Pattern Question)
    (a) Hyperkalemia (b) Nausea
    (c) Arrhythmias (d) All of the above

19. In LVF, drug which can be administered is:
    (Recent NEET Pattern Question)
    (a) Propranolol (b) Morphine
    (c) Amlodipine (d) Epinephrine

20. Digitalis has positive inotropic effect-by the virtue of its effect on: *(Recent NEET Pattern Question)*
    (a) $Na^+ K^+$ ATPase pump
    (b) Na Glucose channels
    (c) H^+K^+ ATPase pump
    (d) Calcium Pump

Cardiovascular System

21. Drugs causing afterload reduction is:
    (Recent NEET Pattern Question)
    (a) Digoxin (b) Captopril
    (c) Dobutamine (d) Frusemide

22. The biochemical mechanism of action of digitalis is associated with: *(Recent NEET Pattern Question)*
    (a) An increase in conduction from atrium to ventricle
    (b) An increase in ATP synthesis
    (c) An increase in systolic intracellular calcium levels
    (d) A block of calcium channels

23. Best treatment of severe digitalis toxicity is:
    (Recent NEET Pattern Question)
    (a) Potassium supplements
    (b) Diphenyl hydantoin
    (c) Quinidine
    (d) Fab fragments of digitalis antibodies

24. Which one of the following is the most characteristic arrhythmia with digitalis toxicity?
    (Recent NEET Pattern Question)
    (a) Atrial fibrillation (b) Extrasystoles
    (c) NPAT with block (d) Auricular flutter

25. Digoxin toxicity produce all of the following changes in ECG *except*: *(Recent NEET Pattern Question)*
    (a) Inverted T waves (b) Prolonged QT interval
    (c) ST depression (d) Prolonged PR interval

26. Mechanism of action of levosimendan include:
    (Recent NEET Pattern Question)
    (a) Na channel opener (b) K channel opener
    (c) Beta blocker (d) Beta 1 agonist

27. Important adverse effect of nesiritide is:
    (Recent NEET Pattern Question)
    (a) Dysgusea (b) Hypotension
    (c) Cough (d) Angioedema

28. Half-life of digoxin is: *(Recent NEET Pattern Question)*
    (a) 24 hrs (b) 40 hrs
    (c) 48 hrs (d) 60 hrs

29. Mechanism of action of digitalis is:
    (Recent NEET Pattern Question)
    (a) Inhibits Na$^+$K$^+$ATPase pump
    (b) Inhibits Na$^+$H$^+$ATPase pump
    (c) Active metabolites are produced in the liver
    (d) Inhibits calcium concentration in blood

30. Which of the following potassium sparing diuretic reduces cardiac mortality? *(Recent NEET Pattern Question)*
    (a) Spironolactone (b) Amiloride
    (c) Triamterene (d) All of these

31. Anti-androgen used in heart failure is:
    (Recent NEET Pattern Question)
    (a) Carvedilol (b) Sampatrilat
    (c) Spironolactone (d) Abiraterone

32. Digoxin can accumulate to toxic levels in patients with:
    (Recent NEET Pattern Question)
    (a) Renal insufficiency (b) Chronic hepatitis
    (c) Advanced cirrhosis (d) Chronic pancreatitis

33. Drug used to reverse remodeling of heart in congestive cardiac failure are all *except*:
    (Recent NEET Pattern Question)
    (a) Beta blocker (b) ACE inhibitor
    (c) Digoxin (d) Aldosterone antagonist

34. Which of the following drug decreases plasma renin activity? *(Recent NEET Pattern Question)*
    (a) Enalapril (b) Nifedipine
    (c) Hydralazine (d) Clonidine

35. Which of the following does not contribute to digoxin toxicity? *(Recent NEET Pattern Question)*
    (a) Hyperkalemia (b) Hypercalcemia
    (c) Renal failure (d) Hypomagnesemia

36. Which of the following is not an inotropic drug?
    (Recent NEET Pattern Question)
    (a) Amrinone (b) Isoprenaline
    (c) Amiodarone (d) Dopamine

37. Dobutamine is preferred over dopamine in cardiogenic shock because of its effect related to:
    (Recent NEET Pattern Question)
    (a) Better cardiac stimulation
    (b) Less peripheral vasoconstriction
    (c) Lower risk of cardiac arrhythmias
    (d) More CNS stimulation

38. All of the following drugs can cause gynaecomastia *except*: *(Recent NEET Pattern Question)*
    (a) Digoxin (b) Amiloride
    (c) Cimetidine (d) Spironolactone

39. Drug to be avoided in hypertrophic obstructive cardiomyopathy is: *(Recent NEET Pattern Question)*
    (a) Amiodarone (b) Verapamil
    (c) Digoxin (d) Beta-blockers

40. Digitalis acts in CHF by: *(Recent NEET Pattern Question)*
    (a) Na$^+$ K$^+$ ATPase inhibition
    (b) Na$^+$ K$^+$ ATPase stimulation
    (c) Blockade of calcium channels
    (d) Increasing the refractory period of AV node

41. Treatment of digitalis toxicity includes:
    (a) Stoppage of drug *(Recent NEET Pattern Question)*
    (b) Potassium supplements
    (c) FAB fragments of digitalis antibodies
    (d) All of the above

42. Which of the following is false about digoxin?
    (Recent NEET Pattern Question)
    (a) Dosage reduction is required in hepatic disease
    (b) Dosage reduction is required in renal failure
    (c) It can cause bradycardia
    (d) It increases the force of contraction in CHF

43. Drug of choice for pregnancy induced hypertension is:
    (AIIMS Nov 2015)
    (a) Methyl dopa (b) Atenolol
    (c) Nitroprusside (d) Enalapril

44. Diuretic that is useful in mild to moderate hypertension is: *(AIIMS May 2015)*
    (a) Loop diuretics
    (b) Thiazides
    (c) Osmotic diuretics
    (d) Potassium sparing diuretics

45. Which of the following antihypertensive drugs is contraindicated in pregnancy? *(AIIMS May 2015)*
    (a) Amlodipine (b) Labetalol
    (c) Enalapril (d) Hydralazine

46. Best antihypertensive drug in pulmonary hypertension is: *(AIIMS May 2015)*
    (a) Bosentan (b) Amlodipine
    (c) Furosemide (d) Digoxin

HYPERTENSION

47. Preferred drug for the treatment of a 48-year-old man with uncomplicated grade 2 hypertension without any associated co-morbidity is: *(NEET Pattern 2020)*
    (a) Chlorthalidone
    (b) Triamterene
    (c) Spironolactone
    (d) Furosemide

48. Which of the following drug should not be used in pregnant woman with hypertension?
    (NEET Pattern Question 2017-2018)
    (a) Labetalol (b) Propranolol
    (c) Methyl dopa (d) Hydralazine

49. Nitric oxide acts: *(NEET Pattern Question 2017-2018)*
    (a) By increasing cAMP (b) By increasing cGMP
    (c) By increasing DAG (d) By increasing IP3

50. Which of the following is NOT a centrally acting antihypertensive agent? *(NEET Pattern Question 2016-17)*
    (a) Methyldopa (b) Moxonidine
    (c) Minoxidil (d) Clonidine

51. Drug of choice for hypertension in eclampsia is:
    (NEET Pattern Question 2016-17)
    (a) MgSO$_4$ (b) Nifedipine
    (c) Hydralazine (d) Labetalol

52. Which of the following statements about clonidine is NOT true? *(NEET Pattern Question 2016-17)*
    (a) Sudden withdrawal will leads to rapid rise in BP
    (b) Plasma half life is 8-12 hours
    (c) It acts through alpha 2a receptor in brainstem
    (d) It does not cause postural hypotension

53. Which of the following antihypertensives is not given in pregnancy? *(AIIMS May 2014)*
    (a) Enalapril (b) α-methyldopa
    (c) Labetalol (d) Nifedipine

54. All of the following can be administrated in acute hypertension during labour *except*: *(AIIMS May 2014)*
    (a) IV Labetalol (b) IV Nitroprusside
    (c) IV Hydralazine (d) IV Esmolol

55. Systemic vascular resistance is twice that of normal, treatment should be: *(AIIMS Nov 2013)*
    (a) Adrenaline (b) Nor-adrenaline
    (c) Sodium nitroprusside (d) Isoprenaline

56. Calcium channel blocking agents of use in the treatment of hypertension include:
    (Recent NEET Pattern Question)
    (a) Prazosin (b) Lidoflazine
    (c) Captopril (d) Nifedipine

57. Which of the following is NOT a frontline antihypertensive agent? *(Recent NEET Pattern Question)*
    (a) Enalapril
    (b) Hydrochlorthiazide
    (c) Amlodipine
    (d) Atenolol

58. Which of the following drugs should NOT be used in setting of severe hypertension in elderly on empirical basis?
    (Recent NEET Pattern Question)
    (a) Enalapril (b) Amlodipine
    (c) Chlorthiazide (d) Prazosin

59. Which of the following antihypertensive drug does not alter serum glucose and lipid levels?
    (Recent NEET Pattern Question)
    (a) Propranolol (b) Prazosin
    (c) Thiazide diuretics (d) None of the above

60. Drug not useful in hypertensive emergency is:
    (Recent NEET Pattern Question)
    (a) IV hydralazine (b) Indapamide
    (c) Sublingual nifedipine (d) Sodium nitroprusside

61. Which of the following is not an adrenergic neuron blocking drug? *(Recent NEET Pattern Question)*
    (a) Reserpine (b) Guanethidine
    (c) Bretylium (d) Minoxidil

62. Which of the following drug has a favourable effect on lipid metabolism? *(Recent NEET Pattern Question)*
    (a) Atenolol (b) Chlorothiazide
    (c) Clonidine (d) Torsemide

63. The choice of antihypertensive medication also depends upon the co-morbid illness of the patient and all of the following recommendations have been made *except*:
    (Recent NEET Pattern Question)
    (a) In hypertensive patients with heart failure, ACE inhibitors may be preferred
    (b) In hypertensive patients with migraine, beta blockers are an excellent choice
    (c) In hypertensive patients with gout, diuretics are particularly useful
    (d) In hypertensive patients with peripheral vascular disease, calcium channel blockers are recommended

64. An anti-hypertensive drug that causes positive Coomb's test is: *(Recent NEET Pattern Question)*
    (a) Methyldopa (b) Clonidine
    (c) Hydralazine (d) Sodium-nitroprusside

65. The drug of choice in digitalis induced ventricular arrhythmias is: *(Recent NEET Pattern Question)*
    (a) IV Lignocaine (b) Phenytoin
    (c) Quinidine (d) Procainamide

66. Centrally acting sympatholytic agent used as antihypertensive agent is: *(Recent NEET Pattern Question)*
    (a) Propranolol (b) Clonidine
    (c) Prazosin (d) Phenoxybenzamine

67. All of the following are vasodilators *except*:
    (Recent NEET Pattern Question)
    (a) Methyl dopa (b) Nitroprusside
    (c) Hydralazine (d) Diazoxide

68. Treatment of choice in hypertension with diabetes mellitus is: *(Recent NEET Pattern Question)*
    (a) Beta-blockers
    (b) Thiazides
    (c) ACE inhibitors
    (d) Calcium channel blockers

69. Which of the following antihypertensives causes sedation? *(Recent NEET Pattern Question)*
    (a) Clonidine   (b) Hydralazine
    (c) Losartan   (d) Amlodipine

70. Centrally acting antihypertensive drug is: *(Recent NEET Pattern Question)*
    (a) Phenoxybenzamine
    (b) Methyl dopa
    (c) Propranolol
    (d) Prazosin

71. All are true about guanethidine *except*: *(Recent NEET Pattern Question)*
    (a) It prevents exocytosis of norepinephrine
    (b) Used for treatment of erectile dysfunction
    (c) Side effects include diarrhea
    (d) No CNS related side effects seen with its use

72. Antihypertensive which can be used in patients with gout and diabetes mellitus is: *(Recent NEET Pattern Question)*
    (a) Thiazide   (b) Enalapril
    (c) Propranolol   (d) Diazoxide

73. Antihypertensive may act by blocking all of the following *except*: *(Recent NEET Pattern Question)*
    (a) Alpha-adrenoceptors
    (b) ATP dependent K$^+$ channels
    (c) Nor adrenaline release
    (d) Beta adrenoceptors

74. Which of the following is a K$^+$ channel opener? *(Recent NEET Pattern Question)*
    (a) Nifedipine   (b) Minoxidil
    (c) Enalapril   (d) Atenolol

75. Which of the following is not a Ca^{++} channel blocker? *(Recent NEET Pattern Question)*
    (a) Enalapril   (b) Nifedipine
    (c) Diltiazem   (d) Verapamil

ANGINA AND MI

76. Major mechanism of action of nitrates in acute attack of angina is: *(AIIMS Nov 2018)*
    (a) Coronary vasodilation
    (b) Decrease in preload
    (c) Decrease in afterload
    (d) Decrease in heart rate

77. A patient of prinzmetal's angina is started on isosorbide mononitrate. What is the mechanism of action of nitrates in this condition? *(AIIMS Nov 2017)*
    (a) Reduced cardiac contractility
    (b) Increased left ventricular end diastolic volume
    (c) Decreased diastolic perfusion pressure
    (d) Endothelium independent coronary vasodilation

78. Nitric oxide acts via: *(AIIMS May 2016)*
    (a) cAMP   (b) cGMP
    (c) Ca   (d) K

79. Nimodipine is given in: *(AIIMS May 2016)*
    (a) Extradural hemorrhage
    (b) Subdural hemorrhage
    (c) Intracerebral
    (d) Subarachnoid hemorrhage

80. Which of the following agent is a rho kinase inhibitor? *(AIIMS Nov 2013, May 2013)*
    (a) Fasudil   (b) Ranolazine
    (c) Amiloride   (d) Nicorandi

81. Glyceryl trinitrate is given by sublingual route because of: *(Recent NEET Pattern Question)*
    (a) Short $t_{1/2}$ in plasma
    (b) High hepatic first pass metabolism
    (c) High bioavailability by oral route
    (d) Extensive protein binding

82. Calcium channel blockers are useful in all, *except*: *(Recent NEET Pattern Question)*
    (a) Angina
    (b) Supraventricular arrhythmia
    (c) Sick sinus syndrome
    (d) Hypertension

83. Which of the following statements is true about nitrates? *(Recent NEET Pattern Question)*
    (a) Acts by raising cGMP which causes dephosphorylation of MLCK
    (b) Metabolized by glutathione reductase
    (c) Used in achalasia cardia
    (d) All of the above

84. Nimodipine is used in: *(Recent NEET Pattern Question)*
    (a) Sub-arachnoid hemorrhage
    (b) Intra cerebral hemorrhage
    (c) Extra dural hemorrhage
    (d) Sub-dural hemorrhage

85. Nitrates decrease myocardial oxygen consumption by all of the following mechanisms *except*: *(Recent NEET Pattern Question)*
    (a) By increasing the left ventricular end diastolic pressure
    (b) By direct reduction of oxygen consumption of the myocardial cell
    (c) By dilation of the capacitance vessels
    (d) By decreasing the size of heart

86. Nitrate causes all of the following *except*: *(Recent NEET Pattern Question)*
    (a) Decrease in heart size
    (b) Increase in cardiac work
    (c) Preload reduction
    (d) Dilatation of cutaneous blood vessels

87. Calcium channel blockers are used in all *except*: *(Recent NEET Pattern Question)*
    (a) Angina
    (b) Arrhythmia
    (c) Congestive heart failure
    (d) Hypertension

88. Drug not to be given in ischemic heart disease is: *(Recent NEET Pattern Question)*
    (a) Atenolol   (b) ACE inhibitor
    (c) Isoproterenol (d) Streptokinase

89. Potassium channel opener with anti-anginal activity is:
 (Recent NEET Pattern Question)
 (a) Nicorandil (b) Dipyridamole
 (c) Trimetazidine (d) Oxyphedrine

90. All of the following drugs act by blocking calcium channels *except*: *(Recent NEET Pattern Question)*
 (a) Dantrolene (b) Nicardipine
 (c) Diltiazem (d) Verapamil

91. Amyl nitrite is used by which route?
 (Recent NEET Pattern Question)
 (a) Oral (b) Inhalation
 (c) IV (d) IM

92. Propranolol should not be given to a patient on treatment with which of the following drug?
 (Recent NEET Pattern Question)
 (a) Nifedipine (b) Nitrates
 (c) ACE inhibitors (d) Verapamil

93. Verapamil is contraindicated in:
 (Recent NEET Pattern Question)
 (a) Hypertesion
 (b) Complete heart block
 (c) Paroxysmal supraventricular tachycardia
 (d) Angina pectoris

94. All are dihydropyridines *except*:
 (Recent NEET Pattern Question)
 (a) Nifedipine
 (b) Nimodipine
 (c) Verapamil
 (d) Felodipine

95. The major clinical use of nimodipine is in:
 (Recent NEET Pattern Question)
 (a) Hypertension
 (b) Angina pectoris
 (c) Subarachnoid haemorrhage
 (d) Raynaud's phenomenon

96. When nitrates are combined with calcium channel blockers: *(Recent NEET Pattern Question)*
 (a) Arterial pressure will decrease
 (b) Heart rate will increase
 (c) Ejection time will decrease
 (d) End-diastolic volume will increase

97. Calcium channel blocker with maximum effect on conduction in heart is: *(Recent NEET Pattern Question)*
 (a) Phenylamine (b) Nifedipine
 (c) Diltiazem (d) Verapamil

98. Mechanism of action of NO is:
 (Recent NEET Pattern Question)
 (a) ↑cAMP (b) ↑cGMP
 (c) ↑PGE_2 (d) ↑PGD_4

99. Treatment of choice for cyanide poisoning is:
 (Recent NEET Pattern Question)
 (a) $NaHCO_3$
 (b) $KMnO_4$
 (c) NaCl
 (d) Sodium nitrite followed by thiosulphate

100. Coronary steal phenomenon is caused by which drug?
 (Recent NEET Pattern Question)
 (a) Disopyramide (b) Verapamil
 (c) Nitroglycerine (d) Dipyridamol

101. Which of the following drugs is used in MI?
 (Recent NEET Pattern Question)
 (a) Cocaine (b) Pethidine
 (c) Morphine (d) Butorphanol

ARRHYTHMIA

102. Which of the following antiarrhythmic drugs is contraindicated in a patient with interstitial lung disease?
 (NEET Pattern 2020)
 (a) Amiodarone (b) Sotalol
 (c) Quinidine (d) Lignocaine

103. Drug of choice for ventricular tachycardia in a patient with myocardial ischemia is: *(NEET Pattern Question 2019)*
 (a) Lignocaine (b) Propranolol
 (c) Diltiazem (d) Digoxin

104. Side effects of amiodarone are all *except*:
 (NEET Pattern Question 2016-17)
 (a) Pulmonary fibrosis (b) Nephrotoxicity
 (c) Hepatotoxicity (d) Hypothyroidism

105. All of the following antiarrhythmic drugs are correctly matched to the group: *(Recent NEET Pattern Question)*
 (a) Procainamide: class I (b) Amiodarone: class III
 (c) Esmolol: class IV (d) Diltiazem: class IV

106. The drug of choice for rapid correction of PSVT in known asthmatic is: *(Recent NEET Pattern Question)*
 (a) Adenosine (b) Esmolol
 (c) Neostigmine (d) Verapamil

107. All of the following drugs are Class I anti-arrhythmic drugs *except*: *(Recent NEET Pattern Question)*
 (a) Quinidine (b) Procainamide
 (c) Flecainide (d) Propranolol

108. Which of the following antiarrhythmic drug decreases the action potential duration in purkinje fibers?
 (Recent NEET Pattern Question)
 (a) Quinidine (b) Flecainide
 (c) Amiodarone (d) Lignocaine

109. All of the following decrease AV conduction *except*:
 (Recent NEET Pattern Question)
 (a) Esmolol (b) Digitalis
 (c) Lignocaine (d) Verapamil

110. Class III antiarrhythmic drug is:
 (Recent NEET Pattern Question)
 (a) Amiodarone (b) Phenytoin
 (c) Propafenone (d) Pindolol

111. A sixteen-year-old girl is found to have paroxysmal attacks of rapid heart rate. The antiarrhythmic of choice in most cases of acute AV nodal tachycardia is:
 (Recent NEET Pattern Question)
 (a) Adenosine (b) Amiodarone
 (c) Propranolol (d) Quinidine

Cardiovascular System

112. Drug of choice for paroxysmal supraventricular tachycardia (PSVT) is: *(Recent NEET Pattern Question)*
    (a) Verapamil
    (b) Digitalis
    (c) Quinidine
    (d) Diphenylhydantoin

113. Drug of choice for ventricular arrhythmias due to myocardial infarction (MI) is:
    (Recent NEET Pattern Question)
    (a) Quinidine   (b) Amiodarone
    (c) Xylocaine   (d) Diphenylhydantoin

114. Drug of choice for ventricular premature beats (VPC) due to digitalis toxicity is:
    (Recent NEET Pattern Question)
    (a) Diphenylhydantoin (b) Quinidine
    (c) Amiodarone   (d) Verapamil

115. Arrhythmias refractory to the treatment of lignocaine can be treated by: *(Recent NEET Pattern Question)*
    (a) Sotalol   (b) Diltiazem
    (c) Amiodarone   (d) Quinidine

116. Quinidine exerts its action on heart by:
    (Recent NEET Pattern Question)
    (a) Ca^{2+} channel blockade (b) Na^+ channel blockade
    (c) K^+ channel opening   (d) Cl^- channel opening

117. All of the following are anti arrhythmic drugs *except*:
    (Recent NEET Pattern Question)
    (a) Lidocaine   (b) Enalapril
    (c) Atenolol   (d) Sotalol

118. Iodine content in amiodarone is:
    (Recent NEET Pattern Question)
    (a) 10-20%   (b) 20-40%
    (c) 40-60%   (d) 60-80%

119. Beta blockers are antiarrhythmic agents of class:
    (Recent NEET Pattern Question)
    (a) I   (b) II
    (c) III   (d) IV

120. Which of the following drug has longest half life?
    (Recent NEET Pattern Question)
    (a) Amiodarone   (b) Quinidine
    (c) Diltiazem   (d) Procainamide

121. Dofetilide is which class of antiarrhythmic drug?
    (Recent NEET Pattern Question)
    (a) Class I   (b) Class II
    (c) Class III   (d) Class IV

122. All of the following are used in atrial arrhythmias *except*: *(Recent NEET Pattern Question)*
    (a) Digoxin   (b) Verapamil
    (c) Quinidine   (d) Lignocaine

123. All the following statements regarding adenosine are true *except*: *(Recent NEET Pattern Question)*
    (a) Dipyridamole potentiates its action
    (b) Used to produce controlled hypotension
    (c) Administered by slow IV injection
    (d) Administered by rapid IV injection

124. Which of the following calcium channel blocker would be useful in the treatment of supra-ventricular tachycardia by suppressing AV node conduction?
    (Recent NEET Pattern Question)
    (a) Amlodipine1   (b) Nimodipine
    (c) Verapamil   (d) Nifedipine

125. Which of the following drugs is a class III antiarrhythmic agent? *(Recent NEET Pattern Question)*
    (a) Quinidine   (b) Amiodarone
    (c) Propranolol   (d) Lignocaine

126. Treatment of choice in ventricular fibrillation is:
    (Recent NEET Pattern Question)
    (a) Sotalol   (b) Cardioversion
    (c) Ibutilide   (d) Adenosine

127. Antiarrhythmic drug is: *(Recent NEET Pattern Question)*
    (a) Phentolamine   (b) Phenobarbitone
    (c) Procainamide   (d) Pentamidine

128. Side effect of corneal microdeposits is seen most commonly with which of the following drugs?
    (Recent NEET Pattern Question)
    (a) Esmolol   (b) Amiodarone
    (c) Adenosine   (d) Bretylium

129. Drug of choice for termination of paroxysmal supra-ventricular ventricular tachycardia is:
    (Recent NEET Pattern Question)
    (a) Calcium channel blocker
    (b) Beta blocker
    (c) Digoxin
    (d) Adenosine

DYSLIPIDEMIA

130. Niacin must be used in diabetics cautiously because:
    (NEET Pattern Question 2017-2018)
    (a) It causes hypoglycemia
    (b) It impairs insulin sensitivity
    (c) It increases skin thickness so difficult to find site for injectable drugs
    (d) Increase metabolism of oral hypoglycemic agents

131. The most potent HMG CoA reductase inhibitor is:
    (NEET Pattern Question 2016-17)
    (a) Simvastatin   (b) Atorvastatin
    (c) Rosuvastatin   (d) Pitavastatin

132. Atorvastatin acts by which of the following mechanism?
    (NEET Pattern Question 2016-17)
    (a) Lipoprotein lipase inhibitor
    (b) Bile acid sequestrants
    (c) HMG-CoA reductase inhibitor
    (d) Cholesterol absorption inhibitor

133. Mechanism of action of Ezetimibe is:
    (NEET Pattern Question 2016-17)
    (a) Interferes with the absorption of bile acids
    (b) Inhibits CETP
    (c) Interferes with absorption of cholesterol by inhibiting NPCIL1
    (d) Inhibitor of PPAR alpha

134. A patient of coronary artery disease with diabetes mellitus has a history of myocardial infarction 2 months back. Lipid profile of the patient is serum triglyceride of 234 mg/dL, LDL 124 mg/dL and HDL 32 mg/dL. Which of the following drugs will you like to administer?
    (AIIMS May 2017)
    (a) Fenofibrate
    (b) Rosuvastatin plus fenofibrate
    (c) Atorvastatin 80 mg
    (d) Rosuvastatin 10 mg

135. The rate-limiting step in cholesterol synthesis is inhibited by: *(Recent NEET Pattern Question)*
    (a) Probucol
    (b) Cholestyramine
    (c) Statins
    (d) Gemfibrozil

136. Lipid lowering drug that significantly reduces lipoprotein-a [Lp (a)] levels is:
    (Recent NEET Pattern Question)
    (a) Fenofibrate
    (b) Gemfibrosil
    (c) Rosuvastatin
    (d) Nicotinic acid

137. Clofibrate, a lipid lowering agent inhibits both cholesterol and triglyceride synthesis by:
    (Recent NEET Pattern Question)
    (a) Inhibiting HMG CoA reductase
    (b) Binding to bile acids and preventing its reabsorption
    (c) Inhibiting VLDL production
    (d) Activating lipoprotein lipase, resulting in VLDL degradation

138. In a patient with hypertriglyceridemia and low HDL, which of the following drug will be best without risk of myopathy as side effect? *(Recent NEET Pattern Question)*
    (a) Fibric acid derivatives
    (b) Nicotinic acid
    (c) Atrovastatin
    (d) Clofibrate

139. HDL is specifically increased by:
    (Recent NEET Pattern Question)
    (a) Lovastatin
    (b) Niacin
    (c) Gemfibrozel
    (d) Probucol

140. The most potent drugs to reduce plasma LDL- cholesterol level are: *(Recent NEET Pattern Question)*
    (a) Plant sterols
    (b) Fibrates
    (c) Anion exchange resins
    (d) Statins

141. Mechanism of action of fibrates is:
    (Recent NEET Pattern Question)
    (a) They increase lipoprotein lipase activity through PPAR alpha and cause increased lipolysis of triglycerides
    (b) Inhibit lipolysis in adipose tissue
    (c) Inhibit HMG CoA reductase
    (d) Bind bile acids and bile salts in small intestine

142. Statins act on which enzyme?
    (Recent NEET Pattern Question)
    (a) Acyl CoA synthetase
    (b) Acyl CoA reductase
    (c) HMG CoA synthetase
    (d) HMG CoA reductase

143. Which of the following drug has maximum oral bioavailability? *(Recent NEET Pattern Question)*
    (a) Fluvastatin
    (b) Atorvastatin
    (c) Pravastatin
    (d) Simvastatin

144. Drug that prevents hypercholesterolemia by inhibiting absorption of cholesterol is:
    (Recent NEET Pattern Question)
    (a) Ezetimibe
    (b) Orlistat
    (c) Cholestyramine
    (d) Statins

145. Mechanism of action of lovastatin is:
    (Recent NEET Pattern Question)
    (a) HMG CoA reductase inhibitor
    (b) Decarboxylase inhibitor
    (c) Activate lipoprotein lipase
    (d) Inhibits lipolysis

146. Most potent statin is: *(Recent NEET Pattern Question)*
    (a) Simvastatin
    (b) Pitavastatin
    (c) Atorvastatin
    (d) Rosuvastatin

147. Which of the following 'statins' has the longest half life?
    (Recent NEET Pattern Question)
    (a) Cerivastatin
    (b) Rosuvastatin
    (c) Atorvastatin
    (d) Simvastatin

148. The vitamin which can be used for treatment of hypercholesterolemia is: *(Recent NEET Pattern Question)*
    (a) Thiamine
    (b) Niacin
    (c) Pyridoxine
    (d) Vitamine B_{12}

RAAS AND MISCELLANEOUS

149. Which of the following is a late inward sodium channel blocker? *(NEET Pattern 2020)*
    (a) Ivabradine
    (b) Ranolazine
    (c) Trimetazidine
    (d) Fasudil

150. Which of the following is a potassium channel opener?
    (NEET Pattern Question 2019)
    (a) Nicorandil
    (b) Ranolazine
    (c) Ivabradine
    (d) Nitroprusside

151. Tadalafil should not be used in:
    (NEET Pattern Question 2017-2018)
    (a) Diabetics
    (b) Patient on vasodilator therapy
    (c) Pulmonary hypertension
    (d) Erectile dysfunction

152. Which of the following drug is contraindicated in a case of bilateral renal artery stenosis?
    (NEET Pattern Question 2016-17)
    (a) Hydralazine
    (b) Enalapril
    (c) Methyldopa
    (d) Dopamine

153. Which of the following angiotensin receptor antagonist contains additional PPAR gamma agonistic activity?
    (AIIMS May 2016)
    (a) Olmesartan
    (b) Telmisartan
    (c) Candesartan
    (d) Losartan

154. Which of the following drug is associated with highest cardiac mortality? *(AI 2012)*
    (a) Rofecoxib
    (b) Nicorandil
    (c) Losartan
    (d) Metoprolol

155. Which of the following drug is used for reversal of cerebral vasospasm and infarct following subarachnoid hemorrhage? *(AI 2012)*
    (a) Nimodipine
    (b) Amlodipine
    (c) Diltiazem
    (d) Verapamil

Cardiovascular System

156. Ivabradine is indicated in the management of: *(AI 2012)*
    (a) PSVT
    (b) Angina pectoris
    (c) Cardiomyopathy
    (d) Irritable bowel syndrome

157. Which of the following drugs is best for reducing proteinuria in a diabetic patient?
    (Recent NEET Pattern Question)
    (a) Metoprolol (b) Perindopril
    (c) Chlorthiazide (d) Clonidine

158. A 50 years old male with type 2 diabetes mellitus is found to have 24 hour urinary albumin of 250 mg. Which of the following drugs may be used to retard progression of renal disease? *(Recent NEET Pattern Question)*
    (a) Hydrochlorthiazide (b) Enalapril
    (c) Amiloride (d) Aspirin

159. Angiotensin II causes all *except*:
    (Recent NEET Pattern Question)
    (a) Stimulates release of ADH
    (b) Increases thirst
    (c) Vasodilation
    (d) Stimulates aldosterone release

160. All are used for treatment of pulmonary hypertension *except*: *(Recent NEET Pattern Question)*
    (a) Endothelin receptor antagonists
    (b) Phosphodiesterase inhibitors
    (c) Calcium channel blockers
    (d) Beta blockers

161. Angiotensin converting enzyme inhibitors when used for a long time in patients with hypertension, cause:
    (Recent NEET Pattern Question)
    (a) Rightward shift in renal pressure-natriuresis curve
    (b) Reduction in filtration fraction
    (c) Significant increase in heart rate
    (d) No change in compliance of large arteries

162. A 30-year-old male presents with severe chest pain, breathlessness, hypotension and ECG shows ST elevation in V3, V4, V5 and V6 leads. He will be best treated with: *(Recent NEET Pattern Question)*
    (a) Streptokinase (b) t-PA
    (c) Heparin (d) PTCA

163. Which among the following is an angiotensin receptor antagonist? *(Recent NEET Pattern Question)*
    (a) Losartan (b) Enlapril
    (c) Ramipril (d) Captopril

164. Drug contraindicated in bilateral renal artery stenosis is:
    (Recent NEET Pattern Question)
    (a) Propranolol (b) Guanethidine
    (c) Captopril (d) Amlodipine

165. Which of the following drugs is deposited in the muscles?
    (Recent NEET Pattern Question)
    (a) Verapamil (b) Digoxin
    (c) Adenosine (d) Phenytoin

166. ACE inhibitors are contraindicated in:
    (Recent NEET Pattern Question)
    (a) Diabetes mellitus
    (b) Hypertension in old age groups
    (c) Scleroderma
    (d) Bilateral renal artery stenosis

167. Indication of ACE inhibitor in diabetes mellitus is:
    (Recent NEET Pattern Question)
    (a) Diabetic nephropathy
    (b) Nephropathy unrelated to diabetes
    (c) Both
    (d) None

168. Cough and angioedema in a patient receiving ACE inhibitors is due to: *(Recent NEET Pattern Question)*
    (a) Bradykinin (b) Renin
    (c) Angiotensin-II (d) All

169. About quinidine, which of the following statements is correct? *(Recent NEET Pattern Question)*
    (a) High doses cause increase in blood pressure
    (b) It inhibits vagus
    (c) It decreases automaticity in heart
    (d) It has antianginal property

170. Food reduces the oral bioavailability of the following angiotensin converting enzyme inhibitors *except*:
    (Recent NEET Pattern Question)
    (a) Enalapril (b) Captopril
    (c) Ramipril (d) Fosinopril

171. Captopril can cause all *except*:
    (Recent NEET Pattern Question)
    (a) Decrease in K^+ concentration
    (b) Decrease in afterload
    (c) Proteinuria
    (d) Blood dyscrasia

172. Which of the following antidotes is used for calcium channel blockers overdose?
    (Recent NEET Pattern Question)
    (a) Atropine (b) Calcium gluconate
    (c) Adrenaline (d) Digoxin

173. Sudden withdrawal of which of the following drugs could result in serious adverse cardiovascular changes in a patient taking the drug over long time?
    (Recent NEET Pattern Question)
    (a) Phenelezine (MAO inhibitor)
    (b) Enalapril (ACE inhibitor)
    (c) Clonidine (α_2 agonist)
    (d) Fluoxetine (serotonin reuptake inhibitor)

174. ACE inhibitors are contraindicated in all of the following *except*: *(Recent NEET Pattern Question)*
    (a) Pregnancy
    (b) Diabetes
    (c) Bilateral renal artery stenosis
    (d) Renal failure

175. Which of the following causes increased renin on prolonged use? *(Recent NEET Pattern Question)*
    (a) Clonidine (b) Enalapril
    (c) Methyldopa (c) Beta Blockers

176. Dialysis is not indicated in toxicity of:
    (Recent NEET Pattern Question)
    (a) Lithium (b) Methanol
    (c) Salicylates (d) Digitalis

177. Cough is an adverse reaction seen with intake of:
 (Recent NEET Pattern Question)
    (a) Thiazide   (b) Nifedipine
    (c) Enalapril   (d) Prazosin

178. Adverse effect of losartan are all *except*:
 (Recent NEET Pattern Question)
    (a) Fetopathic   (b) Cough
    (c) Hyperkalemia   (d) Headache

179. Most effective method of treatment of digitalis toxicity is:
 (Recent NEET Pattern Question)
    (a) Hemodialysis   (b) Cardioversion
    (c) Digoxin antibody (d) Atropine

180. Spironolactone should not be given with:
 (Recent NEET Pattern Question)
    (a) Chlorothiazide   (b) Beta blockers
    (c) ACE inhibitors   (d) Amlodipine

181. Telmisartan lowers blood pressure by:
 (Recent NEET Pattern Question)
    (a) Inhibiting formation of angiotensin I to angiotensin II
    (b) Inhibiting conversion of renin to angiotensin I
    (c) Blocking AT_1 receptors
    (d) Interfering with degradation of bradykinin

182. The drug of choice in scleroderma induced hypertensive crisis is: *(Recent NEET Pattern Question)*
    (a) ACE inhibitors   (b) Thiazides
    (c) β-blockers   (d) Sodium nitroprusside

183. An increase in heart rate and renin release seen in patients of CHF can be overcome by which of the following drugs? *(Recent NEET Pattern Question)*
    (a) Minoxidil   (b) Metoprolol
    (c) Metolazone   (d) Milrinone

184. Coronary vasodilatation is caused by:
 (Recent NEET Pattern Question)
    (a) Adenosine   (b) Bradykinin
    (c) Histamine   (d) Ergotamine

Cardiovascular System

1. **Ans. (b) Trimetazidine** *(Ref: KDT 8th/e p599,600)*
   - **Beta blockers in heart failure**: Beta blockers are contraindicated in acute heart failure but they can be used in chronic heart failure. Beta blockers should be started at low dose, dose should be increased gradually to prevent decompensation.
   - **Beta blockers used are** — Carvedilol, metoprolol and bisoprolol.
   - **Sacubitril**: It acts by inhibiting neutral endopeptidase (NEP), which is required for metabolism of BNP (brain natriuretic peptide). Due to inhibition of NEP, BNP levels are increased resulting in natriuresis and vasodilation. Thus, sacubitril can be used in CHF.
   - **Nesiritide**: It is **recomb**inant BNP. It is given through subcutaneous route.
   - **Trimetazidine**: It is a metabolic modulator. It partially inhibits beta oxidation of fatty acids which results in shifting of metabolism of heart muscles from fatty acids to glucose. This decreases oxygen requirement of heart. It is therefore used in angina pectoris.

2. **Ans. (a) T, (b) T, (c) T, (d) T, (e) T** *(Ref: KDT 8th/e p560)*
   Explanation:
   - Most common and earliest adverse effect of digoxin is nausea and vomiting (option a).
   - Most common arrhythmia seen in digoxin overdose is ventricular bigeminy.
   - Other adverse effects of digoxin include Gynecomastia and Vision defects (initially non-specific and later yellow vision): Option b
   - Early toxicity may not correlate with serum levels because Digoxin has very high volume of distribution (~450L); So when digoxin reaches heart the plasma concentration may not be high.: Option c
   - Hypokalemia increases the risk of toxicity as the binding site of digoxin and K^+ are same on the $Na^+ K^+$ pump. So, normally K inhibits the binding of digoxin to Na K pump. When K is less (hypokalemia), binding of digoxin increases and toxicity can result.
   - However, note that Digoxin toxicity causes hyperkalemia (due to inhibition of Na K pump, K^+ cannot enter inside cells and remain in blood, hence hyperkalemia occurs).

3. **Ans. (c) Guanylate cyclase** *(Ref: KDT 8th/e p613)*
   - **Sodium nitroprusside** and **hydralazine** act by releasing nitric oxide from the endothelium, which in turn increase intracellular cGMP by stimulation of guanylyl cyclase leading to vasodilation.
   - **Nitroprusside, in addition can directly stimulate guanylyl cyclase** to cause increase in cGMP.
   - Nitroprusside is a **very short acting drug**; therefore has to be administered by *constant IV infusion* for the treatment of **hypertensive emergencies**.
   - Its solution should be freshly prepared because it is unstable and *sensitive to light*.
   - Prolonged administration of this drug can result in accumulation of *cyanide* leading to *toxicity* particularly in patients with renal disease.
   - It can also result in *hypothyroidism* due to the accumulation of thiocyanate (antithyroid compound).
   - It is *contraindicated in pregnancy*.

4. **Ans. (d) NEP inhibitor**
   (Ref: CMDT 2018/414, KDT 8th/e p553)
   Neprilysin or Neutral Endo Peptidase (NEP) breaks down BNP. Sacubitril act by inhibiting this enzyme and is useful in CHF.

5. **Ans. (b) Loop diuretic**
   (Ref: Harrison 19th/e p1509; KDT 8th/e p563)

6. **Ans. (d) Hypertrophic obstructive cardiomyopathy**
   (Ref: KDT 6th/e p560)

7. **Ans. (a) Lisinopril** *(Ref: KDT 8th/e p534)*

8. **Ans. (a) Adrenaline** *(Ref: KDT 8th/e p556, 563)*

9. **Ans. (d) Hyperkalemia** *(Ref: KDT 8th/e p561)*

10. **Ans. (b) 0.8-1.5 ng/mL** *(Ref: KDT 8th/e p559)*

	Digitoxin	Digoxin
Therapeutic plasma conc.	15-30 ng/mL	0.5-1.4 ng/mL
Toxic plasma conc.	> 35 ng/mL	> 2.5 ng/mL

11. **Ans. (c) Treat digoxin toxicity** *(Ref: KDT 8th/e p560)*

12. **Ans. (c) It is 95% plasma protein bound**
    (Ref: KDT 8th/e p559)
    Plasma protein binding of digitoxin is high (95%) whereas it is low (70-80%) for digoxin.

13. **Ans. (b) Propranolol** *(Ref: KDT 8th/e p565-566)*
    Afterload is reduced by the drugs having arteriolar dilating property. Propranolol is a non-selective β-blocker. It can cause vasoconstriction by antagonizing $β_2$ mediated vasodilatation. It, therefore do not decrease afterload.

14. **Ans. (a) Guanylate cyclase** *(Ref: KDT 8th/e p613)*
    Nitroprusside generates NO that relaxes vascular smooth muscles by activating guanylate cyclase.

15. **Ans. (d) Na^+K^+ ATPase** *(Ref: KDT 8th/e p558)*
16. **Ans. (c) 5 day** *(Ref: KDT 8th/e p559)*
17. **Ans. (a) Hydralazine** *(Ref: KDT 8th/e p612)*
18. **Ans. (d) All of the above** *(Ref: KDT 8th/e p560)*
19. **Ans. (b) Morphine** *(Ref: KDT 8th/e p506)*
20. **Ans. (a) $Na^+ K^+$ ATPase pump** *(Ref: KDT 8th/e p558)*
21. **Ans. (b) Captopril** *(Ref: Katzung 11th/e p219)*
22. **Ans. (c) An increase in systolic intracellular calcium levels**
    (Ref: Katzung 11th/e p214)
23. **Ans. (d) Fab fragments of digitalis antibodies**
    (Ref: KDT 8th/e p560)
24. **Ans. (c) NPAT with block** *(Ref: KDT 8th/e p560)*

25. **Ans. (b) Prolonged QT interval** *(Ref: KDT 8th/e p557-558)*
    Digoxin increases contractility that manifests as shortening of QT interval.

26. **Ans. (b) K channel opener** *(Ref: Katzung 11th/e p.221)*
    Levosimendan is an inodilator that act by
    - Ca^{2+}-sensitizing action by binding to troponin-C (inotropic action)
    - K^+ Channel opening action – (responsible for vasodilation)

27. **Ans. (b) Hypotension**
    (Ref: Goodman and Gilman 12th/e p696)

28. **Ans. (b) 40 hrs** *(Ref: KDT 8th/e p.559)*

29. **Ans. (a) Inhibits Na^+K^+ATPase pump**
    (Ref: KDT 8th/e p558)

30. **Ans. (a) Spironolactone** *(Ref: KDT 8th/e p567)*

31. **Ans. (c) Spironolactone** *(Ref: KDT 8th/e p567)*

32. **Ans. (a) Renal insufficiency** *(Ref: KDT 8th/e p560)*

33. **Ans. (c) Digoxin** *(Ref: KDT 8th/e p563)*

34. **Ans. (d) Clonidine** *(Ref: KDT 8th/e p529, 530)*

35. **Ans. (a) Hyperkalemia** *(Ref: KDT 8th/e p560-561)*

36. **Ans. (c) Amiodarone** *(Ref: KDT 8th/e p563)*

37. **Ans. (b) Less peripheral vasoconstriction**
    (Ref: KDT 8th/e p147)

38. **Ans. (b) Amiloride** *(Ref: KDT 8th/e p635, 618)*

39. **Ans. (c) Digoxin** *(Ref: KDT 8th/e p560, 561)*
    - Drugs increasing cardiac contractility should be avoided in HOCM.

40. **Ans. (a) $Na^+ K^+$ ATPase inhibition** *(Ref: KDT 8th/e p558)*

41. **Ans. (d) All of the above** *(Ref: KDT 8th/e p560)*

42. **Ans. (a) Dosage reduction is required in hepatic disease**
    (Ref: KDT 8th/e p560)

43. **Ans. (a) Methyl dopa**
    (Ref: Goodman Gilman 12th/e p773, 774; Katzung 12th/e p176)
    Alpha methyl dopa is drug of choice for pregnancy induced hypertension. However, these days labetalol is preferred for this indication.

44. **Ans. (b) Thiazides** *(Ref: Harrison 19th/e p1623)*
    Thiazides are not only diuretics of choice for mild to moderate hypertension but also the first line antihypertensive drugs in these patients.

45. **Ans. (c) Enalapril**
    (Ref: Goodman and Gilman 12th/e p736; Katzung 12th/e p299)
    ACE inhibitors and ARBs are absolutely contraindicated in pregnancy

46. **Ans. (a) Bosentan** *(Ref: Harrison 19th/e p1659)*
    Among the given options, only 2 drugs *i.e.* bosentan and amlodipine are indicated in pulmonary hypertension. Calcium channel blockers like amlodipine are indicated only in those patients which has positive intravenous vasodilator challenge (less than 5 % patients). If the patient has negative test, then endothelin antagonists are indicated like bosentan, macitentan and ambrisentan.
    Non selective Endothelin antagonists (ETA and ETB): Bosentan and Ambrisentan
    ET_A selective antagonist: Ambrisentan

Drugs for pulmonary hypertension:	
Most commonly used drug:	Anticoagulants like warfarin
Drug of choice or best drug:	ET antagonists like bosentan
Most efficacious drug:	Prostacyclins like epoprostenol
Drugs useful in patients with positive IV vasodilator challenge:	Calcium channel blockers

47. **Ans. (a) Chlorthalidone** *(Ref: KDT 8th/e p615)*
    - According to ACC Guidelines and JNC 8 Guidelines, the DOC for hypertension is Thiazides (preferred diuretic).
    - Apart from thiazides, the other first line drugs for hypertension are:
      - ACE inhibitors
      - Angiotensin receptor blockers
      - Calcium channel blockers
    - Triamterene and Spironolactone are K^+ sparing diuretics. These are mainly used along with other diuretics to prevent hypokalemia.
    - Furosemide is a loop diuretic and is used for conditions like congestive heart failure.

48. **Ans. (b) Propranolol** *(Ref: KDT 8th/e p618)*

49. **Ans. (b) By increasing cGMP** *(Ref: KDT 8th/e p586)*

50. **Ans. (c) Minoxidil** *(Ref: KDT 8th/e p613)*

51. **Ans. (d) Labetalol** *(Ref: KDT 8th/e p620)*

52. **Ans. (d) It does not cause postural hypotension**
    (Ref: KDT 8th/e p611)

53. **Ans. (a) Enalapril** *(Ref: Goodman and Gilman 12th/e p736)*
    ACE inhibitors like enalapril are contraindicated in pregnancy. These are teratogenic drugs. Other drugs given in the options are safe in pregnancy.

54. **Ans. (b) IV Nitroprusside** *(Ref: KDT 8th/e p618)*
    Sodium nitroprusside is contra-indicated in eclampsia.

55. **Ans. (c) Sodium nitroprusside** *(Ref: KDT 8th/e p613)*
    Increase in systemic vascular resistance means vasoconstriction, thus a vasodilator drug like nitroprusside should be used. Adrenaline and nor-adrenaline act as vasopressors whereas isoprenaline increases systolic blood pressure by acting on heart.

56. **Ans. (d) Nifedipine**
    (Ref: Katzung 10/e p175; KDT 8th/e p605)
    Nifedipine, amlodipine like calcium channel blockers can be used for hypertension.

57. **Ans. (d) Atenolol** *(Ref: CMDT-2014/429)*
    - Beta blockers are no longer considered to be the first line antihypertensive agents. According to JNC-8, ACE inhibitors, calcium channel blockers and diuretics are first line agents.

58. **Ans. (d) Prazosin** *(Ref: CMDT-2010/409)*
    - Prazosin should be avoided as first choice because of risk of postural hypotension.

59. **Ans. (b) Prazosin** *(Ref: KDT 8th/e p610-611)*

60. **Ans. (b) Indapamide** *(Ref: KDT 8th/e p618,619)*
Indapamide is a thiazide like diuretic, having mild diuretic effect, not used in emergency situations.

61. **Ans. (d) Minoxidil** *(Ref: KDT 8th/e p613)*

62. **Ans. (c) Clonidine** *(Ref: KDT 8th/e p611)*

63. **Ans. (c) In hypertensive patient with gout, diuretics are particularly useful** *(Ref: KDT 8th/e p605)*

> **Antihypertensive in special situations**
> - In patients with CHF or LV systolic dysfunction, ACE inhibitors are antihypertensive of choice.
> - In hypertensive patients with migraine, CCBs are DOC. Beta-Blockers (e.g. propranolol) is also effective.
> - In hypertensive patients with gout, PVD, DM, post MI, hyperlipidemia, ACE inhibitors are preferred.
> - In hypertensive patients with Raynaud's phenomena and other peripheral vascular diseases and migraine CCBs are especially suitable.
>   - Diuretics such as thiazides and frusemide are contraindicated in patients with hyperuricemia.

64. **Ans. (a) Methyldopa** *(Ref: KDT 8th/e p612)*
65. **Ans. (a) IV Lignocaine** *(Ref: CMDT 2010/364)*
66. **Ans. (b) Clonidine** *(Ref: KDT 8th/e p611)*
67. **Ans. (a) Methyl dopa** *(Ref: KDT 8th/e p612)*
68. **Ans. (c) ACE inhibitors** *(Ref: KDT 8th/e p616)*
69. **Ans. (a) Clonidine** *(Ref: KDT 8th/e p611)*
70. **Ans. (b) Methyl dopa** *(Ref: KDT 8th/612)*
71. **Ans. (b) Used for treatment of erectile dysfunction** *(Ref: KK Sharma 2nd/e p195)*

Guanethidine
- Acts by inhibiting exocytosis of NA.
- Does not cross blood brain barrier.
- Postural hypotension, delayed ejaculation and diarrhea are important adverse effects.

72. **Ans. (b) Enalapril** *(Ref: KDT 8th/e p615)*
73. **Ans. (b) ATP dependent K⁺ channels** *(Ref: KDT 8th/e p605)*
74. **Ans. (b) Minoxidil** *(Ref: KDT 8th/e p613)*
75. **Ans. (a) Enalapril** *(Ref: KDT 8th/e p608)*
76. **Ans. (b) Decrease in preload** *(Ref: KDT 8th/586)*
- Beneficial effect of nitrates in classical angina is through the reduction of preload that leads to less end diastolic pressure and in variant angina is via dilation of coronary artery. If type of angina is not mentioned, we will assume it to be classical.
- Beta blockers and calcium channel blockers act by decreasing the heart rate and contractility.
- Mechanism of action of all the drugs used in variant angina (nitrates, calcium channel blockers) is coronary vasodilation.

77. **Ans. (d) Endothelium independent coronary vasodilation** *(Ref: KDT 7th/e p541)*
Predominant mechanism of action of nitrates in angina:
- In Classical angina: Decrease in preload
- In Variant angina: Coronary vasodilation

78. **Ans. (b) cGMP** *(Ref: Katzung 13th/e p329-330)*
Nitric oxide stimulates guanylate cyclase, that increases cGMP. Later is a powerful vasodilator.

79. **Ans. (d) Subarachnoid hemorrhage** *(Ref: Katzung 13th/e p202)*
Nimodipine is a cerebroselective calcium channel blocker indicated in subarachnoid hemorrhage.

80. **Ans. (a) Fasudil** *(Ref: Katzung 12th/e p206)*
- Rho kinase (ROCK) is a major downstream effector of the small GTPase RhoA. ROCK plays central roles in the organization of the actin cytoskeleton and is involved in a wide range of fundamental cellular functions such as contraction, adhesion, migration, proliferation and gene expression.
- **Fasudil** is an experimental drug that acts by inhibiting the rho kinase and is found to be effective in animal models for treatment of:

> - Hypertension
> - Pulmonary Hypertension
> - Coronary artery disease
> - Diabetic cardiomyopathy
> - Vasospastic angina
> - Ischemic stroke
> - Heart failure
> - Erectile dysfunction
> - Cardiac remodeling

81. **Ans. (b) High hepatic first pass metabolism** *(Ref: KDT 8th/e p588)*
Main advantage of sublingual route of drug administration is that liver is bypassed and drugs with high first pass metabolism are absorbed directly into systemic circulation.

82. **Ans. (c) Sick sinus syndrome** *(Ref: KDT 8th/e p597)*
CCBs are contra-indicated in the sick sinus syndrome and along with β-blockers.

83. **Ans. (d) All of the above** *(Ref: KDT 8th/e p586, 587, 590)*
Nitrates act by releasing NO which increases cGMP that cause dephosphorylation of myosin light chain kinase. These are preferential dilator of venules because glutathione reductase (enzyme that releases NO from nitrates) is principally present at these sites. These agents are smooth muscle relaxants and can be used in colics and in achlasia cardia.

84. **Ans. (a) Sub-arachnoid hemorrhage** *(Ref: KDT 8th/e p596)*

85. **Ans. (a) By increasing the left ventricular end diastolic pressure** *(Ref: KDT 8th/e p590)*
Nitrates decreases end diastolic pressure by causing venodilation. For details, see text

86. **Ans. (b) Increase in cardiac work** *(Ref: KDT 8th/e p589-590)*
87. **Ans. (c) Congestive heart failure** *(Ref: KDT 8th/e p597)*
88. **Ans. (c) Isoproterenol** *(Ref: KDT 8/e p585)*
Isoproterenol is a β adrenergic agonist and is C/I in IHD as it can increase myocardial oxygen demand by causing tachycardia.

89. **Ans. (a) Nicorandil** *(Ref: Katzung 11/e p198, KDT 8th/e p598)*

90. Ans. (a) Dantrolene (Ref: KDT 8th/e p592)
91. Ans. (b) Inhalation
    (Ref: Katzung 11th/e p195, KDT, 8th/e p544)
92. Ans. (d) Verapamil (Ref: KDT 8th/e p594)
93. Ans. (b) Complete heart block (Ref: KDT 8th/e p594)
94. Ans. (c) Verapamil (Ref: KDT 8th/e p594-595)
95. Ans. (c) Subarachnoid haemorrhage (Ref: KDT 8th/e p596)
96. Ans. (a) Arterial pressure will decrease
    (Ref: KK Sharma, 1st/e p276)
    Combined use of calcium channel blockers and nitrates enhances the therapeutic effects of each and minimizes the adverse effects.

Parameter	Nitrate	CCB	Combined efficacy
Heart rate	↑	↓	↓ or ±
Contractility	↑	↓	±
Arterial pressure	↓	↓	↓↓
Preload	↓↓	±	↓↓
Afterload	↓	↓↓	↓↓
End diastolic volume	↓	↑	↓ or ±
Ejection time	↓	↑	±
Coronary blood flow	↑	↑	↑↑
Collateral blood flow	↑	↑	↑↑
Endocardial ischemic area blood flow		↑	↑↑
Myocardial wall tension	↓	↓	↓↓
Ventricular volume	↓	±	↓
Heart size	↓	±	↓

97. Ans. (d) Verapamil (Ref: Katzung. 11th/e p181)
98. Ans. (b) ↑cGMP (Ref: KDT 8th/e p587)
99. Ans. (d) Sodium nitrite followed by thiosulphate
    (Ref: KDT 6th/e p527)
100. Ans. (d) Dipyridamol (Ref: KDT 8th/e p598)
101. Ans. (c) Morphine (Ref: KDT 8th/e p602)
102. Ans. (a) Amiodarone Ref: KDT 8th/e p578
   - Amiodarone can result in pulmonary fibrosis. It is therefore, contraindicated in patients with interstitial lung disease
   - Sotalol, Quinidine and Lignocaine does not cause interstitial lung disease

   Adverse effects of amiodarone
The -	Hyper or hypo thyroidism
Periphery of –	Peripheral neuropathy
My –	Myocardial depression
Lung -	Lung fibrosis
&	
Cornea is –	Corneal deposits
Photosensitive –	Photosensitivity

103. Ans. (a) Lignocaine (Ref: CMDT 2019/389)

   Post MI ventricular tachycardia
   - Routine prophylaxis is not recommended.
   - Treat stable patients of sustained ventricular tachycardia with drugs and unstable patients with cardioversion.
   - Drug of choice for treatment of sustained ventricular tachycardia after MI is lignocaine. If it is not effective then amiodarone or procainamide can be used. If the patient still does not respond, then cardioversion should be done.
   - If the arrhythmia is refractory to shock, then amiodarone followed by repeat cardioversion should be done

104. Ans. (b) Nephrotoxicity (Ref: KDT 8th/e p578)
105. Ans. (c) Esmolol: Class IV (Ref: KDT 8th/e p577)
    Beta blockers are classified as class II anti-arrhythmics.
106. Ans. (d) Verapamil
    (Ref: KDT 8th/e p580; Katzung 11th/e p243-244)

   - Adenosine is the DOC for acute termination of PSVT. Esmolol and verapamil are alternative 2nd choice drugs.
   - However adenosine may precipitate bronchospasm in asthmatics, so not preferred in asthmatics.
   - Beta-blockers should be avoided in asthmatics, however if absolutely necessary, cardioselective β blockers (e.g. esmolol) should be used.
   - Further in asthmatic patients, verapamil (as well as nifedipine) given by inhalation significantly inhibits the bronchoconstriction induced by variety of stimuli.

107. Ans. (d) Propranolol
    (Ref: Katzung 11th/e p235,237,239,240, KDT 8th/e 1577)
108. Ans. (d) Lignocaine (Ref: KDT 8th/e p575)
109. Ans. (c) Lignocanine (Ref: KDT 8th/e p575)
110. Ans. (a) Amiodarone (Ref: KDT 8th/e p577)
111. Ans. (a) Adenosine (Ref: KDT 8th/e p581-582)
112. Ans. (a) Verapamil (Ref: KDT 8th/e p580)
113. Ans. (c) Xylocaine (Ref: KDT 8th/e p582, CMDT 2014/362)
   - DOC for ventricular arrhythmias after MI is lignocaine (lidocaine; xylocaine).
   - DOC for supraventricular arrhythmias after MI is beta blockers if cardiac function is adequate.
114. Ans. (a) Diphenylhydantoin (Ref: KDT 6th/e p498)
    Phenytoin is an alternative to lignocaine for digitalis induced ventricular arrhythmia.
115. Ans. (c) Amiodarone (Ref: Katzung 11th/e p241)
116. Ans. (b) Na⁺ channel blockade (Ref: Katzung 11th/e p237)
117. Ans. (b) Enalapril (Ref: KDT 8th/e p573)
118. Ans. (b) 20-40% (Ref: KDT 8th/e p577, 578)
119. Ans. (b) II (Ref: KDT 8th/e p573)
120. Ans. (a) Amiodarone (Ref: kDT 8th/e p578)

Cardiovascular System

121. Ans. (c) Class III *(Ref: KDT 8th/e p579)*
122. Ans. (d) Lignocaine *(Ref: KDT 8th/e p575)*
123. Ans. (c) Administered by slow IV injection
    (Ref: KDT 8th/e p581)
124. Ans. (c) Verapamil *(Ref: KDT 8th/e p580)*
125. Ans. (b) Amiodarone *(Ref: KDT 8th/e p513)*
126. Ans. (b) Cardioversion *(Ref: KDT 8th/e p583)*
127. Ans. (c) Procainamide *(Ref: KDT 8th/e p574)*
128. Ans. (b) Amiodarone *(Ref: KDT 8th/e p578)*
129. Ans. (d) Adenosine *(Ref: KDT 8th/e p581)*
130. Ans. (b) It impairs insulin sensitivity
    (Ref: KDT 8th/e p689, KK Sharma 2nd/e p339)
    Niacin can result in insulin resistance and hyperglycemia, thus should be avoided in diabetic patients.
131. Ans. (d) Pitavastatin *(Ref: KDT's 8th/e pg685)*
132. Ans. (c) HMG-CoA reductase inhibitor
    (Ref: KDT 8th/e p683)
133. Ans. (c) Inteferes with absorption of cholesterol by inhibiting NPCIL1 *(Ref: KDT 8th/e p689)*
134. Ans. (c) Atorvastatin 80 mg *(Ref: CMDT 2017/1263-64)*
    Treatment of hypertriglyceridemia is required only if serum triglycerides are more than 500 mg/dL, so fibrates are not indicated in this person.

> **Indication of statins according to Acc/Aha 2013 guidelines are:** High intensity statins (Atrovastatin 80 mg or rosuvastatin 40 mg)
> - Presence of clinical atherosclerotic cardiovascular disease (irrespective of LDL levels)
> - LDL ≥ 190 mg/dL
> - Age 40–75 years with diabetes mellitus and LDL ≥ 70 mg/dL with 10 year CVD risk ≥ 7.5%
>
> **Low intensity statins (atorvastatin 20 mg, rosuvastatin 10 mg or other statins)**
> - Presence of clinical atherosclerotic cardiovascular disease (irrespective of LDL levels) if age more than 75 years
> - Age 40–75 years with diabetes mellitus and LDL ≥ 70 mg/dL
> - Age 40–75 years with LDL 70-189 mg/dL and 10 year CVD risk ≥7.5%

135. Ans. (c) Statins *(Ref: KDT 8th/e p683)*
136. Ans. (d) Nicotinic acid *(Ref: Katzung 11th/e p613)*
137. Ans. (d) Activating lipoprotein lipase, resulting in VLDL degradation *(Ref: KDT 8th/e p687)*
    Fibrates activate PPAR-α that results in the increased transcription of genes for lipoprotein lipase.
138. Ans. (b) Nicotinic acid *(Ref: KDT 8th/e p689)*
139. Ans. (b) Niacin *(Ref: KDT 8th/e p688)*
140. Ans. (d) Statins *(Ref: KDT 8th/e p685)*
141. Ans. (a) They increase lipoprotein lipase activity through PPAR alpha and cause increased lipolysis of triglycerides
    (Ref: KDT 8th/e p687)
142. Ans. (d) HMG CoA reductase *(Ref: KDT 8th/e p683)*
143. Ans. (a) Fluvastatin
144. Ans. (a) Ezetimibe *(Ref: KDT 8th/e p689)*
145. Ans. (a) HMG CoA reductase inhibitor
    (Ref: KDT 8th/e p683, 684)
146. Ans. (b) Pitavastatin *(Ref: KDT 8th/e p685)*
147. Ans. (b) Rosuvastatin *(Ref: KDT 8th/e p685)*
148. Ans. (b) Niacin *(Ref: KDT 8th/e p688)*
149. Ans. (b) Ranolazine *Ref: KDT 8th/e p600*
    - Ranolazine acts by blocking Na^+ channels along with fatty acid metabolism inhibition. This novel anti-anginal drug primarily acts by inhibiting a late Na^+ current in the myocardium which indirectly facilitates Ca^{2+} entry through Na^+/Ca^{2+} exchanger.
    - Ivabradine selectively inhibits the funny current. It acts by blocking a hyperpolarization activated sodium channel (Known to carry funny current)
    - Trimetazidine is an anti-anginal agent that improves myocardial glucose utilization through inhibition of fatty acid metabolism. It is also known as partial fatty acid oxidation inhibitor.
    - Fasudil is a potent Rho-kinase inhibitor and vasodilator.
150. Ans. (a) Nicorandil *(Ref: Harrison 19th/e p.1862)*
    Nicorandil is the agent that causes coronary dilation by activating myocardial ATP sensitive K^+ channels. In addition it possesses NO releasing property; to which tolerance does not develop.
151. Ans (b) Patient on vasodilator therapy
    (Ref: KDT 8th/e p328)
    Sildenafil should not be combined with vasodilators like nitrates due to risk of development of severe hypotension.
    Sildenafil should be used cautiously in:
    - Presence of liver or kidney disease
    - Peptic ulcer
    - Bleeding disorders
    - With CYP3A4 inhibitors like erythromycin
    - Patients of leukemia, sickle cell anemia or myeloma
152. Ans. (b) Enalapril *(Ref: KDT 8th/e p532)*
153. Ans. (b) Telmisartan
    Telmisartan is an ARB with additional PPAR-gamma agonistic activity. It can benefit dyslipidemia apart from its inhibitory effect on RAAS.
154. Ans. (a) Rofecoxib *(Ref: KDT 8/e p221, 222)*

> - Angiotensin receptor blockers (like losartan) and beta blockers (like metoprolol) are cardioprotective in congestive heart failure. These decrease the mortality.
> - Nicorandil is a potassium channel opener used in angina. It is cardioprotective by causing ischemic pre-conditioning.
> - Rofecoxib is a selective COX-2 inhibitor that was withdrawn due to increased risk of myocardial infarction.

155. **Ans. (a) Nimodipine**
    (Ref: Katzung 11th/e p202, KDT 8th/e p596)

156. **Ans. (b) Angina pectoris**
    (Ref: Katzung 11th/e p203-204, KDT 8th/e p568, CMDT 2014/393)
    - Ivabradine is a bradycardiac drug. It selectively blocks If sodium channel blocker and reduce heart rate by inhibiting the hyperpolarization-activated sodium channel in the SA node. No other significant hemodynamic effect has been noted. It reduces angina attacks similar to calcium channel blockers and beta blockers. Lack of effect on GI and bronchial smooth muscle is an advantage of ivabradine.
    - It can also be used in CHF although not approved by US-FDA.

157. **Ans. (b) Perindopril**
    (Ref: CMDT 2010/1105, KDT 8th/e p 532,535)
    An ACE inhibitor in normotensive diabetics impedes progression to proteinuria and prevents the increase in albumin excretion rate.

158. **Ans. (b) Enalapril**
    (Ref: Katzung 10/e p281; KDT 8th/e p532, 535)
    ACE inhibitors can retard the progression of diabetic complications like nephropathy, neuropathy and retinopathy.

159. **Ans. (c) Vasodilation** *(Ref: Ganong Review of Medical Physiology 22nd; KDT 8th/e p525)*

> - Angiotensin II binds to AT1 receptors and causes vasoconstriction and release of aldosterone.
> - *Angiotensin II is one of the most potent vasoconstrictors in body.*
> - Angiotensin II increases thirst sensation through the subfornical organ (SFO) of the brain.
> - It increases secretion of ATCH in the anterior pituitary.
> - It also potentiates the release of norepinephrine by direct action on postganglionic sympathetic fibers.

160. **Ans. (d) Beta blockers** *(Ref: Harrison 17/e p1577, 1578)*

161. **Ans. (b) Reduction in filtration fraction**
    (Ref: Goodman & Gilman 11/e p804)

> - Angiotensin II shifts the renal pressure natriuresis curve to right and helps to adjust the sodium level of the body according to dietary intake of sodium (more excretion with more intake and less excretion with less consumption). ACE inhibitors block this action of angiotensin II and cause leftward shift of renal pressure natriuresis curve, so that if sodium intake is decreased much more natriuresis can occur.
> - ACE inhibitors increase renal blood flow without increasing GFR and thus result in reduction of filtration fraction
> - ACE inhibitors do not significantly increase heart rate.
> - There are variable effect on various vascular beds with ACE inhibitors, these can dilate large arteries.

162. **Ans. (d) PTCA** *(Ref: Harrison 17/e p1537; KDT 8th/e p603)*
    - It is a characterstic case of ST elevation MI (STEMI). Treatment of choice for STEMI is percutaneous coronary intervention (PCI). Thrombolytics like t PA may also be employed.

163. **Ans. (a) Losartan** *(Ref: KDT 8th/e p535)*
164. **Ans. (c) Captopril** *(Ref: KDT 8th/e p531)*
165. **Ans. (b) Digoxin** *(Ref: KDT 8th/e p559)*
166. **Ans. (d) Bilateral renal artery stenosis** *(Ref: KDT 8th/e p531)*
167. **Ans. (c) Both** *(Ref: KDT 8th/e p535)*
168. **Ans. (a) Bradykinin** *(Ref: KDT 8th/e p531)*
169. **Ans. (c) It decreased automaticity in heart** *(Ref: KDT 8th/e p573)*
170. **Ans. (a) Enalapril** *(Ref: KDT 8th/e p531)*

Effect of food on bioavailability of ACE inhibitors	
Rate and Extent reduced	Captopril Benazepril Moexipril
Rate of absorption reduced	Fosinopril Quinapril Ramipril
No effect	Enalapril Lisinopril Trandolapril Perindopril

171. **Ans. (a) Decrease in K⁺ concentration**
    (Ref: Katzung 11th/e p183)

172. **Ans. (b) Calcium gluconate** *(Ref: Harrison 17th/e p35)*
    Treatment of Calcium channel blocker poisoning
    - Calcium and glucagon for hypotension and symptomatic bradycardia.
    - Dopamine, epinephrine, norepinephrine, atropine, and isoproterenol are less often effective but can be used adjunctively.
    - Amrinone, high-dose insulin (with glucose and potassium to maintain euglycemia and normokalemia), electrical pacing, and mechanical cardiovascular support for refractory cases

173. **Ans. (c) Clonidine (α_2 agonist)** *(Ref: KDT 8th/e p611,612)*
174. **Ans. (b) Diabetes** *(Ref: KDT 8th/e p531,532)*
175. **Ans. (b) Enalapril** *(Ref: KDT 8th/e p530)*
176. **Ans. (d) Digitalis**
    (Ref: KDT 8th/e p560,571 CMDT 2014/1515)
177. **Ans. (c) Enalapril** *(Ref: KDT 8th/e p531)*
178. **Ans. (b) Cough** *(Ref: KDT 8th/e p536)*
179. **Ans. (c) Digoxin antibody** *(Ref: KDT 8th/e p560)*
180. **Ans. (c) ACE inhibitors** *(Ref: KDT 8th/e p532)*
181. **Ans. (c) Blocking AT$_1$ receptors** *(Ref: KDT 8th/e p508)*
182. **Ans. (a) ACE inhibitors**
    (Ref: KDT 8th/e p535, CMDT 2014/808)
183. **Ans. (b) Metoprolol** *(Ref: KDT 8th/e p566-567)*
184. **Ans. (a) Adenosine** *(Ref: KDT 8th/e p581)*

Kidney

CHAPTER 5

DIURETICS

Diuretics mainly exert their effect by the inhibition of renal tubular reabsorption of sodium and water. These may be classified according to their efficacy as high ceiling (loop and osmotic diuretics), medium ceiling (thiazides) and low ceiling (carbonic anhydrase inhibitors and potassium sparing) diuretics. In this chapter, we will classify diuretics based on their site of action.

DIURETICS ACTING ON THE PROXIMAL TUBULE (PT)

These are **non-competitive but reversible** inhibitors of carbonic anhydrase and act by inhibiting the reabsorption of sodium in the proximal tubular portion of the nephron.

Carbonic Anhydrase (CA) Inhibitors (Fig. 5.1)

Luminal membrane of proximal tubules contain Na^+–H^+ antiporter which helps in the excretion of H^+ in exchange with the reabsorption of Na^+. The H^+ is formed inside the tubular cells due to the action of carbonic anhydrase according to the reaction:

$$H_2O + CO_2 \rightleftharpoons H_2CO_3 \rightleftharpoons H^+ + HCO_3^-$$

The secreted H^+ combines with HCO_3^- in the lumen of PT with the help of carbonic anhydrase to form carbonic acid (H_2CO_3), which is converted to H_2O and CO_2. Latter are absorbed in the tubular cell and again converted to HCO_3^- and H^+. Thus, the *net effect of carbonic anhydrase is to cause the absorption of sodium and bicarbonate*. Inhibitors of this enzyme (*acetazolamide, dichlorphenamide and methazolamide*) result in the excretion of sodium and bicarbonate in the urine. Due to urinary excretion of bicarbonate, *metabolic acidosis (and urinary alkalosis) ensues that result in* reduced filtration of HCO_3^- at the glomerulus. Therefore, *action of these diuretics is self limiting*.

These agents also decrease the secretion of H^+ in the distal tubules and collecting ducts. Due to less reabsorption of sodium in the PT, more is delivered to the distal tubules (DT). At this site (also known as cortical diluting segment), Na^+ is exchanged with K^+ and H^+. Drugs that increase the delivery of Na^+ to this site (thiazides, loop diuretics, CA inhibitors), will result in greater exchange and thus can cause hypokalemia. **At equally natriuretic doses, K^+ excretion is maximum with CA inhibitors because** Na^+ delivered to the distal tubules is exchanged only with K^+ (excretion of H^+ is inhibited by these drugs).

CA inhibitors also *decrease aqueous humor formation* (therefore used in glaucoma) *and raise seizure threshold* (basis of their use in catamenial epilepsy). Acetazolamide can be *used orally for the treatment of glaucoma, catamenial epilepsy, acute mountain sickness and to alkalinize urine* (for excretion of acidic drugs). **Dorzolamide and brinzolamide** are topically acting CA inhibitors for use in glaucoma as eye drops.

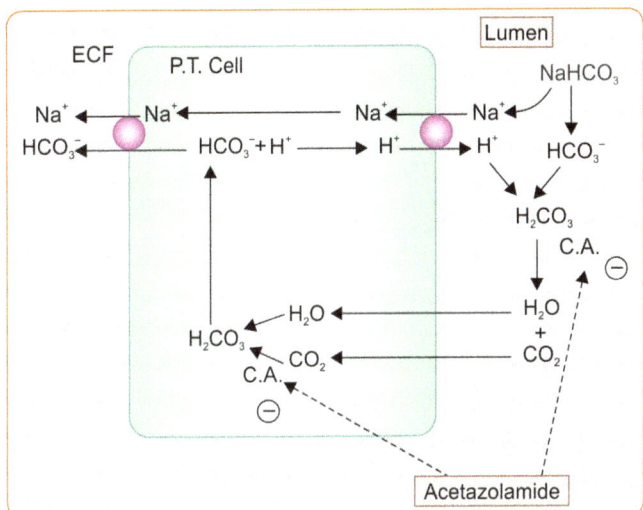

FIG. 5.1: Mechanism of action of carbonic anhydrase inhibitors

> **MNEMONIC**
>
> **Uses of carbonic anhydrase inhibitors**
> **G**laucoma (Angle closure)
> **A**lkalinization of Urine
>   **M**ountain Sickness
>   **E**pilepsy (catamenial)
>
> G A M E

Acetazolamide is a sulfonamide derivative and can result in *bone marrow suppression and hypersensitivity* reactions. Other adverse effects include *metabolic acidosis (urinary alkalosis) and hypokalemia*. These diuretics **should not be used in the presence of liver disease** due to the risk of precipitation of hepatic coma. In liver disease, NH_3 is not converted to urea and if present in excess, can cross the blood brain barrier resulting in encephalopathy. It is excreted through kidney after conversion to NH_4^+ (combines with H^+ in the nephron). CA inhibitors decrease the excretion of H^+ resulting in enhanced reabsorption of ammonia (because it is in non-ionized form in the alkaline medium) and thus more toxicity.

DIURETICS ACTING ON THE LOOP OF HENLE

Loop Diuretics

These act by causing **inhibition of Na^+ K^+ $2Cl^-$ symporter** present at the luminal membrane of the **thick ascending limb of loop of Henle. Furosemide, torsemide, bumetanide, ethacrynic acid, axosemide, piretanide, tripamide and mersalyl** are the important members of this group. These have greater maximal natriuretic effect than all other diuretics (**high ceiling diuretics**). These drugs are *faster acting with short duration of action*. Loop diuretics and thiazides gain access to the tubular lumen through secretion (by organic anion transporter) in the PT.

Loop diuretics *abolish corticomedullary osmotic gradient and decrease positive as well as negative free water clearance*. (details given later in the chapter).

By inhibiting Na^+ K^+ $2Cl^-$ symporter, absorption of Na^+ in loop of Henle decreases. This unabsorbed Na^+ reaches DT, where it is exchanged with K^+ and H^+ resulting in hypokalemia and alkalosis. At equivalent doses, loop diuretics cause less hypokalemia than thiazides. These drugs are also weak CA inhibitors (except ethacrynic acid, it does not increase bicarbonate excretion in the urine). Loop diuretics also change intrarenal hemodynamics resulting in decreased absorption of Na^+ and water in the PT. These changes are mediated by the release of PGs (NSAIDs attenuate diuretic effect). Since GFR is not altered, loop diuretics are the **diuretics of choice in presence of moderate to severe renal failure**.

- **Furosemide** possesses *vasodilatory action which is responsible for the quick relief in LVF and pulmonary edema* (used IV).
- **Bumetanide** is the most potent loop diuretic *(Ref. Goodman & Gilman Pg. 750)* and produces less adverse effects than furosemide.
- **Ethacrynic acid** is *highly ototoxic* with steep DRC.
- **Mersalyl** like organomercurials are not used now due to the risk of kidney damage.
- **Torsemide** has *longest half life (Ref. Goodman & Gilman Pg. 750)*

Uses

Main use of loop diuretics is to remove *the edema fluid* in renal, hepatic or cardiac diseases. These can be administered IV *for prompt relief of acute pulmonary edema* (due to vasodilatory action). These drugs cause excretion of Ca^{++}, therefore can be used for the treatment of hypercalcemia.

Adverse Effects

Hypokalemia, hypomagnesemia, hyponatremia, alkalosis, hyperglycemia (C/I in DM), hyperuricemia (C/I in gout) and dyslipidemia are seen with both thiazides as well as loop diuretics. Effect on Ca^{++} excretion is opposite to thiazides (**LOOP LOOSES CALCIUM**). Loop diuretics cause hypocalcemia by increasing the excretion of Ca^{2+} whereas thiazides cause hypercalcemia by decreasing its excretion. *Ethacrynic acid can cause ototoxicity* more often than other loop diuretics. Furosemide and bumetanide are sulfonamides in chemical structure (should be avoided in persons allergic to sulfonamides).

Osmotic Diuretics

Mannitol, glycerol, urea and isosorbide are inert drugs that can cause osmotic diuresis. **Loop of Henle, is the major site of action of these diuretics**. *(Ref. Goodman & Gilman Pg. 747)* When administered IV, mannitol increases the osmotic pressure in the blood vessels and the consequent removal of excess fluid from the cells (basis of its use in glaucoma and cerebral edema) results in the expansion of extracellular fluid volume. Consequently, renal blood flow and GFR increases. Further, it is filtered at the glomerulus and reaches the proximal tubule (PT) and loop of Henle. Along with water, excretion of all the cations and anions is increased. *Properties* for a substance to act as an *ideal osmotic diuretic* are:

- It *should exert osmotic effect*.
- It should be *pharmacologically inert*.
- It should be *freely filtered* at the glomerulus.
- It *should not be reabsorbed*.

Mannitol is a low molecular weight compound possessing all these properties. It is used IV *for the treatment of glaucoma and cerebral edema* (**drug of choice**). It can also be used to maintain GFR in the impending renal failure. Osmotic diuretics are preferred in prevention of **cisplatin-induced nephrotoxicity** due to their rapid diuretic action. It is *contraindicated in acute renal failure and pulmonary edema* because ECF volume increases but it cannot be filtered. It is **also contraindicated in cerebral hemorrhage (active bleeding)** because in this situation, mannitol can leak from ruptured cerebral blood vessels resulting in the increased ICT (more fluid retention due to its osmotic effect in the cells). If given orally, mannitol can result in osmotic diarrhea. Isosorbide and glycerol can be used orally for the treatment of glaucoma and cerebral edema.

Osmotic Diuretics	
Indications	**Contraindications**
• Cerebral edema	• Pulmonary edema
• Acute congestive glaucoma	• Acute renal failure
• Prevention of cisplatin induced nephrotoxicity	• Active cerebral bleeding
• Impending renal failure	

DIURETICS ACTING ON THE DISTAL TUBULES AND COLLECTING DUCTS

Thiazides

Drugs in this group include *bendroflumethiazide, chlorthiazide, hydrochlorthiazide, methiclothiazide, polythiazide, trichlormethiazide, benzthiazide, hydroflumethiazide, chlorthalidone, metolazone, quinethazone and indapamide*. Chlorthalidone, indapamide, metolazone and quinethazone are thiazide like diuretics whereas other agents in this group are thiazides. These drugs act **by inhibiting Na^+-Cl^- symporter** at the luminal membrane *of early DT (Fig. 5.2)*. This part of DT is impermeable to water and absorbs only solutes. By increasing excretion of solutes, thiazides make the urine concentrated (i.e. *decrease positive free water clearance without affecting negative free water clearance*). These drugs reach the lumen of nephron by secretion through organic acid transporter system. Additional CA inhibitory action is also exhibited by thiazides. Decreased absorption of Na^+ results in its greater delivery to late DT and CD that is responsible for *hypokalemia* (more than loop diuretics). **Chlorthiazide has minimum potency and efficacy** whereas other drugs differ only in potency (efficacy is similar). *Thiazides are moderate efficacy diuretics* with low ceiling effect (**flat DRC**, natriuretic effect does not increase appreciably with increase in dose). These drugs tend to reduce GFR, therefore are *not indicated in renal failure patients*.

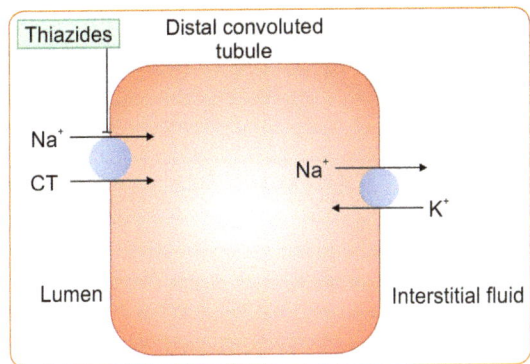

FIG. 5.2: Mechanism of action of thiazides

- Polythiazide and trichloromethiazide are most potent thiazides.
- Chlorthalidone is the longest acting thiazide.
- Metolazone is useful even in severe renal failure.
- Indapamide has no CA inhibitory action. It has vasodilatory property because of which, its antihypertensive effect precedes the natriuretic effect.

Uses

Thiazides are used as first line antihypertensive drugs. These are also used to mobilize the edema fluid in mild to moderate heart failure. Paradoxically, these drugs *decrease urine output in diabetes insipidus*. Thiazides reduce the excretion of Ca^{++} in the kidney, so can be used for the treatment of patients with hypercalciurea and recurrent Ca^{++} stones in the kidney.

Adverse effects

These are similar to loop diuretics except the effect on Ca^{++} excretion. Incidence of *erectile dysfunction* is greater with thiazides than with other antihypertensive drugs (like β blockers, CCBs, ACE inhibitors and α blockers).

Interactions of thiazides and loop diuretics

- Thiazides and loop diuretics enhance digitalis toxicity by causing hypokalemia and hypomagnesemia.
- Loop diuretics can enhance nephrotoxicity and ototoxicity of aminoglycosides.
- NSAIDs attenuate the actions of loop diuretics.
- Lithium toxicity can occur if used with diuretics (due to increased absorption of lithium in the PT).
- Resistance to loop diuretics can be reversed by addition of thiazides and resistance to latter can be decreased by adding potassium sparing diuretics.

POTASSIUM SPARING DIURETICS

These diuretics act in the late DT and CD cells to preserve K^+. Luminal membrane of these portions of renal tubule contains *epithelial Na^+ channels* responsible for reabsorption of Na^+. Due to decreased positive charge in the lumen, a transepithelial potential difference is generated (lumen negative). Under this potential gradient, K^+ and H^+ are secreted. These actions are promoted by aldosterone. Drugs that inhibit the epithelial Na^+ channels or the actions of aldosterone can decrease the reabsorption of Na^+ (diuretic effect) and excretion of K^+ (potassium sparing effect) and H^+.

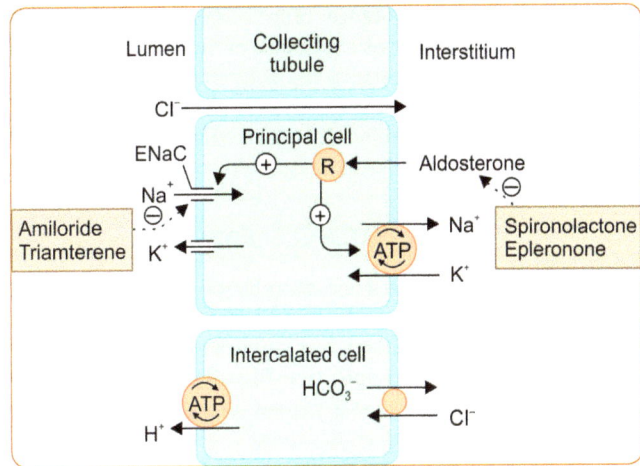

FIG. 5.3: Mechanism of action of K^+ sparing diuretics

(a) Epithelial Na^+ Channel Inhibitors (Fig. 5.3)

These drugs are basic in nature and reach the lumen of PT by **secretion through organic base secretory system**. By travelling through the lumen, these drugs reach its site of action i.e. late DT and CD. Important members of this group are **amiloride and triamterene**. *Pentamidine and high dose trimethoprim (used for pneumocystis) are also weak inhibitors of this channel.*

- Amiloride is more potent and longer acting than triamterene.
- Triamterene is less often used because of incomplete absorption, photosensitivity and impairment of glucose tolerance. It is also associated with interstitial nephritis and renal stones.
- Triameterene is a *weak folic acid antagonist* and can lead to megaloblastic anemia especially in cirrhotic persons.
- **Amiloride** decreases Mg^{++} and Ca^{++} excretion and increases urate excretion.
- Lithium is absorbed through epithelial Na^+ channels in the CD cells and at toxic doses can cause diabetes insipidus. *Amiloride is the drug of choice for this condition*; it acts by blocking the entry of lithium through these channels.
- Amiloride can also be used *as an aerosol to decrease the secretions in cystic fibrosis*.

(b) Aldosterone Antagonists (Fig. 5.3)

Spironolactone, canrenone, potassium canreonate and epleronone antagonize the action of aldosterone and produce effects similar to amiloride. These drugs **act from the interstitial site** of tubular cell (all other diuretics act from luminal side). These agents have *maximum effect when aldosterone levels are high* (e.g. hepatic cirrhosis, CHF, nephrotic syndrome etc.) and are ineffective in its absence (e.g. Addison's disease). **Spironolactone increases Ca^{++} excretion whereas amiloride decreases it**. Spironolactone is converted to canrenone and other active metabolites in the liver.

Uses: These are weak diuretics and are used only in combination with thiazides or loop diuretics to counteract K^+ loss. These can be *used for CHF (decrease mortality), hypertension and cirrhotic edema (diuretic of choice is spironolactone). Spironolactone can be used* *for the treatment of hirsutism because of its anti-androgenic action. (Its structure is similiar to testosterone and thus it acts as a competitive antagonist at testosterone receptors.*

Adverse effects and interactions: Spironolactone can cause **gynaecomastia and impotence**. *Hyperkalemia*, abdominal pain and aggravation of peptic ulcer can also occur. *ACE inhibitors and potassium supplements increase the risk of hyperkalemia*, if used along with these agents. Hyperkalemia and GI disorders are the main adverse effects of eplerenone. It is metabolized by microsomal enzymes; therefore, is prone to drug interactions.

FREE WATER CLEARANCE

- The volume of water in urine, excreted per unit time in excess of that required to excrete the contained solutes isoosmotically with plasma is called free water clearance.
- Free water clearance is **positive for dilute urine, negative when concentrated** urine is passed and zero when isotonic urine is passed.
- To understand the effect of different diuretics on free water clearance one should know the following facts:
  – The nephron of the kidney is arranged in such a way that some portion of it lies in the cortex and some portion of it lies in the **medulla**.

Parts of nephron in the cortex	Parts of nephron in the medulla
Proximal convoluted tubule	Descending thin limb of Henle's loop
Distal convoluted tubule	Ascending limb of Henle's loop
Thick ascending limb of Henle's loop	Medullary collecting duct
Cortical collecting duct	

  – The **cortical portion** of the nephron are responsible for *diluting the urine* (i.e., positive free water clearance).
  – The **medullary portions** of the nephron are responsible for *concentrating the urine* (i.e., negative free water clearance).
  – Thus, the diuretics which act on both medulla and cortex can affect both the positive and negative free water clearance whereas diuretics, which act on either cortex or medulla can affect either the negative or the positive free water clearance.

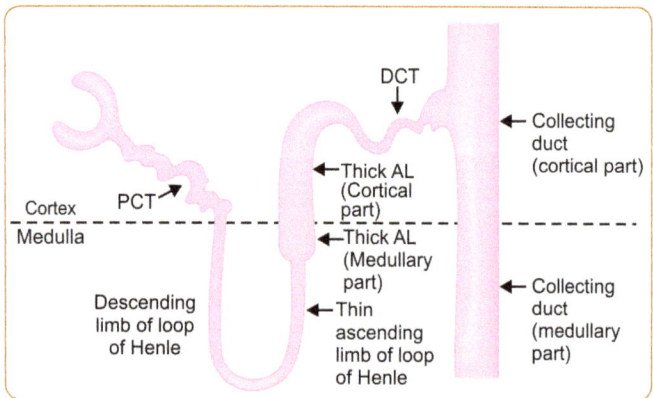

FIG. 5.4: Cortical and medullary portions of nephron

- **Loop diuretics** act on thick ascending limb of Loop of Henle, which has both medullary and cortical parts. Thus, these diuretics **can decrease both positive and negative free water clearance.**

- **Thiazides** act on DCT which is present in cortex. These diuretics therefore, can **decrease positive free water clearance but not negative.**

ANTIDIURETICS

The drugs that decrease urine volume are called antidiuretics. Primary indication of antidiuretics is the treatment of diabetes insipidus (DI).

ANTI-DIURETIC HORMONE (ADH)

Physiological antidiuretic is vasopressin (antidiuretic hormone or ADH) that is synthesized in the hypothalamus and secreted by the posterior pituitary. It is *secreted in response to increased plasma osmolality or decreased volume of extracellular fluid* (ECF). ADH acts via 3 receptors V_1, V_2 and V_3.

Actions of ADH

- In the absence of ADH, collecting ducts (CD) of the nephron are impermeable to water. ADH *increases the permeability of CD by its action on V_2 receptors* **(Fig. 5.5)**. Stimulation of these receptors elevates cAMP levels that increase aquaporins on the apical membrane of CD (by decreasing endocytosis and increasing exocytosis). V_2 receptor activation also increases permeability of CD to urea by stimulating the urea transporter.
- Vasopressin (ADH) as the name suggests is a *potent pressor of blood vessels. Vasoconstrictor action is mediated by the activation of V_1 (also called V_{1a}) receptors. This action requires much higher concentration than V_2 receptor activation. V_2 receptor mediated vasodilatory action (due to the release of NO) has also been demonstrated.*
- ADH is also involved in the *release of vWF and factor VIII from the endothelium. This action is also mediated by V_2 receptors.*
- V_3 receptors (previously known as V_{1b} receptors) are involved in the release of ACTH.

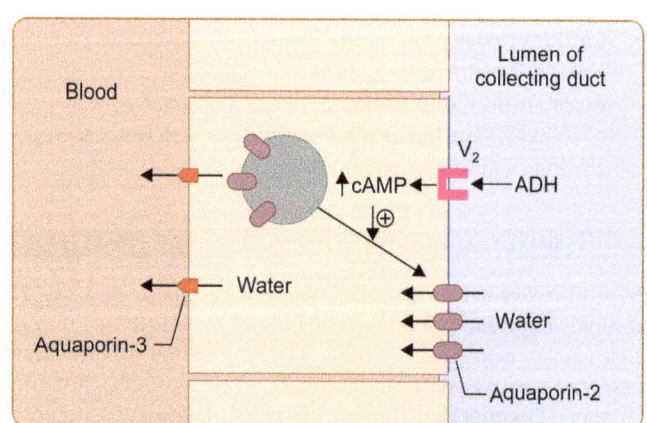

FIG. 5.5: Mechanism of ADH as antidiuretic

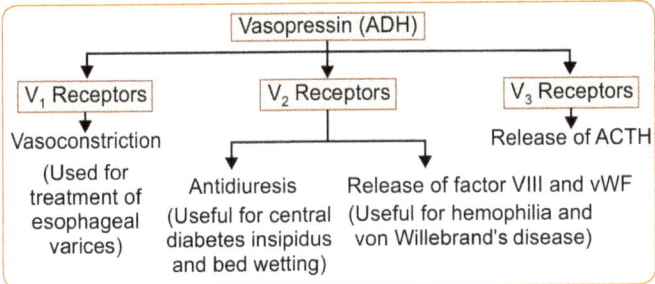

Uses

- Major indication of ADH is central DI. DI is a condition in which there is excessive formation of urine due to decreased activity of ADH. It may be due to decreased production of ADH (central DI) or due to defective receptors in the kidney (nephrogenic DI). **ADH is effective only for central DI.** Use of ADH (arginine vasopressin) for this indication *is limited due to two reasons; its short half life* (require frequent daily dosing) and *non-specific action* on V_1 and V_2 receptors (V_1 mediated vasoconstriction can result in increased BP). Both of these shortcomings have been overcome in **desmopressin**. It is *longer acting and V_2 selective* analogue of vasopressin and is the drug of choice for the treatment of central DI. It can be administered *orally or intranasally*.
- Desmopressin (oral) is also the *drug of choice* for **nocturnal enuresis** and bed wetting in children. Intranasal desmopressin is not used for this indication now because of risk of dilutional hyponatremia
- Another V_2 receptor mediated use of desmopressin is to **check bleeding in patients with hemophilia and von Willebrand's disease**. It acts by releasing factor VIII and vWF from the endothelium.
- Arginine vasopressin (AVP) has vasoconstrictor action that can be utilized **to stop bleeding in esophageal varices.** **Lypressin** *has longer duration of action but is non-specific* (action on both V_1 and V_2). **Terlipressin** (*prodrug of vasopressin) is the preferred agent for this indication.*
- **Felypressin** can also be used along with local anaesthetics to prolong their duration of action (like adrenaline).

Adverse Effects and Contraindications

Intranasal desmopressin can cause *nasal irritation and rhinitis*. AVP can cause *hypertension and precipitation of angina*, so it is contra-indicated in the patients with ischemic heart disease and hypertension.

OTHER ANTIDIURETICS

Thiazides

These drugs are used as diuretics but, **exert paradoxical effect (decrease urine formation) in DI.** This paradoxical effect is believed to be *due to increased formation of cAMP in the distal tubules.* Another proposed mechanism is that thiazides cause dehydration that result in compensatory increase in reabsoprption of Na^+ and water from the proximal portions of nephron. These are low efficacy antidiuretics but are *beneficial in both central as well as nephrogenic DI.*

Chlorpropamide, Clofibrate and Carbamazepine

These drugs increase the action of ADH on the kidney and are *useful only in the central DI.*

Amiloride

It is the agent of choice for *the treatment of Lithium induced DI.*

VASOPRESSIN RECEPTOR ANTAGONISTS

- V_1 receptor antagonists may be useful when total peripheral resistance is increased (e.g. CHF and hypertension) whereas V_2 antagonists may be useful for the treatment of SIADH.
- **Relcovaptan** is *selective V_1 antagonist* whereas **lixivaptan, mozavaptan and tolvaptan** are V_2 *selective antagonists.*
- **Conivaptan** is V_{1a}/V_2 receptor antagonist used as an aquaretic (increase water excretion without affecting electrolytes like sodium) in CHF.
- **Conivaptan** is administered by **IV injection** whereas **lixivaptan and tolvaptan** can be given **orally**.

Tolvaptan is selective V_2 receptor antagonists. It has been approved to slow kidney function decline in adult polycystic kidney disease (APKD) by oral route.

Syndrome of Inappropriate ADH Secretion (SIADH)

ADH is secreted in response to hypovolumeia, in which case its secretion is appropriate. However, if ADH is secreted in high quantities in the presence of euvolemia or hypervolemia, it is called inappropriate secretion (SIADH). The resultant water retention can result in hyponatremia. Thus, SIADH is characterized by normovolemic or hypervolemic hyponatremia.

- **Fluid restriction** is **treatment of choice** for SIADH.
- Hypertonic saline (3% NaCl) + loop diuretics (depending upon volume status) is treatment of choice for severe symptomatic hyponatremia.
- Among drugs, tolvaptan (oral), conivaptan (IV) are preferred for long-term use.
- Alternatives are demeclocycline and lithium (not preferred now).

Golden Points

1. Acetazolamide, dorzolamide and brinzolamide are non-competitive but reversible inhibitors of carbonic anhydrase.

2. Action of carbonic anhydrase inhibitors is self-limiting.

3. At equally natriuretic doses, K+ excretion is maximum with carbonic anhydrase inhibitors.

4. Carbonic anhydrase inhibitors should not be used in the presence of liver disease due to the risk of precipitation of hepatic coma.

5. Loop diuretics decrease positive as well as negative free water clearance whereas thiazides decrease positive free water clearance only.

6. Loop diuretics are the diuretics of choice in the presence of moderate to severe renal failure.

7. Furosemide possesses vasodilatory action which is responsible for the quick relief in LVF and pulmonary edema.

8. Bumetanide is the most potent loop diuretic whereas Torsemide has longest half life.

9. **Ethacrynic acid** is *highly ototoxic* diuretic.

10. Mannitol can be used to maintain GFR in the impending renal failure.

11. Thiazides are used for the treatment of patients with recurrent Ca++ stones in the kidney.

12. *Amiloride is drug of choice for lithium-induced diabetes insipidus.*

13. Aldosterone antagonists **act from the interstitial site** of tubular cell whereas *all other diuretics act from luminal side*.

14. ADH *increases the permeability of collecting ducts by its action on V_2 receptors.*

15. *Vasoconstrictor action of ADH is mediated by the activation of V_1 (also called V_{1a}) receptors.*

16. *ADH-induced release of vWF and factor VIII from the endothelium is mediated by V_2 receptors.*

17. V_3 receptors (previously known as V_{1b} receptors) are involved in the release of ACTH.

18. Desmopressin is longer acting and V_2 selective analogue of vasopressin and is the drug of choice for the treatment of central diabetes insipidus.

19. **Vasopressin receptors**

V_1 (V_{1a})
- Vascular smooth muscle – Vasoconstriction
- Platelets – Aggregation
- Hepatocytes – Glycogenolysis
- Uterus – contraction

V_2
- Collecting tubules – Insersion of AQP2 water channels
- Endothelium – Release of vWF and factor 8
- Vascular smooth muscle – Vasodilation

V_3 (V_{1b})
- Anterior pituitary – ACTH release

Drug of Choice

Condition	Drug of choice
• Edema	
– Due to CHF	Furosemide
– Due to renal disease or nephrotic syndrome	Furosemide
– Pulmonary edema	Furosemide
– Cerebral edema	Mannitol
– Edema due to cirrhosis	Spironolactone
• Diabetes insipidus	
– Central	Desmopressin
– Nephrogenic	Thiazides
– Lithium-induced	Amiloride
• Recurrent calcium stones in kidney due to hypercalciurea	Thiazides
• Acute congestive glaucoma	Acetazolamide
• Acute mountain sickness	Acetazolamide
• Nocturnal enuresis	Desmopressin
• SIADH	Fluid restriction + Hypertonic saline + Furosemide

Image Based Questions

1. A 72-year-old male, Hemraj was admitted to the hospital with severe dyspnoea and orthopnea. On investigations and clinical examination, he was found to be suffering from congestive heart failure. He was given some drug intravenously and the patient experienced brisk diuresis and significant relief of symptoms. This drug acts predominantly on which of the following segments of nephron?

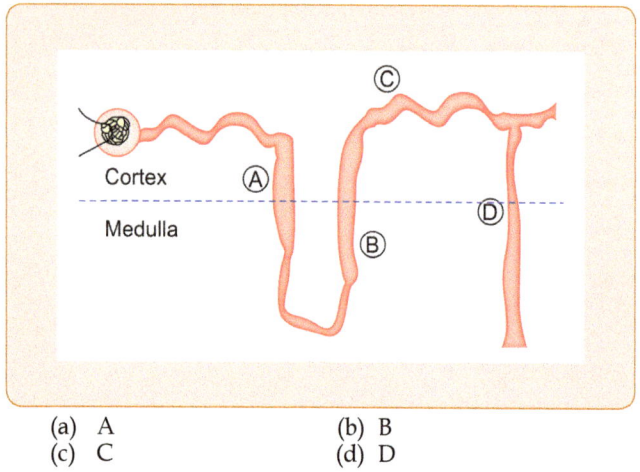

   (a) A
   (b) B
   (c) C
   (d) D

2. Mechanism of action of two diuretics A and B is shown in the image. These are likely to be:

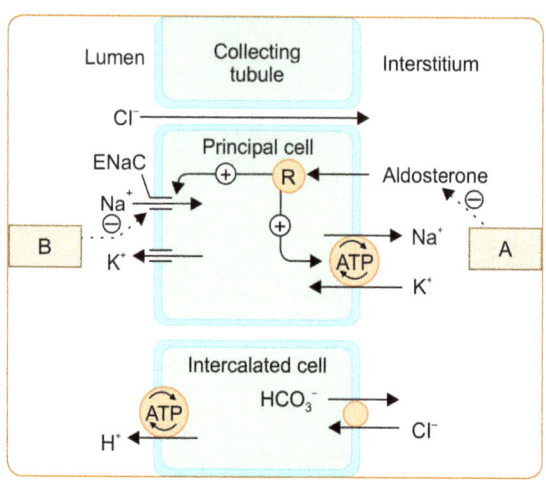

	Drug A	Drug B
(a)	Amiloride	Triamterne
(b)	Amiloride	Spironolactone
(c)	Spironolactone	Amiloride
(d)	Spironolactone	Thiazides

Explanations

1. **Ans. (b) B** *(Ref: KK Sharma 2/e p227)*
   The drug administered to this patient is most likely a loop diuretic that act on ascending limb of the loop of Henle.

2. **Ans. (c)** Drug A is an aldosterone receptor antagonist like spironolactone and epleronone. Drug B is an epithelial sodium channel blocker like amiloride or triamterene.

Multiple Choice Questions

DIURETICS

1. At a high altitude of 3000 m, a person complains of breathlessness. All of the following can be used for the management of this person *except*: *(NEET Pattern 2020)*
   (a) Intravenous digoxin
   (b) Oxygen supplementation
   (c) Immediate descent
   (d) Acetazolamide

2. Drug of choice for prophylaxis of acute mountain sickness: *(AIIMS Nov. 2018)*
   (a) Diltiazem
   (b) Digoxin
   (c) Dexamethasone
   (d) Acetazolamide

3. Mannitol is used for treatment of: *(NEET Pattern Question 2019)*
   (a) Acute congestive glaucoma
   (b) Pulmonary edema
   (c) Acute renal failure
   (d) Congestive heart failure

4. Furosemide causes: *(NEET Pattern Question 2016-17)*
   (a) Metabolic alkalosis
   (b) Respiratory alkalosis
   (c) Metabolic acidosis
   (d) Respiratory acidosis

5. True about Dorzolamide is: *(NEET Pattern Question 2016-17)*
   (a) Carbonic anhyadrase inhibitor
   (b) Na-K-2Cl symporter inhibitor
   (c) Acts on thick ascending limb of loop of Henle
   (d) Used only by parenteral route

6. The site of action of the furosemide is: *(AIIMS May, 2014)*
   (a) Thick ascending limb of loop of Henle
   (b) Descending limb of loop of Henle
   (c) Proximal convoluted tubule
   (d) Distal convoluted tubule

7. Thiazide diuretics can be used for the treatment of all of these conditions *except*: *(AI 2012)*
   (a) Idiopathic hypercalciurea with nephrocalcinosis
   (b) Hyperlipidemia
   (c) Congestive Heart Failure
   (d) Hypertension

8. Which diuretic could be considered appropriate for combining with ACE inhibitors? *(Recent NEET Pattern Question)*
   (a) Spironolactone
   (b) Eplerenone
   (c) Hydrochlorothiazide
   (d) Amiloride

9. Spironolactone is contraindicated with which of the following drugs? *(Recent NEET Pattern Question)*
   (a) Enalapril
   (b) Atenolol
   (c) Verapamil
   (d) Chlorthiazide

10. Furosemide should not be administered with NSAIDs because latter: *(Recent NEET Pattern Question)*
    (a) Prevent platelet aggregation
    (b) Inhibit prostacyclin synthesis
    (c) Decrease sodium reabsorption
    (d) Increase the secretion of furosemide in urine

11. All of the following diuretics inhibit $Na^+ - K^+ - 2Cl^-$ symporter, *except*: *(Recent NEET Pattern Question)*
    (a) Furosemide
    (b) Thiazide
    (c) Ethacrynic acid
    (d) Mersalyl

12. Which of the following statements is not true about diuretics? *(Recent NEET Pattern Question)*
    (a) Acetazolamide is a carbonic acid anhydrase stimulant
    (b) Thiazides act on cortical diluting segment of nephron
    (c) Furosemide is a high ceiling diuretic
    (d) Spironolactone is an aldosterone antagonist

13. Which of the following diuretics cause hypercalcemia and can be used in recurrent renal calcium stones? *(Recent NEET Pattern Question)*
    (a) Spironolactone
    (b) Furosemide
    (c) Chlorthiazide
    (d) Mannitol

14. Which one is a mineralocorticoid antagonist? *(Recent NEET Pattern Question)*
    (a) Thiazide
    (b) Cyproterone acetate
    (c) Furosemide
    (d) Spironolactone

15. In cirrhotic ascites, which diuretic is preferred? *(Recent NEET Pattern Question)*
    (a) Furosemide
    (b) Acetazolamide
    (c) Spironolactone
    (d) Any of the above

16. Aldosterone action is on: *(Recent NEET Pattern Question)*
    (a) Proximal tubule
    (b) Distal tubules
    (c) Loop of Henle
    (d) Collecting duct

17. Thiazide diuretic does not cause: *(Recent NEET Pattern Question)*
    (a) Hyper calcaemia
    (b) Hypo magnesemia
    (c) Hyperkalemia
    (d) Hyperuricemia

18. Potassium sparing diuretics acts on: *(Recent NEET Pattern Question)*
    (a) $Na^+ K^+$ pump
    (b) Aldosterone receptor
    (c) Carbonic anhydrase
    (d) $Na^+ Cl^-$ symporter

19. Drug causing deafness is: *(Recent NEET Pattern Question)*
    (a) Thiazide
    (b) Spiranolactone
    (c) Ethacrynic acid
    (d) Triamterene

20. Drug that can be used for producing alkalinization of urine is: *(Recent NEET Pattern Question)*
    (a) Hydrochlorthiazide
    (b) Furesemide
    (c) Acetazolamide
    (d) Spironolactone

21. Which of the following is aldosterone antagonist? *(Recent NEET Pattern Question)*
    (a) Eplerenone
    (b) Deoxycorticosterone
    (c) Fenoldopam
    (d) Furosemide

22. In a patient on cisplatin therapy, which of the following diuretics would be preferred?
    (Recent NEET Pattern Question)
    (a) Mannitol (b) Acetazolamide
    (c) Thiazide (d) Furosemide

23. Triamterene causes: *(Recent NEET Pattern Question)*
    (a) Hypokalemia (b) Muscle cramps
    (c) Decrease in urea level (d) Better glucose tolerance

24. Acetazolamide side effects include all *except*:
    (Recent NEET Pattern Question)
    (a) Hypokalemia (b) Drowsiness
    (c) Diarrhea (d) Paraesthesia

25. Canrenone is a metabolite of:
    (Recent NEET Pattern Question)
    (a) Ampicillin (b) Spironolactone
    (c) Furosemide (d) Acetazolamide

26. Acetazolamide can be used in all *except*:
    (Recent NEET Pattern Question)
    (a) Epilepsy
    (b) Acute mountain sickness
    (c) Cirrhosis
    (d) Glaucoma

27. Furosemide causes all *except*:
    (Recent NEET Pattern Question)
    (a) Hyperglycemia (b) Hypomagnesemia
    (c) Hypokalemia (d) Acidosis

28. Spirolactone is contraindicated with enalapril because it causes: *(Recent NEET Pattern Question)*
    (a) Hyperkalemia (b) Hypercalcemia
    (c) Hypernatremia (d) Hypokalemia

29. Loop diuretics acts on: *(Recent NEET Pattern Question)*
    (a) PCT
    (b) DCT
    (c) Thick ascending limb of loop of Henle
    (d) Collecting duct

30. Which of the following diuretics is contraindicated in the presence of cardiac failure?
    (Recent NEET Pattern Question)
    (a) Mannitol (b) Spironolactone
    (c) Furosemide (d) Hydrochlorthiazide

31. Thiazide diuretics do not produce ONE of the adverse effects: *(Recent NEET Pattern Question)*
    (a) Hypoglycemia (b) Hyponatremia
    (c) Hypokalemia (d) Hyperuricemia

32. Loop diuretics such as furosemide act by:
    (Recent NEET Pattern Question)
    (a) Decreasing tubular reabsorption of Na^+ and increase GFR
    (b) Decreasing H^+ secretion with resultant increase in Na^+ and K^+ excretion
    (c) Inhibiting Na^+-K^+-$2Cl^-$ cotransporter in the medullary thick ascending limb
    (d) Inhibiting Na^+-K^+ exchange in the collecting duct

33. Side effects of thiazides may include:
    (Recent NEET Pattern Question)
    (a) Hypokalemia (b) Hyperuricemia
    (c) Hyperglycemia (d) All of above

34. Furosemide is useful in: *(Recent NEET Pattern Question)*
    (a) Hypertension (b) Refractory oedema
    (c) Hypocalcemia (d) Hypokalemia

35. Thiazide can cause: *(Recent NEET Pattern Question)*
    (a) Metabolic alkalosis
    (b) Metabolic acidosis
    (c) Respiratory alkalosis
    (d) Respiratory acidosis

36. Side effect of thiazide diuretics are all *except*:
    (Recent NEET Pattern Question)
    (a) Hyponatremia (b) Hypokalemia
    (c) Erectile dysfunction (d) Hypocalcemia

37. True regarding acetazolamide is:
    (Recent NEET Pattern Question)
    (a) Irreversible inhibitor of carbonic anhydrase
    (b) Structural resemblance to sulfonamides
    (c) It decreases potassium excretion
    (d) It cause metabolic alkalosis

38. All of the following adverse effects can be caused by loop diuretics *except*: *(Recent NEET Pattern Question)*
    (a) Hypercalcemia (b) Hyperglycemia
    (c) Hypomagnesemia (d) Hyperuricemia

39. All of the following diuretics cause increase in K^+ excretion *except*: *(Recent NEET Pattern Question)*
    (a) Ethacrynic acid (b) Acetazolamide
    (c) Frusemide (d) Triamterene

40. High ceiling diuretics are useful in the treatment of all of the following conditions *except*:
    (a) Generalized edema *(Recent NEET Pattern Question)*
    (b) Cerebral edema
    (c) Acute pulmonary edema
    (d) Pulmonary hypertension

41. Which one of the following is not a clinical use of spironolactone? *(Recent NEET Pattern Question)*
    (a) Pulmonary edema
    (b) Hypertension
    (c) Congestive heart failure
    (d) To counteract hypokalemia due to thiazide diuretics

42. All of the following are potassium sparing diuretics *except*: *(Recent NEET Pattern Question)*
    (a) Triamterene (b) Spironolactone
    (c) Amiloride (d) Indapamide

43. Site of action of ADH is: *(Recent NEET Pattern Question)*
    (a) PCT (b) DCT
    (c) Collecting tubule (d) Ascending loop

44. Hypercalcemia is caused by which drug?
    (Recent NEET Pattern Question)
    (a) Bumetanide (b) Spironolactone
    (c) Thiazide (d) Furosemide

45. Diuretics that can be used in renal failure is:
    (Recent NEET Pattern Question)
    (a) Furosemide (b) Chlorthiazide
    (c) Mannitol (d) Chlorthalidone

ANTIDIURETICS

46. Tolvaptan is used for: *(NEET Pattern Question 2019)*
    (a) SIADH
    (b) Central DI
    (c) Von Willebrand disease
    (d) Catecholamine resistant shock

47. Treatment of choice for SIADH is:
    (Recent NEET Pattern Question)
    (a) Lithium carbonate (b) Demeclocycline
    (c) Vasopressin (d) Hypertonic saline

48. Vasopressin antagonist acts on: *(AIIMS May, 2013)*
    (a) Proximal convoluted tubule
    (b) Distal convoluted tubule
    (c) Cortical collecting tubule
    (d) Medullary collecting duct

49. Drug used in mild hemophilia is:
    (Recent NEET Pattern Question)
    (a) Corticosteroids (b) DDAVP
    (c) Vitamin K (d) Tranexamic acid

50. All of the following drugs can be used for diabetes insipidus, *except*:
    (Recent NEET Pattern Question)
    (a) Amiloride (b) Furosemide
    (c) Chlorpropamide (d) Carbamazapine

51. Drug causing gynecomastia is:
    (Recent NEET Pattern Question)
    (a) Spironolactone (b) Rifampicin
    (c) Penicillin (d) Bumetanide

52. Which of the following agents will not cause rise in K^+ levels in chronic renal failure?
    (Recent NEET Pattern Question)
    (a) Furosemide (b) Beta blockers
    (c) ACE inhibitors (d) Losartan

53. True regarding conivaptan is:
    (Recent NEET Pattern Question)
    (a) Vasopressin antagonist
    (b) V_2 selective action
    (c) Given orally
    (d) Used in the treatment of hypernatremia

54. In diabetes insipidus, diuretic showing paradoxical antidiuretic activity is: *(Recent NEET Pattern Question)*
    (a) Thiazide (b) Triamterene
    (c) Spironolactone (d) Furosemide

55. Desmopressin is preferred over vasopressin because desmopressin has all the properties *except*:
    (Recent NEET Pattern Question)
    (a) More potent
    (b) More selective for V_1 receptor
    (c) Has little vasoconstrictor activity
    (d) Longer acting

56. Site of action of anti diuretic hormone is:
    (Recent NEET Pattern Question)
    (a) Loop of Henle (b) Proximal tubule
    (c) Distal tubule (d) Cortical collecting duct

57. Drug of choice for neurogenic diabetes insipidus is:
    (Recent NEET Pattern Question)
    (a) Vasopressin (b) Terlipressin
    (c) Desmopressin (d) Pralipressin

Explanations

1. **Ans. (a) Intravenous digoxin** *(Ref: KDT 8th/e p633-634)*
   - Breathlessness at high altitude is suggestive of mountain sickness. This occurs due to very low partial pressure of oxygen in the environment at high altitudes.
   - Acetazolamide is drug of choice for treatment as well as prophylaxis of mountain sickness
   - Oxygen supplementation will help as there is lesser oxygen in environment.
   - Best treatment of mountain sickness is immediate descent to low altitude.
   - Intravenous digoxin is used in CHF. It has no role in mountain sickness.

2. **Ans. (d) Acetazolamide** *(Ref: KDT 8th/e p633-634)*
   - Acetazolamide is drug of choice for prophylaxis and treatment of acute mountain sickness.
   - For severe cases of pulmonary edema due to high altitude sickness, dexamethasone is indicated.
   - Best treatment of all forms of high altitude sickness problems is to descent down.

3. **Ans. (a) Acute congestive glaucoma**
   (Ref: Goodman and Gilman 13th/e p452)
   - Mannitol is an osmotic diuretic and is used for acute congestive glaucoma

Osmotic Diuretics	
Indications	**Contraindications**
• Cerebral edema • Acute congestive glaucoma • Prevention of cisplatin induced nephrotoxicity • Impending renal failure	• Pulmonary edema • Acute renal failure • Active cerebral bleeding

4. **Ans. (a) Metabolic alkalosis** *(Ref: KDT 8th/e p632)*

5. **Ans. (a) Carbonic anhydrase inhibitor**
   (Ref: KDT's 8th/e p634)

6. **Ans. (a) Thick ascending limb of loop of Henle**
   (Ref: Goodman and Gilman 12th/e p678)
   Furosemide is a loop diuretic and this group of drugs act on thick ascending limb of loop of Henle.

7. **Ans. (b) Hyperlipidemia** *(Ref: KK Sharma 2/e p230-231)*
   Thiazides cause hyperlipidemia as adverse effect and thus cannot be used to treat this condition.
   Indications of thiazides:

Diuretic uses	Non-diuretic uses
Hypertension (First line drugs)	Diabetes insipidus
Congestive heart failure	Idiopathic hypercalciurea with Nephrocalcinosis

8. **Ans. (c) Hydrochlorothiazide**
   (Ref: Katzung 10/e p571; KDT 8/e p632)
   - ACE inhibitors are contraindicated in the presence of hyperkalemia. Aldosterone antagonists (like spironolactone and epleronone) and epithelial sodium channel blockers (like amiloride and triamterene) are potassium sparing diuretics and should not be combined with ACE inhibitors. Thiazides on the other hand cause hypokalemia and can be combined with ACE inhibitors.

9. **Ans. (a) Enalapril** *(Ref: KDT 8/e p635)*
   - Spironolactone is a K^+ sparing diuretic. It should be used cautiously if the patient is receiving K^+ salts or drugs increasing serum K^+ levels.
   - ACE inhibitors can also cause hyperkalemia as an adverse effect. If these are combined with K^+ sparing diuretics, cardiac arrhythmia due to high serum K^+ levels may develop.

10. **Ans. (b) Inhibit prostacyclin synthesis**
    (Ref: Goodman & Gilman 11/e p753)

11. **Ans. (b) Thiazide** *(Ref: KDT 8/e p628)*
    - Thiazide diuretics inhibit Na^+-Cl^- symport at the luminal membrane of DCT.
    - All other options are loop diuretics.

12. **Ans. (a) Acetazolamide is a carbonic anhydrase stimulant**
    (Ref: KDT 8/e p633)
    - Acetazolamide is an inhibitor of the enzyme carbonic anhydrase.

13. **Ans. (c) Chlorthiazide** *(Ref: KDT 8/e p672)*
14. **Ans. (d) Spironolactone** *(Ref: KDT 8/e p634)*
15. **Ans. (c) Spironolactone** *(Ref: KDT 8/e p634)*
16. **Ans. (d) Collecting duct** *(Ref: KDT 8/e p634)*
17. **Ans. (c) Hyperkalemia** *(Ref: KDT 8/e p631)*
18. **Ans. (b) Aldosterone receptor** *(Ref: KDT 8/e p634)*
19. **Ans. (c) Ethacrynic acid** *(Ref: Katzung 11/e p259)*
20. **Ans. (c) Acetazolamide** *(Ref: KDT 8/e p633)*
21. **Ans. (a) Eplerenone** *(Ref: KDT 8/e p635)*
22. **Ans. (a) Mannitol** *(Ref: KDT 8/e p638)*
23. **Ans. (b) Muscle cramps** *(Ref: KDT 8/e p637)*
24. **Ans. (c) Diarrhea** *(Ref: KDT 8/e p634)*
25. **Ans. (b) Spironolactone** *(Ref: KDT 8/e p634)*
26. **Ans. (c) Cirrhosis** *(Ref: KDT 8/e p633, 634)*
27. **Ans. (d) Acidosis** *(Ref: KDT 8/e p627)*
28. **Ans. (a) Hyperkalemia** *(Ref: KDT 8/e p635)*
29. **Ans. (c) Thick ascending limb of loop of Henle**
    (Ref: KDT, 8/e p626)
30. **Ans. (a) Mannitol** *(Ref: KDT 8/e p638)*
31. **Ans. (a) Hypoglycemia** *(Ref: KDT 8/e p631-632)*
32. **Ans. (c) Inhibiting Na^+-K^+-$2Cl^-$ cotransporter in the medullary thick ascending limb** *(Ref: Katzung 11/e p258)*
33. **Ans. (d) All of above** *(Ref: KDT 8/e p631-632)*
34. **Ans. (b) Refractory oedema** *(Ref: KDT 8/e p628)*
35. **Ans. (a) Metabolic alkalosis** *(Ref: KDT 8/e p631)*
36. **Ans. (d) Hypocalcemia** *(Ref: KDT 8/e p628)*

37. **Ans. (b) Structural resemblance to sulfonamides**
 (Ref: KDT 8/e p633-634)
 - Acetazolamide is non-competitive but reversible inhibitor of carbonic anhydrase
 - It is a sulfonamide derivative
 - It causes hypokalemia and metabolic acidosis.

38. **Ans. (a) Hypercalcemia** *(Ref: KDT 8/e p628)*
39. **Ans. (d) Triamterene** *(Ref: KDT 8/e p637)*
40. **Ans. (d) Pulmonary hypertension** *(Ref: KDT 8/e p628)*
41. **Ans. (a) Pulmonary edema** *(Ref: KDT 8/e p634-635)*
42. **Ans. (d) Indapamide** *(Ref: KDT 8/e p625)*
43. **Ans. (c) Collecting tubule** *(Ref: KDT 8/e p639)*
44. **Ans. (c) Thiazide** *(Ref: KDT 8/e p632)*
45. **Ans. (a) Furosemide** *(Ref: KDT 8/e p628)*
46. **Ans. (a) SIADH** *(Ref: Harrison 20/e p302)*
 - Vaptans like tolvaptan are vasopressin receptor antagonists.
 - V_1 receptor antagonists may be useful when total peripheral resistance is increased (e.g. CHF and hypertension) whereas V_2 antagonists may be useful for the treatment of SIADH.
 - **Relcovaptan is selective V_1 antagonist** whereas *lixivaptan, mozavaptan and tolvaptan are V_2 selective antagonists.*
 - *Conivaptan* is V_{1a}/V_2 receptor antagonist used as an aquaretic (increase water excretion without affecting electrolytes like sodium) in CHF.
 - **Conivaptan** is administered by *iv injection* whereas *lixivaptan and tolvaptan* can be given *orally*.

47. **Ans. (d) Hypertonic saline** *(Ref: CMDT 2014/842)*
48. **Ans. (d) Medullary collecting duct**
 (Ref: Goodman and Gilman 12/e p707)
 Vaspressin receptors (V2) are present on principal cells of inner medullary collecting tubule. The antagonist like Conivaptan and Tolvaptan may be used in conditions like SIADH and CHF.

49. **Ans. (b) DDAVP** *(Ref: KDT 8/e p643)*
 - DDAVP is an analogue of ADH. It acts on V_2 receptors to cause increased release of factor VIII and vWF from the endothelium. Due to this property, it can be used for the treatment of mild hemophilia.

50. **Ans. (b) Furosemide** *(Ref: KDT 8/e p644)*
51. **Ans. (a) Spironolactone** *(Ref: KDT 8/e p635)*
 Important drugs causing gynaecomastia are:

D	-	Digitalis
I	-	Isoniazid
S	-	Spironolactone
C	-	Cimetidine (and Ketoconazole)
O	-	Oestrogens (and anti-testosterones)

52. **Ans. (a) Furosemide** *(Ref: KDT, 8/e p632)*
53. **Ans. (a) Vasopressin antagonist** *(Ref: CMDT 7th/e p866)*
54. **Ans. (a) Thiazide** *(Ref: KDT 8/e p644)*
55. **Ans. (b) More selective for V_1 receptor** *(Ref: KDT 8/e p642)*
56. **Ans. (d) Cortical collecting duct** *(Ref: KDT 8/e p639)*
57. **Ans. (c) Desmopressin** *(Ref: KDT 8/e p 643)*

CHAPTER 6

Endocrinology

Hormones are the substances which are produced by specific cells in the body and act away from their site of production. These are produced by endocrine glands (Fig. 6.1).

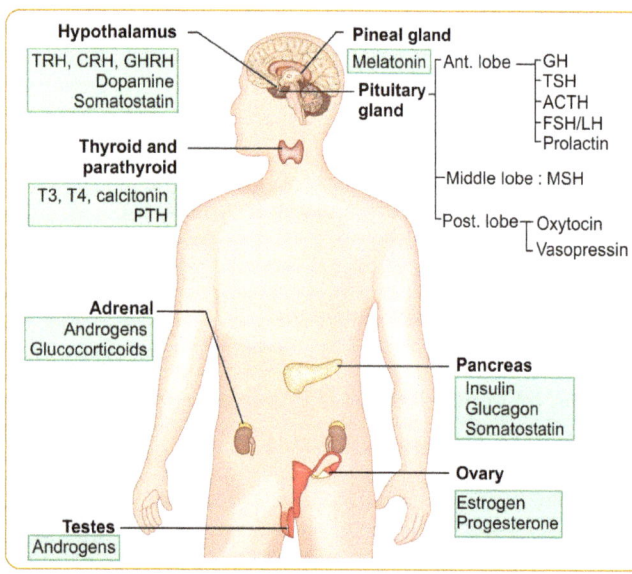

FIG 6.1: Endocrine glands and hormones secreted by them.

MECHANISM OF ACTION OF HORMONES

NUCLEAR RECEPTORS		T_3, T_4, Estrogen, Progesterone, Testosterone
CYTOPLASMIC RECEPTORS		Glucocorticoids Mineralocorticoids
MEMBRANE RECEPTORS		
1. Tyrosine Kinase		Insulin Growth Hormone Prolactin
2. GPCRs	(a) IP_3/DAG/Ca^{2+}	Vasopressin (V_1 receptors) Oxytocin Gonadotropin Releasing Hormone Thyrotropin Releasing Hormone
	(b) K^+ Channel Opening	Somatostatin
	(c) Decrease cAMP	Prolactin Inhibiting Hormone (Dopamine)
	(d) Increase cAMP	Rest all hormones including V_2 receptors of vasopressin

HYPOTHALAMUS AND ANTERIOR PITUITARY HORMONES

Anterior lobe of pituitary secretes several hormones; each of which is under the control of hypothalamus (increases release of all hormones except prolactin).

Gland	Hormones	Controlling Hormones
Anterior pituitary	Growth hormone	GHRH
		Somatostatin (GHIH)
	ACTH	CRH
	TSH	TRH
	FSH/LH	GnRH
	Prolactin	PRIH (Same as dopamine)
Middle lobe	MSH	
Posterior pituitary	Oxytocin Vasopressin	

GROWTH HORMONE (GH) AND GROWTH HORMONE RELEASING HORMONE (GHRH)

GH controls growth of almost all organs of the body except brain and eye. It acts by elaboration of somatomedins, which are also known as insulin like growth factors (IGF-1 and IGF-2). Apart from causing growth, this hormone also increases blood glucose.

- Hypothalamus secretes GHRH (increases GH release) and somatostatin (inhibits GH release).
- Dopamine increases GH release in normal subjects but decreases it in acromegalics. Best response with dopamine agonists is seen in patients secreting both GH and prolactin.
- Excess of GH causes acromegaly and its deficiency results in dwarfism.
- Recombinant growth hormones (**somatrem and somatropin**) are approved for
  - Pituitary dwarfism
  - AIDS related wasting.
  - *Patients with short bowel syndrome who are dependent on total parenteral nutrition.*
- *Fundoscopic examination of children is recommended* at initiation of therapy and at periodic intervals thereafter (because, rarely GH therapy is associated with *intracranial hypertension* with papilledema, visual changes, headache and vomiting).

Somapacitan is a recombinant growth hormone analog. It is used as **once weekly** therapy for GH deficiency by subcutaneous route. All other growth hormone analogs needs to be given daily.

- **Sermorelin and hexarelin** are recombinant GHRH analogs that are used for pituitary dwarfism.
- **Mecasermin rinfabate** is a complex of recombinant human IGF-1 (Insulin-like Growth Factor - 1) and IGF-binding protein-3. It is **indicated for growth failure due to deficiency of IGF-1** that is not responsive to GH. It is administered subcutaneously. IGF-binding protein-3 is needed to maintain adequate half-life of IGF-1. Most important adverse effect of mecasermin is hypoglycemia.

- **Pegvisomant** is a **GH receptor antagonist** indicated for the treatment of acromegaly.

> **MNEMONIC**
>
> Poly Ethylene Glycol (Reduce clearance)
>   VIsual feild defects (adverse effect)
>   SOMatropin (growth hormone)
>   ANTagonist
> **PEGVISOMANT**

SOMATOSTATIN

It is secreted by hypothalamus, GIT as well as by δ-cells of pancreas. It inhibits the secretion of GH, TSH, prolactin, insulin, glucagon, gastrin, and HCl.

- It is indicated for the management of acromegaly, islet cell tumors, bleeding due to esophageal varices and secretory diarrhea but has the disadvantage of short duration of action.
- **Octreotide** is a somatostatin analogue having high potency and *long duration of action*. It is preferred over somatostatin for all the indications.
- Octreotide also inhibits TSH secretion and is the *treatment of choice for TSH-secreting adenoma* in patients who are not the candidates of surgery.
- Lanreotide is another somatostatin analog that can be given i.m. in slow release formulation
- **Vapreotide, pasireotide** and **seglitide** are other somatostatin analogs.

> **MNEMONIC**
>
> Indications of Somatostatin Analogs
> Secretory diarrhea
>   Oesophageal varices
>   Malignancy [Islet cell tumors]
>   Acromegaly
>   TSH-Secreting adenoma
>   Overdose of
>   Sulfonylureas
> **SOMATOStatin**

PROLACTIN

It causes growth and development of breast during pregnancy and induces milk secretion after delivery. It inhibits hypothalamic pituitary-gonadal axis and its excess is responsible for amenorrhea (lactational), inhibition of ovulation and infertility. Excess of this hormone can also cause galactorrhoea in female and infertility in males. Hypothalamus secretes **prolactin release inhibitory hormone (same as dopamine)**. Thus, dopamine agonists like bromocriptine possess inhibitory actions on prolactin and D_2 blockers like antipsychotics and metoclopramide can cause hyperprolactinemia.

- **Bromocriptine** is a dopamine agonist useful in the *treatment of hyperprolactinemia* (amenorrhoea in females, impotence and sterility in males). Although less effective than octreotide, it can also be used in the treatment of *acromegaly*. Other uses of bromocriptine include *Parkinsonism* and *suppression of lactation*. Recently, it has been **approved for treatment of type 2 diabetes mellitus**.
- Nausea, vomiting and postural hypotension are marked at the initiation of therapy with bromocriptine whereas on prolonged use it can result in behavioral alterations, hallucinations and abnormal movements.
- **Cabergoline** is a **longest acting** dopamine agonist (ergot derivative) that is better tolerated than bromocriptine.
- **Quinagolide** is a non-ergot dopamine agonist having less adverse effects.

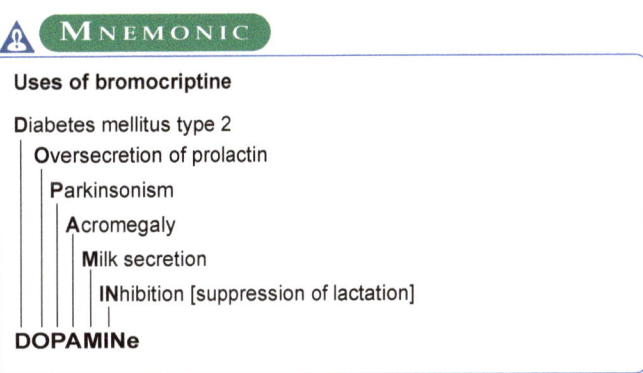

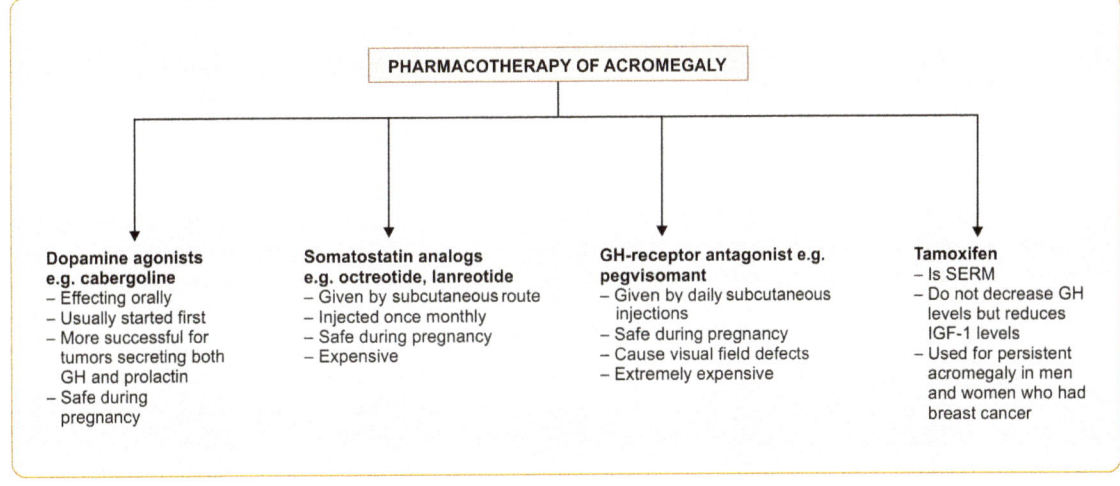

GONADOTROPINS AND GONADOTROPIN RELEASING HORMONE (GNRH)

Follicle stimulating hormone (FSH) and luteinising hormone (LH) are the gonadotropins secreted by anterior lobe of pituitary gland. FSH is involved in spermatogenesis and the secretion of estrogen whereas LH stimulates progesterone and testosterone secretion. *Mid cycle LH surge is responsible for ovulation*. Secretion of these hormones is controlled by GnRH that is secreted from the hypothalamus in a pulsatile manner.

- Deficiency of gonadotropins can lead to anovulatory infertility in females and oligozoospermia and infertility in males (hypogonadotropic hypogonadism). Excessive secretion of these hormones is associated with precocious puberty, endometriosis, prostatic carcinoma, fibroids and polycystic ovarian disease (PCOD).
- Synthetic GnRH (**gonadorelin**) is used *to differentiate between pituitary and hypothalamic defect in patients with hypogonadotropic hypogonadism*. If LH levels increase (> 10 mIU/mL) after administration of GnRH, it indicates that pituitary is normal.

- **GnRH analogues** like *busurelin, goserelin, leuprolide, nafarelin, deslorelin, triptorelin* and *histrelin* are more potent and **longer acting** than natural GnRH. These drugs **stimulate gonadotropin secretion when given in a pulsatile manner whereas inhibit the release on continued administration**. Therefore, these agents can be used in *pulsatile manner* for the treatment of *anovulatory infertility, hypogonadotropic hypogonadism, delayed puberty and cryptorchidism* (these conditions require excess of gonadotropins for treatment). On the other hand, if given *continuously*, reduction in gonadotropin secretion is seen that is beneficial in the conditions like *precocious puberty (drug of choice), endometriosis, prostatic carcinoma, PCOD and uterine fibroids.* Most of these drugs are used by s.c. route whereas *nafarelin* and *busurelin* can be used by nasal route and *goserelin* can be used as *s.c. implant*. Major disadvantage of GnRH analogues is that there is stimulation of gonadotropin release initially (**flare up reaction**) that can be dangerous in conditions like prostatic carcinoma and endometriosis.

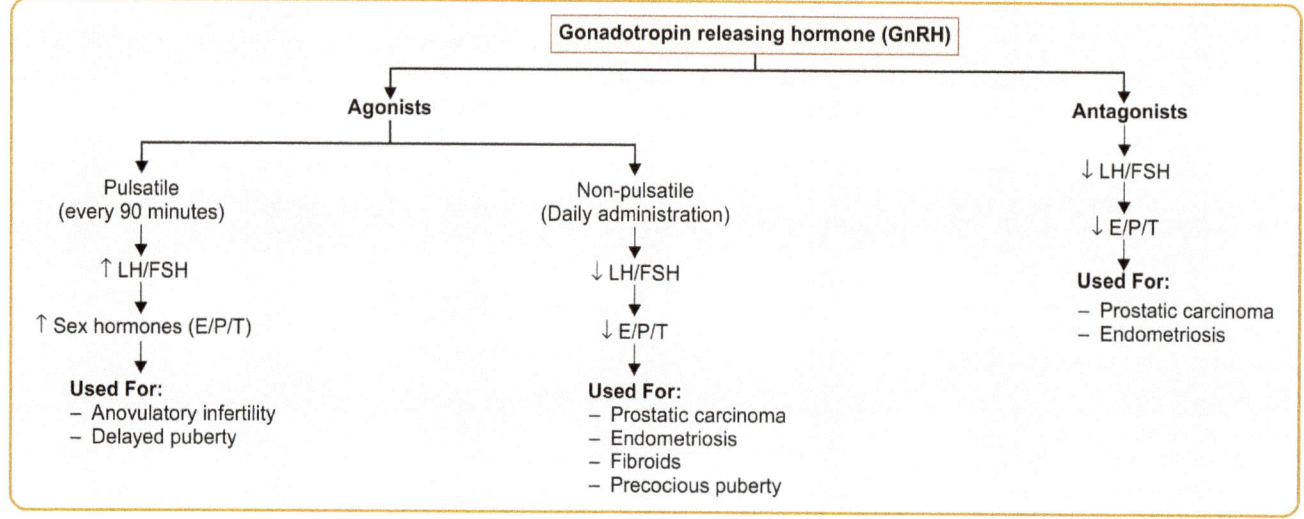

- *Cetrorelix, ganirelix* and *abarelix* are **GnRH antagonists**. These do not cause initial flare up reaction. These are administered subcutaneously for the treatment of uterine fibroids and endometriosis. Another use of these drugs is controlled ovarian stimulation in **in-vitro fertilization**. In this process, recombinant FSH is given to prepare the ova for ovulation induction. Constant monitoring of serum estradiol is done and when sufficient levels are reached, GnRH antagonists are given to prevent premature spontaneous ovulation.
- GnRH agonists as well as antagonists can cause *hot flushes, loss of libido and osteoporosis* as adverse effects.

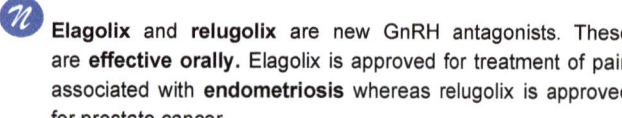 **Elagolix** and **relugolix** are new GnRH antagonists. These are **effective orally**. Elagolix is approved for treatment of pain associated with **endometriosis** whereas relugolix is approved for prostate cancer.

THYROID HORMONES

Thyroid gland contains follicular cells and parafollicular (C) cells. Former secretes thyroid hormones (T_3 and T_4) whereas the latter is responsible for the secretion of calcitonin. Thyroid hormones are synthesized and stored in thyroid follicles in the following manner:

- Iodine is first taken up in the follicular cell with the help of Na^+: I^- symporter (NIS).
- After entry in the follicular cells, iodine is oxidized to form iodinium (I^+) ions. These ions combine with tyrosine residues of thyroglobulin to form mono-iodo tyrosine (MIT) and di-iodo-tyrosine (DIT). This process is known as organification of iodine.
- DIT combines with DIT to form 3, 5, 3', 5' tetra-iodo-thyronine (T_4) and with MIT to form 3, 5, 3' tri-iodo-thyronine (T_3). This process is known as coupling.
- Oxidation, organification and coupling reactions are catalyzed by thyroid peroxidase enzyme.
- After formation, T_3 and T_4 are transported to the follicles where these remain stored as colloid. On stimulation via TSH, these hormones are released in the circulation.
- In the liver and kidney, T_4 is converted to T_3 (peripheral conversion) with the help of 5'-deiodinase and taken up by target tissues *(brain and pituitary take up T_4 and conversion to T_3 takes place in their own cells)*. If 5-deiodinase acts in place

of 5'-deiodinase, reverse T_3 (3, 3', 5'-tri-iodo-thyronine) is formed which is inactive.

Liothyronine (T_3)	l-Thyroxine (T_4)
More potent and more active thyroid hormone.	Less potent but main circulating thyroid hormone.
Short acting, therefore beneficial in emergency situations like myxedema coma.	Long acting, therefore preferred for long term use in hypothyroidism.

Indications

Main indication of thyroid hormones is **hypothyroidism** (cretinism, myxedema and *myxedema coma*). *Levo-thyroxine* (T_4) is *preferred for all these indications* due to its **long half life** and requirement of less frequent dosing. **Myxedema coma** is an emergency situation, in which *liothyronine* (only indication) can also be used (It should be used cautiously in patients with heart diseases like AF).

DRUGS USEFUL FOR HYPERTHYROIDISM

Drugs can inhibit various steps in thyroid hormone synthesis and release **(Fig. 6.2)**.

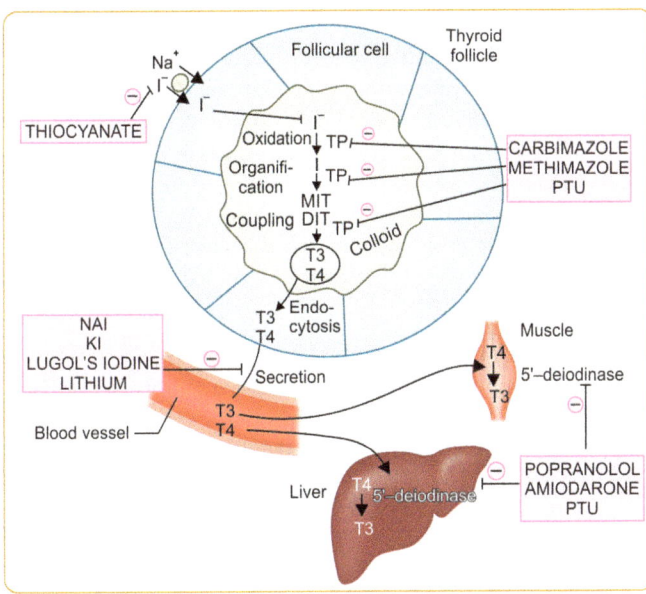

FIG. 6.2: Synthesis and action of thyroid hormones with drug targets

1. Inhibitors of Na⁺–I⁻ Symporter

Iodine is trapped in the follicular cells with $Na^+:I^-$ symporter. **Thiocyanate**, fluoborate, **perchlorate**, pertechtenate and **nitrates** inhibit this transporter and thus thyroid hormone synthesis. These drugs are very toxic and are obsolete now. Thiocyanate is produced by cabbage, cigarette smoking and sodium nitroprusside.

2. Thyroid Peroxidase Inhibitors

Thyroid peroxidase enzyme catalyzes three reactions (oxidation, organification and coupling) in the process of thyroid hormone synthesis. Thioamides like **Carbimazole, methimazole and propylthiouracil** act by inhibiting this enzyme. These drugs inhibit the formation of new thyroid hormones but their action manifests only when already stored pool of T_3 and T_4 is utilized. Thus, a lag period of 1-3 weeks is present. These drugs can rarely cause **reversible agranulocytosis** (most serious adverse effect) whereas most common adverse effect associated with these drugs is maculopapular pruritic rash. Carbimazole is a prodrug and acts after conversion to methimazole.

> **Key Points**
>
> Propylthiouracil is drug of choice for hyperthyroidism in first trimester of pregnancy and in lactation. For all other patients, methimazole is preferred.

	Carbimazole Methimazole	PTU
Potency	High	Low
Plasma $t_{1/2}$	More	Less
Frequency of dosing	Once a day	Thrice a day
Plasma protein binding	Low	High
Transfer across placenta	High	Low
Peripheral conversion	No effect	Inhibits
Hepatotoxicity	Absent	Present

Uses

- Thyroid peroxidase inhibitors are used for the control of thyrotoxicosis in patients with Graves' disease and toxic nodular goiter.
- **Propylthiouracil** is **drug of choice** for hyperthyroidism in **first trimester** of pregnancy and **lactation**. For all other patients, methimazole is preferred.
- These are also used in young patients before performing thyroidectomy.
- Another use of antithyroid drugs is to make the patient euthyroid before application of radioactive iodine.

3. Inhibitors of Thyroid Hormone Release

Sodium iodide, potassium iodide and Lugol's solution (5% iodine in 10% KI) act as **'thyroid constipating agents'** by inhibiting the release of T_3 and T_4. These drugs are the **fastest acting antithyroid drugs**. These agents make thyroid gland *shrink* in size and *decrease its vascularity*. These properties are utilized in preoperative preparation of thyroid gland. Thyroid storm is another indication of these drugs. **Iodine is also used as an antiseptic and expectorant**. Lithium can cause hypothyroidism by inhibiting the release of thyroid hormones.

In sensitive individuals, acute reaction consisting of swelling of lips, angioedema, fever, joint pain and petechial hemorrhages can occur. Chronic overdose of iodides is called **iodism**. Major symptoms are inflamed mucus membranes, increase in secretions (salivation, lacrimation and rhinorrhoea), headache, rashes and gastrointestinal distress. These drugs may also cause *flaring up of acne* in adolescents.

4. Drugs Causing the Destruction of Thyroid Gland

I^{131} **is** the most commonly used radioactive iodine with a **half-life of 8 DAYS** (stable isotope of iodine is I^{127}). When administered (as sodium salts, orally), these are actively taken up by the thyroid gland and stored in the colloid. Here, it emits X-rays and β-particles. Latter can penetrate only 0.5-2 mm of tissue and destroy the gland from within. Concentration of radioactive iodine by the thyroid gland is responsible for its *selective thyroid destroying effect*. I^{131} can be used for the treatment of hyperthyroidism but response is slow (*maximum response may take 3 months*). Thyroid peroxidase inhibitors are administered to make the patient euthyroid. After a gap of 5 days (after stopping anti-thyroid drugs), radioactive iodine is given and thyroid peroxidase inhibitor treatment is resumed till the effect of I^{131} starts. Radioactive iodine therapy is primarily indicated for **patients older than 35 years, those with heart disease** and in the presence of other contraindications of surgery. These drugs **are not suitable for young children and in the pregnancy**. Another disadvantage of radioactive iodine is that if **hypothyroidism** develops, it is **permanent** (requiring life long T_4 therapy). *Coexisting ophthalmopathy* is a *relative contraindication*.

5. Drugs Inhibiting the Peripheral Conversion of T_4 to T_3

Propranolol and propylthiouracil inhibits the generation of more active T_3 from T_4 by inhibiting 5'-deiodinase. These drugs therefore, can be used in the treatment of hyperthyroidism. **Amiodarone** also inhibit this enzyme and thus can result in hypothyroidism.

6. Adjuvant Drugs

- **β-blockers** (propranolol, esmolol, atenolol) antagonize the sympathetic effects of thyrotoxicosis like tremors, tachycardia, palpitations and anxiety.
- Calcium channel blockers like **diltiazem** can also be used for this purpose.
- Steroids (IV methylprednisolone) are used for Graves's ophthalmopathy. Latter can be aggravated by I^{131} and thiazolidinediones (like pioglitazone and rosiglitazone).

Note
1. Beta blockers are drug of choice for thyroid storm.
2. PTU is anti-thyroid drug of choice for thyroid storm

INSULIN AND ORAL HYPOGLYCEMIC AGENTS

Diabetes mellitus (DM) is diagnosed when:
- Fasting blood glucose exceeds 126 mg/dL or
- Postprandial glucose > 200 mg/dL or
- HbA_{1c} > 6.5 g%.

Type I DM (IDDM) is treated only by insulin whereas in the treatment of type II DM (NIDDM), orally active drugs are tried first in uncomplicated cases.

INSULIN

It was discovered by Banting and Best in 1921. It consists of 51 amino acids arranged in two chains; A (21 amino acids) and B (30 amino acids).

SECRETION OF INSULIN

Glucose is the main stimulus for release of insulin. It enters beta cells via GLUT-2. Within beta cells, glucose is metabolized and generates ATP that inhibits ATP sensitive K channels. As K^+ is not able to go out, beta cells get slightly depolarized. This triggers opening of Ca^{2+} channels resulting in secretion of insulin (Fig. 6.3).

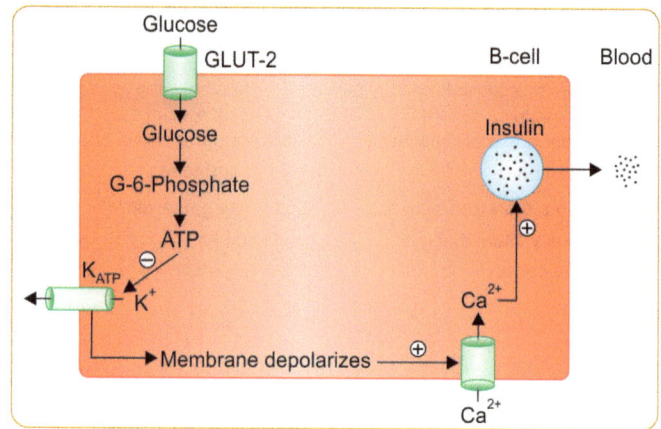

FIG. 6.3: Secretion of insulin

- **Somatostatin** and **$α_2$ agonists** *inhibit* the release of insulin whereas **glucagon, vagus** and **$β_2$ receptor** activation *stimulates* the release of insulin.

Actions

1. It decreases blood glucose by
   - Stimulating the entry of glucose in muscle and fat (by increasing the synthesis of GLUT 4).
   - Inhibiting glycogenolysis (by inhibiting phosphorylase) and gluconeogenesis (by inhibiting phosphoenol pyruvate carboxykinase). These processes are inhibited at lower concentration of insulin.
   - Increasing glycolysis (by stimulation of glucokinase) and glycogenesis (by stimulating glycogen synthase). These require more concentration of insulin.
2. It inhibits lipolysis and thus favors triglyceride deposition.
3. It increases the synthesis and inhibits the breakdown of proteins.

Preparations

Conventional preparations are obtained from pork and beef. Addition of zinc makes it long acting.

Insulin	Type		
	Onset	Duration	Comment
Rapid Acting			
Lispro	15-20 min	3-4 hours	Present as monomers
Apart	15-20 min	3-4 hours	Most rapidly acting
Glulisine	15-20 min	3-4 hours	
Short Acting			
Regular	30-60 min	5-8 hours	Regular insulin can be given IV
Semi-Lente	1-2 hours	8-12 hours	
Intermediate Acting			
NPH or Isophane	2 hours	16-18 hours	
Lente (30% amorphous + 70% crystalline)	2 hours	16-20 hours	
Long Acting			
Ultra–Lente	4-6 hours	20-36 hours	
Glargine	4-6 hours	15-24 hours	Supplied at pH = 4
Detemir	2-4 hours	20-24 hours	
Degludec	2-4 hours	24-40 hours	

Endocrinology

> **Note**
> - All insulin preparations are supplied at neutral pH (7.2.-7.4) except glargine (supplied at pH 4.0). Therefore, glargine cannot be mixed with any insulin.
> - If regular insulin is mixed with lente or ultralente insulin, it can loose its rapidity of action.

Routes of administration

- All preparations can be given by subcutaneous route on abdomen (except 2 inches around umbilicus), thigh, buttocks, or dorsal arms **(Fig. 6.4)**.
- Only regular (crystalline zinc) insulin can be given IV
- Inhalational insulin (exubera) had lead to lung cancers and fibrosis. In june 2014, a new inhalational insulin (Afrezza) was approved by FDA for type-1 DM. It should not be used in patients with chronic lung diseases like asthma.

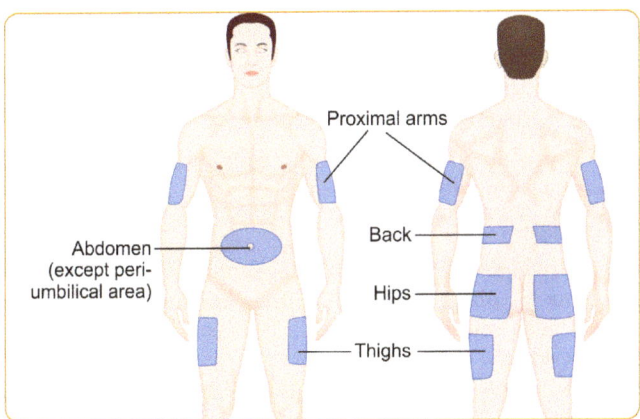

FIG. 6.4: Insulin injection sites

Factors affecting insulin absorption

- *Site* of injection (most rapid from abdomen followed by arm, buttock and thigh).
- *Type* of insulin (Fast with regular, aspart, lispro and glulisine)
- Subcutaneous *blood flow* (rate increases with massage, hot bath or exercise).
- *Depth* of injection (faster with IM than with SC route)

Complications of insulin therapy

- *Most common complication is hypoglycemia* that can be treated by glucose (oral or IV) or glucagon (IV).
- *Lipodystrophy* at the injection site can occur with conventional preparations and the chances are less with highly purified and recombinant forms of insulin.
- Allergic reactions like lipoatrophy can occur with conventional preparations.
- Sodium and water retention leading to edema has been rarely reported.

Drug interactions

- Use of **non-selective beta blockers** in patient on insulin therapy **delays the recovery from hypoglycemia** (less chances with cardioselective beta blockers). These drugs may also *mask the warning signs of hypoglycemia i.e. palpitations, tremors and anxiety*. All the warning signs may be masked **except sweating** (It is mediated by sympathetic cholinergic fibres and not by beta receptors)
- Acute consumption of **alcohol** can precipitate **hypoglycemia**.
- Drugs elevating blood glucose (diuretics, corticosteroids, oral contraceptives and diazoxide etc.) decrease the effectiveness of insulin.

Indications of insulin therapy

- All cases of IDDM
- NIDDM patients
  - Not controlled on OHA
  - In pregnancy
  - In complications like diabetic ketoacidosis and hyperosmolar coma (regular insulin IV is preferred).
  - To tide over stressful conditions like infections and surgery etc.
- Acute hyperkalemia

ORAL ANTI-HYPERGLYCEMIC AGENTS

These drugs may be classified into two groups based on the mechanism of action.

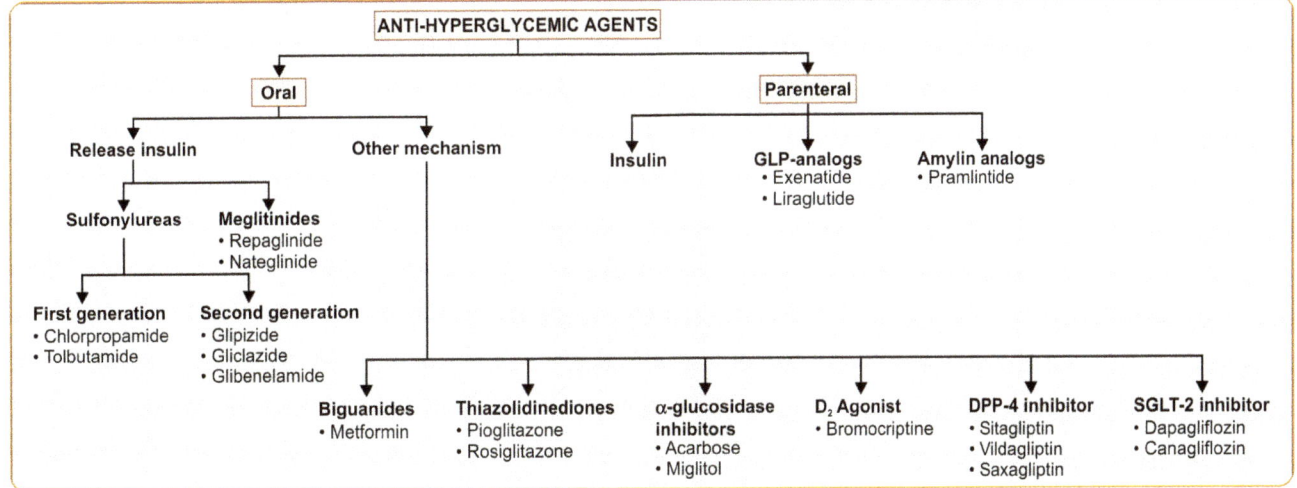

1. Drugs Acting by the Release of Insulin [Insulin Secretagogues]

This group includes sulfonylureas and meglitinides. These drugs **inhibit ATP sensitive K⁺ channels** and cause depolarization of β cells resulting in the release of insulin. These drugs are **effective only if 30% or more of the β cells** in the pancreas are available. **Major limitation** of these drugs is that like insulin, these can also cause **hypoglycemia**.

(a) Sulfonylureas

These may be first generation or second generation:

First Generation	Second Generation
• Chlorpropamide	Glibenclamide
• Tolbutamide	Glipizide
• Tolazamide	Gliclazide
• Acetohexamide	Glimepiride

- *Tolbutamide is the shortest acting whereas chlorpropamide is the longest acting sulfonylurea.*
- *Second generation drugs are more potent than the first generation agents.*
- Sulfonylureas can cause weight gain.
- All these drugs can cause **hypoglycemia** (*maximum with chlorpropamide*)
- **Chlorpropamide** can cause **dilutional hyponatremia** (ADH like action), **cholestatic jaundice and disulfiram like reaction** (intolerance to alcohol).
- Gliclazide has additional antiplatelet action also.
- *Glimepiride exerts beneficial effects with regard to ischemic preconditioning.*
- *Because of lower potency and shorter duration of action, tolbutamide and glipizide are relatively safe in elderly patients and in renal disease.*

> **Note**
> - **Glyburide (Glibenclamide)** has **maximum insulinotropic potency** whereas tolbutamide has least
> - **Half-life of glyburide** is only *1-2 hours*, but its effects persist beyond 24 hours because
>   – It produces an active metabolite
>   – Apart from binding to sulfonylurea receptor at the membrane, it also **gets sequestered within β-cells** of pancreas (only sulfonylurea with this property)
> - **Glimepiride** decreases blood glucose at **lowest dose** among sulfonylureas.
> - **Mitiglinde** is another sulfonylurea approved in **Japan**

(b) Meglitinides

These drugs have similar mechanism to cause release of insulin. *Nateglinide and repaglinide* are the drugs in this group. These drugs are used for the treatment of post prandial hyperglycemia due to their rapid onset and short duration of action. These drugs can also result in **hypoglycemic episodes and weight gain**.

2. Drugs Acting by other Mechanisms

These drugs do not cause hypoglycemia because these are not increasing serum insulin concentration.

(a) Biguanides

- *Metformin and phenformin* are biguanides and are preferred agents for **obese patients** (as these are weight neutral and may even cause weight loss). These can improve hypertriglyceridemia in obese patients.
- These drugs decrease blood glucose **by activating AMPK** (Adenosine Mono Phosphate-activated protein Kinase) that helps in *decreasing the production* (inhibit gluconeogenesis and glycogenolysis) and *increasing the utilization* (stimulation of glycolysis and tissue uptake of glucose). These drugs also inhibit the intestinal absorption of glucose **(Fig. 6.5)**.

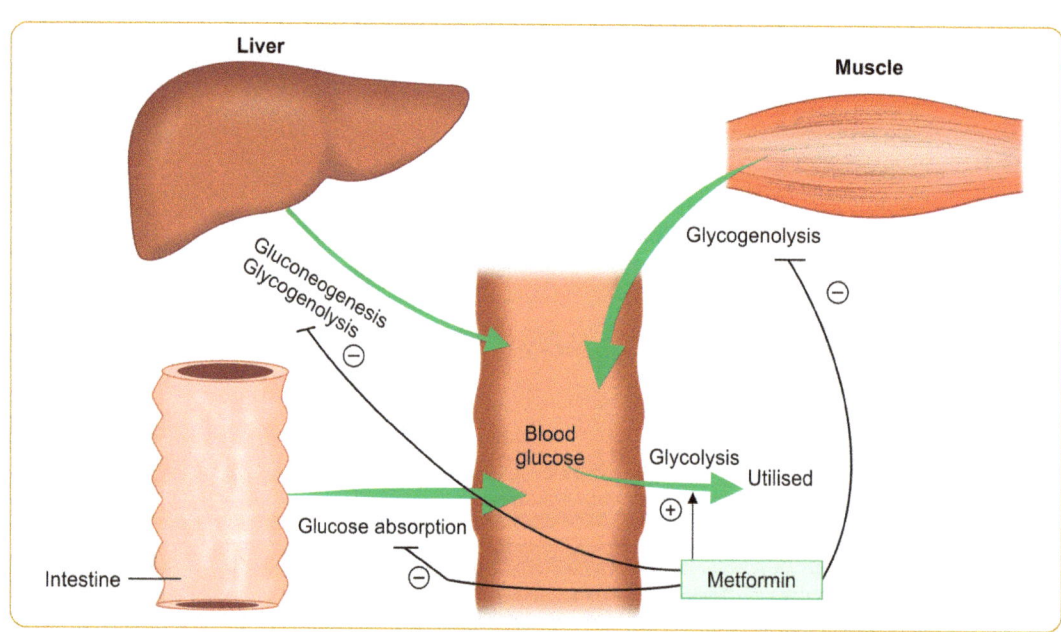

FIG. 6.5: Mechanism of action of metformin

Endocrinology

 Key Points

Recent evidence indicates that metformin reduces hepatic glucose production by antagonizing glucagon's ability to generate cAMP in hepatocytes.

- **Lactic acidosis** (more with phenformin) and **megaloblastic anemia** (more with metformin) due to vitamin B_{12} deficiency are the major adverse effects of these drugs.
- Metformin **interferes with** calcium dependent **absorption of vitamin B_{12}**-intrinsic factor complex in terminal ileum. Long-term use of metformin can result in megaloblastic anemia that may be *prevented by increased in take of dietary calcium*.
- Biguanides increase the intestinal production of lactate by anaerobic glycolysis. In normal individuals, the lactate produced in the intestine is converted to glucose by gluconeogenesis in the liver. Biguanides put patients at risk of lactic acidosis by inhibiting this very same process of gluconeogenesis. **Lactic acidosis** is more likely to occur in the presence of **hepatic and renal impairment or alcohol ingestion**.

Risk factors for lactic acidosis include:
- Elderly
- Renal insufficiency
- Liver disease
- Severe hypoxemia
- Any form of acidosis
- Unstable CHF
- Alcoholic patients

- Other contraindications include **cardiac failure**, and **chronic hypoxic lung disease**.
- Metformin is also useful for **polycystic ovarian disease** (PCOD).
- Metformin is the **only oral agent** that has been demonstrated to **reduce macrovascular events** in type 2 DM.
- Metformin is first-line therapy for type 2 diabetes and cause maximum reduction in HbA1c levels.

MNEMONIC

M	–	**M**etformin preferred in
O	–	**O**bese patients
S	–	**S**ulfonylureas preferred in
T	–	**T**hin Patients

(b) Thiazolidinediones

- Troglitazone, pioglitazone and rosiglitazone are the drugs in this group that act as agonists of a nuclear receptor; peroxisome proliferator activated receptor gamma (PPARγ). It regulates the transcription of genes involved in glucose and lipid metabolism. Important genes that are up regulated by PPAR-γ are:

  - Adiponectin
  - Fatty acid transport protein
  - Insulin receptor substrate
  - GLUT – 4

- These drugs are used to reverse insulin resistance in type II DM. These drugs also tend to increase HDL. *Troglitazone*

was *withdrawn* due to serious *hepatotoxicity* and monitoring of hepatic function is recommended for other glitazones also. Glitazones have been reported to cause *weight gain, edema and plasma volume expansion*. Therefore, these should be avoided in CHF patients. (NYHA class III and IV).
- **Rosiglitazone** *increases total and LDL cholesterol* as well as HDL-cholesterol whereas pioglitazone increases HDL-cholesterol without affecting total and LDL-cholesterol. So, pioglitazone is preferred agent from this group.
- There were concerns of Pioglitazone to be associated with **increased risk of bladder cancer** on long term use. However, long term studies failed to establish this fact.
- **Both of these** can result in:
  - Weight gain
  - Edema
  - New onset or worsening of **macular edema**
  - Increase in fracture risk in women
  - Anemia

 Key Points

Effect of antidiabetic drugs on weight
- **Increase:**
  - Sulfonylureas
  - Insulin
  - Pioglitazone
- **Decrease:**
  - GLP - I agonists
  - Pramlintide
    SGLT2 inhibitors
- **No effect:**
  - DPP-4 inhibitors
  - Metformin

(c) α-Glucosidase inhibitors

- Complex carbohydrates (polysaccharides and sucrose) are absorbed after conversion to simple carbohydrates by α glucosidase.
- Inhibitors of this enzyme (*acarbose, voglibose and miglitol*) decrease carbohydrate absorption from the GIT.
- Major adverse effect of these drugs is *flatulence* due to fermentation of unabsorbed carbohydrates. (therefore, contra-indicated in inflammatory bowel disease)
- These do not cause hypoglycemia. However, if hypoglycemia occurs due to concomitant use of sulfonylureas, simple carbohydrates like glucose (not sucrose or other complex carbohydrates) can be used to reverse it.
- According to some trials, these drugs can help in restoring β-cell function and prevent new cases of type 2 diabetes in pre-diabetics.
- Acarbose can decrease blood glucose in both type 1 as well as type 2 diabetes. However, apart from insulin, **the only drug approved for treatment of both type 1 as well as type 2 diabetes is pramlintide**.
- **Acarbose is not absorbed from GIT** whereas miglitol can be absorbed. Therefore, **miglitol is contra-indicated in renal failure**.

NEW DRUGS FOR DIABETES MELLITUS

1. Incretins

Oral glucose provokes 4 times higher insulin release than intravenous glucose. This is because oral glucose releases GLP-1 (Glucagon like peptide-1) from **L-cells of intestine** that amplifies the glucose-induced insulin release **(Fig. 6.6)**. GLP-1 secretion is reduced in patients with type 2 diabetes. Incretins like GLP-1 has little stimulatory effect on insulin secretion at normoglycemic concentration (Unlike sulfonylureas and other insulin secretagogues). Thus, GLP-1 has lower risk of causing hypoglycemia. Apart from releasing insulin, GLP-1 has following actions:

- Suppresses glucagon secretion
- Preserves islet cell integrity and decreases apoptosis.
- Delays gastric emptying resulting in reduced appetite
- Anorectic effect through CNS

The endogenous GLP-1 is rapidly broken by dipeptidyl peptidase-4 and thus has a half-life of 1-2 minutes only. The two strategies by which incretin effect can be strengthened are:

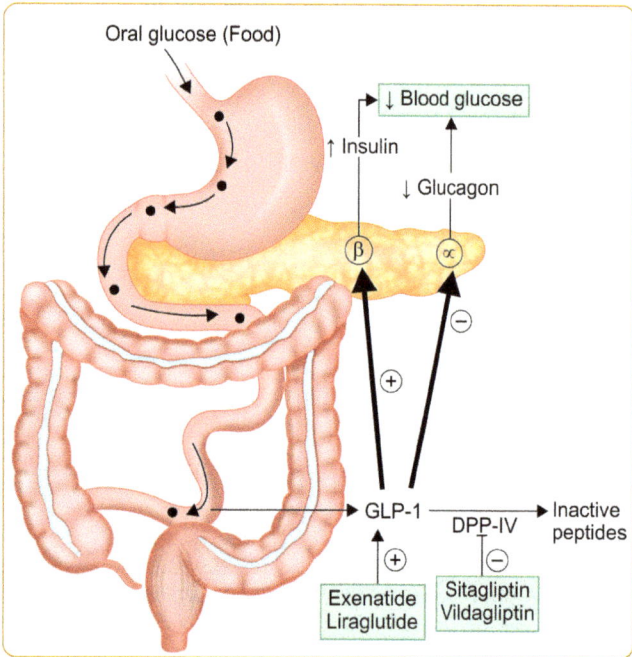

FIG. 6.6: Incretin-mimetic drugs

GLP-1 Receptor Agonists:
Exenatide and liraglutide are GLP-1 receptor agonists. These are administered *subcutaneously* and act by mechansm similar to GLP-1 (as discussed above): New drugs of this category, recently approved are **albiglutide, semaglutide** and **dulaglutide.** These are very long acting drugs that can be given **once weekly**.
Lixisenatide is another GLP-1 agonist which can be given once daily.

- These drugs can promote **weight loss**.
- Most common adverse effect of these drugs is **nausea followed by vomiting**. **Albiglutide has lowest risk** of these.
- These can also result in **acute pancreatitis**
- These are contra-indicated in patients with personal or family history of **medullary thyroid cancer or MEN-2.**
- **Liraglutide** is **longer acting** (once daily) as compared to exenatide (twice daily)
- Liraglutide does not require dose adjustment in renal failure whereas exenatide dose should be reduced.
- Recently, **liraglutide** has been approved for **management of obesity.**
- **Semaglutide** has been approved as an **oral preparation** for type 2 diabetes mellitus

Teduglutide is a long-acting **GLP-2 analogue**. It works by promoting mucosal growth and possibly restoring gastric emptying and secretions. It is indicated for **short bowel syndrome**. It is resistant to DPP-4 and is given by SC route.

DPP-4 Inhibitors:
Sitagliptin, vildagliptin, saxagliptin, alogliptin and linagliptin prolong the action of endogenous GLP-1 by inhibiting its metabolism through DPP-4:

- Unlike incretin-mimetic drugs, these *do not cause nausea or weight loss.*
- **Most common** adverse effect of DPP-4 inhibitors is **nasopharyngitis** and upper respiratory tract infections. These drugs are also associated with **acute pancreatitis**.
    - DPP-4 inhibitors are **effective orally**.
    - These drugs require dose adjustment in renal failure except **linagliptin.**
    - *Vildagliptin can cause hepatitis* and requires dose adjustment in both renal as well as hepatic disease.
    - **Linagliptin and saxagliptin** increase the risk of *heart failure*

2. Sodium Glucose Co-transporter-2 Inhibitors
Glucose is freely filtered across glomerulus and is reabsorbed in proximal tubules by sodium glucose co-transporter-2 [SGLT-2]. **Dapagliflozin, empagliflozin, ertugliflozin and canagliflozin** act by inhibiting this transporter and cause glucosuria in diabetics **(Fig. 6.7)**. These also result in weight loss. These are effective orally.

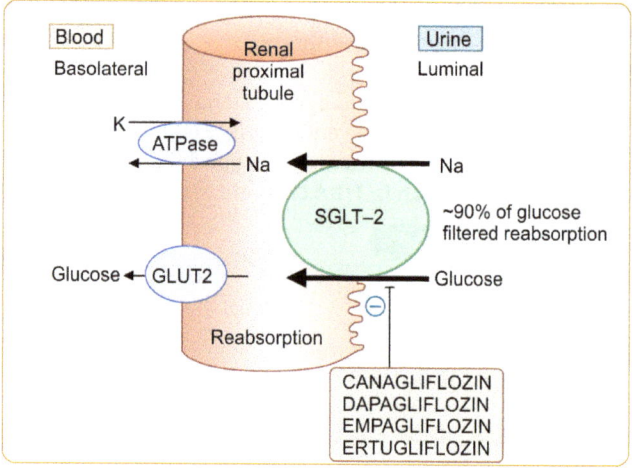

FIG. 6.7: Mechanism of action of SGLT-2 inhibitors

- Efficacy of these drugs is reduced in renal failure.
- Main adverse effects are **increased incidence of urinary tract infections** and genital infections.
- SGLT-2 inhibitors cause decrease in bone mineral density and **increase risk of fractures**
- **Empagliflozin** has been found to *decrease the risk of mortality from cardiovascular causes* in diabetic patients.

3. Amylin Analogs
Pramlintide is a synthetic analog of islet amyloid polypeptide (IAPP) also called amylin. It acts by:

- Decreasing glucagon secretion
- Delaying gastric emptying
- Decreasing appetite

Important points about pramlintide are:

> - It is administered by **subcutaneous** route.
> - It can cause **weight loss**
> - It is **approved for treatment of type 2 as well as type 1 diabetes mellitus** (only drug apart from insulin)
> - It **can cause hypoglycemia**.

4. Bile Acid Binding Resins

Bile acid metabolism is abnormal in patients with type 2 diabetes mellitus and bile acid binding agents have been found to lower blood glucose in these patients. Colesevalam is specifically approved for type 2 diabetes. These drugs can result in hypertriglyceridemia.

5. Bromocriptine

Recently, FDA has approved bromocriptine mesylate as an adjunct to diet and exercise to improve glycemic control in type -2 diabetes. It has been found that dopamine alter insulin resistance by acting on hypothalmus and bromocriptine targets D_2 receptors.

> **Key Points**
>
> Studies in migratory birds revealed that they develop insulin resistance during hibernation stage characterized by increased lipolytic activity, increased hepatic glucose production and gluconeogenesis. Circadian neuroendocrine rhythms may play a vital role in this process. In humans with diabetes mellitus, similar changes have been noted, characterized by early morning decrease in dopaminergic activity and excessive sympathetic activity. **Bromocriptine** acts as a central sympatholytic agent. When given **within 2 hours of awakening**, it augments hypothalamic dopamine levels and inhibits excessive sympathetic activity within CNS. This has been shown to reverse insulin resistance. Bromocriptine has been approved for type 2 diabetes mellitus. It is used in much lesser doses than in Parkinsonism and apart from nausea, it is well tolerated.

GLUCAGON

Glucagon is secreted by **α-cells** of pancreas. It primarily increases blood sugar by promoting glycogenolysis. It is thus indicated for treatment of hypoglycemia. However, glucagon is **ineffective** (for hypoglycemia) in conditions where glycogenolysis is not possible like **in starvation** and hypoglycemia due to **alcoholism**.

- Glucagon is also DOC for treatment of **beta blocker poisoning**. In beta blocker overdose, there is decrease in heart rate and cardiac output due to blockade of cardiac β1 receptors. All drugs acting through β1 (like adrenaline, noradrenaline, dopamine, dobutamine etc.) are likely to be ineffective because β1 receptors are already blocked. Normally, β1 acts via increasing cAMP in heart. When glucagon is administered from outside, it stimulates glucagon receptors present in heart and increase cAMP. It, thus stimulates the heart and reverse β-blocker poisoning.

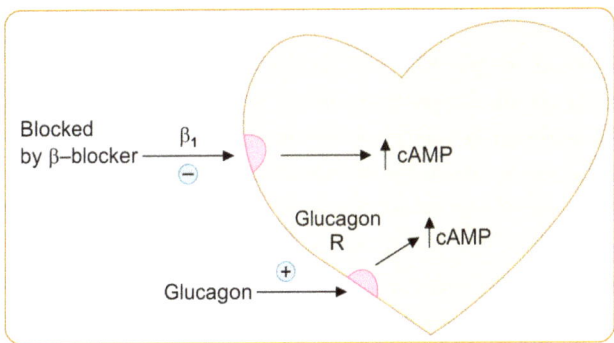

- **Dasiglucagon:** It is an analog of human glucagon and acts by stimulating glucagon receptors. It is approved for treatment of severe **hypoglycemia in diabetic patients**. It is administered by **subcutaneous route**.

CORTICOSTEROIDS

Adrenal cortex consists of three layers; *zona glomerulosa, zona fasciculata and zona reticularis* from outside to within respectively (remembered as GFR). *Mineralocorticoids* are *secreted from zona glomerulosa* whereas inner layers secrete glucocorticoids and sex steroids. Corticosteroids are synthesized from cholesterol. Glucocorticoid secretion is maximum in the early morning.

ACTIONS

Mineralocorticoids

Major endogenous mineralocorticoid is **aldosterone**.

- It acts in DCT of the kidney to cause reabsorption of Na^+ and excretion of K^+ and H^+. Thus, *excess of mineralocorticoids can lead to retention of sodium and water (hypertension and edema), hypokalemia* and *alkalosis* whereas Addison's disease (deficiency of adrenal corticoids) is characterized by hyperkalemia, acidosis and hypotension.
- Aldosterone is also involved **in causing myocardial remodeling** associated with CHF and the drugs blocking this effect [*spironolactone, ACE inhibitors*, angiotensin receptor antagonists (*ARBs*) and β blockers] decrease the mortality in patients with CHF.

Glucocorticoids

Major endogenous glucocorticoid is **hydrocortisone** (cortisol). Many of the effects of glucocorticoids are dose-dependent whereas some are permissive effects (without these, many normal functions become deficient) e.g. response of vascular and bronchial smooth muscle to catecholamines is diminished in the absence of cortisol.

- **Effect on metabolism:** Glucocorticoids are *catabolic* in nature and thus cause breakdown of carbohydrates (hyperglycemia), proteins (muscle wasting) and fat. There is *redistribution of fat*; deposition over face (moon face), mouth (fish mouth) and back (buffalo hump) whereas removal from the extremities is seen. Glucocorticoids cause negative Ca^{2+} balance (by inhibiting intestinal absorption, enhancing renal excretion and causing loss of Ca^{2+} from the bones) and can predispose to osteoporosis.
- **Effect on CVS and CNS:** Glucocorticoids *prevent the increase in the permeability of capillaries*. These have *mild euphoric* effect and high doses can lower seizure threshold.

- **Effect on GIT:** These hormones may *aggravate peptic ulcer* by increasing the secretion of HCl and pepsin in stomach.
- **Effect on hematopoietic system:** Glucocorticoids cause *destruction* of T cells and B cells (less sensitive) in malignancies whereas little effect is exerted on normal cells. These drugs cause *sequestration* of lymphocytes, eosinophils, monocytes and basophils in tissues (and thus decrease circulating levels of these cells) whereas circulating neutrophils are increased due to release from bone marrow.
- **Effect on inflammatory response:** Glucocorticoids are *powerful anti-inflammatory* agents. Most important mechanism is the *inhibition of chemotaxis* (recruitment of the cells at the site of inflammation). These hormones also induce the production of **annexins** (previously called, **lipocortins**) that are responsible for the inhibition of phospholipase A_2 (involved in the production of prostaglandins and leukotrienes). They also delay the healing of wounds and scar formation.
- **Effect on immunity:** These hormones suppress cell mediated immunity (CMI) more than humoral immunity. Main effect is **due to inhibition of recruitment of immune cells**, but they also inhibit the release of IL-1 and IL-2. Antibody production is affected at high doses and continuous administration of glucocorticoids *can result in catabolism of IgG*. Immunosuppressive effect of glucocorticoids is the basis of their use in graft rejection and various hypersensitivity reactions.

Glucocorticoids (G)

Short acting (8–12 hours)
- Hydrocortisone (cortisol) : G with maximum M activity
- Cortisone : Least potent G

Intermediate acting (12–36 hours)
- Prednisone : Prodrug
- Prednisolone
- Meprednisone
- Fluprednisone
- Triamcinolone*
- Methylprednisolone*

Long acting (36–72 hours) :
- Dexamethasone* : Maximum G activity
- Betamethasone* : Maximum G potency
- Paramethasome* :
 :
 :

Mineralocorticoids (M)
- **Aldosterone** : Most potent M
 : Maximum M activity
- **Fludrocortisone** : M with maximum G activity
- **DOCA** : Selective M (Zero G activity)

*Selective G (Zero M activity)

USES OF CORTICOSTEROIDS

1. Replacement Use

(A) *Acute adrenal insufficiency:* It is an emergency condition and requires immediate management with parenteral administration (IV) of hydrocortisone.

(B) *Chronic adrenal insufficiency (Addison's disease):* It is treated with oral doses of **hydrocortisone**. Mineralocorticoids like fludrocortisone may also be required.

(C) *Congenital adrenal hyperplasia (CAH):* This disorder is a result of *congenital deficiency of the enzymes* involved in the synthesis of corticosteroids. Due to decreased adrenal steroids, there is no feedback inhibition of pituitary and consequently ACTH secretion increases. ACTH cannot release corticosteroids (because they are not synthesized) but it results in overgrowth of adrenal glands leading to symptoms. Thus, **treatment** of CAH is **aimed at reducing ACTH secretion**. Exogenous glucocorticoids like hydrocortisone cause feedback inhibition of HPA axis and lead to amelioration of symptoms. **To prevent CAH** (in a pregnant female with history of baby with CAH), **steroids should be administered at 6 weeks period** (i.e. as soon as the pregnancy is diagnosed). The *genotype and sex of the fetus is then determined*. Steroid therapy is stopped if sex is male. If genotyping reveals *female sex*, steroid therapy is *continued till delivery* (to prevent virilization).

2. Diagnostic Use

Dexamethasone suppression test (Fig. 6.8) is used *to test the intactness of HPA axis function* and diagnosis of Cushing's syndrome.
- Dexamethasone (1 mg) is given orally at night (11 PM) and plasma cortisol levels are measured in the morning (8 AM).
- If cortisol levels are less than 3 µg/dL (feedback inhibition is present), it signifies that HPA axis is functioning properly.
- If cortisol in plasma is more than 5 µg/dL (no feedback inhibition), it indicates that there is excessive secretion of cortisol due to adrenal or pituitary tumor (Cushing syndrome).
- Large dose (8 mg) of dexamethasone may be used to differentiate between Cushing's disease (due to pituitary tumor) and other causes (adrenal tumor or ectopic ACTH)

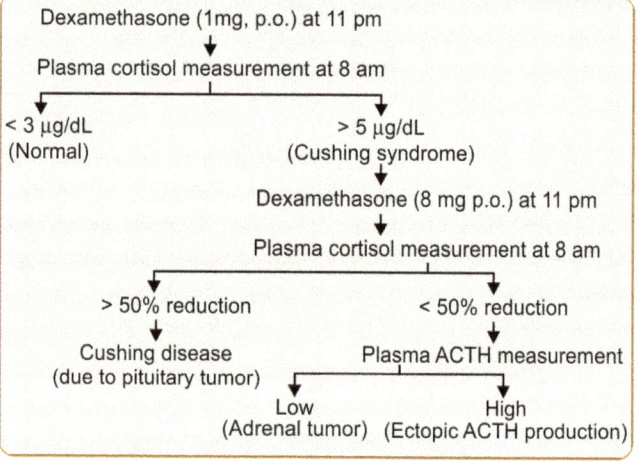

FIG. 6.8: Dexamethasone suppression test

3. Antenatal Use

Betamethasone can be given **to accelerate the fetal lung maturation**, if delivery is anticipated before 32 weeks of gestation. Antenatal steroids may decrease the incidence of respiratory distress syndrome, **PDA, necrotizing enterocolitis** and **periventricular/intraventricular hemorrhage**.

Drug	Route	No. of doses	Interval	Dose	Special points
Dexamethasone	IM	4	12 hourly	6 mg	
Betamethasone acetate-phosphate	IM	2	24 hourly	12 mg	Not available in India

- WHO do not recommend any of the two in preference to other, but mostly betamethasone acetate-phosphate is preferred due to requirement of 2 doses only.
- Betamethasone acetate-phosphate salt is not available in India, so dexamethasone is used.

4. Non-Adrenal Uses

(a) *Anti-inflammatory uses:* Corticosteroids can be useful in rheumatoid arthritis, osteoarthritis (intra-articular) and acute gouty arthritis when NSAIDs fail to provide pain relief. These are also useful in inflammatory conditions of eye like conjunctivitis, iritis, iridocyclitis and keratitis. However, steroids are **contraindicated in herpes simplex keratitis.**

(b) *Anti-allergic uses:* Corticosteroids are useful in the management of anaphylaxis (*DOC is adrenaline*), urticaria, angioedema and serum sickness. These are used by inhalational route in chronic severe asthma and IV (hydrocortisone) route is employed in acute severe asthma (status asthmaticus). Skin conditions like pemphigus vulgaris, exfoliative dermatitis and Steven Johnson syndrome also require systemic steroid therapy.

(c) *Immunosuppressive uses:* High dose corticosteroid therapy is required in the organ transplantation to prevent graft rejection. They are also useful in autoimmune diseases (e.g. myasthenia gravis, hemolytic anemia) and collagen vascular diseases (like SLE, polyarteritis nodosa and nephrotic syndrome). Steroids are also useful in patients with ulcerative colitis and Crohn's disease who are not responding to 5-aminosalicylic acid.

(d) *Anti-cancer uses:* Due to prominent lympholytic action in malignant cells, steroids are essential component of the combination therapy of ALL and lymphomas (both Hodgkin as well as non-Hodgkin). These are also useful in the CLL, multiple myeloma and breast carcinoma. These can also be used with anti-neoplastic agents *to decrease nausea and vomiting*.

(e) *Other uses*

- Steroids with selective glucocorticoid action (without Na⁺ and water retaining activity) like betamethasone and dexamethasone are used *to decrease cerebral edema* due to malignancies or TB.
- Steroids are also useful in severe infective conditions (like TB meningitis and lepra reaction) to tide over the acute crisis. However these are *contra-indicated in intestinal (Ileocaecal) TB* due to the risk of perforation.
- These can be used as a desperate measure in the septicemic shock.
- **Deflazacort** is recently approved for the oral treatment of Duchenne's muscular dystrophy.
- Steroids can also be used for treatment of *sarcoidosis*.
- In *thrombocytopenia*, prednisolone is used to decrease bleeding tendency.
- *Autoimmune hemolytic anemia* is treated with prednisolone.
- Significant decrease in neurological defects have been seen in *spinal cord injury* patients treated with large doses of methylprednisolone (within 8 hours).

POINTS TO REMEMBER FOR SYSTEMIC USE OF STEROIDS

- Long term use (for more than 2 weeks) can lead to HPA axis suppression. Steroids should not be withdrawn abruptly because it may precipitate acute adrenal insufficiency. Many patients recover from *HPA-axis suppression* within several weeks to months but **recovery may take one year or longer in some patients.**
- Large single dose is less harmful than small doses given for long periods. Thus 80 mg prednisolone for 2 days is much less harmful than 20 mg dose for 6 months.
- During condition of stress like infection or trauma, steroid dose should be unchanged or increased (2 to 10 fold). *It should not be reduced.*
- To prevent HPA axis suppression, steroids can be given on alternate days but long acting steroids like betamethasone and dexamethasone cause HPA axis suppression even when administered on alternate days.

ADVERSE EFFECTS AND CONTRAINDICATIONS

- *Hypertension, edema (contra-indicated in CHF and hypertension), alkalosis and hypokalemia* can occur due to mineralocorticoid activity.
- *Cushing's habitus* (characteristic appearance due to redistribution of fat) and *striae* can occur.
- *Hyperglycemia* (C/I in DM), *muscular weakness* and resorption of bones (C/I in *osteoporosis*) can result due to chronic steroid therapy.
- These may cause *posterior subcapsular cataract* (on systemic use) and development of *glaucoma* (topical use) on long term use.
- Due to immunosuppressant action, steroids increase the *susceptibility to infections* and due to anti-inflammatory activity these can *delay wound healing*.
- These are contraindicated in *peptic ulcer disease* because bleeding and perforation can occur.
- Given during pregnancy, steroids can cause fetal abnormalities and given to young children for prolonged periods, these may result in growth retardation.
- Steroids are *contraindicated in psychosis* (due to CNS stimulatory action) *and epilepsy* (due to lowering of seizure threshold).
- *Osteonecrosis* (avascular necrosis), most commonly of hip can occur with high doses of glucocorticoids.

MNEMONIC

Adverse effects and contraindications of steroids:

- G – **G**laucoma (on topical use)
- L – **L**imb muscle atrophy
- U – **U**lcer (peptic ulcer)
- C – **C**ushing syndrome
- O – **O**steoporosis
- C – **C**ataract (on systemic use)
- O – **O**steonecrosis (avascular necrosis)
- R – C/I in **R**enal failure
- T – C/I in **T**uberculosis (particularly ileo-caecal)
- I – **I**mpair healing
- C – C/I in **C**HF
- O – **O**edema
- I – **I**nfections (due to immuno suppressant action)
- D – **D**iabetes mellitus
- S – **S**uppression of HPA-axis

GLUCOCORTICOID SYNTHESIS INHIBITORS

These drugs are useful in the diagnosis of adrenal diseases and in the treatment of Cushing's syndrome.

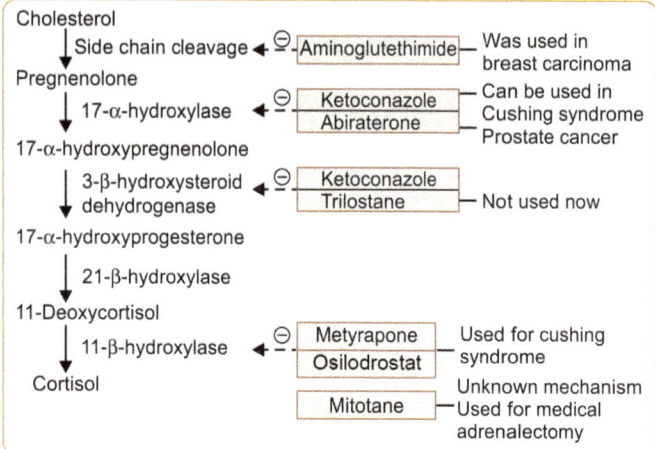

CORTICOSTEROID RECEPTOR ANTAGONISTS

- **Mifepristone** is a long acting *antagonist at the glucocorticoid and progesterone receptors*. It is used for medical termination of pregnancy, as a post-coital contraceptive and rarely for inoperable patients of Cushing's syndrome.
- **Spironolactone and eplerenone** are aldosterone receptor antagonists that are used as K⁺ sparing diuretics.
- **Drospirenone**, a progestin in an oral contraceptive, also antagonizes the effects of aldosterone.
- **Osilodrostat** is a new drug approved for oral treatment of Cushing syndrome. It acts by inhibiting 11-β-hydroxylase and aldosterone synthase.

DRUGS AFFECTING BONE MINERAL HOMEOSTASIS

Calcium and phosphate homeostasis is maintained by the action of vitamin D (active form is **calcitriol**), parathyroid hormone (PTH) and FGF-23 (Fibroblast growth factor-23). Secondary regulators of Ca^{2+} homeostasis include calcitonin, glucocorticoids and estrogens.

	Serum PO_4^{3-}	Serum Ca^{2+}	Mechanism
Vitamin D	↑	↑	↑ Intestinal absorption of both Ca^{2+} and PO_4^{3-} ↓ Renal excretion of both
PTH	↓	↑	↓ Renal excretion of Ca^{2+} and ↑ that of PO_4^{3-} ↑ Resorption of Ca^{2+} from bone ↑ Intestinal absorption of calcium by increasing calcitriol
FGF-23	↓	-	↓ Ca^{2+} and PO_4^{3-} absorption by intestines ↑ PO_4^{3-} excretion by kidneys

Thus **vitamin D and calcitonin can be used to treat osteoporosis whereas PTH excess can result in osteoporosis.**

- *Plasma Ca^{2+} is the major factor regulating PTH secretion.* Hypocalcemia stimulates PTH secretion whereas hypercalcemia inhibits it. Calcium inhibits PTH secretion by stimulating calcium sensing receptor on parathyroid cells.
- *PTH increases circulating calcitriol* by two mechanisms; Directly by stimulating 1α hydroxylase in kidney and indirectly by decreasing serum phosphate.
- Vitamin D_2 is ergocalciferol whereas D_3 is cholecalciferol.
- Vitamin D is converted to 25-OHD (calcifediol) *in the liver* with the help of *25-α-hydroxylase* and then to 1, 25-dihydroxy D_3 (calcitriol) by the action of *1α hydroxylase in kidney*. Calcitriol is inactivated to 1, 24, 25 (OH)₃ D with the help of 24-α-hydroxylase in kidney. **Doxercalciferol and Paricalcitol** have been approved for treatment of secondary hyperparathyroidism in patients with chronic renal disease. These are less likely to cause hypercalcemia than calcitriol.
- Apart from effects on Ca^{2+} and PO_4^{3-}, **calcitriol also affects maturation and differentiation of mononuclear cells** (*possibility of use in cancers*), inhibits epidermal proliferation and promotes epidermal differentiation (*potential treatment of psoriasis vulgaris*). **Topical calcipotriol** (*calcipotriene*) has been **approved for use in psoriasis**. It is slightly more effective than glucocorticoids.
- **Fibroblast growth factor-23** inhibits calcitriol production and phosphate reabsorption in kidney. It is produced by osteoblasts and osteoclasts. Recently, a new drug **burosumab** has been approved for **X-linked hypophosphataemia**. It is a **monoclonal antibody against FGF-23** and thus interferes with phosphaturic action of FGF-23 in kidney. It also decreases the inhibitory effect of FGF-23 on calcitriol production (**Fig. 6.9**).

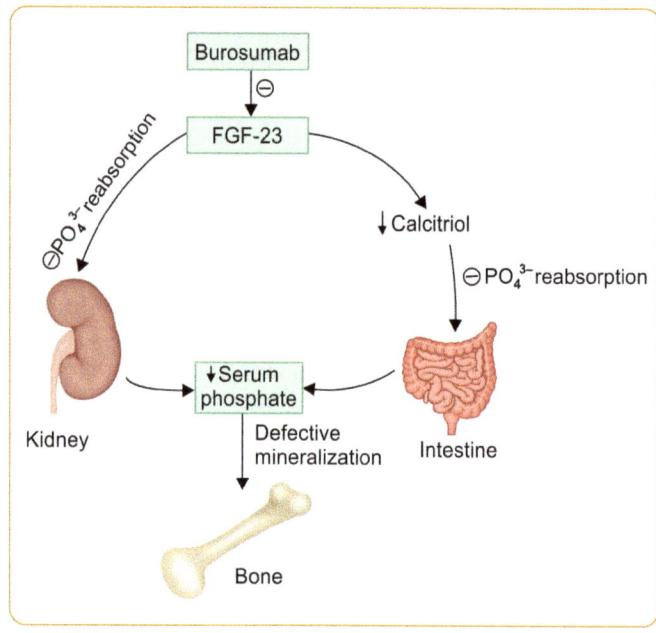

FIG. 6.9: Mechanism of action of burosumab

> Drugs decreasing bone resorption intially increases bone mineral density (BMD), but it reaches a plateu in 2-3 years because bone formation also decreases. On the other hand, drugs promoting bone formation can increase BMD throughout the period of treatment.

Endocrinology

DRUGS USEFUL FOR THE TREATMENT OF OSTEOPOROSIS

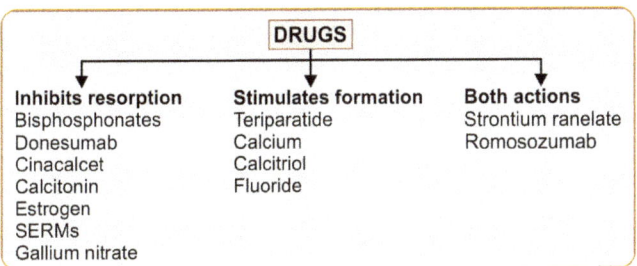

DRUGS

- **Inhibits resorption**: Bisphosphonates, Donesumab, Cinacalcet, Calcitonin, Estrogen, SERMs, Gallium nitrate
- **Stimulates formation**: Teriparatide, Calcium, Calcitriol, Fluoride
- **Both actions**: Strontium ranelate, Romosozumab

> **Note**
> - Main contraindications of bisphosphonates are renal dysfunction, esophageal motility disorders and peptic ulcer.
> - Zoledronate infusion of 5 mg once yearly has been approved for treatment of osteoporosis.

Bisphosphonates

- These agents are used for the treatment of osteoporosis due to their *inhibitory effect on osteoclast mediated bone resorption*. These drugs accelerate **apoptosis of osteoclasts** and also **suppress differentiation of osteoclast precursors to mature osteoclasts** (by inhibiting IL-6). This results due to reduction in cholesterol synthesis via inhibition of farnesyl pyrophosphate synthase by bisphosphonates.
- Drugs in this group include:
  - **First generation** agents (least potent) like *medronate, clodronate and etidronate*,
  - **Second generation** drugs like *alendronate, ibadronate and pamidronate*
  - **Third generation compounds** like *risedronate and zoledronate (most potent)*.
- These are used for the treatment of *post-menopausal and steroid induced osteoporosis, Paget's disease and hypercalcemia of malignancy* (pamidronate and zoledronate by i.v route are preferred).
- Bisphosphonates can also be used in malignancies. **Zoledronate** has been used successfully as an adjunct in treating philadelphia-chromosome positive **CML**.
- Distinctive toxicity of these agents is **esophageal irritation** that can lead to ulceration as well. To prevent this complication, patients taking bisphosphonates are advised to **take nothing by mouth except full glass of water** and not to lie down at least for half an hour. This minimizes the chances of the drug touching the esophagus.
- *Zoledronate* has been associated with *renal toxicity* and *first generation* bisphosphonates can result in *osteomalacia*.
- Recently, **osteonecrosis of jaw** has been noted with use of bisphosphonates particularly zolendronate. Patients receiving bisphosphonates must receive regular dental care and try to avoid dental extraction.
- Long-term use of bisphosphonates increases the risk of **atypical 'chalkstick' fracture of femur (subtrochantric or shaft)**. Risk increases with concurrent high dose steroid therapy.
- Long-term use of bisphosphonates increase the risk of **esophageal cancer**.
- Bisphosphonates **can result in hypocalcemia as well as hypercalcemia**.
- Half-life of alendronate in bone is 10 years.

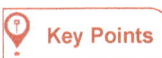 **Key Points**

Bisphosphonates are drug of choice for the treatment of:
- Post-menopausal osteoporosis
- Steroid induced osteoporosis
- Paget's disease
- Hypercalcemia of malignancy

Selective Estrogen Receptor Modulators

- Estrogens inhibit bone resorption directly by inhibiting osteoclasts and indirectly by modulating paracrine factors.
- It **increases anti-resorptive [IGF-1 and TGF-β] and suppresses pro-resorptive [IL-1, IL-6, TNF-α and osteocalcin]** factor synthesis by osteoblasts.
- Estrogen increases bone formation and its deficiency in the old age may result in post-menopausal osteoporosis. Use of hormone replacement therapy for this condition predisposes the patients to the adverse effects of estrogens on breast and endometrium (increased incidence of breast and endometrial carcinoma).
- **Raloxifene** is a selective estrogen receptor modulator with estrogen agonistic action on bone and antagonistic action on breast and endometrium. It is therefore the preferred drug for the treatment and prevention of *post-menopausal osteoporosis*. Major adverse effect of this agent is increased risk of **thromboembolism**.
- **Bazedoxifene** is another SERM that has been approved recently for prevention of post menopausal osteoporosis and to treat vasomotor symptoms of menopause.

Teriparatide and Abaloparatide

Teriparatide and abaloparatide can stimulate osteoblasts whereas most other agents used for osteoporsis act by inhibiting osteoclasts.

These are **recombinant PTH$_{1-34}$**. In low and pulsatile dose, these stimulate bone formation (**Fig. 6.10**) whereas in excess, these cause resorption of bones. These are available for the treatment of osteoporosis by intermittent subcutaneous administration.

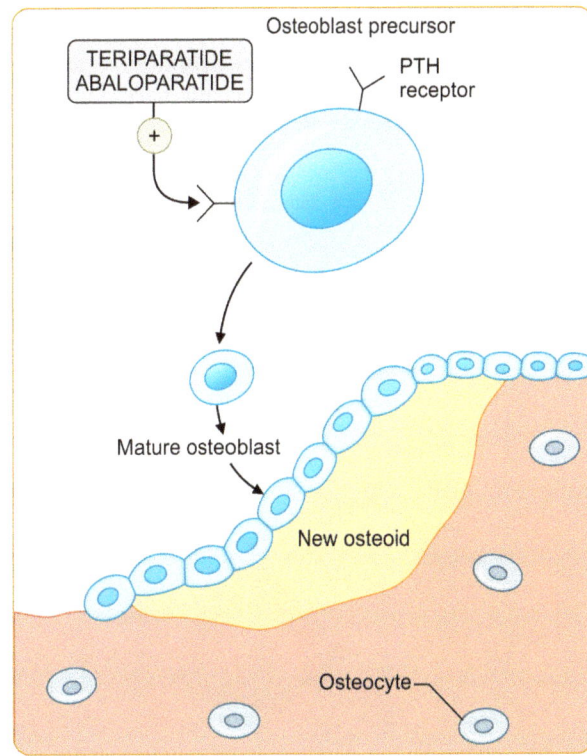

FIG. 6.10: Mechanism of action of PTH analogs

- These stimulate the production of new collagenous bone matrix that must be mineralized. Therefore, patients receiving these drugs must have sufficient intake of vitamin D and calcium.
- When administered to patients with osteoporosis in doses of 20 mcg/d subcutaneously for 2 years, teriparatide dramatically improves bone density in most bones **except the distal radius**.
- The recommended dose should not be exceeded, since teriparatide and abaloparatide has caused osteosarcoma in rats when administered in very high doses. Due to **potential risk of osteosarcoma**, these drugs should be avoided in:
  - *Paget's disease* of bone
  - *Prior radiotherapy* to bone
  - *Past history of osteo or chondrosarcoma*
  - *Unexplained increase in alkaline phosphatase*
- Teriparatide should be used with caution in patients if they also taking corticosteroids and thiazide diuretics along with oral calcium supplementation because **hypercalcemia may develop**.
- Following a course of Teriparatide, a course of bisphosphonates should be considered in order to retain the improved bone density.
- Other adverse effects have included exacerbation of nephrolithiasis and elevation of serum uric acid levels.
- Teriparatide may be **used for healing of chalkstick fractures associated with bisphosphonate therapy**.

Denosumab

Osteoclasts express a receptor called receptor for activated nuclear factor κ B (RANK) on its surface. When this receptor is stimulated by RANK ligand (secreted by obsteoblasts). Bone resorption results due to activation of osteoclasts. **Denosumab is a monoclonal antibody against this ligand and is useful for the treatment of osteoporosis (Fig. 6.11)**. It can also prevent osteoporosis. It **can decrease serum calcium** therefore *avoided in patients with hypocalcemia*. It has recently been approved for unresectable **giant cell tumor** of bone.

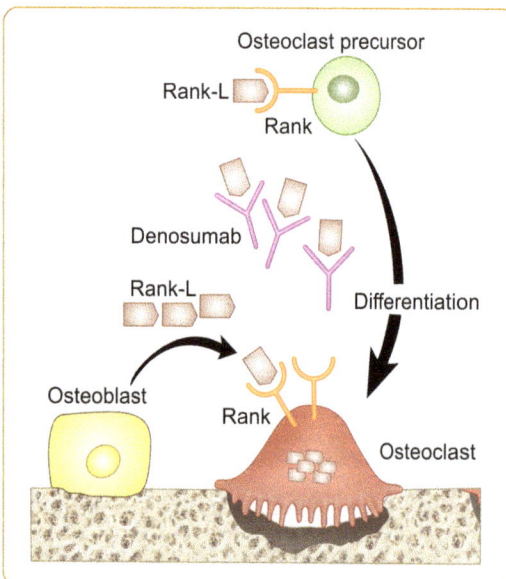

FIG. 6.11: Mechanism of action of denosumab

Romosozumab

It is a monoclonal antibody **against sclerostin**. Latter stimulates bone resorption and inhibits bone formation. Thus, romosozumab acts by **dual mechanism** of inhibiting osteoclast as well as stimulating osteoblasts. It is given by **subcutaneous route**.

Cinacalcet

Calcium sensing receptors (CaSR) are present on parathyroid gland that regulates the secretion of PTH. Ca^{2+} activates these receptors and decreases PTH secretion. Hypocalcemia will have opposite effect i.e. increased PTH secretion. Cinacalcet acts as a **calcimimetic drug** by directly *activating calcium sensing receptors on parathyroid gland*. It has been *approved for* the treatment of *secondary hyperparathyroidism* (due to chronic renal disease) and for patients with hypercalcemia associated with *parathyroid carcinoma*.

Etelcalcetide is a new **CaSR agonist**. It is indicated for intravenous treatment of secondary hyperparathyroidism with CKD on hemodialysis.

Strontium Ranelate

It has a novel mechanism of action as it **inhibits bone resorption as well as stimulates bone formation**. Strontium is incorporated into hydroxyapatite, replacing calcium. Small increased risk of venous thrombosis, seizures and abnormal cognition have been seen and require further studies.

Other Drugs

- **Calcium and calcitriol** (vitamin D) can be used in the *prophylaxis and treatment of osteoporosis*. Calcium can be life saving in *extreme hyperkalemia (> 7 mEg/L)*. It can reverse some of the cardiotoxic effects of K^+. Calcium is also approved for *IV treatment of black widow spider envenomation and magnesium toxicity*.
- **Thiazides** inhibit the renal excretion of Ca^{2+} and thus can be used for the treatment of osteoporosis (apart from their use in recurrent calcium stones due to hypercalciurea).
- **Calcitonin** and **Salcatonin** (Salmon calcitonin) inhibit resorption of bone and thus can be used for the treatment of osteoporosis. These can be administered by *nasal route* for this indication. Calcitonin possess **analgesic effects** on bone pain from fractures.

GONADAL HORMONES

Estrogen, progesterone and testosterone are principal gonadal hormones. Estrogen and progesterone are produced by ovaries whereas testosterone is mainly formed by testes.

ESTROGENS

- Natural estrogens include **estradiol (principal and most potent estrogen)**, estrone and estriol (weakest).
- **Natural estrogens** are ineffective orally due to **extensive first pass metabolism**. Estrogens *undergo enterohepatic circulation* that is also responsible for hepatic adverse effects (hepatic adenoma and thromboembolism).

Estrogen	Estrone	Estradiol	Estriol
Known as	E1	E2	E3
Potency	Intermediate	Maximum	Minimum
Main estrogen in	Menopause	Reproductive age group	Pregnancy
Major site of production	Fat cells	Ovaries	Liver

Effects of Female Sex Hormones

Parameter	Estrogen	Progesterone
Menstrual cycle	Proliferatory endometrium	Secretory endometrium
Lipid profile	↓ LDL, ↑ HDL, ↑ TG	↑ LDL, ↓ HDL
Glucose tolerance	Impair	↑ Insulin response
Fluid balance	Retain Na⁺ and water	↓ Sodium reabsorption
Thromboembolism	↑ risk by ↑ Factor VII, VIII, IX, X ↓ Antithrombin	–
Risk of breast cancer	Increase	Increase
Risk of endometrial cancer	Increase	Decrease
Bone	↓ Resorption	–
Bile lithogenicity	Increase	–

Indications

Deficiency of this hormone as seen in postmenopausal females may result in osteoporosis, hot flushes, urogenital atrophy and increased risk of cardiovascular diseases. *Major use of estrogen is for hormone replacement therapy (HRT) in post menopausal females.* **Progesterone is added to HRT to decrease the risk of endometrial carcinoma.** Estrogens can reverse all the features of its deficiency.

- Another important use of estrogens is as a *component of oral contraceptives.*
- These can be used in the treatment of dysfunctional uterine bleeding *(DUB), if it is due to estrogen withdrawal.*
- Estrogens reduce testosterone production due to feed back inhibition of LH secretion. This property has been utilized for the treatment of *testosterone dependent tumors like prostatic carcinoma.* But now a days, GnRH agonists and antagonists are preferred for this indication.

Adverse effects and interactions

- Treatment with estrogen can result in *feminization, gynaecomastia and decreased libido in males and nausea, migraine and increased risk of carcinomas (endometrial and breast) in females.*
- *Diabetes, fluid retention, hepatic adenoma, cholelithiasis and predisposition to thromboembolism* can be seen in both the sexes.
- Increased incidence of *vaginal and cervical adenocarcinoma* was noted in the *female offsprings* of mothers who have taken *diethylstilbesterol (DES) during first trimester of pregnancy.* Intake of DES during pregnancy has also been associated with development of hypospadias in new born babies.
- Antimicrobials like *ampicillin* and enzyme inducers like *rifampicin decrease the effect of estrogen;* former by inhibiting enterohepatic cycling and latter by increasing the metabolism of estrogen.

SELECTIVE ESTROGEN RECEPTOR MODULATORS (SERMs)

These are the agents that act as estrogen agonists in some tissues and antagonists in other tissues. *Agonistic action is beneficial in tissues like bone (decreased resorption) and blood (better lipid profile) whereas it is deleterious in endometrium, breast (increased risk of carcinoma) and liver (predisposition to thromboembolism).*

- SERMs are targeted to provide beneficial effect of estrogen as well as to antagonize its adverse effects. **Clomiphene, tamoxifen, doloxifene, toremifene, fulvestrant, raloxifene, bazedoxifene, ospemifene and ormeloxifene** are now classified as SERMs.
- In humans **clomiphene** has *estrogen antagonistic action in hypothalamus* (reduces feedback inhibition of GnRH secretion). It is used for the treatment of **anovulatory infertility** by increasing GnRH release. Major adverse effect is *hyperstimulation syndrome (polycystic ovarian disease) and multiple pregnancy.*
- **Tamoxifen, doloxifene and toremifene** possess estrogen antagonistic activity in the breast and blood whereas agonistic activity in bone, uterus and liver. Their major indication is in the treatment of **breast carcinoma.** *These have beneficial effect on bone and lipid profile but increase the risk of endometrial carcinoma and thromboembolism.*

> ⚠️ **MNEMONIC**
>
> **Tamoxifen has**
> Beneficial effect on three **B**
> Bone (↓ resorption)
> Breast (↓ carcinoma)
> Blood (↑ HDL & ↓ LDL)

- **Raloxifene and bazedoxifene are** used for **osteoporosis.** Raloxifene also possesses beneficial effects on lipid profile, breast and endometrium. *Major adverse effect is increased predisposition to thromboembolism.*

Ospemifene is a new SERM indicated for dyspareunia due to menopause.

- **Centchroman (ormeloxifene)** is used as a **non hormonal oral contraceptive (Saheli).** It is also approved for the treatment of DUB.

Prasterone is an inactive steroid that is converted to estrogens and androgens in the body. It is indicated for treatment of **dyspareunia due to vulvovaginal atrophy**

SELECTIVE ESTROGEN RECEPTOR DOWNREGULATORS (SERD)

Fulvestrant is the first FDA approved agent in the new class of drugs that are called **selective estrogen-receptor downregulators (SERDs).** It has an *improved safety profile, faster onset, and longer duration of action than the SERMs* due to its pure ER antagonist activity. It was approved for postmenopausal women with **hormone receptor-positive metastatic breast cancer that has progressed despite antiestrogen therapy.** It binds to the estrogen receptor (ER).

Contd...

Contd...

with an affinity more than 100 times that of tamoxifen, inhibits its dimerization, and increases its degradation. As a consequence of this ER "downregulation," ER-mediated transcription is abolished, completely suppressing the expression of estrogen-dependent genes. This difference in the activity of fulvestrant likely explains why fulvestrant **demonstrates efficacy against tamoxifen- resistant breast cancer.** Fulvestrant is administered *intramuscularly at monthly intervals*. Most common adverse effects of this drug include *nausea, asthenia, pain, vasodilation (hot flushes), and headache.*

SELECTIVE TISSUE ESTROGEN ACTIVITY REGULATOR (STEAR)

STEAR are the compounds with estrogenic activity, tissue-selective mode of action and particular metabolism that regulates ligand levels. **Tibolone** belongs to this group. It is considered as a designer HRT and is used for preventing vasomotor symptoms and osteoporosis in menopause.

AROMATASE INHIBITORS

Androgens are converted to estrogen in the peripheral tissue of post-menopausal females with the help of an enzyme, aromatase. The drugs inhibiting this enzyme *decrease the formation of estrogen and are beneficial in the treatment of breast carcinoma.* These are useful for the treatment of **tamoxifen resistant breast carcinoma.** Common side effects of these drugs include bone pain, hot flushes and thromboembolism.

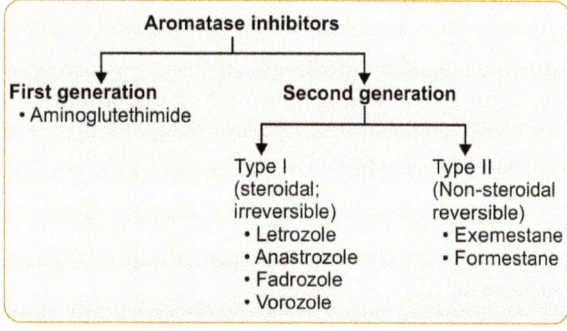

PROGESTINS

Progesterone is the most important progestin in humans. It is primarily secreted by corpus luteum. Synthetic progestins may be classified as:

Generation	Properties
1st Generation (Estranes) • Norethindrone • Norethinodrel • Lynestrenol	• Weak estrogenic, androgenic and anabolic • Potent antiovulatory
2nd Generation (Gonanes) • Norgestrel • Levonorgestrel	• More potent than 1st generation • Reduced androgenic activity • Levonorgestrel is more potent than norgestrel

3rd Generation
• Desogestrel
• Norgestimate
• Gestodene
	• Very potent
	• strong antiovulatory
	• Reduced androgenic effects; thus
	  – ↓ risk of acne
	  – ↓ hirsutism

Contd...

Contd...

Generation	Properties
4th Generation • Nomegestrol • Drospirenone	• Weak anti-androgenic • Less anti-ovulatory • Strong antiestrogenic on endometrium • No adverse effect on lipid profile or glucose tolerance • **Drospirenone** possess aldosterone receptor antagonistic activity; preferred in woman who have fluid retention after taking OCPs

Uses

Major indications of progesterone are for **oral contraception** and **hormone replacement therapy,** for which these are combined with estrogens. Progestins are **added to decrease the risk of endometrial and ovarian carcinoma.** Progestins are also used for secondary amenorrhea, abnormal uterine bleeding, premature labour and luteal phase support to treat infertility.

SELECTIVE PROGESTERONE RECEPTOR MODULATOR (SPRM)

Mifepristone, onapristone, ulipristal and asoprisnil are the drugs affecting progesterone receptors.

- **Mifepristone** is a SPRM with mainly antagonistic activity and some agonistic activity on progesterone receptors. It also has **glucocorticoid and androgen receptor blocking activity.** It has a long $t_{1/2}$ of 20 hours. Its uses are:
  - **Medical termination of pregnancy**: Oral dose of 600 mg mifepristone with oral misoprostol (400 µg) effectively terminates pregnancy upto 49 days in 95% of patients. Most severe adverse effect is vaginal bleeding. *Recently, low dose mifepristone (200 mg) with oral misoprostol (800 µg) is indicated for termination of pregnancy upto 63 days.*
  - Single 600 mg dose is an effective **emergency contraceptive.**
  - It is recommended for treatment of **Cushing's syndrome** for patients with ectopic ACTH secretion or adrenal inoperable carcinoma who failed to respond to other treatments.
  - Other potential uses include **endometriosis, breast cancer, meningioma** (containing glucocorticoid or progesterone receptors), and **fibroids.**

⚠ MNEMONIC

Uses of mifepristone

M – Morning after pill
I – Induction of abortion
F – Fibroid
E – Endometriosis
P – Progesterone
R – Receptor +ve breast cancer and meningioma
I – Increased
S – Steroids (Cushing)
TONE

- **Onapristone** is a pure progesterone antagonist in contrast to mifepristone.
- **Ulipristal** acts as partial agonist on progesterone receptors. It does not block glucocorticoid receptors. It acts by inhibiting ovulation. A 30 mg dose is used as

emergency contraceptive that can be taken within 120 hours (5 days) after unprotected intercourse. If taken withing 72 hours, it is as effective as levonorgestrel whereas it is more effective than levonorgestrel if taken within 72-120 hours of unprotected intercourse. Major adverse effects are headache and abdominal pain.
- **Asoprisnil** is an investigational SPRM, tested for treatment of progesterone sensitive myomata. Clinical trials were discontinued due to endometrial changes in patients.

HORMONAL CONTRACEPTIVES

Hormonal contraceptives can be used *orally (combined oral contraceptive, progestin only pills and emergency pills) or by implants*.

Combined Oral Contraceptives

- These contain both estrogen and progestin. Most commonly used estrogen in combined OCPs is ethinyl estradiol. On the basis of amount of estrogen, combined OCPs can be classified as

Type of OCP	Amount of ethinyl estradiol
Standard dose	50 µg
Low dose	30-35 µg
Very low dose	20 µg

- Most commonly used progesterone in combined OCPs is levonorgestrel (LNG)
- Combined OCPs may be:
    - *Monophasic*: Content of estrogen and progesterone remain same in all the pills (for 21 days).
    - *Biphasic*: Content of progesterone is different in pills for first 10 days and that for 11-21 days
    - *Triphasic*: Content of progesterone is gradually increased. It is lowest in first phase (1-6 days), moderate in second phase (7-11 days) and further increased in third phase (12-21 days).

- **Biphasic and triphasic pills** permit reduction in progesterone content without compromising efficacy. These pills **decrease the risk of breakthrough bleeding**.
- Main mechanism of combined OCPs is to cause **feedback inhibition of pituitary** (causing abolition of LH surge) *resulting in inhibition of ovulation*. Other mechanisms include *thickening of cervical mucus, decreased motility and secretions of the fallopian tubes and making endometrium unfavourable for implantation*.

📍 Key Points

Major mechanism of different OCPs	
Combined OCP	**Inhibit ovulation**
Mini-pills	Cervical mucus thickening
Emergency Contraceptive	Inhibit implantation

- Combined OCPs are started on first day of menstrual cycle and given for 21 days. To allow withdrawl bleeding, iron tablets are given (without hormones) for next seven days.

- Ovulation returns within 3 months of stopping OCP use in 90% of cases
- OCPs are **contraceptives of choice for:**
    - Newly married couples
    - After evacuation of molar pregnancy

Segesterone plus ethinyl estradiol combination has been approved as vaginal ring for reuse as contraceptive. It can be used for one year.

Progesterone Only Pills (Minipills)

- These contain low dose of progestin without any estrogen. These are less effective than combined OCPs.

- Minipills are preferred in women where estrogen is contraindicated e.g.
    - Smokers
    - >35 years of age
    - Risk factors of thromboembolism

- Minipills are oral contraceptives of choice for
    - Lactating women
    - Sickle cell anemia
    - Seizure disorder
- Progesterone only pills are given daily without any break.
- Thickening of cervical mucus is major mechanism of minipills.

Emergency Contraceptives (Post-Coital Pills; Morning-After Pills)

Method	Use within	Dose and Duration
1. Levonorgestrel (LNG)	72 hours*	1.5 mg (oral) single dose
2. OC pills	72 hours	2 tablets followed by another 2 within 12 hours
3. Mifepristone	72 hours	600 mg oral single dose
4. Ulipristal	120 hours	30 mg oral single dose
5. IUD	5 days	–

*LNG and ulipristal can be used up to 120 hours, however LNG has very low efficacy.

Parenteral Contraceptives

- These can be used in females with contraindication to estrogens.
- Major problem with these methods is prolonged infertility after their use.
- Most common adverse effects of parenteral contraceptives is irregular bleeding.
- **DMPA** (Depot Medroxy Progesterone Acetate) and **NET-EN** (Nor-ethindrone Enanthate) are implanted **intramuscularly**.
- **Norplant and capranor** are LNG **subcutaneous implants**. **Norplant is longest acting** implant (replaced after 5 years) whereas *capranor is biodegradable implant*.
- *Implanon* (Etonorgestrel) and *uniplant* (nomegestrel) are also implanted *subcutaneously*.

Adverse Effects

- *Nausea*, mastalgia, *breakthrough bleeding* and edema are related to the amount of estrogen in the preparation.

- *Migraine* is made worse with the use of OCPs.
- *Failure of withdrawal bleeding* is another important adverse effect.
- **Breakthrough bleeding is the most common problem with the use of progesterone only pills.** Chances of this bleeding decrease with biphasic and triphasic pills.
- Weight gain can occur *with* the use of progestins containing androgenic properties. **Desogestrel and norgestimate cause less weight gain.**
- **Acne and hirsutism may worsen by progestins containing androgenic properties.**
- **Risk of venous thromboembolism**, MI and stroke is increased with the use of OCPs because estrogen increases the clotting factors (VII, VIII, IX and X) and decreases anticlotting factors (antithrombin III).
- *Cholestatic jaundice, gall bladder disease and incidence of hepatic adenomas* are increased with OCP use.
- Chances of **breast and cervical carcinoma** are **increased whereas endometrial and ovarian carcinomas are decreased** by OCP use. *Progesterone is responsible for decreasing the risk of these cancers.*

Non-Contraceptive Benefits of OCPs

> **MNEMONIC**
>
> OCPs decrease the risk of:
> Other – Ovarian cyst
> B – Benign breast disease
> E – Ectopic pregnancy
> N – Neoplasia (Ovarian, Endometrial, Colon cancer)
> E – Endometriosis
> F – Fibroid
> I – Iron deficiency anemia
> T – Tension (Pre-menstrual tension syndrome)
> S – Skeletal (RA and Osteoporosis)

ANDROGENS

Most important androgens are *testosterone and dihydrotestosterone (DHT).* Less potent androgens include androstenidione and de-hydroepiandrostenidione (DHEA). **Testosterone is converted to DHT by 5-α reductase and to estradiol by aromatase.**

Uses

- Long acting derivatives like testosterone enanthate (i.m.) are indicated for *hypogonadal men* to compensate for the decreased endogenous secretion. Long term oral therapy is associated with liver adenomas and carcinomas. It can *also be administered by transdermal route.* Polycythemia and hypertension (due to erythropoietic action) may be a problem.
- These can also be used *to reduce breast engorgement* during postpartum period.
- Sometimes, these are used for *chemotherapy of breast tumors* in premenopausal females.
- These are frequently *abused by athletes* due to their anabolic properties.
- These agents have been used *to stimulate growth in boys with delayed puberty.*
- Androgens have been used in the *treatment of osteoporosis.*

Adverse Effects

- *Masculinising* actions (hirsutism, amenorrhoea, clitoral enlargement and deepening of voice) in females.
- *Increased risk of atherosclerosis* due to decrease in HDL and increase in LDL cholesterol.
- Use of androgens during pregnancy may result in masculinization of the female fetus and under-masculinization of the male fetus.
- *Sodium retention and edema* can occur rarely, so caution is advised in patients with heart and kidney disease.
- 17-alkyl substituted compounds (**methyltestosterone and fluoxymestrane**) are more likely to cause **cholestatic jaundice and peliosis hepatica.**
- Increased chances of *acne, erythrocytosis, gynaecomastia and azoospermia.*
- Androgens are contraindicated in pregnant females, infants, carcinoma of the male breast and prostate and patients with cardiac and renal diseases.

Danazol

It is a compound with **weak androgenic, progestational and glucocorticoid activities**. It decreases the secretion of gonadotropins from the pituitary by causing feedback inhibition. Its major use is in the **treatment of endometriosis**. Other uses include fibrocystic disease of breast, hemophilia, Christmas disease, ITP and angioneurotic edema. *Weight gain, edema, acne, increased hair growth, hot flushes and changes in libido are the major adverse effects* of this drug. *It can also produce mild to moderate hepatocellular damage.*

ANTI-ANDROGENS

Drugs in this group can act **by inhibiting the synthesis, activation or action of androgens**.

- **Steroid synthesis inhibitors: Ketoconazole** inhibits the synthesis of adrenal and gonadal hormones but its usefulness in the treatment of prostatic carcinoma is limited by serious toxicity on prolonged use. It can cause *gynaecomastia* due to increase in estradiol: testosterone ratio. **Abiraterone** is an *orally active prodrug* that acts by inhibiting 17-α-hydroxylase and 17, 20-lyase. It reduces the synthesis of cortisol and androgens, and is approved for castration resistant refractory *prostate cancer.*
- **5-α reductase inhibitors:** Most of the actions of testosterone are mediated by its conversion to DHT by 5-α reductase. Important amongst these are growth of prostate, male pattern baldness and hirsutism in females. **Finasteride and dutasteride** are 5-α reductase inhibitors useful in the *treatment of BHP, male pattern baldness and hirsutism* by reducing the production of DHT.
- **Androgen receptor antagonists: Cyproterone and cyproterone acetate** act as antagonists of androgen receptors. Latter compound has marked progestational activity that inhibits feedback enhancement of LH and FSH. These drugs are useful in the **treatment of hirsutism** and as a component of **contraceptive** pills. **Flutamide, bicalutamide, enzalutamide, nilutamide, apalutamide** and **darolutamide** are other anti-androgens that act by same mechanism. These are useful for the treatment of *prostatic carcinoma. Flutamide can cause gynaecomastia and reversible liver damage. These drugs can also be combined with GnRH agonists (like leuprolide) to reduce the initial flare up reaction.*
- **Spironolactone:** It is an aldosterone antagonist that also competes with DHT for its receptor. It can be used for the *treatment of hirsutism.*

Endocrinology

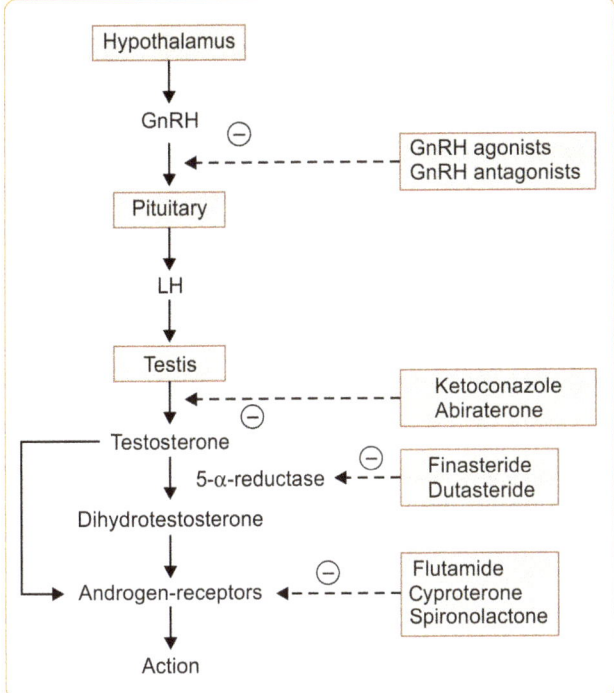

UTERINE STIMULANTS

These drugs increase uterine contractions and are known as **oxytocics or ecbolics.**

OXYTOCIN

It is secreted by *posterior pituitary* along with ADH. It *increases the uterine contractions with complete relaxation in between*. It *increases the contraction of upper segment* (fundus and body) of uterus *whereas lower segment is relaxed* facilitating the expulsion of the fetus. *Estrogen increases whereas progesterone decreases the sensitivity of uterus to oxytocin.*

- Oxytocin is involved in milk ejection reflex whereas prolactin causes milk secretion.
- High doses of oxytocin cause fall in BP (due to *vasodilation*) resulting in reflex tachycardia.
- It *also has ADH like action* in high dose and can result in fluid retention.

Uses

It is used for the **induction of labor** in post-maturity and uterine inertia. It is now drug of choice for the *treatment as well as prevention of* **postpartum hemorrhage. Methyergometrine** and **misoprostol** are alternative drugs for this indication. *Oxytocin challenge test* is performed to know the adequacy of uteroplacental circulation in high risk pregnancies.

Adverse effects

Injudicious use may result in *rupture of uterus* due to powerful uterine contractions. It may also cause *water intoxication* due to ADH like action. Oxytocin **should not be used** in cases of *contracted pelvis, obstructed labour, malpresentation, history of LSCS, hypovolemic states and cardiac disease.*

ERGOT DERIVATIVES

Ergometrine is derived from *Claviceps purpura* and is used as an oxytocic agent. It produces uterine *contractions in the upper as well as lower segment and is used to control postpartum hemorrhage*. Its derivative, **methylergometrine is more potent** oxytocic and is preferred for this indication. Latter is *administered at the delivery of anterior shoulder*. These drugs are preferred over oxytocin for this indication. *Hypertension and sepsis are contraindications* for their use.

> **Post Partum Hemorrhage (PPH)**
> - **Oxytocin is drug of choice** for treatment (10 IU, iv) as well as prevention (10 IU, iv or im) of PPH. **Carbetocin** is a long acting oxytocin that can be used as single intravenous bolus dose of 100 microgram for treatment.
> - Alternatives are methylergometrine and misoprostol.
> - Misoprostol is used as 600 microgram orally for prevention of PPH and 800 microgram sublingually for treatment of PPH.
> - Tranexamic acid is indicated if above measures fail.

UTERINE RELAXANTS

These drugs decrease uterine contractions and are known as **tocolytics.** These are mainly used *to delay labour* when premature contractions are present.

Beta Agonists

Ritodrine, isoxsuprine and **terbutaline** are the *selective* β_2 *agonists* useful as tocolytic agents. These drugs should not be used in mother having heart disease or diabetes mellitus. **Pulmonary edema** is a serious complication of these drugs at high doses. β_2 agonists can also produce tachycardia, palpitations, tremors, hyperglycemia and hypokalemia.

Magnesium Sulphate

It is mainly used *to control convulsions in eclampsia*. It also possesses tocolytic activity and can be used. It is preferred over β_2 agonists in patients with cardiac problems, diabetes, hyperthyroidism and hypertension. Toxicity is manifested initially as *loss of patellar reflex* followed by respiratory depression and finally cardiac arrhythmias and arrest. *Magnesium sulphate by IV or inhalational route has also been utilized in the treatment of acute severe asthma.*

Other Drugs

Calcium channel blockers like nifedipine and **oxytocin antagonist 'atosiban'** can also be used to delay premature labour. *Ethyl alcohol* (IV infusion), *NSAIDs and progesterone* also suppress uterine contractions but are rarely used for this indication. 'Halothane' is an efficacious tocolytic agent and is the *anaesthetic of choice for version (external or internal)*. **Hydroxyprogesterone** has been used prophylactically to *prevent pre-term labour*; however, teratogenic potential limits its use. Calcium channel blockers and atosiban provides the best balance of successful delayed delivery with lesser risk to mother and baby.

Golden Points

1. GH controls growth of almost all organs of the body except brain and eye.

2. Mecasermin rinfabate is a complex of recombinant human IGF-1 (Insulin-like Growth Factor- 1) and IGF-binding protein-3. It is indicated for growth failure due to deficiency of IGF-1 that is not res-ponsive to GH.

3. **Pasireotide** is a new somatostatin analog approved for treatment of Cushing's disease.

4. GnRH agonists stimulate gonadotropin secretion when given in a pulsatile manner whereas inhibit the release on continued administration.

5. *Nafarelin* and *busurelin* can be administered by *nasal* route

6. *Levo-thyroxine (T_4) is preferred over liothyronine (T_3) for treatment of hypothyroidism* due to its **long half life**

7. Iodides are the **fastest acting anti-thyroid drugs**.

8. I^{131} is the most commonly used radioactive iodine with a half-life of 8 DAYS

9. α_2 receptor stimulation inhibits insulin secretion whereas β_2 agonists and vagal stimulation enhances insulin release.

10. Advantage of rapid acting insulins (lispro etc) is that their duration of action remain constant (~ 4 hours) irrespective of dose. This contrasts with all other insulins (including regular) where duration of action is prolonged with increase in dose

11. **Insulin degludec** is longest acting insulin and unlike insulin glargine, it can be mixed with other insulins too.

12. Beta blockers mask all the warning signs of hypoglycemia expect **sweating** (It is mediated by sympathetic cholinergic fibres and not by beta receptors).

13. Rapid acting insulins (lispro, aspart and glulisine) are preferred for use in CSII (continous subcutaneous insulin infusion) devices

14. **Afrezza** is commercial name of long acting **inhaled insulin**. It is used with long acting insulin in patients with IDDM

15. Sulfonylureas (except glyburide) and meglitinides (nateglinide and repaglinide) are safe in renal failure.

16. **Metformin is drug of choice for type 2 diabetes mellitus**

17. **Metformin** is the **only oral agent** that has been demonstrated to **reduce macrovascular events** in type 2 DM.

18. Hypoglycemia in the presence of α-glucosidase inhibitors can be reversed by simple carbohydrates like glucose (not sucrose or other complex carbohydrates).

19. Acarbose can decrease blood glucose in both type 1 as well as type 2 diabetes. However, apart from insulin, the only drug approved for treatment of both type1 as well as type 2 diabetes is pramlintide

20. **Dexamethasone suppression test** is used *to test the intactness of HPA axis function* and diagnosis of Cushing's syndrome.

21. **Antenatal Use of Steroids**
    - Accelerate fetal lung maturation
    - Decrease incidence of PDA
    - Decrease risk of intraventricular hemorrhage
    - Decrease risk of necrotizing enterocolitis

22. **Antenatal Steroids for fetal lung maturation**
    - **Betamethasone**: 12 mg i.m. 2 doses at 24 hours interval
    - **Dexamethasone**: 6 mg i.m. 4 doses at 12 hours interval

23. Distinctive toxicity of bisphosphonates is **esophageal irritation** that can lead to ulceration as well

24. Teriparatide and strontium ranelate can stimulate osteoblast whereas most other agents used for osteoporosis act by inhibiting osteoclast

25. Denosumab has recently been approved for giant cell tumor of bone

26. Cinacalcet acts as a **calcimimetic drug** by directly *activating calcium sensing receptors on parathyroid gland. It has been approved for* the treatment of *secondary hyper-parathyroidism*

27. Strontium ranelate inhibits bone resorption as well as stimulates bone formation.

28. Progesterone is added to hormone replacement to decrease the risk of endometrial carcinoma.

29. **Fulvestrant** is a **selective estrogen-receptor downregulator (SERD).** It has *improved safety profile, faster onset, and longer duration of action than the SERMs* due to its pure ER antagonist activity.

30. Chances of breast and cervical carcinoma are increased whereas endometrial and ovarian carcinomas are decreased by OCP use.

31. *Biphasic and triphasic pills decrease the breakthrough bleeding without increasing the total hormone content.*

32. **Danazol** is a compound with **weak androgenic, progestational and glucocorticoid activities**. It decreases the secretion of gonadotropins from the pituitary by causing feedback inhibition. Its major use is in the **treatment of endometriosis**.

33. DOC for treatment as well as prevention of post partum hemorrhage is oxytocin

34. Dose of misoprostol for treatment of PPH is 800 µg sublingually whereas for prevention of PPH, it is given 600 µg orally

35. Toxicity of magnesium sulfate manifests initially as *loss of patellar reflex* followed by respiratory depression and finally cardiac arrhythmias and arrest.

Endocrinology

Drug of Choice

Condition	Drug
Infantile spasms	ACTH
Hypothyroidism	Levo-thyroxine
Myxedema coma	Levo-thyroxine
Hyperthyroidism	Carbimazole or methimazole
– In lactation	Propylthiouracil
– In 1st trimester of pregnancy	Prophylthiouracil
– In 2nd and 3rd trimester of pregnancy	Carbimazole or methimazole
– Graves' opthalmopathy	Methylprednisolone
Thyroid storm	Propranolol (life saving) + Propylthiouracil
Diabetes mellitus	
Type 1 (IDDM)	Insulin
Type 2 (NIDDM)	Metformin
– In obese	Metformin
– Uncontrolled	Insulin
– Pregnancy	Insulin
– To tide over stress	Insulin
Diabetic ketoacidosis	Insulin (Regular)
Post prandial hyperglycemia	Nateglinide
Acute hyperkalemia	Calcium gluconate
Beta blocker poisoning	Glucagon
Hypoglycemia	Glucose (oral or IV)
Adrenal insufficiency	
– Acute	Hydrocortisone
– Chronic (Addison's disease)	Hydrocortisone

Condition	Drug
Erectile dysfunction	Sildenafil
Contraceptive	
– Newly married	Combined oral contraceptives
– In lactation	Mini pills
– Emergency contraceptive	Levonorgestrel
Anovulatory infertility	Clomiphene
Osteoporosis	
– Post menopausal	Alendronate
– Steroid-induced	Alendronate
– In women with risk factors for breast cancer	Raloxifene
Hypercalcemia of malignancy	Bisphosphonates
Paget's disease of bone	Bisphosphonates
Tetany	Calcium
Induction of labour	Oxytocin
Post partum hemorrhage	Oxytocin
Acromegaly	Cabergoline
Esophageal varices	Terlipressin (if not available, octreotide)
Hyperprolactinemia	Cabergoline
Androgenital alopecia	Finasteride
Dysfunctional uterine bleeding	
– Light bleeding	Medroxyprogesterone acetate
– Heavy bleeding	Combined oral contraceptives
– Intractable bleeding	Leuprolide
Endometriosis	Combined oral contraceptives
Ectopic pregnancy	Methotrexate

Image Based Questions

1. The only oral drug (among the given options) effective for the treatment of the condition shown in the below is:

   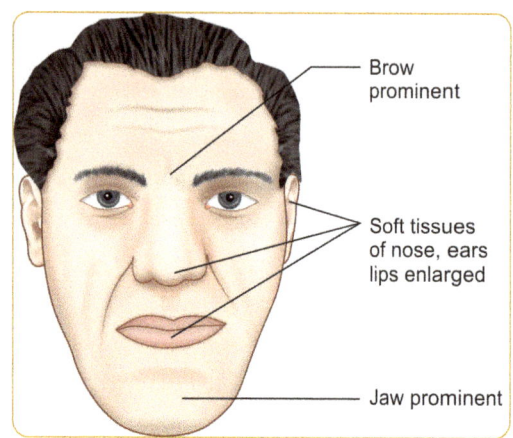

   (a) Octretide
   (b) Cabergoline
   (c) Pegvisomant
   (d) L- thyroxine

2. A 40-year-old male presented to emergency (as shown in Figure) with fever, extreme restlessness, confusion and marked weakness. On examination, severe tachycardia and BP of 170/110 mmHg was noted. ECG revealed the presence of atrial fibrillation. Which among the following is the only life saving drug that should be given immediately to this person?

   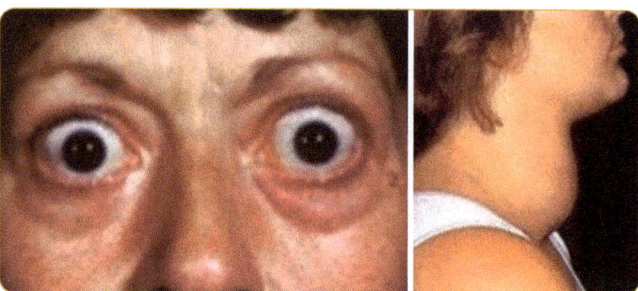

   (a) Carbimazole
   (b) Radioactive iodine
   (c) Propranolol
   (d) Liothyronine

3. A patient presented to OPD with swelling in the neck as shown in the below figure. He complains of decreased appetite, fatigue and cold intoerance. He has gained 8 kg of weight in last 4 months. Thyroid function tests revealed normal T4 but elevated TSH. The patient should be treated with:

   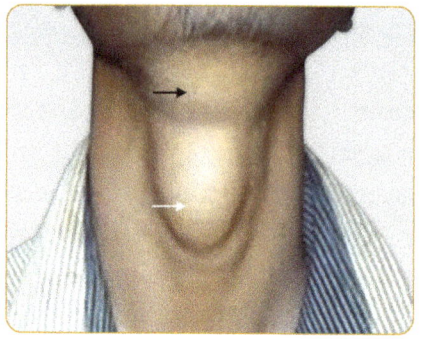

   (a) Liothyronine   (b) L-thyroxine
   (c) Carbimazole   (d) Steroids

4. A 40-year-old male suffering from a chronic disease presents to OPD with the features shown in the below figure. This is likely to be adverse effect of:

   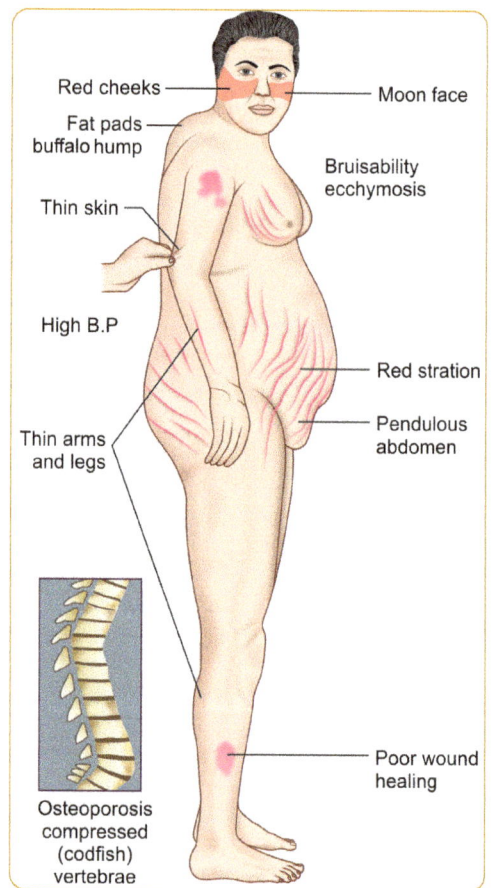

   (a) Corticosteroids   (b) NSAIDs
   (c) Infliximab   (d) Androgens

5. The medicine shown in the below figure is used for:

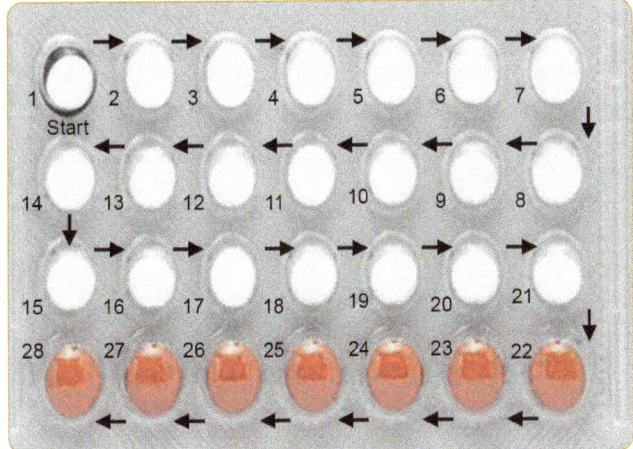

(a) Multibacillary leprosy
(b) Paucibacillary leprosy
(c) Tuberculosis
(d) Contraception

6. The oral contraceptives shown in the below figure are:

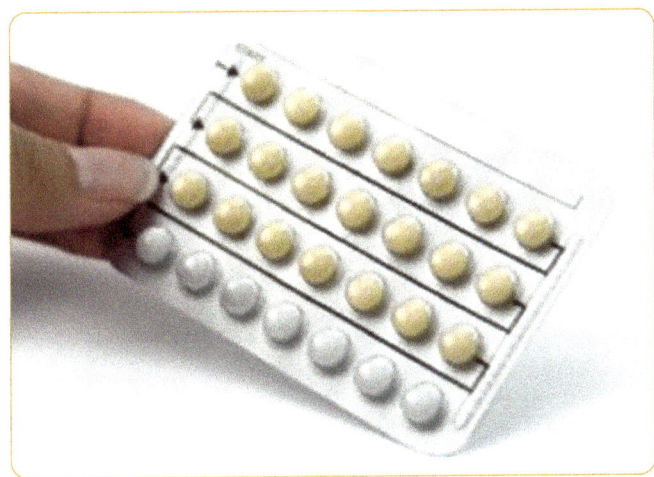

(a) Monophasic combined OCPs
(b) Biphasic combined OCPs
(c) Triphasic combined OCPs
(d) Emergency Pills

7. The oral contraceptives shown in the below figure are:

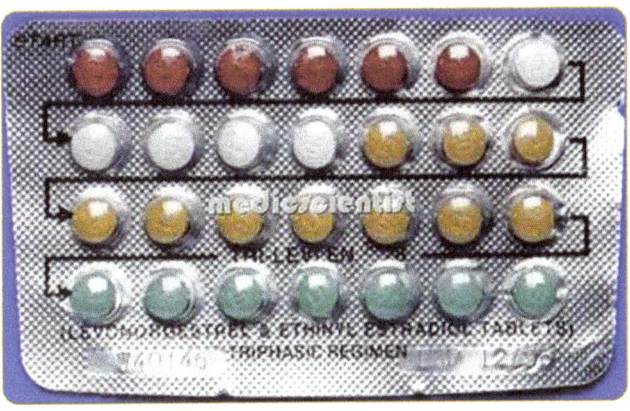

(a) Monophasic combined OCPs
(b) Biphasic combined OCPs
(c) Triphasic combined OCPs
(d) Emergency Pills

8. The drug Z shown in the below figure is likely to be:

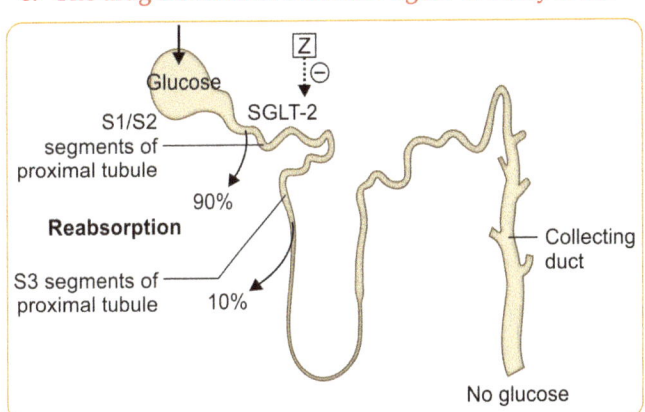

(a) Pramlintide
(b) Exenatide
(c) Canagliflozin
(d) Sitagliptin

9. Based on the given mechanism of action as shown in below figure, Drug A is likely to be:

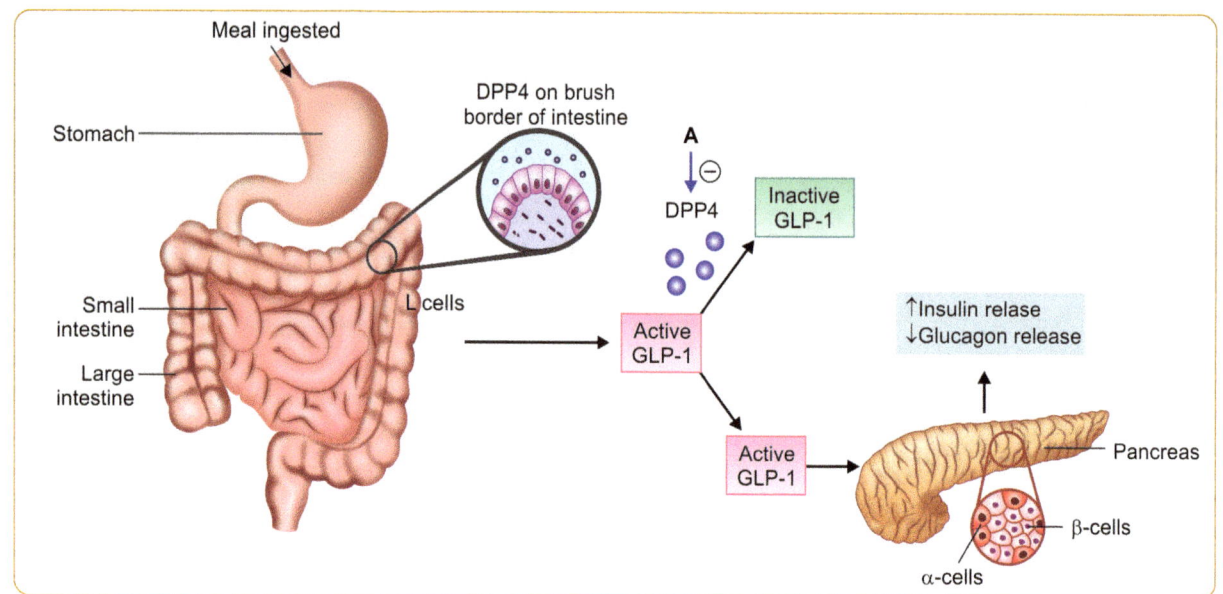

(a) Exenatide
(b) Vildagliptin
(c) Canagliflozin
(d) Pramlintide

10. The drug X used in osteoporosis has the mechanism shown in the below figure is likely to be:

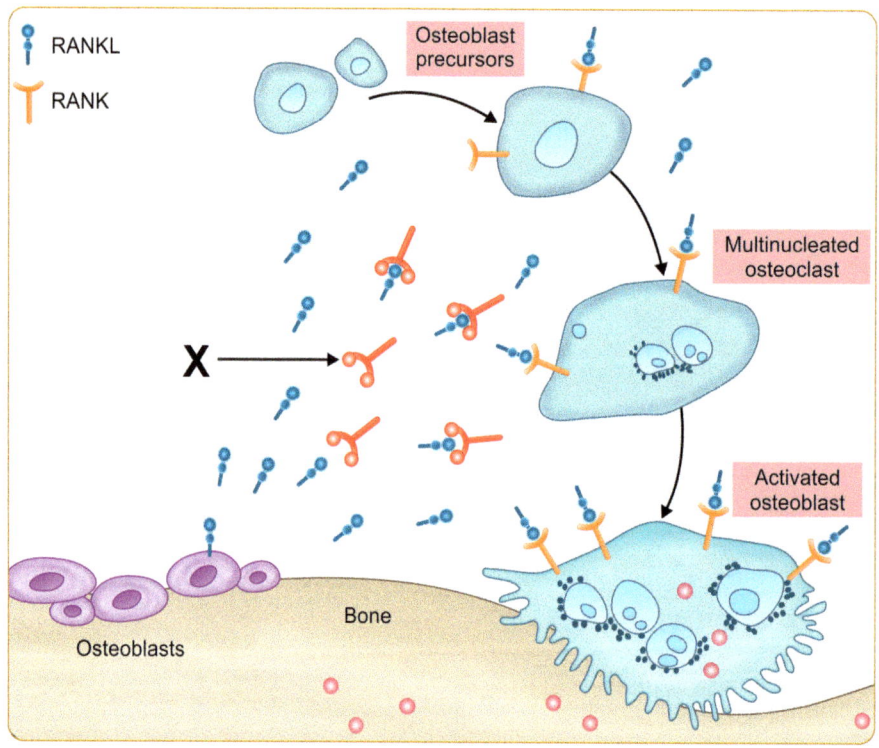

(a) Teriparatide
(b) Alendronate
(c) Denosumab
(d) Estrogen

11. A 15-year-old female, Rashmi presents to the emergency in comatose state. She is a known case of type 1 diabetes mellitus. Immediate blood sugar is measured by glucometer and found to be 658 mg/dL. Urine is found to be positive for glucose as well as ketone bodies. Which of the following insulin types depicted in the figure below is most appropriate for the treatment of this patient's condition?

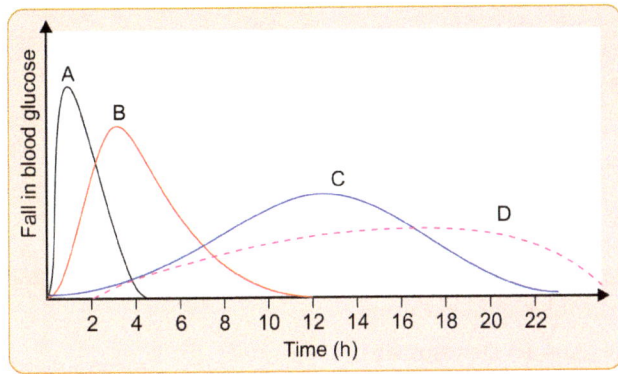

(a) A
(b) B
(c) C
(d) D

12. Amarnath, a 58-year-old businessman is a known case of type 2 diabetes and was well controlled on metformin. But since last 5 years the different combinations of oral antidiabetic drugs were tried and still the blood sugar was not controlled. So, the physician thought of giving him insulin. Which of the following insulin (From below figure) can be used to maintain the basal levels of insulin without producing significant risk of hypoglycemia in this patient?

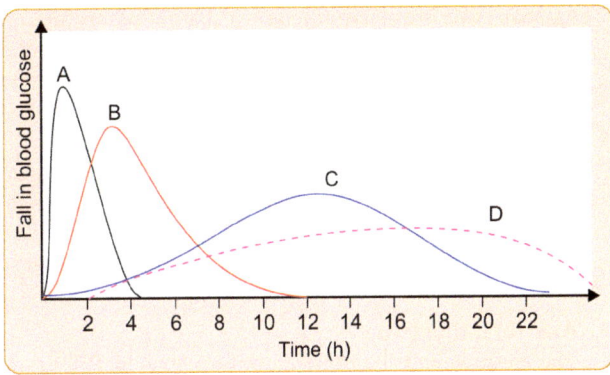

(a) A
(b) B
(c) C
(d) D

Explanations

1. **Ans. (b) Cabergoline**
   The figure shows the features of acromegaly. Dopamine agonists like bromocriptine and cabergoline are the only oral drugs for acromegaly. Octreotide and pegvisomant are injectable drugs for acromegaly. L-thyroxine has no role in acromegaly.

2. **Ans. (c) Propranolol**
   The features given in the question, points towards thyrotoxic crisis. To save the life, we need to immediately reverse cardiovascular symptoms. It can be done by beta blockers like propranolol or by calcium channel blockers like verapamil or diltiazem.

3. **Ans. (b) L-thyroxine**
   The features and the investigations (elevated TSH) points towards hypothyroidism. L-thyroxine is drug of choice for this condition.

4. **Ans. (a) Corticosteroids**
   The figure shows the characteristic "Cushing's Habitus". It is the adverse effect of prolonged use of corticosteroids.

5. **Ans. (d) Contraception**
   The figure shows the 28 day pills with 21 of different colour and 7 of different. These are combined oral contraceptive pills which are given for 21 days and last 7 days are hormone free tablets (containing only iron) are given.

6. **Ans. (a) Monophasic pills**
   The strip shows 28 tablets with 21 on one colour and 7 of different colour. These are monophasic combined OCPs. Here the hormone content of 21 tablets is same whereas 7 tablets contains only iron without any hormone. As all the tablets containing hormone are same (the content is not changed), these are called monophasic pills. On the other hand in biphasic pills the first 11 tablets have lesser progesterone and next 10 have higher progesterone. Similiarly in triphasic pills hormone content is changed thrice ie less hormone for first 6 days then slightly more progesterone for 7-11 days and still higher progesterone in 12-21 day tablet.

7. **Ans. (c) Triphasic pills**

8. **Ans. (c) Canagliflozin**
   The figure shows the mechanism of drug action to be sodium glucose cotransporter 2 (SGLT2) inhibition. This is done by canagliflozin, dapagliflozin and empagliflozin.

9. **Ans. (b) Vildagliptin**
   The figure shows the drug action to be inhibition of enzyme DPP4. This mechanism is possessed by sitagliptin, vildagliptin like drugs.

10. **Ans. (c) Denosumab**
    Denosumab is a monoclonal antibody against RANK ligand. It inhibit interaction of RANK with its ligand on the surface of osteoclasts and thus prevents its activation.

11. **Ans. (a) A**
    The patient is having neutropenia and the drug most likely being discussed about is ticlopidine. Clopidogrel and ticlopidine act as ADP antagonists. Ticlopidine is rarely used due to the occurrence of serious side effects like neutropenia that typically presents with fever and mouth ulcers. Though this is rare, it is a serious complication and complete blood count should be monitored biweekly for the first three months.

12. **Ans. (b) B**
    This is a case of diabetic coma due to diabetic ketoacidosis (DKA). The insulin of choice for DKA is regular insulin by intravenous route. Curve A shows rapidly acting inslulins like aspart, glulisine and lispro (onset in 15-20 min.). However, these are given by subcutaneous route and not the first choice in diabetic ketoacidosis. Curve B represents regular insulin that can be given IV and is insulin of choice for DKA. Curve C represents ultralente and curve D represents insulin glargine.

Endocrinology

Multiple Choice Questions

PITUITARY AND HYPOTHALAMUS

1. Nonpulsatile dose of GnRH agonist is used in all of the following conditions *except*: *(NEET Pattern 2020)*
   (a) Endometriosis   (b) Male infertility
   (c) Central precocious puberty
   (d) Prostate cancer

2. Which of the following hormone is/are under inhibitory control of hypothalamus? *(AIIMS Nov. 2018)*
   (a) Prolactin
   (b) Only prolactin
   (c) Only growth hormone
   (d) Both prolactin and growth hormone

3. Bromocriptine can be used in all of the following conditions *except*: *(NEET Pattern Question 2016-17)*
   (a) Hyperprolactinoma   (b) Acromegaly
   (c) Parkinsonism   (d) Diabetes insipidus

4. Bromocriptine is used in treatment of: *(NEET Pattern Question 2016-17)*
   (a) Diabetes mellitus   (b) Epilepsy
   (c) Schizophrenia   (d) Esophageal varices

5. Octreotide is used for: *(NEET Pattern Question 2016-17)*
   (a) Acromegaly   (b) Osteoarthritis
   (c) Pancreatitis   (d) Constipation

6. A 27-year-old female presented to OPD of infertility clinic. She was prescribed bromocriptine. What could be the possible reason? *(AIIMS Nov 2017)*
   (a) Hyperprolactinemia
   (b) Polycystic ovarian disease
   (c) Hypogonadotropic hypogonadism
   (d) Pelvic inflammatory disease

7. Drug of choice for precocious puberty in girls is:
   (a) GnRH analogue   *(AIIMS Nov 2016)*
   (b) Danazol
   (c) Cyproterone acetate
   (d) Medroxy progesterone acetate

8. Which of the following pairs of drug and its indications is matched incorrectly? *(AIIMS May 2014)*
   (a) Carbamazepine — Syndrome of inappropriate ADH secretion
   (b) Octreotide — Treatment of diarrhea associated with vasoactive intestinal peptide tumors
   (c) Desmopressin — Treatment of diabetes insipidus
   (d) hCG — Treatment of infertility in men and women

9. Which of the following is not an adverse effect of growth hormone therapy? *(AIIMS May 2012)*
   (a) Carpal tunnel syndrome
   (b) Hypoglycemia
   (c) Intracranial hypertension
   (d) Slipped femoral epiphysis

10. Which of the following is used in the treatment of hyperprolactinemia? *(AIIMS May 2012)*
    (a) Cimetidine   (b) Methysergide
    (c) Bromocriptine   (d) Ondansetron

11. Long acting dopamine agonist is: *(Recent NEET Pattern Question)*
    (a) Bromocriptine   (b) Lisuride
    (c) Cabergoline   (d) Apomorphine

12. Bromocriptine is useful in all *except*:
    (a) Parkinsonism   *(Recent NEET Pattern Question)*
    (b) Prolactinoma
    (c) Endogenous depression
    (d) Infertility

13. Drugs used for treatment of acute variceal bleeding are all *except*: *(Recent NEET Pattern Question)*
    (a) Octreotide   (b) Somatostatin
    (c) Desmopressin   (d) Terlipressin

14. GnRH analogue used in hormonal treatment of carcinoma prostate is: *(Recent NEET Pattern Question)*
    (a) Goserelin   (b) Nilutamide
    (c) Cyproterone acetate   (d) Finasteride

15. Which of the following is given at intervals as a pulsatile therapy? *(Recent NEET Pattern Question)*
    (a) GnRH   (b) GH
    (c) FSH   (d) Estrogen

16. True regarding use of bromocriptine for suppression of lactation includes: *(Recent NEET Pattern Question)*
    (a) It can cause deep vein thrombosis
    (b) It can cause hypotension
    (c) Metoclopramide potentiates the action of bromocriptine
    (d) It is given for 1 week only

17. The clinical use of leuprolide include all the following *except*: *(Recent NEET Pattern Question)*
    (a) Endometriosis   (b) Osteoporosis
    (c) Prostate cancer   (d) Precocious puberty

18. LHRH analogue used in breast cancer is: *(Recent NEET Pattern Question)*
    (a) Cetrorelix   (b) Anastrozole
    (c) Leuprolide   (d) Tamoxifen

19. Which of the following drug is a dopamine receptor agonist? *(Recent NEET Pattern Question)*
    (a) Methyl dopa   (b) Bromocriptine
    (c) Haloperidol   (d) Morphine

20. All are true statements regarding octreotide *except*: *(Recent NEET Pattern Question)*
    (a) Somatostatin analogue
    (b) Used in refractory diarrhea in AIDS
    (c) Used in carcinoid syndrome
    (d) An absorbent

21. cAMP is second messenger for the following *except*:
 (Recent NEET Pattern Question)
 (a) TSH (b) Insulin
 (c) LH (d) FSH

22. Which of the following is preferred for infertility treatment of a female with increased prolactin levels?
 (Recent NEET Pattern Question)
 (a) Dopamine (b) Carbidopa
 (c) Cabergoline (d) Bromocriptine

23. Female with secondary amenorrhea with serum prolactin level 75 ng/mL is to be treated with:
 (Recent NEET Pattern Question)
 (a) Cabergoline (b) Ganirelix
 (c) Clomiphene (d) Estradiol

24. Bromocriptine is indicated in the following conditions *except*: *(Recent NEET Pattern Question)*
 (a) Prolactin—secreting adenomas
 (b) Prolactin deficiency
 (c) Amenorrhea—Galactorrhea
 (d) Acromegaly

25. Bromocriptine: *(Recent NEET Pattern Question)*
 (a) Inhibits prolactin release
 (b) Inhibits adrenalin synthesis
 (c) Inhibits insulin synthesis
 (d) Inhibits thyroid synthesis

26. Somatostatin secreted by which type of cells in pancreas?
 (Recent NEET Pattern Question)
 (a) Gamma cells (b) Delta cells
 (c) Alpha cells (d) Beta cells

27. Bromocriptine is indicated in the following *except*:
 (Recent NEET Pattern Question)
 (a) Parkinsonism (b) Galactorrhoea
 (c) Acromegaly (d) Hypothyroidism

28. Octreotide is given in all the following conditions *except*:
 (Recent NEET Pattern Question)
 (a) Bleeding esophageal varices
 (b) Secretory diarrhea
 (c) Infective diarrhea
 (d) Acromegaly

29. Drug of choice for bleeding oesophageal varices is:
 (Recent NEET Pattern Question)
 (a) Ethanolamine oleate (b) Octreotide
 (c) Propranolol (d) Phytonadione

THYROID

30. What is the major mechanism of action of propylthiouracil in hyperthyridism? *(NEET Pattern Question 2016-17)*
 (a) Helps in peripheral conversion of T4 to T3
 (b) Inhibit the enzyme thyroid peroxidase
 (c) Inhibits the hormone release
 (d) Inhibits iodine uptake

31. Anti-thyroid drug comparatively safe in 1st trimester of pregnancy is: *(NEET Pattern Question 2016-17)*
 (a) Propylthiouracil (b) Carbimazole
 (c) Methimazole (d) Amiodarone

32. All of the following are rare but life-threatening adverse effects of thioamide group of anti-thyroid drugs *except*:
 (AIIMS Nov 2016)
 (a) Agranulocytosis (b) Aplasia anemia
 (c) Liver toxicity (d) Lung fibrosis

33. Which of the following statements about iodine is false?
 (AIIMS Nov 2013)
 (a) Contraindicated in hyperthyroidism
 (b) Causes iodism
 (c) Inhibits the release of thyroxine
 (d) Inhibits the synthesis of iodo thyroxine and iodo thyronine

34. Which of the following is not used in the management of thyroid storm? *(Recent NEET Pattern Question)*
 (a) Potassium iodide
 (b) Reserpine
 (c) Propranolol
 (d) Calcium channel blockers

35. Plasma half life of carbimazole is:
 (Recent NEET Pattern Question)
 (a) 4 hours (b) 8 hours
 (c) 16 hours (d) 24 hours

36. All are antithyroid drugs *except*:
 (Recent NEET Pattern Question)
 (a) Propylthiouracil (b) Methimazole
 (c) Carbimazole (d) Carbamazepine

37. L-Thyroxine is used in: *(Recent NEET Pattern Question)*
 (a) Thyroid storm (b) Cretinism
 (c) Endemic goiter (d) Grave's disease

38. Safest treatment of hyperthyroidism in pregnant women is: *(Recent NEET Pattern Question)*
 (a) Radioactive iodine (b) Methimazole
 (c) Carbimazole (d) Propylthiouracil

39. All can cause hypothyroidism *except*:
 (Recent NEET Pattern Question)
 (a) PAS (b) Captopril
 (c) Lithium (d) Amiodarone

40. Conversion of T_4 to T_3 inhibition is associated with:
 (Recent NEET Pattern Question)
 (a) Propylthiouracil (b) Ampicillin
 (c) Lithium (d) Carbimazole

41. Drug which inhibits conversion of T_4 to T_3 is:
 (Recent NEET Pattern Question)
 (a) Carbimazole (b) Methimazole
 (c) Propylthiouracil (d) Lugol's iodine

42. Which of the following decreases thyroid hormone on a long term basis? *(Recent NEET Pattern Question)*
 (a) T_4 (b) I^{131}
 (c) Calcitriol (d) Fluorouracil

43. Fastest acting antithyroid drug is:
 (Recent NEET Pattern Question)
 (a) Potassium iodide (b) Propylthiouracil
 (c) Carbimazole (d) Cholestyramine

44. Lugol's Iodine contains: *(Recent NEET Pattern Question)*
 (a) 5% iodine & 10% KI (b) 10% iodine & 20% KI
 (c) 10% iodine & 15% KI (d) 5% iodine & 15% KI

Endocrinology

45. Thyroid gland function is best monitored by which of the following? *(Recent NEET Pattern Question)*
    (a) Basal metabolic rate (BMR)
    (b) Thyroxine and tri-iodothyronine uptake
    (c) Level of thyroid stimulating hormone
    (d) Level of protein bound iodine

46. The management of thyrotoxic crisis includes all the following *except*: *(Recent NEET Pattern Question)*
    (a) Propranolol (b) Hydrocortisone
    (c) Oral I^{131} (d) Propylthiouracil

47. Which of the following drugs is used to control tachycardia and palpitations in persons with acute symptoms of hyperthyroidism? *(Recent NEET Pattern Question)*
    (a) Liothyronine
    (b) Propranolol
    (c) Methimazole
    (d) Potassium iodide solution

48. Deaths from lactic acidosis in diabetes mellitus is associated with therapy with which one of the following? *(Recent NEET Pattern Question)*
    (a) Metformin (b) Tolbutamide
    (c) Phenformin (d) Glipizide

49. Lugol's iodine is given to the patient: *(Recent NEET Pattern Question)*
    (a) Before surgery (b) After surgery
    (c) During surgery (d) Adjuvant therapy

50. Orally active hormone is: *(Recent NEET Pattern Question)*
    (a) TSH (b) Thyroxine
    (c) GH (d) Prolactin

51. Drug of choice for the treatment of hyperthyroidism in pregnancy is: *(Recent NEET Pattern Question)*
    (a) Propylthiouracil (b) Radio iodine
    (c) Carbimazole (d) Iodides

52. Thyroxine is used in the treatment of which thyroid cancer? *(Recent NEET Pattern Question)*
    (a) Medullary (b) Radiation induced
    (c) Anaplastic (d) Papillary

53. All of the following reduce T_4 absorption *except*: *(Recent NEET Pattern Question)*
    (a) Metformin (b) Iron salts
    (c) Raloxifene (d) Colsevelam

PANCREAS AND DIABETES MELLITUS

54. Which of the following is/are adverse effect of SGLT2 inhibitors? *(AIIMS Nov. 2019)*
    1. Ketoacidosis 2. Urosepsis
    3. Fourniers gangrene 4. Angioedema
    (a) 1, 2 and 4 are correct (b) 1, 2 and 3 are correct
    (c) Only 4 is correct (d) All are correct

55. True statement about teduglutide is: *(Recent Question 2019)*
    (a) It is effective orally
    (b) It is GLP2 agonist
    (c) It is a pancreatic enzyme
    (d) It is shorter acting because of degradation by dipeptidylpeptidase 4.

56. Mechanism of action of Sulfonylureas is: *(Recent Question 2016-17)*
    (a) Increases insulin release from pancreas
    (b) Increases insulin sensitivity
    (c) Increases to glucose uptake from blood
    (d) Decreases glucose absorption

57. Which of the following drug is used mainly to lower post-prandial blood glucose levels? *(Recent Question 2016-17)*
    (a) Sitagliptin (b) Acarbose
    (c) Repaglinide (d) Sulfonylurea

58. Which of the following drug can be used in treatment of both type 1 as well as type 2 diabetes mellitus? *(Recent Question 2016-17)*
    (a) Metformin (b) Rapaglinide
    (c) Pramlintide (d) Sitagliptin

59. Insulin of choice in a patient with diabetic ketoacidosis is: *(Recent Question 2016-17)*
    (a) Lispro (b) Aspart
    (c) Regular insulin (d) Glargine

60. Which of the following is the advantage of GLP-1 analogues over sulfonylureas? *(Recent Question 2016-17)*
    (a) They provide better glycemic control
    (b) They induce insulin release at low glucose concentration
    (c) These are effective orally
    (d) These have lesser risk of precipitating hypoglycemia in normoglycemic patients

61. Among anti-diabetic drugs which DPP-4 inhibitor requires dose reduction in both liver as well as renal disease? *(Recent Question 2016-17)*
    (a) Vildagliptin (b) Sitagliptin
    (c) Saxagliptin (d) Linagliptin

62. A diabetic and hypertensive patient taking several drugs presented with septicemia. Serum creatinine levels are 5.7 mg/dL. Which of the following drug should be stopped? *(AIIMS Nov 2017)*
    (a) Insulin (b) Metoprolol
    (c) Linagliptin (d) Metformin

63. A diabetic patient presented with uncontrolled blood sugar level. He has history of pancreatitis and family history of urinary bladder carcinoma. He is allergic to sulfonylureas and do not want to take injectable drugs. Which of the following drug can be added to control his blood sugar? *(AIIMS Nov 2017)*
    (a) Liraglutide (b) Sitagliptin
    (c) Canagliflozin (d) Glipizide

64. A 70-year-old patient has diabetes mellitus and hypertension. He presents with renal failure and does not want to take injectable drugs. Which anti-diabetic drug will you prefer in this patient that does not require dose modification in renal disease? *(AIIMS May 2017)*
    (a) Linagliptin (b) Vildagliptin
    (c) Exenatide (d) Metformin

65. **Components of lente insulin are:** *(AIIMS May 2017)*
    (a) 30% amorphus + 70% crystalline
    (b) Amorphous
    (c) 30% crystaline + 70% amorphus
    (d) Same as NPH insulin

66. **All are preferred sites of insulin administration** *except*:
    (AIIMS Nov 2016)
    (a) Thigh   (b) Buttocks
    (c) Dorsum of arm   (d) Around umbilicus

67. **A well-known complication of metformin therapy is lactic acidosis. All are risk factors for increased lactic acidosis in patient on metformin therapy** *except*:
    (AIIMS Nov 2016)
    (a) Advanced age   (b) Liver dysfunction
    (c) Renal dysfunction (d) Smoking

68. **Which of the following anti-diabetic drugs does not need dose reduction in a patient with renal disease?**
    (AIIMS Nov 2016)
    (a) Sitagliptin   (b) Linagliptin
    (c) Vildagliptin (d) Saxagliptin

69. **All of the following antidiabetic drugs act by enhancing insulin secretion** *except*: *(AIIMS May 2015)*
    (a) Exenatide   (b) Sitagliptin
    (c) Rosiglitazone (d) Repaglinide

70. **Which of the following is secreted by beta cells of pancreas along with insulin?** *(AIIMS May 2015)*
    (a) Somatostatin   (b) Amylin
    (c) Pancreatic polypeptide (d) Glucose like peptide

71. **Which of the following anti-diabetic drugs can cause vitamin B_{12} deficiency?** *(AI 2012)*
    (a) Glipizide   (b) Acarbose
    (c) Metformin   (d) Pioglitazone

72. **Insulin causes:** *(Recent NEET Pattern Question)*
    (a) Na^+ entry into cells   (b) K^+ exit from cells
    (c) Na^+ exit/K^+ entry   (d) K^+ entry into cells

73. **Which of the following is not used for the treatment of insulin induced hypoglycemia?**
    (Recent NEET Pattern Question)
    (a) Intravenous glucose (b) Glucagon
    (c) Adrenaline   (d) Oral carbohydrates

74. **Sulfonylureas act by:** *(Recent NEET Pattern Question)*
    (a) Decreasing glucagon secretion from pancreas
    (b) Decreasing insulin secretion from pancreas
    (c) Increasing gluconeogenesis
    (d) Increasing insulin secretion from pancreas

75. **Flushing is common in patient taking which of the following oral hypoglycemic drug with alcohol?**
    (Recent NEET Pattern Question)
    (a) Chlorpropamide (b) Phenformin
    (c) Glibenclamide (d) Tolazamide

76. **Anti-diabetic effect of sulfonylureas is by reducing:**
    (a) Glucagon production *(Recent NEET Pattern Question)*
    (b) Insulin secretion
    (c) Tissue sensitivity to insulin
    (d) Tissue sensitivity to glycogen

77. **Lactic acidosis is common in:**
    (Recent NEET Pattern Question)
    (a) Metformin   (b) Phenformin
    (c) Repaglinide (d) Rosiglitazone

78. **Tolbutamide acts by increasing:**
    (Recent NEET Pattern Question)
    (a) Insulin receptors   (b) Glucose entry
    (c) Glucose absorption (d) Insulin secretion

79. **Adverse effects of insulin include all of the following** *except*: *(Recent NEET Pattern Question)*
    (a) Edema   (b) Hyperglycaemia
    (c) Lipodystrophy (d) Allergy

80. **Long acting insulin is:** *(Recent NEET Pattern Question)*
    (a) Lente   (b) Semilente
    (c) Ultralente (d) Lispro insulin

81. **2nd generation sulfonylurea drugs are all** *except*:
    (Recent NEET Pattern Question)
    (a) Glipizide   (b) Gliclazide
    (c) Tolbutamide (d) Glibenclamide

82. **Which of the following drug is alpha-glucosidase inhibitor?** *(Recent NEET Pattern Question)*
    (a) Pioglitazone (b) Miglitol
    (c) Metformin   (d) Nateglinide

83. **Monotherapy with which of the following antidiabetic drug can cause hypoglycemia?**
    (Recent NEET Pattern Question)
    (a) Metformin   (b) Glibenclamide
    (c) Pioglitazone (d) All of the above

84. **Which of the following is not a starting criteria for sulfonylurea therapy?** *(Recent NEET Pattern Question)*
    (a) Total pancreatectomy (b) NIDDM
    (c) Diabetes after 60 years (d) None

85. **Oral hypoglycemic drug that is less likely to cause hypoglycemia is:** *(Recent NEET Pattern Question)*
    (a) Repaglinide   (b) Gliclazide
    (c) Rosiglitazone (d) Glimipiride

86. **All of the following are true regarding chlorpropamide** *except*: *(Recent NEET Pattern Question)*
    (a) It is short acting
    (b) It can cause hypoglycemia in elderly
    (c) Causes weight gain
    (d) Associated with alcoholic flush

87. **Common side effect of thiazolidinediones is:**
    (a) Dysguesia *(Recent NEET Pattern Question)*
    (b) Hypoglycemia
    (c) Water retention with weight gain
    (d) Anemia

88. **Long acting insulin preparations are frequently administered by:** *(Recent NEET Pattern Question)*
    (a) Oral route   (b) Intramuscular route
    (c) Intradermal route (d) Subcutaneous route

89. **Glipizide, the oral hypoglycaemic drug acts by:**
    (Recent NEET Pattern Question)
    (a) Improving insulin resistance
    (b) Inhibiting brush border enzyme
    (c) Helps in insulin secretion
    (d) Increased glucose uptake by fat cells

Endocrinology

90. Which is an intermediate acting insulin?
    (Recent NEET Pattern Question)
    (a) Insulin lispro   (b) Regular insulin
    (c) NPH insulin   (d) Insulin glargine

91. Which of the following does not cause insulin release?
    (Recent NEET Pattern Question)
    (a) Rosiglitazone   (b) Nateglinide
    (c) Glimipiride   (d) Tolbutamide

92. Which of the following can cause lactic acidosis?
    (Recent NEET Pattern Question)
    (a) Biguanides   (b) Glibenclamide
    (c) Tolbutamide   (d) Chlorpropamide

93. Glucagon is most effective for which of the following conditions? *(Recent NEET Pattern Question)*
    (a) Cocaine intake with BP of 180/110 mmHg
    (b) Old man with decreased BP/decreased heart rate due to atenolol
    (c) Old man with type 2 diabetes mellitus and no glipizide for 4 days
    (d) Female with lactic acidosis due to shock

94. Which insulin is never mixed with other insulins?
    (a) Lente   *(Recent NEET Pattern Question)*
    (b) Aspart
    (c) Lispro
    (d) Glargine

95. Insulin release due to closure of K⁺ channels is seen with:
    (Recent NEET Pattern Question)
    (a) Nateglinde   (b) Acarbose
    (c) Exenatide   (d) Sitagliptin

96. Drug used to control postprandial hyperglycemia is:
    (Recent NEET Pattern Question)
    (a) Acarbose   (b) Biguanides
    (c) Sulfonylurea   (d) Repaglinide

97. Long acting insulin is: *(Recent NEET Pattern Question)*
    (a) Insulin glargine   (b) Insulin lispro
    (c) Insulin aspart   (d) Insulin glulisine

98. Which of the following is not an insulin analogue?
    (Recent NEET Pattern Question)
    (a) Insulin glargine   (b) Insulin lispro
    (c) Actrapid   (d) Insulin aspart

99. Which of the following does not cause hypoglycemia?
    (Recent NEET Pattern Question)
    (a) Insulin   (b) Glimepiride
    (c) Metformin   (d) Gliclazide

100. Sulphonylureas act by: *(Recent NEET Pattern Question)*
    (a) Reducing the absorption of carbohydrate from the gut
    (b) Stimulating the beta islet cells of pancreas to release insulin
    (c) Increasing the uptake of glucose in peripheral tissue
    (d) Reducing the hepatic gluconeogenesis

101. All of the following drugs used in the management of diabetes mellitus cause hypoglycemia *except*:
    (Recent NEET Pattern Question)
    (a) Metformin   (b) Tolbutamide
    (c) Glibenclamide   (d) Glipizide

102. Which of the following drugs used to treat type II diabetes mellitus causes weight loss?
    (Recent NEET Pattern Question)
    (a) Metformin   (b) Glimepiride
    (c) Repaglinide   (d) Gliclazide

103. Most important step in management of diabetic ketoacidosis is administration of:
    (Recent NEET Pattern Question)
    (a) Insulin
    (b) Intravenous fluids (saline)
    (c) Soda-bicarbonate
    (d) Potassium

104. The following insulin can be given intravenously:
    (Recent NEET Pattern Question)
    (a) Protamine zinc insulin
    (b) Ultra lente insulin
    (c) Semi lente insulin
    (d) Regular insulin

CORTICOSTEROIDS

105. An 18-month-old child with ambiguous genitalia presented to the hospital, his BP is 118/78 mm Hg, Serum K is 6 mEq/L, serum sodium is 120 mEq/L. Patient was started on intravenous fluids. What additional specific therapy will you add? *(AIIMS Nov. 2019)*
    (a) Hydrocortisone
    (b) Potassium binding resin
    (c) Digoxin
    (d) Calcium gluconate

106. Which of the following drug is a corticosteroid synthesis inhibitor? *(NEET Pattern Question 2017-2018)*
    (a) Metyrapone   (b) Finasteride
    (c) Flutamide   (d) Mifepristone

107. Which of the following drug is not used in treatment of Cushing's disease? *(NEET Pattern Question 2016-17)*
    (a) Ketoconazole   (b) Spironolactone
    (c) Metyrapone   (d) Mifepristone

108. Which of the following is a non-inhalational steroid?
    (NEET Pattern Question 2016-17)
    (a) Budesonide   (b) Fluticasone
    (c) Mometasone   (d) Dexamethasone

109. Least glucocorticoid activity is found in:
    (NEET Pattern Question 2016-17)
    (a) Fludrocortisone   (b) Dexamethasone
    (c) Aldosterone   (d) DOCA

110. Which of the following regimen of antenatal steroids is preferred for fetal lung maturation? *(AIIMS Nov 2016)*
    (a) Dexamethasone 6 mg 12 hourly 4 doses
    (b) Betamethasone 6 mg 12 hourly 4 doses
    (c) Dexamethasone 12 mg 12 hourly 4 doses
    (d) Betamethasone 12 mg 12 hourly 4 doses

111. Steroids are used in all of the following conditions *except*:
    (AIIMS Nov 2015)
    (a) Chronic Lymphoid Leukemia
    (b) Hodgkin's lymphoma
    (c) Multiple myeloma
    (d) Kaposi's sarcoma

112. All of the following are seen in adrenal insufficiency except: *(AIIMS Nov 2015)*
    (a) Hyperkalemia   (b) Fever
    (c) Weight gain   (d) Postural hypotension

113. Dose of dexamethasone given to mother in anticipated preterm delivery: *(AIIMS May 2015)*
    (a) 12 mg 12 hourly 2 doses
    (b) 12 mg 24 hourly 4 doses
    (c) 6 mg 24 hourly 2 doses
    (d) 6 mg 12 hourly 4 doses

114. The most potent topical corticosteroid is: *(Recent NEET Pattern Question)*
    (a) Hydrocortisone butyrate cream 0.1%
    (b) Betamethasone valerate cream 0.5%
    (c) Clobetasol propionate cream 0.5%
    (d) Clobetasone butyrate cream 0.5%

115. Steroids are indicated in all of the following forms of tuberculosis except: *(Recent NEET Pattern Question)*
    (a) Meningitis   (b) Pericarditis
    (c) Ileo-caecal tuberculosis (d) Adrenal involvement

116. Which is not true about beclomethasone? *(Recent NEET Pattern Question)*
    (a) Indicated for chronic use
    (b) Inhalational steroid
    (c) Effective in acute asthma
    (d) Predispose to fungal infections

117. Most potent mineralocorticoid is: *(Recent NEET Pattern Question)*
    (a) Aldosterone   (b) DOCA
    (c) Fludrocortisone (d) Triamcinolone

118. All are side effects of steroids except: *(Recent NEET Pattern Question)*
    (a) Skin atrophy   (b) Telengectasia
    (c) Folliculitis   (d) Photosensitivity

119. Systemic steroids can cause all of the following except: *(Recent NEET Pattern Question)*
    (a) Hypertension   (b) Glaucoma
    (c) Cataract   (d) Osteoporosis

120. Compared to hydrocortisone maximum glucocorticoid action is found in: *(Recent NEET Pattern Question)*
    (a) Dexamethasone   (b) Prednisolone
    (c) Methyl prednisolone (d) Cortisone

121. Steroids are contraindicated in all, except: *(Recent NEET Pattern Question)*
    (a) Diabetes mellitus
    (b) Hypertension
    (c) Eczematous skin disease
    (d) Peptic ulcer disease

122. In Addison's disease drug to be given is: *(Recent NEET Pattern Question)*
    (a) Hydrocortisone   (b) Betamethasone
    (c) Prednisolone   (d) DOCA

123. Corticosteroids cause all except: *(Recent NEET Pattern Question)*
    (a) Muscular hypertrophy
    (b) Peptic ulceration
    (c) Psychosis
    (d) Suppression of pituitary-adrenal axis

124. Glucocorticoids with mineralocorticoids activity is seen in: *(Recent NEET Pattern Question)*
    (a) Triamcinolone   (b) Betamethasone
    (c) Cortisol   (d) Dexamethosone

125. Which of the following antifungal drug can be used in the treatment of Cushing syndrome? *(Recent NEET Pattern Question)*
    (a) Ketoconazole   (b) Fluconazole
    (c) Itraconazole   (d) Miconazole

126. All of the following glucocorticoids lack mineralocorticoid activity, except: *(Recent NEET Pattern Question)*
    (a) Beclomethasone   (b) Triamcinolone
    (c) Prednisolone   (d) Dexamethasone

127. All of the following are side effects of steroids except: *(Recent NEET Pattern Question)*
    (a) Hyperglycemia   (b) Infection
    (c) Osteomalacia   (d) Peptic ulcer

128. All are side effects of steroids except: *(Recent NEET Pattern Question)*
    (a) Diabetes   (b) Osteoporosis
    (c) Fragile skin   (d) Hypotension

129. Anti-inflammatory action of corticosteroids is due to blocking of: *(Recent NEET Pattern Question)*
    (a) 15 lipoxygenase
    (b) Prostaglandin synthetase
    (c) Thromboxane synthetase
    (d) Break down of phospholipids

130. Which of the following is used for medical adrenalectomy? *(Recent NEET Pattern Question)*
    (a) Mitotane   (b) Methotrerate
    (c) Doxorubicin   (d) 5-Fluorouracil

131. Which of the following is the side effect of steroids due to its mineralocorticoid component? *(Recent NEET Pattern Question)*
    (a) Skin striae   (b) Hypertension
    (c) Osteoporosis   (d) Moon face

132. Side effect of steroids are all except: *(Recent NEET Pattern Question)*
    (a) Hypoglycemia
    (b) Hypertension
    (c) Psychosis
    (d) Growth retardation

133. Which one has least mineralocorticoid activity? *(Recent NEET Pattern Question)*
    (a) Cortisol   (b) Prednisolone
    (c) Fludrocortisone (d) Methyl prednisolone

134. Steroids cause: *(Recent NEET Pattern Question)*
    (a) Increased TSH
    (b) Increased FSH
    (c) Prevent de-iodination
    (d) All of the above

135. In which of the following disease is corticosteroids indicated? *(Recent NEET Pattern Question)*
    (a) Osteoporosis
    (b) Peptic ulcer
    (c) Collagen vascular diseases
    (d) Tuberculosis

136. Long-term ingestion of steroids lead to all of the following except: *(Recent NEET Pattern Question)*
    (a) Avascular necrosis of head of femur
    (b) Cataract
    (c) Glaucoma
    (d) Growth retardation

137. Which of the following agents has the least glucocorticoid action? *(Recent NEET Pattern Question)*
    (a) Fludrocortisone (b) Cortisone
    (c) Dexamethasone (d) Betamethasone

138. Steroid with 12-36 hrs half life is: *(Recent NEET Pattern Question)*
    (a) Betamethasone (b) Prednisolone
    (d) Hydrocortisone (d) Dexamethasone

139. Compared to hydrocortisone, maximum glucocorticoid activity is seen in: *(Recent NEET Pattern Question)*
    (a) Cortisone (b) Prednisolone
    (c) Dexamethasone (d) Methylprednisolone

140. Drug of choice for acute adrenal insufficiency is: *(Recent NEET Pattern Question)*
    (a) Oral prednisone (b) IV hydrocortisone
    (c) IV betamethasone (d) IV dexamethasone

141. All of the following are topical steroids except: *(Recent NEET Pattern Question)*
    (a) Hydrocortisone valerate
    (b) Fluticasone propionate
    (c) Triamcinolone
    (d) Prednisolone

142. Corticosteroid with maximum sodium retaning potential is: *(Recent NEET Pattern Question)*
    (a) Dexamethasone (b) Prednisolone
    (c) Aldosterone (d) Betamethasone

143. Long term administration of glucocorticoids can cause all of the following except: *(Recent NEET Pattern Question)*
    (a) Proximal myopathy (b) Hyperkalemia
    (c) Hypertension (d) Cataract

144. The primary goal of glucocorticoid treatment in rheumatoid arthritis is: *(Recent NEET Pattern Question)*
    (a) Suppression of inflammation and improvement in functional capacity
    (b) Reversal of the degenerative process
    (c) Development of a sense of well-being in the patient
    (d) Prevention of suppression of the hypothalamic-pituitary-adrenal axis

145. Which of the following drugs causes osteoporosis on long term use? *(Recent NEET Pattern Question)*
    (a) Etidronate (b) Prednisolone
    (c) Phenytoin (d) Calcitriol

146. All of the following therapeutic uses of corticosteroids are appropriate except: *(Recent NEET Pattern Question)*
    (a) Beclomethasone in bronchial asthma
    (b) Cortisone for Cushing's syndrome
    (c) Prednisolone for Rheumatoid arthritis
    (d) Dexamethasone for reducing intracranial pressure

147. A 35 years old male with long standing disseminated TB presents in a emaciated state with following features:
    • BP = 85/60 mmHg
    • Low volume pulse of 100 BPM
    • Diffuse hyperpigmentation that involves hand creases
    • Serum Na^+ = 120 mEq/L (N = 136-146 mEq/L)
    • Serum K^+ = 6.6 mEq/L)
    Your most immediate response would be: *(Recent NEET Pattern Question)*
    (a) To suspect secondary hyperaldosteronism and start IV steroids
    (b) To suspect gram negative sepsis and start IV antibiotics
    (c) To suspect adrenocortical insufficiency and start IV steroids
    (d) To suspect massive pulmonary thromboembolism and start IV Heparin

148. The most potent topical corticosteroid is: *(Recent NEET Pattern Question)*
    (a) Betamethasone valerate
    (b) Triamcinolone acetonide
    (c) Hydrocortisone acetate
    (d) Clobetasol butyrate

149. Longest acting glucocorticoids is: *(Recent NEET Pattern Question)*
    (a) Prednisone (b) Prednisolone
    (c) Cortisone (d) Dexamethasone

OSTEOPOROSIS AND CALCIUM METABOLISM

150. Drug of choice for postmenopausal osteoporosis is: *(NEET Pattern 2020)*
    (a) Estrogen (b) Bisphosphonates
    (c) Teriparatide (d) Thyroxine

151. Bone resorption is not decreased by: *(NEET Pattern Question 2017-2018)*
    (a) Teriparatide (b) Strontium ranelate
    (c) Alendronate (d) Raloxifene

152. Which of the following drug is not used in osteoporosis? *(AIIMS Nov 2016)*
    (a) PTH (b) Milnacipran
    (c) Strontium ranelate (d) Denosumab

153. Immediate treatment of hypercalcemia of malignancy is: *(AIIMS May 2016)*
    (a) IV fluids (b) Bisphosphonates
    (c) Calcitonin (d) Glucocorticoids

154. Bisphosphonates are prescribed to a patient with the following advice: *(AIIMS Nov 2015)*
    (a) Take empty stomach with plenty of water
    (b) Take after meals
    (c) Discontinue if gastritis develops
    (d) Discontinue if severe bone pain occurs

155. Bone resorption is enhanced by: *(Recent NEET Pattern Question)*
    (a) PGD_2 (b) PDF_2
    (c) PGE_2 (d) PGI_2

156. Calcitonin causes hypocalcemia by: *(Recent NEET Pattern Question)*
    (a) Inhibiting bone resorption
    (b) Promoting osteolysis
    (c) Decreasing renal tubular reabsorption of calcium
    (d) Decreasing absorption of phosphorus

157. Correct statement about mode of administration of pamidronate: *(Recent NEET Pattern Question)*
    (a) IV
    (b) Orally
    (c) IM
    (d) SC

158. Bisphosphonates act by: *(Recent NEET Pattern Question)*
    (a) Increasing the osteoid formation
    (b) Infreasing the mineralization of osteoid
    (c) Decreasing the osteoclast mediated resorption of bone
    (d) Decreasing the parathyroid hormone secretion

159. Which is the fastest calcium lowering agents?
    (Recent NEET Pattern Question)
    (a) Calcitonin
    (b) Plicamycin
    (c) Etidronate
    (d) Zoledronate

160. Prevention or treatment of osteoporosis in post-menopausal women may be achieved by all *except*:
    (a) Estrogen and progesterone hormone replacement therapy *(Recent NEET Pattern Question)*
    (b) Calcium and vitamin D supplementation
    (c) Bisphosphonates
    (d) Multivitamins

161. Which of the following is a topical vitamin D analogue?
    (Recent NEET Pattern Question)
    (a) Cholecalciferol
    (b) Doxercalciferol
    (c) Calcipotriol
    (d) Paricalcitol

162. rPTH used in osteoporosis is:
    (Recent NEET Pattern Question)
    (a) Teriparatide
    (b) Denosumab
    (c) Calcitriol
    (d) Calcipotriol

163. Intranasal calcitonin is used for:
    (a) Paget's disease *(Recent NEET Pattern Question)*
    (b) MEN Syndrome
    (c) Hypercalcemia
    (d) Postmenopausal osteoporosis

164. Parathormone is useful in which of the following?
    (Recent NEET Pattern Question)
    (a) Hyperparathyroidism
    (b) Paget's disease
    (c) Osteoporosis
    (d) Osteomalacia

165. Bisphosphonates are not used in:
    (a) Paget's disease *(Recent NEET Pattern Question)*
    (b) Osteoporosis
    (c) Cancer induced osteolysis
    (d) Vitamin D intoxication

166. Bisphosphonate-induced osteomalacia is commonly seen with: *(Recent NEET Pattern Question)*
    (a) Alendronate
    (b) Pamidronate
    (c) Zolendronate
    (d) Etidronate

167. Vitamin beneficial in osteoporosis in combination with Vitamin D is: *(Recent NEET Pattern Question)*
    (a) Vitamin E
    (b) Vitamin A
    (c) Vitamin K
    (d) Vitamin B

168. Which of the following is not a treatment of osteoporosis?
    (Recent NEET Pattern Question)
    (a) Calcitriol
    (b) Androgen
    (c) Estrogen
    (d) Vitamin D

GONADAL HORMONES AND CONTRACEPTIVES

169. Which of the following is not used as emergency contraceptive? *(NEET Pattern 2020)*
    (a) Danazol
    (b) Levonorgestrel
    (c) Mifepristone
    (d) IUCD

170. Dose of ulipristal for emergency contraception is:
    (NEET Pattern Question 2019)
    (a) 30 mg
    (b) 30 mcg
    (c) 300 mg
    (c) 300 mcg

171. Fulvestrant is used in the treatment of:
    (NEET Pattern Question 2016-17)
    (a) ALL
    (b) Multiple myeloma
    (c) Breast Carcinoma
    (d) Prostate Carcinoma

172. Total dose of levnorgestrol for emergency contraception:
    (NEET Pattern Question 2016-17)
    (a) 1.5 mg single pill
    (b) 1.5 mg two pills
    (c) 7.5 mg single pills
    (d) 0.25 mg two pills

173. Most potent progesterone is:
    (NEET Pattern Question 2016-17)
    (a) Estranes
    (b) Levonorgestrel
    (c) Desogestrel
    (d) Gestodene

174. Tibolone is: *(NEET Pattern Question 2016-17)*
    (a) Estrogen receptor agonist that act on ER Alfa receptor
    (b) Estrogen receptor antagonist
    (c) Used in hormone replacement therapy designed to relieve menopausal symptoms
    (d) Aromatase inhibitor

175. Fulvestrant is used: *(NEET Pattern Question 2016-17)*
    (a) For hormone receptor (HR)-positive metastatic breast cancer in postmenopausal women
    (b) As a selective progesterone receptor modulator
    (c) In HRT
    (d) In male breast cancer

176. Which of the following drug can decrease the size of prostate? *(AIIMS Nov 2017)*
    (a) Tamsulosin
    (b) Sildenafil
    (c) Finasteride
    (d) Prazosin

177. WHO recommended dose of misoprostol for prophylaxis of post-partum hemorrhage is: *(AIIMS Nov 2016)*
    (a) 400 micrograms
    (b) 600 micrograms
    (c) 800 micrograms
    (d) 1000 micrograms

178. Ulipristal acetate is: *(AIIMS Nov 2015)*
    (a) GnRH agonist
    (b) Androgen antagonist
    (c) Selective estrogen receptor modulator
    (d) Selective progesterone receptor modulator

179. Which of these is not a non-contraceptive use of levonorgestrel? *(AIIMS Nov 2015)*
    (a) Endometriosis
    (b) Pre-menstrual Tension
    (c) Complex endometrial hyperplasia
    (d) Emergency contraception

180. All of these can be used for post-coital contraception except: *(AIIMS Nov 2015)*
    (a) Desogestrel
    (b) Copper-T
    (c) Levonorgestrel
    (d) Combined oral contraceptive pills

181. Which of the following drug is not used in the management of polycystic ovarian disease? *(AIIMS May 2015)*
    (a) Clomiphene
    (b) Tamoxifen
    (c) Oral contraceptives
    (d) Metformin

182. Hormone replacement therapy is beneficial for all of the following conditions except: *(AIIMS May 2013)*
    (a) Vaginal atrophy
    (b) Flushing
    (c) Osteoporosis
    (d) Coronary heart disease

183. Use of tamoxifen in carcinoma of breast patients does not lead to the following side effects: *(Recent NEET Pattern Question)*
    (a) Thromboembolic events
    (b) Endometrial carcinoma
    (c) Cataract
    (d) Cancer in opposite breast

184. Oral contraceptive pills can cause all except: *(Recent NEET Pattern Question)*
    (a) Mastalgia
    (b) Dysmenorrhea
    (c) Chloasma
    (d) Breakthrough bleeding

185. Side effects of oral contraceptives are all except: *(Recent NEET Pattern Question)*
    (a) Irregular bleeding
    (b) Headache
    (c) Thrombosis
    (d) Increased risk of ovarian cancer

186. All of the following are natural estrogens except: *(Recent NEET Pattern Question)*
    (a) Estradiol
    (b) Ethinylestradiol
    (c) Estriol
    (d) Estrone

187. Mechanism of action of tamoxifen is: *(Recent NEET Pattern Question)*
    (a) Has androgenic receptor blocking action
    (b) Inhibits enzyme 5 α-reductase
    (c) Has partial agonist and antagonist action on estrogen receptors
    (d) Inhibition of FSH and LH release from the pituitary

188. The progestogenic emergency contraceptive pills act by: *(Recent NEET Pattern Question)*
    (a) Altered cervical secretion
    (b) Inhibition of ovulation
    (c) Anti-implantation effect
    (d) Inhibition of LH secretion

189. Which one of the following agents inhibits spermatogenesis? *(Recent NEET Pattern Question)*
    (a) Gelusil
    (b) Gemcadiol
    (c) Gestodene
    (d) Gossypol

190. Which one of the following has both estrogenic and anti-estrogenic property? *(Recent NEET Pattern Question)*
    (a) Chlorpromazine
    (b) Clofibrate
    (c) Clomiphene
    (d) Clonidine

191. Tamoxifen is useful in: *(Recent NEET Pattern Question)*
    (a) Carcinoma prostate
    (b) Carcinoma ovary
    (c) Estrogen receptor positive breast carcinoma
    (d) Seminoma

192. Thromboembolism is due to which component of oral contraceptive pills? *(Recent NEET Pattern Question)*
    (a) Progesterone
    (b) Estrogen
    (c) Iron
    (d) FSH

193. An example of antiprogesterone is: *(Recent NEET Pattern Question)*
    (a) Gossypol
    (b) Atosiban
    (c) Clomiphene
    (d) Mifepristone (RU 486)

194. The drug used for first trimester abortion is: *(Recent NEET Pattern Question)*
    (a) Oral mifepristone
    (b) Intra-amniotic saline
    (c) Extra-amniotic ethacrydine lactate
    (d) Oxytocin infusion

195. "Oral contraceptive pills" protect against: *(Recent NEET Pattern Question)*
    (a) Thrombosis
    (b) Ovarian cancer
    (c) Cancer cervix
    (d) Hepatocellular adenoma

196. Mifepristone is a: *(Recent NEET Pattern Question)*
    (a) Progesterone antagonist
    (b) Oestrogen antagonist
    (c) Both
    (d) None

197. All are anti-androgens except: *(Recent NEET Pattern Question)*
    (a) Finasteride
    (b) Flutamide
    (c) Cyproterone acetate
    (d) Dihydrotestosterone

198. Oral contraceptive pill is useful in preventing all of the following except: *(Recent NEET Pattern Question)*
    (a) Carcinoma breast
    (b) Carcinoma ovary
    (c) Pelvic inflammatory disease
    (d) Anaemia

199. Oral contraceptive failure occurs with: *(Recent NEET Pattern Question)*
    (a) Phenytoin
    (b) Phenobarbitone
    (c) Rifampicin
    (d) All

200. Clomiphene citrate is used for: *(Recent NEET Pattern Question)*
    (a) Mania
    (b) Induction of ovulation
    (c) Depression
    (d) Psychosis

201. Which of the following is role of progestogens? *(Recent NEET Pattern Question)*
    (a) Inhibits ovulation
    (b) Protects against endometrial cancer
    (c) Causes prompt withdrawal bleeding
    (d) All

202. Which of the following is anti-androgenic drug? *(Recent NEET Pattern Question)*
    (a) Bicalutamide
    (b) Oxymetholone
    (c) Raloxifene
    (d) Stanozolol

203. Which among the following is not a SERM? *(Recent NEET Pattern Question)*
    (a) Flutamide (b) Ormeloxifen
    (c) Tamoxifen (d) Raloxifen

204. Following are the adverse effects of estrogens *except*: *(Recent NEET Pattern Question)*
    (a) Supression of libido
    (b) Fusion of epiphyses
    (c) Hot flushes
    (d) Gynaecomastia in males

205. All of the following are recognized effects of combined oral contraceptive *except*: *(Recent NEET Pattern Question)*
    (a) Breakthrough bleeding
    (b) Decreased risk of endometrial cancer
    (c) Increased risk of ischemic stroke
    (d) Increased risk of ovarian cancer

206. Which of the following is a selective progesterone receptor modulator? *(Recent NEET Pattern Question)*
    (a) Tamoxifen (b) Ulipristal
    (c) Nomegestrol (d) Toremifene

207. Combined oral contraceptive pills act mainly by: *(Recent NEET Pattern Question)*
    (a) Production of cervical mucus hostile to sperm penetration
    (b) Inhibition of ovulation
    (c) Making endometrium unsuitable for implantation
    (d) Enhancing uterine contractions to dislodge the fertilized ovum.

208. Which of the following is an anabolic steroid? *(Recent NEET Pattern Question)*
    (a) Methyltestosterone (b) Fluoxymesterone
    (c) Nandrolone (d) Danazol

209. Tibolone is a: *(Recent NEET Pattern Question)*
    (a) SSRI (b) SPRM
    (c) STEAR (d) SERM

210. Adverse effects of diethylstilbesterol when used in pregnant woman is: *(Recent NEET Pattern Question)*
    (a) Deep vein thrombosis in pregnant woman
    (b) Feminization of external genitalia of male offspring
    (c) Development of vaginal carcinoma in female offspring
    (d) Virilization of the external genitalia of female offspring

211. Which of the following is a synthetic estrogen? *(Recent NEET Pattern Question)*
    (a) Estrone (b) Estriol
    (c) Estradiol (d) Diethylstilbestrol

212. All are true about estrogen *except*: *(Recent NEET Pattern Question)*
    (a) Causes cholestasis
    (b) Used in treatment of gynaecomastia
    (c) Used in hormone replacement therapy
    (d) Increased risk of breast cancer

213. All of the following are uses of mifepristone *except*: *(Recent NEET Pattern Question)*
    (a) Termination of pregnancy
    (b) Post coital contraception
    (c) Post partum hemorrhage
    (d) Cushing's syndrome

214. Bicalutamide is a specific inhibitor of: *(Recent NEET Pattern Question)*
    (a) 5-alpha reductase (b) Androgen receptors
    (c) Aromatase (d) Estorgen receptor

215. An old man has enlarged prostate. Which of the following may be use to suppress his prostatic growth? *(Recent NEET Pattern Question)*
    (a) Spironolactone (b) Ketoconazole
    (c) Finasteride (d) Flutamide

216. Absolute contraindication of combined oral contraceptive pill is: *(Recent NEET Pattern Question)*
    (a) Epilepsy (b) Obesity
    (c) Smoking 10 cigars/day (d) Active liver disease

217. Which of the following is the principle disadvantage of depot progestin? *(Recent NEET Pattern Question)*
    (a) Weight gain
    (b) Breast tenderness
    (c) Depression
    (d) Irregular menstrual bleeding and prolonged anovulation

218. Combined oral pill reduces the risk of: *(Recent NEET Pattern Question)*
    (a) Breast cancer (b) Ovarian cancer
    (c) Cervical cancer (d) Vaginal cancer

219. Which one of the following is an adverse effect associated with combined oral contraceptives? *(Recent NEET Pattern Question)*
    (a) Cerebral stroke
    (b) Aggravation of asthma
    (c) Peripheral neuropathy
    (d) Nephrotic syndrome

220. Mifepristone (RU-486) is: *(Recent NEET Pattern Question)*
    (a) Anti-androgen (b) Anti-estrogen
    (c) Anti-progestin (d) Androgen

221. Which of the following is not a steroid? *(Recent NEET Pattern Question)*
    (a) 17 α Hydroxyprogesterone
    (b) Estrone
    (c) Pregnenolone
    (d) Relaxin

222. Hormone replacement therapy in postmenopausal women can aggravate: *(Recent NEET Pattern Question)*
    (a) Osteoporosis (b) Migraine
    (c) Hot flushes (d) All of the above

223. What is the correct administration of oral pills for post coital contraception? *(Recent NEET Pattern Question)*
    (a) Combined pills 2 immediately and 2 after 12 hrs
    (b) Combined pills 2 immediately and 2 after 48 hrs
    (c) Progesterone pills 2 immediately and 2 after 12 hrs
    (d) Progesterone pills 2 immediately and 2 after 48 hrs

DRUGS ACTING ON UTERUS AND MISCELLANEOUS

224. Mechanism of action of sildenafil is:
    (a) Aromatase inhibitor *(NEET Pattern Question 2016-17)*
    (b) 5 alpha reductase inhibitor
    (c) Phosphodiesterase 5 inhibitor
    (d) SERM

Endocrinology

225. Finasteride, a 5- alpha reductase inhibitor is used for the treatment of: *(NEET Pattern Question 2016-17)*
    (a) Impotance
    (b) Benign prostatic hyperplasia
    (c) Gynaecomastia
    (d) Depression

226. WHO recommended dose of misoprostol in the treatment of post partum hemorrhage is: *(AIIMS Nov 2015)*
    (a) 400 mcg oral
    (b) 600 mcg sublingual
    (c) 800 mcg sublingual
    (d) 1000 mcg oral

227. Dose of carbetocin for post partum hemorrhage is: *(AIIMS May 2015)*
    (a) 100 microgram intramuscular
    (b) 50 microgram intravenous
    (c) 150 microgram intravenous
    (d) 200 microgram intramuscular

228. All of these hormones use cAMP as second messenger *except*: *(AIIMS Nov 2009)*
    (a) Corticotropin
    (b) Dopamine
    (c) Glucagon
    (d) Vasopressin

229. Hypospadias in the baby is caused by maternal use of which of the following drug? *(AI 2012)*
    (a) Diethylstilbestrol
    (b) Tolbutamide
    (c) Clomiphene
    (d) Clobazam

230. Oxytocin causes all *except*: *(Recent NEET Pattern Question)*
    (a) Lactogenesis
    (b) Milk ejection
    (c) Contraction of uterine muscle
    (d) Myoepithelial cell contraction

231. Drug of choice for polycystic ovarian disease is: *(Recent NEET Pattern Question)*
    (a) Metformin
    (b) Estrogen
    (c) Estrogen and progesterone combination pill
    (d) Dopamine antagonist

232. Which of the following is not administered by intradermal route ? *(Recent NEET Pattern Question)*
    (a) BCG
    (b) Insulin
    (c) Mantoux
    (d) Drug sensitivity injection

233. Which of the following is not an indication for oxytocin? *(Recent NEET Pattern Question)*
    (a) Spontaneous premature labour
    (b) Post partum haemorrhage
    (c) Uterine inertia
    (d) Breast engorgement due to inefficient milk ejection reflex

234. Hirsutism producing drugs include all *except*: *(Recent NEET Pattern Question)*
    (a) Methyldopa
    (b) Corticosteroids
    (c) Phenytoin
    (d) Minoxidil

235. All of the following drugs are oxytocics *except*: *(Recent NEET Pattern Question)*
    (a) Oxytocin
    (b) Ergometrine
    (c) Prostaglandin
    (d) Orciprenaline

236. Norplant contains how many capsule of levonorgesterol? *(Recent NEET Pattern Question)*
    (a) 4
    (b) 6
    (c) 8
    (d) 10

237. Mechanism of Calcitriol is: *(Recent NEET Pattern Question)*
    (a) Decreased calcium resorption calcium from bone
    (b) Increase calcium absorption from intestine
    (c) Decreased calcium absorption from kidney
    (d) Decrease calcium absorption from intestine

238. What is the action of oxytocin in small doses, when used as intravenous infusion in a full term uterus? *(Recent NEET Pattern Question)*
    (a) Relaxes uterus
    (b) Induces uterine contractions
    (c) Causes cervical dilatation
    (d) All

239. True about atosiban is that it: *(Recent NEET Pattern Question)*
    (a) Is an oxytocin receptor antagonist
    (b) Is an progesterone receptor antagonist
    (c) Is least effective in inhibiting preterm uterine contractions
    (d) Is a anti-tocolytic drug

240. Beta agonist which is used for stopping premature labor is: *(Recent NEET Pattern Question)*
    (a) Carvedilol
    (b) Terbutaline
    (c) Pindolol
    (d) Nadolol

241. Which one of the following drugs is not a uterine relaxant? *(Recent NEET Pattern Question)*
    (a) Isoxsuprine
    (b) Dopamine
    (c) Salbutamol
    (d) Terbutaline

242. A 46-years-old male patient has Cushing's syndrome that is due to the presence of adrenal tumor. Which of the following drugs would be expected to reduce the signs and symptoms of the man's disease? *(Recent NEET Pattern Question)*
    (a) Betamethasone
    (b) Cortisol
    (c) Fludrocortisone
    (d) Ketoconazole

243. Side effects of oxytocin are all *except*: *(Recent NEET Pattern Question)*
    (a) Placental abruption
    (b) Fetal distress
    (c) Peripheral vascular disease
    (d) Water intoxication

244. Which of the following is a tocolytic agent? *(Recent NEET Pattern Question)*
    (a) Prazosin
    (b) Ritodrine
    (c) Yohimbine
    (d) Propranolol

245. Which of the following is an oxytocin antagonist? *(Recent NEET Pattern Question)*
    (a) Ritodrine
    (b) Atosiban
    (c) Isoxsuprine
    (d) Methergine

246. The following drugs are used in the management of Post-partum Hemorrhage, *except*: *(Recent NEET Pattern Question)*
    (a) Oxytocin
    (b) Methyl ergometrine
    (c) Mifepristone
    (d) Carboprost

Explanations

1. **Ans. (b) Male infertility** *(Ref: KDT 8th/e p262,263)*
   Pulsatile exposure to GnRH induces FSH/LH secretion while sustained exposure desensitizes the receptors resulting in decrease in secretion of gonadotropins. Therefore, nonpulsatile (continuous) GnRH agonists are given when we want to decrease the sex hormones.
   Indications:
   - Prostatic carcinoma
   - Endometriosis
   - Precocious puberty
   - Fibroid

   But in case of male infertility, more testosterone is required to induce spermatogenesis, so GnRH agonists are given in pulsatile manner.

2. **Ans. (d) Both Prolactin and Growth hormone** *(Ref: KDT 8th/e p258)*
   Hypothalamus secretes inhibitory hormones for prolactin (Prolactin Inhibitory Hormone) and growth hormone (somatostatin). However, for growth hormone, hypothalamus also secrete stimulatory hormone called Growth Hormone Releasing Hormone.
   Read the question carefully! If it is asked which hormone is under inhibitory control only? Then answer would be prolactin. However, in this question, they are asking which hormones are under inhibitory control? So, both prolactin and GH will be the answer.

3. **Ans. (d) Diabetes insipidus** *(Ref: KDT 8th/e p261)*
   Bromocriptine is approved in diabetes mellitus not diabetes insipidus

4. **Ans. (a) Diabetes mellitus** *(Ref: KDT's 8th/e p261)*

5. **Ans. (a) Acromegaly** *(Ref: KDT's 8th/e p260)*

6. **Ans. (a) Hyperprolactinemia** *(Ref: KDT 7/e p239)*
   Bromocriptine is a dopamine agonist which is used in hyperprolactinemia, which is a well-known cause of infertility.

7. **Ans. (a) GnRH analogue**
   (Ref: Harrison 19th/e p2380, KDT 8/e p264)
   - Long-acting gonadotropin releasing hormone (GnRH) agonists are the current therapy of choice for central precocious puberty. In girls, mostly central precocious puberty is seen.
   - GnRH agonists are not effective as therapy for peripheral precocious puberty. Androgen antagonists, spironolactone, aromatase inhibitors (Anastrozole and Letrozole), ketoconazole, and medroxy-progesterone acetate are used to treat peripheral precocious puberty.

8. **Ans. (a) Carbamazepine- Syndrome of inappropriate ADH secretion**
   (Ref: Goodman and Gilman 12th/e p712, 1338, KDT 8/e 260, 643, 644)
   - Carbamazepine releases ADH from hypothalamus and is used for treatment of diabetes insipidus as an alternative to desmopressin. It is not indicated in SIADH.
   - Octreotide is a long acting somatostatin used for secretory diarrhea due to carcinoid syndrome and VIPoma.
   - Desmopressin is drug of choice for diabetes insipidus.
   - Human chorionic gonadotropin can be used for induction of ovulation in female infertility and treatment of oligospermia and thus male infertility.

9. **Ans. (b) Hypoglycemia**
   (Ref: Goodman and Gilman 12/e p1116-1117)
   Growth hormone therapy commonly leads to hyperglycemia (not hypoglycaemia)

10. **Ans. (c) Bromocriptine** *(Ref: KDT 8/e p261)*
    It is an ergot alkaloid and is a dopamine agonist. Dopamine acts as prolactin inhibiting hormone in the brain. Agonism of dopamine receptors by bromocriptine is responsible for its use in hyperprolactinemia.

11. **Ans. (c) Cabergoline** *(Ref: KDT 8/e p261)*

12. **Ans. (c) Endogenous depression** *(Ref: KDT 8/e p261)*

13. **Ans. (c) Desmopressin** *(Ref: KDT 8/e p260, 643)*

14. **Ans. (a) Goserelin** *(Ref: KDT 8/e p264)*

15. **Ans. (a) GnRH** *(Ref: KDT 8/e p264)*

16. **Ans. (b) It can cause hypotension** *(Ref: KDT 8/e p261)*
    - For suppression of lactation, D_2 agonists like bromocriptine can be used. In hyperprolactinemia, these are given for long periods.
    - Metoclopramide being a D_2 antagonist will stop the action of bromocriptine.
    - Adverse effects of bromocriptine include nausea, vomiting, postural hypotension, digital vasospasm and CNS effects like hallucinations, psychosis etc.

17. **Ans. (b) Osteoporosis** *(Ref: KDT 8/e p264, 265)*
    GnRH agonists as well as antagonists can cause *hot flushes, loss of libido and osteoporosis* as adverse effects.

18. **Ans. (c) Leuprolide** *(Ref. KDT 8th/e p264)*

19. **Ans. (b) Bromocriptine** *(Ref: KDT 8th/e p261)*

20. **Ans. (d) An absorbent** *(Ref: KDT 8/e p260)*

21. **Ans. (b) Insulin** *(Ref: KDT 8/e p55)*

22. **Ans. (c) Cabergoline** *(Ref: KDT 8/e p261)*

23. **Ans. (a) Cabergoline** *(Ref: KDT 8/e p261)*

24. **Ans. (b) Prolactin deficiency** *(Ref: KDT 8/e p261)*

25. **Ans. (a) Inhibits prolactin release** *(Ref: KDT 8/e p261)*

26. **Ans. (b) Delta cells** *(Ref: KDT 7/e p261)*

27. **Ans. (d) Hypothyroidism** *(Ref: KDT 8/e p261)*

28. **Ans. (c) Infective diarrhea** *(Ref: KDT 8/e p260)*

29. **Ans. (b) Octreotide** *(Ref: KDT 8/e p260)*

30. **Ans. (b) Inhibit the enzyme thyroid peroxidase**
    (Ref: KDT's 8th/e p 275)

Endocrinology

31. **Ans. (a) Propylthiouracil** *(Ref: KDT's 8th/e p275)*
32. **Ans. (d) Lung fibrosis** *(Ref: KDT 8th/e p275-276)*
    Thioamides include drugs like methimazole, carbimazole and propylthiouracil.
    - Agranulocytosis and aplastic anemia is serious side effect of all of these drugs but it is seen rarely.
    - Propylthiouracil is associated with hepatotoxicity.
    - All the 3 drugs are teratogenic. Least teratogenic is propylthiouracil.
33. **Ans. (a) Contraindicated in hyperthyroidism** *(Ref: KDT 8/e p276-277)*
    Iodine and iodides are useful in Graves' disease and make the gland shrink, firm and less vascular. These can inhibit all facets of thyroid function. Chronic iodine overdose is called iodism.
34. **Ans. (b) Reserpine** *(Ref: Katzung 11/e p677, CMDT 2010/1015, KDT 8/e p278-279)*
    Thyroid storm is an extreme form of thyrotoxicosis. The drugs used in thyroid storm are:
    - Propranolol to control severe cardiovascular manifestations.
    - Calcium channel blockers like diltiazem are used if β-blockers are contra-indicated as in asthmatics.
    - Iodides (NaI, KI, Lugol's iodine) to inhibit the release of thyroid hormones from the gland.
    - Propylthiouracil or methimazole to reduce the synthesis of thyroid hormones.
    - Hydrocortisone to protect the patient against shock.

    > **Note**
    > Aspirin should be avoided as it may displace T_4 from thyroid binding globulin resulting in elevated levels of free T_4

35. **Ans. (b) 8 hours** *(Ref: KDT 8/e p275)*
    Half-life of carbimazole is around 8 hours whereas propylthiouracil has t½ of 2 hours.
36. **Ans. (d) Carbamazepine** *(Ref: Katzung 11/e p671-673, KDT 8/e p274)*
37. **Ans. (b) Cretinism** *(Ref: CMDT 2010/1005, KDT 8/e p273)*
38. **Ans. (d) Propylthiouracil** *(Ref: KDT 8/e p276)*
39. **Ans. (b) Captopril** *(Ref: KDT 8/e p531)*
40. **Ans. (a) Propylthiouracil** *(Ref KDT 8/e p276)*
41. **Ans. (c) Propylthiouracil** *(Ref. KDT 8th/276)*
42. **Ans. (b) I^{131}** *(Ref: KDT 8/e p278)*
43. **Ans. (a) Potassium iodide** *(Ref: KDT 8/e p276)*
44. **Ans. (a) 5% iodine & 10% KI** *(Ref: KDT 8/e p277)*
45. **Ans. (c) Level of thyroid stimulating hormone** *(Ref: KDT 8/e p270)*
46. **Ans. (c) Oral I^{131}** *(Ref: CMDT 2014/ p1078)*
47. **Ans. (b) Propranolol** *(Ref: KDT 8/e p278)*
48. **Ans. (c) Phenformin** *(Ref: KDT 8/e p298)*
49. **Ans. (a) Before surgery** *(Ref: KDT 8/e p277)*
50. **Ans. (b) Thyroxine** *(Ref: KDT 8/e p272)*
51. **Ans. (a) Propylthiouracil** *(Ref: KDT 8/e p276)*
52. **Ans. (d) Papillary** *(Ref: KDT 8/e p274)*
53. **Ans. (a) Metformin** *(Ref: Goodman Gilman 12/e p1136)*

    > - **Absorption of T_4 is reduced by:**
    >   - Antacids
    >   - Bile acid binding agents
    >   - Calcium carbonate
    >   - Iron salts
    >   - Proton pump inhibitors
    >   - Raloxifene
    >   - Sucralfate

    - Metformin may decrease TSH without changing free T_4 in levothyroxine-treated patients.

54. **Ans. (b) 1, 2 and 3 are correct** *(Ref: KDT 8th/e p301)*
    SGLT-2 Inhibitors
    - Sodium Glucose Transporter 2 (also called SGLT2) is a transporter for reabsorption of glucose and Na⁺. It is present in PCT of nephrons. Drugs inhibiting this transporter are Canagliflozin, Dapagliflozin, Empagliflozin, Ertugliflozin etc.
    - By inhibiting the reabsorption of glucose, these drugs result in glucosuria. This can result in urinary tract infections (including Urosepsis) and genital tract infections like Fournier's gangrene.
    - If used in type 1 diabetes, these decrease the blood sugar by causing glucosuria. The patient usually decreases the dose of insulin or may altogether stop using insulin as blood sugar levels are within required range. However, type 1 diabetes has absolute insulin deficiency. Insulin not only controls blood sugar but is also required for metabolism of ketone bodies. If the person stops using insulin, it may result in Ketoacidosis. Hence, SGLT-2 inhibitors are contra-indicated in Type 1 diabetes mellitus.

55. **Ans. (b) It is GLP2 agonist** *(Ref: Harrison 20th/e p2255)*
    Teduglutide:
    - It is a recombinant analog of human glucagon like peptide 2.
    - It is used for the treatment of adults with **short bowel syndrome.**
    - It works by promoting mucosal growth and possibly restoring gastric emptying and secretion.
    - It is given by subcutaneous route.
    - It is long acting drug because it is resistant to degradation by DPP-4

56. **Ans. (a) Increases insulin release from pancreas** *(Ref: KDT's 8th/e p.294)*
57. **Ans. (c) Repaglinide** *(Ref: KDT's th/e p296)*
58. **Ans. (c) Pramlintide** *(Ref: KDT's 8th/e p293)*
59. **Ans. (c) Regular insulin** *(Ref: KDT's 8th/e pg.286)*
60. **Ans. (d) These have lesser risk of precipitating hypoglycemia in normoglycemic patients** *(Ref: KDT's 8th/e pg.293)*
61. **Ans. (a) Vildagliptin** *(Ref: KDT 8th/e p298)*
62. **Ans. (d) Metformin** *(Ref: KDT 7/e p276)*

    > Metformin should be avoided in the following patients because of risk of lactic acidosis:
    > - Renal disease
    > - Liver disease
    > - COPD
    > - Heart failure
    > - Elderly

All DPP-4 inhibitors require dose adjustment in renal failure except linagliptin

63. **Ans. (c) Canagliflozin** *(Ref: KDT 7/e p270,274,275)*
    - As the patient is allergic to sulfonylureas, so glipizide (second generation sulfonylurea) cannot be given.
    - Liraglutide is a GLP agonist and is given subcutaneously. As the patient is not willing to take injectable drugs, this cannot be added.
    - Sitagliptin is a DPP-4 inhibitor and increase the risk of pancreatitis, so it should also be avoided.
    - Pioglitazone increase the risk of urinary bladder carcinoma

    So, among the given options, the best drug to add is canagliflozin.

64. **Ans. (a) Linagliptin** *(Ref: CMDT 2017/e p1227)*
    All DPP-4 inhibitors require dose adjustment in renal failure except linagliptin.

65. **Ans. (a) 30% amorphus + 70% crystalline** *(Ref: KDT 7/e p264)*
    Lente insulin is a mixture of amorphous (30%) and crystalline (70%) insulin.

66. **Ans. (d) Around umbilicus** *(Ref: CMDT 2017/1231, Fundamental nursing skills and concepts 831)*
    Any part of the body covered by loose skin can be used for insulin administration such as

    - Abdomen (except 2 inches around umbilicus)
    - Thighs
    - Dorsum of Upper arms
    - Flanks
    - Buttocks

67. **Ans. (d) Smoking** *(Ref: KDT 8th/e p299)*
    Risk factors for increased lactic acidosis due to metformin are:

    - Advanced age
    - Kidney disease
    - Liver disease
    - Cardio-respiratory insufficiency (Tissue hypoxia)
    - Alcoholism

68. **Ans. (b) Linagliptin** *(Ref: Katzung 13th/e p740, KDT 8/e p298)*
    - All DPP-4 inhibitors are require dose reduction in renal failure except Linagliptin
    - Vildagliptin requires dose reduction in both renal as well as hepatic disease

69. **Ans. (c) Rosiglitazone** *(Ref: KDT 8th/e p294; Goodman Gillman 12th/e p1260; Katzung 12th/e p757)*
    Rosiglitazone does not act by increasing insulin secretion. Rosiglitazone is an oral antihyperglycemic agent that acts primarily by decreasing insulin resistance.

70. **Ans. (b) Amylin** *(Ref: KDT 8th/e p293)*
    Amylin is secreted along with insulin from beta cells of pancreas. Like insulin, it also help in decreasing blood sugar. Analog of this substance, Pramlintide, is approved for both type 1 as well as type 2 diabetes mellitus.

71. **Ans. (c) Metformin** *(Ref: Goodman Gilman 12/e p1259, KDT 8/e p299)*
    - **Lactic acidosis** (more with phenformin) and **megaloblastic anemia** (more with metformin) due to vitamin B_{12} deficiency are the major adverse effects of these drugs. Lactic acidosis is more likely to occur in the presence of hepatic and renal impairment or alcohol ingestion.

72. **Ans. (d) K⁺ entry into cells** *(Ref: CMDT-2010/798)*
    - Insulin, bicarbonate and b-agonists shift K⁺ intracellularly within minutes of administration. Thus, these drugs can be used for treatment of acute hyperkalemia

73. **Ans. (c) Adrenaline** *(Ref: Harrison 16/e p2185)*
    - Hypoglycemia is treated urgently by oral glucose.
    - It neuroglucopenia precludes oral feeding, IV glucose (25 g) should be given.
    - If IV therapy is not practical, s.c. or i.m. glucagon should be given. Because glucagon primarily acts by glycogenolysis, it is ineffective in glycogen depletion states (e.g. alcohol induced hypoglycemia).

74. **Ans. (d) Increasing insulin secretion from pancreas** *(Ref: KDT 8/e p294)*
    - Sulfonylureas stimulate the release of insulin by the beta cells of the islets of Langerhans by blocking K⁺ channels. Glucagon secretion is also reduced by sulfonylureas, but it is a minor action.

75. **Ans. (a) Chlorpropamide** *(Ref: KDT 8/e p296)*
    - Intolerance to alcohol with flushing (disulfiram like reaction) occurs with chlorpropamide.
    - Chlorpropamide, tolbutamide, tolazamide and acetohexamide are first generation sulfonylureas.

76. **Ans. (a) Glucagon production** *(Ref: KDT 8/e p294)*
    Sulfonylureas act by
    - Increasing insulin release from pancreas (not by decreasing insulin secretion), so 'option b' ruled out.
    - A minor action reducing glucagon and increasing somatostatin release has been demonstrated.

77. **Ans. (b) Phenformin** *(Ref: Katzung 11/e p741; KDT 8/e p299)*
78. **Ans. (d) Insulin secretion** *(Ref: KDT 8/e p294)*
79. **Ans. (b) Hyperglycemia** *(Ref: KDT 8/e p288)*
80. **Ans. (c) Ultralente** *(Ref: KDT 8/e p285)*
81. **Ans. (c) Tolbutamide** *(Ref: KDT 6/e p266)*
82. **Ans. (b) Miglitol** *(Ref: KDT 8/e p294)*
83. **Ans. (b) Glibenclamide** *(Ref: KDT 8/e p296)*
84. **Ans. (a) Total pancreatectomy** *(Ref: KDT 8/e p294)*
85. **Ans. (c) Rosiglitazone** *(Ref: Katzung 11/e p739-740: KDT 8/e p300)*
86. **Ans. (a) It is short acting** *(Ref: KDT 8/e p664)*
87. **Ans. (c) Water retention with weight gain** *(Ref: Katzung 11/e p743; KDT 8e p300)*
88. **Ans. (d) Subcutaneous route** *(Ref: KDT 8/e p287)*
89. **Ans. (c) Helps in insulin secretion** *(Ref. KDT 8th/294)*
90. **Ans. (c) NPH insulin** *(Ref: KDT 8th/e p285)*
91. **Ans. (a) Rosiglitazone** *(Ref: KDT 8th/e p300)*
92. **Ans. (a) Biguanides** *(Ref: KDT 8/e p298-299)*
93. **Ans. (b) Old man with decreased BP/decreased heart rate due to atenolol** *(Ref: KDT 8/e p304)*
94. **Ans. (d) Glargine** *(Ref: KDT 8/e p287)*
95. **Ans. (a) Nateglinde** *(Ref: KDT 8/e p297)*

Endocrinology

96. **Ans. (d) Repaglinide** *(Ref: KDT 8/e p297)*
97. **Ans. (a) Insulin glargine** *(Ref: KDT 8/e p285)*
98. **Ans. (c) Actrapid** *(Ref: KDT 8/e p285)*
    - Actrapid (regular insulin) and monotard (Lente-insulin) are unmodified insulins with same amino acid squence as natural insulin
    - Lispro, aspart, glulisine and glargine are insulin analogues in which slightly different amino acid sequence is present to modify pharmacokinetics.
99. **Ans. (c) Metformin** *(Ref: KDT 8/e p299)*
100. **Ans. (b) Stimulating the beta islet cells of pancreas to release insulin** *(Ref: KDT 8/e p294)*
101. **Ans. (a) Metformin** *(Ref: KDT 8/e p299)*
102. **Ans. (a) Metformin** *(Ref: KDT 8/e p299)*
103. **Ans. (b) Intravenous fluids (saline)** *(Ref: CMDT 2014 p1190, KDT 8/e p291)*
104. **Ans. (d) Regular insulin** *(Ref: KDT 8/e p286)*
105. **Ans. (a) Hydrocortisone** *(Ref: KDT 8th/e p314)*
    Normal serum K$^+$ level is 3.5–5.0 mEq/L.
    Normal Na$^+$ level is 136-152 mEq/L.
    So, the patient in the question has hyperkalemia and hyponatremia. This together with ambiguous genitalia suggests the diagnosis of CAH (Congenital adrenal hyperplasia).
    In CAH, there is deficiency of glucocorticoids and mineralocorticoids
    Hydrocortisone is the glucocorticoid with maximum mineralocorticoid activity, so it is the preferred drug for treatment of this patient.
    K$^+$ binding resins and Calcium gluconate are used in treatment of hyperkalemia.
106. **Ans. (a) Metyrapone** *(Ref: KDT 8th/e p319)*
107. **Ans. (b) Spironolactone** *(Ref: KDT's 8th/e p319)*
108. **Ans. (d) Dexamethasone** *(Ref: KDT's 8th/e p314)*
109. **Ans. (d) DOCA** *(Ref: KDT's 8th/e p314; From ROAMS 13th/e p349)*
110. **Ans. (a) Dexamethasone 6 mg 12 hourly 4 doses** *(Ref: Dutta 7th/e p316, Nelson 20th/e p852)*

    Antenatal steroids
    - Total dose of 24 mg of dexamethasone or betamethasone is used in 48 hours
    - Total dose of 24 mg of dexamethasone or betamethasone is used in 48 hours
    - Dexamethasone is given in 4 divided doses (Mnemonic: starts with letter D, which is fourth letter), whereas betamethasone is given in 2 divided doses (Mnemonic: Starts with letter B, which is second letter).
    - Thus dose of dexamethasone is 6 mg 12 hourly for 4 doses and dose of betamethasone is 12 mg 24 hourly for 2 doses.

111. **Ans. (d) Kaposi's Sarcoma** *(Ref Harrison's 19th/e p1269-1270)*
    Steroids are used in CLL, Hodgkin lymphoma and multiple myeloma. However these should be avoided in Kaposi Sarcoma.

112. **Ans. (c) Weight gain** *(Ref: Harrison 19th/e p2325)*
    Adrenal insufficiency results in weight loss.
113. **Ans. (d) 6 mg 12 hourly 4 doses** *(Dutta 7th/e p316; Nelson 20th/e p852)*
    Dose of dexamethasone given to mother in anticipated preterm delivery is 6 mg 12 hourly 4 doses.
    Antenatal Corticosteroids

Steroid	Dose
Betamethasone (Steroid of choice)	12 mg IM 24 hours apart (two doses)
Dexamethasone	6 mg IM every 12 hours (four doses)

114. **Ans. (b) Betamethasone valerate cream 0.5%** *(Ref: Katzung 10/e p102; KDT 8/e p313)*
    Betamethasone is most potent and hydrocortisone is least potent topical steroid.
115. **Ans. (c) Ileo-caecal tuberculosis** *(Ref: Katzung 10/e p1263; KDT 8/e p319)*
    - If used in intestinal tuberculosis, steroids can result in silent perforation, therefore are contra-indicated in ileo-caecal tuberculosis.
116. **Ans. (c) Effective in acute asthma** *(Ref: Katzung 11/e p348)*

    - Beclomethasone is an inhalational steroid useful in prophylaxis of asthma. Like other inhalational steroids, it can also cause oropharyngeal candidiasis.
    - For acute attack of asthma, bronchodilators are used. Steroid are slow to act, therefore are not effective in acute attack. Prednisolone or hydrocortisone can be used along with bronchodilators for acute severe asthma.

117. **Ans. (a) Aldosterone** *(Ref: KDT 8/e p308)*
    Aldosterone is most potent mineralocorticoid whereas betamethasone is most potent glucocorticoid.
118. **Ans. (d) Photosensitivity** *(Ref: KDT 8/e p317-319)*
    - Steroids are used for treatment of photosensitivity.
    - Other effects i.e. skin atrophy, telangiectasia and folliculitis can be caused by steroids.
119. **Ans. (b) Glaucoma** *(Ref: KDT 8/e p318)*
    - Glaucoma occurs after the use of prolonged **topical** therapy in susceptible individuals.
120. **Ans. (a) Dexamethasone** *(Ref: KDT 8/e p314)*
    For details, refer to text.
121. **Ans. (c) Eczematous skin disease** *(Ref: KDT 8/e p319)*
    Hypertension and diabetes are aggravated by steroids. In peptic ulcer, bleeding and silent perforation may occur. Thus, steroids are contraindicated in these conditions. However, since steroids may have to be used as a life saving measure, all of these are relative contraindications. Topical corticosteroids are highly effective in eczematous skin diseases.
122. **Ans. (a) Hydrocortisone** *(Ref: KDT 8/e p314, CMDT 2014/1116)*
    - In chronic adrenal insufficiency or Addison's disease, hydrocortisone given orally is the drug of choice.
    - Hydrocortisone is a glucocorticoid with maximum mineralocorticoid action.

123. **Ans. (a) Muscular hypertrophy** *(Ref: KDT 8/e p317-318)*
 "Muscle weakness occurs in both hypo or hypercorticism"
124. **Ans. (c) Cortisol** *(Ref: KDT 8/e p313)*
125. **Ans. (a) Ketoconazole** *(Ref: Katzung 11/e p693; KDt 8/e p844)*
126. **Ans. (c) Prednisolone** *(Ref: KDT 8/e p313)*
127. **Ans. (c) Osteomalacia** *(Ref: KDT 8/e p317-318)*
128. **Ans. (d) Hypotension** *(Ref: KDT 8/e p317-318)*
129. **Ans. (d) Break down of phospholipids** *(Ref: KDT 8/e p311)*
130. **Ans. (a) Mitotane** *(Ref: Katzung 11/e p695)*
131. **Ans. (b) Hypertension** *(Ref: KDT 8/e p317)*
132. **Ans. (a) Hypoglycemia** *(Ref: KDT 8/e p317)*
133. **Ans. (d) Methyl prednisolone** *(Ref: KDT 8/e p313)*
134. **Ans. (c) Prevent de-iodination** *(Ref: Katzung 11/e p670, 686)*
 Glucocorticoids on long term use suppress the release of ACTH, GH, TSH and LH. These also inhibit the activity of 5'- deiodinase and thus inhibit the peripheral conversion of T4 to T3. These also decrease thyroid binding globulin.
135. **Ans. (c) Collagen vascular diseases** *(Ref: KDT 8/e p315)*
136. **Ans. (c) Glaucoma** *(Ref. KDT 8th/e p318)*
 Glaucoma occurs on long-term topical use, not due to ingestion.
137. **Ans. (b) Cortisone** *(Ref. KDT 8th/e p314)*
138. **Ans. (b) Prednisolone** *(Ref. KDT 8th/e p313)*
139. **Ans. (c) Dexamethasone** *(Ref: KDT 8/e p314)*
140. **Ans. (b) IV hydrocortisone** *Ref: KDT 8/e p313)*
141. **Ans. (d) Prednisolone** *(Ref: KDT 8/e p313,314)*
142. **Ans. (c) Aldosterone** *(Ref: KDT 8/e p313)*
143. **Ans. (b) Hyperkalemia** *(Ref: KDT 8/e p317-318)*
144. **Ans. (a) Suppression of inflammation and improvement in functional capacity** *(Ref: KDT 8/e p315)*
145. **Ans. (b) Prednisolone** *(Ref: KDT 8/e p318)*
 - Etidronate and phenytoin cause osteomalacia whereas calcitriol is used in treatment of osteoporosis.
146. **Ans. (b) Cortisone for Cushing's syndrome** *(Ref: KDT 8/e p315-317)*
147. **Ans. (c) To suspect adrenocortical insufficiency and start IV steroids** *(Ref: KDT 8/e p314)*
148. **Ans. (a) Betamethasone valerate** *(Ref: KDT 8/e p954)*
149. **Ans. (d) Dexamethasone** *(Ref: KDT 8/e p314)*
150. **Ans. (b) Bisphosphonates** *(Ref: KDT 8th/e p370)*
 - Bisphosphonates are drug of choice for post-menopausal as well as steroid induced osteoporosis.
 - These act by inhibiting the action of osteoclasts.
 - These can result in esophageal toxicity.
151. **Ans. (a) Teriparatide** *(Ref. CMDT 2018/1173; KDT 8/e p365)*
 Drugs used in osteoporosis may act by inhibiting osteoclast (inhibiting resorption) of bone or by stimulating osteoblasts (increasing formation of bone).

Drugs inhibiting osteoclast:	Drug stimulating osteoblast
Bisphosphonates	Teriparatide
Estrogen	Strontium ranelate
Raloxifene	
Strontium ranelate	
Denosumab	

152. **Ans. (b) Milnacipran** *(Ref: Katzung 13th/e p754-756)*
 Milnacipran is an SNRI used for severe depression.
 - Teriparatide is a recombinant PTH_{1-34} that is indicated in osteoporosis. It acts by stimulating osteoblasts
 - Strontium ranelate acts by dual mechanism in osteoporosis. It inhibits osteoclasts as well as stimulates osteoblasts.
 - Denosumab is monoclonal antibody against RANK receptor and prevent activation of osteoclasts. It is indicated in osteoporosis and giant cell carcinoma of bone.
153. **Ans. (a) IV fluids** *(Ref: Harrison 19th/e p610; KDt 8/e p370)*
 Management of hypercalcemia of malignancy

Drug of choice	Bisphosphonates
Immediate treatment	IV fluids with furosemide
Fastest calcium lowering drug	Calcitonin

154. **Ans. (a) Take empty stomach with plenty of water** *(Ref: KDT 8th/e p370)*
 Bisphosphonates are to be taken empty stomach in the morning with full glass of water and patient is instructed not to lie down or take food for at least 30 min. These measures are required to prevent contact of the drug with esophageal mucosa which result in esophagitis.
155. **Ans. (c) PGE_2** *(Ref: Katzung 11/e p321-322)*
 Major effect of prostaglandins especially PGE2 is to increase bone turnover. PGs may contribute to the bone loss that occurs at menopause, it has been speculated that NSAIDs may be of therapeutic value in osteoporosis, however clinical evaluation is required.
156. **Ans. (a) Inhibiting bone resorption** *(Ref: KDT 6/e p330; Ganong 22/e p394; KDT 8/e p365)*
 - Calcitonin inhibits bone resorption by *direct action* on osteoclasts. Calcitonin receptors are present on osteoclasts (inhibits osteoclastic activity → hypocalcemia)
 - It also inhibits proximal tubular calcium and phosphate reabsorption by direct action on kidney. However, hypocalcemia which occurs overrides the direct action by decreasing the total Ca^{++} filtered at the glomerulus → urinary Ca^{++} actually decreased.
157. **Ans. (a) IV** *(Ref: KDT 8/e p371)*
158. **Ans. (c) Decreasing the osteoclast mediated resorption of bone** *(Ref: KDT 8/e p369)*
159. **Ans. (a) Calcitonin** *(Ref: CMDT 2010/801; KDt 8/e p365)*
 Bisphosphonates are the treatment of choice for hypercalcemia of malignancy but require 48-72 hours before reaching full therapeutic effect. Calcitonin may be helpful to treat hypercalcemia before the onset of action of bisphosphonates.
160. **Ans. (d) Multivitamins** *(Ref: Katzung. 11/e p765-766)*
161. **Ans. (c) Calcipotriol** *(Ref. KDT 8th/e p368)*

Endocrinology

162. Ans. (a) Teriparatide *(Ref: KDT 8/e p365)*
163. Ans. (d) Postmenopausal osteoporosis *(Ref: KDT 8/e p366)*
164. Ans. (c) Osteoporosis *(Ref: KDT 8/e p365)*
165. Ans. (d) Vitamin D intoxication *(Ref: KDT 8/e p370-370)*
166. Ans. (d) Etidronate *(Ref: KDT 8/e p371)*
167. Ans. (c) Vitamin K *(Ref: CMDT 2014 p712)*
168. Ans. (b) Androgen *(Ref: KDT 8/e p365-371)*
169. Ans. (a) Danazol *(Ref: KDT 8th/e p348, 344)*
    - Danazol is an androgen used for treatment of endometriosis. It has no role in prevention of pregnancy after unprotected intercourse.
    - The drugs used as emergency contraceptives are:
        - Combined oral contraceptives
        - Levonorgestrel
        - Mifepristone
        - Ulipristal
        - Intra-uterine contraceptive devices

170. Ans (a) 30 mg *(Ref: Harrison 20th/e p2815)*
    Ulipristal
    - **Ulipristal is** one of the selective progesterone receptor modulators **(SPRM).**
    - It acts as partial agonist on progesterone receptors.
    - It does not block glucocorticoid receptors.
    - It acts by inhibiting ovulation.
    - A 30 mg dose is used as **emergency contraceptive** that can be taken within 120 hours (5 days) after unprotected intercourse.
    - If taken within 72 hours, it is as effective as levonorgestrel whereas it is more effective than levonorgestrel if taken within 72-120 hours of unprotected intercourse.
    - **Major adverse effects are headache and abdominal pain.**

171. Ans. (c) Breast Carcinoma *(Ref: Harrison's 19th/e p530)*
172. Ans. (a) 1.5 mg single pill *(Ref: KDT's 8th/e p347)*

    Levonorgestrel 0.75mg two doses 12 hours apart or 1.5 mg single dose should be taken within 72 hours of unprotected intercourse for emergency contraception

173. Ans. (d) Gestodene *(Ref: KDT's 8th/e p341)*
174. Ans. (c) Used in **hormone replacement therapy designed to relieve menopausal symptoms** *(Ref: KDT 8th/e p335)*
175. Ans. (a) For hormone receptor (HR)-positive metastatic breast cancer in postmenopausal women
    (Ref: KDTs 8th/e p337)
176. Ans. (c) Finasteride *(Ref: KDT 7/e p302)*

    - Finasteride is a 5 alpha reductase inhibitor. It can decrease the size of prostate in BHP. It, thus can affect the static component in BHP. Another drug in this group is dutasteride.
    - Tamsulosin and prazosin are alpha 1 blockers. They relax the urethra and provided symptomatic relief (dynamic component) from urinary retention. These do not affect the size of the prostate.

177. Ans. (b) 600 micrograms *(Ref: WHO recommendations for prevention and treatment of PPH 2012)*

Dose of misoprostol for PPH is
- For treatment: 800 microgram sublingually
- For prophylaxis: 600 microgram orally

178. Ans. (d) Selective progesterone receptor modulator
    (Ref: Harrison's 19/e p2391; Goodman Gilman 12th/e p1185)
    Ulipristal is a selective progesterone receptor modulator (SPRM) like mifepristone. It is used as an emergency contraceptive that can be used within 120 hours of unprotected intercourse.

179. Ans. (d) Emergency contraception
    (Ref: Goodman Gilman 12th/e p1184, 1190)
    Emergency contraception is the contraceptive use of levonorgestrel.

180. Ans. (a) Desogestrel
    (Ref: Williams Obstetrics 24/e p714; Dutta 7th/e p551)
    Desogestrel is not used as post-coital contraceptive.
    Drugs used for Emergency Contraception
    - Levonorgestrel (0.75 mg stat and after 12 hours)
    - Ethinyl estradiol 50 µg + Norgestrel 0.25 mg (2 tab stat and 2 after 12 hours)
    - Mifepristone (10 mg single dose)
    - Copper IUDs
    - Centchroman (60 mg to be taken twice at an in interval of 12 hours within 24 hours of intercourse)
    - Ulipristal (30 mg)

181. Ans. (b) Tamoxifen *(Ref: Dutta Gynae 6th/e p470)*
    Tamoxifen has no role in treatment of PCOD.
    Treatment of PCOD
    - Weight loss of more than 5% of previous weight is important.
    - Cigarette smoking should be avoided.
    - Estrogen in combination with progesterone (lacking androgenic properties).
    - Dexamethasone 0.5 mg at bedtime also reduces androgen production.
    - Hirsutism is treated with cyproterone acetate or spironolactone.
    - Infertility is treated with Clomiphene. Ovulation is induced in around 80% of patients and about 40% conceive. However, abortion rate of 25-40% is due to corpus luteal phase defect manifested by Clomiphene.
    - In Clomiphene failed group, ovulation can be induced with FSH or GnRH analogues.
    - Metformin treats the root cause of PCOD, rectifies endocrine and metabolic functions and improves fertility and is drug of choice.

182. Ans. (d) Coronary heart disease
    (Ref: CMDT 2014/1140-1141)
    Combined estrogen plus progesterone hormone replacement therapy increases the risk of coronary artery disease and breast cancer.
    Estrogen alone has no effect or protective effect on CAD whereas combination with progesterone increases the risk. Vaginal atrophy, hot flushes and osteoporosis are decreased by hormone replacement therapy

183. Ans. (d) Cancer in opposite breast
    (Ref: Goodman and Gilman 12/e p1179, CMDT 2010/1505)

Tamoxifen is a SERM that acts as antagonist at estrogen receptors in the breast. It decreases the risk of contralateral breast cancer and is approved for primary prevention of breast cancer in women at high risk.

Adverse effects of Tamoxifen include:

- Hot flashes
- Vaginal discharge or bleeding
- Menstrual irregularities
- Thromboembolic events (rare)
- Endometrial hyperplasia
- Cataract
- Hepatotoxicity
- Tumor flare

184. **Ans. (b) Dysmenorrhea**
 (Ref: Katzung 11/e p713, CMDT-2010/697)
 - Oral contraceptive pills cause amenorrhea but not dysmenorrhea.
 - Mastalgia, breakthrough bleeding and chloasma all can be seen due to OCP use.
 - Breakthrough bleeding is more common with progesterone only pills.

185. **Ans. (d) Increased risk of ovarian cancer**
 (Ref: KDT 8/e p352)
 - Ovarian carcinoma risk is decreased by oral contraceptives due to progestin component.

186. **Ans. (b) Ethinylestradiol** *(Ref: KDT 8/e p330)*

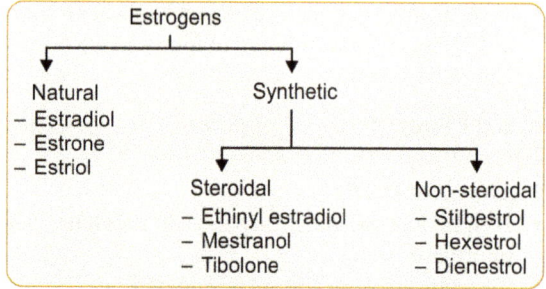

187. **Ans. (c) Has partial agonist and antagonistic action on estrogen receptors** *(Ref: KDT 8/e p337)*
 - Tamoxifen is used for the treatment of breast carcinoma.
 - It acts as estrogen receptor antagonist in the breast tissue and as partial agonist in uterus, bone, liver and pituitary.

188. **Ans. (c) Anti-implantation effect** *(Ref: KDT 8/e p345)*

189. **Ans. (d) Gossypol** *(Ref: KDT 8/e p353)*
 Gossypol is a non-steroidal compound obtained from cotton seed. It causes suppression of spermatogenesis in 99.9% of men and reduces sperm motility. Most important adverse effect of this drug is hypokalemia and resultant muscles weakness.
 Gelusil is an antacid containing aluminium-hydroxide
 Gestedone is newer 19-testosterone derivative. It is a potent progestin with strong anti-ovulatory action.

190. **Ans. (c) Clomiphene** *(Ref: KDT 8/e p336)*
 Clomiphene citrate is an estrogen antagonist with weak agonistic action.
 - It increases gonadotropin secretion by blocking estrogenic feed back. Its chief use in ovulation induction.

191. **Ans. (c) Estrogen receptor positive breast carcinoma**
 (Ref: KDT 8/e p337)
 Tamoxifen is used as a hormonal therapy by breast cancer in both pre and post menopausal women. Response is better in ER +ve breast cancers.

192. **Ans. (b) Estrogen** *(Ref: KDT 8/e p351)*
 "Estrogen component of OCPs has been mainly responsible for venous thromboembolism, while both estrogen and progesterone have been blamed for the arterial phenomena.
 - Estrogen tend to ↑ HDL/LDL ratio but progestin nullifies this benefits.

193. **Ans. (d) Mifepristone (RU 486)** *(Ref: KDT 8/e p345)*
194. **Ans. (a) Oral mifepristone** *(Ref: KDT 8/e p345)*
195. **Ans. (b) Ovarian cancer** *(Ref: KDT 8/e p352)*
196. **Ans. (a) Progesterone antagonist** *(Ref: KDT 8/e p345)*
197. **Ans. (d) Dihydrotestosterone** *(Ref: KDT 8/e p320)*
198. **Ans. (a) Carcinoma breast** *(Ref: KDT 8/e p352)*
199. **Ans. (d) All** *(Ref: KDT 8/e p352)*
200. **Ans. (b) Induction of ovulation** *(Ref: KDT 8/e p337)*
201. **Ans. (d) All** *(Ref: KDT 8/e p341, 342)*
202. **Ans. (a) Bicalutamide** *(Ref: KDT 8/e p326)*
203. **Ans. (a) Flutamide** *(Ref: KDT 8/e p326)*
204. **Ans. (c) Hot flushes** *(Ref: KDT 8/e p334)*

- Suppression of libido and gynaecomastia are well recognized adverse effects of estrogens.
- Fusion of epiphyses are not mentioned anywhere as the action of estrogens but definitely estrogen deficiency results in hot flushes and these are used for treatment of these vasomotor symptoms in post menopausal females. Therefore, according to us, the best answer should be 'hot flushes'

205. **Ans. (d) Increased risk of ovarian cancer**
 (Ref: KDT 8/e p350-351)
206. **Ans. (b) Ulipristal** *(Ref: KDT 8th/e p346)*
207. **Ans. (b) Inhibition of ovulation** *(Ref: KDT 8th/e p349)*
208. **Ans. (c) Nandrolone** *(Ref: KDT 8th/e p325)*
209. **Ans. (c) STEAR** *(Ref: KDT 8th/e p335)*
201. **Ans. (c) Development of vaginal carcinoma in female offspring** *(Ref: KDT 8th/e p350-351)*
211. **Ans. (d) Diethylstilbestrol** *(Ref: KDT 8th/e p330)*
212. **Ans. (b) Used in treatment of gynaecomastia**
 (Ref: KDT 8/e p334-355)
- Estrogens can result in suppression of libido, gynaecomastia and feminization as adverse effects when given to males.

213. **Ans. (c) Post partum hemorrhage** *(Ref: KDT 8/e p345-346)*
214. **Ans. (a) 5-alpha reductase** *(Ref: KDT 8/e p326)*
215. **Ans. (c) Finasteride** *(Ref: KDT 8/e p326)*
216. **Ans. (d) Active liver disease** *(Ref: KDT 8/e p351)*
217. **Ans. (d) Irregular menstrual bleeding and prolonged anovulation** *(Ref: KDT 8/e p349)*
218. **Ans. (b) Ovarian cancer** *(Ref: KDT 8/e p352)*
219. **Ans. (a) Cerebral stroke** *(Ref: KDT 8/e p351)*
220. **Ans. (c) Anti-progestin** *(Ref: KDT 8/e p345)*
221. **Ans. (d) Relaxin** *(Ref: KDT 8/e p330)*

222. Ans. (b) Migraine *(Ref: KDT 8/e p335)*
223. Ans. (a) **Combined pills 2 immediately and 2 after 12 hrs** *(Ref: KDT 8/e p348)*
224. Ans. (c) **Phosphodiesterase 5 inhibitor** *(Ref: KDT's 8th/e p327)*
225. Ans. (b) **Benign prostatic hyperplasia** *(Ref: KDT 8th/e p326)*
226. Ans. (c) **800 mcg sublingual**
    (Ref: WHO recommendations for prevention and treatment of PPH 2012)
    According to WHO 2012 recommendations
    - Oxytocin is drug of choice for treatment and well as prevention of post partum hemorrhage.
    - Alternatives are ergometrine, fixed dose combination of oxytocin and ergometrine and misoprostol
    - Misoprostol is recommended as 600 microgram orally for prevention of PPH and 800 microgram sublingually for treatment of PPH.
    - The use of tranexamic acid is recommended for the treatment of PPH if oxytocin and other uterotonics fail to stop bleeding or if it is thought that the bleeding may be partly due to trauma.
227. Ans. (a) **100 microgram IM** *(Ref: Goodman Gillman 12th/e p1851; Dutta 7th/e p412; Williams 24/e p547, 595)*
    Carbetocin is a long acting Oxytocin that is useful to prevent post-partum hemorrhage when given intramuscularly or intravenously in a dose of 100 microgram.
228. Ans. (d) **Vasopressin** *(Ref: Katzung 11/e p301, Ganong 22/e p41-43)*
    Vasopressin acts via V_1 and V_2 receptors. V_1 receptors use IP_3-DAG-Ca^{2+} pathway whereas V_2 use cAMP as second messenger. All other drugs mentioned in the question [corticotrophin, glucagon and dopamine] act by cAMP pathway only. Thus, all of these use cAMP as second messenger, but if we need to choose one option we can answer vasopressin as it is acting through IP_3 – DAG – Ca^{2+} pathway also.
229. Ans. (c) **Clomiphene** *(Ref: Goodman Gilman 12/e p1846)*
    The drugs that have been associated with high incidence of hypospadias include:
    - Valproic acid
    - Phenytoin
    - Progesterone (often given to mothers as part of IVF treatment)
    - Diethylstilbestrol (prescribed up until the 1970s to prevent miscarriage)
    - Clomiphene (used to induce ovulation during IVF treatment)

    From the above information, in this question also there are two answers i.e. DES and clomiphene. As we have to choose one, we will go with clomiphene because it is being commonly used these days for fertility induction whereas diethylstilbestrol is rarely used now-a-days.
230. Ans. (a) **Lactogenesis** *(Ref: Katzung 11/e p657; KDT 8/e p355)*
    - Important actions of oxytocin are:
    - Contraction of uterine smooth muscle (directly by acting on GPCR and indirectly by release of PG and LTs).
    - Milk ejection by contraction of myoepithelial cells surrounding mammary alveoli.
    - At high concentration; anti-diuretic and vasopressor action can be seen.

    > **Note**
    > Lactogenesis is the action of prolactin (not oxytocin)

231. Ans. (c) **Estrogen and Progesterone combination pill** *(Ref: CMDT 2014/744)*
    - Oral contraceptives are used for the treatment of menstrual irregularity. These are drug of choice for PCOD
    - PCOD is also known as Stein-Leventhal syndrome
    - Weight loss by regular exercise, low glycemic index diet combined with insulin lowering drugs like metformin can restore fertility in 85% of females.
    - For females who don't respond to weight loss, metformin therapy may be helpful.
    - Clomiphene is even more effective to restore fertility.
    - Cyproterone acetate, flutamide or spironolactone can be used for the treatment of hirsutism and acne.

232. Ans. (b) **Insulin** *(Ref: KDT 8/e p286)*
    Insulin is administered by s.c. route.
233. Ans. (a) **Spontaneous premature labour** *(Ref: KDT 8/e p356)*

    > **Note**
    > Spotaneous premature labour is an indication for use of tocolytics and not oxytocin.

234. Ans. (a) Methyldopa *(Ref: KDT 8/e p317,441, 613)*
235. Ans. (d) Orciprenaline *(Ref: KDT 8/e p354)*
236. Ans. (b) 6 *(Ref: KDT 8/e p349)*
237. Ans. (b) **Increase calcium absorption from intestine** *(Ref: KDT 8/e p366)*
238. Ans. (b) **Induces uterine contractions** *(Ref: KDT 8/e p356)*
239. Ans. (a) **Is an oxytocin receptor antagonist** *(Ref: KDT 8/e p359)*
240. Ans. (b) Terbutaline *(Ref: KDT 8/e p359)*
241. Ans. (b) Dopamine *(Ref: KDT 8/e p358)*
242. Ans. (d) Ketoconazole *(Ref: KDT 8/e p319)*
243. Ans. (c) **Peripheral vascular disease** *(Ref: KDT 8th/e p356)*
244. Ans. (b) Ritodrine *(Ref: KDT 8/e p358)*
245. Ans. (b) Atosiban *(Ref: KDT 8/e p359)*
246. Ans. (c) Mifepristone *(Ref: KDT 8/e p45,357)*

Central Nervous System

CHAPTER 7

SEDATIVE HYPNOTIC DRUGS

Sedative is a drug that calms a person whereas hypnotics induce sleep. CNS depressant drugs can produce sedation, hypnosis, anaesthesia and coma depending on the dose. Major group of drugs useful for the treatment of insomnia include barbiturates, benzodiazepines and newer drugs.

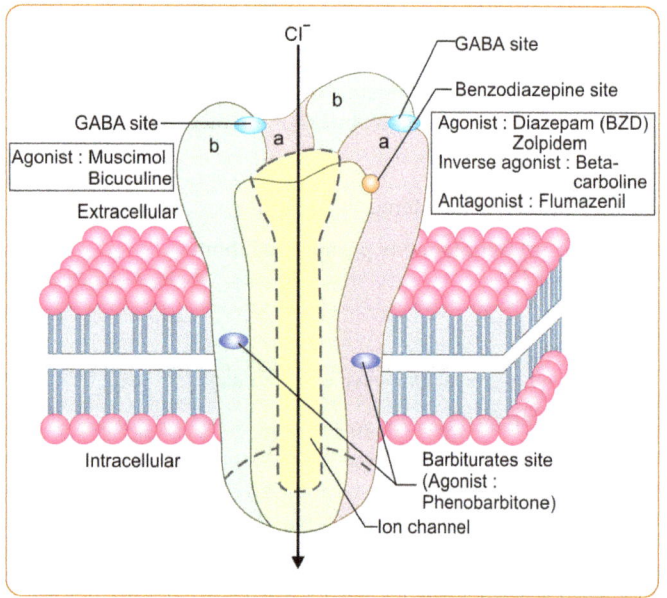

FIG. 7.1: GABA-BZD-Chloride channel complex

- $GABA_A$-BZD-Cl^- channel complex (Fig. 7.1) is an ion channel, which on opening increases the conductance of chloride ions resulting in CNS depression. Several compounds can modulate the effect of this channel.
- GABA increases the duration of channel opening by directly binding to $GABA_A$ receptor site.
- **Barbiturates** bind to another site on this channel to exert **GABA mimetic** (direct activation of $GABA_A$ receptors) as well as **GABA facilitatory** (increase the binding of GABA to $GABA_A$ receptors) actions.
- **Benzodiazepines** bind to a different site (BZD receptor) and increase the binding of GABA to $GABA_A$ receptor (**GABA facilitatory** action). These drugs increase the frequency of Cl^- channel opening.
- **Bicuculline** binds to $GABA_A$ receptor and acts as a competitive inhibitor of GABA and **non competitive inhibitor of benzodiazepines**.
- **β-carboline** acts as an **inverse agonist** at benzodiazepine site and *thus produces convulsions* due to stimulation of the brain.
- **Flumazenil** acts as a **competitive antagonist at BZD site** and therefore **inhibits the action of benzodiazepines as well as β-carboline**.

1. BARBITURATES

These are the derivatives of barbituric acid and act by increasing the Cl^- conductance across $GABA_A$-BZD-Cl^- channel complex. These drugs have GABA mimetic as well as GABA facilitatory action to increase the **duration of Cl^- channel opening** (no effect on frequency). Important indications of barbiturates in clinical practice are epilepsy (phenobarbitone) and anaesthesia (thiopentone as inducing agent). These are generally not used for other purposes because

- These have narrow therapeutic index due to **steep dose response curve** (with slight increase in dose, severe CNS depression leading to coma can occur).
- These are **powerful enzyme inducing agents** and are prone to several drug interactions.
- These have **high abuse liability** and may precipitate withdrawal symptoms.
- If poisoning occurs, **no specific antidote** is available.

Adverse effects and contraindications

- Due to the long duration of action, **hangover** is common. Barbiturates can cause distortion of sleep architecture by *decreasing the duration of REM* and *stage 3 and 4 sleep and increasing the duration of stage 2 sleep*.
- **Learning and memory impairment** can occur.
- **Idiosyncratic reaction** resulting in excitement can occur in some patients.
- These are **absolutely contraindicated in acute intermittent porphyria** (because porphyrin synthesis is increased due to induction of δ-ALA synthase; rate limiting enzyme in porphyrin synthesis, by barbiturates).
- At high doses, acute poisoning may occur (manifests as coma, depressed respiration, hypotension, cardiovascular collapse and *barbiturate blisters*). It is treated by gastric lavage, symptomatic treatment and with **forced alkaline diuresis**. Hemodialysis can also be done.

2. BENZODIAZEPINES

These drugs act by **GABA facilitatory** action. These also possess *anxiolytic, anticonvulsant and skeletal muscle relaxant properties*.

Benzodiazepines used for various indications are:

Hypnotic:	Diazepam, Flurazepam, Nitrazepam, Flunitrazepam, Temazepam, Triazolam, Quazepam and Midazolam
Anti-convulsants:	Diazepam, Clonazepam, Clobazam, Lorazepam
Anti-anxiety:	Diazepam, Oxazepam, Lorazepam, Alprazolam, Chlordiazepoxide
Muscle Relaxant:	Diazepam

Benzodiazepines are preferred over barbiturates as hypnotic drugs due to several reasons:

- BZDs have **flat dose response curves (Fig. 7.2).** These have high therapeutic index and require high dose to produce coma.
- These cause **less hangover** and **less distortion of sleep architecture**. Duration of REM sleep is shortened but increase in the number of REM cycles compensate for that. **Nitrazepam** actually **increases REM sleep.**
- These are **less prone to drug interactions** (because they do not induce microsomal enzymes).
- Abuse liability is less.
- BZD poisoning can be treated with **specific antidote, flumazenil.**
- Diazepam can produce analgesia whereas *barbiturates may even cause hyperalgesia.*

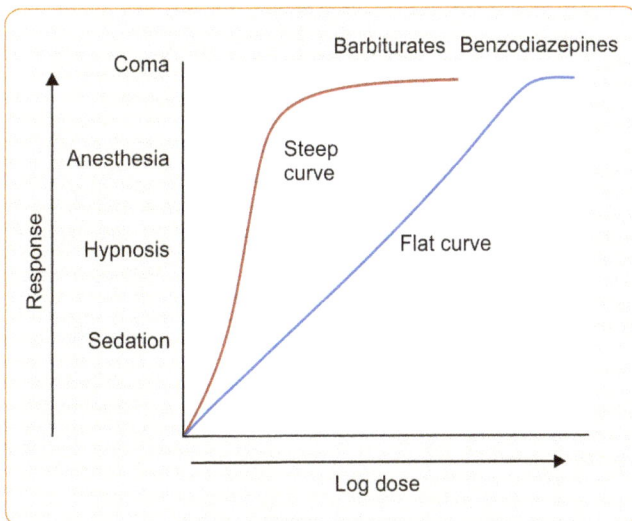

FIG. 7.2: Log DRC of barbiturates and benzodiazepines

Pharmacokinetics

Most of the BZDs are metabolized in the liver to *produce active products* (thus long duration of action). *Active metabolites may result in cumulative effects.* After metabolism these are conjugated and are excreted via kidney. **Estazolam, lorazepam, oxazepam, temazepam and triazolam** are **directly conjugated without metabolism** to active products. These drugs are thus **short acting** and do not accumulate on repeated administration. Further these drugs can be **safely** administered **in liver failure and in elderly** because these are conjugated directly without undergoing metabolism in the liver. Compounds with *shorter half life* are favored in patients with *sleep onset insomnia* whereas *longer acting BZDs* are favored in patients with *day time anxiety.*

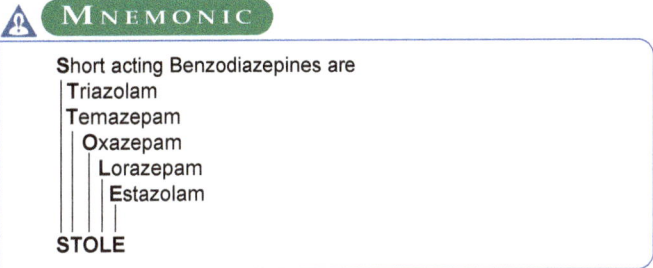

MNEMONIC

Short acting Benzodiazepines are
Triazolam
Temazepam
Oxazepam
Lorazepam
Estazolam
STOLE

Adverse effects

- Benzodiazepines are much safer than barbiturates (less chances of respiratory depression and coma) and also have less abuse potential. However, these drugs can also **impair learning and memory.**
- **Flunitrazepam** is a tasteless BZD and is implicated as a **date rape drug** due to its propensity to cause dose dependent amnesic effects.
- **Paranoia and other psychiatric distrubances can occur with triazolam.**
- **Midazolam** can cause *ataxia and blackouts in elderly.*
- **Flurazepam** results in *paradoxical stimulation and increase in nightmares* in some persons.

Benzodiazepine Antagonist

Flumazenil is the substance that acts as a competitive antagonist at BZD receptor.

- It *blocks the depressant action of benzodiazepines, zolpidem and zaleplon as well as the convulsant action of inverse agonists (like β carboline).*
- It is administered i.v. **for the treatment of BZD poisoning** (specific antidote) and can also be used to reverse BZD anaesthesia.
- Its **duration of action** is *approximately 30-40 minutes* and **half life** is 1 hour.

3. NEWER HYPNOTIC DRUGS

A. Zopiclone

It stimulates $GABA_A$ receptors by binding to a site different than benzodiazepines. It prolongs stage 3 and 4 sleep and does not affect REM sleep. Chances of **rebound insomnia and hangover are less** than benzodiazepines and barbiturates. It is used for the treatment of insomnia. It is also **indicated in the patients taking benzodiazepines** regularly for induction of sleep. It helps in **weaning off** hypnotic medications in such patients. The active enantiomer, **eszopiclone** is also available now.

B. Zolpidem

It binds selectively to ω_1 **subtype of benzodiazepine receptors** and increases GABA mediated neuronal inhibition. It possesses pronounced hypnotic and amnesic effects but **lacks anti-anxiety, muscle relaxant and anticonvulsant actions.** It has **little effect on sleep architecture** and **does not produce hangover and rebound insomnia.** Abuse potential of zolpidem is very low. It is also **indicated for the short term treatment of insomnia.**

C. Zaleplon

It also acts by selectively binding to ω_1 **subtype of benzodiazepine receptors.** It **decreases sleep latency** without affecting total sleep time or sleep architecture (therefore useful in persons having difficulty to fall asleep). Other properties are similar to zolpidem.

D. Suvorexant and Lemborexant

These are **orexin receptor antagonists**. Orexin acts as a central promotor of wakefulness. Therefore, its antagonists have been approved for insomnia.

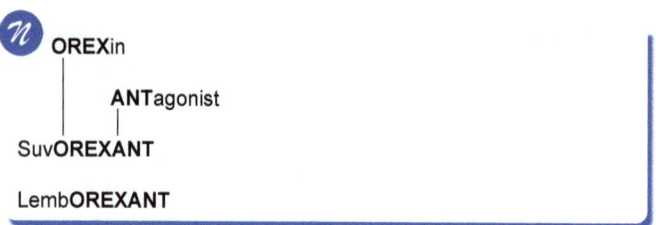

4. MELATONIN AGONISTS

MELATONIN is a hormone of pineal gland that synchronizes the circadian rhythm. It increases the sleep during night but has no effect on latency or duration of sleep. It is **used to reduce symptoms of jet lag**. It can also synchronize the sleep wakefulness cycle in **shift workers** and is also used in **elderly hypnotic dependent insomniacs**. **Lowering of seizure threshold** and **psychiatric changes** are the possible adverse effects.

- **Ramelteon** is agonist of MT_1 and MT_2 receptors of melatonin in suprachiasmatic nucleus. It is approved for long term use in treatment of sleep onset insomnia. It **do not possess addictive property** but causes hyperprolactinemia, dizziness, somnolence and fatigue as adverse effects. It is metabolized by *microsomal enzymes* (CYP1A2) and should not be given with enzyme inducers (e.g. rifampicin) or inhibitors (e.g. ciprofloxacin)

MNEMONIC

```
        R A M E L T E O N
        └─┘   └─┘     └─┘
     Receptor Agonist Melatonin
```

- **Tasimelteon** is melatonin receptor agonist (like ramelteon) indicated for treatment of non-24 hour sleep-wake disorder in totally blind.

5. OTHER HYPNOTICS

Chloral hydrate (active metabolite is trichloroethanol), **glutethimide** and **meprobamate** (a metabolite of carisoprodol, a skeletal muscle relaxant) have CNS depressant properties but are rarely used in clinical practice.

Trazodone is an antidepressant that can be used for insomnia at low doses. **Priapism** is a rare side effect of this agent.

PARKINSONISM

It is a neurodegenerative disease characterized by rigidity, bradykinesia, dyskinesia, tremor, mask like facies and unstable gait (**Fig. 7.3**). Idiopathic Parkinsonism is known as Parkinson's disease.

In basal ganglia, the output neurons are controlled by dopamine and acetylcholine. Due to their opposite action, a balance is required between these two neurotransmitters for proper functioning of basal ganglia.

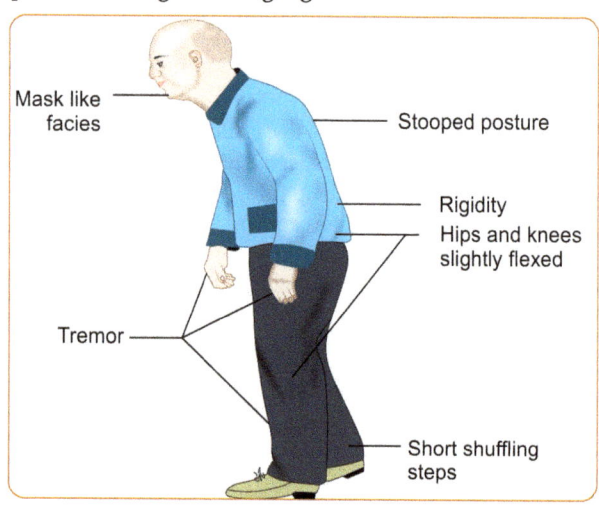

FIG. 7.3: Clinical features of Parkinsonism

Major pathology in Parkinsonism is decrease in nigrostriatal dopaminergic neurons, (with appearance of **Lewy bodies**) consequently cholinergic activity becomes dominant. Thus, **two major strategies** for the treatment of Parkinsonism are to *increase* brain *dopaminergic activity* or to *decrease central cholinergic activity*.

DRUGS INCREASING BRAIN DOPAMINERGIC ACTIVITY

Brain dopaminergic activity can be increased by precursors of dopamine, inhibitors of dopamine metabolism, dopamine receptor agonists and drugs increasing presynaptic release of dopamine (**Fig. 7.4**).

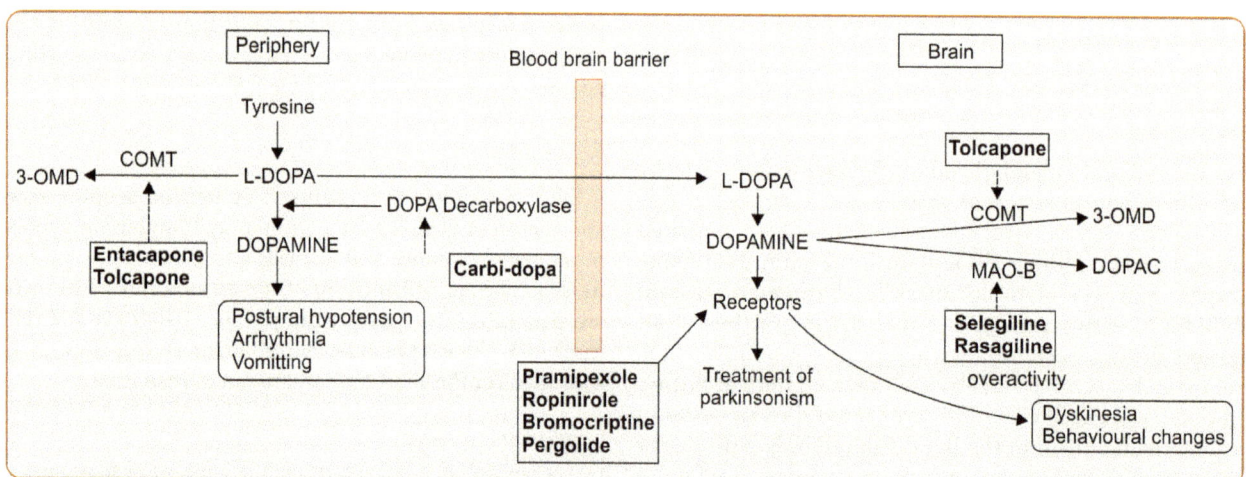

FIG. 7.4: Site of action of anti-Parkinsonian drugs

A. Dopamine Precursors

Dopamine itself cannot cross blood brain barrier (BBB) but its precursor levo-dopa can cross BBB. Levo-dopa is metabolized by **dopa decarboxylase** (contains pyridoxine as co-factor) to dopamine. This conversion occurs both in periphery as well as in the brain. Peripheral conversion is undesirable due to two reasons:

- It forms dopamine peripherally that cannot cross BBB, therefore only about 1-3% of l-dopa can reach its target site (brain).
- Peripherally formed dopamine will result in adverse effects like postural hypotension.

Therefore *levo-dopa is always given in combination with* peripheral dopa decarboxylase inhibitors like *carbidopa or benserazide*. This combination has beneficial effects on all symptoms of Parkinsonism, although **tremors respond less well than rigidity or bradykinesia.**

Adverse Effects

- Peripherally formed dopamine can lead to **postural hypotension** and **arrhythmias**. **Nausea and vomiting** occurs commonly due to CTZ stimulation by dopamine (*Domperidone but not metoclopramide can be used for the treatment of this vomiting*). On long term use **"wearing off"** effect and **on-off phenomenon** can result. 'On' means patient is having no symptoms of Parkinsonism (but abnormal movements are present) and 'off' means patient has full blown symptoms of Parkinsonism (like no treatment is given). This effect is **due to short half life** (1-2hrs) of l-dopa and is reduced by carbidopa. **Long acting dopamine agonists show little tendency to cause on-off phenomenon.**
- **Abnormal choreiform movements** (dyskinesia) of limbs, trunk and tongue can occur with prolonged high dose treatment. **Carbidopa does not prevent** or decrease this adverse effect. This adverse effect **responds to amantadine and possibly levetiracetam.**
- L-dopa especially in elderly can result in **hallucinations, vivid dreams, sleep disturbances** and even **psychosis** (thus C/I in psychosis). These behavioural disturbances are not prevented by carbidopa. Clozapine and quetiapine can be used to treat levodopa induced psychosis.
- It may even cause **mydriasis** (C/I in angle closure glaucoma).
- Vitamin complexes containing **pyridoxine decrease the effectiveness** of levo-dopa (pyridoxine is a cofactor of dopa decarboxylase and increases the formation of dopamine in the periphery. This results in decrease in l-dopa's central penetration).
- *Abrupt withdrawal* of levodopa may precipitate *neurolept malignant syndrome.*
- Levo-dopa should be given **carefully** in patients with **active peptic ulcer** (increased risk of bleeding) and **malignant melanoma** (levo-dopa is a precursor of melanin).

Adverse effect of L-dopa

Adverse Effect	Mechanism	Remarks
1. Nausea, Vomiting	CTZ stimulation	Reduced by carbi-dopa
2. Postural hypotension	D_1 stimulation	Reduced by carbi-dopa
3. Arrhythmias	β_1 stimulation	Reduced by carbi-dopa
4. Hypertension	α_1 stimulation	Reduced by carbi-dopa More likely when combined with MAO inhibitors
5. Mydriasis	α_1 stimulation	Contraindicated in acute angle closure glaucoma
6. Dyskinesia	↑Activity of DA in Brain	Not reduced by carbi-dopa
7. Psychotic symptoms	↑Activity of DA in Brain	Not reduced by carbi-dopa

B. Drugs Inhibiting Metabolism of Dopamine

Dopamine is metabolized by MAO and COMT (catechol-o-methyl transferase).

(i) COMT Inhibitors

This enzyme metabolizes dopamine as well as l-dopa to form 3-O-methyldopa. **Tolcapone, entacapone** and **opicapone** (act by inhibiting this enzyme) help in Parkinsonism because:

- Metabolism of l-dopa is inhibited, so more is able to cross BBB. These can be given in combination with l-dopa + carbidopa (*inhibition of dopa decarboxylase diverts the metabolism of l-dopa to methylation by COMT*)
- 3-O-methyl dopa formed by metabolism of l-dopa competes with it for entry in the brain. Tolcapone and entacapone decrease this interaction.
- By inhibiting dopamine metabolism in brain (tolcapone only), its duration of action is increased.

Tolcapone inhibits COMT in periphery as well as brain whereas entacapone acts only in the periphery. **Major beneficial effect** of these drugs in Parkinsonism is due to **peripheral inhibition** of COMT. **Tolcapone** is more potent and longer acting than entacapone but is not preferred because of **hepatotoxic** effects. **Opicapone** is a new drug recently approved for treatment of off episodes in Parkinson's disease.

Key Points

Tolcapone inhibits COMT in periphery as well as brain whereas entacapone acts only in the periphery.

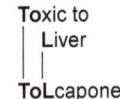
MNEMONIC

Toxic to
Liver
ToLcapone

(ii) MAO-B Inhibitors

Selegiline and rasagiline are irreversible and **selective inhibitors of MAO-B**. These drugs can be given in combination with levo-dopa + carbidopa to decrease the dose of levo-dopa (and thus decreased abnormal movements). At normal doses these inhibit only MAO-B and thus have no interaction with cheese or tricyclic antidepressants. However, at high doses, they also inhibit MAO-A and can lead to hypertensive crisis (**cheese reaction**) with tyramine containing foods and serotonin syndrome with TCAs. Rasagiline is more potent than selegiline. These drugs are thought to **reduce the disease progression.**

Safinamide is a new MAO-B inhibitor. It is used with levo-dopa/carbidopa in patients of Parkinson's disease experiencing 'off' episodes.

C. Dopamine Agonists

These drugs directly activate D_2 receptors and can be used as monotherapy in Parkinsonism.

- **Ergot derived** dopamine agonists include **bromocriptine and pergolide**. These drugs are **short acting** and can cause digital **vasospasm** (leading to gangrene) and erythromelalgia. These drugs can also result in *pleural, peritoneal and cardiac fibrosis*. Ergot alkaloids require slow upward titration of dose. Long term use of *pergolide* is associated with *cardiac valvular defects*.
- Newer **non-ergot dopamine agonists**; **pramipexole** and **ropinirole** do not have these limitations (these are **long acting** and **do not cause gangrene**). These are now the **first choice drugs for Parkinsonism** (preferred over levodopa). **Ropinirole** has also been approved for **restless leg syndrome**. Pramipexole is excreted mainly by kidney whereas ropinirole is metabolized by liver. Rare but important adverse effect of these drugs is **excessive day time sleepiness**. Recently, **dopamine agonists** have been associated with **impulse-control disorders** including *pathological gambling, hypersexuality,* etc.
- **Rotigotine** is a dopamine agonist that can be administered through a **transdermal patch** but was discontinued due to crystal formation on the patches.
- **Apomorphine** can be given subcutaneously for *temporary relief of off-periods*. However, it cause *troublesome nausea*.

D. Drugs Increasing Dopamine Level at Synapse

- **Amantadine** is an **antiviral drug** that is also useful in Parkinsonism.
- It increases synaptic dopamine level by increasing presynaptic release and decreasing its reuptake.
- It also possesses anticholinergic and antiglutaminergic (NMDA blocking) activity.
- Adverse effects of this drug include nausea, insomnia, **ankle edema and livedo reticularis** (Fig. 7.5).
- It is indicated for treatment of **dyskinesia associated with chronic levo-dopa therapy**.

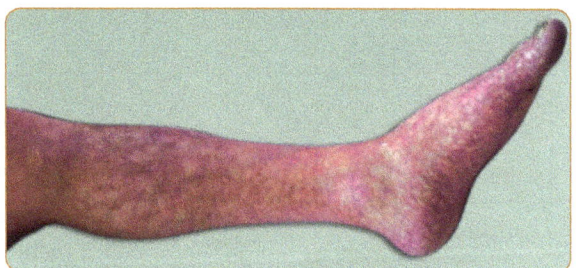

FIG. 7.5: Livedo reticularis caused by amantadine

- **Istradefylline** is a selective antagonist at adenosine A_{2A} receptors (A2AR). Normally, adenosine binds to A2AR and inhibits the function of D_2 receptors of dopamine. Therefore, istradefylline activities D_2 receptors by antagonizing this effect of adenosine. It is approved for treatment of 'off' episodes of Parkinsonism.

DRUGS INHIBITING BRAIN CHOLINERGIC TRANSMISSION

Drugs that act by blocking D_2 receptors in the brain (like antipsychotics, metoclopramide etc.) can cause Parkinsonism. In this condition, increasing dopamine level is not effective because the receptors on which it has to act (D_2) are already occupied, therefore anticholinergics are preferred.

- **Central anticholinergic** drugs like **trihexiphenidyl (benzhexol), procyclidine, benztropine, orphenadrine** and **biperiden** are **the drugs of choice for drug induced Parkinsonism**.
- **First generation antihistaminics** with high antimuscarinic activity like **promethazine** and **diphenhydramine** can also be used for this indication.
- Adverse effects of antimuscarinic drugs include urinary retention, blurred vision, dry mouth and constipation.

OTHER NEURODEGENERATIVE DISEASES

ALZHEIMER'S DISEASE (AD)

- It is a form of senile dementia that is due to the deposition of amyloid plaques in the hippocampus (Presence of neurofibrillary tangles). There is loss of cholinergic neurons in the brain. Anticholinesterases that can cross the blood brain barrier are the mainstay of treatment of this disease.
- **Tacrine** was used previously but its use has declined due to its **hepatotoxic** potential and the need of frequent (four times a day) dosing.
- **Donepezil, rivastigmine** and **galantamine** are newer cholinesterase inhibitors useful in AD that are **less toxic** than tacrine. *Donepezil* can be administered *once daily*, offering an advantage over other anticholinesterases. **Rivastigmine** is approved for treatment of **dementia due to Alzheimer's disease as well as due to Parkinsonism**.
- **Acetyl-l-carnitine** (structural analogue of ACh) has **antioxidant property** apart from **increasing cholinergic transmission**. It shows promise in decreasing symptoms and slowing the progression of AD.
- **Memantine is an NMDA antagonist** approved by FDA for the treatment of advanced AD in combination with cholinesterase inhibitors.
- **Aducanumab:** It is a new drug recently approved for treatment of Alzheimer's disease. Aducanumab is the only drug that targets the underlying cause of Alzheimer's disease i.e. Aβ amyloid. It is a monoclonal antibody against amyloid Aβ and is approved as intravenous therapy for Alzheimer's disease.

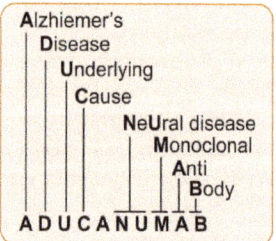

HUNTINGTON'S CHOREA

It is due to loss of GABAergic neurons in the striatum that lead to dopaminergic overactivity (opposite to Parkinsonism). Thus D_2 **blockers** like chlorpromazine, haloperidol as well as olanzapine are useful in the treatment of this disease. **Tetrabenazine** (dopamine depleter) is **drug of choice** for this indication. **Deutetrabenazine is** a new vesicular monoamine transporter-2 (VMAT-2) inhibitors like tetrabenazine. It can also be used for Huntington's chorea. **Reserpine** also act by depleting central monoamines.

AMYOTROPHIC LATERAL SCLEROSIS (ALS)

This disease is due to degeneration of neurons in spinal cord, medulla or cortex. Spasticity is the major presenting feature. **Riluzole** is an **NMDA antagonist** that is useful in ALS. Most useful agent for symptomatic treatment of spasticity in ALS is *baclofen*. **Edaravone** is a free radical scavenger recently approved for ALS.

MULTIPLE SCLEROSIS (MS)

It is an autoimmune disease resulting in demyelination of neurons.
- Drug of choice for **acute episode** is **corticosteroids**. Treatment with steroids hasten the recovery but extent of *recovery remains unchanged*. Long-term treatment with steroids provide no benefit.
- First line drugs **for relapse prevention** are **interferons** (β-1a and β-1b), *glatiramer and fingolimod*. Teriflunomide and dimethylfumarate are less efficacious. **Fingolimod** can cause **bradycardia** and heart block, therefore monitoring of heart rate is required.
- If disease activity continues despite first-line drugs, then natalizumab, alemtuzumab and mitoxantrone can be used.
- **Natalizumab** is highly effective but increases the **risk of** progressive multifocal leukoencephalopathy (**PML**). Therefore, it is used in patients with negative JC virus testing. *PML is also associated with dimethylfumarate.*
- **Sphingosine-1-phosphate (S1P) receptor modulators:** The drugs in this group include **fingolimod, siponimod, ponesimod and ozanimod**. These drugs stimulate S1P receptors and prevent egress of lymphocytes from lymph nodes. These drugs can cause bradycardia as an adverse effect. Fingolimod is also associated with lymphopenia. These drugs are given orally.

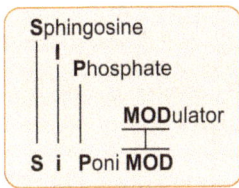

- **Fumarates: Dimethylfumarate** and **diroximel fumarate** (active metabolite is monomethylfumarate) are the drugs in this group. These act by activating nuclear factor like 2 (Nrf2) pathway and produce beneficial immune and neuroprotective pathway. These drugs are effective orally. Both drugs are associated with **Progressive Multifocal Leucoencephalopathy**. Dimethylfumarate is commonly associated with GI adverse effects like diarrhea, nausea, vomiting etc. There are less likely with diroximelfumarate.
- **Fingolimod** and **alemtuzumab** are associated with disseminated *varicella-zoster* infection.
- **Mitoxantrone** is *cardiotoxic* whereas **teriflunomide** can cause *liver damage*.
- **Dalfampridine** is an oral K⁺ channel blocker indicated to improve walking in patients with multiple sclerosis. It can cause seizures
- **Modafinil** is approved for improving fatigue in multiple sclerosis.
- **Ocrelizumab** is a CD-20 directed monoclonal antibody. It is approved for relapsing as well as primary progressive multiple sclerosis.

Amifampridine is a new K channel blocker (similar to dalfampridine) that is recent approved for oral treatment of **Lambert-Eaton Myasthenic syndrome**.

Drugs Used for Multiple Sclerosis

Drug	Route	Frequency	Major adverse effects
1. Interferon-β 1a	i.m.	Once a week	• Flu-like symptoms
Interferon β 1b	S.C	Thrice a week	• Neutralizing antibodies
2. Glatiramer	S.C.	Thrice a week	• Lipoatrophy
3. Natalizumab	i.v. infusion	Once a month	**PML**, if used for > 2 years
4. Fingolimod	Oral	Once a day	• First degree **heart block** • Bradycardia • Herpes zoster
5. Mitoxantrone	i.v.	Once in 3 months	• Cardiotoxicity • Acute leukemia
6. Dimethyl fumarate	Oral	Twice a day	PML
7. Teriflunomide	Oral	Once a day	Hepatotoxicity
8. Alemtuzumab	i.v.	Once daily for 5 days	• Herpes zoster
9. Dalfampridine (4-Aminopy-ridine)	Oral	Once a day	• Seizures

Key Points

Mitoxantrone has broadest indication in multiple sclerosis (RRMS, SPMS and worsening RRMS) but not used as first-line drug because of cardiotoxicity

WILSON'S DISEASE

It is characterized by hepatolenticular degeneration due to excessive accumulation of copper.
- **d-Penicillamine** can be used as a copper chelating agent but it can cause lupus like syndrome, optic neuritis and blood dyscrasias.
- **Trientine** is another copper chelating agent with much less toxicity but very high cost.
- *Zinc sulphate and potassium sulfide decrease intestinal absorption of copper and induce hepatic metallothinein synthesis, that sequester additional toxic copper. Zinc acetate can be used for maintenance therapy and is much safer than other drugs.*

Wilson's disease	Drug of choice
1. Hepatitis or cirrhosis without decompensation	Zinc
2. Mild to moderate hepatic decompensation	Trientine + zinc
3. Neurological or psychiatric symptoms	Tetrathiomolybdate + zinc
4. For maintenance, children, regnancy	Zinc

ANTIEPILEPTIC DRUGS

Epilepsy is the condition characterized by recurrent episodes of seizures. Seizures may be generalized, focal or unclassified. Generalized seizures include tonic clonic (grand mal), absence (petit mal), myoclonic, tonic, atonic and clonic seizures. Focal seizures may be simple partial (jacksonian) or complex partial (psychomotor or temporal lobe epilepsy). Febrile seizures and infantile spasms are unclassified forms of seizures. Lennox Gestaut syndrome is a form of epilepsy with impaired cognitive function.

Adenosine is an endogenous antiepileptic substance.

MECHANISM OF ACTION (FIG. 7.6)

Drugs useful for epilepsy act by various mechanisms like:

(a) **Inhibition of Use Dependent Na+ Channels:**
Phenytoin, carbamazepine, valproate, topiramate, lamotrigine, zonisamide, rufinamide, cenobamate and lacosamide act by inhibiting the sodium channels when these are open. These drugs also *prolong the inactivated stage* of these channels (Na+ channels are refractory to stimulation till these reach the closed/resting phase from inactivated phase).

(b) **Increase in Inhibitory Neurotransmission (Fig. 7.7):**
GABA is a major inhibitory neurotransmitter in the brain. *Barbiturates* (phenobarbitone, primidone) and *benzodiazepines* (diazepam, clonazepam, clobazam) activate GABAA receptors by binding to GABA-BZD-Cl- channel complex. *Ganaxolone* (a neurosteroid) also acts by activating this channel but the binding site is different. Drugs can also act by increasing the release (*Gabapentin*), decreasing the metabolism (*Vigabatrin*) or inhibiting the reuptake in neurons (*Tiagabine*).

(c) **Decrease in Excitatory Neurotransmission:**
Glutamate and aspartate are major excitatory amino acids in the brain. Glutamate can act by stimulating metabotropic (GPCRs) or ionotropic receptors (kainate, NMDA and AMPA). *Felbamate* acts by inhibiting NMDA receptors. **Topiramate** act by inhibiting kainate receptors. Perampanel is AMPA receptor antagonist.

(d) **Inhibition of Ca^{2+} Channels:**
T-type Ca^{2+} channels are **important in absence seizures**. Drugs inhibiting these channels (*ethosuximide, valproate, lamotrigine*) are useful in petit mal epilepsy. **Gabapentin and pregabalin** bind to $\alpha_2\delta_1$ subunit of presynaptic calcium channels and act by unknown mechanism.

Mechanism of action of antiepileptic drugs

1. **Prolong inactivated state of Na+ channels**
   - Phenytoin
   - Fosphenytoin
   - Carbamazepine
   - Oxcarbazepine
   - Valproate
   - Divalproex
   - Lamotrigine
   - Topiramate
   - Zonisamide
   - Lacosamide
   - Rufinamide
   - Cenobamate

2. **K+ channel openers**
   - Retigabine (Ezogabine)
   - Topiramate

3. **↓ Glutamate activity**
   - Lamotrigine
   - Topiramate
   - Perampanel
   - Felbamate

4. **↑ GABA activity**
   - Valproate
   - Topiramate
   - Tiagabine
   - Barbiturates
   - Benzodiazepines
   - Stiripentol

5. **T-Ca^{2+} channel blocker**
   - Valproate
   - Ethosuximide
   - Zonisamide

6. **Incompletely understood mechanism**
   - Levetiracetam (binds to SV_2A)
   - Brivaracetam (binds to SV_2A)
   - Gabapentin, Pregabalin (bind Ca^{2+} channel)
   - Lacosamide (CRMP-2 inhibitor)
   - Cannabidiol (CB_1 receptor agonist)

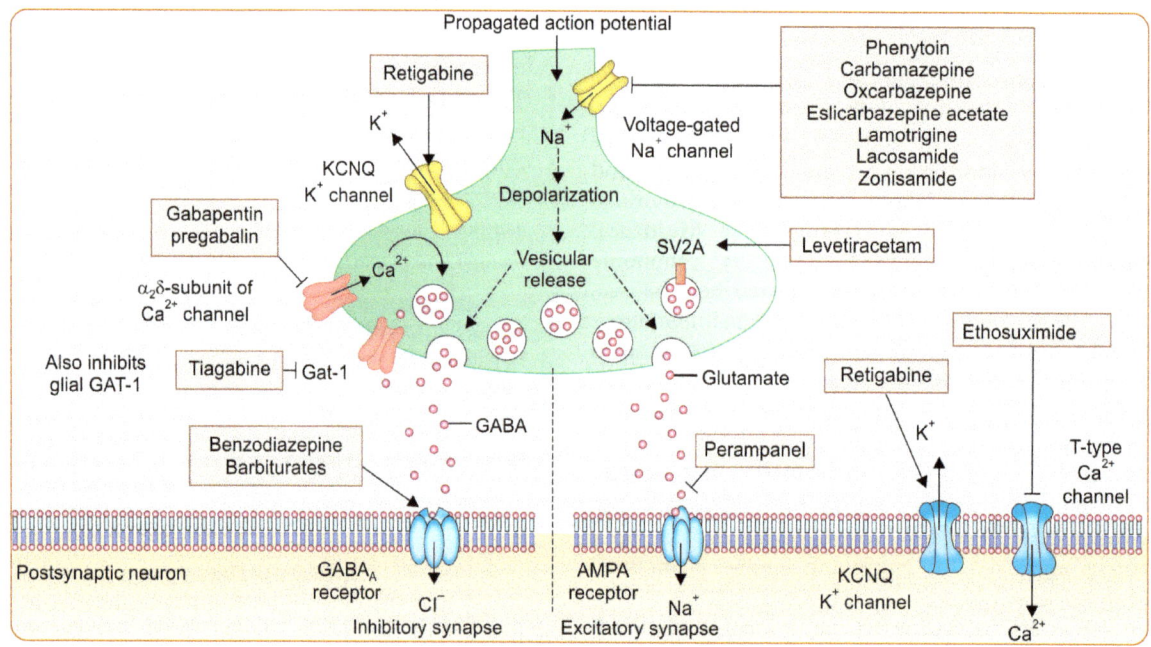

FIG. 7.6: Mechanism of action of anti-epileptic drugs

Central Nervous System

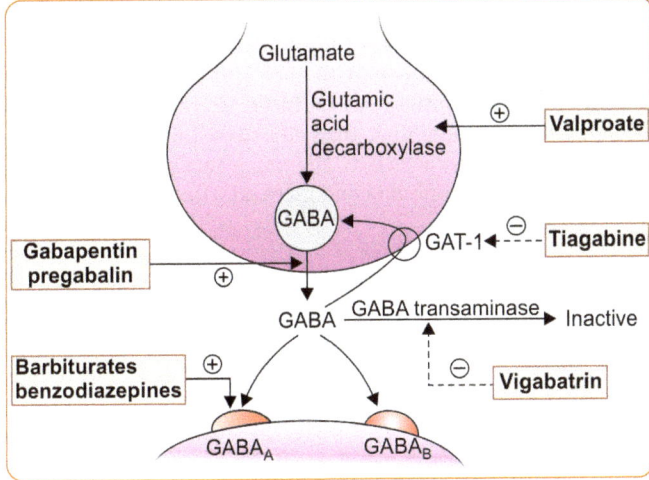

FIG. 7.7: GABAergic transmission and drug targets

IMPORTANT DRUGS

1. Barbiturates

Phenobarbitone and primidone act as anticonvulsant drugs due to GABA mimetic as well as GABA facilitatory properties. These drugs increase the duration of opening of chloride channels. These drugs are useful in generalized tonic clonic seizures (GTCS) and partial seizures. These drugs are *highly sedating* but tolerance develops to this effect. Barbiturates are *contraindicated in acute intermittent porphyria*. These drugs can cause *paradoxical excitation* in some patients. *Phenobarbitone is drug of choice for GTCS in infants but can cause hyperkinesia in older children.*

2. Benzodiazepines

Diazepam, clonazepam, lorazepam and clobazam are benzodiazepines that act by GABA facilitatory activity. These drugs increase the frequency of Cl⁻ channel opening. Diazepam, lorazepam and clonazepam are useful for the management of acute seizures. These can also be used IV for **status epilepticus (Lorazepam is DOC).** *Diazepam given by per rectal route is DOC for febrile seizures.* Benzodiazepines also have prominent **sedative** effects like barbiturates. Tolerance develops to the antiepileptic effect so these are not indicated for long term use.

3. Phenytoin

It is a **non sedating oral** antiepileptic drug. **Fosphenytoin** is a water soluble prodrug of phenytoin that can be administered **parenterally** (IV or IM) for acute attack of seizures (status epilepticus). These drugs act by blocking the use dependent Na⁺ channels. Phenytoin is useful in GTCS and partial seizures.

- It can also be used as an **anti-arrhythmic drug (class Ib)** for the treatment of digitalis induced arrhythmia.
- **Recently** it has been found to **enhance wound healing**.
- This drug **follows saturation kinetics** (kinetics changes from first order to zero order within therapeutic concentrations).
- Phenytoin from different manufacturers (different brands) have different bioavailability and therefore **brand change can lead to toxicity** or suboptimal levels.
- At toxic plasma levels *oral dose of phenytoin* can result in **cerebellar symptoms** (ataxia, vertigo, nystagmus, diplopia).

Contd...

Contd...

- Fosphenytoin should be given by slow *i.v.* infusion because *fast* administration of high doses can lead to *arrhythmias, cardiovascular collapse and coma.*
- **Prolonged use** of phenytoin can result in **gingival hyperplasia** (gum hypertrophy). It results due to overexpression of platelet-derived growth factor (PDGF). It may regress after discontinuation of phenytoin. Other adverse effects on long-term use include **hirsutism, coarsening of facial features, megaloblastic anemia** (treated with folic acid), **vitamin D deficiency** (rickets and **osteomalacia**), vitamin K deficiency, **hyperglycemia** (due to inhibition of insulin release), **hypersensitivity** and **teratogenicity** (**fetal hydantoin syndrome**; hypoplastic phalanges, cleft lip, cleft palate and microcephaly).

> **MNEMONIC**
>
> **Fetal Hydantoin syndrome:**
> P – Hypoplastic Phalanges
> C – Cleft Lip and palate
> M – Microcephaly

- **Osteomalacia** may not always be ameliorated by administration of vitamin D because some *vitamin K dependent proteins* also play a role in Ca²⁺ metabolism in bone.
- **Lymphadenopathy (pseudolymphoma) and malignant lymphoma** (associated with reduced IgA) *and inhibition of ADH release* (in SIADH patients) has also been reported.
- Phenytoin should be stopped gradually because sudden discontinuation may result in precipitation of seizures.
- It is also a **potent enzyme inducer** and can increase the metabolism of various drugs.

> **MNEMONIC**
>
> **Adverse effect of phenytoin:**
> H – Hirsutism
>   Hypertrophy of gums
> O – Osteomalacia
> T – Teratogenicity
> M – Megaloblastic anemia
> A – Ataxia and nystagmus
> L – Lymphadenopathy
> I – Inhibits insulin release (hyperglycemia)
> K – Vitamin K deficiency
> A – Arrhythmias

4. Carbamazepine and Oxcarbazepine

These drugs act by blocking the use dependent sodium channels. Oxcarbazepine has similar efficacy but less toxicity than carbamazepine (CBZ). These are the **drugs of choice for partial seizures** and can also be used in GTCS. *Carbamazepine is DOC for trigeminal neuralgia* and can also be used for glossopharyngeal and post herpetic neuralgia. Another use of carbamazepine is in the treatment of **bipolar disorder** (manic depressive psychosis) and as an **antidiuretic in DI**. It is a potent enzyme inducer and can **induce its own metabolism** (thus requiring more dose if used for long term). Major adverse effects of these drugs include dizziness, headache, ataxia, vertigo and diplopia. It can also cause **rash, leukopenia, aplastic anemia, Steven Johnson syndrome and hepatotoxicity**. Congenital malformations are induced in children delivered to females taking this drug during pregnancy.

Eslicarbazepine is a Na⁺ channel blocker (like carbamazepine) indicated for adjunctive treatment of focal seizures.

5. Valproic Acid

It is a broad spectrum antiepileptic drug effective in all types of seizures. It acts by several mechanisms including blockade of use dependent Na⁺ channels, increased activity of GABA (by increasing synthesis due to stimulation of glutamic acid decarboxylase and decreasing metabolism by inhibiting GABA transaminase), inhibition of T type Ca²⁺ channels and decrease in release of glutamate in the brain. It is the **DOC in GTCS, myoclonic, atonic, atypical absence, clonic and tonic seizures**. It is also effective in Lennox Gestaut syndrome, absence seizures, infantile spasms and partial seizures.

It should be gradually stopped to avoid withdrawl seizures. Other uses of this drug include **bipolar disorder, prophylaxis of migraine** and as an alternative to carbamazepine in **trigeminal neuralgia**. Recently it has also been used in tardive dyskinesia. It is also the **drug of choice for bipolar disorder in patient having rapid cycles** (4 or more cycles per year).

> **Key Points**
>
> **Valproate is drug of choice for**
> - GTCS
> - Myoclonic Seizures
> - Atonic Seizures
> - Absence Seizures
> - Clonic Seizures
> - Tonic Seizures
> - Lennox Gastaut Syndrome

Valproic acid is a potent microsomal **enzyme inhibitor**. Adverse effect of this drug includes weight gain, alopecia, tremors, carnitine deficiency and **irreversible hepatic necrosis (more in children < 2 yrs old)**. The risk of **hepatotoxicity increases** when combined **with** enzyme inducers like **carbamazepine** (due to more production of hepatotoxic metabolite of valproate). It is **DOC for absence seizures** (petit mal epilepsy). However, it should be avoided in children <2 years due to risk of irreversible hepatic necrosis. As absence seizures rarely develop before 5 years of age, valproate may be considered as drug of choice for majority of absence seizures. In rare cases of absence seizure in young children (<2 years), ethosuximide should be used. **Acute pancreatitis and hyperammnonemia** have been frequently associated with valproic acid. If used during pregnancy, it can result in **neural tube defects in the baby** (prevented by folic acid administration during pregnancy). It is a associated with **polycystic ovarian disease** in girls.

MNEMONIC

Adverse effects of valproate
- V – Vomiting
- A – Alopecia
- L – Liver damage
- P – Pancreatitis, PCOD
- R – Rash
- O – Obesity
- A – Agranulocytosis
- T – Tremors
- E – Epigastric pain

6. Ethosuximide and Trimethadione

These drugs act by inhibiting T type Ca²⁺ channels and are **useful only in absence seizures** (petit mal epilepsy). Ethosuximide is **DOC for this condition in children less than 2 years old**. Trimethadione is more toxic than ethosuximide and is therefore no longer used. **Characteristic adverse effect of trimethadione is hemarlopia** (photophobia and glare effect).

7. Other Antiepileptic Drugs

- **Vigabatrin** is an irreversible **inhibitor of GABA transaminase**, thus increases GABAergic activity. It is the *DOC for infantile spasms associated with tuberous sclerosis (ACTH is DOC for all other cases)*. It can result in **irreversible visual field defects** due to retinal atrophy.

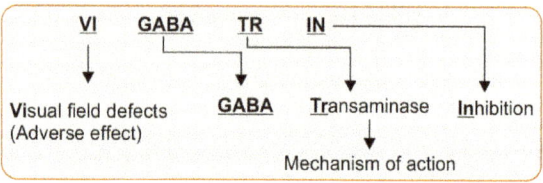

- **Lamotrigine is a broad spectrum** antiepileptic drug useful for various seizures including absence seizures and myoclonic epilepsy. It is **specifically indicated for depressive phase of manic depressive psychosis. Steven Johnson syndrome and toxic epidermal necrolysis** are important adverse effects of this drug.
- **Gabapentin** acts by inhibiting presynaptic calcium channels by binding to $α_2δ_1$ subunits. Its absorption from GIT is saturable, therefore it is safe even after overdosing. It is useful in GTCS and partial seizures. Non epileptic uses include **diabetic and post herpetic neuralgia** (DOC for both of these conditions) and pain associated with multiple sclerosis. Another drug similar to gabapentin is **pregabalin**.
- **Ganaxolone** is a **neurosteroid** (synthesized in the brain) and is effective for absence seizures, infantile spasms and catamenial epilepsy (seizures occurring during menstruation).
- **Topiramate** acts by blocking Na⁺ channels, increasing GABA transmission and inhibiting kainate receptors. It is useful in GTCS, partial seizures and Lennox Gestaut syndrome. **It can cause weight loss. Zonisamide** (another antiepileptic drug) and **topiramate** can cause **renal stones** due to their carbonic anhydrase inhibitory activity.
- **Felbamate** is an NMDA blocker useful in drug resistant epilepsies but its use is limited due to hepatotoxicity and **aplastic anemia**.
- **Perampanel** is a new selective AMPA-type glutamate receptor antagonist. It is indicated for focal seizures.
- **Levetiracetam** and **brivaracetam** are antiepileptic drugs useful for focal seizures. These modify synaptic release of GABA and glutamate by *binding to synaptic vesicular protein SV2A*. These drugs can cause **CNS adverse effects like irritability, aggression and lability of mood**.
- **Magnesium sulphate** is **DOC for treating the convulsions during labour (eclampsia)**. Its toxicity is monitored by *patellar reflex* (knee jerk).
- **Tiagabine** is indicated for adjunctive treatment of partial seizures. It is a **rationally designed** drug as an inhibitor of GABA uptake (by inhibiting GAT-1).
- **Lacosamide** is a recently approved drug for the adjunctive therapy of partial-onset seizures. It acts by blocking Na⁺ channels and CRMP-2 (Collapsin-Response Mediator Protein). Blockade of CRMP-2 result in stopping the effect of neurotrophic factors like BDNF and NT3 on axonal and dendritic growth.

Central Nervous System

- **Stiripentol** is a new oral antiepileptic drug. It increases GABAergic activity. It has recently been approved for oral treatment of **Dravet syndrome**.
- **Rufinamide** is another recently approved drug for adjunctive treatment of seizures associated with Lennox-Gastaut syndrome. It is thought to act by inhibiting Na⁺ channels.
- **Retigabine** (also called **ezogabine**) is approved as add-on drug for partial seizures in adults. **Urinary retention,** blue pigmentation of skin and retinal toxicity are major adverse effects.

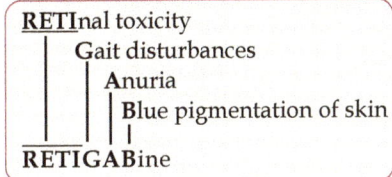

- **Cenobamate** is recently approved Na⁺ channel blocker for focal seizures

- **Cannabidiol** is a CB_1 receptor agonist. It is recently approved for Lennox Gastaut syndrome and Dravet syndrome. It is first drug approved by FDA containing a purified marijuana derivative.

Epilepsy in Pregnancy

- Most important step in management is to control the seizure.
- If a female is already on antiepileptic drugs, the **same drug should be continued** in pregnancy. *Folic acid should be added* to prevent neural tube defects (particularly with valproate). If phenytoin is being taken, vitamin K should be given during labour and to baby after delivery. Regular ultrasound and other assessments should be done to know the fetal malformations.
- If a female is planning to become pregnant, she should be *stabilized on minimum number of antiepileptic drugs.*
- *Newer antiepileptic drugs* are assumed to have *lesser teratogenicity* as compared to older ones (valproate being most tetratogenic). However, the choice of drug depends primarily on type of seizure.
- Among the older drugs, *carbamazepine is assumed to be relatively safer.* However, *Lamotrigine has widest spectrum* (GTCS, typical Absence, atypical absence, myoclonic, atonic, focal seizures) and is *preferred drug in pregnancy.* Topiramate can also be used for all of these except typical absence seizures.
- Folic acid (400 μg or 0.4 mg) should be prescribed to all females of reproductive age group who are on antiepileptic drugs.
- If pregnancy is planned in high-risk women (previous child with neural tube defects), 4000 μg (4 mg) folic acid should be given daily, beginning 1 month before the time of the planned conception.

Selection of Antiepileptic Drugs

	Seizure	First-Line drugs	Alternatives
1.	GTCS	Valproate (DOC) Lamotrigine	Phenytoin Carbamazepine Oxcarbazepine Topiramate Felbamate Barbiturates

Contd...

Contd...

	Seizure	First-Line drugs	Alternatives
2.	Focal	Carbamazepine (DOC) Lamotrigine Phenytoin Levetiracetam	Most other drugs except ethosuximide and benzodiazepines
3.	Absence	Valproate (DOC) Ethosuximide	Lamotrigine Clonazepam
4.	Myoclonic Atonic	Valproate (DOC) Lamotrigine Topiramate	Clonazepam Clobazam Felbamate Rufinamide
5.	Infantile spasms	ACTH (DOC)	Vigabatrin Corticosteroids
6.	Febrile	Diazepam	
7.	Status epilepticus	Lorazepam	Diazepam
8.	Lennox-Gastaut Syndrome	Valproate (DOC) Rufinamide Clobazam	Felbamate Lamotrigine Topiramate
9.	Eclamptic seizures	Magnesium sulphate	

> **Note**
> In a patient with first episode of epilepsy, treatment can be discontinued after tapering the drug, if patient is seizure-free for 2 years.

LENNOX GASTAUT SYNDROME

It is a difficult-to-treat form of childhood-onset epilepsy that most often appears between 2 to 6 years of age. It is characterized by frequent occurrence of different seizure types associated with developmental delay and psychological and behavioural problems. EEG shows characteristic slow spike-wave complexes. **First-line drugs** for treatment are **rufinamide, valproate and benzodiazepines** (clonazepam and clobazam). Second-line drugs are *felbamate* and *topiramate*

DRUGS FOR PSYCHIATRIC ILLNESS

Two major types of psychiatric disorders are psychosis and neurosis.

1. **Psychosis**: Patient is not aware of his illness (*insight is absent*) and refuses to take treatment. It includes major psychosis like schizophrenia as well as mood disorders (like mania, depression and bipolar disorder).
2. **Neurosis**: It is less serious and insight is present. It includes anxiety, obsessive compulsive disorder (OCD), phobias, eating disorders and post traumatic stress disorder (PTSD).

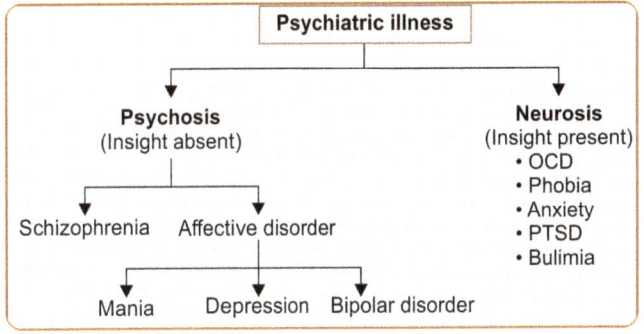

ANTIPSYCHOTIC DRUGS

Schizophrenia is a severe psychiatric illness and is thought to be *due to dopaminergic overactivity in the limbic system* of brain. Other neurotransmitters like 5-HT and NA also probably play a role in this disorder. All drugs for schizophrenia have equal efficacy, these *mainly differ in potency* and can be classified as typical (D_2 blockers) and atypical (acting via other mechanisms) antipsychotics.

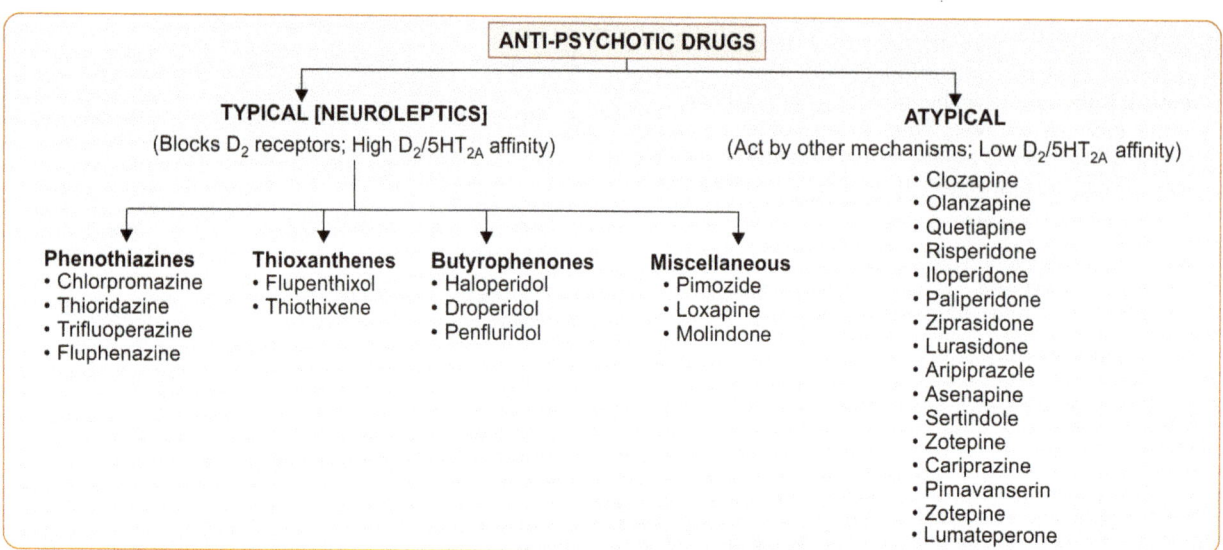

Actions of Typical Antipsychotics

- These drugs act by **blocking D_2 receptors** and differ significantly in potency. **Low potency drugs (like chlorpromazine)** are highly sedative whereas high potency drugs cause less sedation.
- High potency drugs are more likely to cause **extrapyramidal symptoms (maximum with haloperidol)** whereas it is **least common with thioridazine**.
- High potency drugs have low anticholinergic and autonomic side effects as compared to low potency drugs.
- These drugs **lower seizure threshold** and can precipitate convulsions in an epileptic patient.
- All of these agents are **potent antiemetic drugs except thioridazine**.
- **Low potency drugs** possess significant **α blocking** (maximum with chlorpromazine) **and anticholinergic** (maximum with thioridazine) properties. High potency compounds have less activity on these receptors.
- Due to blockade of D_2 receptors in hypothalamus and pituitary, these drugs can **increase prolactin release** resulting in *galactorrhoea and amenorrhea*.

Actions of Atypical Antipsychotics

These drugs act by *antagonistic actions at 5-HT$_2$ and α receptors* and may or may not possess D_2 blocking activity. These drugs are *less likely to cause extrapyramidal symptoms*. However, most of these agents *(except ziprasidone and aripiprazole)* can result in **weight gain, hyperlipidemia and new-onset diabetes mellitus**.

Individual Drugs

- **Thioridazine:** It has *least incidence of extrapyramidal symptoms among typical antipsychotic* drugs due to low potency D_2 blocking action and presence of central anticholinergic activity.
  - It interferes with male sexual function by *inhibiting ejaculation* (due to α blocking action)
  - It can cause cardiac arrhythmia (Prolongation of QT interval).
  - *Retinal damage* limits long term administration.

- **Trifluperazine, fluphenazine and haloperidol**
  - These are high potency drugs and have *least α blocking, anticholinergic, sedative and proconvulsant actions*. However, extrapyramidal symptoms are marked.
- **Penfluridol** is the *longest acting* antipsychotic drug.
- **Pimozide** selectively blocks D_2 receptors without affecting α and muscarinic receptors. It also possesses long duration of action. It carries the risk of arrhythmias due to *QT prolongation*.
- **Clozapine** is an *atypical antipsychotic* drug having weak D_2 blocking action. It mainly acts by blocking 5-HT$_2$, α adrenergic and D_4 receptors.
  - It *suppresses both positive as well as negative symptoms* (First FDA approved drug for antisuicide indication) of schizophrenia.
  - It is used only as a reserve drug due to the *risk of precipitation of seizures* (even in non-epileptics) and **agranulocytosis**.
  - Convulsions are dose-dependent adverse effect seen only in high doses whereas agranulocytosis is independent of dose.
  - Because of association with **myocarditis**, clozapine is *contra-indicated in patients with severe heart disease*.
  - **Most common adverse effect** of clozapine is **sedation**.
  - It has powerful anticholinergic effects (equivalent to chlorpromazine and thioridazine).
  - Risk of *extrapyramidal symptoms is least* with the use of this drug.
  - It specifically has two risks of intestinal dysfunction; *potentially severe ileus and sialorrhea*.
- **Risperidone:** It acts by blocking 5-HT$_2$, α adrenergic and D_2 receptors. It is more potent D_2 blocker than clozapine and can cause extrapyramidal symptoms at high dose. Risk of precipitation of seizures is less than clozapine. **Hyperprolactinemia** has been reported more commonly with risperidone than other atypical antipsychotics. Its active metabolite (paliperidone) has lesser risk of causing metabolic adverse effects.

> **Key Points**
>
> **Long-acting Injectable anti-psychotics for un-cooperative patients.**
> - Fluphenazine decanoate
> - Haloperidol decanoate
> - Risperidone microspheres
> - Paliperidone palmitate

- **Olanzapine**: It has similar mode of action as risperidone. It is also a potent anticholinergic drug and can cause dry mouth and constipation. It can cause seizures and *weight gain*. Apart from its use in schizophrenia, it is also used in *acute mania and bipolar disorder*. It has been associated with significantly **higher risk of stroke and death** in elderly patients.
- **Ziprasidone**: It causes *QT prolongation* and carries risk of arrhythmias. Unlike other atypical antipsychotics, it is not associated with weight gain, hyperlipidemia or diabetes.
- **Quetiapine**: Can cause *cataract formation*. It has *shortest half life*.
- **Aripiprazole**: Acts as a partial agonist at $5\text{-}HT_{1A}$ and D_2 receptors and antagonist at $5\text{-}HT_{2A}$ receptors. It is also known as *dopamine- serotonin stabilizer*. It has quite long half life. It has also been approved for treatment of *irritability associated with autistic disorders in children*.
- **Asenapine** is used **sublingually** for schizophrenia and acute mania.
- **Iloperidone** has less risk of extrapyramidal adverse effects but cause orthostatic hypotension and can prolong QT interval.
- **Brexipiprazole** and **cariprazine** are new drugs approved for schizophrenia.
- **Pimavanserin** is a new atypical antipsychotic drug. It is indicated for oral treatment of **hallucinations** and **delusions** associated with **Parkinson's disease**.
- **Lumateperone** is antagonist at $5HT_{2A}$ receptor and several dopamine receptor subtypes. It also inhibits reuptake of serotonin. Additional action of this drug is alpha 1 receptor antagonism without significant antimuscarinic or antihistaminic properties. It has recently been approved for treatment of schizophrenia.

Adverse Effects

- Sedation (maximum with chlorpromazine; minimum with ziprasidone and aripiprazole), weight gain (with all, less with ziprasidone) and aggravation of seizures (more with clozapine, olanzapine and chlorpromazine; less chances with risperidone and quetiapine).
- Postural hypotension and inhibition of ejaculation (α blocking property).
- Weight gain (with all *except haloperidol*). All atypical antipsychotics may result in **weight gain, hyperlipidemia and new-onset diabetes** except ziprasidone. According to their potential to cause **adverse metabolic side effects**, antipsychotics can be classified as:

High potential:	Clozapine, Olanzapine
Intermediate potential:	Quetiapine
Low potential:	Risperidone, Paliperidone
Least potential:	Ziprasidone, Aripiprazole, Iloperidone, Asenapine

- Retinal degeneration with thioridazine.
- Agranulocytosis with clozapine.
- Cataract formation with quetiapine.
- Cholestatic jaundice with chlorpromazine.
- Dry mouth, blurred vision, constipation, urinary retention (due to anticholinergic effects; maximum with thioridazine).
- Hyperprolactinemia, amenorrhoea and galactorrhoea (due to D_2 blockade in pituitary).
- **Extrapyramidal symptoms** (due to D_2 blockade in nigrostriatal pathway) are closely **related to antipsychotic potency** of typical antipsychotic drugs

> - **Acute muscular dystonia**: It is the *earliest appearing symptom* (within hours) and may manifest as torticollis, locked jaw, oculogyric crisis or spasm of other muscles. *Central anticholinergics* are useful in the treatment.
> - **Parkinsonism**: It appears between 1-4 weeks of therapy. *Central anticholinergics* like benzhexol are drug of choice for drug induced Parkinsonism.
> - **Akathisia**: It is an irresistible desire to move about in the absence of anxiety. It is the **most common extrapyramidal symptom**. Cigarette smoking is associated with increased risk of akathisia. *Propranolol is the preferred drug for this condition*; however central anticholinergics are also useful in the treatment.
> - **Malignant neuroleptic syndrome**: It presents as hyperthermia, extreme generalized rigidity, autonomic instability and altered mental status. It can be treated by *i.v. dantrolene or bromocriptine*.
> - **Tardive dyskinesia**: It occurs late in therapy and is characterized by purposeless involuntary movements like chewing or puffing of cheeks. It is assumed to occur due to supersensitivity of dopamine receptors. Therefore, *central anticholinergics are contraindicated*. Recently, valbenazine (a VMAT2 inhibitor) is approved for Tardive dyskinesia.

Extrapyramidal Symptoms (EPS)

Disorder	Special feature	Treatment
1. Acute muscular dystonia	Earliest to appear	Benzhexol is drug of choice
2. Akathisia	Most common EPS	Propranolol is drug of choice; Benzhexol can be used
3. Parkinsonism		Benzhexol is drug of choice
4. Tardive dyskinesia	Very late to appear; Due to supersensitivity to dopaminergic receptors	Valbenazine is only drug approved; Benzhexol is contra-indicated
5. Malignant neuroleptic syndrome	Can be life-threatening	Dantrolene is used to relax muscle spasms; Benzhexol and bromocriptine are also indicated

Other Uses

> **MNEMONIC**
>
> Use of antipsychotics
> **ANTI**-emetics
> **Psy**chosis
>   **CHO**rea
>   **TIC** disorders (Gille de la Tourette syndrome)
>
> ANTI PSY CHO TIC

- Antipsychotics are used in acute mania and bipolar disorder. **Atypical antipsychotics (like olanzapine) are drug of choice for acute mania in pregnancy.** Haloperidol is also safe in pregnancy
- These agents can be used as an alternative to ECT in *severe depression with psychotic features.*
- Alcoholic hallucinosis.
- Gilles de la Tourette's syndrome and Huntington's disease.

 Key Points

Treatment of Tic Disorders
- **Tetrabenazine** is drug of choice
- Antipsychotics, both typical (haloperidol, pimozide) as well as atypical (aripiprazole, risperidone) can also be used.
- Alpha 2 agonists like clonidine are most commonly used agents
- Clonazepam, carbamazepine and local injection of botulinum toxin are also indicated

Note

1. **Haloperidol and fluphenazine are most potent typical** antipsychotic drugs whereas **risperidone is most potent atypical antipsychotic agent.**
2. Risk of extrapyramidal adverse effects is negligible with clozapine, quetiapine and aripiprazole.
3. **Chlorpromazine, thioridazine and clozapine possess strongest anticholinergic** activity.
4. **Fluphenazine** (enanthate and decanoate) **and haloperidol** (decanoate) are long-acting **injectable** (s.c. or i.m) forms of typical antipsychotics. **Risperidone** and paliperidone are *atypical antipsychotics available* in long-acting **injectable** form.
5. Most commonly used antipsychotic by intravenous route is haloperidol
6. **Ziprasidone, aripiprazole, asenapine and iloperidone** has negligible risk to cause metabolic adverse *effects* (weight gain, hyperlipidemia and new onset diabetes mellitus)
7. **Asenapine, paliperidone and ziprasidone** has greatest potential to *prolong QT interval.*

Samidorphan is a new drug that acts by μ–receptor antagonism. It has been found to reduce weight gain caused by olanzapine. It is recently approved in combination with olanzapine for treatment of Schizophrenia and bipolar disorder.

ANTIDEPRESSANT DRUGS

According to latest research, depression is **associated with decreased levels** of brain derived neurotrophic factor (**BDNF**) which is critical for regulation of neural plasticity and neurogenesis. Chronic activation of monoamine receptors (5HT and NA receptors) by antidepressants result in increase in BDNF transcription. Another method for treatment of depression is to inhibit the metabolism of BDNF by inhibiting the enzyme glycogen synthase kinase-3 (GSK-3). This action is produced by lithium.

Till date, the best hypothesis assumed is that the depression results due to decreased monoaminergic (*5-HT and NA*) activity in the brain, therefore drugs *increasing* their activity are called **typical anti-depressants (Fig. 7.8).** Drugs acting by other mechanisms are called **atypical anti-depressants.**

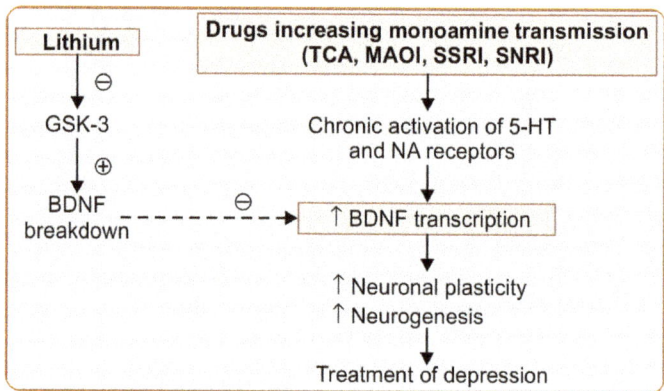

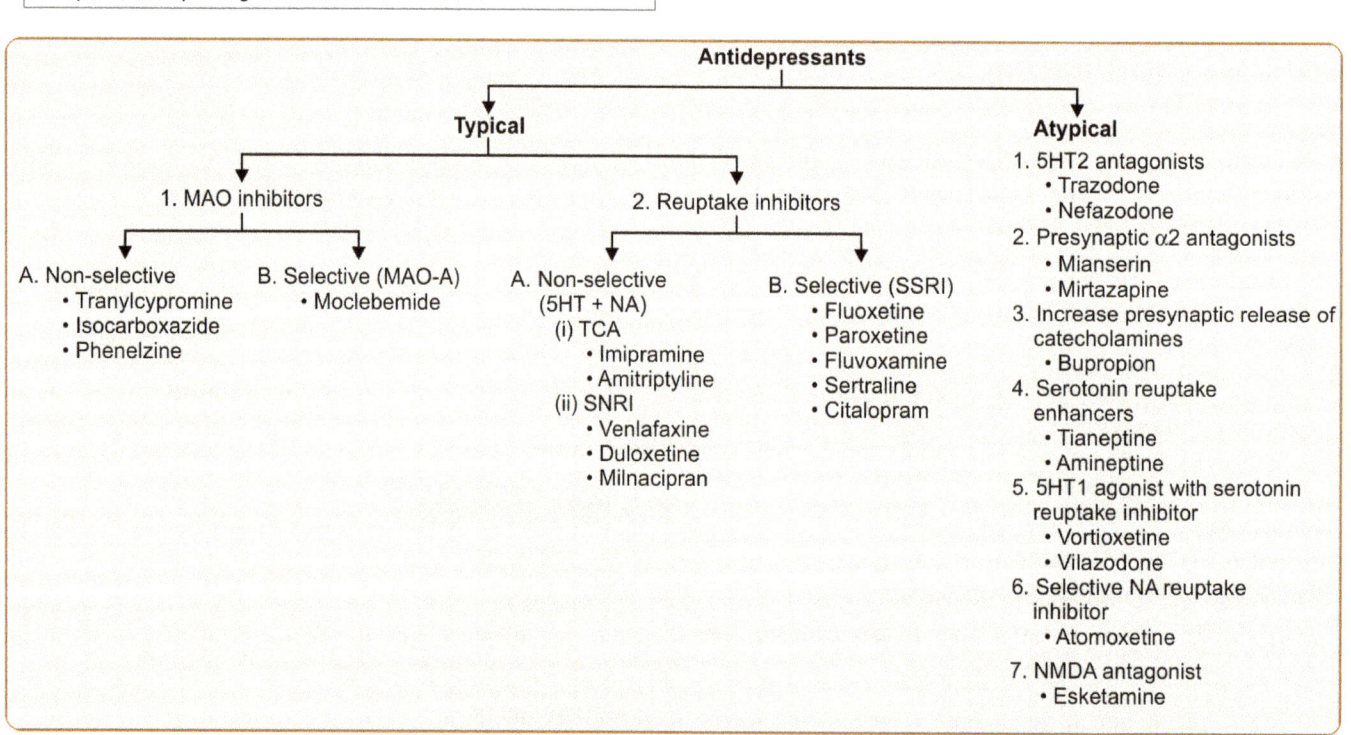

A. TYPICAL ANTIDEPRESSANTS

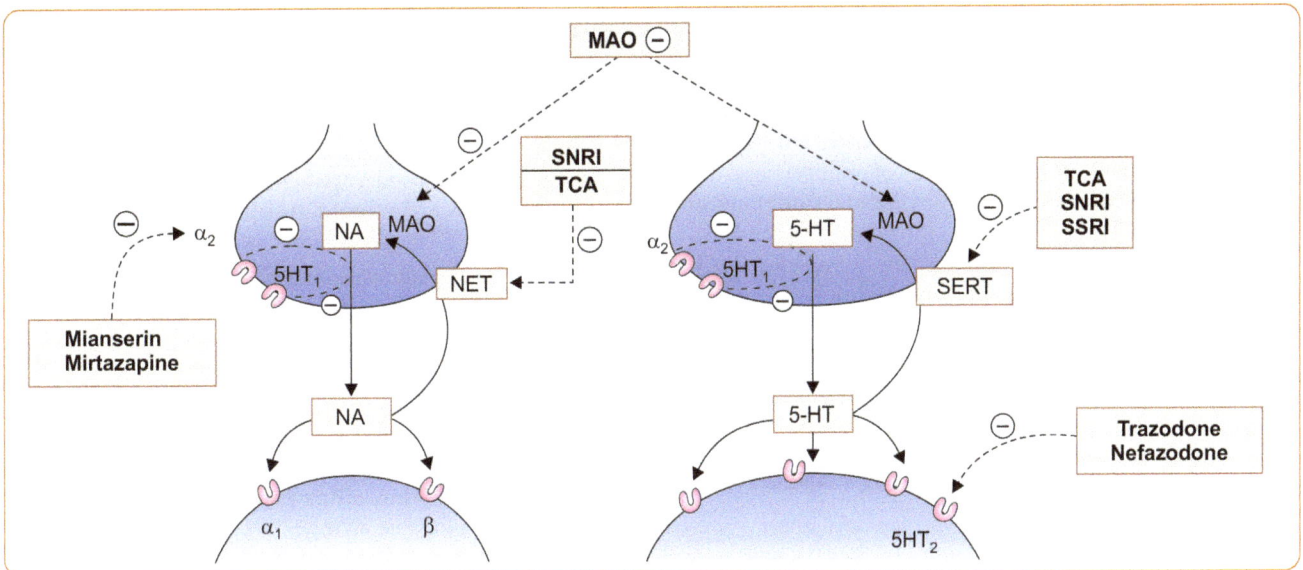

FIG. 7.8: Site of action of antidepressants

Drugs may increase monoaminergic transmission by *inhibiting the metabolism* (MAO inhibitors) or reuptake of 5-HT or NA.

1. MAO Inhibitors

Two types of monoamine oxidase enzymes (MAO-A and MAO-B) are involved in the metabolism of monoamines.

- **MAO-A** predominantly metabolizes **NA, 5-HT and DA** and is present in the intestine, peripheral nerve endings and liver.
- **MAO-B** preferentially metabolizes **dopamine** and is present in the brain, platelets and liver.

Non-selective MAO inhibitors

Tranylcypromine, isocarboxazid and phenelzine inhibits both isoforms of MAO irreversibly. Their anti-depressant effect takes 3-4 weeks to develop. These drugs exhibit a large number of drug and food interactions. The important ones are:

- **Cheese reaction**: *Cheese, beer and red wine contain tyramine* (indirectly acting sympathomimetic). Normally it is metabolized by MAO-A present in the intestine and is not absorbed. In persons taking non-selective MAO inhibitors, tyramine escapes degradation and can lead to **hypertensive crisis**. It is known as cheese reaction. So, cheese etc. should not be given to patients on long term non-selective MAO inhibitor therapy. **Phentolamine** is the drug of choice for cheese reaction.
- Non-selective MAO inhibitors **increase the risk of seizures** if given along with pethidine due to enhanced generation of excitatory metabolite normeperidine.
- **Serotonin syndrome**: If given along with or just after discontinuation of MAO inhibitors, **SSRIs** can result in serotonin syndrome. To avoid this fatal condition, SSRIs should be started at least 14 days after discontinuation of MAO inhibitors. It allows sufficient time for regeneration of MAO.

Reversible inhibitors of MAO-A (RIMA)

Moclebemide inhibits MAO-A selectively and reversibly. Because of its reversible and short action, it **does not exhibit cheese reaction** with foods. It can be used as an alternative to TCAs for the treatment of depression.

Selective MAO-B inhibitors

Selegiline inhibits only MAO-B and is useful in **Parkinsonism**. It is available as a *transdermal patch* for treatment of depression.

2. Reuptake Inhibitors

Drugs may inhibit the reuptake of both serotonin and nor-adrenaline (non-selective reuptake inhibitors, e.g. tricyclic antidepressants) or only serotonin (selective serotonin reuptake inhibitors).

(i) Non-Selective Reuptake Inhibitors

These are further divided into tricyclic antidepressants and serotonin noradrenaline reuptake inhibitors (SNRI).

A. Tricyclic Antidepressants (TCA)

These drugs act by inhibiting the reuptake of **both serotonin and noradrenaline**. This results in increased concentration of these transmitters in the synaptic cleft. *Bupropion also inhibits dopamine reuptake.* NA and serotonin *initially act on presynaptic α_2 and $5HT_{1A}$ receptors respectively and decrease the firing of locus ceruleus (NA) and nucleus raphe magnus (5HT). On long term administration, desensitization of these receptors occurs and enhanced transmission is seen. This explains the *long latency (2-3 weeks)* for the anti-depressant action of TCA and SSRIs despite immediate inhibition of reuptake process.

Adverse effects

- **Sedative** action of TCAs appears immediately and these drugs (particularly clomipramine, maprotiline and bupropion) **lower the seizure threshold.**
- **Weight gain** is another problem with the use of TCAs.
- Most TCAs possess **powerful anticholinergic and weak α blocking property**. Overdose manifestations are mainly

anticholinergic (delirium, urinary retention, blurred vision and constipation) in nature. These also cause postural hypotension (due to α blockade) and cardiac arrythmias at toxic levels.
- TCAs have **low safety margin**.
- **Amoxapine** acts by **blocking D_2 receptors** in addition to the inhibition of NA reuptake. It **possesses antipsychotic properties as well** (It is a metabolite of antipsychotic drug; loxapine). However, risk of extrapyramidal symptoms and convulsions is also present.
- *TCAs (imipramine) are also indicated for nocturnal enuresis in children* (**However, DOC is desmopressin**).

Mechanism of adverse effects of TCA

S.No.	Inhibition of	Adverse Effects
1	Presynaptic NT reuptake	Tremors, Insomnia
2	Cardiac fast Na⁺ channels	Conduction defects, arrhythmias, hypotension
3	Muscarinic ACh receptors	Hyperthermia, flushing, mydriasis, Paralytic ileus, urinary retention, sinus tachycardia
4	α_1 Adrenergic receptors	Postural hypotension
5	H_1 histamine receptors	Sedation

Tricyclic Antidepressant Poisoning

Clinical Presentation

The presenting signs of a TCA overdose include cardiac arrhythmias, hypotension, and anticholinergic signs (hyperthermia, flushing, dilated pupils, intestinal ileus, urinary retention, and sinus tachycardia). Central nervous system signs, such as confusion, delirium, and hallucinations, typically occur before the onset of seizures or coma. Cardiotoxic effects are responsible for the mortality in TCA overdose.

Treatment

- **Intravenous sodium bicarbonate** is the single most effective intervention for the management of TCA cardiovascular toxicity. This agent can reverse QRS prolongation, ventricular arrhythmias, and hypotension. Intravenous sodium bicarbonate is the treatment of choice for sudden-onset ventricular tachycardia, ventricular fibrillation, or cardiac arrest.
- **Lignocaine is the drug of choice for TCA-induced ventricular dysrhythmias.** However, care must be taken to avoid precipitation of seizures. In comparison, many antiarrhythmic drugs should not be used with TCA overdoses. Propranolol, for example, depresses myocardial contractility and conduction while procainamide, disopyramide, and quinidine, via membrane stabilizing effects, may enhance tricyclic toxicity.
- **Intravenous fluids** are the preferred therapy in hypotensive patients. Dopamine can be used if needed because it has both inotropic and vasoconstrictor activity. On the other hand, sympathomimetic vasopressor agents carry the risk of precipitating tachyarrhythmias.
- **Diazepam** is the drug of choice in the management of acute-onset seizures. Phenytoin or phenobarbital may be used as second-line drugs.

- **Physostigmine,** a short-acting cholinesterase inhibitor, has been referred to as the antidote for TCAs because of its ability to increase cholinergic tone and reverse anticholinergic effects. It can, however, causes severe bradycardia, seizures, and asystole by overcompensating for cholinergic tone and suppressing supraventricular and ventricular pacemakers. As a result, physostigmine should only be used in patients with coma or those with convulsion or arrhythmias resistant to standard therapy.

B. Serotonin Noradrenaline Reuptake Inhibitors (SNRI)

- These are also non-selective reuptake inhibitors of both 5-HT and NA like TCAs. However, these *donot possess other properties of TCAs* (like α-blocking, anticholinergic, anti-histaminic, etc). Therefore, SNRI are much safer than TCAs and are currently considered **drug of choice for severe depression.**
- These include **venlafaxine, desvenlafaxine** (longer acting d-isomer), **duloxetine, milnacipran** and **levo-milnacipran**
- **Duloxetine is longest acting** SNRI.
- **Milnacipran and duloxetine** are also indicated in *fibromyalgia*.
- **Venlafaxine** has *faster onset* of action and minimum drug-drug interactions.
- **Duloxetine** is indicated in *neuropathic pain* also.

(ii) Selective Serotonin Reuptake Inhibitors (SSRI)

These drugs inhibit the reuptake of **5-HT only** (not NA) and lack anticholinergic and α blocking properties. SSRIs are now the **first choice drugs** for *depression, phobias, OCD, PTSD, bulimia, premenstrual tension syndrome and panic attacks* because they offer several advantages over TCAs:
- No anticholinergic adverse effects
- No sedation or weight gain
- No propensity to cause seizures or arrhythmias

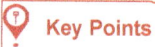 **Key Points**

SSRIs are now the first choice drugs for
- Depression
- Obsessive-Compulsive Disorder
- Post-Traumatic Stress Disorder
- Bulimia
- Premenstrual Tension Syndrome
- Panic Disorder

Adverse Effects

Nausea is the **most frequent complaint** with the use of SSRIs. Anxiety is the next most common adverse effect followed by diarrhea. Other CNS problems like headache, insomnia, etc. are also common. These can **also** cause **inhibition of ejaculation and anorgasmia.** Coadministration of SSRIs with MAO inhibitors can result in *serotonin syndrome*. SSRIs can cause akathisia. Because SSRIs affect platelet serotonin levels, abnormal bleeding can occur. *Sertraline and citalopram appear to be safest SSRIs to be used with warfarin.*

Important compounds

- **Fluoxetine:** It is a prototype SSRI and is **longest acting** drug in this group. It is metabolized to nor-fluoxetine that retains the anti-depressant activity.
- **Fluvoxamine** is the **shortest acting** SSRI.
- **Paroxetine, sertraline** and **citalopram** are other SSRIs.
- **Escitalopram** is *most specific* SSRI.
- **Paroxetine is most teratogenic among SSRIs.**

Central Nervous System

B. ATYPICAL ANTIDEPRESSANTS

These drugs may or may not increase monoaminergic levels and possess different anti-depressant mechanisms.

- **Trazodone** is a prominent α blocker and weak 5-HT$_2$ antagonist. It produces *sedation, priapism* (prolonged and painful erection) and *postural hypotension* as adverse effects.
- **Mianserin** acts by **blocking presynaptic α$_2$ receptors** but *seizure* augmenting and *bone marrow depressant* actions restrict its use.
- **Tianeptine and amineptine** acts by **enhancing** the serotonin reuptake (*action opposite to SSRI*).
- **Mirtazapine:** It inhibits presynaptic α$_2$ receptors and thus increases NA and 5-HT release due to inhibition of auto- and hetero-receptors respectively. Although it increases serotonin levels in synapse, there is selective activation of 5-HT$_1$ receptors due to antagonistic activity at 5-HT$_2$ and 5-HT$_3$ receptors. Therefore it is also known as **nor-adrenergic and specific serotonergic anti-depressant (NSSA)**. It has **minimal sexual side effects** compared with SSRIs. It commonly causes sedation, weight gain, lipid abnormalities and dizziness.
- **Vortioxetine** is a serotonin reuptake inhibitor with 5HT3 antagonistic and 5HT1A receptor agonistic action. It is indicated for major depressive disorder.
- **Bupropion:** It inhibits the uptake of NA and DA. More significant effect of bupropion is **presynaptic release of catecholamines**. It is metabolized to amphetamine like compound and possesses excitatory property. It is **used for smoking cessation** as sustained release formulation. It can precipitate **seizures** at high dose.
- **Nafazodone:** It blocks serotonin reuptake and antagonizes 5-HT$_2$ receptors. It lacks antichelinergic effects (of TCAs) and agitation (seen with SSRI). It has very short half life and is hepatotoxic.
- **Atomoxetine:** It is a selective inhibitor of NA reuptake and is useful for **Attention Deficit Hyperkinetic Disorder** (efficacy similar to methylphenidate).
- **Vilazodone** is a serotonin reuptake inhibitor and partial agonist at 5HT$_{1A}$ receptors.
- **Esketamine** is S-enantiomer of ketamine. It is a non-competitive antagonist of NMDA-receptors. It also inhibits reuptake of dopamine. However, unlike ketamine, it **does not interact with sigma receptors**. It is approved for treatment of patients with treatment resistant depression. It is given by **intranasal route**.
- **Brexanolone** (Also called Allopregnanolone) is a neurosteroid. It is approved for treatment of **post-partum depression** by intravenous route. Like neurosteroids, it acts as a positive allosteric modulator of GABA$_A$ receptors.

> ⚠️ **MNEMONIC**
>
> **Uses of anti-depressants**
> D - Depression
> E - Enuresis (Imipramine)
> P - Phobia
> R - Recurrent panic attacks
> E - Eating disorders (Bulimia)
> S - Smoking cessation (Bupropion)
> S - Stress disorder (Post-traumatic)
> I - Impulse disorder (Kleptomania)
> O - Obsessive compulsive disorder
> N - Neuropathic pain

ANTI MANIC DRUGS

Lithium

It is a small monovalent cation that *does not produce any acute effect* but on prolonged use, acts as a mood stabilizer. It has no psychotropic effect in normal persons.

Mechanism of Action

Some neurotransmitters in the brain act on G-protein coupled receptors. They use IP3 and DAG (formed from PIP2) as second messengers. IP3 is metabolized to regenerate PIP2 **(Fig. 7.9)**. Activity of these pathways is postulated to be markedly increased during a manic episode. **Lithium** *inhibits the regeneration of PIP2* by inhibiting an enzyme inositol monophosphatase, thereby decreasing this activity.

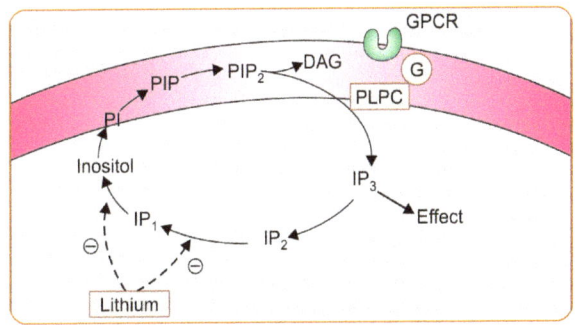

FIG. 7.9: Mode of action of lithium

In addition, lithium (and valproate) inhibit glycogen synthase kinase 3 (GSK3), an enzyme involved in degradation of BDNF. This action is likely to be involved in the use of lithium for unipolar depression.

Uses and Adverse Effects

- It has **narrow margin of safety** (low therapeutic index) and therapeutic drug monitoring (TDM) is essential.
- It takes 1-2 weeks to exert its maximum effect. It is the **drug of choice for the prophylaxis of bipolar disorder. Its t1/2 is 24 hours**. Lithium is the only drug used in bipolar disorder which has **documented anti-suicide properties**.
- It can be used in **acute mania** but *benzodiazepines* like lorazepam must be added (due to slow action of Li). In patients not controlled by BZDs, antipsychotics like olanzapine may be added.
- Plasma concentration of lithium should be **0.5-0.8 mEq/L for maintenance** therapy of bipolar disorder and **0.8-1.2 mEq/L for acute mania.** Toxic symptoms are seen if plasma concentration exceeds 1.5 mEq/L.
- **Diuretics** (particularly thiazides) decrease the renal excretion of lithium and thus **may result in toxicity.** This is due to increased reabsorption of Na$^+$ and lithium ions (as a compensatory response to excessive loss of Na$^+$).

Other effects of lithium are
L – Leucocytes
I – Increased
T – Tremors (Most common side effect)
H – Hypothyroidism
I – Increased ⎤ Nephrogenic diabetes insipidus, can be used for the treatment of SIADH.
U – Urine ⎦ *Amiloride is DOC for lithium induced DI.*
M should be avoided in expectant **Mothers** as it causes *Ebstein's anomaly*

- Acne and weight gain (due to Na⁺ and water retention) are the other adverse effects.
- It can cause benign and reversible elevation of T waves in ECG.

Alternatives to Lithium
- **Carbamazepine and valproate** are useful in manic depressive psychosis (bipolar disorder). These can also be used for acute mania. **Valproic acid is the drug of choice for treatment of rapid cyclers** (> 4 cycles/year).
- **Benzodiazepines like lorazepam** are the **drugs of choice for acute mania** when combined with lithium. Olanzapine and other atypical antipsychotics show efficacy in bipolar disorder as well as acute mania.
- **Lamotrigine is specifically useful for depressive phase of bipolar disorder.** It is the first agent to be *approved* by FDA *for bipolar disorder without* an indication for *acute mania*.

Lithium Toxicity

- Acute intoxication is characterized by vomiting, diarrhea, coarse tremor (fine tremor in mild intoxication), ataxia, coma and convulsions.
- More serious effects involve mental confusion, hyperreflexia, dysarthria, seizures, and cranial and focal neurological signs progressing to coma and death.
- Other toxic effects are cardiac arrhythmias, hypotension and albuminuria.
- There is **no specific antidote** for lithium. **Dialysis** is most effective means of removing Li from body. It is indicated at serum Li levels of **> 4 mEq/L in acute overdose or > 1.5 mEq/L in chronic overdose.**

ANTI ANXIETY DRUGS

Reduction in the GABAergic activity or increase in serotonergic activity may result in anxiety. It is due to mild CNS stimulation. Drugs commonly used for anxiety are CNS depressants (like benzodiazepines) or those decreasing serotonin level (like buspirone).

Benzodiazepines

Chlordiazepoxide is used for **chronic** anxiety states whereas *oxazepam, lorazepam, alprazolam and diazepam* are indicated for *short lasting anxiety states. Oxazepam and lorazepam are safe in elderly and in patients with liver disease.* Benzodiazepines are most commonly used anxiolytic drugs; however sedation, cognitive impairment and abuse liability are potential limitations in their use.

Azapirones

Buspirone, gepirone and ipsapirone act as *partial agonists of presynaptic 5-HT₁ₐ receptors* and decrease the release of serotonin. These drugs *do not cause sedation* or cognitive impairment and are *devoid of abuse potential, muscle relaxant and anticonvulsant activity.* Therapeutic effect of these drugs takes up to 2 weeks and therefore these are **ineffective in acute anxiety states** like panic attacks. These are indicated for mild to moderate generalized anxiety states.

Beta Blockers

Propranolol is indicated for **performance anxiety** where it decreases the sympathetic manifestations of anxiety.

Other Drugs
- **Hydroxyzine** is H₁ antihistaminic having anti-anxiety activity but profound sedation limits its usefulness.
- **SSRIs** like fluoxetine are agents of choice for panic disorder whereas benzodiazepines are drug of choice for panic attacks and generalized anxiety disorder.

 Key Points
- DOC for acute management of generalized anxiety is benzodiazepines
- SSRI are first line medications for sustained treatment of generalized anxiety disorders.

Key Points
- Lorazepam is DOC for acute treatment of panic attacks whereas for sustained treatment, SSRIs are preferred.

ALCOHOLS

Ethyl Alcohol (Ethanol)

It is a CNS depressant drug that can result in psychological as well as physical dependence. It is an *imperfect food* because it lacks essential constituents and it *cannot be stored*. It follows **zero order kinetics** and plasma concentration >300 mg/dL may result in death. **Acute ingestion** of large quantities may result in **fall in blood pressure** whereas **chronic alcohol** consumption may contribute to **hypertension and dilated cardiomyopathy.** *Moderate consumption* of alcohol (18-20 g daily, roughly equivalent to 50-100 mL of whiskey) *decreases the risk of coronary artery disease* by increasing HDL and decreasing LDL cholesterol. Ethanol is **metabolized to acetaldehyde** (by alcohol dehydrogenase) and **finally to acetic acid** (by aldehyde dehydrogenase). **Disulfiram** (antabuse) and several drugs (*chlorpropamide, cefoperazone, moxalactam, cefamandole, metronidazole, griseofulvin* etc.) cause inhibition of aldehyde dehydrogenase resulting in accumulation of acetaldehyde. Acetaldehyde may lead to severe distressing symptoms known as *disulfiram like reaction*.

- **Chronic alcohol** consumption **induces microsomal enzymes.** More generation of toxic metabolite (NAPQI) of **acetaminophen** is responsible for increased risk of **hepatotoxicity** in alcoholics.
- Alcohol **increases** the chances of **hypoglycemia** in diabetic patients taking insulin and other oral hypoglycemic agents.

 MNEMONIC

Disulfiram like reaction is caused by:
Cyclic :	Chlorpropamide
	Cefoperazone
	Cefomandole
	Cefotetan
G :	Griseofulvin
M :	Metronidazole
	Moxalactam
P :	Procarbazine

Treatment of Alcohol Dependence

Alcohol can produce physical and psychological dependence. In the treatment of alcohol dependence, major aim is to prevent withdrawal symptoms first and to avoid relapse of addiction thereafter.

- **Benzodiazepines** (chlordiazepoxide and diazepam) are given to **prevent withdrawal**. These are long acting CNS depressants and can be withdrawn gradually.
- **Naltrexone** is an opioid antagonist that can be used to **reduce alcohol craving**.
- **Acamprosate** is an **NMDA antagonist** that can be used for **maintenance therapy of alcohol abstinence.**
- **Disulfiram** can be used in psychologically dependent persons who are motivated to quit alcohol. It is **contraindicated in physically dependent** individuals. Disulfiram produces severe distressing symptoms (like flushing, headache, vomiting, visual disturbances and mental confusion) after intake of alcohol. These symptoms are due to accumulation of acetaldehyde. Due to these symptoms, individual's resolution to quit alcohol is strengthened.
- **Topiramate and ondansetron** can also *decrease alcohol craving*.

> **MNEMONIC**
>
> Drugs decreasing alcohol craving
> None – Naltrexone
> Of – Ondansetron
> The – Topiramate
> Above – Acamprosate

Methyl Alcohol (Methanol)

It is metabolized to formaldehyde (by alcohol dehydrogenase) and finally to formic acid (by aldehyde dehydrogenase). Accumulation of **formic acid** may **result in lactic acidosis (high anion gap metabolic acidosis), blindness and death. Specific toxicity of formic acid is retinal damage** leading to blindness. Methanol poisoning can be treated by supportive measures, gastric lavage and sodium *bicarbonate* (to treat acidosis). **Ethanol** is useful because it **competitively inhibits the conversion of methanol to formic acid. Fomepizole (4-Methylpyrazole)** can also be used in methanol poisoning because it is a **specific inhibitor of alcohol dehydrogenase. Folic acid or folinic acid** can also be used because folate dependent systems are responsible for conversion of formic acid to CO_2.

Ethylene Glycol

It is used as a solvent and as an **anti-freeze** in industry. It is metabolized to glycolaldehyde and glycolic acid. At toxic levels, it can cause renal tubular acidosis with **excretion of oxalate crystals in the urine. Fomepizole is the drug of choice** for the treatment of ethylene glycol poisoning.

OPIOIDS

These are the substances obtained from the crude extract of *Papaver somniferum* (poppy plant). Morphine is the prototype opioid and acts by agonistic activity on μ, κ and δ receptors.

Actions Mediated by Opioid Receptors

μ	κ	δ
Sedation	Dysphoria (Psychomimetic effects)	Spinal Analgesia
Analgesia	Constipation	Modulation of hormone and NT release
Constipation	Analgesia	
Respiratory depression		
truncal Rigidity		
eUphoria		
Miosis		

Certain endogenous peptides (endorphins, dynorphins and enkephalins) act on these opioid receptors to produce analgesic effects. Recently a **new endogenous peptide, nociceptin** is isolated that acts on nociceptin/orphanin FQ (N/OFQ) or orphanin like receptors (ORL_1).

Endogenous peptide	Major action on receptors
Endorphin	μ
Dynorphin	k
Enkephalin	δ
Nociceptin	N/OFQ

Pharmacokinetics

- **Sufentanil** is the **most potent** whereas meperidine (**pethidine**) and **propoxyphene** are the **least potent** opioids.
- Morphine is metabolized mainly to morphine-3-glucuronide (**M3G**) that has **neuroexcitatory** properties. Approximately 10% of morphine is metabolized to active product M6G. **Renal failure** can lead to **accumulation** of these metabolites and can result in **seizures** (due to M3G) or prolonged opioid action (due to M6G).
- **Pethidine** is metabolized mainly to meperidinic acid by MAO and very little is demethylated to **norpethidine**. Latter has **seizure inducing and cumulative properties**. Pethidine can result in **seizures if used** for prolonged periods, in patients with **renal failure or** those taking **MAO inhibitors** (due to accumulation of norpethidine).

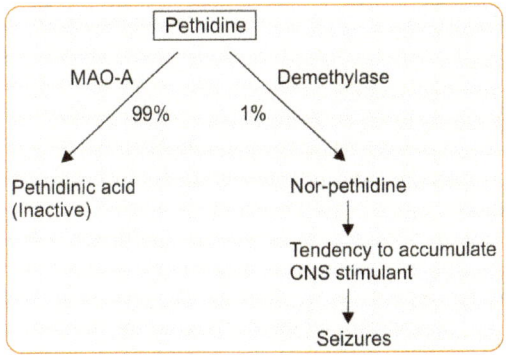

Actions of Pure Opioids

Pure agonists include *morphine, methadone, pethidine, levorphanol, codeine, hydrocodone, oxycodone and propoxyphene*. Actions of these drugs are:

1. **CNS Actions**

- Morphine produces spinal and supraspinal analgesia by acting on **μ, κ and δ receptors.**

- μ receptor opioids have **dependence** producing actions due to euphoric action. κ receptors mediate **psychomimetic** effects (dysphoria). Tolerance develops to all actions of opioids except 3C (**C**onstipation, **c**onvulsions and **c**onstriction of pupil)
- Opioids produce **marked sedation** but chances of sedation are less with pethidine and fentanyl.
- Opioids can produce **respiratory depression and cough suppression.**
- Miosis can occur with morphine use and **pin point pupil** is a valuable sign in diagnosis of opioid poisoning.
- Highly lipid soluble drugs like **fentanyl, alfentanyl and sufentanil** can result in **truncal rigidity** on rapid i.v. infusion.
- By stimulating CTZ, opioids can result in **nausea and vomiting.**

Key Points

Fentanyl is responsible for post operative muscle rigidity whereas succinylcholine causes post operative muscle pain and fasciculations.

2. Peripheral Effects

- Opioids have no direct effect on heart except **pethidine and pentazocine** (that **increase heart rate**). Blood pressure may decrease due to depression of vasomotor system and release of histamine.
- Constipation can result due to decreased motility and increased tone of GIT. Alvimopan is a peripheral opioid antagonist developed for **paralytic ileus.**
- Opioids **increase intrabiliary pressure** by constricting biliary smooth muscle. (C/I in biliary colic).
- These may **aggravate bronchoconstriction** in asthmatics by releasing histamine. (C/I in asthmatics).
- **Spinal or epidural** administration of opioids may result in **intense pruritus** over lips and torso (due to histamine release).

Actions of Mixed Agonists-antagonists

- **Buprenorphine** is partial agonist at μ receptor with κ and δ antagonistic property. It is useful as an analgesic and as an **alternative to methadone** for the management of opioid withdrawal.
- **Nalbuphine, pentazocine and dezocine** are κ agonists and μ receptor antagonists. These drugs can produce **psychomimetic effects** with hallucinations, nightmares and anxiety.
- **Butorphanol** is a predominant κ agonist that produces **equivalent analgesia but more sedation than morphine.**

Clinical Uses

- These are used as **analgesic** agents. Visceral, dull and constant pain is relieved more effectively than inflammatory pain. Opioids are however **contraindicated in biliary colic.**
- Morphine (IV) is useful in **myocardial infarction** as well as in **acute pulmonary edema.**
- **Codeine, pholcodeine, dextromethorphan and noscapine** are effective **cough suppressants.** *Dextromethorphan is devoid of constipating action* unlike other drugs in this group.
- **Loperamide and diphenoxylate** can be used for the treatment of non-infective **diarrhea.**
- Morphine is useful as a pre-anaesthetic medication whereas highly lipid soluble drugs (like **fentanyl, alfentanyl, sufentanil** etc) are used as adjuncts to other **anaesthetic agents.**
- **Pethidine** is used to *reduce shivering* after anaesthesia [by its *action on* α_2 *receptor*]

Routes of Administration

- **Morphine** can be administered by **oral, rectal, IV, IM, intrathecal or epidural routes.**
- **Fentanyl** can be applied as **transdermal patch** or can be administered by **buccal transmucosal** route.
- **Butorphanol** is the only opioid available in **nasal** formulation.

Adverse Effects and Toxicity

- **Respiratory depression, nausea, vomiting, constipation, urinary retention, itching and dysphoria** are important adverse effects of opioids.
- **Tolerance** develops to most of the actions of opioids **except miosis, constipation and convulsions.**
- Opioids are **highly addictive** substances and can lead to development of psychological as well as physical dependence. Sudden discontinuation of these drugs in a dependent subject may lead to **withdrawal syndrome** characterized by **rhinorrhoea**, lacrimation, **yawning**, chills, mydriasis, vomiting, diarrhea and anxiety. Most of these symptoms are opposite to the normal actions of opioids.

Contraindications and Precautions

- **Morphine** is absolutely contraindicated in **head injury** because it increases intracranial tension by causing retention of CO_2 (due to respiratory depression). It also interferes with the assessment of neurological function by masking the important pupillary signs (causes miosis).
- These drugs should be used cautiously in patients with pulmonary, hepatic or renal dysfunction.
- Use of opioids in infants and elderly also require caution.
- Patients of hypothyroidism may show exaggerated response to opioids.
- Prolonged use of opioids in pregnancy may lead to in-utero physical dependence of fetus and severe withdrawal symptoms may be precipitated after birth.

Important Points about Specific Agents

- Morphine, hydromorphone and oxymorphone are strong opioid agonists useful as analgesics.
- Heroin (diacetylmorphine) is a potent and fast acting opioid but carries high risk of abuse potential.
- **Methadone** is a long acting opioid analgesic that can be administered by oral, IV, SC and rectal routes. Apart from potent agonistic actions at μ receptors, it **also blocks NMDA** receptors and reuptake of monoamines.
  These properties explain its ability to **relieve neuropathic and cancer pain** that are not controlled with morphine. Due to its **long $t_{1/2}$**, development of dependence and tolerance is very slow, making it **useful for the treatment of opioid abuse**. It is also useful for opioid rotation therapy.
- **Pethidine and pentazocine** possess anticholinergic activity (can result in **tachycardia**). **These drugs are therefore C/I in MI.** Because of anticholinergic properties, these are **relatively safer in biliary colic** as compared to other agents. Accumulation of active metabolite of pethidine (**norpethidine**) can produce **seizures.**
- Levorphanol is similar to morphine in its actions.
- **Propoxyphene** is a *least potent and least efficacious* analgesic agent.
- **Diphenoxylate** and its active metabolite **difenoxin**, as well as **loperamide** are useful for diarrhea.
- **Buprenorphine exhibits ceiling effect to its respiratory depressant action.**

- **Buprenorphine** dissociates slowly from μ receptors and is thus **resistant to naloxone reversal**.
- **Butorphanol, pentazocine and dezocine** possess **psychomimetic** effects due to κ agonistic activity.
- **Ziconotide** is approved for intrathecal analgesia. It acts by blocking voltage-gated N type Ca^{2+} channels.
- **Tramadol** is a weak m receptor agonist. It also inhibits reuptake of **NA and 5-HT**. These effects are responsible for its **analgesic action**, which can be **abolished by 5-HT3 antagonists** like ondansetron. **At high doses**, it can lead to **seizures**.
- **Tapentadol** is a new analgesic drug with μ-receptor agonistic action and NA reuptake inhibiting action.
- **Eluxadoline** is a m-agonist and d-receptor antagonist. It is approved for oral treatment of diarrhea dominant irritable bowel syndrome.

OPIOID ANTAGONISTS

Naloxone, naltrexone and **nalmefene** are potent m receptor antagonists with significant blocking action at k and d receptors also. **Alvimopan** and **methylnaltrexone** are peripheral opioid antagonists.

- **Naloxone** is given parenterally (**ineffective orally**) and is a **very short acting** drug.
- **Nalmefene** is also given **parenterally** but has a **longer half life**.
- **Naltrexone** is **long acting orally** effective opioid antagonist.
- **Samidorphan** is a μ-receptor antagonist. It is more potent, longer acting and has higher oral bioavailability than naltrexone.

Actions

These have no action in the absence of agonists but promptly **reverses the opioid effects** when administered IV. They **can precipitate withdrawal** symptoms **in** opioid **dependent** subjects

Uses

- **Naloxone** is the **drug of choice for acute opioid poisoning** but it has to be repeated frequently.
- **Naltrexone** is used as a **maintenance drug for opioid poisoning**. It is also used **to prevent relapse after opioid de-addition**. It is **also** used to **decrease craving** in chronic alcoholics. However, naltrexone **DOES NOT DECREASE CRAVING FOR OPIOIDS.**
- **Naltrexone plus bupropion** has recently been approved for **treatment of obesity**
- **Naloxone** is also used in **neonatal resuscitation** to reverse the effects of opioids (if used during labour). However, it should **not be used** for this purpose **if mother is dependent** on opioids. (*Baby is also dependent in utero and naloxone can precipitate withdrawal*).
- Naloxone is being added to opioids meant for oral use to minimize their addictive potential. If the patient takes the combination orally, only opiod is absorbed not naloxone. Thus, it will produce the desired action. However, if the person takes it by i.v. route for addiction, naloxone also reaches the blood and stops euphoria.

- **Methylnaltrexone, naldemedine** and **naloxegol** are peripheral opioid antagonists indicated for **opioid-induced constipation. Alvimopan** is another peripheral μ-receptor antagonist. It is used for postoperative ileus.
- **Samidorphan** is given in combination with olanzapine for schizophrenia and bipolar disorder. It prevents the weight gain caused by olanzapine due to μ receptor antagonism.

  Key Points

Uses of opioid antagonists

Naloxone
- Acute opioid poisoning
- Neonatal resuscitation
- With opioids (oral)

Naltrexone
- Maintenance drug is opioid poisoninig
- To prevent relapse in opioid de-addiction
- To decrease craving in alcoholics.

OPIOID DE-ADDICTION

Chronic intake of opioids can result in physical and psychological dependence. If suddenly stopped, the person may develop severe withdrawal symptoms, which may be life threatening. For de-addiction of opioids (or any addictive drug), first aim is to stop the further use of the drug by the patient followed by maintainance of de-addiction (i.e., to prevent relapse).

- If addiction is of short duration and with small doses of addictive drug, sudden stoppage of drug therapy can be attempted and the *mild withdrawal symptoms can be treated with β-blockers or clonidine (or lofexidine)*.
- If addiction is of long duration or with large dose of opioids, sudden withdrawal of the offending drug may be dangerous (due to severe withdrawal symptoms). In such patients, the addictive drug is replaced by equivalent dose of *methadone* (known as methadone maintenance). It *prevents withdrawal symptoms* by stimulating opioid receptors but is much less addictive. The dose of methadone is then gradually decreased and finally stopped.
- To prevent relapse after de-addiction, naltrexone is used. Naltrexone prevents euphoric action by blocking μ receptors. If the person again takes opioids (after de-addiction), there will be no euphoria and the person's resolution to quit addiction will be strengthened.

Note
- β-blockers and clonidine treat withdrawal symptoms.
- Methadone prevents withdrawal symptoms.
- Naltrexone is used to prevent relapse.
- Methadone is used as maintenance therapy in opioid dependence whereas naltrexone is used as maintenance therapy in opioid poisoning.

Golden Points

1. GABA$_C$ receptors are present in retina and are ionotropic mediating influx of chloride (like GABA$_A$) whereas GABA$_B$ receptors are G-protein coupled receptors.

2. Barbiturates are absolutely contraindicated in acute inter-mittent porphyria.

3. Ramelteon is agonist of MT$_1$ and MT$_2$ receptors of melatonin in suprachiasmatic nucleus. It is approved for long term use in treatment of sleep onset insomnia.

4. **Addition of carbi-dopa to l-dopa therapy**
   - Increase entry of L-dopa in brain
   - Decrease adverse effects due to peripherally formed dopamine.

5. Carbi-dopa decrease all adverse effects of l-dopa therapy except:
   - Abnormal movements
   - Behavioural Changes.

6. **Ergot alkaloids** are short acting and can cause digital **vasosopasm** (leading to gan-grene) and pleural, peritoneal and cardiac **fibrosis**.

7. **Pramipexole and ropinirole** are long acting and do not cause gangrene. These are now the **first choice drugs** for Parkinsonism.

8. **Pramipexole and Ropinirole** are drug of choice for treatment of restless leg syndrome.

9. **Rotigotine** is a dopamine agonist that can be administered through a **transdermal patch** but was discontinued due to crystal formation on the patches.

10. **Central anticholinergic** drugs like trihexiphenidyl (benzhexol), procyclidine, benztropine, orphenadrine and biperiden are the drugs of choice for **drug induced Parkinsonism**.

11. Drug of choice for acute attacks in MS is steroids whereas interferon-β is DOC for preventing the relapse in RRMS.

12. Penicillamine and trientine can worsen neurological symptoms in Wilson disease, therefore are not recommended for initial neurological therapy.

13. Benzodiazepines (preferably lorazepam) are drug of choice for status epilepticus.

14. Carbamazepine is drug of choice for partial seizures and trigeminal neuralgia.

15. Phenytoin and carbamazepine can worsen generalized seizures including absence, myoclonic, tonic and atonic seizures.

16. Drug of choice for infantile spasms is ACTH whereas infantile spasms associated with tuberous sclerosis is treated with vigabatrin.

17. Zonisamide and topiramate can cause renal stones.

18. **Retigabine** (also called **ezogabine**) is approved as add-on drug for partial seizures in adults.

19. Magnesium sulphate is DOC for treating the convulsions during labour (eclampsia). Its toxicity is monitored by patellar reflex (knee jerk).

20. Clozapine induced convulsions are dose-dependent adverse effect whereas agranulocytosis is independent of dose.

21. Ziprasidone can cause QT prolongation and Quetiapine can cause cataract formation.

22. Asenapine is used sublingually.

23. Acute muscular dystonia is the earliest appearing symptom whereas akathisia is the most common extrapyramidal symptom.

24. **Prazosin** decreases nightmares and improves quality of sleep in post-traumatic stress disorder.

25. SSRIs should be started at least 14 days after dis-continuation of MAO inhibitors to avoid the risk of serotonin syndrome.

26. Imipramine, amitryptiline, trimipramine and clomipramine inhibit the uptake of both 5-HT and NA whereas desipramine, nortryptiline and amoxapine are predominantly NA reuptake inhibitors.

27. Systematic densensitization by gradual exposure to feared situation is used for management of specific phobias. **Cycloserine** enhances extinction of fear responses with exposures.

28. **Venlafaxine, milnacipran, levo-milnacipran and duloxetine** inhibit reuptake of serotonin and NA but lack anticholinergic and α blocking properties. These are also referred to as serotonin and nor-adrenaline reuptake inhibitors (**SNRI**).

29. **Mirtazapine** is also known as nor-adrenergic and specific serotonergic anti-depressant (**NSSA**).

30. **Bupropion** is used for **smoking cessation**.

31. Half-life of lithium is 24 hours.

32. Naltrexone is an opioid anta-gonist that can be used to reduce alcohol craving.

33. Pethidine can result in seizures if used for prolonged periods, in patients with renal failure or those taking MAO inhibitors (due to accumulation of norpethidine).

34. **Nalbuphine, pentazocine and dezocine** are κ agonists and μ receptor antagonists. These drugs can produce psychomimetic effects with hallucinations, nightmares and anxiety.

35. Pethidine is used to reduce shivering after anaesthesia [by its action on α$_2$ receptor].

36. Morphine is absolutely contraindicated in head injury because it increases intracranial tension by causing retention of CO_2 (due to respiratory depression). It also interferes with the assessment of neurological function by masking the important pupillary signs (causes miosis).

37. Buprenorphine exhibits ceiling effect to its respiratory depressant action.

Drug of Choice

Condition	Drug of choice
Alcohol dependence	
– Withdrawl symptoms (including seizures)	Benzodiazepines like chlordiazepoxide or diazepam
– Maintenance therapy	Chlordiazepoxide
– To prevent craving	Naltrexone
Methanol poisoning	Fomepizole
Ethylene glycol poisoning	Fomepizole
Anxiety disorders	
– Performance anxiety	Propranolol
– Generalized anxiety disorder (GAD)	
- Acute attacks	Benzodiazepines
- Sustained treatment	Antidepressants (venlafaxine/duloxetine)
– Panic disorder	
- Acute panic attacks	Benzodiazepines
- Sustained treatment	SSRI (Sertraline)
Insomnia	Zolpidem
Benzodiazepine poisoning	Flumazenil
Epilepsy/seizure disorders	
– Grand mal (GTCS)	Valproate
– Petit mal (Absence)	Valproate
– Focal	Carbamazepine/Oxcarbazepine
– Myoclonic	Valproate
– Atonic	Valproate
– Infantile spasms	
- Without tuberous sclerosis (TS)	ACTH
- With TS	Vigabatrin
– Febrile seizures	Diazepam
– Status epilepticus	Lorazepam
– Eclamptic seizures	Magnesium sulphate
– Epilepsy in pregnancy	Lamotrigine/Topiramate/levetiracetam
– Lennox-Gastaut syndrome	Valproate/Rufinamide/Clonazepam
Neuropathic pain	
– Trigeminal neuralgia	Carbamazepine
– Post-herpetic neuralgia	Pregabalin or gabapentin
– Diabetic neuropathic pain	Pregabalin or gabapentin
Parkinsonism	
– Early	Pramipexole/Ropinirole
– Late	Pramipexole/Ropinirole
– Drug induced	Anticholinergics (Benzhexol)
Levo-dopa induced	
– Vomiting	Domperidone
– Psychosis	Atypical antipsychotics (olanzapine)
Schizophrenia	Olanzapine
– In non-compliant patients	Risperidone LAI (long acting injection)
– Refractory	Clozapine
Manic disorder	
– Acute mania	Benzodiazepines/Antipsychotics (olanzapine) + lithium
– Prophylaxis of mania	Lithium
– Bipolar disorder	Lithium
– Rapid cyclers	Valproate
Gille de la Tourette syndrome	• Haloperidol (FDA-approved) • Clonidine/guanafacine (off label)
Relapsing remitting multiple sclerosis	Beta-interferon
Huntington's disease	Tetrabenazine
Wilson disease	Zinc
Depression	SSRI
– Mild to moderate	SSRI (Fluoxetine)
– Severe	SNRI (Venlafaxine)
Neurotic disorders	
– Obsessive compulsive disorder	SSRI (Fluoxetine)
– Post-traumatic stress disorder	SSRI (Sertraline)
– Bulimia	SSRI (Fluoxetine)
– Phobia	SSRI (Sertraline)
– Impulse-control disorders	SSRI (Fluoxetine)
Attention deficit hyperkinetic disorder	Methylphenidate
Nocturnal enuresis	Desmopressin
Severe (cancer) pain	Opioids (morpine)
Neurolept analgesia	Droperidol + fentanyl
Neurolept anaesthesia	Droperidol + Fentanyl + N_2O
Opioid poisoning	Naloxone
– Acute	Naloxone
– Maintenance	Naltrexone
Opioid de-addiction	
– Maintenance therapy	Methadone
– To prevent relapse	Naltrexone
– To treat withdrawl symptoms	Beta blockers/clonidine
Alzhiemer's dementia	Donepezil
Amyotrophic lateral sclerosis	Riluzole
Extrapyramidal symptoms	
– Acute muscular dystonias	Benzhexol
– Parkinsonism	Benzhexol
– Akathisia	Propranolol
– Neurolept malignant syndrome	Dantrolene
– Tardive dyskinesia	No treatment (benzodiazepines may help)
Restless leg syndrome	Pramipexole

Image Based Questions

1. A 50 year old male presented with suicidal overdose of a drug. Patient is flabby and comatose with shallow failing respiration. The BP of the person is 80/40 mm Hg and the lesion on the right is shown in the image. The likely poisoning is:
   (a) Heroin
   (b) Phenobarbitone
   (c) Imipramine
   (d) Phenytoin

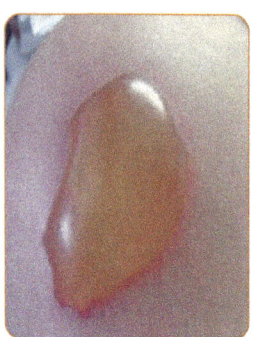

2. Which antiepileptic drug can lead to this adverse effect?

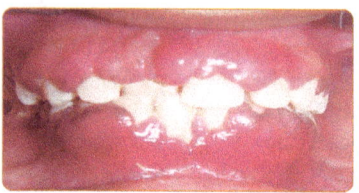

   (a) Phenytoin
   (b) Carbamazepine
   (c) Valproate
   (d) Lamotrigine

3. Drug E is likely to be:

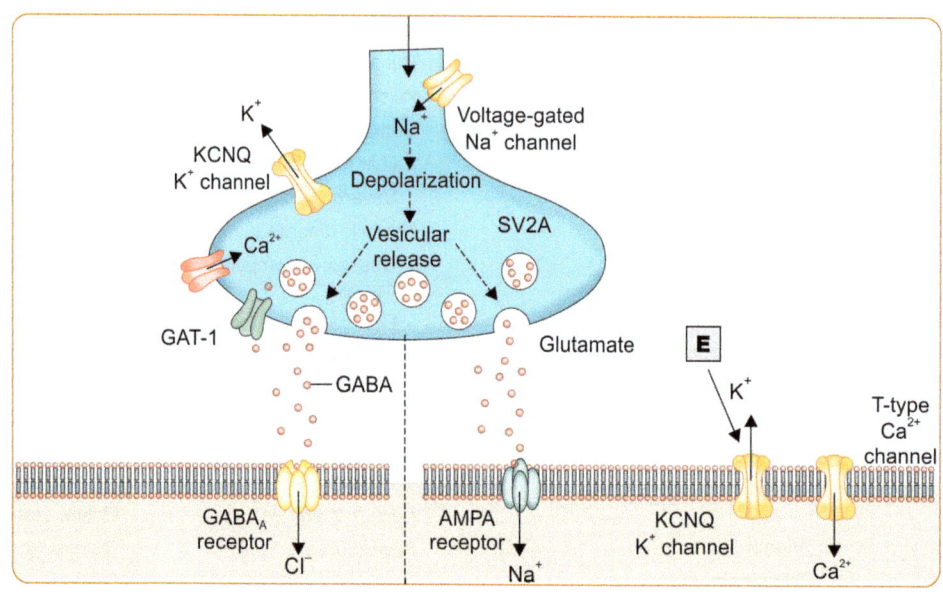

   (a) Retigabine
   (b) Lamotrigine
   (c) Levetiracetam
   (d) Topiramate

4. A patient of Parkinsonism developed this condition after treatment. Which of the following drugs is likely to cause this adverse effect?

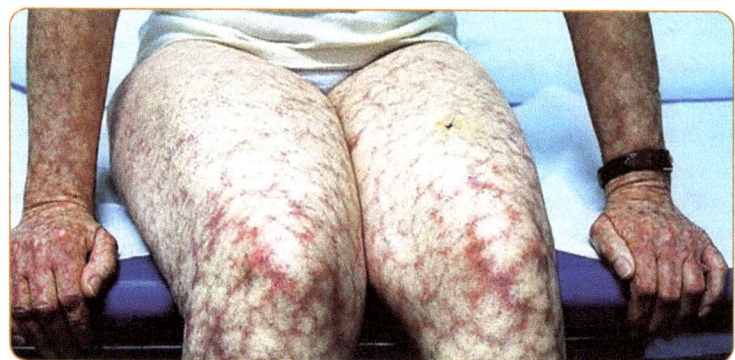

   (a) Levo-dopa
   (b) Amantadine
   (c) Selegiline
   (d) Pramipexole

Central Nervous System

5. A patient with Schizophrenia was prescribed haloperidol. Next day she returned with the features shown in the image. What should be the treatment?

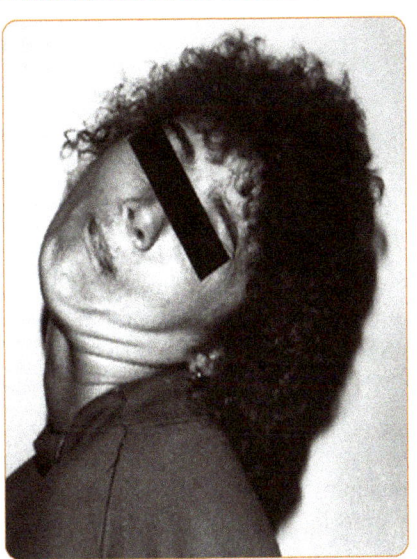

   (a) Increase the dose of haloperidol
   (b) Give Propranolol
   (c) Give Benzhexol
   (d) Reassurance is enough

6. A female patient on several antiepileptic drugs presented with hair growth as shown in figure. The likely drug responsible for this pattern of hair growth is:

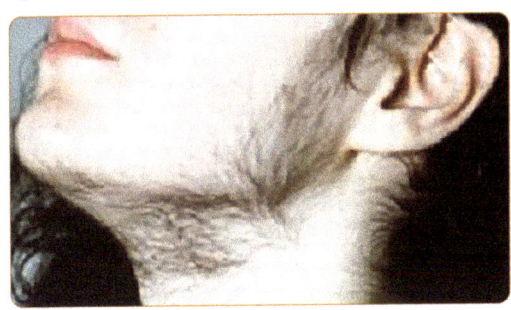

   (a) Phenytoin   (b) Valproate
   (c) Levetiraetam   (d) Lamotrigine

Explanations

1. **Ans. (b) Phenobarbitone**
   The clinical features points towards poisoning caused by CNS depressant drug. The figure shows the characteristic barbiturate blisters. So it is phenobarbitone poisoning.

2. **Ans. (a) Phenytoin**
   The figure shows the gum hypertrophy which is caused by phenytoin
   The mechanism of action of antiepileptic drugs

Main mechanism	Drug
Na Channel blockers	Phenytoin Carbamazepine Lamotrigine Valproate
Stimulate GABA-BZD Cl channel complex	Barbiturates Benzodiazepines
Inhibit GABA transaminase	Vigabatrin
Inhibit GAT-1	Tiagabine
Act on SV2A	Levetiracetam
Open K+ Channels	Retigabine
Block NMDA receptors	Felbamate
Block AMPA receptors	Perampanel
Block L type Ca Channels	Ethosuximide

3. **Ans. (a) Retigabine**

4. **Ans. (b) Amantadine**
   The figure shows the livedo reticularis, a type of skin pigmentation in the form of mesh (reticular). It is characteristic adverse effect of amantadine

5. **Ans. (c) Give Benzhexol**
   The figure shows the torticollis. This is an extrapyramidal adverse effect caused by antipsychotics. Benzhexol is drug of choice for this adverse effect.

6. **Ans. (a) Phenytoin**
   Male pattern hair growth in females is called hirsutism. It is caused by
   Phenytoin
   Cyclosporine
   Minoxidol

Multiple Choice Questions

SEDATIVE HYPNOTICS

1. Benzodiazepines act on: *(NEET Pattern 2016-17)*
   - (a) GABA-A receptor
   - (b) GABA-B receptor
   - (c) Both GABA-A and GABA-B
   - (d) Calcium channels

2. Duration of action of flumazenil is: *(AIIMS Nov 2013)*
   - (a) 5 minute
   - (b) 10 minute
   - (c) 20 minute
   - (d) 30 minute

3. The effect of thiopentone on the CNS is quickly terminated because of: *(Recent NEET Pattern Question)*
   - (a) Rapid metabolism in the CNS
   - (b) Quick first-pass elimination
   - (c) Redistribution
   - (d) Rapid metabolism in systemic circulation

4. Which of the following drugs is contra-indicated in acute intermittent porphyria? *(Recent NEET Pattern Question)*
   - (a) Thiopentone
   - (b) Midazolam
   - (c) Propofol
   - (d) Etomidate

5. Action of flumazenil on benzodiazepine receptor is: *(Recent NEET Pattern Question)*
   - (a) Agonist
   - (b) Partial agonist
   - (c) Inverse agonist
   - (d) Antagonist

6. Both barbiturates and salicylates are maximally absorbed in stomach because: *(Recent NEET Pattern Question)*
   - (a) They are weakly basic and so highly ionised in stomach
   - (b) They are highly basic and so less isonized in stomach
   - (c) They are weakly acidic and do not ionise in stomach
   - (d) They are highly acidic and are highly ionised in stomach

7. Which of the following drug is not metabolized by liver? *(Recent NEET Pattern Question)*
   - (a) Flunitrazepam
   - (b) Diazepam
   - (c) Oxazepam
   - (d) Nitrazepam

8. Shortest acting benzodiazepine is: *(Recent NEET Pattern Question)*
   - (a) Midazolam
   - (b) Alprazolam
   - (c) Lorazepam
   - (d) Diazepam

9. Shortest acting benzodiazepine among these is: *(Recent NEET Pattern Question)*
   - (a) Flurazepam
   - (b) Alprazolam
   - (c) Triazolam
   - (d) Diazepam

10. Most effective non habit forming sedative is: *(Recent NEET Pattern Question)*
    - (a) Lorazepam
    - (b) Zolpidem
    - (c) Flurazepam
    - (d) Trazadone

11. Antagonist of benzodiazepine is: *(Recent NEET Pattern Question)*
    - (a) Naltrexone
    - (b) Flumazenil
    - (c) Naloxone
    - (d) N-Acetyl-cysteine

12. Which of the following drug does not affect $GABA_A$ gated chloride channel? *(Recent NEET Pattern Question)*
    - (a) Muscimol
    - (b) Alcohol
    - (c) Picrotoxin
    - (d) Buspirone

13. The specific antidote for benzodiazepine poisoning is: *(Recent NEET Pattern Question)*
    - (a) Naloxone
    - (b) Flumazenil
    - (c) Fomepizole
    - (d) Pralidoxime

14. Which one of the following drug is effective in painful tingling sensation due to diabetic neuropathy? *(Recent NEET Pattern Question)*
    - (a) Aspirin
    - (b) Ibuprofen
    - (c) Gabapentin
    - (d) Tramodol

15. One of the following is not true about melatonin: *(Recent NEET Pattern Question)*
    - (a) Induces sleep
    - (b) Used in treatment of jet lag syndrome
    - (c) Is secreted by pituitary
    - (d) Is a pineal hormone

16. All of the following are CNS stimulants *except*: *(Recent NEET Pattern Question)*
    - (a) Amphetamines
    - (b) Benzodiazepines
    - (c) Cocaine
    - (d) Methylphenidate

NEURODEGENERATIVE DISORDERS

17. A female developed pain and insect crawling like sensation on legs at night which is relieved by shaking her legs. Which of the following is drug of choice for this condition? *(NEET Pattern Question 2020)*
    - (a) Pramipexole
    - (b) Gabapentin
    - (c) Vit B12
    - (d) Iron tablets

18. New drug recently approved for Amyotrophic Lateral Sclerosis is: *(AIIMS May 2018)*
    - (a) Edaravone
    - (b) Piracetam
    - (c) Ceftriaxone
    - (d) Doxycycline

19. Drug of choice for drug-induced Parkinsonism is: *(NEET Pattern 2016-17)*
    - (a) Tolcapone
    - (b) Selegiline
    - (c) Amantadine
    - (d) Biperidin

20. Tolcapone is: *(NEET Pattern 2016-17)*
    - (a) Ototoxic
    - (b) Nephrotoxic
    - (c) Hepatotoxic
    - (d) All of the above

Central Nervous System

21. A popular anti-Parkinsonism drug, Bromocriptone acts as:
    (NEET Pattern 2016-17)
    (a) Dopamine agonist
    (b) Peripheral carboxylase inhibitor
    (c) COMT inhibitor
    (d) MAO inhibitor

22. Selegiline is an example of: *(NEET Pattern 2016-17)*
    (a) COMT inhibitor
    (b) Peripheral decarboxylase inhibitor
    (c) Peripherial carboxylase inhibitor
    (d) MAO inhibitor

23. Peripheral vasospasm is observed with which of the following anti-Parkinsonian drugs? *(AIIMS May 2014)*
    (a) Ropinirole   (b) Levodopa
    (c) Bromocriptine   (d) Entacapone

24. Which of the following agents enhances the bio-availability of levodopa in patients with Parkinson's disease? *(Recent NEET Pattern Question)*
    (a) Amantadine   (b) Ropinirole
    (c) Entacapone   (d) Selegiline

25. Which of the following drug should not be given along with levodopa? *(Recent NEET Pattern Question)*
    (a) Carbidopa   (b) MAO inhibitors
    (c) Vitamin B complex   (d) Benserazide

26. Drug of choice in drug induced parkinsonism is:
    (Recent NEET Pattern Question)
    (a) Levodopa   (b) Benzhexol
    (c) Amantidine   (d) Carbidopa

27. Which of the following abolishes the therapeutic effect of levodopa? *(Recent NEET Pattern Question)*
    (a) Thiamine   (b) Carbidopa
    (c) Pyridoxine   (d) Benzerazide

28. Which one of the following drug is used in Alzheimer's disease? *(Recent NEET Pattern Question)*
    (a) Donepezil   (b) Pemoline
    (c) Doxapram   (d) Methylphenidate

29. Which drug is not used in Alzheimer disease?
    (Recent NEET Pattern Question)
    (a) Memantine   (b) Galantamine
    (c) Ropinirole   (d) Donepezil

30. In treatment of Parkinsonism, L-Dopa is combined with carbidopa mainly: *(Recent NEET Pattern Question)*
    (a) To decrease the treatment duration
    (b) To decrease central side effects of L-Dopa
    (c) To decrease effectiveness of L-Dopa
    (d) To increase crossing of L-Dopa through BBB

31. Which of the following is a 'nootropic' drug?
    (Recent NEET Pattern Question)
    (a) Rivastigmine   (b) Tacrine
    (c) Amantadine   (d) Piracetam

32. Mechanism of action of donepezil is:
    (Recent NEET Pattern Question)
    (a) Centrally acting reversible anticholinesterase
    (b) Centrally acting irreversible anticholinesterase
    (c) Irreversible cholinergic action
    (d) Reversible anticholinesterase

33. Anti-Parkinsonism drug that is a selective COMT inhibitor: *(Recent NEET Pattern Question)*
    (a) Entacapone   (b) Ropinirole
    (c) Pergolide   (d) Pramipexole

34. True statement about drugs used in Parkinsonism is:
    (Recent NEET Pattern Question)
    (a) Amantadine is a cholinergic drug
    (b) Vitamin B6 enhances the L-Dopa action
    (c) COMT inhibitors prolong the action of L-dopa
    (d) None

35. A 72-year-old patient with Parkinsonism presents with swollen feet. They are red, tender and very painful. You could clear up these symptoms within a few days if you tell the patient to stop taking: *(Recent NEET Pattern Question)*
    (a) Amantadine   (b) Benztropine
    (c) Bromocriptine   (d) Levodopa

36. The drug found to be beneficial in amyotrophic lateral sclerosis is: *(Recent NEET Pattern Question)*
    (a) Riluzole   (b) Methylprednisolone
    (c) Hydroxyurea   (d) None of the above

37. All of the following are side efffect of ropinirole *except*:
    (Recent NEET Pattern Question)
    (a) Sedation   (b) Nausea
    (c) Retroperitoneal Fibrosis (d) Hallucination

38. Anti-Parkinson's drug known to cause cardiac valvular fibrosis is: *(Recent NEET Pattern Question)*
    (a) Levo-dopa   (b) Ropinirole
    (c) Pramipexole   (d) Pergolide

39. All are dopaminergic agonists used for Parkinsonism *except*: *(Recent NEET Pattern Question)*
    (a) Bromocriptine   (b) Ropinirole
    (c) Pramipexole   (d) Selegiline

40. Which of the following anti-Parkinson drugs has the potential to cause retro peritoneal fibrosis?
    (Recent NEET Pattern Question)
    (a) Pramipexole   (b) Entacapone
    (c) Bromocriptine   (d) Ropinirole

41. Drug of choice in drug induced Parkinsonism is:
    (Recent NEET Pattern Question)
    (a) Levodopa   (b) Carbidopa
    (c) Amantadine   (d) Benzhexol

ANTIEPILEPTIC DRUGS

42. Which of the following adverse effect is likely to increase when carbamazepine is added to valproate?
    (AIIMS Nov. 2018)
    (a) Hepatotoxicity   (b) Thrombocytopenia
    (c) Pancreatitis   (d) Hyperammonemia

43. Lorazepam is preferred over Diazepam in treatment of status epilepticus as:
    (NEET Pattern 2016-17)
    (a) It has longer half life than diazepam
    (b) It has more sustained action because of lower lipid solubility and slower redistribution
    (c) Faster clearance
    (d) More bioavailability

44. Drug which should NOT be used in absence seizure:
    (NEET Pattern 2016-17)
    (a) Ethosuximide   (b) Valproate
    (c) Vigabatrin   (d) Phenytoin

45. An epileptic adult man is on levetiracetam 1 g twice a day therapy. He is seizure free for 2 years. Now, he started developing irritability, aggression and liability of mood that is affecting his daily life. What should the doctor do?
    (AIIMS May, 2017)
    (a) Stop the drug and start another antiepileptic
    (b) Taper the drug over 6 months
    (c) Continue the medication for another 3 years
    (d) Decrease the dose of levetiracetam

46. All are idiosyncratic reactions to carbamazepine *except*:
    (a) Rash   *(AIIMS May 2017)*
    (b) Steven Johnson syndrome
    (c) Blurred vision
    (d) Agranulocytosis

47. Given below is a list of first line and second line drugs for the management of seizures. Which of the following is wrong regarding seizure and its treatment?
    (AIIMS Nov 2016)

Option	Seizure Type	First line drugs	Second line drugs
(a)	Focal seizure	Valproate Carbamazepine Lamotrigine	Phenytoin Topiramate
(b)	GTCS	Valproate Lamotrigine	Phenytoin Topiramate
(c)	Absence seizure	Lamotrigine Carbamazepine	Ethosuximide Valproate
(d)	Myoclonic seizures	Valproate	Lamotrigine

48. Gender specific adverse effect of valproate is:
    (AIIMS Nov-2015)
    (a) Weight gain   (b) Tremors
    (c) Alopecia   (d) Polycystic ovarian disease

49. A-22-year-old female on antiepileptic therapy got married. When should the folic acid supplementation be advised to this female?   *(AIIMS Nov-2015)*
    (a) 3 months before pregnancy
    (b) All women who could become pregnant
    (c) As soon as pregnancy is confirmed
    (d) After delivery

50. Anticonvulsant causing visual field contraction is:
    (AIIMS Nov-2015)
    (a) Vigabatrin   (c) Levetiracetam
    (d) Ethosuximide   (e) Phenytoin

51. A 26-year-old female presents for ante natal visit. She has a history of abortion in last pregnancy due to neural tube defect in the fetus. What is the amount of folic acid that should be prescribed to this female?
    (AIIMS May-2015)
    (a) 4 micrograms per day
    (b) 40 micrograms per day
    (c) 400 micrograms per day
    (d) 4000 micrograms per day

52. All of the following adverse effects are associated with carbamazepine *except*:   *(AIIMS Nov 2013)*
    (a) Teratogenicity
    (b) Neurotoxicity
    (c) Decrease in antidiuretic hormone
    (d) Hypersensitivity

53. Which is a treatment of juvenile myoclonic epilepsy in pregnancy?   *(AIIMS Nov 2013)*
    (a) Levetiracetam   (b) Carbamazepine
    (c) Vigabatrin   (d) Phenytoin

54. Which of the following statements about anti-epileptics is false?   *(AIIMS Nov 2013)*
    (a) Phenytoin and carbamazepine act by prolonging the inactivated state of Na+ channels
    (b) Carbamazepine can be used in trigeminal neuralgias
    (c) Diazepam is an anticonvulsant drug
    (d) Lamotrigine mainly acts by causing GABA mediated Cl- channel opening

55. Carbamazepine in elderly causes:
    (Recent NEET Pattern Question)
    (a) Hypernatremia   (b) Hyponatremia
    (c) Hyperkalemia   (d) Hypokalemia

56. Pseudolymphoma can result from long-term use of:
    (Recent NEET Pattern Question)
    (a) Phenytoin   (b) Carbamazepine
    (c) Sodium valproate (d) Phenobarbital

57. Management of typical febrile seizures include all the following *except*:   *(Recent NEET Pattern Question)*
    (a) Tepid sponging
    (b) Paracetamol and ibuprofen
    (c) Intermittent diazepam
    (d) Prophylactic phenobarbitone

58. The drug of choice in treatment of infantile spasms is:
    (Recent NEET Pattern Question)
    (a) ACTH   (b) Phenobarbitone
    (c) Carbamazepine   (d) Phenytoin

59. Which of the following is not a side effect of phenytoin?
    (Recent NEET Pattern Question)
    (a) Hypoglycemia   (b) Osteomalacia
    (c) Gum hypertrophy (d) Lymphadenopathy

60. Drug of choice for Trigeminal neuralgia is:
    (Recent NEET Pattern Question)
    (a) Carbamazepine   (b) Phenobabitone
    (c) Phenytoin   (d) Valproic acid

61. Myoclonus in children is best treated by:
    (Recent NEET Pattern Question)
    (a) Clonazepam   (b) Sodium Valproate
    (c) Phenobarbitone   (d) Ethosuccimide

62. DOC for myoclonic seizure is:
    (Recent NEET Pattern Question)
    (a) Phenobarbitone   (b) Ethosuximide
    (c) Lamotrigine   (d) Valproic acid

63. All are the side effects of prolonged phenytoin therapy *except*:   *(Recent NEET Pattern Question)*
    (a) Osteomalacia   (b) Gynaecomastia
    (c) Megaloblastic anemia (d) Gum hyperplasia

64. Antiepileptic drug that can cause folate deficiency anemia is: *(Recent NEET Pattern Question)*
    (a) Valproate (b) Phenytoin
    (c) Phenobarbitone (d) Carbamazepine

65. Which of the following antiepileptic drugs acts by affecting the levels of GABA? *(Recent NEET Pattern Question)*
    (a) Sodium valproate (b) Ethosuximide
    (c) Phenytoin sodium (d) Carbamazepine

66. Which one of the following drugs is used to treat status epilepticus? *(Recent NEET Pattern Question)*
    (a) Primidone (b) Carbamazepine
    (c) Diazepam (d) Sodium valporate

67. The antiepileptic drug which does not produce enzyme induction is: *(Recent NEET Pattern Question)*
    (a) Phenobarbitone (b) Sodium valproate
    (c) Phenytoin sodium (d) Carbamazepine

68. Osteomalacia is adverse effect of: *(Recent NEET Pattern Question)*
    (a) Primidone (b) Phenytoin
    (c) Carbamazepine (d) Valproic acid

69. Among the following structures which one is not used in the treatment of epilepsy? *(Recent NEET Pattern Question)*
    (a) Barbiturates (b) Hydantoins
    (c) Acetylurea (d) Atropine

70. Gum hypertrophy is an adverse effect of the following drug when used at therapeutic levels: *(Recent NEET Pattern Question)*
    (a) Phenobarbitone (b) Phenytoin
    (c) Carbamazepine (d) Sodium evaporate

71. Drug of choice in complex partial seizure is: *(Recent NEET Pattern Question)*
    (a) Phenytoin (b) Valproate
    (c) Carbamazepine (d) Phenobarbitone

72. Which drug should be avoided in pregnancy? *(Recent NEET Pattern Question)*
    (a) Phenytoin (b) Insulin
    (c) Heparin (d) All

73. Which of the following antiepileptic agent does not act via Na⁺ channel modulation? *(Recent NEET Pattern Question)*
    (a) Vigabatrin (b) Phenytoin
    (c) Valproate (d) Lamotrigne

74. Side effects of phenytoin are all *except*: *(Recent NEET Pattern Question)*
    (a) Osteomalacia (b) Maculopapular rash
    (c) Sedation (d) Megaloblastic anaemia

75. Antiepileptics used as analgesics are: *(Recent NEET Pattern Question)*
    (a) Carbamazepine and valproate
    (b) Phenytoin and valproate
    (c) Carbamazepine and phenytoin
    (d) Diazepam and Chlorpromazine

76. A patient on anticonvulsant therapy took 20 tablets at a time following which he developed hyponatremia and BP of 160/100 mm of Hg. Which of the following anticonvulsant toxicity is most likely responsible for this? *(Recent NEET Pattern Question)*
    (a) Carbamazepine (b) Phenytoin sodium
    (c) Phenobarbital (d) Sodium valproate

77. The side effect of phenytoin when its plasma concentration is above therapeutic level is: *(Recent NEET Pattern Question)*
    (a) Ataxia (b) Gum hypertrophy
    (c) Osteomalacia (d) Hirsutism

78. Neural tube defect is an adverse effect of: *(Recent NEET Pattern Question)*
    (a) Valproate (b) Phenytoin
    (c) Diazoxide (d) None

79. False about mechanism of action of anticonvulsants is: *(Recent NEET Pattern Question)*
    (a) Ethosuximide – K⁺ channel opener
    (b) Phenytoin – Na⁺ channel blocker
    (c) Diazepam – Facilitates GABA action
    (d) Gabapentin – Increase GABA release

80. Folate deficiency occurs due to: *(Recent NEET Pattern Question)*
    (a) Phenytoin (b) Phenobarbitone
    (c) Primidone (d) All

81. Drug of choice for absence seizures is: *(Recent NEET Pattern Question)*
    (a) Valproate (b) Phenytoin
    (c) Diazepam (d) Ethosuximide

82. Weight gain is not seen with: *(Recent NEET Pattern Question)*
    (a) Chlorpromazine (b) Sodium valproate
    (c) Carbamazepine (d) Phentermine

83. Renal stones are seen as a complication by using the following drug: *(Recent NEET Pattern Question)*
    (a) Tiagabine (b) Oxcarbamazepine
    (c) Zonisamide (d) Phenytoin

84. Lamotrigine has common side effects of: *(Recent NEET Pattern Question)*
    (a) Rash (b) Irritability
    (c) Nephrotoxicity (d) Behavioral disturbances

85. With chronic use in seizure state, the adverse effects of this drug include coarsening of facial features, hirsutism, gingival hyperplasia and osteomalacia: *(Recent NEET Pattern Question)*
    (a) Carbomazepine (b) Ethosuccimide
    (c) Gabapentin (d) Phenytoin

86. Which one of the following statements about phenytoin is accurate? *(Recent NEET Pattern Question)*
    (a) It is not effective orally
    (b) Drug of choice in myoclonic seizures
    (c) Half-life is increased if used with phenobarbital
    (d) Toxicity may occur with only small increments in dose

87. The drug of choice for a patient with a combination of primary generalized tonic clonic seizure and absence seizures is: *(Recent NEET Pattern Question)*
    (a) Ethosuximide (b) Carbamazepine
    (c) Valproic acid (d) Phenytoin sodium

88. Side effects of diphenyl hydantoin may include all except: *(Recent NEET Pattern Question)*
    (a) Gingival hyperplasia
    (b) Acute cerebellar syndrome
    (c) Inter-nuclear ophthalmoplegia
    (d) Megaloblastic anaemia

89. The drug of choice to control convulsions in eclampsia is: *(Recent NEET Pattern Question)*
    (a) Pethidine   (b) Diazepam
    (c) Magnesium sulphate (d) Phenytoin

90. 'Vigabatrin' a new antiepileptic agent acts by: *(Recent NEET Pattern Question)*
    (a) GABA – antagonism
    (b) GABA – agonism
    (c) NMDA antagonism
    (d) Carbonic anhydrase inhibition

91. Off label use of topiramate is: *(Recent NEET Pattern Question)*
    (a) Alcohol de-addiction
    (b) Extrapyramidal symptoms on anti-psychotic use
    (c) Opioid withdrawal
    (d) Sedative agent

92. Fosphenytoin is different from phenytoin in which of the following aspect? *(Recent NEET Pattern Question)*
    (a) Can be used in absence seizures
    (b) Can be mixed with dextrose
    (c) Can be given orally
    (d) It is the drug of choice for myoclonic seizures

93. Drug of choice for infantile spasms in a patient with tuberous sclerosis is: *(Recent NEET Pattern Question)*
    (a) Vigabatrin   (b) Tiagabine
    (c) Lamotrigine   (d) Levetiracetam

94. Valproic acid causes all except: *(Recent NEET Pattern Question)*
    (a) It is an enzyme inducer
    (b) It causes obesity
    (c) It causes hepatotoxicity
    (d) It causes neural tube defects

95. Regarding phenytoin, all of the following are correct except: *(Recent NEET Pattern Question)*
    (a) It acts on voltage sensitive neuronal Na+ channels
    (b) Used by slow IV injection in status epilepticus
    (c) Kinetics change form 1st order to zero order over therapeutic range
    (d) It inhibits microsomal enzymes

96. Not true about fosphenytoin is: *(Recent NEET Pattern Question)*
    (a) Used for GTCS   (b) Prodrug of phenytoin
    (c) Lipid soluble   (d) Highly protein bound

97. All of the following are side effects of valproic acid, except: *(Recent NEET Pattern Question)*
    (a) Alopecia   (b) Hepatitis
    (c) Nephrotoxicity   (d) Skin rashes

98. Drug of choice for tonic-clonic seizures is: *(Recent NEET Pattern Question)*
    (a) Sodium valproate   (b) Carbemazepine
    (c) Phenobarbitone   (d) Felbamate

99. The drug of choice for status epilepticus is: *(Recent NEET Pattern Question)*
    (a) Propofol   (b) Lorazepam
    (c) Thiopentone   (d) Haloperidol

100. Drug of choice for treatment of absence seizures is: *(Recent NEET Pattern Question)*
    (a) Phenytoin   (b) Valproate
    (c) Ethosuximide   (d) Carbamazepine

101. A 20 years old female with generalized tonic clonic epilepsy is well controlled of Tab. phenytoin 300 mg/day, becomes pregnant. Pick the correct advise you would give her: *(Recent NEET Pattern Question)*
    (a) Stop Phenytoin + start Phenobarbitone and Folic acid
    (b) Stop Phenytoin + start Lamotrigine and Folic acid
    (c) Stop Phenytoin + start Magnesium infusion
    (d) Continue with Phenytoin and add Tab. Folic acid and during the last 2 weeks of pregnancy give oral Vitamin K too

102. Administration of which antiepileptic drug is associated with development of hyperkinesia in children? *(Recent NEET Pattern Question)*
    (a) Phenytoin sodium   (b) Sodium valproate
    (c) Carbamazepine   (d) Phenobarbitone

103. GABA transmission is facilitated by: *(Recent NEET Pattern Question)*
    (a) Vigabatrin   (b) Carbamazepine
    (c) Phenytoin   (d) Buspirone

104. Drug of choice for myoclonic seizures is: *(Recent NEET Pattern Question)*
    (a) Valproic acid   (b) Phenytoin
    (c) Ethosuximide   (d) Carbamazepine

DRUGS FOR PSYCHIATRIC ILLNESS

105. A patient on lithium therapy developed hypertension. He was started on thiazides for hypertension. After few days, he developed coarse tremors and other symptoms suggestive of lithium toxicity. Explain the likely mechanism of this interaction: *(NEET Pattern Question 2020)*
    (a) Thiazides inhibit the metabolism of lithium
    (b) Thiazides act as an add on drug to lithium
    (c) Thiazides increase the tubular reabsorption of lithium
    (d) Thiazides cause loss of water thereby increase serum lithium levels.

106. A female patient was on lithium therapy for bipolar disorder for 6 months. She kept the fast for few days due to religious reasons and presented with seizures, coarse tremors, confusion and weakness of limbs. Which of the following should be done to diagnose her condition? *(NEET Pattern Question 2020)*
    (a) Serum electrolytes (b) Serum lithium levels
    (c) ECG   (d) MRI

107. A patient was recently started on Fluphenazine. Few weeks later, he developed tremors, rigidity, bradykinesia and excessive salivation. First line of management for this patient is: *(NEET Pattern Question 2020)*
    (a) Selegiline   (b) Trihexyphenidyl
    (c) Pramipexole   (d) Amantadine

Central Nervous System

108. Chlorpromazine is an antipsychotic drug. It also produces sedation and adverse effects like dry mouth and hypotension. All these actions result due to action on which of the following receptors? *(AIIMS May 2019)*
    1. D2 and 5HT2 receptors
    2. GABA and beta-adrenergic receptors
    3. Muscarinic and alpha-adrenergic receptors
    4. H1 receptors
    (a) 1, 3 and 4 are correct
    (b) Only 2 is correct
    (c) 1 and 2 are correct
    (d) All are correct

109. A bank employee, felt depressed with no interest in activities, came to AIIMS OPD. He was started on escitalopram. Which of these adverse effects cannot be explained with escitalopram? *(AIIMS May 2019)*
    (a) Sialorrhea
    (b) Anorgasmia
    (c) Nausea
    (d) Vivid dreams

110. Use of lithium during pregnancy increases the risk of development of which of the following malformations in the baby? *(AIIMS May 2018)*
    (a) Facial defects
    (b) Cardiac defects
    (c) Neural tube defects
    (d) Urogenital defects

111. Which of the following is not an adverse effect of escitalopram? *(AIIMS May 2018)*
    (a) Sialorrhea
    (b) Insomnia
    (c) Nausea
    (d) Anorgasmia

112. Discontinuation of which of the following drugs can result in anxiety and insomnia? *(AIIMS May 2018)*
    (a) Venlafaxine
    (b) Imipramine
    (c) Valproate
    (d) Olanzapine

113. Mechanism of action of Mianserin: *(NEET Pattern 2016-17)*
    (a) Inhibits alpha-adrenergic, H1, and some types of serotonin receptors.
    (b) Inhibits alpha-adrenergic, H2, and some types of serotonin receptors.
    (c) Inhibits beta-adrenergic, H1, and some types of serotonin receptors.
    (d) Inhibits alpha-adrenergic and H1 receptors.

114. Among the following antipsychotic drugs, the sedation is maximum with: *(NEET Pattern 2016-17)*
    (a) Asenapine
    (b) Aripiprazole
    (c) Thioxanthine
    (d) Olanzapine

115. Which of the following drug can be used for treatment of premature ejaculation? *(NEET Pattern 2016-17)*
    (a) Nitric oxide inhibitor
    (b) SSRI
    (c) SNRI
    (d) Phosphodiesterase inhibitor

116. First line treatment for arrhythmias due to amitriptyline is: *(NEET Pattern 2016-17)*
    (a) $CaCl_2$
    (b) Amiodarone
    (c) IV $NaHCO_3$
    (d) Insulin + glucagon

117. Which of the following mood stabilizers has anti-suicide properties? *(AIIMS May 2017)*
    (a) Lithium
    (b) Carbamazepine
    (c) Valproate
    (d) Lamotrigine

118. A 30-year-old female, married since one year, presents to the psychiatry clinic with hyperactivity since 2 weeks. A diagnosis of mania is made. She had 3 prior episodes of mania in last 5 years and every time after taking medication she goes to premorbid state. Her urine pregnancy test is positive. Which is the preferred drug for management of this patient? *(AIIMS Nov 2015)*
    (a) Promethazine
    (b) Haloperidol
    (c) Clonazepam
    (d) Lithium

119. A 21-year-old student is taking 3 mg risperidone for schizophrenia since 2 months. It was the first episode and the patient is asymptomatic now. There is no family history of any psychiatric disease. How long risperidone should be continued in this patient? *(AIIMS Nov 2015)*
    (a) At least 6 months of symptom remission
    (b) At least 12 months of symptom remission
    (c) 2 years
    (d) 5 years

120. A young girl on antidepressant therapy presented to emergency with palpitations, altered sensorium and hypotension. There is wide QRS interval and right axis deviation in ECG. Next best step in the management of this patient is: *(AIIMS Nov 2015)*
    (a) Physostigmine
    (b) $NaHCO_3$
    (c) Dialysis
    (d) Flumazenil

121. A patient with violent behavior and agitation was diagnosed as Schizophrenia and was prescribed haloperidol. On third day he developed rigidity and was unable to move his neck that fixed his stare to one side. Which of the following drugs can be used for treatment of this patient?
    (a) Increase dose of haloperidol *(AIIMS May 2015)*
    (b) Promethazine
    (c) Risperidone
    (d) Diazepam

122. A 30 year old male presents with history of abnormal excessive blinking and grunting sounds. He has no control of these symptoms which have increased in frequency. Which of the following medications can be used for treatment of this person? *(AIIMS May 2015)*
    (a) Carbamazepine
    (b) Imipramine
    (c) Risperidone
    (d) Methylphenidate

123. Which of the following serum concentration of lithium indicates lithium toxicity? *(AIIMS Nov 2014)*
    (a) 2 m Eq/L
    (b) 4 m Eq/L
    (c) 6 m Eq/L
    (d) 8 m Eq/L

124. A patient of schizophrenia was started on haloperidol 5 mg. Next day, he presented with uprolling of eyes. Complete neurological examination revealed no spasticity or any other abnormality. Visual acuity and opthalmoscopic findings are normal. Most likely diagnosis is: *(AIIMS Nov 2014)*
    (a) Akathisia
    (b) Acute dystonia
    (c) Seizure
    (d) Tardive dyskinesia

125. A person taking tricyclic antidepressants presents with blurred vision and dry mouth. These adverse effects result due to blockade of: *(AIIMS Nov 2013)*
    (a) M_3 muscarinic receptors
    (b) $GABA_A$ receptors
    (c) H_1 histamine receptors
    (d) $5HT_2$ receptors

126. A patient of depression is stabilized on selective serotonin reuptake inhibitor (SSRI). This group of drugs produced withdrawal symptoms when stopped. Which of the following drugs has minimum risk of causing drug discontinuation symptoms? *(AIIMS Nov 2013)*
    (a) Paroxetine   (b) Fluoxetine
    (c) Sertraline   (d) Fluvoxamine

127. Best agent for premenstrual syndrome management is: *(AIIMS May 2013)*
    (a) Progesterone   (b) Anxiolytic
    (c) SSRI   (d) Vitamin E

128. Which of the following antipsychotic drugs is available as a depot injection? *(AIIMS May 2013)*
    (a) Fluphenazine   (b) Ziprasidone
    (c) Trifluperazine   (d) Aripiprazone

129. All are true about Clozapine *except*: *(AI 2012)*
    (a) More potently blocks D_2 as compared to D_1 receptors
    (b) Blood level below 350 ng/mL should be maintained to avoid agranulocytosis
    (c) Should not be used along with Carbamazepine
    (d) Should be discontinued if the WBC count is below 3,000/mm³ cells

130. Which of the following agent is not a serotonin and dopaminergic blocker? *(AI 2012)*
    (a) Doxepin   (b) Amisulpiride
    (c) Sertindole   (d) Zotepine

131. Which of the following has highest potential to cause metabolic syndrome? *(Recent NEET Pattern Question)*
    (a) Clozapine   (b) Risperidone
    (c) Quetiapine   (d) Aripiprazole

132. Which of the following is not a serotonin-norepinephrine reuptake inhibitor? *(Recent NEET Pattern Question)*
    (a) Venlafaxine   (b) Duloxetine
    (c) Milnacipran   (d) Tianeptin

133. Which of the following is not a side effect of paroxetine? *(Recent NEET Pattern Question)*
    (a) Premature ejaculation   (b) Erectile dysfunction
    (c) Decreased libido   (d) Diarrhea

134. Which of the following is not a mood stabilizer? *(Recent NEET Pattern Question)*
    (a) Lithium   (b) Valproate
    (c) Carbamazepine   (d) Fluoxetine

135. Correct about the use of lithium as an important component of management of manic-depressive psychosis is: *(Recent NEET Pattern Question)*
    (a) Is associated with delayed (>2 weeks) electrolyte disturbances
    (b) Can be given alone for acute episodes
    (c) Monitoring of serum concentration is seldom useful for guiding dose adjustment
    (d) Cause benign and reversible depression of T wave on ECG

136. In depression, there is deficiency of: *(Recent NEET Pattern Question)*
    (a) 5-HT   (b) Acetylcholine
    (c) Dopamine   (d) GABA

137. Lithium is used in the prophylactic treatment of: *(Recent NEET Pattern Question)*
    (a) Schizophrenia   (b) MDP
    (c) Acute depression   (d) Conversion reaction

138. Risperidone is most commonly used to treat which of the following disorders? *(Recent NEET Pattern Question)*
    (a) Dementia
    (b) Depression
    (c) Schizophrenia
    (d) Obsessive-compulsive disorder

139. As a side effect the metabolic syndrome is most commonly associated with which of the following group of medications? *(Recent NEET Pattern Question)*
    (a) Anti-anxiety drugs
    (b) Anti-depressant drugs
    (c) Anti-psychotic drugs
    (d) Anti-cholinergic drugs

140. Drug of choice in intractable hiccups is: *(Recent NEET Pattern Question)*
    (a) Metoclopramide   (b) Fluoxetine
    (c) Selegiline   (d) Chlorpromazine

141. All of the following drugs cause hyperprolactinemia *except*: *(Recent NEET Pattern Question)*
    (a) Haloperidol   (b) Chlorpromazine
    (c) Bromocriptine   (d) Metoclopramide

142. Dryness of mouth caused by antipsychotic drug is caused by blockade of: *(Recent NEET Pattern Question)*
    (a) Muscarinic ACh receptors
    (b) GABA receptors
    (c) Serotonergic receptors
    (d) Dopaminergic receptors

143. Selective serotonin reuptake inhibitors are drug of choice for all of the following conditions *except*: *(Recent NEET Pattern Question)*
    (a) Acute panic attack
    (b) Social phobia
    (c) Post traumatic stress disorder
    (d) Generalized anxiety disorder

144. Prophylactic plasma concentration range of lithium in mEq does not include: *(Recent NEET Pattern Question)*
    (a) 0.5   (b) 0.8
    (c) 0.6   (d) 1.0

145. Drug having proven efficacy in bipolar depression is: *(Recent NEET Pattern Question)*
    (a) Carbamazepine   (b) Valproate
    (c) Tiagabine   (d) Lamotrigine

146. Drug of choice for rapid cyclers in manic-depressive psychosis is: *(Recent NEET Pattern Question)*
    (a) Carbamazepine   (b) Valproate
    (c) Phenytoin   (d) Lithium

147. Akathisia is treated by all *except*: *(Recent NEET Pattern Question)*
    (a) Trihexyphenidyl   (b) Propranolol
    (c) Haloperidol   (d) Promethazine

148. Which of the following drug causes sedation but no extra pyramidal side effect? *(Recent NEET Pattern Question)*
    (a) Clozapine   (b) Pimozide
    (c) Fluphenazine   (d) Haloperidol

Central Nervous System

149. Akathisia is seen with the use of: *(Recent NEET Pattern Question)*
 (a) Clozapine (b) Propranolol
 (c) Benztropine (d) Haloperidol

150. Which of the following is not a side effect of clozapine? *(Recent NEET Pattern Question)*
 (a) Agranulocytosis (b) Seizure
 (c) Sialosis (d) Weight loss

151. With MAO inhibitors, food not given is: *(Recent NEET Pattern Question)*
 (a) Cheese (b) Beer
 (c) Fish (d) All of the above

152. Which of the following has least extrapyramidal side effect? *(Recent NEET Pattern Question)*
 (a) Haloperidol (b) Fluphenazine
 (c) Clozapine (d) Flupenthioxol

153. Buspirone as compared to benzodiazepines: *(Recent NEET Pattern Question)*
 (a) Is more potent anticonvulsant
 (b) Does not interfere with GABAergic transmission
 (c) More effective in severe anxiety with panic attacks
 (d) Produces significantly more sedation

154. Depression is not a side effect of: *(Recent NEET Pattern Question)*
 (a) Propranolol (b) Oral contraceptives
 (c) Reserpine (d) Flupenthixol

155. Schizophrenia can be treated with all the following *except*: *(Recent NEET Pattern Question)*
 (a) Pemoline (b) Olanzapine
 (c) Sulpiride (d) Chlorpromazine

156. Which of the following is not a side effect of amitriptyline? *(Recent NEET Pattern Question)*
 (a) Constipation (b) Fine tremors
 (c) Weight loss (d) Dry mouth

157. Which of the following drug may cause hypertensive crisis in a patient on MAO inhibitor therapy? *(Recent NEET Pattern Question)*
 (a) Tyramine (b) Guanethidine
 (c) Phenobarbitone (d) Nor-epinephrine

158. Antipsychotic drug with least extra pyramidal side effect is: *(Recent NEET Pattern Question)*
 (a) Triflupromazine (b) Thioridazine
 (c) Pimozide (d) Trifluoperazine

159. Which of the following drug treatment increases thirst and causes dilute diuresis? *(Recent NEET Pattern Question)*
 (a) Phenobarbitone (b) Lithium
 (c) Chlorpromazine (d) Clozapine

160. False statement regarding Lithium is: *(Recent NEET Pattern Question)*
 (a) Maximum plasma concentration is avoided due to low therapeutic index
 (b) Contraindicated in pregnancy
 (c) No individual variation in the rate of excretion
 (d) 80% reabsorbed in the proximal convoluted tubule

161. Extrapyramidal symptoms are a complication of treatment with following drugs: *(Recent NEET Pattern Question)*
 (a) Antipsychotics (b) Anti anxiety drugs
 (c) Anti depressants (d) Anti malarial drugs

162. Which of the following is an atypical antipsychotic? *(Recent NEET Pattern Question)*
 (a) Clozapine (b) Chlorpromazine
 (c) Thiothixene (d) Haloperidol

163. Drug useful in malignant hyperthermia is: *(Recent NEET Pattern Question)*
 (a) Halothane (b) Succinyl choline
 (c) Dantrolene (d) Haloperidol

164. Risperidone acts on which receptor? *(Recent NEET Pattern Question)*
 (a) D_2 (b) $5 HT_2$
 (c) Both (d) NA

165. Neuroleptic malignant syndrome is caused by: *(Recent NEET Pattern Question)*
 (a) Carbamazepine (b) Clonazepam
 (c) Haloperidol (d) Fluoxetine

166. Non-selective serotonin and nor-adrenaline reuptake inhibitor is: *(Recent NEET Pattern Question)*
 (a) Sertraline (b) Citalopram
 (c) Venlafaxine (d) Paroxetine

167. Half-life of lithium is: *(Recent NEET Pattern Question)*
 (a) 8 hours (b) 16 hours
 (c) 24 hours (d) 36 hours

168. Therapeutic levels of lithium (in mEq/l) in a patient of acute mania is: *(Recent NEET Pattern Question)*
 (a) 0.4-0.8 (b) 0.8-1.2
 (c) 1.2-1.6 (d) 1.6-2.0

169. Which of the following drugs should not be given with tyramine as it may result in dangerous reaction? *(Recent NEET Pattern Question)*
 (a) Selegiline (b) Meperidine
 (c) Tranylcypromine (d) Dextromethorphan

170. Drug used to treat extrapyramidal syndrome due to phenothiazines: *(Recent NEET Pattern Question)*
 (a) Diphenhydramine
 (b) Benzhexol
 (c) Clonidine
 (d) Promethazine

171. True statement regarding lithium toxicity is: *(Recent NEET Pattern Question)*
 (a) Increased by increased serum sodium levels
 (b) Increased by decreased serum sodium levels
 (c) Increased in acute tubular necrosis
 (d) Appears when the serrum levels become triple the dose of therapeutic levels

172. Which of the following antidepressants causes urine retention? *(Recent NEET Pattern Question)*
 (a) Imipramine (b) Fluoxetine
 (c) Dothiepin (d) Respiridone

173. Anti-depressant drug that can be safely used in children is: *(Recent NEET Pattern Question)*
    (a) Imipramine   (b) Fluoxetine
    (c) Dothiepin   (d) Respiridone

174. Coarse tremors, dysarthria and ataxia are side effects of: *(Recent NEET Pattern Question)*
    (a) Lithium   (b) Haloperidol
    (c) Imipramine   (d) None

175. Tranylcypromine (MAO Inhibitor) should be avoided with .... as it causes dangerous drug interaction: *(Recent NEET Pattern Question)*
    (a) Morphine   (b) Amitriptyline
    (c) Alprazolam   (d) Any of the above

176. Which among the following is not an antipsychotic? *(Recent NEET Pattern Question)*
    (a) Risperidone   (b) Haloperidol
    (c) Fluoxetine   (d) Clozapine

177. Galactorrhoea is caused by: *(Recent NEET Pattern Question)*
    (a) Phenothiazines (b) Bromocriptine
    (c) Pyridoxine   (d) None

178. Common side effects of chlorpromazine are all *except*: *(Recent NEET Pattern Question)*
    (a) Osteoporosis   (b) Parkinson's disease
    (c) Skin rash   (d) Amenorrhoea

179. All are selective serotonin reuptake inhibitor *except*: *(Recent NEET Pattern Question)*
    (a) Fluoxetine   (b) Fluvoxamine
    (c) Paroxetine   (d) Amoxapine

180. All are atypical antipsychotic drugs *except*: *(Recent NEET Pattern Question)*
    (a) Clozapine   (b) Risperidone
    (c) Olanzapine   (d) Loxapine

181. Treatment of malignant neuroleptic syndrome include all *except*: *(Recent NEET Pattern Question)*
    (a) Chlorpromazine (b) Dantrolene
    (c) Peripheral cooling (d) Diazepam

182. Long-term antipsychotic use may cause: *(Recent NEET Pattern Question)*
    (a) Depression   (b) Mania
    (c) Schizophrenia   (d) Tardive dyskinesia

183. Moclebemide is: *(Recent NEET Pattern Question)*
    (a) SSRI   (b) Antipsychotic drug
    (c) MAO inhibitor   (d) Tricyclic antidepressant

184. Which of the following is not associated with increase in prolactin? *(Recent NEET Pattern Question)*
    (a) Haloperidol   (b) Chlorpromazine
    (c) Hydroxysulpiride (d) Quetiapine

185. Pimozide belongs to class of: *(Recent NEET Pattern Question)*
    (a) Thiothixene   (b) Phenothiazine
    (c) Butyrophenone   (d) Diphenyl butyl piperidine

186. Antipsychotic drug with the longest elimination half life is: *(Recent NEET Pattern Question)*
    (a) Aripriprazole   (b) Loxapine
    (c) Quetiapine   (d) Ziprasidone

187. Which of the following is NOT a MAO inhibitor? *(Recent NEET Pattern Question)*
    (a) Tranylcypromine (b) Isocarboxazide
    (c) Phenelzine   (d) Maprotiline

188. Which of the following statements is NOT correct of Tardive dyskinesia? *(Recent NEET Pattern Question)*
    (a) It is an unwanted effect of antipsychotics
    (b) Levodopa exacerbates the symptoms
    (c) Antimuscarinic drug reduces its severity
    (d) Often diazepam is used to bring improvement

189. Which of the following medication is associated with an increased risk of agranulocytosis? *(Recent NEET Pattern Question)*
    (a) Clozapine   (b) Imipramine
    (c) Lithium   (d) Haloperidol

190. The side effects of lithium used in psychiatry practice include all *except*: *(Recent NEET Pattern Question)*
    (a) Nausea, vomiting (b) Tremors
    (c) Hypothyroidism (d) Hypercalcemia

191. Drug of choice for the treatment of negative symptoms of schizophrenia is: *(Recent NEET Pattern Question)*
    (a) Chlorpromazine (b) Haloperidol
    (c) Clozapine   (d) Doxepin

192. Which among the following medications has been found to be effective in smoking cessation? *(Recent NEET Pattern Question)*
    (a) Bupropion   (b) Buspirone
    (c) Paroxetine   (d) Venlafaxine

193. Drug of choice in nocturnal enuresis is: *(Recent NEET Pattern Question)*
    (a) Desmopressin   (b) Diazepam
    (c) Amoxapine   (d) Reboxetine

194. A patient presents with malignant hyperthermia and metabolic acidosis. Immediate treatment should be started with: *(Recent NEET Pattern Question)*
    (a) Intravenous Dantrolene
    (b) Sodium bicarbonate
    (c) Intravenous fluids
    (d) Paracetamol

195. Which is a late side effect of typical anti-psychotics?
    (a) Parkinsonism   *(Recent NEET Pattern Question)*
    (b) Tardive dyskinesia
    (c) Acute muscular dystonia
    (d) Akathisia

196. Use of Buspirone is: *(Recent NEET Pattern Question)*
    (a) Anxiolytic   (b) Sedative
    (c) Acute panic attacks (d) Muscle relaxant

197. Weight gain caused by antipsychotics is due to antagonism of: *(Recent NEET Pattern Question)*
    (a) $5\,HT_3$ (b) $5\,HT_{2A}$
    (c) $5\,HT_{2B}$ (d) $5\,HT_{2C}$

198. Drug of choice in lithium induced polyuria is: *(Recent NEET Pattern Question)*
    (a) Amiloride   (b) Demeclocycline
    (c) Thiazide diuretics (d) Indomethacin

Central Nervous System

199. Which of the following is not a SSRI?
 (Recent NEET Pattern Question)
 (a) Escitalopram (b) Sertraline
 (c) Paroxetine (d) Amitriptyline

200. Drug with both antidepressant and antipsychotic properties is: *(Recent NEET Pattern Question)*
 (a) Buspirone (b) Amoxapine
 (c) Trazodone (d) Minaserine

201. The drug of choice in obsessive compulsive disorder is which one of the following? *(Recent NEET Pattern Question)*
 (a) Sertraline (b) Amoxapine
 (c) Hydroxyzine (d) Alprazolam

202. Which of the following is the treatment of choice for patients with schizophrenia, who refuse to take treatment? *(Recent NEET Pattern Question)*
 (a) Clozapine (b) Thioridazine
 (c) Olanzapine (d) Fluphenazine

203. Which is the drug of choice for maintenance therapy in uncomplicated bipolar disorder?
 (Recent NEET Pattern Question)
 (a) Sodium valproate (b) Carbamazepine
 (c) Lithium (d) Lamotrigine

204. A 25 years old male started taking antipsychotic (haloperidol) since last three days. He presented to the emergency department with protruded tongue, breathing difficulty along with spasm of neck and jaw muscles. What could be the most likely diagnosis? *(Recent NEET Pattern Question)*
 (a) Drug hypersensitivity reaction
 (b) Acute dystonia
 (c) Neuroleptic malignants
 (d) Tardive dystonia

205. Which drug is the most useful in treating an episode of antipsychotic induced acute dystonia?
 (Recent NEET Pattern Question)
 (a) Lorazepam (b) Haloperidol
 (c) Promethazine (d) Phenobarbitone

206. Drug of choice for manic depressive psychosis is:
 (Recent NEET Pattern Question)
 (a) Lithium (b) Diazepam
 (c) Olanzapine (d) Carbamazepine

207. Extrapyramidal symptoms are seen with the use of:
 (Recent NEET Pattern Question)
 (a) Metoclopramide (b) Domperidone
 (c) Prolactin (d) All of the above

208. Which of the following is not an antidepressant?
 (Recent NEET Pattern Question)
 (a) Amitriptyline (b) Fluoxetine
 (c) Imipramine (d) Chlorpromazine

209. Drug of choice for obsessive compulsive disorder is:
 (Recent NEET Pattern Question)
 (a) Clozapine (b) Alprazolam
 (c) Amoxapine (d) Fluoxetine

210. Which of the following drugs is not used for anxiety?
 (Recent NEET Pattern Question)
 (a) Propranolol (b) Alprazolam
 (c) Buspirone (d) Haloperidol

211. Drug of chocie for schizophrenia is:
 (Recent NEET Pattern Question)
 (a) Olanzapine (b) Haloperidol
 (c) Lithium (d) Chlorpromazine

212. Drugs which can be used to treat mania in ICU are all *except*: *(Recent NEET Pattern Question)*
 (a) Carbamazepine (b) Lithium
 (c) Diazepam (d) Lorazepam
 (e) Opioids and Drug Addiction

OPIOIDS AND DRUG ADDICTION

213. A patient of biliary colic presented to hospital. Intern gave an injection and the pain worsened. Which is the most likely injection given? *(NEET Pattern Question 2020)*
 (a) Morphine (b) Diclofenac
 (c) Nefopam (d) Etoricoxib

214. Like all the opioids, tramadol acts as an analgesic drug by stimulating μ opioid receptors. Apart from this, the additional analgesic mechanism of tramadol is:
 (AIIMS May 2019)
 (a) Serotonin and noradrenaline reuptake inhibition
 (b) Anticholinergic
 (c) Antihistaminic
 (d) Serotonin and dopamine reuptake inhibition

215. Morphine should not be used in the treatment of:
 (AIIMS May 2018)
 (a) Ischemic pain (b) Biliary colic
 (c) Cancer pain (d) Postoperative pain

216. Drug of choice for alcohol withdrawal is:
 (NEET Pattern 2016-17)
 (a) Disulfiram (b) Naltrexone
 (c) Diazepam (d) Chlordiazepoxide

217. Acamprostate given to prevent: *(NEET Pattern 2016-17)*
 (a) Alcohol intoxication
 (b) Opioid withdrawal
 (c) Alcohol craving
 (d) Opioid intoxication

218. In opioid addiction, drug used in maintenance therapy is:
 (NEET Pattern 2016-17)
 (a) Methadone (b) Clonidine
 (c) Naloxone (d) Naltrexone

219. Heroine is: *(NEET Pattern 2016-17)*
 (a) Diacetyl morphine
 (b) Dimethoxymethyl amphetamine
 (c) Methylene dioxy methamphetamine
 (d) Methylene dioxy amphetamine

220. Angel dust is : *(NEET Pattern 2016-17)*
 (a) Phenylbutazone
 (b) Dimethoxymethyl amphetamine
 (c) Phentolamine
 (d) Phencyclidine

221. A female in labor ward was administered opioid analgesic. Which of the following drugs should be kept ready for emergency? *(AIIMS Nov 2017)*
 (a) Lignocaine (b) Naloxone
 (c) Diphenhydramine (d) Fentanyl

222. A patient presented with pain in the right lower quadrant of abdomen. He has history of renal stones in right kidney. He was prescribed an opioid which is agonist at kappa receptors and antagonist at mu receptors. The likely drug given was: *(AIIMS Nov 2017)*
    (a) Pentazocine
    (b) Buprenorphine
    (c) Tramadol
    (d) Fentanyl

223. A patient presented with vomiting and ataxia. There were oxalate crystals in the urine. The patient was given ethanol and 4 methyl pyrazole for treatment. The likely diagnosis of the patient was: *(AIIMS May, 2017)*
    (a) Methanol poisoning
    (b) Ethanol poisoning
    (c) Ethylene glycol poisoning
    (d) Diazepam poisoning

224. Which of the following is not used for alcohol detoxification? *(AIIMS Nov 2015)*
    (a) Disulfiram
    (b) Flumazenil
    (c) Acamprosate
    (d) Naltrexone

225. A person consumes large quantities of alcohol daily since 20 years. He is physically dependent on alcohol. Drug that should not be given to this person is: *(AIIMS Nov 2014)*
    (a) Disulfiram
    (b) Acamprosate
    (c) Naltrexone
    (d) Chlordiazepoxide

226. True statement regarding methadone are all *except*: *(AIIMS May 2014)*
    (a) It is a long acting µ-receptor agonist
    (b) It is rapidly absorbed from the gastrointestinal tract and is detected in plasma 30 minutes after oral administration
    (c) The primary use of methadone is relief of chronic pain
    (d) The onset of analgesia is 30–60 minutes after parenteral administration and 1–2 hours after oral administration

227. Dysphoria caused by opiates is mediated by which receptor? *(AIIMS May 2013)*
    (a) mu
    (b) kappa
    (c) delta
    (d) sigma

228. Preferred drug for alcohol withdrawal seizures is: *(AIIMS May 2013)*
    (a) Diazepam
    (b) Valproate
    (c) Phenobarbitone
    (d) Carbamazepine

229. All are true regarding METHANOL poisoning *except*: *(AIIMS May 2013)*
    (a) Hemodialysis should be done when serum methanol concentration is above 50 mg/dL
    (b) Fomepizole acts by inhibiting aldehyde dehydrogenase
    (c) High anion gap metabolic acidosis is seen in severe cases
    (d) Visual disturbances are commonly seen

230. A young man is with known heroin addiction is brought in the emergency in unconscious state. On examination, the patient has decreased bowel sounds, depressed respiration and pin point pupil. The treatment of choice for this patient is: *(AIIMS Nov 2012)*
    (a) Oral natrexone
    (b) IV naloxone
    (c) Oral diazepam
    (d) Oral Buprenorphine

231. Which among the following drug is contra-indicated in renal failure? *(AI 2012)*
    (a) Pethidine
    (b) Morphine
    (c) Fentanyl
    (d) Atracurium

232. Naltrexone is used to maintain abstinence following opioid withdrawal in addicts. It blocks all of the following features of opioid use, *except*:
    (a) Euphoriant effects of opioids
    (b) Craving for opioids *(Recent NEET Pattern Question)*
    (c) Miosis
    (d) Respiratory depression

233. The following symptoms may be seen in opium withdrawal: *(Recent NEET Pattern Question)*
    (a) Constipation
    (b) Lacrimation
    (c) Dry nose and mouth
    (d) Constipation

234. In alcohol withdrawal, drug of choice is: *(Recent NEET Pattern Question)*
    (a) TFP
    (b) Chlormethazole
    (c) Chlordiazepoxide
    (d) Buspirone

235. Which of the following is used to maintain abstinence in alcohol dependence? *(Recent NEET Pattern Question)*
    (a) Naltrexone
    (b) Clonidine
    (c) Disulfiram
    (d) Naloxone

236. In methyl alcohol poisoning there is CNS depression, cardiac depression and optic nerve atrophy. These effects are produced due to: *(Recent NEET Pattern Question)*
    (a) Formaldehyde and formic acid
    (b) Acetaldehyde
    (c) Pyridine
    (d) Acetic acid

237. Drugs used in alcohol withdrawal are all, *except*: *(Recent NEET Pattern Question)*
    (a) Naltrexone
    (b) Naloxone
    (c) Acamprosate
    (d) Disulfiram

238. Characterstic features of opioid withdrawal is: *(Recent NEET Pattern Question)*
    (a) Rhinorrhea and lacrimation
    (b) Seizures
    (c) Delirium Tremors
    (d) Transient visual, tactile or auditory hallucinations

239. Drug of choice for controlling severe pain in cancer patients is: *(Recent NEET Pattern Question)*
    (a) Morphine
    (b) Diclofenac
    (c) Ibuprofen
    (d) Codiene

240. Which of the following statement is FALSE about Naltrexone? *(Recent NEET Pattern Question)*
    (a) Parenterally administered
    (b) Used to prevent relapse of heavy drinking
    (c) Long acting
    (d) Cause hepatotoxicity

241. Dysphoria is mediated by which opioid receptor: *(Recent NEET Pattern Question)*
    (a) Mu
    (b) Kappa
    (c) Delta
    (d) None

Central Nervous System

242. In acute morphine poisoning, the drug of choice is:
 (Recent NEET Pattern Question)
 (a) Atropine (b) Methadone
 (c) Naloxone (d) Alcohol

243. Naltrexone is used for which of the following poisoning? *(Recent NEET Pattern Question)*
 (a) Heroin (b) Atropine
 (c) Cannabis (d) Diazepam

244. Disulfiram like reaction is not seen with:
 (Recent NEET Pattern Question)
 (a) Amoxicillin (b) Metronidazole
 (c) Cefoperazone (d) Disulfiram

245. Regarding opioid induced seizures:
 (Recent NEET Pattern Question)
 (a) They usually occur at therapeutic doses
 (b) Children are more susceptible
 (c) Seizures occur only with m-opioid agonists
 (d) Diazepam is the drug of choice in treatment

246. Antabuse: *(Recent NEET Pattern Question)*
 (a) Inhibits glucuronide conjugation
 (b) Inhibits oxidation of alcohol
 (c) Inhibits excretion of alcohol through kidney
 (d) None of the above

247. The drug acamprosate is therapeutically used for:
 (a) Cough *(Recent NEET Pattern Question)*
 (b) Rickets
 (c) Thrombolysis
 (d) Maintenance therapy of alcohol abstinence

248. Which one of the following drug is contraindicated in acute myocardial infarction?
 (Recent NEET Pattern Question)
 (a) Morphine (b) Pentazocine
 (c) Nitroglycerin (d) Beta blockers

249. The most important feature of the following opioid analgesic is high oral parenteral activity ratio (1:2):
 (Recent NEET Pattern Question)
 (a) Morphine (b) Oxymorphine
 (c) Methadone (d) Diacetylmorphine

250. Actions of opiates in man include all except:
 (Recent NEET Pattern Question)
 (a) Constipation (b) Vomiting
 (c) Analgesia (d) Mydriasis

251. Disulfiram and acamprosate are used for:
 (Recent NEET Pattern Question)
 (a) Alcohol abstinence
 (b) Cocaine abuse
 (c) Opium poisoning
 (d) Atropine over dose

252. Which drug has more analgesic effects than morphine?
 (Recent NEET Pattern Question)
 (a) Heroin (b) Apomorphine
 (c) Codeine (d) Pethidine

253. Ethanol is given in methyl alcohol poisoning poisoning because: *(Recent NEET Pattern Question)*
 (a) It inhibit alcohol dehydrogenase
 (b) It inhibit aldehyde synthetase
 (c) It binds to aldehyde dehydrogenase 100 times stronger than methanol
 (d) None

254. Which of the following is not an opioid peptide?
 (Recent NEET Pattern Question)
 (a) β-Endorphin (b) Epinephrine
 (c) Leu5-encephalin (d) Met5-encephalin

255. In liver, which of the following is responsible for metabolism of alcohol? *(Recent NEET Pattern Question)*
 (a) Alcohol dehydrogenase (ADH)
 (b) Aldehyde dehydrogenase (ALDH)
 (c) Microsomal ethanol-oxidizing system (MEOS)
 (d) All of the above

256. Pure opiate antagonists are all of the following except:
 (Recent NEET Pattern Question)
 (a) Naloxone (b) Nalorphine
 (c) Nalmefene (d) Naltrexone

257. Endogenous opioid peptide includes:
 (Recent NEET Pattern Question)
 (a) Encephalin (b) Endorphins
 (c) Dynorphins (d) All of the above

258. Antidote of methyl alcohol poisoning is:
 (Recent NEET Pattern Question)
 (a) Barbiturate (b) Fomepizole
 (c) Phenytoin (d) Lamotrigne

259. Which of the following opioid analgesic is suitable for haemodynamically unstable patients?
 (Recent NEET Pattern Question)
 (a) Morphine (b) Meperidine
 (c) Fentanyl (d) Pentazocine

260. Tramadol is: *(Recent NEET Pattern Question)*
 (a) Antiflatulent (b) Antireflux drug
 (c) Beta-blocker (d) Opioid analgesic

261. Opioid analgesic used in treatment of cough is:
 (Recent NEET Pattern Question)
 (a) Loperamide (b) Diphenoxylate
 (c) Codeine (d) Meperidine

262. True about naltrexone is all except:
 (Recent NEET Pattern Question)
 (a) Acts on opioid receptors
 (b) Is used in treatment of alcohol dependence
 (c) Is used to reduce craving in dependence
 (d) Is an opioid agonist

263. Dextromethorphan differs from codeine in:
 (Recent NEET Pattern Question)
 (a) Its antitussive action can be blocked by naloxone
 (b) Depresses mucocilliary function of the airway mucosa
 (c) Addiction common
 (d) Causes no constipation

264. Which of the following is 100 times more potent than morphine? *(Recent NEET Pattern Question)*
 (a) Pethidine (b) Fentanyl
 (c) Pentazocin (d) Meperidine

265. Drugs that can be used in opioid de-addiction are:
 (Recent NEET Pattern Question)
 (a) Clonidine (b) Diazepam
 (c) Methadone (d) All of the above

266. Site of action of opioid receptor is:
    (Recent NEET Pattern Question)
    (a) Area postrema   (b) Dorsal horn
    (c) Injury site   (d) Brain

267. Opium is a derivative of:
    (Recent NEET Pattern Question)
    (a) Solanum tuberosum   (b) Datura stromonium
    (c) Papaver somniferum (d) Nicotiana tobacum

268. The most potent analgesic agent is:
    (Recent NEET Pattern Question)
    (a) Fentanyl   (b) Sufentanil
    (c) Remifentanil   (d) Alfentanil

269. Morphine can be given by all the following routes *except*:
    (Recent NEET Pattern Question)
    (a) Intravenous   (b) Intramuscular
    (c) Subcutaneous   (d) Sublingual

270. "Opioids" differ from "opiates" in that they are:
    (Recent NEET Pattern Question)
    (a) More powerful in action
    (b) More long acting
    (c) Synthetic derivatives
    (d) Derived directly from opium

271. Which of the following is a naturally occurring opioid?
    (Recent NEET Pattern Question)
    (a) Pentazocine   (b) Heroin
    (c) Fentanyl   (d) Morphine

272. Toxic dose of lithium is: *(Recent NEET Pattern Question)*
    (a) 0.6 mEq/L   (b) 1.2 mEq/L
    (c) 2.0 mEq/L   (d) <0.6 mEq/L

273. Which drug is used for pain control in cancer patients?
    (Recent NEET Pattern Question)
    (a) Pethidine   (b) Fentanyl
    (c) Methadone   (d) Remifentanil

274. The effect of morphine which has least tolerance is?
    (Recent NEET Pattern Question)
    (a) Analgesis   (b) Respiratory depression
    (c) Constipation   (d) Bradycardia

275. Opioid that activates monoamine action is:
    (Recent NEET Pattern Question)
    (a) Tramadol   (b) Pentazocine
    (c) Pethidine (d) Meperidine

276. Which of the following drugs does not possess even slightest agonist action? *(Recent NEET Pattern Question)*
    (a) Buprenorphine   (b) Butorphanol
    (c) Nalbuphine   (d) Nalmefene

277. Methadone is used in the management of opioid addiction because: *(Recent NEET Pattern Question)*
    (a) Its analgesic activity is less than that of morphine
    (b) It is an opioid receptor antagonist
    (c) It is not addictive
    (d) It is longer acting and causes milder withdrawal symptoms

278. Fomepizole is a selective antidote for poisoning with:
    (Recent NEET Pattern Question)
    (a) MAO inhibitors
    (b) Ethyl alcohol
    (c) Methyl alcohol
    (d) Tricyclic antidepressants

279. Morphine is used in the treatment of which one of the following: *(Recent NEET Pattern Question)*
    (a) Asthma   (b) Kyphoscoliosis
    (c) Chronic cor pulmonale (d) Left ventricular failure

280. All of the following may be used for detoixification therapy of chronic alcoholism *except*:
    (Recent NEET Pattern Question)
    (a) Naltrexone   (b) Disulfiram
    (c) Flumazenil   (d) Acamprostate

281. Hallucinations, psychosis, hypertension and tachycardia are adverse effects typically associated with which of the following narcotics?
    (Recent NEET Pattern Question)
    (a) Morphine   (b) Meperidine
    (c) Pentazocine (d) Buprenorphine

282. Features of opioid intake are all of the following *except*:
    (Recent NEET Pattern Question)
    (a) Feeling of relaxation   (b) Euphoria
    (c) Analgesia   (d) Dilated pupils

283. The disulfiram alcohol reaction occurs due to inhibition of which enzyme? *(Recent NEET Pattern Question)*
    (a) Alcohol reductase   (b) Alcohol dehydrogenase
    (c) Aldehyde reductase (d) Aldehyde dehydrogenase

284. Which of the following analgesics should not be given in acute MI? *(Recent NEET Pattern Question)*
    (a) Methadone   (b) Morphine
    (c) Buprenorphine (d) Pentazocine

285. Drug of choice for prophylaxis of mania is:
    (Recent NEET Pattern Question)
    (a) Lithium   (b) Haloperidol
    (c) Clozapine (d) Carbamazepine

286. Derivative of morphine used for diarrhea is:
    (Recent NEET Pattern Question)
    (a) Oxymorphine (b) Diphenoxylate
    (c) Pethidine   (d) Codeine

287. Drug used for cessation of smoking are all *except*:
    (NEET Pattern 2016-17)
    (a) Buspirone   (b) Bupropion
    (c) Varenecilline (d) Nicotine

Explanations

1. **Ans. (a) GABA- A receptor** *(Ref: KDT 8/e p429)*

2. **Ans. (d) 30 minute**
   (Ref: Goodman and Gilman 12/e p469; KDT 8/e p435)
   Duration of action of flumazenil is 30-60 min. So the best answer seems to be 30 min.

3. **Ans. (c) Redistribution** *(Ref: Katzung 10/e p407; KDT 8/e p24)*
   Thiopentone is highly lipid soluble drug. On i.v. administration, it quickly reaches the brain and cause anaesthesia. But due to high lipid solubility, it again crosses the membranes of brain and diffuses to other tissues like fat and muscle. As it is not present in brain, its action is terminated. This is known as re-distribution.

4. **Ans. (a) Thiopentone** *(Ref: KDT 8/e p427)*
   Barbiturates are contra-indicated in acute intermittent porphyria.

5. **Ans. (d) Antagonist** *(Ref: KDT 8/e p435)*

6. **Ans. (c) They are weakly acidic and do not ionise in stomach** *(Ref: KDT 8/e p17)*
   Barbiturates and salicylates are maximally absorbed in stomach because these are weakly acidic and do not ionize in stomach.

7. **Ans. (c) Oxazepam** *(Ref: KDT 8/e p494)*

8. **Ans. (a) Midazolam** *(Ref: Goodman and Gilman 11/e p411)*

9. **Ans. (c) Triazolam** *(Ref: KDT 8/e p431)*

10. **Ans. (b) Zolpidem** *(Ref: KDT 8/e p433)*

11. **Ans. (b) Flumazenil** *(Ref: KDT 8/e p435)*

12. **Ans. (d) Buspirone** *(Ref: KDT 8/e p435)*

13. **Ans. (b) Flumazenil** *(Ref: KDT 8/e p435)*

14. **Ans. (c) Gabapentin** *(Ref: KDT 8/e p446)*

15. **Ans. (c) Is secreted by pituitary** *(Ref: KDT 8/e p436)*

16. **Ans. (b) Benzodiazepines** *(Ref: KDT 8/e p425)*

17. **Ans. (a) Pramipexole** *(Ref: KDT 8th/e p458)*
    Restless legs syndrome (RLS)
    - It is a condition that causes an uncontrollable urge to move the legs, usually because of an uncomfortable sensation. It typically happens in the evening or night hours when a person is sitting or lying down. Moving eases the unpleasant feeling temporarily. It is also known as Ekboom syndrome
    - Ropinirole, rotigotine and pramipexole are approved by the Food and Drug Administration for the treatment of moderate to severe RLS.
    - Gabapentin and pregabalin may work for some people with RLS.
    - Opioids can relieve mild to severe symptoms, but they may be addicting if used in high doses.

18. **Ans. (a) Edaravone** *(Ref: Harrison 20th/e p3146)*

    Edaravone
    - It is a free radical scavenger specifically indicated for the treatment of **amyotrophic lateral sclerosis** (ALS) by intravenous infusion.
    - It is believed to relieve effects of oxidative stress, a likely key factor in the onset and progression of ALS. Oxidative stress is thought to be an imbalance between the production of free radicals (unpaired, reactive electrons) and the ability of the body to counteract or detoxify their harmful effects. In patients with ALS, there are consistent increases in oxidative stress biomarkers.

    HOW TO REMEMBER
    - Name contains A and O (edarAvOne) means it is **Anti-Oxidant**
    - Name starts with **EDA** means it is **E**ffective **D**rug for **A**myotrophic lateral sclerosis.

19. **Ans. (d) Biperidin** *(Ref: KDT 8/e p460)*

20. **Ans. (c) Hepatotoxic** *(Ref: KDT 8th/e p459)*

21. **Ans. (a) Dopamine agonist** *(Ref: KDT 8/e p453)*

22. **Ans. (d) MAO inhibitor** *(Ref: KDT 8/e p453)*

23. **Ans. (c) Bromocriptine**
    (Ref: KDT 8/e p191; Goodman and Gilman 12th/e p1114)
    Ergot derivatives like bromocriptine can lead to worsening of vasospasm especially in patients of peripheral vascular disease due to their strong vasoconstrictor activity.

24. **Ans. (c) Entacapone** *(Ref: Katzung 10/e p448-449; KDT 8/e p459)*
    Levo-dopa etabolized in the body by two enzymes; MAO and COMT. Thus MAO inhibitors like selegiline and COMT inhibitors like entacapone and tolcapone can increase the bioavailability of dopa.

25. **Ans. (c) Vitamin B complex** *(Ref: KDT 8/e p456)*

26. **Ans. (b) Benzhexol** *(Ref: KDT 8/e p460)*
    Central anticholinergics like trihexy phenydyl (Benzhexol) are the only drugs effective in drug induced Parkinsonism.

27. **Ans. (c) Pyridoxine** *(Ref: KDT 8/e p456)*
    'Pyridoxine abolishes therapeutic effect of levodopa by enhancing peripheral decarboxylation of levodopa, less is available to cross to the brain.

28. **Ans. (a) Donepezil** *(Ref: KDT 8/e p122)*

29. **Ans. (c) Ropinirole** *(Ref: KDT 8/e p122, 519)*

30. **Ans. (d) To increase crossing of L-Dopa through BBB** *(Ref: KDT 8/e p456-457)*

31. **Ans. (d) Piracetam** *(Ref: KDT 8/e p519)*
    Nootropic drugs are those that enhance memory. Piracetam is used for this function in patients with head injury.

32. Ans. (a) Centrally acting reversible anticholinesterase
    (Ref: KDT 8/e p122)
33. Ans. (a) Entacapone (Ref: KDT 8/e p459)
34. Ans. (c) COMT inhibitors prolong the action of L-dopa
    (Ref: KDT 8/e p459)
35. Ans. (a) Amantadine (Ref: KDT 8/e p459, 460)
36. Ans. (a) Riluzole (Ref: KDT 6/e p464-465)
37. Ans. (c) Retroperitoneal Fibrosis (Ref: KDT 8/e p 458)
    - Adverse effects of ropinirole and pramipexole include nausea, dizzinesss, hallucinations, postural hypotension and excessive day time sleepiness
    - Their advantage over ergot derivatives like bromocriptine is lack of retroperitoneal fibrosis and gangrene and long duration of action.
    - Ropinirole has been approved by FDA for restless leg syndrome
38. Ans. (d) Pergolide (Ref: KDT 7/e p 430)
39. Ans. (d) Selegiline (Ref: KDT 8/e p458)
40. Ans. (c) Bromocriptine (Ref: KDT 7/e p430)
41. Ans. (d) Benzhexol (Ref: KDT 8/e p460)
42. Ans. (a) Hepatotoxicity
    (Ref: Modern concepts of acute and chronic hepatitis, p209)
    - Valproate is metabolized to a hepatotoxic metabolite.
    - Enzyme inducers like carbamazepine induce the formation of this metabolite and increase the risk of hepatotoxicity.
43. Ans. (b) It has more sustained action because of lower lipid solubility and slower redistribution (Ref: KDT 8th/e p450)
44. Ans. (d) Phenytoin (Ref: Harrison's 19/e p2543)
45. Ans. (b) Taper the drug over 6 months
    (Ref: CMDT 2017/e p988)
    CMDT mentions that gradual withdrawal (over weeks or months) of anti-epileptics can be considered if the patient is seizure free for minimum 2 years. CNS adverse effects like aggression and irritability are well known adverse effects of levetiracetam. As the patient is seizure free for 2 years, gradual withdrawal over a period of months can be carried out
46. Ans. (c) Blurred vision (Ref: KDT 7/e p416)

    Carbamazepine can cause
    - Steven Johnson syndrome
    - Rash
    - Allergy
    - Bone marrow suppression (Agranulocytosis)
    - Neurotoxicity

47. Ans. (c) (Ref: Harrison 19th/e p2552; KDT 8/e p449)
    DOC for absence seizures is valproate. Another first line drug is ethosuximide.
48. Ans. (d) Polycystic ovarian disease (Ref: KDT 8/e p417)
    Long term use of valproate in young girls is associated with higher incidence of polycystic ovarian disease and menstrual irregularities.
49. Ans. (b) All women who could become pregnant
    (Ref: Nelson 19th/e p2001)

"The U.S. Public Health Service has recommended that all women of childbearing age and who are capable of becoming pregnant take **0.4 mg of folic** acid daily. If, however, a pregnancy is planned in high-risk women (previously affected child), supplementation should be started with 4 mg (= 4000 microgram) of folic acid daily, beginning 1 month before the time of the planned conception."

50. Ans. (a) Vigabatrin (Ref: KDT 8/e p448)
    Vigabatrin can cause visual field contraction, production of behavioural changes, depression or psychosis as adverse effects.
51. Ans. (d) 4000 micrograms per day
    (Ref: Williams Obstetrics 24th/e p1104; Nelson 19th/e p2001)
    - All women of childbearing age and who are capable of becoming pregnant should take 0.4 mg (=400 mcg) of folic acid daily.
    - If pregnancy is planned in high-risk women (previously affected child), supplementation should be started with 4 mg (= 4000 microgram) of folic acid daily, beginning 1 month before the time of the planned conception.
52. Ans. (c) Decrease in antidiuretic hormone (Ref: KDT 8/e p442)
    - Carbamazepine like other antiepileptic drugs is teratogenic.
    - It can cause neurotoxicity manifested as dizziness, sedation, vertigo, diplopia and ataxia
    - It can result in hypersensitivity reactions like rash, photosensitivity, hepatitis and rarely agranulocytosis
    - It increases the release of ADH from the hypothalamus and thus can result in dilutional hyponatremia particularly in elderly people.
53. Ans. (a) Levetiracetam (Ref: KDT 8/e p447)
    - Levetiracetam, lamotrigine, valproate and topiramate are useful in myoclonic epilepsy. Valproate should be avoided in pregnancy.
    - Vigabatrin has no role in this condition whereas carbamazepine and phenytoin are contra-indicated in myoclonic epilepsy.
54. Ans. (d) Lamotrigine mainly acts by causing GABA mediated CI- channel opening (Ref: Goodman Gilman 12th/e p600)
    Lamotrigine mainly acts by inhibiting Na$^+$ and prolonging their recovery from inactivated state. It can also increase GABA- ergic activity, decrease glutamatergic activity and block Ca^{2+} channels.
55. Ans. (b) Hyponatremia (Ref: Katzung 11/e p406; KDT 8/e p442)
    Carbamazepine can cause hyponatremia and water intoxication at high doses. This adverse effect appears to be due to its ADH releasing property (resulting in dilutional hyponatremia). The same adverse effect can be utilized for treatment of diabetes insipidus.
56. Ans. (a) Phenytoin (Ref: Katzung 11/e p405)
    Phenytoin on long term administration can lead to lymphadenopathy which is sometimes difficult to distinguish from malignant lymphoma. It is known as pseudolymphoma.
57. Ans. (d) Prophylactic phenobarbitone
    (Ref: Current Pediatrics diagnosis and treatment 18th/e p722,726)
    Prophylactic phenobarbitone is indicated for atypical febrile seizures only.

Central Nervous System

58. Ans. (a) ACTH (Ref: Katzung 11/e p418)
59. Ans. (a) Hypoglycemia (Ref: KDT 8/e p441)
    - Phenytoin cause hyperglycemia.
60. Ans. (a) Carbamazepine (Ref: KDT 8/e p442)
61. Ans. (b) Sodium Valproate (Ref: KDT 8/e p444)
    - Juvenile myoclonic epilepsy (also known as Janz syndrome) occurs in 12-18 years old children.
    - Valproic acid is drug of choice for this condition whereas carbamazepine can worsen it.
62. Ans. (d) Valproic acid (Ref: KDT 8/e p444)
63. Ans. (b) Gynaecomastia (Ref: KDT 8/e p441)
64. Ans. (b) Phenytoin (Ref: KDT 8th/441)
65. Ans. (a) Sodium valproate (Ref: KDT 8/e p444)

- It acts by various mechanisms like increase in GABA, blockade of Na^+ channels and inhibition of T-type Ca^{2+} currents. Valproate increases the formation of GABA (by stimulating glutamic acid decarboxylase) and inhibits the degradation of GABA (by inhibiting GABA transaminase and succinic semialdehyde dehydrogenase).
- Phenytoin and carbamazepine acts by affecting neuronal Na^+ channels.
- Ethosuximide acts by affecting T-type Ca^{2+} currents.

66. Ans. (c) Diazepam (Ref: KDT 8/e p450)
67. Ans. (b) Sodium valproate (Ref: KDT 8/e p444)
    Most anticonvulsants are enzyme inducers except valproate (inhibitor).
68. Ans. (b) Phenytoin (Ref: Katzung 11th./405; KDT 8/e p441)
69. Ans. (d) Atropine (Ref: KDT 8/e p449)
70. Ans. (b) Phenytoin (Ref: KDT 8/e p441)
71. Ans. (c) Carbamazepine (Ref: KDT 8/e p442)
72. Ans. (a) Phenytoin (Ref: KDT 8/e p441)
73. Ans. (a) Vigabatrin (Ref: KDT 8/e p448)
74. Ans. (c) Sedation (Ref: KDT 8/e p441)
75. Ans. (c) Carbamazepine and phenytoin (Ref: KDT 8/e p442)
76. Ans. (a) Carbamazepine (Ref: KDT 8/e p442)
    Carbamazepine releases ADH and causes dilutional hyponatremia.
77. Ans. (a) Ataxia (Ref: KDT 8/e p441)
78. Ans. (a) Valporate (Ref: KDT 8/e p444)
79. Ans. (a) Ethosuximide – K⁺ channel opener (Ref: KDT 8/e p443)
80. Ans. (d) All (Ref: KDT 8/e p656)
81. Ans. (a) Valporate (Ref: KDT 8/e p444)
82. Ans. (d) Phentermine (Ref: CMDT 2010/1137)
    Phentermine was used for treatment of obesity. It decreases appetite and causes weight loss.
83. Ans. (c) Zonisamide (Ref: Goodman and Gilman 11/e p521; KDT 8/e p447)
84. Ans. (a) Rash (Ref: Katzung 11/e p409; KDt 8/e p446)
85. Ans. (d) Phenytoin (Ref: KDT 8/e p441)
86. Ans. (d) Toxicity may occur with only small increment in dose (Ref: KDT 8/e p440)
87. Ans. (c) Valproic acid (Ref: KDT 8/e p444)
88. Ans. (c) Inter-nuclear ophthalmoplegia (Ref: KDT 8/e p441)
89. Ans. (c) Magnesium sulphate
    (Ref: Principles of pharmacology 1st/e p542)
90. Ans. (b) GABA – agonism (Ref: KDT 8/e p448)
91. Ans. (a) Alcohol de-addiction (Ref: KDT 8/e p421)
92. Ans. (b) Can be mixed with dextrose (Ref: KDT 8/e p441)
93. Ans. (a) Vigabatrin (Ref: KDT 8/e p448)
94. Ans. (a) It is an enzyme inducer (Ref: KDT 8/e p444)
95. Ans. (d) It inhibits microsomal enzymes
    (Ref: KDT 8/e p440-441)
96. Ans. (c) Lipid soluble (Ref: KDT 8/e p441)
    - Fosphenytoin is water soluble prodrug of phenytoin developed to overcome the difficulties in IV administration of phenytoin.
97. Ans. (c) Nephrotoxicity (Ref: KDT 8/e p444)
98. Ans. (a) Sodium valproate
    (Ref: CMDT 2014/ p937; KDT 8/e p 444)
99. Ans. (b) Lorazepam (Ref: KDT 8/e p450)
100. Ans. (b) Valproate (Ref:CMDT 2014/ p938; KDT 8/e p 444)
101. Ans. (d) Continue with Phenytoin and add Tab. Folic acid and during the last 2 weeks of pregnancy give oral Vitamin K too (Ref: KDT 8/e p449)
102. Ans. (d) Phenobarbitone (Ref: KDT 8/e p443)
103. Ans. (a) Vigabatrin (Ref: KDT 8/e p448)
104. Ans. (a) Valproic acid (Ref: KDT 8/e p444)
105. Ans. (c) Thiazides increase the tubular reabsorption of lithium (Ref: KDT 8th/e p477)
    Diuretics like thiazides cause loss of Na^+ through the kidney. Therefore, kidney tends to retain sodium by increasing its tubular reabsorption. As lithium is also a monovalent cation similar to Na (belong to same group in periodic table), kidney handles it similar to sodium. Therefore, tubular reabsorption of lithium also increases and its plasma level rises.
106. Ans. (b) Serum lithium levels (Ref: KDT 8th/e p476)
    The features in the question (seizures, coarse tremors, confusion, and weakness of limbs) point towards lithium toxicity. Therefore, serum lithium level should be measured immediately.
    - When the patient was fasting for few days, there will be decreased salt (sodium) intake that would have led to decrease in sodium levels. To maintain serum sodium levels, kidney increases the reabsorption of sodium. As, lithium is handled in same way as sodium by kidney, its reabsorption also increases. Therefore, lithium toxicity could have resulted. This is the reason that patients on lithium therapy are advised to take fixed dose of salt per

day and also should avoid drugs causing sodium loss from body like thiazides.
- Serum electrolytes is not the answer here because body maintains the level of serum sodium and therefore its level most likely will be normal in the investigations

107. **Ans. (b) Trihexyphenidyl** *(Ref: KDT 8th/e p460)*
- The features given in the question are suggestive of drug induced Parkinsonism.
- Parkinsonism is an EPS caused by antipsychotic drugs like fluphenazine.
- Trihexyphenidyl (benztropine) is an anticholinergic agent and is the most commonly used as well as drug of choice for drug induced Parkinsonism.
- Selegiline, Pramipexole and Amantadine are used in Parkinson's disease but not effective in drug induced Parkinsonism.

108. **Ans. (a) 1, 3 and 4 are correct** *(Ref: KDT 8th/e p470-471)*
Chlorpromazine is a typical anti-psychotic drug having main mechanism of antipsychotic action as D2 blockade and minor as 5HT2 blockade. However, it also blocks many other receptors that can result in adverse effects.

D2 and 5HT2 blocking action	Anti-psychotic effect
H1 blockade	Sedation
Muscarinic blockade	Dry mouth
Alpha blockade	Hypotension.
D2 blockade	Extra pyramidal symptoms (EPS) and hyperprolactenemia

109. **Ans. (a) Sialorrhea** *(Ref: KDT 8th/e p488)*
- Escitalopram is a selective serotonin reuptake inhibitor (SSRI).
- Other SSRIs include Fluoxetine, Paroxetine, Fluvoxamine etc.
- Side-effects of SSRI include:
  - Most common: Nausea, Vomiting
  - Next most common: Anxiety
  - Other side effects: Delayed ejaculation, anorgasmia, diarrhea, vivid dreams etc.
- Main drug which causes sialorrhoea is clozapine (an atypical anti-psychotic drug)

110. **Ans. (b) Cardiac defects** *(Ref: KDT 8th/e p477)*
Lithium, if taken during pregnancy, can cause Ebstein's anomaly in the fetus, which is a congenital heart disease presenting as tricuspid atresia.
- Lithium is the drug of choice for prophylaxis of bipolar disorder. For acute mania, usually a sedatives like antipsychotics or benzodiazepines need to be added because the action of lithium takes minimum one week to manifest.
  - Lithium has narrow therapeutic index and therefore therapeutic drug monitoring is done for dose adjustment.
  - Electrolyte disturbances particularly sodium depletion can precipitate lithium toxicity.
  - It cause benign and reversible depression of T wave on ECG.

111. **Ans. (a) Sialorrhea**
(Ref: Katzung 13th/e p525, Harrison 20th/e p3264)
- Escitalopram is an SSRI used for depression
  - Nausea, vomiting
  - Diarrhea
  - Headache
  - Insomnia
  - Sexual dysfunction (anorgasmia, delayed ejaculation)

112. **Ans. (a) Venlafaxine** *(Ref: KDT 8th/e p489)*
- All antidepressants including SSRIs and SNRIs can result in discontinuation syndrome. The symptoms of withdrawal include dizziness, headache, nervousness, nausea and insomnia.
- This withdrawal is more intense with paroxetine and venlafaxine because these are relatively short acting.

113. **Ans. (a) Inhibits alpha-adrenergic, H1, and some types of serotonin receptors** *(Ref: KDT 8/e p490)*

114. **Ans. (c) Thioxanthine**
(Ref: KDT 8/e p470; Kaplan and Saddock 1297)

115. **Ans. (b) SSRI** *(Ref: KDT's 8/e p492)*

116. **Ans. (c) IV NaHCO$_3$**
(Ref: Harrison's 19/e p2716, KDT's 8th/e p487)

117. **Ans. (a) Lithium** *(Ref: Harrison 19/e p2718)*
Both lamotrigine and lithium can reduce the depressive phase of bipolar disorder. However, lithium consistently shows the decreased risk of suicides whereas lamotrigine is found to be effective in some studies and not in others. Other antiepileptic drugs may actually increase the risk of depressive episodes.

118. **Ans. (b) Haloperidol** *(Ref: Niraj Ahuja 7/e p79)*
- Benzodiazepine plus lithium is drug of choice for acute mania. However both of them are avoided in pregnancy because of teratogenic effects.
- Antipsychotics are preferred drugs for mania in pregnancy. Atypical antipsychotics like olanzapine are preferred over typical antipsychotics like haloperidol.
- As olanzapine is not in the options, next best answer to choose is haloperidol

119. **Ans. (b) At least 12 months of symptom remission**
(Ref: Clinical Practice Guidelines by APA)
American Psychiatry Association recommendations for duration of antipsychotic treatment:
- For first episode, medication discontinuation can be done (after at least 1 year of symptom remission or optimal response while taking medication) with close follow-up and with a plan to reinstitute antipsychotic treatment on symptom recurrence.
- Indefinite maintenance antipsychotic medication is recommended for patients who have had multiple prior episodes or two episodes within 5 years.

120. **Ans. (b) NaHCO$_3$** *(Ref: Harrison 19/e p172)*
- The clinical features and ECG findings typically suggest a diagnosis of tricyclic antidepressant (TCA) poisoning.
- Antidote for TCA poisoning is sodium bicarbonate
- Hemodialysis is not effective is TCA poisoning

121. **Ans. (b) Promethazine** *(Ref: KDT 8/e p471)*
The given history suggests the presence of acute muscular dystonia induced by haloperidol. Anticholinergics like benzhexol are drug of choice for this condition. However,

first generation antihistaminics like promethazine and hydroxyzine can also be used for the same.

122. Ans. (c) Risperidone *(Ref: Katzung 12th/e p484)*
The history of the patient suggests the presence of tic disorder.

> **Treatment of Tic Disorder:**
> - Dopamine depleter: Tetrabenazine (drug of choice)
> - Dopamine receptor blockers: Haloperidol, Fluphenazine, Pimozide
> - Atypical antipsychotics: Aripiprazole, Risperidone
> - Alpha 2 agonists: Clonidine, Guanafacine
> - Clonazepam
> - Carbamazepine
> - Botulinum toxin (Local injection)

123. Ans. (a) 2 mEq/L *(Ref: KDT 8/e p476, Katzung 12th/e p517)*

Important serum levels of lithium

For bipolar disorder	0.5–0.8 mEq/L
For acute mania	0.8–1.2 mEq/L
Lithium toxicity	> 2 mEq/L
Dialysis done if level	> 4 mEq/L

124. Ans. (b) Acute dystonia *(Ref: Harrison 18th/e p3544)*
Acute muscular dystonia is the earliest appearing extrapyramidal symptom caused by antipsychotic drugs like haloperidol.

125. Ans. (a) M_3 muscarinic receptors *(Ref: KDT 8/e p486)*
Anticholinergic adverse effects of TCAs include dry mouth, constipation, blurring of vision, urinary retention, etc.

126. Ans. (b) Fluoxetine *(Ref: Goodman and Gilman 12/e p411)*
- All antidepressants including SSRIs and SNRIs can result in discontinuation syndrome. The symptoms of withdrawal include dizziness, headache, nervousness, nausea and insomnia.
- This withdrawal is more intense with paroxetine and venlafaxine because these are relatively short acting.
- This is unlikely with fluoxetine as it produces a very long acting metabolite.

127. Ans. (c) SSRI *(Ref: Katzung 12th ed. Pg 533)*
Premenstrual syndrome (PMS) is a collection of emotional symptoms, with or without physical symptoms, related to a woman's menstrual cycle.

> - SSRIs can be used to treat severe PMS. Fluoxetine and sertraline have been approved for this indication. Treating for 2 weeks out of a month in luteal phase may be as effective as continuous treatment. The rapid effects of SSRIs in PMS may be associated with rapid increases in pregnenolone levels.
> - Hormonal contraception is commonly used as combined oral contraceptive pills and the contraceptive patch. This class of medication may cause PMS-related symptoms in some women, and may reduce physical symptoms in other women. They do not relieve emotional symptoms. Progesterone support has been used for many years but evidence of its efficacy is inadequate.

128. Ans. (a) Fluphenazine
(Ref: Goodman Gilman 12th ed/e p424-426; KDT 8/e p467)
- The common problem of medication nonadherence among schizophrenia patients has led to the development of long-acting injectable (LAI) antipsychotic medications, often referred to as depot antipsychotics.
- There are currently four available LAI forms

> - Fluphenazine decanoate
> - Haloperidol decanoate
> - Risperidone-impregnated microspheres
> - Paliperidone palmitate.

129. Ans. (b) Blood level below 350 mg/mL should be maintained to avoid agranulocytosis *(Ref: Drug Facts and Comparisons 2006/1205-1206, Goodman Gilman 12th/427,432)*
High plasma concentration of Clozapine increases the risk of seizures (not agranulocytosis). However, usual plasma concentration required in many persons is 300-600 ng/ml.
- Clozapine is an atypical antipsychotic drug that has high potency to block $5HT_2$ receptors as compared to D_2 receptors. It has high potency to block D_2 as compared to D_1 receptors.
- It should not be used with Carbamazepine due to two reasons:
  - Carbamazepine induces its metabolism and thus decreases the plasma concentration.
  - Carbamazepine has bone marrow suppressant action and can add to agranulocytosis caused by Clozapine.
- Clozapine should be started at low doses (12.5 mg) and gradually dose should be increased. Baseline WBC counts should be measured and then weekly counts should be done atleast for first 6 months. When WBC count becomes less than 3000/mm³ or absolute neutrophil count becomes less than 1500/mm³, Clozapine should be discontinued. After discontinuation, weekly WBC counts should be measured for additional 4 weeks.
- Patients discontinued for WBC count less than 2000/mm³ or absolute neutrophil count below 1000/mm³ should not be started on Clozapine again.

130. Ans. (a) Doxepin *(Ref: Katzung 11/e p519)*
- Serotonin and dopaminergic receptor blocking drugs are used for treatment of psychosis. Amisulpiride, sertindole and zotepine are antipsychotic drugs acting by this mechanism. On the other hand, doxepin is an antidepressant and do not block serotonin and dopaminergic receptors, rather it can inhibit the reuptake of serotonin and noradrenaline. It also has strong antihistaminic and anticholinergic property.

131. Ans. (a) Clozapine
(Ref: Goodman and Gilman 12th/440-441; KDT 8/e p 468)

132. Ans. (d) Tianeptin *(Ref: KDT 8/e p481)*
- Tianeptin enhances the reuptake of serotonin rather than inhibiting it whereas the other drugs mentioned in the options inhibit the reuptake of serotonin and norepinephrine.

133. Ans. (a) Premature ejaculation
(Ref: Goodman and Gilman 12th/e p410-411)

- SSRIs can result in adverse effects like insomnia, anxiety, irritability and decreased libido due to excessive stimulation of brain 5-HT$_2$ receptors.
- Excessive activity at spinal 5-HT$_2$ receptors causes sexual side effects including erectile dysfunction, anorgasmia and ejaculatory delay, these are more prominent with paroxetine.
- Stimulation of 5-HT$_3$ receptors in the CNS and periphery contributes to GI effects which are usually limited to nausea but can also result in diarrhea and emesis.
- Unlike other SSRIs, paroxetine is associated with an increased risk of congenital cardiac malformations.

134. **Ans. (d) Fluoxetine** *(Ref: Goodman and Gilman 12th/e p444-445)*
   - Fluoxetine is an anti-depressant drug of SSRI category whereas lithium, valproate and carbamazepine are used for mania and bipolar disorder as mood stabilizers.

135. **Ans. (d) Cause benign and reversible depression of T wave on ECG** *(Ref: Katzung 10/e p472)*

   - Lithium is the drug of choice for prophylaxis of bipolar disorder. For acute mania, usually a sedative agent like lorazepam has to be added because the action of lithium takes minimum one week to manifest.
   - Lithium has narrow therapeutic index and therefore therapeutic drug monitoring is done for dose adjustment.
   - Electrolyte disturbances particularly sodium depletion can precipitate lithium toxicity.
   - It cause benign and reversible depression of T wave on ECG.

136. **Ans. (a) 5-HT** *(Ref: Katzung 10/e p475; KDT 8/e p483)*
   Monoamines like serotonin and nor-adrenaline are deficient in depressive patients, therefore reuptake inhibitors of these monoamines are used for treatment of depression.

137. **Ans. (b) MDP** *(Ref: Katzung 10/e p470; KDT 8/e p447)*

138. **Ans. (c) Schizophrenia**
   (Ref: Katzung 10/e p465; KDT 8/e p472, 473)

139. **Ans. (c) Anti-psychotic drugs**
   (Ref: Katzung 10/e p467; KDT 8/e p471)
   Atypical antipsychotic drugs are known to cause hyperglycemia, hyperlipidemia, insulin resistance and weight gain. Minimum risk of these metabolic adverse effects is with ziprasidone.

140. **Ans. (d) Chlorpromazine** *(Ref: CMDT-2010/506)*
   Chlorpromazine is most commonly used drug for intractable hiccups.
   Other drugs that can be used are:
   - Anticonvulsants (Phenytoin, carbamazepine)
   - Benzodiazepines (Lorazepam, diazepam)
   - Metoclopramide
   - Baclofen
   - Gabapentin

141. **Ans. (c) Bromocriptine** *(Ref: KDT 8/e p191)*
   Bromocriptine is used for treatment of hyperprolactenemia (do not cause it).

142. **Ans. (a) Muscarinic ACh receptors** *(Ref: Katzung 10/e p468)*

143. **Ans. (a) Acute panic attack** *(Ref: KDT 8/e p489)*
   - SSRIs are drug of choice for depression, sustained treatments of panic disorder and generalized anxiety disorder, obsessive compulsive disorder, post-traumatic stress disorder, social and other phobias and bulimia.
   - In acute panic attacks and for acute treatment of generalized anxiety disorder, benzodiazepines are preferred.

144. **Ans. (d) 1.0** *(Ref: KDT 8/e p476)*
   Therapeutic plasma concentration of lithium for acute therapy is 0.8-1.2 mEq/L whereas for prophylaxis, its concentration should be 0.5-0.8 mEq/L.

145. **Ans. (d) Lamotrigine** *(Ref: KDT 8/e p478)*
   Lamotrigine is specifically indicated for depressive phase of bipolar disorder.

146. **Ans. (b) Valproate** *(Ref: KDT 8/e p478)*

147. **Ans. (c) Haloperidol** *(Ref: KDT 6/e p471)*
   - Akathisia is a side effect of antipsychotic drugs like haloperidol: It is treated with:

   - Central anticholinergics like Trihexyphenidyl
   - First generation antihistaminics like promethazine
   - Propranolol
   - Diazepam

148. **Ans. (a) Clozapine** *(Ref: KDT 8/e p468)*

149. **Ans. (d) Haloperidol** *(Ref: KDT 8/e p467, 468)*

150. **Ans. (d) Weight loss** *(Ref: KDT 8/e p468)*
   Clozapine and other atypical antipsychotics result in wieght gain.

151. **Ans. (d) All of the above** *(Ref: KDT 8/e p482)*
   Cheese, beer, wine, pickled meat, fish and yeast extract are rich in sympathomimetic amines (e.g., tyramine). In MAO inhibited patients, these indirectly acting sympathomimetic amines are not degraded in the intestinal wall and liver and reach into systemic circulation where they cause release of large amounts of norepinephrine from adrenergic nerve endings, thus precipitating hyperensive crisis. It is known as cheese reaction.

152. **Ans. (c) Clozapine** *(Ref: KDT 8/e p468)*
   Clozapine is an atypical neuroleptic with least extrapyramidal side effects among all antipsychotics.

153. **Ans. (b) Does not interfere with GABAergic transmission** *(Ref: KDT 8/e p495)*

154. **Ans. (d) Flupenthixol** *(Ref: KDT 8/e p468)*
   - Flupenthixol is sometime used for treatment of depression, whereas other drugs mentioned in question can cause depression.

155. **Ans. (a) Pemoline** *(Ref: KDT 5th/471)*
   Pemoline is used for ADHD whereas other drugs mentioned are antipsychotics.

156. **Ans. (c) Weight loss.** *(Ref: KDT 8/e p486, 487)*
   'Weight gain (not weight loss) in seen with TCAs.

157. **Ans. (a) Tyramine** *(Ref: KDT 8/e p482)*

158. **Ans. (b) Thioridazine** *(Ref: KDT 8/e p467)*

159. **Ans. (b) Lithium** *(Ref: KDT 8/e p476)*

160. **Ans. (c) No individual variation in the rate of excretion**
   (Ref: KDT 8/e p476-477)

161. Ans. (a) Antipsychotics *(Ref: KDT 8/e p471)*
162. Ans. (a) Clozapine *(Ref: KDT 8/e p464)*
163. Ans. (c) Dantrolene *(Ref: KDT 8/e p472)*
164. Ans. (c) Both *(Ref: KDT 8/e p468)*
165. Ans. (c) Haloperidol *(Ref: KDT 8/e p467, 471)*
166. Ans. (c) Venlafaxine *(Ref: KDT 8/e p489)*
167. Ans. (c) 24 hours *(Ref: Katzung 11/e p500)*
168. Ans. (b) 0.8-1.2 *(Ref: KDT 8/e p476)*
169. Ans. (c) Tranylcypromine *(Ref: KDT 8/e p482)*
170. Ans. (b) Benzhexol *(Ref: KDT 8/e p471)*
171. Ans. (b) Inceased by decreased serum sodium levels
(Ref: KDT 8/e p477)
172. Ans. (a) Imipramine *(Ref: KDT 8/e p486)*
173. Ans. (b) Fluoxetine *(Ref: KDT 8/e p488)*
174. Ans. (a) Lithium *(Ref: KDT 8/e p476)*
175. Ans. (b) Amitriptyline *(Ref: KDT 8/e p482)*
176. Ans. (c) Fluoxetine *(Ref: KDT 8/e p464)*
177. Ans. (a) Phenothiazines *(Ref: KDT 8/e p466)*
178. Ans. (a) Osteoporosis *(Ref: KDT 8/e p466)*
179. Ans. (d) Amoxapine *(Ref: KDT 8/e p481)*
180. Ans. (d) Loxapine *(Ref: KDT 8/e p464)*
181. Ans. (a) Chlorpromazine *(Ref: Katzung 11/e p482)*
182. Ans. (d) Tardive dyskinesia *(Ref: KDT 8/e p472)*
183. Ans. (c) MAO inhibitors *(Ref: KDT 8/e p482)*
184. Ans. (d) Quetiapine *(Ref: KDT 8/e p469)*
All other drugs are typical antipsychotics except quetiapine and release prolactin by blocking hypothalamic dopamine receptors.
185. Ans. (d) Diphenyl butyl piperidine
(Ref: Goodman and Gilman 11/e p467)
186. Ans. (a) Aripriprazole *(Ref: KDT 8/e p469)*
187. Ans. (d) Maprotiline *(Ref: KDT 8/e p482)*
Maprotiline is a tricyclic antidepressant.
188. Ans. (c) Antimuscarinic drugs reduces its severity
(Ref: Principles of Pharmacology by KK Sharma and HL Sharma 1st/466; KDT 8/e p472)

- **Tardive dyskinesia** occurs due to increased sensitivity of dopaminergic receptors (due to chronic presence of D_2 antagonists i.e. antipsychotics). Due to increased dopaminergic activity, cholinergic activity decreases that ultimately results in decreased release of GABA from striatal neurons.
- Thus dopaminergic drugs like levo-dopa and anticholinergic drugs like trihexyphenydil will worsen the symptoms.
- A reduction in dose of the dopamine receptor blocker will also worsen the dyskinesia due to same reason, while an increase in dose may suppress it.
- The management of Tardive dyskinesia may involve the following strategies:
  - To decrease dopaminergic activity by increasing the dose of anti-psychotic but it is not advisable as these drugs themselves have resulted in supersensitivity of receptors
  - To increase cholinergic activity by choline or lecithin but the doses required are very high and success rate is limited (only 20%)
  - To increase the GABA activity by diazepam along with neurolept holiday (i.e. stopping anti-psychotic and anticholinergic medications).

189. Ans. (a) Clozapine *(Ref: KDT 8/e p468)*
190. Ans. (d) Hypercalcemia *(Ref: KDT 8/e p476)*
191. Ans. (c) Clozapine *(Ref: KDT 8/e p468)*
192. Ans. (a) Bupropion *(Ref: Katzung 11/e p562; KDT 8/e p492)*
193. Ans. (a) Desmopressin *(Ref: KDT 8/e p643)*
194. Ans. (a) Intravenous dantrolene *(Ref: Harrison 18th/e p147)*
The current treatment of choice for malignant hyperthermia is the intravenous administration of dantrolene.
Other important measures are:
- Discontinuation of triggering agents
- Supportive therapy directed at correcting hyperthermia, acidosis, and organ dysfunction.

195. Ans. (b) Tardive dyskinesia *(Ref: KDT 8/e p472)*
196. Ans. (a) Anxiolytic *(Ref: KDT 8/e p187)*
197. Ans. (d) 5 HT_{2C} *(Ref: Goodman Gilman 12/e p435)*
- Antipsychotics cause weight gain due to their antagonistic action on H_1 and $5HT_{2C}$ receptors.

198. Ans. (a) Amiloride *(Ref: KDT 8/e p644)*
199. Ans. (d) Amitriptyline *(Ref: KDT 8/e p481)*
200. Ans. (b) Amoxapine *(Ref: KDT 8/e p491)*
201. Ans. (a) Sertraline *(Ref: KDT 8/e p489, 492)*
202. Ans. (d) Fluphenazine *(Ref: KDT 8/e p4467)*
203. Ans. (c) Lithium *(Ref: KDT 8/e p477)*
204. Ans. (b) Acute dystonia *(Ref: KDT 8/e p471)*
205. Ans. (c) Promethazine *(Ref: KDT 8/e p471)*
206. Ans. (a) Lithium *(Ref: KDT 8/e p477)*
207. Ans. (a) Metoclopramide *(Ref: KDT 8/e p714)*
208. Ans. (d) Chlorpromazine *(Ref: KDT 8/e p481)*
209. Ans. (d) Fluoxetine *(Ref: KDT 8/e p488)*
210. Ans. (d) Haloperidol *(Ref: KDT 8/e p493)*
211. Ans. (a) Olanzapine *(Ref: KDT 8/e p473)*
212. Ans. (b) Lithium *(Ref: KDT 8/e p437-478)*
213. Ans. (a) Morphine *(Ref: KDT 8th/e p502)*
Morphine is used for treatment of severe pain.
- It is contraindicated in biliary colic. It increases the risk of rupture of bile duct by causing spasm of sphincter of Oddi.
- Diclofenac, Nefopam and Etoricoxib are NSAIDs and can be used for treatment of pain in biliary colic.

214. Ans. (a) Serotonin and noradrenaline reuptake inhibition
(Ref: KDT 8th/e p504)
- Tramadol is an atypical opioid which relieves pain by opioid as well as additional mechanisms.
- Like all other opioids, It is μ opioid receptor agonist and relieves pain.
- Unlike other opioids, it inhibits reuptake of NA and 5-HT and thus activates mono-aminergic spinal inhibition of pain (descending inhibitory pathway).
- Its analgesic action is only partially reversed by the opioid antagonist naloxone.

215. Ans. (b) Biliary colic *(Ref: KDT 8th/e p502)*
- Opioids **increase intrabiliary pressure** by constricting biliary smooth muscle. Therefore contraindicated in biliary colic.

216. **Ans. (d) Chlordiazepoxide**
 (Ref: KDT 8/e p421; From ROAMS 13/e p954)

217. **Ans. (c) Alcohol craving** *(Ref: KDT 8/e p421)*

218. **Ans. (a) Methadone** *(Ref: KDT 8/e p504)*

219. **Ans. (a) Diacetyl morphine** *(Ref: KDT 8/e p503)*

220. **Ans. (d) Phencyclidine** *(Ref: Reddy's 23rd/e)*

221. **Ans. (b) Naloxone** *(Ref: KDT 7/e p483)*
 When opioids are given, we must have opioid antagonist ready to manage opioid poisoning if any. Naloxone is an opioid antagonist used for this purpose.

222. **Ans. (a) Pentazocine** *(Ref: KDT 7/e p480)*
 The opioids which are agonist at kappa and antagonist at mu receptors are called agonist-antagonists. These include:

223. **Ans. (c) Ethylene glycol poisoning** *(Ref: Harrison 19/e p319)*
 Symptoms of alcohol overdose along with oxalate crystalluria points towards ethylene glycol poisoning. It is confirmed because the patient is being treated with antidotes like ethanol and fomepizol (4 methyl pyrazole).

224. **Ans. (b) Flumazenil** *(Ref: KDT 8/e p421)*
 Flumazenil is a benzodiazepine antagonist. It has no role in alcohol detoxification.

225. **Ans. (a) Disulfiram** *(Ref: KDT 8/e p422)*
 The aim of treatment in alcohol dependence is to prevent withdrawl symptoms first and to avoid relapse thereafter.

 - Drugs to reduce craving are:
   - N- Naltrexone
   - O- Ondansetron
   - T- Topiramate
   - A- Acamprosate
 - Disulfiram is used in psychological dependent persons who are motivated to quit alcohol. It is contraindicated in physically dependent persons.

226. **Ans. (d) The onset of analgesia is 30-60 minutes after parenteral administration and 1-2 hours after oral administration** *(Ref: Goodman and Gilman 12th/e p506-507)*

 Methadone
 - The onset of analgesia occurs 10-20 minutes after parenteral administration of methadone and 30-60 minutes after oral administration.
 - Methadone is a long-acting µ opioid receptor agonist with pharmacological properties qualitatively similar to those of morphine.
 - It is well absorbed from the GI tract and can be detected in plasma within 30 minutes of oral ingestion.
 - Primary uses are relief of chronic pain and in maintenance therapy of opioid addiction.

227. **Ans. (b) Kappa** *(Ref: KDT 8/e p507)*
 Dysphoria and psychomimetics effects are caused by kappa receptors.

228. **Ans. (a) Diazepam** *(Ref: CMDT 2014/939; KDT 8/e p421)*
 Treatment with anticonvulsants is generally not required for alcohol withdrawal seizures, since they are self limited. Benzodiazepines (diazepam or lorazepam) are effective and safe for preventing further seizures.

229. **Ans. (b) Fomepizole acts by inhibiting aldehyde dehydrogenase** *(Ref: Katzung 12/e p398: KDT 8/e p423)*
 Fomepizole inhibits alcohol dehydrogenase and not aldehyde dehydrogenase
 - Serum methanol concentration above 20 mg/dL is an indication to start treatment and above 50 mg/dL is for hemodialysis.
 - Metabolic product formaldehyde and formic acid is responsible for blindness and high anion gap metabolic acidosis
 - Three specific modalities of treatment are:
   - Inhibit formation of toxic metabolites by inhibiting alcohol dehydrogenase by fomepizole or ethanol
   - Hemodialysis
   - Alkalinization to counter metabolic acidosis.

230. **Ans. (b) IV naloxone** *(Ref: Kaplan & Sadock's Comprehensive Textbook of Psychiatry 9th/e p1375-76, 1384; KDT p511-512)*
 The decreased bowel sounds (constipation), respiratory depression, pin point pupil and history of heroin addiction strongly points toward the diagnosis of acute opioid poisoning. The drug of choice for acute opioid poisoning is intravenous naloxone.

231. **Ans. (a) Pethidine**
 (Ref: Goodman Gilman 12th/499, 504; KDT 8/e p503)
 - Pethidine (meperidine) is metabolized to form norpethidine which is excreted by kidneys. It has long half life (15-20 hours) as compared to pethidine (3 hours). Accumulation of this metabolite resulting in excitatory syndrome including hallucinations, tremors, muscle twitches, dilated pupils, hyperactive reflexes and convulsions. Renal failure increases the likelihood of toxicity and thus pethidine should be avoided.
 - Morphine produces morphine-6-glucuronide which can accumulate in renal failure. The actions of this metabolite are similar to morphine. In patients with renal failure morphine has more potency and longer duration of action due to accumulation of morphine-6-glucuronide and thus need to be given in lower doses

232. **Ans. (b) Craving for opioids**
 (Ref: Goodman and Gilman 12th/e p661)
 - Naltrexone has no action in the absence of agonists but promptly reverses the opioid effects when administered i.v.
 - It can reverse all effects of opioids like sedation, analgesia, constipation, respiratory depression and miosis etc but it do not reduce craving.

233. **Ans. (b) Lacrimation** *(Ref: Katzung 10/e p502; KDT 8/e p501)*
 Opioid withdrawal is characterized by yawning, rhinorrhea and lacrimation along with diarrhea.

234. **Ans. (c) Chlordiazepoxide** *(Ref: Katzung 10/e p370)*
 Long acting benzodiazepines like diazepam and chlordiazepoxide are drug of choice for alcohol withdrawal.

235. **Ans. (a) Naltrexone** *(Ref: Katzung 10/e p371; KDT 8/e p481)*

236. **Ans. (a) Formaldehyde and formic acid**
 (Ref: Katzung 11/e p1024; KDT 8/e p422)
 Methyl alcohol (methanol) is metabolized to formaldehyde by alcohol dehydrogenase and then to formic acid by aldehyde dehydrogenase. These compounds are responsible for the toxicity. Formic acid can lead to coma and blindness also. Therefore, inhibitor of alcohol dehydrogenase, **Fomepizole** is used for treatment of methanol overdose.

Central Nervous System

237. **Ans. (b) Naloxone** (Ref: Katzung 11/e p395; KDT 8/e p 421)
Naloxone is an i.v. opioid antagonist used for acute opioid poisoning. It has no role in alcoholism.

238. **Ans. (a) Rhinorrhea and lacrimation** (Ref: KDT 8/e p501)
- Withdrawal symptoms are opposite of the acute effect of drug. For opioids, these include lacrimation, rhinorrhea, lacrimation, yawning, piloerection, diarrhea, nausea, coughing, mydriasis, sweating and twitching of muscles.

239. **Ans. (a) Morphine** (Ref: Katzung 10/e p499, KDT 8/e p506)
Opioids like morphine can be used to treat severe pain associated with terminal cancers.

240. **Ans. (a) Parenterally administered** (Ref: KDT 8/e p512)

- Naltrexone is chemically related to naloxone and is a pure opioid antagonist. It is more potent than Naloxone.
- It differs from Naloxone in being orally active and having a long duration of action (1-2 days) which is used to prevent relapse of heapy drinking.
- Side effects are nausea and headache; high doses can cause hepatotoxicity.

241. **Ans. (b) Kappa** (Ref: KDT 8/e p507)

242. **Ans. (c) Naloxone** (Ref: KDT 8/e p501)

243. **Ans. (a) Heroin** (Ref: KDT 8/e p512, 502)
Naltrexone is an orally effective opioid antagonist. It is useful for the maintenance of the patient of opioid poisoning once it has been treated with naloxone. Heroin is an opioid, whose poisoning can be treated by naloxone and naltrexone.

244. **Ans. (a) Amoxicillin** (Ref: KDT 8/e p422, 778, 895)

245. **Ans. (b) Children are more susceptible**
(Ref: Goodman & Gillman's Pharmacology 10/e p583)

Opioid induced seizures

- In animals high dose of morphine and related opioids can produce convulsions.
- Morphine excites hippocampal pyramidal cells
- Selective δ-agonists produce similar effect.
- These action may contribute to seizures that are produced by some agents at doses only moderately higher than those required for analgesia, esp. in children. However with most opioids seizures occur only at doses far in excess of therapeutic dose.
- Seizures are not seen when potent μ-agonists are used.
- Naloxone is potent drug for treatment of opioid poisoning.
- Anticovulsants (like diazepam) are not always effective in supressing opioid induced seizures.
- So the best answer is (b)

246. **Ans. (b) Inhibits oxidation of alcohol** (Ref: KDT 8/e p385)
Antabuse (disulfiram) inhibits the enzyme aldehyde dehydrogenase, which causes oxidation of aldehyde.

247. **Ans. (d) Maintenance therapy of alcohol abstinence**
(Ref: KDT 8/e p422)

248. **Ans. (b) Pentazocine** (Ref: KDT 8/e p510)

249. **Ans. (c) Methadone** (Ref: KDT 8/e p506)

250. **Ans. (d) Mydriasis** (Ref: KDT 8/e p507)

251. **Ans. (a) Alcohol abstinence** (Ref: KDT 8/e p421)

252. **Ans. (a) Heroin** (Ref: KDT 8/e p503)

253. **Ans. (a) It inhibit alcohol dehydrogenase**
(Ref: KDT 8/e p423)

254. **Ans. (b) Epinephrine** (Ref: KDT 8/e p513)

255. **Ans. (d) All of the above** (Ref: KDT 8/e p418)

256. **Ans. (b) Nalorphine** (Ref: KDT 8/e p509)

257. **Ans. (d) All of the above** (Ref: KDT 8/e p513)

258. **Ans. (b) Fomepizole** (Ref: KDT 8/e p423)

259. **Ans. (c) Fentanyl** (Ref: KDT 8th/503)
In analgesic doses, fentanyl produces little cardiovascular effects. It has less propensity to release histamine.

260. **Ans. (d) Opioid analgesic** (Ref: KDT 8/e p504)

261. **Ans. (c) Codeine** (Ref: KDT 8/e p502)

262. **Ans. (d) Is an opioid agonist** (Ref: KDT 8/e p512)

263. **Ans. (d) Causes no constipation** (Ref: KDT 8/e p239, 503)

264. **Ans. (b) Fentanyl** (Ref: KDT 8/e p503)

265. **Ans. (d) All of the above** (Ref: KDT 8/e p399, 460, 546)

266. **Ans. (b) Dorsal horn** (Ref: KDT 8/e p498)

267. **Ans. (c) Papaver somniferum** (Ref: KDT 8/e p497)

268. **Ans. (b) Sufentanil** (Ref: Goodman Gilman 11/e p571)

269. **Ans. (d) Sublingual** (Ref: KDT 8/e p458, KK Sharma 2nd/e p500)

270. **Ans. (c) Synthetic derivatives** (Ref: Principles of Pharmacology by HL Sharma and KK Sharma, 1st/509; KDT 8/e p497)
Term Opiate means from 'opium' whereas opioid means opium like analgesics.

271. **Ans. (d) Morphine** (Ref: Principles of Pharmacology by HL Sharma and KK Sharma 1st/509; KDT 8/e p497)

272. **Ans. (c) 2.0 mEq/L** (Ref: KDT 8/e p476)

273. **Ans. (b) Fentanyl** (Ref: KDT 8/e p504)

274. **Ans. (c) Constipation** (Ref: KDT 8/e p500)

275. **Ans. (a) Tramadol** (Ref: KDT 8/e p504)
- Tramadol inhibits re-uptake of NA and 5-HT and thus activates monoaminergic spinal inhibition of pain.

276. **Ans. (d) Nalmefene** (Ref: KDT 8/e p512)

277. **Ans. (d) It is longer acting and causes milder withdrawal symptoms** (Ref: KDT 8/e p504)

278. **Ans. (c) Methyl alcohol** (Ref: KDT 8/e p423)

279. **Ans. (d) Left ventricular failure** (Ref: KDT 8/e p499)

280. **Ans. (c) Flumazenil** (Ref: KDT 9/e p421, 435)

281. **Ans. (c) Pentazocine** (Ref: KDT 8/e p510)

282. **Ans. (d) Dilated pupils** (Ref: KDT 8/e p507)

283. **Ans. (d) Aldehyde dehydrogenase** (Ref: KDT 8/e p421)

284. **Ans. (d) Pentazocine** (Ref: KDT 8/e p510)

285. **Ans. (a) Lithium** (Ref: KDT 8/e p477)

286. **Ans. (b) Diphenoxylate** (Ref: KDT 8/e p733)

287. **Ans. (a) Buspirone** (Ref: KDT's 8/e p187)

Anaesthesia

CHAPTER 8

LOCAL ANAESTHETICS

These drugs act by blocking the conduction of nerve impulse along the axon. Small diameter fibres (Types B and C) are more sensitive to blockade than large diameter fibres (Type A) with similar diameter, myelinated fibres are blocked first than unmyelinated fibres. Thus, the **order of blockade of fibres is B, C, Aδ and then Aβ and Aγ and Aα at last. Autonomic fibres are blocked first, then sensory and finally motor** are blocked at last. *Order of recovery is in the reverse order.*

Local anaesthetics (LAs) can be **classified into amide and ester types**. Amides are usually long acting and chances of allergic reactions are less whereas esters are short acting (due to metabolism by esterases present in the plasma). **Ester LAs** can cause allergic reactions and also **antagonize** the action of **sulfonamides** due to degradation of PABA.

Amide class	Ester class
• Lignocaine	• Cocaine
• Prilocaine	• Procaine
• Bupivacaine	• Chlorprocaine (Shortest acting)
• Dibucaine (Longest acting)	• Tetracaine (Amethocaine)
• Mepivacaine	• Benzocaine
• Etidocaine	
• Ropivacaine	

Mechanism of Action

All LAs are **weak bases**. These drugs act by penetrating the axonal membrane (in unionized form) and **blocking the voltage gated sodium channels from within (in ionized form)**. **Sodium bicarbonate speeds the onset of action** of LAs by increasing the unionized form (weak bases are unionized in the alkaline medium) that can penetrate the axonal membrane. Vasoconstrictors like **adrenaline** can **prolong the duration of action and decrease the systemic toxicity**. Alternative vasoconstrictor **felypressin** (synthetic vasopressin) can also be used with LAs in order to avoid cardiovascular complications due to adrenaline.

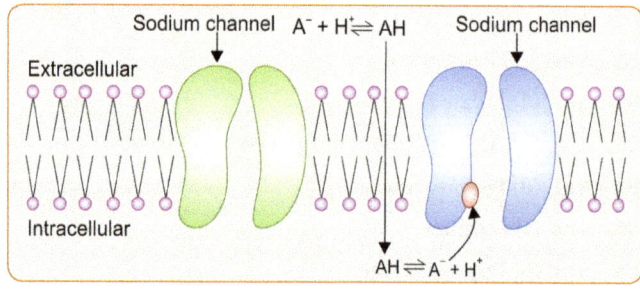

FIG. 8.1: Mechanism of action of local anaesthetics

Key Points

Lignocaine with adrenaline SHOULD NOT be used for:
- Areas with **end arteries**, e.g. for ring block of fingers, toes, penis, pinna (absolute contraindication)
- When an inhalational agent especially **halothane** which sensitizes myocardium to adrenaline is used.
- **Myocardial ischemic** patients
- **Hyperthyroid** patient
- Severe **hypertensives**
- Intravenous regional anaesthesia *hesia (**Bier's block**)

IMPORTANT POINTS

- **Small** diameter axons are **more susceptible** to block than large diameter fibres.
- **Myelinated fibres are more sensitive than non-myelinated.**
- **Sequence of block is type Aγ > Aδ > Aα = Aβ > B > C.**
- In functional terms: **Autonomic > sensory > motor**.
- Among sensory fibres sequence of block is *pain > temperature (cold before heat) > touch > deep pressure > proprioception.*
- **All LAs are vasodilators except cocaine** (act as sympathomimetic due to inhibition of noradrenaline reuptake) which is a vasoconstrictor. Therefore all LAs decrease BP except cocaine (increases).
- **Cocaine** should **NEVER** be given by **intravenous route** or with adrenaline.
- **Cocaine** is the only ester which is *not* metabolized by pseudocholinesterase. It is metabolized in the liver.
- **Procaine** is the **local anaesthetic of choice** in *malignant hyperthermia*.
- **Chlorprocaine** is the **shortest acting** local anaesthetic and is **contraindicated in spinal anaesthesia** (It may cause paraplegia due to the presence of sodium metabisulphite as preservative, which is neurotoxic).
- **All LAs** if absorbed in systemic circulation can cause **CNS toxicity** that manifests as excitation followed by depression. Initial excitation is due to inhibition of inhibitory neurons. Thus LAs may lead to **seizures followed by coma** at high doses.
- **Dibucaine** is the most potent, longest acting and most toxic LA whereas chlorprocaine is the shortest acting LA.
- **Lignocaine is the most commonly used LA** and is **the drug of choice for ventricular tachycardia**. It **can precipitate malignant hyperthermia** due to release of calcium. Dose is limited to 7 mg/kg with adrenaline or 4 mg/kg without adrenaline.

- **Bupivacaine is the best drug for regional block** but it is also the **most cardiotoxic LA**. Due to cardiotoxic effect, it **should not be used for Bier's block**. It is more potent and longer acting than lignocaine. Addition of adrenaline does not significantly increase the duration of action of this drug. For spinal anaesthesia, 0.5% solution is made hyperbaric with 8.25% dextrose in water. Its *maximum dose is 2 mg/kg*. Most common ECG changes in bupivacaine toxicity are slow idioventricular rhythm with broad QRS complex. **Bretylium** is the drug of choice for bupivacaine induced ventricular tachycardia.
- Ropivacaine is less cardiotoxic congener of bupivacaine.
- **Prilocaine** produces a metabolite "**O-toluidine**" which is an oxidizing agent. Latter can oxidize hemoglobin to methemoglobin that can cause **methemoglobinemia**. It is **the most suitable LA for Bier's block**.

  MNEMONIC

LA causing methemoglobinemia
B – Benzocaine
P – Prilocaine (Max)
L – Lignocaine

- **Oxethazaine** (mucaine) can be used to provide symptomatic relief in gastritis (it **remains unionized in the acidic pH of stomach**).

Uses of Local Anaesthetics

These agents can be used for following types of anaesthesia.

1. Surface Anaesthesia

It is the topical application of LA to mucous membranes and abraded skin. Only superficial area is anaesthetized. **Lignocaine** is the commonly used agent for topical anaesthesia of mucous membranes of nose, ear, eye, mouth and pharynx. It is also used during proctoscopy, catheterization and per rectal examinations. Lignocaine is **ineffective on intact skin**. However a mixture of **2.5% prilocaine and 2.5% lignocaine** in 1:1 ratio can anaesthetize even unbroken skin. Combination of these two agents lowers the melting point of individual drugs and helps to form a semi-solid ointment. This mixture is known as **Eutectic mixture**. Oxethazaine (mucaine) can be used to provide symptomatic relief in gastritis (it remains unionized in the acidic pH of stomach).

2. Infiltration Anaesthesia

LA is infiltrated S.C. in the area of operation site for blocking the sensory nerve endings. It is used in minor surgeries like incisions, excisions, suturing, hydrocele etc. **Adrenaline** can be added to the LA to prolong its duration of action and to prevent systemic side effects.

3. Nerve Blocks

LA is injected around the nerve trunks supplying a particular area to anaesthetize all the nerves coming to or leaving that area. It includes blocks of head and neck (stellate ganglion, trigeminal nerve, cervical plexus and phrenic nerve block), upper limbs (brachial plexus and wrist block), thorax and abdomen (intercostal nerve, celiac plexus, lumbar sympathetic chain, ilioinguinal nerve, iliohypogastric nerve, penile and paravertebral block) and lower limbs (psoas compartment and perivascular block). Pneumothorax is the most common complication of brachial plexus block.

4. Intravenous Regional Block (Bier's Block)

Intravenous regional anaesthesia (IVRA) is indicated for any procedure on the arm below the elbow or leg below the knee that will be completed within 40-60 minutes. An intravenous cannula is inserted in a distal vein in the limb scheduled for surgery. The tourniquet is then applied to the upper arm or thigh. The local anaesthetic solution is then slowly injected into the cannula. Analgesia will occur within 3-4 minutes and surgery can then commence. The **pressure in the tourniquet must be maintained at least 50 mm Hg above the patient's systolic blood pressure**. The **drug of choice for IVRA is prilocaine** as it is the least toxic local anaesthetic and has the largest therapeutic index. If prilocaine is not available, lignocaine is an acceptable alternative. It is essential that *plain and not adrenaline-containing solutions are used*. **Bupivacaine should never be employed** as it is too toxic, particularly to the myocardium.

 Key Points

IVRA should be avoided in a patient with sickle cell disease.

5. Spinal Anaesthesia

It is the injection of LA in the subarachnoid space (between pia and arachnoid; also known as intrathecal space) in lumbar spinal cord. **Spinal cord ends at lower border of L_3 vertebrae in children and at lower border of L_1 vertebrae in adults**. Thus, spinal anaesthesia can be performed safely in L_{2-3} intervertebral space in adults and L_{4-5} space in children. Spinal anaesthesia leads to creation of a **zone of differential blockade** in which autonomic fibres are blocked at two segments higher and motor fibres are blocked at two levels lower than sensory blockade. It is due to different sensitivity of various types of nerve fibres.

Structures encountered during lumbar puncture
1. Skin
2. Subcutaneous tissue
3. Supraspinous ligament
4. Interspinous ligament
5. Ligamentum flavum
6. Dura mater
7. Arachnoidmater

Drugs Used for Spinal Anaesthesia

- *Lignocaine* – 5% in 7.5% dextrose (heavy or hyperbaric)
- *Bupivacaine* – 0.5% in 8% dextrose

 Key Points

Maximum dose of lignocaine
- With adrenaline   : 7 mg/kg
- Without adrenaline : 4.5 mg/kg
- For IVRA   : 4 mg/kg

Indications

- Orthopaedic surgery of lower limbs and pelvis.
- Surgery of lower abdomen (all pelvic and perineal surgeries, hernia, hydrocele, appendix, testicular surgeries).
- Gynaecological and obstestrics surgeries (hysterectomy, myomyectomy, cervical surgeries, tubectomy, tuboplasty, caesarean section).

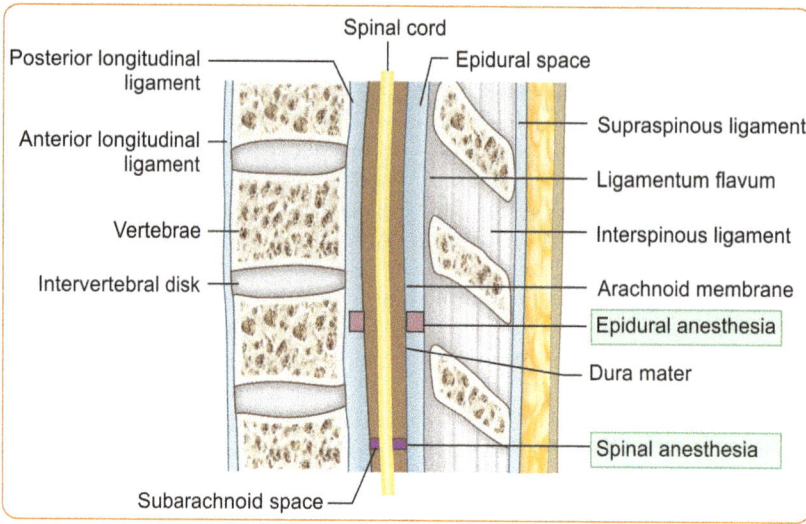

FIG. 8.2: Sites of epidural and spinal anesthesia

Complications

- **Hypotension** is the **most common intraoperative complication**. It can be prevented by preloading with crystalloids or colloids and treated by head low position (**Trendlenburg position**), fluids, vasopressors and inotropic agents. Other intraoperative complications include bradycardia, respiratory depression, and cardiac arrest.
- **Most common postoperative complication is headache**, known as **post dural puncture headache (PDPH)**. It is mainly occipital headache that occurs **after 12-24 hours**. It is different from any headache previously experienced by the patient and is initiated or **made worse by** the adoption of **sitting or erect posture**. It is **relieved by abdominal compression**, which raises the venous pressure. Most common cause of PDPH is **leakage of CSF** through the hole in the dura mater. It can be **prevented by using small bore needle** (25G). Treatment of PDPH consists of lying down for 24 hours, plenty of fluids, abdominal compression and sealing the hole by epidural blood patch. Other postoperative complications include *urinary retention, paralysis of cranial nerves (most commonly involved nerve is abducens, sixth cranial nerve), meningitis, arachnoiditis, paraplegia and cauda equina syndrome.*

Contraindications	
Absolute	Relative
• Raised intracranial tension • Uncooperative patient • Shock • Bleeding disorders/coagulopathy • Patients on anticoagulants, thrombolytic therapy • Infection at local site • Septicemia	• Aortic stenosis • Mitral stenosis • Recent MI, heart block • Spinal deformity • Pyschiatric disorders • CNS disorders

Key Points

Management of LA Toxicity

(*ASRA guidelines)

1. 20% Intralipid IV at first sign of toxicity
2. Benzodiazepines are DOC for seizures. If not able to control, give SCh. If not available, use propofol.
3. Lignocaine and other class Ib drugs avoided for arrhythmias.
4. $NaHCO_3$ for severe acidosis.

*ASRA: American Society of Regional Anesthesia

6. Epidural Anaesthesia

Epidural anaesthesia is given in **epidural space** (between dura mater and bone) with **Tuohy's needle**. Epidural space extends from foramen magnum to sacral hiatus (triangular in shape) and contains anterior and posterior nerve roots, epidural veins, spinal nerves, lymphatics and fat.

Indications

- **Mainly used for controlling postoperative pain** (by continuous epidural through a catheter).
- All surgeries which can be performed under spinal anaesthesia.
- Upper abdominal surgeries, thoracic surgeries and even neck surgeries.
- Painless labour.
- Chronic pain due to cancer and other conditions.

Spinal versus Epidural Anaesthesia

- **Spinal anaesthesia** is *highly reliable, easier* to place (because it can be confirmed by the presence of CSF in the needle and loss of resistance) and has *very quick onset*. However, it can be performed *only for the surgeries of limited duration. Re-dosing cannot be done* if the procedure takes longer time than expected. *PDPH is a very common problem.*
- **Epidural anaesthesia** is *difficult* to perform (requires expert persons) and therefore is less reliable. Further, onset of analgesic effect is *slower*. But it can be used for *surgeries of any duration* by inserting an epidural catheter. Chances of *PDPH is very less* because it is quite superficial procedure (no CSF leak).

Key Points

Concentration (in %) of LA for different uses		
	Lignocaine	Bupivacaine
Infiltration	0.5 – 2	0.25 – 0.5
Spinal	5	0.5
Epidural	2	0.5

Anaesthesia

SKELETAL MUSCLE RELAXANTS

These drugs are used in anesthesia to relax lower limbs and abdominal wall muscles so that operative manipulation becomes easy. These can also be used to facilitate endotracheal intubation by relaxing laryngeal musculature. Some of these drugs are useful in the spastic conditions also. Skeletal muscle relaxants may be **divided into centrally acting and peripherally acting agents.**

CENTRALLY ACTING MUSCLE RELAXANTS

These drugs cause muscle relaxation by their action in the CNS. All these drugs can cause **sedation**. Important drugs in this class are:

- **Mephenesin** group includes *carisoprodol* (its metabolite meprobamate is used as a CNS depressant), *chlorzoxazone, chlormezanone and methocarbamol*. These drugs **selectively inhibit polysynaptic reflexes** and are useful in local muscle spasms like sprains and spasms due to spondylitis.
- **Benzodiazepines** like diazepam and clonazepam **inhibit both polysynaptic** as well as **monosynaptic reflexes** and are useful in muscle spasms of almost any origin. They are mainly used in spinal injuries and tetanus.
- **$GABA_B$** (It is a G protein coupled receptor unlike $GABA_A$, which is an ionotropic receptor) **agonists** like *baclofen increase K^+ conductance and can inhibit monosynaptic as well as polysynaptic reflexes*. Baclofen is used to relieve spasticity in multiple sclerosis and spinal injuries. It is **not useful in cerebral palsy**.
- **Tizanidine** is a centrally acting α_2 **agonist** but unlike clonidine, has **no effect on blood pressure**. It inhibits the release of excitatory neurotransmitters in the spinal cord (by its presynaptic action). It can be used to relieve spasms in multiple sclerosis, amyotrophic lateral sclerosis, other neurological disorders and spinal injuries.
- **Thiocolchicoside** is a muscle relaxant with anti-inflammatory and analgesic effects. It acts as a **$GABA_A$ and glycine receptor antagonist**. It has **pro-convulsant** action and is avoided in epileptic patients.

PERIPHERALLY ACTING MUSCLE RELAXANTS

These drugs do not enter the CNS and cause muscle relaxation by blocking neuromuscular junction (neuromuscular blockers) or by acting directly on the muscle.

A. Directly Acting Skeletal Muscle Relaxants

- **Dantrolene** and **quinine** act directly on the skeletal muscles.
- Dantrolene inhibits the release of Ca^{++} from sarcoplasmic reticulum via inhibition of *ryanodine receptors*. It is used to relieve spasticity due to multiple sclerosis, cerebral palsy and spinal cord injuries but is ineffective in spasms due to musculoskeletal injuries. It is **the drug of choice** for the treatment of **malignant hyperthermia** and is also useful in **neurolept malignant syndrome**. Major adverse effects of this drug are **muscle weakness** and **hepatitis**.
- **Quinine** acts by decreasing the excitability of motor end plate and can be used in patients with **nocturnal leg cramps**.

B. Drugs Acting on Neuromuscular Junction (NMJ)

These drugs decrease the transmission of impulse across NMJ either by inhibiting nicotinic N_M receptors or by consistently depolarizing the muscle end plate.

(a) Depolarizing Blockers

Succinylcholine (SCh) or suxamethonium is the only depolarizing SMR in use at present. It is an ACh analogue and thus **stimulates nicotinic N_M receptors** resulting in depolarization of the membrane. This effect is responsible for **initial fasciculations** seen on administration of this agent (results in post operative muscle pain or soreness). Constant depolarization makes the end plate refractory to other impulses and muscle relaxation results. It is a type of **flaccid paralysis** that **cannot be reversed with neostigmine (Phase I block)**. On prolonged use, this block may be converted to **phase II block** that can be **reversed with anticholinesterases**.

- *SCh is the shortest and the fastest acting SMR*. Due to its quick onset of action, it is **the preferred SMR for endotracheal intubation**. It is metabolized by pseudocholinesterase that may be non-functioning (**atypical pseudocholinesterase**) in some individuals. This is a **genetic condition** and may result in **prolonged apnea on SCh administration** (due to decreased metabolism, action of SCh is prolonged). **Activity of atypical enzyme can be assessed by dibucaine number**.
- SCh can **stimulate the autonomic ganglia** whereas non-depolarizing blockers inhibit the ganglia.
- It can cause **hyperkalemia** especially in patients with **nerve and muscle disorders**. Therefore it is **contraindicated in** patients with nerve diseases (like *paraplegia, hemiplegia and Guillain barre syndrome*) and muscle diseases (*muscular dystrophy, myasthenia gravis, crush injury, burns and rhabdomyolysis*).
- **SCh increases all pressures** i.e. intraocular pressure (**C/I in glaucoma**), intracranial tension (**C/I in head injury**), blood pressure (due to **stimulation of sympathetic ganglia**) and intragastric pressure (responsible for **nausea and vomiting**).
- It **may trigger malignant hyperthermia** specially when given in combination *with halothane*.

(b) Non-depolarizing Blockers or Competitive Skeletal Muscle Relaxants

These drugs act by **competitively inhibiting N_M receptors** and thus cause muscle relaxation without any fasciculations (no postoperative muscle soreness). Further, due to competitive nature of inhibition, effect of these drugs can be **reversed by anticholinesterases** like neostigmine. These are divided into two major groups (benzylisoquinolines and steroidal) on the basis of chemical structure.

(i) Steroidal skeletal muscle relaxants

Pancuronium, vecuronium, pipecuronium, rocuronium and rapacuronium are the drugs in this group. These drugs have very little histamine releasing action and no effect on autonomic ganglia.

- **Pancuronium** can produce **tachycardia** due to its **vagolytic action** (M_2 blocker).

- **Rocuronium** is the **fastest acting non-depolarizing skeletal muscle relaxant** and can be used for rapid sequence endotracheal intubation as an alternative to SCh.
- **Rapacuronium** has been withdrawn due to reports of **severe bronchoconstriction**. It was the **fastest acting** non-depolarizing skeletal muscle relaxant.
- **Vecuronium** is preferred in cardiac patients because of better cardiovascular stability. It is contra indicated in hepatic disease and biliary obstruction.
- **Gantacurium** is *shortest (< 10 min) and fastest* acting non-depolarizing neuromuscular blocker in phase 3 clinical trials. It is being investigated as an alternative to sch. It causes less release of histamine. Its metabolism is carried out non-enzymatically by cysteine.

> **Sugammadex** is a modified gamma cyclodextrin that can be used to reverse neuromuscular blockade by rocuronium. It is the first **selective relaxant binding agent** (SRBA). It encapsulates rocuronium and inhibits its access to N_M receptors at neuromuscular junction. It can also be used to reverse vecuromium and pancuronium induced muscle relaxation. *It is ineffective against SCh and benzylisoquinolines (curiums).* Major advantage of sugammadex over neostigmine is that it produces **reliable and rapid reversal** without producing autonomic instability.

(ii) Benzylisoquinoline derivatives

This group includes d-Tubocurarine **(d-TC)**, metocurine, doxacurium, atracurium, cis-atracurium and mivacurium.

> - These drugs **release histamine (maximum with d-TC** and minimum with cis-atracurium) and block autonomic ganglia (maximum with d-TC and metocurine).
> - and ganglionic blockade property. It can also cause **bronchospasm** due to histamine release.
> - **Doxacurium** is the **longest acting** and most potent SMR.
> - **Mivacurium** is the **shortest acting** non-depolarizing SMR because it is **metabolized by an esterase**. It can be used as an alternative to SCh for endotracheal intubation.
> - **Atracurium and cis-atracurium** undergo **Hoffmann's elimination** (spontaneous non-enzymatic molecular rearrangement) and are the **agents of choice for patients**
>
> *Contd...*

Contd...

> with hepatic or renal insufficiency. Atracurium is metabolized to laudanosine that is responsible for seizures. Cis-atracurium is relatively safe in this regard. Cis-atracurium release **much less histamine** as compared to atracurium.
> - **d-TC** causes **hypotension** due to histamine releasing
> - **Gantacurium** is undergoing phase III clinical trials. It is **fastest** (even rapid than rapacuronium) **and shortest** (shorter than mivacurium) acting non-depolarizing neuromuscular blocker. If approved, it can be used as an alternative to succinylcholine for endotracheal intubation.

Elimination of muscle relaxants:

Renal	Hepatic	Both	None
Doxacurium	Rapacuronium	Pipecuronium	Atracurium
Tubocurarine		Vecuronium	Cis-atracurium
Pancuronium		Rocuronium	Mivacurium
			SCh

(iii) Gallamine

The **least potent** skeletal muscle relaxant. It is rarely used now a days because of its **nephrotoxic and teratogenic** potential. It possesses **vagolytic** action and can lead to **tachycardia**.

> **Note**
> - Shortest acting SMR is succinylcholine whereas *shortest acting non-depolarizing SMR is mivacurium.*
> - Fastest acting SMR is succinylcholine whereas *fastest acting non-depolarizing SMR is rapacuronium* but next is rocuronium (because rapacuronium has been withdrawan).
> - Doxacurium is the longest acting and most potent skeletal muscle relaxant whereas gallamine is the least potent skeletal muscle relaxant.
> - Neostigmine reverses the effect of non-depolarizing SMRs whereas it potentiates the effects of depolarizing SMRs.

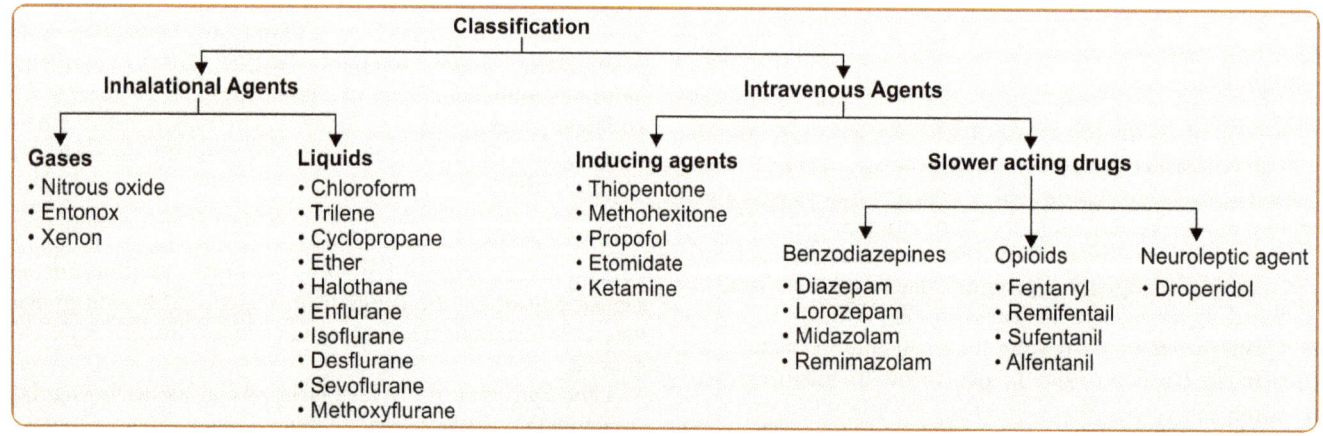

GENERAL ANAESTHETICS

Anaesthesia is the reversible loss of response to a noxious stimuli. It may be **general anaesthesia** (if associated with loss of consciousness) or **local anaesthesia** (consciousness is maintained). Four main features of balanced anaesthesia are:

Unconsciousness	Muscle relaxation
Analgesia	Abolition of compensatory reflex responses

INHALATIONAL AGENTS

These agents are stored in cylinders and are delivered to the patient through Boyle's machine. *Colour coding of the cylinders (for identification) and the Pin index system* is present for the **safety** (so that only the required cylinder can fit in the machine at that site).

Colour Coding of Cylinders

N_2O	Blue
Cyclopropane	Orange
Air	**Grey body with white shoulders**
O_2	Black body with white shoulders
CO_2	Grey
Helium	Brown
Entonox	**Blue body with white shoulders**

> **Key Points**
>
> **Pin Index System**
> | | |
> |---|---|
> | Air | 1,5 |
> | O_2 | 2,5 |
> | N_2O | 3,5 |
> | CO_2 (>7.5%) | 1,6 |
> | CO_2 (<7.5%) | 2,6 |
> | Cyclopropane | 3,6 |
> | Entonox | 7 |

Properties

Two important properties of an inhalational agent is its minimum alveolar concentration (MAC) and blood gas partition coefficient.

- **Minimum Alveolar Concentration (MAC):** It is the minimum concentration of an inhalational agent required in the alveoli to produce unresponsiveness to the skin incision in 50% of the patients. It is the **measure of potency** of an agent. *Greater is the MAC, lesser is the potency.*

> - **Nitrous oxide** is a gas with **maximum MAC** and thus **least potency**. Its MAC is 104% i.e. even with pure (100%) nitric oxide alone, we cannot get complete anaesthesia. This is thus, not a complete anaesthetic agent.
> - **Methoxyflurane** is the **most potent** agent (having least MAC).

- **Blood gas partition coefficient:** It is determined by solubility of an agent in the blood. It **determines the speed of onset and recovery** of an anaesthetic drug. *Greater is blood gas partition coefficient, lesser is the speed of onset and recovery and vice versa.*

> - **Xenon** is the **fastest acting** agent as it has *minimum blood gas partition coefficient.* Next fastest acting agent is desflurane.
> - **Methoxyflurane** is the **slowest acting** agent (*maximum blood gas partition coefficient*).
> - **Ether** also has a very high value of this coefficient; therefore it is also a **slow acting** agent. Due to its slow onset of action, we can differentiate the four stages of general anaesthesia whereas with modern anaesthetics like desflurane, these stages are hardly discernible.

Anaesthetic	MAC (% atm)	Blood gas partition coefficient
Halothane	0.74	2.3
Enflurane	1.68	1.8
Isoflurane	1.15	1.4
Desflurane	6.0	**0.42**
Sevoflurane	2.05	0.69
Cyclopropane	9.2	0.44
Nitrous oxide	**104**	0.47
Trilene	0.2	9
Ether	1.92	12
Chloroform	0.8	8
Methoxyflurane	**0.16**	**15**
Xenon	70	0.115

Systemic Effects

Respiratory System

- All inhalational anaesthetic agents result in **respiratory depression (maximum with Enflurane)**. These also *blunt the ventilatory response to hypercapnea and hypoxia (maximum with halothane)*.
- All inhalational agents cause **bronchodilation** (thus increase anatomical dead space). **Maximum** bronchodilation is seen **with halothane** in asthmatics and with sevoflurane in non-asthmatics.
- All of these agents **reduce** the **ciliary activity** in respiratory system **except ether**.

Cardiovascular System

- All inhalational agents **reduce cardiac output except isoflurane and desflurane. Maximum** decrease in cardiac output is seen **with enflurane**.
- Blood pressure is reduced by all of these agents. **Maximum reduction in blood pressure** is seen with **isoflurane**. It is therefore used as an **agent of choice for producing controlled hypotension. Cyclopropane** results in increase in blood pressure. It is therefore **preferred in patients having shock.**
- All agents reduce cardiac contractility (maximum with halothane).
- **Baroreceptor reflexes** are also **blunted** by all inhalational anaesthetic agents (*maximum with halothane*). **Isoflurane** does not blunt these reflexes; therefore is the **drug of choice for cardiac patients**.

Liver

- **Halothane, chloroform and methoxyflurane** can result in hepatotoxicity on long term use.

Kidney

- **Methoxyflurane** can result in **vasopressin resistant polyuric renal failure** due to the presence of high content of *fluoride* in it (*maximum*). *Fluoride is added to decrease the inflammability* of these agents.

Blood

- **Nitrous oxide** can result in **megaloblastic anemia** due to vitamin B_{12} **deficiency**. It can also lead to *bone marrow suppression*.

Skeletal Muscles

- All inhalational agents are good **skeletal muscle relaxants except nitrous oxide. Maximum** muscle relaxation is caused **by ether.**

Analgesia

- Newer anaesthetic agents like halothane and isoflurane **are not** very good **analgesic** agents. **Maximum analgesia** is caused **by trilene** (*ether is also a good analgesic agent*).

Metabolic Effects

- Chloroform (*maximum*), ether and cyclopropane can cause hyperglycemia.

Inflammability

- **Ether and cyclopropane** are highly **inflammable** agents. *Cautery should not be used* when these agents are used to induce the anaesthesia.
- **Reaction with soda lime**
- Sevoflurane, trilene and methoxyflurane should not be used in closed circuit.
- **Sevoflurane** reacts with soda lime to produce **compound A**, which is highly **nephrotoxic**.
- **Trilene** reacts with soda lime in the closed circuit to produce **dichloroacetylene (neurotoxic) and phosgene (can cause ARDS).**
- **Methoxyflurane** reacts **with rubber tubing** of the closed **circuit.**

Individual Drugs

Nitrous Oxide

- It is also called '**laughing gas**'.
- It is colourless, non-irritating and non-inflammable.
- Colour of N_2O cylinder is **blue.**
- It is a very **good analgesic** but *weak* anaesthetic agent (**Highest MAC**).
- It is a **poor muscle relaxant.**
- It shows **faster induction & recovery** of anaesthesia (low blood gas partition coefficient).
- It is used in a concentration of 50 to 65% with 33% oxygen.
- **Entonox** is a *mixture of 50% N_2O + 50% O_2.*

> - **Concentration effect** is seen with agents like N_2O, which are administered in high concentrations. Due to high concentration, when diffusion occurs from alveoli to blood, there is generation of negative pressure in the alveoli that leads to more removal of anaesthetic gas from the cylinder.
> - **Second gas effect** is seen when another inhalational agent (like halothane) is administered along with N_2O. Due to generation of negative pressure, second gas is also taken in from the cylinder.
> - **Diffusion hypoxia** occurs when supply of N_2O is stopped **while recovery** from anaesthesia. It can be **prevented by 100% oxygen** inhalation for a few minutes before discontinuing N_2O.

Methemoglobinemia and laryngospasm may occur due to the presence of impurities like nitric oxide (NO) and nitrogen dioxide (NO_2).

- Bone marrow depression and megaloblastic anemia due to vitamin B_{12} deficiency may also occur. Latter can result in subacute combined degeneration of spinal cord.
- N_2O use is **contraindicated in pneumothorax and volvulus** because it may lead to development of high pressure in the closed cavities in the body (like gut, pneumothorax and pneumoperitoneum).
- It is used as a supplement to anaesthesia (because it is not a complete anaesthetic).
- It is also used as a carrier gas for inhalational agents like halothane.

Halothane

- It is a colourless, volatile liquid.
- It is a non-irritant, non-explosive and pleasant smelling agent.
- It is stored in amber coloured bottles and contains thymol (0.01%) as preservative.
- It is a **good anaesthetic but very poor analgesic** agent.
- It can cause **hepatitis** on repeated use.
- It can also result in **malignant hyperthermia**, which can be treated with dantrolene.
- It can result in **post-anaesthetic chills and shivering. Pethidine is used for treatment** of this condition.
- Halothane relaxes the uterus. Due to this property, it is the **agent of choice in internal version and manual removal of placenta** (version can be accomplished easily in a relaxed uterus). However due to its uterine relaxing property, it is **contraindicated in labour**, because if post-partum hemorrhage results, it will be difficult to control (contraction of uterus stops bleeding after labour).
- It sensitizes heart to the arrhythmogenic action of catecholamines. It is therefore **contraindicated in** patients with **pheochromocytoma.**
- It is also a cardiodepressant drug that causes hypotension, bradycardia and arrhythmias.
- It is the inhalational **agent of choice in bronchial asthma** due to its bronchodilator action.
- It is an excellent agent for induction in **children.**

> ⚠️ **MNEMONIC**
>
> **Properties of Halothane**
> H – Hyperthermia [malignant hyperthermia]
> A – Arrhythmias (sensitize heart to adrenaline)
> L – Liver toxic
> O – Orthostatic hypotension
> T – Tocolytic
> H – Heart [inhibits heart; decreases cardiac output]
> A – Asthma [bronchodilator]
> N Non-explosive
> E
> C – Chills [post-anaesthetic shivering]
> C – Catecholamines [sensitizes heart to arrhythmogenic action]
> C – Children [safe in children]

Ether

- It is a **pungent smelling and irritant** liquid (can result in excessive secretions).
- It is a highly **inflammable and explosive** agent. Cautery should not be used with ether anaesthesia.
- It is a **very good analgesic and muscle relaxant**.
- It is very **slow in induction** of anaesthesia. Guedel's four stages of anaesthesia are based on ether.
- It **does not affect the ciliary action and is also a good bronchodilator**. Therefore it is safe in asthmatic patients.
- It is **very economical** and can be used as a sole agent for anaesthesia.
- It is the **safest agent in unskilled hands**.
- It can result in **hyperglycemia**, therefore is contra-indicated in diabetic patients.

Enflurane

- It is a halogenated ether.
- It is inflammable at high concentrations (> 5%)
- It is **contraindicated in epilepsy** as it can raise intracranial tension and produce tonic clonic seizures.
- Like other newer agents, it is also **not a good analgesic**.

Isoflurane

- It is an isomer of enflurane.
- It is not a good analgesic agent.
- Cardiac output is maintained with isoflurane. Therefore, it is the inhalational **agent of choice for cardiac surgery.**
- It produces least increase in intracranial tension, therefore is the **agent of choice for neurosurgery**.
- It produces maximum decrease in blood pressure, therefore is inhalational **agent of choice for producing controlled hypotension**.
- It can be used in **day care surgery**.
- It is **safe in pheochromocytoma** (does not sensitize the heart to catecholamines).
- It **can cause coronary steal phenomenon**.

MNEMONIC

Inhalational anaesthetics that can precipitate seizures
S – Sevoflorane
E – Enflurane (Maximum)
I – Isoflurane
ZURE

Desflurane

- It has minimum blood gas partition coefficient and therefore is the **fastest** inducing agent.
- It has **very high vapour pressure**. Its boiling point is 23°C; therefore it boils at room temperature. It requires special vaporizers due to this property.
- It produces cardiovascular effects similar to isoflurane except coronary steal phenomenon.
- Induction with desflurane is unpleasant. It causes **maximum irritation to airways**. As it can lead to coughing, breath holding and laryngospasm.
- It **can also be used in day care surgery**.

 Key Points

Desflurane has lowest boiling temperature (~24°C) whereas methoxyflurane has highest boiling point (~104°C).

Sevoflurane

- It is the inhalational **agent of choice for induction in children**.
- It is a very good muscle relaxant but poor analgesic agent.
- It should not be used in **closed circuit** because it can produce a **nephrotoxic metabolite, Compound A.**

Key Points

Sevoflurane should not be used in closed circuit because it can produce a nephrotoxic metabolite, **Compound A**.

Methoxyflurane

- It is the **most potent** inhalational agent (least MAC).
- It has the **slowest induction and recovery** (highest B/G partition coefficient).
- It can lead to **high output renal failure** (highest amount of fluoride content).
- **It should not be used in closed circuit** (reacts with rubber tubing of the closed circuit).

Trielene (Trichlorethylene)

- It is the **most potent analgesic** agent.
- It should not be used in **closed circuit** because reaction with soda lime can result in the production of **phosgene gas** (responsible for Acute Respiratory Distress Syndrome), and **dichloroacetylene** (neurotoxic to Vth and VIIth cranial nerves).
- It can be used for analgesia in labour.

Cyclopropane

- It is **highly inflammable and explosive** agent.
- Colour of its **cylinder is orange**
- It is the **inhalational agent of choice in hemorrhagic shock** (increases BP by increasing sympathetic tone).
- It should be stopped slowly because sudden discontinuation may result in hypotension (**cyclopropane shock**).

Chloroform

- It is a cardiotoxic agent and can result in **ventricular fibrillation**.
- It is also a **hepatotoxic** drug.
- It can cause profound **hyperglycemia**.

Carbon Dioxide

- 5% concentration is used for creating **pneumoperitoneum in laparoscopy**.
- Colour of its cylinder is **grey**.

Helium

- It is **lighter than air**.
- Mixture of 80% helium and 20% oxygen is used in cases of **tracheal obstruction**.

Xenon

Xenon is Greek for stranger. It was discovered in 1898 and found to be the **only noble gas to be anaesthetic under normobaric conditions**. Xenon is *extremely scarce* with an average room containing only 4ml. It is *very close to the 'ideal agent'*.

- It is a *colourless and odourless* gas with no irritation to the respiratory tract. Well tolerated with gas induction.
- It has **lowest blood/gas partition co-efficient** (0.115) allowing rapid induction and reversal of anaesthesia.
- It produces unconsciousness with analgesia and a degree of muscle relaxation
- It has a MAC of 60-70% that allows a reasonable inspired oxygen concentration
- It **does cause respiratory depression**, to the point of apnoea.
- It is has **no effect on cardiovascular function**.
- It is *not metabolised in the body* and is eliminated rapidly and completely via the lungs.
- It is *non toxic* and is not associated with allergic reactions
- It is *stable in storage*, has *no interaction with anaesthesia circuits or soda lime*. However, it should not be used with rubber anaesthesia circuits as there is a high loss through the rubber.
- It is *non-inflammable*
- Major problem with xenon is that is **highly expensive** and routine usage will only be possible with a closed circuit delivery system that recycles xenon.

 Key Points

Xenon can be considered as an ideal inhalational anaesthetic.

Note
- Trielene has maximum analgesic activity.
- Ether has maximum muscle relaxant activity.
- All inhalational agents increase cerebral blood flow (maximum with halothane) as well as intracranial tension (maximum with halothane and ether).
- Halothane, chloroform and methoxyflurane are hepatotoxic whereas methoxyflurane and sevoflurane are nephrotoxic.

INTRAVENOUS AGENTS

These may be fast acting (used for induction) or may be slow acting.

1. Inducing Agents

A. Thiopentone

- It is an *ultra short acting barbiturate* and is the *most commonly used intravenous inducing agent*. It is used as a 2.5% solution.
- *Sulphur* is added to pentobarbitone to *increase the lipid solubility*.
- Due to high lipid solubility, it is very fast acting drug.
- Action of this drug terminates very quickly due to **redistribution** (although half life is longer).
- It also possesses **anticonvulsant** action (another barbiturate methohexitone increases the risk of convulsions, therefore *used for electroconvulsive therapy*).
- It is the *agent of choice for cerebral protection* (decreases cerebral oxygen consumption, decreases intra-cranial tension and decreases cerebral metabolic rate).
- It causes peripheral vasodilatation and also depresses cardiovascular system, therefore can cause *hypotension*.
- Instead of producing analgesic effect, it can *produce hyperalgesia* at subanaesthetic doses.
- *Respiratory depression* and transient apnea are other problems seen with this agent.
- On **accidental injection** of thiopentone **in the arteries**, it can lead to thrombosis and vasoconstriction that may progress to **ischemia and gangrene**. It is accompanied by very severe pain. This condition is treated by **leaving the needle in situ** (*needle should not be withdrawn*), dilution of injected thiopentone with saline, immediate heparinization and papaverine injection to relieve spasm. Vasodilators, steroids, lignocaine and urokinase can also be employed. Brachial plexus and stellate ganglion block should be performed.
- Barbiturates are absolutely **contra-indicated in acute intermittent porphyria**.

B. Methohexitone

- It is also an ultra short acting barbiturate.
- It is 3 times more potent than thiopentone.
- It induces seizures; therefore, it is the agent of choice for electroconvulsive therapy.

C. Ketamine

- It is a *phencyclidine (hallucinogenic) derivative* that is administered in a dose of 2 mg/kg.
- Its onset of action is 30-60s whereas action terminates in 15-20 min due to *redistribution*.
- It acts by **blocking NMDA receptors** of glutamate.
- It is a **very strong analgesic** agent but *lacks muscle relaxant property*.
- It is used for producing **dissociative anaesthesia** (state of profound analgesia, amnesia with light sleep, immobility, feeling of dissociation from one's own body and the surroundings).
- It does not depress pharyngeal and laryngeal reflexes; therefore is the **agent of choice for** emergency anaesthesia with **full stomach** (because vomiting will prevent aspiration).
- It **increases all pressures** (blood pressure, intracranial tension, intraocular pressure) in the body. It is therefore intravenous *anaesthetic of choice for shock* (increases blood pressure). Further it is *contraindicated in glaucoma* (increases IOP) *and head injuries* (increases ICT).
- It is a powerful bronchodilator agent and is therefore **intravenous anaesthetic of choice in bronchial asthma** (*halothane is the inhalational* anaesthetic agent of choice for bronchial asthma).
- It is the **intravenous anaesthetic agent of choice for induction in children** (*Sevoflurane is inhalational* agent of choice in children).
- On discontinuation of ketamine anaesthesia, several adverse effects may be seen (known as **emergence reaction**). **Hallucinations are the most common side effect**. Other effects include *vivid dreams, illusions and excitement*.

Anaesthesia

> **MNEMONIC**
>
> K — Kids (IV anaesthetic of choice in children)
> E — Emergence reaction [hallucinations, illusions, vivid dreams etc. seen while recovery from anaesthesia]
> T — Thalamocortical junction [site of action, responsible for dissociative anaesthesia]
> A — Analgesic [maximum among anaesthetics]
> M — Meals [can be given in full stomach]
> I — Increases all pressures [BP, IOP, ICT]
> N — NMDA antagonist
> E — Excellent for asthmatics.

D. Propofol

- It is a **milky white powder** that is **preservative free**. Therefore, it must be used within 6 hours.
- It is an **oil based preparation**, therefore injection is *painful*.
- Its onset of action is within 15 seconds and last for 5-10 min (due to redistribution)
- It possesses very **strong antiemetic and antipruritic action**.
- It *decreases blood pressure* and impairs baroreceptor reflexes.
- It produces more severe and prolonged *respiratory depression* than thiopentone.
- It has *no muscle relaxant property*.
- It has cerebroprotective activity but does not possess anticonvulsant activity. Rather, **myoclonic jerking and muscle twitching** can be seen with the use of propofol.
- It is the intravenous anaesthetic of choice for **day care surgery**.

Key Points

Drugs Useful for Day Care Surgery	
Dr	Desflurane
Manmohan	Midazolam (Benzodiazepine)
Singh	Sevoflurane
Is	Isoflurane
A	Alfentanil
Prime	Propofol
Minister	Mivacurium (Muscle relaxant)

- It is also the intravenous anaesthetic of *choice for sedation in ICU*.
- Propofol is the intravenous anaesthetic of choice in the patients with **malignant hyperthermia**.
- This agent is intravenous anaesthetic of choice, and is used with alfentanil for **total intravenous anaesthesia** (TIVA).

Key Points

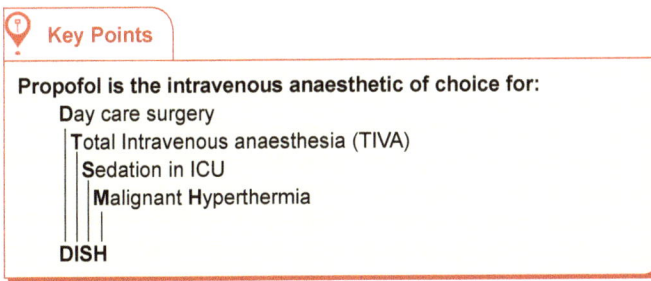

E. Etomidate

- It does not interfere with cardiovascular functions; therefore is **the agent of choice for aneurysm surgeries and cardiac disease**.
- It causes minimal respiratory depression.
- Maximum incidence of **nausea and vomiting** is seen with the use of this agent.
- It can also produce **myoclonus**.
- Injection of etomidate is **painful** and may result in thrombophlebitis.
- It can lead to **adrenocortical suppression**.
- **Vitamin C deficiency** can also develop with the use of etomidate.

2. Slow Acting Agents

A. Benzodiazepines

- Important benzodiazepines are diazepam, lorazepam, midazolam and remimazolam.
- These are not analgesic agents.
- However, these possess muscle relaxing and anticonvulsant property.
- Lorazepam is the most commonly used benzodiazepine in pre-anaesthetic medication.
- Midazolam is used for day care surgery.
- These agents may cause sedation and anterograde amnesia.
- **Remimazolam** is a new drug which is **rapid and short acting than midazolam**. It is used to induce sedation for short procedures.

B. Opioids

- **Fentanyl, alfentanil, sufentanil and remifentanil** are the opioids used in anaesthesia.
- These are 100 times **more potent than morphine. Sufentanil is the most potent** opioid.
- These drugs possess very **strong analgesic** activity.
- Fentanyl is used along with droperidol for **neurolept analgesia**.
- If nitrous oxide is also added, the combination can be used as **neurolept anaesthesia** (N_2O + fentanyl + droperidol).
- These agents can lead to **postoperative muscle rigidity** (SCh causes post operative muscle pain and fasciculations).
- **Alfentanil** is used for day care surgery and for **total intravenous anaesthesia**.
- **Remifentanil is the shortest acting** opioid (due to its metabolism by esterases).

C. Neuroleptic agent

- **Droperidol** is a D_2 receptor blocker.
- It is used along with fentanyl to produce **neurolept analgesia and neurolept anaesthesia**.
- It can produce **extrapyramidal symptoms**.

Anaesthetic agents of choice for various conditions	
Day care:	Propofol
Ischemic heart disease:	Etomidate
Congenital heart disease	
• Left to right shunt:	Isoflurane
• Right to left shunt:	Ketamine
CHF:	Ketamine
Shock:	Ketamine
To produce delibrate hypotenion:	Isoflurane
Asthma and COPD:	Ketamine
Epilepsy:	Thiopentone
For electroconvulsive therapy:	Methohexitone
Thyrotoxicosis:	Thiopentone
Cardiac surgery:	Isoflurane
Neurosurgery:	Isoflurane

Golden Points

1. Adrenaline is added to LA to make them long acting whereas sodium bicarbonate makes them fast acting.

2. A mixture of 2.5% prilocaine and 2.5% lignocaine in 1:1 ratio can anaesthetize even unbroken skin. Combination of these two agents lowers the melting point of individual drugs and helps to form a semi-solid ointment. This mixture is known as **Eutectic mixture**.

3. The drug of choice for **IVRA** is **prilocaine**.

4. Hypotension is the most common intraoperative complication of spinal anaesthesia whereas most common postoperative complication is headache, known as post dural puncture headache (PDPH).

5. Dantrolene is the drug of choice for the treatment of malignant hyperthermia and is also useful in neurolept malignant syndrome.

6. Succinylcholine can cause hyperkalemia especially in patients with nerve and muscle disorders. Therefore it is contraindicated in patients with nerve diseases (like paraplegia, hemiplegia and Guillain barre syndrome) and muscle diseases (muscular dystrophy, myasthenia gravis, crush injury, burns and rhabdomyolysis).

7. Rapacuronium has been withdrawn due to reports of severe bronchoconstriction.

8. Sugammadex is first selective relaxant binding agent (SRBA).

9. Atracurium and cis-atracurium undergo Hoffmann's elimination (spontaneous non-enzymatic molecular rearrangement) and are the agents of choice for patients with hepatic or renal insufficiency.

10. Mac is inversly related to potency whereas blood gas partition coefficient is inversly related to speed of onset and recovery of an inhalational agent.

11. Nitrous oxide is a gas with maximum MAC (least potent) whereas methoxyflurane is the most potent agent (having least MAC).

12. Maximum bronchodilation is seen with halothane in asthmatics and with sevoflurane in non-asthmatics.

13. Halothane sensitizes the heart to arrhythmogenic action of adrenaline and noradrenaline. It is therefore contraindicated in patients with pheochromocytoma.

14. Sevoflurane, trilene and methoxyflurane should not be used in closed circuit.

15. Diffusion hypoxia occurs when supply of N_2O is stopped during recovery from anaesthesia. It can be prevented by 100% oxygen inhalation for a few minutes before discontinuing N_2O.

16. N_2O use is contraindicated in pneumothorax and volvulus because it may lead to development of high pressure in the closed cavities in the body.

17. Halothane can result in post-anaesthetic chills and shivering. Pethidine is used for treatment of this condition.

18. **Enflurane** is contraindicated in **epilepsy** as it can raise intracranial tension and produce tonic clonic seizures.

19. **Isoflurane** is inhalational agent of choice for producing **controlled hypotension**.

20. Thiopentone is used as a 2.5% solution for IV induction of anaesthesia

21. Action of thiopentone terminates very quickly due to redistribution.

Drug of Choice

Condition	Drug of choice
• Neurolept analgesia	Droperidol + Fentanyl
• Neurolept anaesthesia	Droperidol + Fentanyl + N_2O
• GA for internal version	Halothane
• GA for asthma	
– Inducing agent	Ketamine
– Inhalational	Halothane
• GA to produce controlled hypotension	Isoflurane
• GA for cardiac surgery	
– Inducing agent	Etomidate
– Inhalational	Isoflurane
• GA for neurosurgery	Isoflurane/Sevoflurane
• Day care surgery	Propofol
• Total Intravenous Anaesthesia	Propofol

Condition	Drug of choice
• GA for malignant hyperthermia	Propofol
• GA in patients with shock	Ketamine
• LA in patients with malignant hyperthermia	Procaine
• Intravenous Regional Anaesthesia (IVRA; Bier's block)	Prilocaine
• Malignant hyperthermia	Dantrolene
• MR in patients with asthma	Vecuronium
• MR in liver and kidney disease	Atracurium or Cis-atracurium
• MR for endotracheal intubation	Succinylcholine

Note

- GA : General Anaesthetic
- LA : Local Anaesthetic
- MR : Muscle Relaxant

Image Based Questions

1. A new inhaled anesthetic has been developed and tested in a series of experiments. Anesthetic tension in the arterial blood is shown on the graph below as a function of time after inhalation (Drug A). A similar curve for nitrous oxide is also shown:

   Which of the following best describes the properties of the new anesthetic compared to nitrous oxide'?
   (a) High blood: Gas partition coefficient
   (b) Low solubility in the blood
   (c) Rapid onset of action
   (d) Low potency

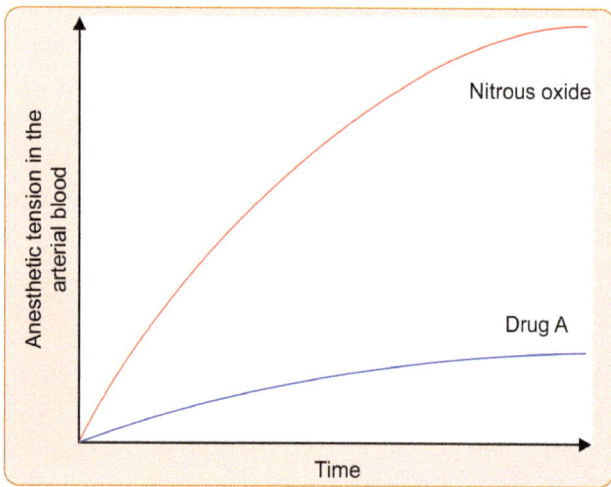

2. A 53-year-old male Arjun presented to emergency with blunt injury to abdomen and crushing of his left leg under the tyres of a bus in a road traffic accident. His blood pressure was 80/40 mmHg. Emergency laparotomy was planned to repair the ruptured viscera and to know the cause of internal bleeding. Succinylcholine was used for intubation and vecuronium for maintenance of muscle relaxation. Anaesthesia was induced by thiopentone and maintained by halothane. However, during intraoperative period, the patient developed arrhythmias as shown in ECG below. Which of the following is the likely cause of this ECG finding?
   (a) Presence of atypical pseudocholinesterase in this patient
   (b) Succinylcholine induced hyperkalemia
   (c) Vecuronium overdose
   (d) Accident intra-arterial injection of thiopentone

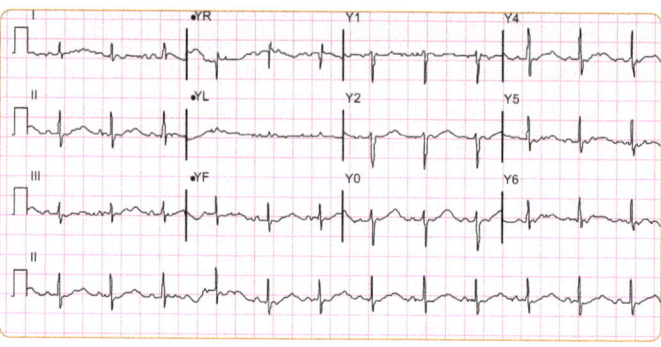

3. You are studying pharmacokinetic properties of thiopentone. A dose-time relationship in various tissues after a single bolus of thiopentone is shown in the graph below. Curves A, B and C in the graph represent:

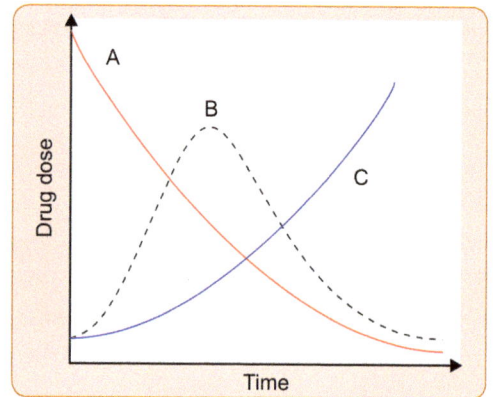

	Curve A	Curve B	Curve C
(a)	Brain	Blood	Adipose tissue
(b)	Blood	Brain	Adipose tissue
(c)	Brain	Adipose tissue	Blood
(d)	Adipose tissue	Brain	Blood

4. The given image is of which cylinder?

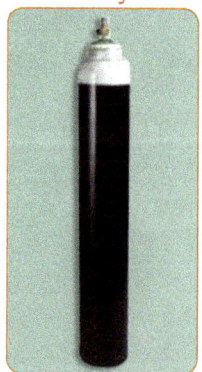

(a) Oxygen
(b) Nitrons oxide
(c) Cyclopropane
(d) Entonox

5. The cylinder shown in the figure contain which gas?

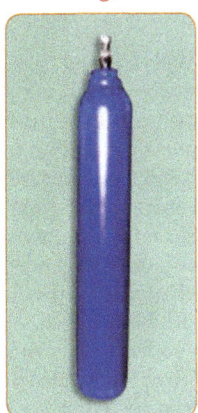

(a) Oxygen
(b) Nitrous oxide
(c) Cyclopropane
(d) Entonox

6. Which of the following statements regarding the pin-index system of cylinders shown below is not true?

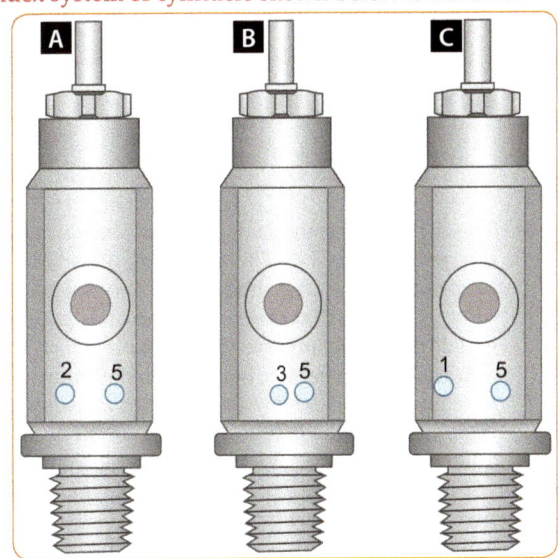

(a) Colour of cylinder A is black with white shoulders
(b) Gas in cylinder B has highest MAC
(c) Cylinder C may contain air
(d) Entonox is a mixture of gases from cylinder A and cylinder C

Explanations

1. **Ans. (a) High blood: Gas partition coefficient**
   (Ref:Katzung 11th/e p427)
   - The depth of anesthesia depends on the partial pressure of anesthetic in CNS. The transfer of anesthetic into the brain starts only after the blood is fully saturated (or, in other words partial pressure of the anesthetic in blood equals the partial pressure in the inspired air). The speed of transfer of anesthetic to the brain determines its onset of action (rapid vs slow induction of anesthesia) and is dependent on the solubility of anesthetic in the blood. Solubility of an anesthetic is directly related to its blood/gas partition coefficient: highly soluble anesthetics have high blood/gas partition coefficient.
   - If the agent is poorly soluble the amount of gas needed to saturate the blood is small and saturation occurs fairly quickly. Nitrous oxide is an example of poorly soluble gas with a blood/gas partition coefficient of 47. On the graph above the curve of partial pressure of NO in blood rises rapidly. In the highest point on the curve the partial pressure on NO in blood equals that in the inspired air, and the transfer to brain occurs.
   - The second curve (drug A) portrays the process of blood saturation for a highly soluble gas. The higher the solubility the more gas can be taken up by blood before it is saturated. Note that the curve of the partial pressure of drug A in blood rises slower than that for NO. When the blood is fully saturated with NO the partial pressure of drug A in blood is approximately 25% of that in inspired air. For drug A, it takes a longer time to fully saturate the blood and to start transfer in tissues. Drug A, therefore is characterized with high blood/gas partition coefficient and slower onset of action.

Effect	Poorly soluble gas NO	Highly soluble gas (Halothane)
Amount needed to saturate the blood	Small	Large
Rise in tension of gas in blood	Rapid	Slow
Equilibrium with the brain	Rapid	Slow
Onset of action	Rapid	Slow

2. **Ans. (b) Succinylcholine induced hyperkalemia**
   (Ref: Katzung 11th/e p460)
   Succinylcholine has high risk of causing hyperkalemia if used in patients with injury to muscles and nerves. The ECG shows changes characteristic of hyperkalemia and the patient also has crush injury, so this seems to be the most likely hyperkalemia caused by succinylcholine.

3. **Ans. (b) Blood, Brain, Adipose tissue**
   (Ref:Katzung 11/e p434)
   Thiopentone is a short-acting barbiturate used for induction of anesthesia. After equilibration with the brain it rapidly redistributes into skeletal muscles and adipose tissue, which results in rapid recovery from.

4. **Ans a. Oxygen**
   The color of oxygen cylinder is black body with white shoulder.

5. **Ans. b. Nitrous oxide**
   The color of nitrous oxide cylinder is blue.

6. **Ans. d. Entonox is mixture of gases from cylinder A and cylinder C.**
   - Cylinder A is oxygen. It is pin-index is 2,5. The colour of oxygen cylinder is black with white shoulders
   - Cylinder B is nitrous oxide. Its colour is blue. It has highest MAC (104%)
   - Cylinder C with pin-index 1,5 is air
   - Entonox is a mixture of 50% N_2O with 50% O_2.

Multiple Choice Questions

LOCAL ANAESTHESIA

1. All of the following statements about lignocaine are true *except*: *(AIIMS Nov 2012)*
   (a) It blocks active sodium channels with more affinity than resting sodium channels
   (b) It can cause cardiotoxicity
   (c) It is given orally for treatment of cardiac arrhythmias
   (d) Adrenaline increases the duration of action of lignocaine when used for infiltration anaesthesia

2. Maximum dose of lignocaine given with adrenaline for infiltration anaesthesia is: *(AIIMS May 2012)*
   (a) 3 mg/kg   (b) 5 mg/kg
   (c) 7 mg/kg   (d) 10 mg/kg

3. Bupivacaine poisoning is treated with all of the following *except*: *(Recent NEET Pattern Question)*
   (a) Esmolol   (b) Sotalol
   (c) Lignocaine   (d) Diazepam

4. All are vasodilators *except*: *(Recent NEET Pattern Question)*
   (a) Procaine   (b) Lidocaine
   (c) Cocaine   (d) Chlorprocaine

5. Which of the following local anaesthetics belongs to the ester group? *(Recent NEET Pattern Question)*
   (a) Procaine   (b) Bupivacaine
   (c) Lignocaine   (d) Mepivacaine

6. The following statements about Bupivacaine are true *except*: *(Recent NEET Pattern Question)*
   (a) Must never be injected into a vein
   (b) More cardiotoxic than lignocaine
   (c) 0.5 percent is effective for sensory block
   (d) It produces methaemoglobinemia

7. Local anesthetics act by: *(Recent NEET Pattern Question)*
   (a) Affecting at the spinal level
   (b) Affecting the Na^+ channels
   (c) Affecting the K^+ channels
   (d) Blocking axonal transport

8. Local anesthetics: *(Recent NEET Pattern Question)*
   (a) Block the release of neurotransmitters
   (b) Blocks the influx of sodium into the cell
   (c) Increase the release of inhibitory neurotrans-mitters
   (d) Inhibit the efflux of sodium from neurons

9. All are true about bupivacaine *except*: *(Recent NEET Pattern Question)*
   (a) Less cardiotoxic than lignocaine
   (b) Dose increases with adrenaline
   (c) Long acting
   (d) Cannot given in vein

10. Post dural (Spinal) puncture headache is due to: *(Recent NEET Pattern Question)*
    (a) Seepage of CSF   (b) Fine needle
    (c) Toxic effects of the drugs
    (d) Traumatic damage to nerve roots

11. True statement regarding Bupivacaine is: *(Recent NEET Pattern Question)*
    (a) Used intravenously along with lignocaine
    (b) More cardiotoxic than lignocaine
    (c) Contraindicated in pregnancy
    (d) All of the above

12. Percentage of lignocaine used in spinal anesthesia is: *(Recent NEET Pattern Question)*
    (a) 0.5%   (b) 1%
    (c) 2%   (d) 5%

13. The mechanism of action of local anesthetics is that they act on Na^+ channels in their: *(Recent NEET Pattern Question)*
    (a) Activated state   (b) Inactivated state
    (c) Resting state   (d) Any state

14. The most potent and longest acting anaesthetic agent is: *(Recent NEET Pattern Question)*
    (a) Dibucaine   (b) Tetracaine
    (c) Bupivacaine   (d) Lignocaine

15. Adrenaline is added to lignocaine to prolong its effect and decrease its absorption into bloodstream in a ratio of: *(Recent NEET Pattern Question)*
    (a) 1:50,000   (b) 1:100,000
    (c) 1:200,000   (d) 1:500,000

16. Eutectic mixture of local anaesthetic (EMLA) cream is: *(Recent NEET Pattern Question)*
    (a) Bupivacaine 2.0% + Prilocaine 2.5%
    (b) Lidocaine 2.5% + Prilocaine 2.5%
    (c) Lidocaine 2.5% + Prilocaine 5%
    (d) Bupivacaine 0.5% + Lidocaine 2.5%

17. Cocaine overdose presents with all of the following *except*: *(Recent NEET Pattern Question)*
    (a) Diaphoresis   (b) Hypertension
    (c) Constricted pupils (d) Agitation

18. All of the following are the true for post lumbar puncture headache *except*: *(Recent NEET Pattern Question)*
    (a) Presents 12 hours after procedure
    (b) Pain is relieved in standing position
    (c) Pain is worsened by headshaking
    (d) Pain is occipito-frontal in location

19. Local anaesthetic used as an antiarrhythmic agent is: *(Recent NEET Pattern Question)*
    (a) Bupivacaine   (b) Lignocaine
    (c) Cocaine   (d) Chlorprocaine

SKELETAL MUSCLE RELAXANTS

20. A person was given a muscle relaxant that competitively blocks nicotinic receptors. Which of the following drug is used for reversal of muscle relaxation caused by this agent after surgery? *(NEET Pattern Question 2020)*
    (a) Neostigmine   (b) Carbachol
    (c) Succinylcholine   (d) Physostigmine

21. Advantage of cisatracurium over atracurium is:
    (NEET Pattern Question 2019)
    (a) Short duration of action
    (b) Rapid onset
    (c) Less allergic
    (d) Releases less histamine

22. Mechanism of action of curare type drugs is:
    (NEET Pattern Question 2019)
    (a) Competitive inhibitor of ACh receptors
    (b) Calcium channel blockade
    (c) Persistent depolarization of receptors
    (d) Blocking release of ACh

23. Centrally acting muscle relaxant with alpha 2 adrenergic agonist activity is: (NEET Pattern Question 2017-2018)
    (a) Chlorzoxazone   (b) Baclofen
    (c) Tizanidine   (d) Pirenzepine

24. Mechanism of action of tubocurarine is:
    (NEET Pattern Question 2017-2018)
    (a) Cholinesterase inhibitor
    (b) Cause membrane depolarization
    (c) Competitive antagonist of acetylcholine receptor
    (d) Inhibit opening of chloride channels

25. Which of the following drug undergoes Hoffman's elimination? (AIIMS May, 2016)
    (a) Atracurium   (b) Pancuronium
    (c) Mivacurium   (d) Vecuronium

26. Which of the following drug does not act on neuromuscular junction? (AIIMS May, 2016)
    (a) Succinylcholine   (b) Dantrolene
    (c) Vecuronium   (d) Mivacurium

27. Muscle relaxant of choice in a patient with serum bilirubin of 6 mg/dL and serum creatinine of 4.5 mg/dL is:
    (AIIMS May, 2015)
    (a) Vecuronium   (b) Atracurium
    (c) Pancuronium   (d) Mivacurium

28. Which of the following skeletal muscles is relaxed first by tubocurarine? (AIIMS Nov, 2013)
    (a) Respiratory   (b) Fingers
    (c) Limbs   (d) Head and neck

29. Which of the following drugs has spasmolytic activity and could also be used in the management of seizure caused by overdose of a local anesthetic? (AIIMS May 2012)
    (a) Baclofen   (b) Dantrolene
    (c) Diazepam   (d) Tizanidine

30. Which one of the following skeletal muscle relaxants causes pain on injection? (AIIMS Nov 2011) (AI 2012)
    (a) Succinyl choline   (b) Vecuronium
    (c) Rocuronium   (d) Pancuronium

31. The administration of succinylcholine to a paraplegic patient led to appearance of dysarrythmias, conduction abnormalities and finally cardiac arrest. The most likely cause is: (Recent NEET Pattern Question)
    (a) Hypercalcemia   (b) Hyperkalemia
    (c) Anaphylaxis   (d) Hypermagnesemia

32. d-Tubocurarine acts by: (Recent NEET Pattern Question)
    (a) Inhibiting nicotinic receptors at myoneural junction
    (b) Inhibiting nicotinic receptors at autonomic ganglion
    (c) Producing depolarizing block
    (d) By inhibiting reuptake of acetylcholine

33. The enzyme pseudocholinesterase acts on:
    (Recent NEET Pattern Question)
    (a) Decamethonium   (b) Tubocurarine
    (c) Gallamine   (d) Suxamethonium

34. Hoffman's elimination is seen with:
    (Recent NEET Pattern Question)
    (a) Atracurium   (b) Vecuronium
    (c) Pancuronium   (d) Rocuronium

35. Non-depolarizing blockade is potentiated by:
    (a) Hyperkalemia   (Recent NEET Pattern Question)
    (b) Hypomagnesemia
    (c) Chronic phenytoin therapy
    (d) Quininidine

36. The drug causing curare like effect are all, except:
    (Recent NEET Pattern Question)
    (a) Chloramphenicol   (b) Polymyxin
    (c) Tetracycline   (d) Streptomycin

37. Which of the following muscle relaxants is free of cardiovascular effects over the entire clinical dose range?
    (Recent NEET Pattern Question)
    (a) Pancuronium   (b) Vecuronium
    (c) Atracurium   (d) Pipecuronium

38. Suxamethonium is: (Recent NEET Pattern Question)
    (a) Non depolarizing muscle relaxant
    (b) Depolarising muscle relaxant
    (c) Direct acting muscle relaxant
    (d) All of the above

39. Baclofen is: (Recent NEET Pattern Question)
    (a) Centrally acting muscle relaxant
    (b) Peripherally acting muscle relaxant
    (c) Both centrally and peripherally acting muscle relaxant
    (d) Direct acting muscle relaxant

40. True statement regarding depolarizing neuromuscular blocking drugs is: (Recent NEET Pattern Question)
    (a) The depolarized muscles fibres are unresponsive to other stimuli
    (b) Causes muscular fasciculations
    (c) Not reversed by neostigmine
    (d) All of the above

41. Shortest acting neuromuscular blocker is:
    (Recent NEET Pattern Question)
    (a) Gallamine   (b) Pancuronium
    (c) Succinylcholine   (d) d-TC

42. Long acting non-depolarizing muscle relaxants is:
    (Recent NEET Pattern Question)
    (a) Succinylcholine   (b) Mivacurium
    (c) Pancuronium   (d) Phenylephrine

43. In case of spasticity, the drug not used is:
    (Recent NEET Pattern Question)
    (a) Diazepam   (b) Baclofen
    (c) Tizanidine   (d) Amitriptyline

44. The drug inactivated in plasma by spontaneous non-enzymatic degradation is: (Recent NEET Pattern Question)
    (a) Atracurium   (b) Vecuronium
    (c) Pipecuronium   (d) Pancuronium

45. Which one of the following drugs is not a long acting neuromuscular blocking agent?
    (Recent NEET Pattern Question)
    (a) Doxacurium (b) Mivacurium
    (c) Pancuronium (d) Pipecuronium

46. The following is the feature of depolarizing blockade:
    (a) Tetanic fade *(Recent NEET Pattern Question)*
    (b) Post tetanic potentiation
    (c) Progression to dual blockade
    (d) Antagonism by anticholinesterases

47. Drug not acting on neuromuscular junction is:
    (Recent NEET Pattern Question)
    (a) Baclofen (b) Carisoprodol
    (c) Haloperidol (d) All of the above

48. Short acting non-depolarizing blocker is:
    (Recent NEET Pattern Question)
    (a) Rocuronium
    (b) Suxamethonium
    (c) Mivacurium
    (d) Pancuronium

49. In pseudocholinesterase deficiency, drug to be used cautiously is: *(Recent NEET Pattern Question)*
    (a) Barbiturate (b) Succinylcholine
    (c) Halothane (d) Gallamine

50. Mechanism of action of curare is:
    (Recent NEET Pattern Question)
    (a) Reducing end plate potential
    (b) Reducing presynaptic potential
    (c) Inhibits K^+ channels
    (d) Inhibits Na^+ channels

51. Baclofen is used in the treatment of:
    (Recent NEET Pattern Question)
    (a) Schizophrenia (b) Depression
    (c) Anxiety (d) Spasticity

52. Regarding muscle relaxants which one of the following is true? *(Recent NEET Pattern Question)*
    (a) Atracurium is contraindicated in renal failure
    (b) Pancuronium causes bradycardia
    (c) Cis-atracurium is a depolarizing muscle relaxant
    (d) Vecuronium induced muscle relaxation can be reversed by neostigmine

GENERAL ANAESTHESIA

53. A patient was schedule for surgery. Before giving anesthesia, he was administered glycopyrrolate. What is rationale of giving glycopyrrolate before anesthesia?
    (AIIMS Nov. 2019)
    (a) To allay anxiety (b) To decrease secretions
    (c) As inducing agent (d) For muscle relaxation

54. Injection of all of the following drugs is painful *except*:
    (NEET Pattern Question 2019)
    (a) Propofol (b) Etomidate
    (c) Ketamine (d) Methohexitone

55. Which intravenous anaesthetic agent does not cause cardiac depression? *(NEET Pattern Question 2019)*
    (a) Etomidate (b) Midazolam
    (c) Propofol (d) Thiopentone

56. Which of the following inhalational anaesthetic agent causes maximum respiratory irritation?
    (NEET Pattern Question 2019)
    (a) Enflurane (b) Halothane
    (c) Sevoflurane (d) Desflurane

57. Injection of all of the following drugs is painful *except*:
    (NEET Pattern Question 2019)
    (a) Propofol (b) Etomidate
    (c) Ketamine (d) Methohexitone

58. Which intravenous anaesthetic agent does not cause cardiac depression? *(NEET Pattern Question 2019)*
    (a) Etomidate (b) Midazolam
    (c) Propofol (d) Thiopentone

59. Which of the following inhalational anaesthetic agent causes maximum respiratory irritation?
    (NEET Pattern Question 2019)
    (a) Enflurane (b) Halothane
    (c) Sevoflurane (d) Desflurane

60. A female presents with placenta previa with active bleeding and blood pressure of 80/50 mm Hg and pulse rate of 140 bpm. The choice of anaesthesia for emergency cesarean section in this female is: *(AIIMS Nov 2015)*
    (a) General anaesthesia with intravenous propofol
    (b) General anaesthesia with intravenous ketamine
    (c) Spinal anaesthesia
    (d) Epidural anaesthesia

61. Color of oxygen cyclinder is: *(AIIMS Nov 2015)*
    (a) Black body with white shoulder
    (b) Black body with grey shoulder
    (c) Grey body with white shoulder
    (d) Grey body with black shoulder

62. Which of the following agents can be used in day care surgery? *(AIIMS May 2015)*
    (a) Fentanyl, midazolam and propofol
    (b) Morphine, midazolam and propofol
    (c) Midazolam, alfentanil and propofol
    (d) Morphine, diazepam and ketamine

63. Anaesthetic agent causing pain on intravenous administration is: *(AIIMS May 2015)*
    (a) Thiopentone (b) Propofol
    (c) Ketamine (d) Midazolam

64. Which of the following agents is used for day care surgery? *(AIIMS Nov 2014)*
    (a) Propofol (b) Thiopentone
    (c) Diazepam (d) Ketamine

65. The plane of surgical anesthesia during ether anesthesia is defined as: *(AIIMS May 2014)*
    (a) Loss of consciousness
    (b) Loss of consciousness to the onset of spontaneous respiration
    (c) From onset of regular respiration to cessation of spontaneous breathing
    (d) Absence of reflexes

66. Which of the following intravenous anesthetic agents is contraindicated in epileptic patients posted for general anesthesia? *(AIIMS May 2014)*
    (a) Ketamine
    (b) Thiopentone
    (c) Propofol
    (d) Midazolam

67. A patient with ruptured spleen is taken for laparotomy. His blood pressure is 80/50 and heart rate is 125/min. Induction agent of choice for this patient is: *(AIIMS May 2012)*
    (a) Sodium Thiopentone
    (b) Fentanyl
    (c) Ketamine
    (d) Halothane

68. Which of these can be safely stopped before an abdominal surgery? *(AI 2012)*
    (a) ACE inhibitors
    (b) Beta blocker
    (c) Statins
    (d) Steroids

69. Xenon anesthesia all are true *except*: *(AI 2012)*
    (a) Slow induction and recovery
    (b) Non explosive
    (c) Minimal cardiovascular side-effects
    (d) Low blood solubility

70. The following causes increased intra ocular pressure: *(Recent NEET Pattern Question)*
    (a) Thiopentone
    (b) Althesin
    (c) Ketamine
    (d) Barbiturate

71. Nitrous oxide is contraindicated in patients with pneumothorax, pneumopericardium or intestinal obstruction, because it: *(Recent NEET Pattern Question)*
    (a) Depresses an already compromised myocardium
    (b) Permits the use of limited FIO_2 only
    (c) Is less soluble than nitrogen
    (d) Causes the expansion of air filled body cavities

72. Anaesthesia contraindicated in volvulus of gut is: *(Recent NEET Pattern Question)*
    (a) Halothane
    (b) Nitrous oxide
    (c) Ketamine
    (d) Pancuronium

73. A 5 years old child is suffering from cyanotic heart disease. He is planned for corrective surgery. The induction agent of choice would be: *(Recent NEET Pattern Question)*
    (a) Thiopentone
    (b) Ketamine
    (c) Halothane
    (d) Midazolam

74. Which of the following induction agent produce cardiac stability? *(AIIMS May 2009)*
    (a) Ketamine
    (b) Etomidate
    (c) Propofol
    (d) Midazolam

75. Anaesthetic agent which is explosive in the presence of cautery: *(Recent NEET Pattern Question)*
    (a) Nitrous oxide
    (b) Ether
    (c) Trilene
    (d) Halothane

76. Best uterine relaxation is seen with: *(Recent NEET Pattern Question)*
    (a) Chloroform
    (b) Nitrous oxide
    (c) Ether
    (d) Halothane

77. Hallucinations are seen after .... anaesthesia: *(Recent NEET Pattern Question)*
    (a) Ketamine
    (b) Thiopentone
    (c) Fentanyl
    (d) Nitrous oxide

78. Anaesthetic that has a smooth induction is: *(Recent NEET Pattern Question)*
    (a) Diethyl ether
    (b) Isoflurane
    (c) N_2O
    (d) Halothane

79. Which of the following drugs are believed to be effective in the treatment of post operative shivering? *(Recent NEET Pattern Question)*
    (a) Ondansetron
    (b) Diclofenac sodium
    (c) Pethidine
    (d) Paracetamol

80. "MAC" of desflurane is: *(Recent NEET Pattern Question)*
    (a) 1.15
    (b) 2
    (c) 4
    (d) 6

81. Which of the following should be considered as the cause of generalized convulsions 20 minutes postoperatively? *(Recent NEET Pattern Question)*
    (a) Halothane
    (b) Enflurane
    (c) Isoflurane
    (d) Sevoflurane

82. Ketamine should be avoided in: *(Recent NEET Pattern Question)*
    (a) The presence of increased arterial pressure
    (b) Pregnancy
    (c) Hypovolemic shock
    (d) Asthmatic

83. The drug for OPD analgesia is: *(Recent NEET Pattern Question)*
    (a) Morphine
    (b) Pethidine
    (c) Fentanyl
    (d) Alfentanil

84. "Shivering" is observed in the early part of postoperative period due to: *(Recent NEET Pattern Question)*
    (a) Chloroform
    (b) Halothane
    (c) Trichloroethylene
    (d) Ether

85. Following accidental intra-arterial injection of thiopentone, which should not be done? *(Recent NEET Pattern Question)*
    (a) Remove the needle
    (b) Intra-arterial heparin
    (c) Intra-arterial papaverine
    (d) Do a stellate ganglion block

86. An anaesthetic agent with boiling temperature more than 75°C is: *(Recent NEET Pattern Question)*
    (a) Ether
    (b) Halothane
    (c) Cyclopropane
    (d) Methoxyflurane

87. True statement about sevoflurane is: *(Recent NEET Pattern Question)*
    (a) It is nephrotoxic at high doses
    (b) It has maximum risk of causing convulsions
    (c) It is cardiostable
    (d) It can cause fulminant hepatitis

88. Which of the following does not have analgesic action? *(Recent NEET Pattern Question)*
    (a) Ether
    (b) Ketamine
    (c) Halothane
    (d) Morphine

89. Induction agent of choice in day care surgery is: *(Recent NEET Pattern Question)*
    (a) Ketamine
    (b) Propofol
    (c) Methohexitone
    (d) Thiopentone sodium

Anaesthesia

90. True statements regarding halothane is:
    (Recent NEET Pattern Question)
    (a) Hepatitis occurs in susceptible individuals after repeated dose
    (b) It potentiates competitive neuromuscular blockers
    (c) Causes respiratory depression
    (d) All of the above

91. Which of the following agents is most commonly used to induce anaesthesia? *(Recent NEET Pattern Question)*
    (a) Thiopentone sodium (b) Methohexitone sodium
    (c) Propofol (d) Etomidate

92. All of the following are halogenated anaesthetic agents *except*: *(Recent NEET Pattern Question)*
    (a) Halothane (b) Propofol
    (c) Enflurane (d) Isoflurane

93. In raised ICT, anesthetic agent of choice is:
    (Recent NEET Pattern Question)
    (a) Enflurane (b) Isoflurane
    (c) Ketamine (d) Ether

94. Which anesthetic agent is contraindicated in epilepsy?
    (Recent NEET Pattern Question)
    (a) Xenon (b) Enflurane
    (c) Halothane (d) Ether

95. In patients with liver disease, anesthetic of choice is:
    (Recent NEET Pattern Question)
    (a) Halothane (b) Ether
    (c) Isoflurane (d) None

96. Dissociative anesthesia is seen on administration of:
    (Recent NEET Pattern Question)
    (a) Ether (b) Halothane
    (c) Enflurane (d) Ketamine

97. Profound analgesia is produced by which parenteral anesthetic? *(Recent NEET Pattern Question)*
    (a) Thiopental (b) Propofol
    (c) Ketamine (d) Etomidate

98. Thiopental sodium is administered intravenously as:
    (Recent NEET Pattern Question)
    (a) 25% solution (b) 2.5% solution
    (c) 0.25% solution (d) 0.025% solution

99. Which of the following increase the speed of induction with an inhalational agent?
    (a) Opiate pre-medication *(Recent NEET Pattern Question)*
    (b) Increased alveolar ventilation
    (c) Increased cardiac output
    (d) Reduced FIO_2

100. The recommended time for prophylactic antibiotic is:
     (Recent NEET Pattern Question)
     (a) 30 min prior to induction of anaesthesia
     (b) 15 min after the initiation of surgery
     (c) At the time of induction
     (d) At the time of skin incision

101. Trilene when used with sodalime causes:
     (Recent NEET Pattern Question)
     (a) Renal damage
     (b) ARDS
     (c) Myocardial depression
     (d) Reaction with rubber tubing of closed circuit

102. Drug used in day care anaesthesia is:
     (Recent NEET Pattern Question)
     (a) Propofol (b) Enflurane
     (c) Xenon (d) Thiopentone

103. Which opioid does not require kidney and liver for metabolism? *(Recent NEET Pattern Question)*
     (a) Remifentanil (b) Sufentanil
     (b) Alfentanil (d) Fentanyl

104. The term "balanced anaesthesia" has been given by:
     (Recent NEET Pattern Question)
     (a) Simpson (b) Fischer
     (c) Lundy (d) Mortan

105. Regarding propofol, which one of the following is false?
     (Recent NEET Pattern Question)
     (a) It is used as an intravenous induction agent
     (b) It causes severe vomiting
     (c) It is painful on injecting intravenously
     (d) It has no muscle relaxant property

106. Ketamine produces: *(Recent NEET Pattern Question)*
     (a) Emergence delirium
     (b) Pain on injection
     (c) Bronchoconstriciton
     (d) Depression of cardiovascular system

107. Which one of the following inhalational anesthetics is most likely to cause fluoride ion nephrotoxicity?
     (Recent NEET Pattern Question)
     (a) Methoxyflurane (b) Enflurane
     (c) Halothane (d) Isoflurane

108. Pin index of oxygen is which one of the following:
     (Recent NEET Pattern Question)
     (a) 2, 5 (b) 3, 5
     (c) 1, 5 (d) 3, 6

109. All of the following are intravenous anesthetic induction agents *except*: *(Recent NEET Pattern Question)*
     (a) Thiopentone sodium (b) Ketamine
     (c) Etomidate (d) Bupivacaine

Explanations

1. **Ans. (c) It is given orally for treatment of cardiac arrhythmias** *(Ref: Katzung 12th/e p453, 457, 458)*
   - All local anaesthetics (LA) are weak bases. These drugs act by penetrating the axonal membrane (in unionized form) and **blocking the voltage gated sodium channels from within (in ionized form).** Resting sodium channels are less sensitive to block than active and inactive channels.
   - Vasoconstrictors like **adrenaline can prolong the duration of action and decrease the systemic toxicity.**
   - **Lignocaine is the most commonly used LA** and is **the drug of choice for ventricular tachycardia.** However because of very high first pass metabolism, it is not effective orally.
   - All LA can cause cardiotoxicity and neurotoxicity. Bupivacaine is most cardiotoxic LA.

2. **Ans. (c) 7 mg/kg** *(Ref: Goodman and Gilman 12th/e p576)*
   - For normal healthy adults, the individual maximum recommended dose of lignocaine HCl with epinephrine should not exceed **7 mg/kg** of body weight, and in general it is recommended that the maximum total dose not exceed 500 mg.
   - When used without epinephrine the maximum individual dose should not exceed **4.5 mg/kg** of body weight, and in general it is recommended that the maximum total dose does not exceed 300 mg.
   - For **intravenous** regional anaesthesia, the dose administered should not exceed **4mg/kg** in adults.

3. **Ans. (c) Lignocaine** *(Ref: Ajay yadav 2nd/e p110)*

   - Bupivacaine is most cardiotoxic local anaesthetic.
   - At toxic doses, local anaesthetics can result in CNS (convulsions) or CVS (hypotension, bradycardia, arrhythmias) symptoms.
   - Diazepam is used to treat convulsions. If not responding, thiopentone may be used.
   - Arrhythmias should be promptly treated using bretylium, amiodarone, disopyramide, magnesium sulphate, esmolol or sotalol.
   - Lignocaine should be avoided as anti-arrhythmic because it can exacerbate the CNS toxicity.
   - In refractory arrhythmias, intravenous lipid emulsion (like intralipid) has been found to be extremly useful.
   - Bupivacaine induced cardiotoxicity is enhanced by acidosis, hypercarbia and hypoxemia.

4. **Ans. (c) Cocaine** *(Ref: Katzung 11th/e p448)*
   All local anaesthetics cause vasodilation *except* cocaine. It blocks reuptake of nor-adrenaline and result in sympathetic overactivity. Therefore, cocaine can cause hypertension and cardiac arrhythmias.

5. **Ans. (a) Procaine** *(Ref: Katzung 11th/e p441)*

6. **Ans. (d) It produces methemoglobinemia** *(Ref: Katzung 11th/e p448-450)*
   - Bupivacaine is the most cardiotoxic local anaesthetic, therefore should never be given intravenously. Most common ECG findings in patients with bupivacaine toxicity are slow idioventricular rhythm with broad QRS complexes and eventually electromechanical dissociation.
   - Methemoglobinemia is caused by prilocaine and not by bupivacaine.

7. **Ans. (b) Affecting the Na⁺ channels** *(Ref: KDT 8th/e p388, 389)*

8. **Ans. (b) Blocks the influx of sodium into the cell** *(Ref: KDT 8th/e p388,389)*
   LA block nerve conduction by inhibiting Na⁺ entry during upstroke of action potential.

9. **Ans. (a) Less cardiotoxic than lignocaine** *(Ref: KDT 8th/e p393)*

10. **Ans. (a) Seepage of CSF** *(Ref: KDT 8th/e p396)*

11. **Ans. (b) More cardiotoxic than lignocaine** *(Ref: Katzung 11/e p448)*

12. **Ans. (d) 5%** *(Ref: KDT 8th/e p396)*

13. **Ans. (a) Activated state** *(Ref: Katzung 11th/e p443)*

14. **Ans. (a) Dibucaine** *(Ref: KDT 8th/e p393)*

15. **Ans. (c) 1:200,000** *(Ref: KDT 8th/e p150,389)*

16. **Ans. (b) Lidocaine 2.5% + Prilocaine 2.5%** *(Ref: KDT 8th/e p392)*

17. **Ans. (c) Constricted pupils** *(Ref: KDT 8th/e p391)*

18. **Ans. (b) Pain is relieved in standing position** *(Ref: Evidence-Based obstetric Anesthesia p75)*
    - Post-dural-puncture headache (PDPH) or post-lumbar-puncture headache occurs 12-24 hours after dural puncture.
    - It presents with headache (occipito frontal) and nausea that typically worsens when the patient assumes upright position.
    - Incidence is higher in younger patients.

19. **Ans. (b) Lignocaine** *(Ref: KDT 8th/e p392)*

20. **Ans. (a) Neostigmine** *(Ref: KDT 8th/e p122)*
    - Neostigmine is a water soluble reversible anti-cholinesterase. It is used to reverse muscle paralysis induced by competitive neuromuscular blockers
    - Carbachol is a parasympathomimetic agent that mimics the effect of acetylcholine on both the muscarinic and nicotinic receptors. This drug is used to induce miosis in patients with closed angle glaucoma.
    - Succinyl choline is a depolarizing muscle relaxant.
    - Physostigmine is a lipid soluble reversible anti-cholinesterase. It can cross blood brain barrier and result in central adverse effects. It is therefore not used in reversal of action of muscle relaxants.

21. **Ans. (d) Releases less histamine** *(Ref: Goodman and Gilman 13th/e p182)*

- Both atracurium and cis-atracurium are non-depolarizing neuromuscular blockers.
- Both of these are intermediate acting agents (both have same duration of action).
- Both of these agents are cardiostable
- Atracurium has faster onset of action as compared to cis-atracurium.
- Both are eliminated by Hoffman's elimination. Atracurium is also metabolized by liver to some extent and result in production of a metabolite laudanosine that can cause CNS toxicity including seizures. On the other hand cis-atracurium is almost completely eliminated by Hoffman's elimination and produce negligible laudanosine.
- Major advantage of cis-atracurium over atracurium is that the former do not release histamine.

22. **Ans. (a) Competitive inhibitor of ACh receptors** *(Ref: Goodman and Gilman 13th/e p179)*
D-tubocurarine is a skeletal muscle relaxant that acts by competitive inhibition of NM receptors at neuromuscular junction.

23. **Ans. (c) Tizanidine** *(Ref: KDT 8th/e p384)*

24. **Ans. (c) Competitive antagonist of acetylcholine receptor** *(Ref: KDT 8th/e p374)*

25. **Ans. (a) Atracurium** *(Ref: KDT 8th/e p380)*
- Atracurium and cis-atracurium undergo Hoffmann's elimination (spontaneous non-enzymatic molecular rearrangement) and are the agents of choice for patients with hepatic or renal insufficiency.
- Atracurium is metabolized to laudanosine that is responsible for seizures. Cis-atracurium is relatively safe in this regard.

26. **Ans. (b) Dantrolene** *(Ref: Katzung 13th/e p467-468)*
Dantrolene is a directly acting muscle relaxant. It does not act at neuromuscular junction

Neuromuscular blockers

Depolarising	Non-depolarising
SCh	Tubocurarine
	Atracurium
	Cis-atracurium
	Mivacurium
	Pancuronium
	Vecuronium
	Pipecuronium

27. **Ans. (b) Atracurium** *(Ref: KDT 8th/e p380)*
Atracurium is eliminated by Hoffman's elimination. It means it neither require liver for metabolism, nor kidney for excretion. Its molecules spontaneously rearrange to make it inactive. Thus it is safest muscle relaxant in a patient with liver and kidney disease.

28. **Ans. (b) Fingers** *(Ref: KDT 8th/e p376)*
- Tubocurarine is a Non-depolarizing muscle relaxant (NDMR). The order of relaxation of muscles with NDMR like d-Tubocurarine is
- Fingers, Eye > Limbs> Neck> Trunk> Respiratory

29. **Ans. (c) Diazepam** *(Ref: KDT 8th/e p381)*

Diazepam possesses following activities:
• Muscle relaxing
• Anticonvulsant
• Antianxiety
• Sedative-hypnotic

30. **Ans. (c) Rocuronium** *(Ref: Pharmacology for Nurse Anaesthesiology/110)*
- Rocuronium causes pain on injection. It can be minimized by alkalinizing the solution.
- Propofol is also responsible for pain on injection
- Remember, post-operative muscular pain is caused by succinylcholine and post-operative muscle rigidity is caused by fentanyl group of drugs.

31. **Ans. (b) Hyperkalemia** *(Ref: Katzung 11th/e p460)*
Succinylcholine can cause hyperkalemia especially in patients with nerve and muscle disorders. Therefore it is contraindicated in patients with nerve diseases (like paraplegia, hemiplegia and Guillain barre syndrome) and muscle diseases (muscular dystrophy, myasthenia gravis, crush injury, burns and rhabdomyolysis).

32. **Ans. (a) Inhibiting nicotinic receptors at myoneural junction** *(Ref: Katzung 10/e p429; KDT 8th/e p374)*
D-tubocurarine is a skeletal muscle relaxant that acts by competitive inhibition of NM receptors at neuron-muscular junction.

33. **Ans. (d) Suxamethonium** *(Ref: Katzung 11th/e p454)*
Suxamethonium is the other name of succinylcholine. It is the shortest acting muscle relaxant due to metabolism by pseudocholinesterase

34. **Ans. (a) Atracurium** *(Ref: KDT 8th/e p380)*

35. **Ans. (d) Quinidine** *(Ref: Clinical Anesthesiology by Murray and Morgan/189; KDT 8th/e p381)*
Non-depolarizing blockade is potentiated by:

Hypothermia	Respiratory acidosis
Hypokalemia	Hypocalcemia
Hypermagnesemia	Neonatal period
Aminoglycosides, Tetracyclines, Polymyxin B	Quinine, Lignocaine, CCBs, Procainamide
Trimethaphan	Dantrolene
MgSO$_4$	Local Anaesthetics
Ketamine	

36. **Ans. (a) Chloramphenicol** *(Ref: KDT 8th/e p381)*

Drugs causing curare like effect are:
• Aminoglycosides
• Polypeptide antibiotics:
– Polymyxin B
– Bacitracin
– Colistin
– Tyrothricin
• Tetracycline
• Clindamycin, lincomycin

37. **Ans. (b) Vecuronium** *(Ref: KDT 8th/e p379)*
It does not cause ganglion blockade or histamine release and is having good cardiovascular stability.

38. **Ans. (b) Depolarising muscle relaxant** *(Ref: KDT 8th/e p373)*

39. **Ans. (a) Centrally acting muscle relaxant** *(Ref: Katzung 11th/e p463)*

40. Ans. (d) All of the above (Ref: Katzung 11th/e p457)
41. Ans. (c) Succinylcholine (Ref: KDT 8th/e p379)
42. Ans. (c) Pancuronium (Ref: KDT 8th/e p379)
43. Ans. (d) Amitrypityline (Ref: Katzung 11/e p462-464)
44. Ans. (a) Atracurium (Ref: KDT 8th/e p380)
45. Ans. (b) Mivacurium (Ref: KDT 8th/e p380)
46. Ans. (c) Progression to dual blockade
    (Ref: Katzung 11th/e p457; KDT 8th/e p375)
47. Ans. (d) All of the above (Ref: KDT 8th/e p373)
48. Ans. (c) Mivacurium (Ref: KDT 8th/e p380)
49. Ans. (b) Succinylcholine (Ref: KDT 8th/e p379)
50. Ans. (a) Reducing end plate potential (Ref: KDT 8th/e p374)
51. Ans. (d) Spasticity (Ref: KDT 8th/e p384)
52. Ans. (d) Vecuronium induced muscle relaxation can be reversed by neostigmine (Ref: KDT 8th/e p379)
53. Ans. (b) To decrease secretions (Ref: KDT 8th/e p413,414)
    - Preanesthetic medication refers to the use of drugs before anesthesia to make it safe and less unpleasant.
    - When inhalation anesthetic agents are given, they inhibit the ciliary function resulting in accumulation of secretions in the respiratory pathway. Therefore anti-cholinergic drugs like atropine or glycopyrrolate are used as preanesthetic medication for their anti-secretory action.
    - Glycopyrrolate is twice as potent and longer acting quaternary anti-muscarinic which does not produce central effects. Anti-secretory action is more marked than atropine and tachycardia is less marked. It acts rapidly when given IV and is the preferred anti-muscarinic in anesthetic practice.
54. Ans. (c) Ketamine (Ref: Goodman and Gilman 13th/e p391)
    - Ketamine is a strong analgesic drug and is water soluble. Its injection is not painful.
    - Propofol and etomidate solutions has to be made in oil due to poor water solubility, so these injections are quite painful.
    - Methohexitone can cause hyperalgesia.
55. Ans. (a) Etomidate (Ref: Goodman and Gilman 13th/e p391)
    Etomidate
    - It does not interfere with cardiovascular functions; therefore is **the agent of choice for aneurysm surgeries and cardiac disease**.
    - It causes minimal respiratory depression.
    - Maximum incidence of **nausea and vomiting** is seen with the use of this agent.
    - It can also produce **myoclonus**.
    - Injection of etomidate is **painful** and may result in thrombophlebitis.
56. Ans. (d) Desflurane (Ref: Goodman and Gilman 13th/e p395)
    Desflurane
    - It has minimum blood gas partition coefficient and therefore is the **fastest** inducing agent.
    - It has **very high vapor pressure**. Its boiling point is 23°C; therefore it boils at room temperature. It requires special vaporizers due to this property.
    - It produces cardiovascular effects similar to isoflurane except coronary steal phenomenon.
    - Induction with desflurane is unpleasant due to respiratory irritation. It can lead to coughing, breath holding and laryngospasm.
    - It can **also be used in day care surgery**.
57. Ans. (c) Ketamine (Ref: Goodman and Gilman 13th/e p391)
    - Ketamine is a strong analgesic drug and is water soluble. Its injection is not painful.
    - Propofol and etomidate solutions has to be made in oil due to poor water solubility, so these injections are quite painful.
    - Methohexitone can cause hyperalgesia.
58. Ans. (a) Etomidate (Ref: Goodman and Gilman 13th/e p391)
    Etomidate
    - It does not interfere with cardiovascular functions; therefore is **the agent of choice for aneurysm surgeries and cardiac disease**.
    - It causes minimal respiratory depression.
    - Maximum incidence of **nausea and vomiting** is seen with the use of this agent.
    - It can also produce **myoclonus**.
    - Injection of etomidate is **painful** and may result in thrombophlebitis.
59. Ans. (d) Desflurane (Ref: Goodman and Gilman 13th/e p395)
    Desflurane
    - It has minimum blood gas partition coefficient and therefore is the **fastest** inducing agent.
    - It has **very high vapour pressure**. Its boiling point is 23°C; therefore it boils at room temperature. It requires special vaporizers due to this property.
    - It produces cardiovascular effects similar to isoflurane except coronary steal phenomenon.
    - Induction with desflurane is unpleasant due to respiratory irritation. It can lead to coughing, breath holding and laryngospasm.
    - It can **also be used in day care surgery**.
60. Ans. (b) General anaesthesia with intravenous ketamine
    (Ref: Williams Obstetrics 24th/e p518; Morgan 4th/e p197-199)
    The patient is presenting with shock, so spinal anaesthesia cannot be used. Among the general anaesthetics, ketamine is drug of choice for induction in patients with low blood pressure.
61. Ans. (a) Black body with white shoulder (Ref: Anaesthetic Equipments & Procedures, Practical Approach/p37, 38;)
    The color of a medical oxygen cylinder is a black body with a white shoulder.

Medical Gas	Colour
Oxygen	Black body with white shoulder
Carbon dioxide	Grey
Nitrous oxide	Blue
Cyclopropane	Orange
Helium	Brown
Entonox	Blue body with white shoulder

62. Ans. (c) Midazolam, alfentanil and propofol

Drugs used for day care surgery are	
Dr	Desflurane
Manmohan	Midazolam
Singh	Sevoflurane
Is	Isoflurane
A	Alfentanil
Prime	Propofol
Minister	Mivacurium

63. Ans. (b) Propofol *(Ref: Katzung 12th/e p431)*
Propofol is highly lipid soluble. Its solution is made in oil (oily liquid employed as 1% emulsion), thus it is painful on injection.

64. Ans. (a) Propofol *(Ref: Katzung 12th/e p440)*
Propofol is drug of choice for day care surgery.

65. Ans. (c) From onset of regular respiration to cessation of spontaneous breathing *(Ref: KDT 8th/e p406)*
The plane of surgical anesthesia during ether anesthesia is defined as from onset of regular respiration to cessation of spontaneous breathing.

Guedel's Stages of Anesthesia
- Guedel described four stages with ether anesthesia, dividing the stage III into four planes.

I: Stage of analgesia
- It starts from beginning of anesthetic inhalation and lasts up to the loss of consciousness.
- Pain is progressively abolished.
- Patient remains conscious, can hear and see, and feels a dream-like state; amnesia develops by the end of this stage.
- Reflexes and respiration remain normal.
- Though some minor operations can be carried out during this stage, it is rather difficult to maintain. The use is thus limited to short procedures.

II: Stage of delirium
- It lasts from loss of consciousness to the beginning of regular respiration.
- Apparent excitement is seen – patient may shout, struggle and hold his breath.
- Muscle tone increases.
- Jaws are tightly closed
- Breathing is jerky.
- Vomiting, involuntary micturition or defecation may occur.
- Heart rate and BP may rise and pupils dilate due to sympathetic stimulation.
- No stimulus should be applied or operative procedure carried out during this stage.
- This stage is inconspicuous in modern anesthesia.

III: Stage of surgical anesthesia
- It extends from onset of regular respiration to cessation of spontaneous breathing.
- This has been divided into four planes, which may be distinguished as:
  - Plane I: Roving eyeballs
  - Plane II: Loss of corneal and laryngeal reflexes
  - Plane III: Pupil starts dilating and light reflex is lost
  - Plane IV: Intercostal paralysis, shallow abdominal respiration, dilated pupil

IV: Stage of medullary paralysis
- It lasts from cessation of spontaneous breathing to failure of circulation and death.
- Pupil is widely dilated, muscles are totally flabby, pulse is thready or imperceptible and BP is very low.

66. Ans. (a) Ketamine *(Ref: Morgan 4th/e p197-199)*
Ketamine should be avoided in patients with history of seizures as it further increases ICP and also causes delirium and hallucinations.

Contraindications of Ketamine:
- Head injury, intracranial space occupying lesion, eye injury (increases ICT, IOT).
- Ischemic heart disease, vascular aneurysm and hypertension (increases myocardial oxygen demand and blood pressure.
- Psychiatric diseases and drug addicts (more incidence of hallucination and emergence reaction).

67. Ans. (c) Ketamine *(Ref: Goodman and Gilman 12th/e p538-39)*
Ketamine increases all pressures (blood pressure, intracranial tension, intraocular pressure) in the body. It is therefore intravenous anaesthetic of choice for shock (increases blood pressure).

68. Ans. (a) ACE inhibitors *(Ref: CMDT 2014/45-47)*
- All antihypertensives should be continued in perioperative period except ACE inhibitors, Angiotensin receptor blockers and diuretics. ACE inhibitors and ARBs should be stopped 24 hours before surgery to prevent intraoperative hypotension. Diuretics should be stopped once the patient is kept NPO (Nil per oral) to prevent intraoperative volume depletion and electrolyte abnormalities.
- Statins should be continued if the patient is taking them.
- Corticosteroid therapy in excess of prednisone 5 mg/day or equivalent for more than five days in the 30 days preceding surgery might predispose patients to acute adrenal insufficiency in the perioperative period. Therefore, the recommendation is to continue a patient's baseline steroid dose and supplement it with stress-dose steroids tailored to the severity of operative stress.

69. Ans. (a) Slow induction and recovery
(Ref: Goodman and Gilman 12th/e p547-548)
Xenon is very close to the 'ideal agent'.

Advantages of Xenon Anesthesia

- Inert (probably nontoxic to liver and kidney with no metabolism)
- Minimal effect on CVS function
- Lowest blood solubility (Lowest blood gas partition coefficient) therefore rapid induction and recovery.
- Does not trigger malignant hyperthermia
- Environmental friendly
- Non-explosive.

70. Ans. (c) Ketamine *(Ref: Goodman and Gilman 12/e p538)*

71. Ans. (d) Causes the expansion of air filled body cavities
(Ref: Goodman and Gilman 12/e p547)
N_2O use is contraindicated in pneumothorax and volvulus because it may lead to development of high pressure in the closed cavities in the body (like obstructed loop of bowel, intraocular air bubble, a pulmonary bulla, pneumothorax, obstructed middle ear, air embolus, intracranial air and pneumoperitoneum).

72. Ans. (b) Nitrous oxide *(Ref: Goodman and Gilman 12/e p547)*

73. Ans. (b) Ketamine *(Ref: Ajay Yadav 2/e p215)*

74. Ans. (b) Etomidate *(Ref: Katzung 11/e p437; KDT 8th/e p410)*

- 'Major advantage of etomidate over other intravenous anaesthetics is that it causes minimum cardiovascular and respiratory depression.'
- Propofol has greatest negative inotropic action among all intravenous anaesthetics.
- Ketamine has cardiostimulatory properties and can cause hypertension.
- Midazolam is not used as an inducing agent.

75. **Ans. (b) Ether**
    (Ref: Goodman & Gilman 11th/e p341; KDT 8th/e p405)
    Ether is an explosive agent and should not be used with cautery.

76. **Ans. (d) Halothane**
    (Ref: Katzung 10th/e p405; KDT 8th/e p407)
    Halogenated inhalational anaesthetic agents like halothane are powerful tocolytic agents. Halothane is anaesthetic of choice for internal version and manual removal of placenta.

77. **Ans. (a) Ketamine** *(Ref: Katzung 10th/e p409; KDT 8th/e p411)*

78. **Ans. (d) Halothane**
    (Ref: Katzung 10th/e p404; KDT 8th/e p407)
    Halothane and sevoflurane have smooth induction, so these are preferred agents for anaesthesia in children.

79. **Ans. (c) Pethidine**
    (Ref: Anaesthesiology by Longnecker/1485; KDT 8th/e p503)
    Pethidine is most effective drug for treatment of post-operative shivering. Other drugs that can be used for this purpose are clonidine, doxapram, ketanserin and alfentanil.

80. **Ans. (d) 6**
    (Ref: Anaesthesiology by Longnecker/744; KDT 8th/e p405)

81. **Ans. (b) Enflurane** *(Ref: Anaesthesiology by Longnecker/761; KDT 8th/e p407)*
    Enflurane is known to produce seizures.

82. **Ans. (a) The presence of increased arterial pressure**
    (Ref: Katzung 11th/e p437)

83. **Ans. (d) Alfentanil** *(Ref: Katzung 11th/e p546)*

84. **Ans. (b) Halothane** *(Ref: Ajay yadav 2nd/e p61)*
    Postoperative shivering (halothane shakes) and hypothermia is maximum with halothane. Pethidine is used for treatment of this condition.

85. **Ans. (a) Remove the needle** *(Ref: Ajay yadav 2nd/e p73)*
    Treatment of accidental intra-arterial injection of thiopentone is:

- Immediately stop further injection.
- Leave the needle at site.
- Inject heparin through this needle.
- Inject papaverine through this needle.
- If vasodilators like papaverine are not available, xylocaine can be used.
- Brachial plexus or stellate ganglion block should be done to relieve vasospasm.

86. **Ans. (d) Methoxyflurane**
    (Ref: Anaesthesiology by Longnecker 2008/777)
    Boiling point of methoxyflurane is 104.7°C whereas other fluorinated inhalational anaesthetics have boiling point between 50°C and 60°C (except desflurane: 22.9°C).

87. **Ans. (a) It is nephrotoxic at high doses**
    (Ref: Goodman & Gilman 11th/e p360)

- Sevoflurane is a general anaesthetic used by inhalational route.
- It is very good agent for children and asthmatic patients.
- It can produce dose dependent hypotension and decrease in cardiac output.
- It high doses, it can release fluoride resulting in nephrotoxicity. Also, it can interact with soda lime (in closed circuit) to produce nephrotoxic, compound A.
- It is not known to cause hepatotoxicity.
- Enflurane has maximum potential to induce seizures.

88. **Ans. (c) Halothane** *(Ref: KDT 8th/e p407)*
    Halothane and newer flourinated inhalation anaesthetic agent are devoid of analgesic property.

89. **Ans. (b) Propofol** *(Ref: KDT 8th/e p410)*

90. **Ans. (d) All of the above** *(Ref: Katzung 11th/e p432,461)*

91. **Ans. (a) Thiopentone sodium** *(Ref: Katzung 11th/e p434)*

92. **Ans. (b) Propofol** *(Ref: KDT 8th/e p406,407,409)*

93. **Ans. (b) Isoflurane** *(Ref: KDT 8th/e p407)*

94. **Ans. (b) Enflurane** *(Ref: KDT 8th/e p407)*

95. **Ans. (c) Isoflurane** *(Ref: KDT 8th/e p407)*

96. **Ans. (d) Ketamine** *(Ref: KDT 8th/e p411)*

97. **Ans. (c) Ketamine** *(Ref: KDT 8th/e p411)*

98. **Ans. (b) 2.5% solution** *(Ref: Morgan 4th/e p187)*

99. **Ans. (b) Increased alveolar ventilation**
    (Ref: Katzung 11th/e p427)

100. **Ans. (a) 30 min prior to induction of anaesthesia**
     (Ref: Katzung 11th/e p898)
- Antibiotic should be present in adequate concentration at the operative site before incision and throughout the procedure.
- Parenteral agents should be administered during the interval begining 60 minutes before incision; administration up to the time of incision is preferred.

101. **Ans. (b) ARDS** *(Ref: KK Sharma 2nd/e p122)*

102. **Ans. (a) Propofol** *(Ref: KDT 8th/e p409-410)*

103. **Ans. (a) Remifentanil** *(Ref: KK Sharma 2nd/e p440)*

104. **Ans. (c) Lundy** *(Ref: Goodman Gilman 12th/e p528)*
     Term 'balanced anaesthesia' was introduced by Lundy in 1926.

105. **Ans. (b) It causes severe vomiting** *(Ref: KDT 8th/e p410)*

106. **Ans. (a) Emergence delirium** *(Ref: KDT 8th/e p411)*

107. **Ans. (a) Methoxyflurane**
     (Ref: Nurse Anaesthesia by John J. Nagelhout p77)

108. **Ans. (a) 2, 5** *(Ref: KDT 7/e p513)*

109. **Ans. (d) Bupivacaine** *(Ref: KDT 8th/e p392)*

CHAPTER 9

Hematology

HAEMATINICS

These are the agents required for the formation of blood and treatment of anemia. Main haematinics include iron, folic acid and vitamin B_{12}. Other substances like copper, pyridoxine etc. are also required in small quantities for the formation of blood.

IRON

- Daily requirement of iron is:

Adult male	1 mg
Menstruating female	2 mg
Pregnant female	3-5 mg

- Liver, egg yolk, beans and dry fruits are good source of iron whereas **milk and its products are poor sources**.
- Iron is **absorbed** mostly **in the duodenum** in the **ferrous form (Fe^{2+})**. Heme contains the iron in ferrous form and most of the inorganic iron is in ferric form (Fe^{3+}). This must be reduced to ferrous form for absorption. Thus reducing substances like **ascorbic acid** and also gastric acid **(HCl) increases the absorption**. On the other hand, substances like *alkalies, phosphates, phytates and tetracyclines decrease the absorption*.
- After absorption, iron can either be stored as ferritin or it is transported with transferrin to be utilized in the formation of blood. When there is **excess of iron** in the body, it combines with apoferritin to form **ferritin,** which remains stored in the mucosal cells and is removed from the body when these cells are shed. In case of **iron deficiency, number of transferrin receptors increase** on erythropoietic cells (so, iron selectively goes to these cells) resulting in brisk erythropoiesis.
- Iron is used for *prophylaxis or treatment of* iron deficiency anemia (*microcytic hypochromic anemia*). It can be given by oral route or parenteral route. **Parenteral route (IV, IM) is indicated only when oral iron is not tolerated**, not absorbed or along with erythropoietin. *Rate of hematopoietic response with parenteral iron is not faster* than that with optimal doses of oral iron therapy.
- Oral preparations include ferrous sulphate, gluconate, succinate etc. **Ferrous sulphate** contains **20% elemental iron**. For treatment of iron deficiency, the dosage recommended is 200 mg elemental iron daily that can be obtained by giving 1000 mg of ferrous sulphate in three divided doses providing around 60 mg elemental iron per dose [maximum tolerated dose]. Iron *absorption increases in response to low iron stores* or increased iron requirements. The *reticulocyte count should begin to increase in two weeks* and peak in 4 weeks. This suggests good response to treatment. Treatment with oral iron should be **continued for 3–6 months**. This will correct the anemia and *replenish iron stores*.
- **Rise of** hemoglobin level of blood by **0.5-1 g/dL per week** is considered **adequate response** to iron therapy. For prophylaxis of iron deficiency, 200 mg ferrous sulphate once daily is enough. In pregnancy, iron should be started in the **second trimester**.
- Major *adverse effects* of oral iron that result in poor compliance are gastrointestinal problems like *epigastric pain, nausea, vomiting and metallic taste,* etc. These are **related to elemental iron content in the iron preparation**.
- **Ferric citrate has the capacity to bind phosphate and form non-absorbable complex. It is indicated to control hyperphosphatemia in patients with chronic kidney disease on dialysis. It is given orally.**
- **Parenteral** iron preparations are **iron-dextran and iron-sorbitol-citrate**. Former can be given by either IV or IM routes whereas the **latter should not be used intravenously** because it will cause rapid saturation of transferrin receptors, which can cause iron toxicity due to more free iron. **Total iron requirement** can be calculated by the formula:

  $$4.3 \times \text{Body weight (kg)} \times \text{Hemoglobin deficit (g/dL)}$$

  This formula includes iron required for replenishment of stores also.
- Intramuscular injections are usually given by **z-track technique** to avoid staining and pigmentation of skin **(Fig. 9.1)**. Major problem with parenteral route is pain at injection site and pigmentation of skin.

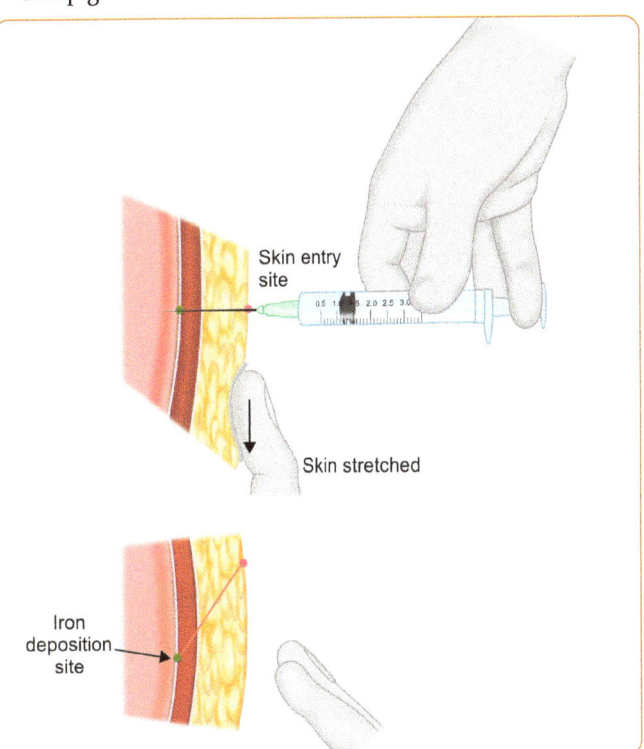

FIG. 9.1: Z-track technique.

Iron-dextran	Iron-sorbitol-citrate
1. Can be given IV or IM	• Only IM
2. Not excreted	• About 30% excreted in urine
3. Absorbed through lymphatics	• Absorbed directly in the circulation
4. Not bound to transferrin	Not bound to transferrin

Iron Poisoning

- Acute iron poisoning can occur in children due to accidental intake of large number of the iron tablets. The **antidote** of acute iron poisoning is **desferrioxamine**. It is given by IM injection. DTPA and calcium disodium EDTA may also be used but dimercaprol **(BAL) is contraindicated** because its complex with iron is itself toxic.
- For **chronic iron overload**, as occurs in thalassemia patients, oral chelating agent like **deferiprone** is preferred.

FOLIC ACID

It consists of pteridine, para-aminobenzoic acid (PABA) and glutamic acid. Dietary folic acid is in the form of polyglutamates and these are cleaved off in the intestine before absorption. Maximum **absorption** occurs in **jejunum**. It is *reduced to first* dihydrofolic acid (*DHFA*) and *then to* tetrahydrofolic acid (*THFA*), which is methylated *to form methyl tetrahydrofolate*. Latter compound is the main form in which it is transported in blood. **THFA** participates in many **one carbon transfer** reactions. Important among these are conversion of **homocysteine to methionine** (which releases THFA from its methylated form) with vitamin B_{12} as the intermediary carrier **and generation of thymidylate**.

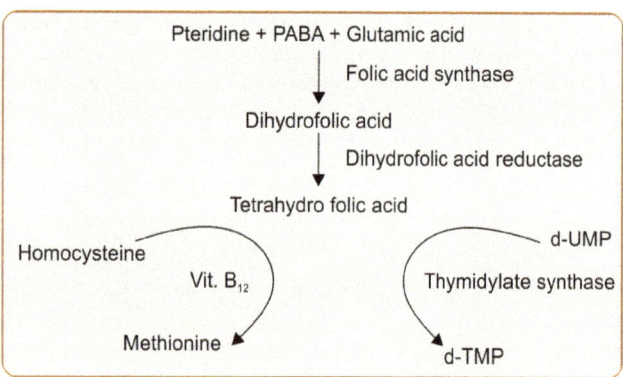

- **Deficiency** of folic acid results in **megaloblastic anemia** that is indistinguishable from that due to vitamin B_{12} deficiency.
- Main uses of folic acid are in the treatment of megaloblastic anemia due to folic acid deficiency (dietary, due to malabsorption, phenytoin therapy, chronic alcoholism etc.). It is also indicated in **pregnancy** to **prevent neural tube defects** in the fetus. It should be started as soon as the pregnancy is diagnosed.
- **Leucovorin** (folinic acid, formyl THFA or citrovorum factor) can be used to **prevent the toxicity of methotrexate**.

VITAMIN B_{12}

- This vitamin *contains cobalt and cyanocobalamin and hydroxocobalamin are the two forms that are present in diet*.
- It is present in animal foods (liver, kidney, meet, cheese, egg yolk etc.) and the **only vegetable source is legumes** (microorganisms in the nodules synthesize it).

- Vitamin B_{12} is released from the foods with the help of gastric acid and then it combines with intrinsic factor (secreted by stomach), and the combination is **absorbed in terminal ileum**. After absorption, it is transported in the blood in combination with transcobalamin II. **Active forms** of this vitamin are **deoxyadenosyl-cobalamin** and **methyl-cobalamin**.
- It serves several functions like **conversion of homocysteine to methionine** (folic acid is also required) which is essential for one carbon transfer reactions, **conversion of methylmalonyl CoA to succinyl CoA** (this reaction is required for myelin formation and methylcobalamin is utilized, folic acid is not required for this reaction) and also conversion of **methionine to S-adenosyl methionine**.
- **Deficiency** of vitamin B_{12} leads to **megaloblastic anemia** which is indistinguishable from folic acid deficiency. **Deficiency** also have manifestations related to loss of myelin like **subacute combined degeneration of spinal cord** (symptoms of *lesions of posterior column* like loss of vibration and proprioception, paraesthesia, depressed stretch reflexes and mental changes like poor memory and hallucinations, etc.)
- Vitamin B_{12} is used for **treatment** of megaloblastic anemia (**IM or SC for pernicious anemia** due to deficiency of intrinsic factor and **orally for other causes**), **for correcting neurological abnormalities in diabetics** etc. (methylcobalamin is used) and also for treatment of **tobacco amblyopia** (*hydroxocobalamin is used*, it combines with cyanide to form cyanocobalamin).
- If the cause of megaloblastic anemia is not known, **folic acid alone should not be given** because it will correct the blood picture of anemia but neurological deficits due to vitamin B_{12} deficiency may be aggravated (due to diversion of small amount of B_{12} left, in correcting anemia instead of utilization in myelin formation).

HEMATOPOIETIC GROWTH FACTORS

- Apart from nutritional agents, certain endogenous substances are required for proper hematopoiesis; these substances are known as growth factors. **Growth factor** for **RBCs** is **erythropoietin**, for **WBCs**, it is granulocyte colony stimulating factor (**G-CSF**) and granulocyte monocyte colony stimulating factor (**GM-CSF**) and for **platelets** these are **thrombopoietin and IL-11**.
- Erythropoietin is secreted from kidney and helps in the formation of red blood cells. Recombinant human erythropoietin (**Epoietin**) is mainly useful for anemia due to **chronic renal failure** and also due to bone marrow suppressing drugs like zidovudine and anticancer drugs. Response is manifested as elevated hematocrit and reticulocyte count. Major *adverse effect* is *polycythemia* and *hypertension*. **Darbopoietin alpha** is long acting derivative having similiar indications.

Peginesatide is a new drug called erythropoiesis stimulating agent (ESA). It acts by stimulating erythropoietin receptors. It is indicated for treatment of anemia due to CRF in patients on dialysis.

- **Recombinant G-CSF is filgrastim** and recombinant **GM-CSF is sargramostim**. These are **used for leucopenia** induced by cancer chemotherapy and are also useful **for harvesting peripheral blood stem cells** (these substances result in mobilization of stem cells from bone marrow to peripheral blood, which can be utilized for transplantation). Filgrastim is better tolerated although both can cause bone pain. **GM-CSF** is associated with *capillary leak syndrome*.

- **Oprelvekin** is the drug, which is **recombinant IL-11** and is used for the prevention and treatment of **thrombocytopenia induced by cancer chemotherapy**.
- **Romiplostim** is a new class of drugs called **"PEPTIBODIES"**. These are peptides (containing biological activity) linked to antibody fragments (increase the half-life of peptide). It acts as an **agonist of thrombopoietin** receptor and is **indicated for chronic idiopathic thrombocytopenic purpura (ITP)** by *subcutaneous route*. Its half-life is inversely proportional to serum platelet count (Longer in patients with thrombocytopenia and shortest in patients whose platelet count has recovered to normal).
- All of these growth factors (erythropoietin, G-CSF, GM-CSF and IL-11 derivatives) are administered by **subcutaneous route**.

In patients with ITP, antibody coated platelets are engulfed and destroyed by macrophages. Spleen tyrosine kinase (Syk) is required for making cytoskeletal re-arrangements necessary for this phagocytosis. **Fostamatinib** is a Syk inhibitor that can inhibit this phagocytosis and prevent platelet destruction. It is recently approved for oral treatment of ITP.

- **Eltrombopag** is a new **orally** active thrombopoietin agonist **approved for ITP**.

Avatrombopag and lusutrombopag are new **oral** platelet thrombopoietin receptor agonists. These are approved for thrombocytopenia in adults with chronic liver disease who are scheduled to undergo a surgical procedure.

Luspatercept is a new drug which is approved **for treatment of anemia** in patients with β-thalassemia and myelodysplastic syndromes. It is a fusion protein **against** Transforming Growth Factor beta **(TGF-β)**. Normally, TGF-β binds to its receptors to activate SMAD signalling pathway that inhibits maturation of erythroid precursors. Luspatercept inhibit SMAD signalling and thus activates erythroid maturation.

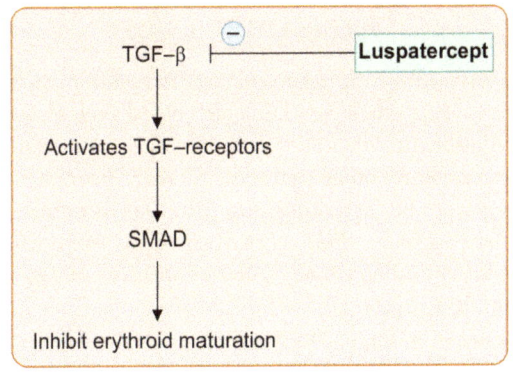

Blood cell	Growth factor	Drug	Indications
1. RBC	Erythropoietin	Epoietin Darbopoietin Peginesatide	Anemia in CRF, myelosuppressive drug use [zidovudine and cancer chemotherapy]
2. WBC	G-CSF	Filgrastim Peg-filgrastim Lenograstim	Neutropenia due to anti-cancer drugs Severe chronic neutropenia, Stem cell transplantation, Mobilization of peripheral blood stem cells.
	GM-CSF	Sargramostim Molgramostim	
3. Platelets	IL-11	Oprelvekin	Thrombocytopenia due to anti-cancer drugs
	Thrombo-poietin	Romiplostim Eltrombopag Avatrombopag Lusutrombopag	ITP ITP Thrombocytopenia in patients with chronic liver disease

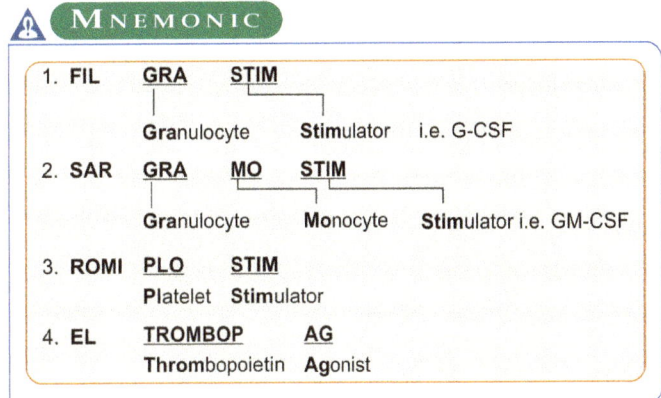

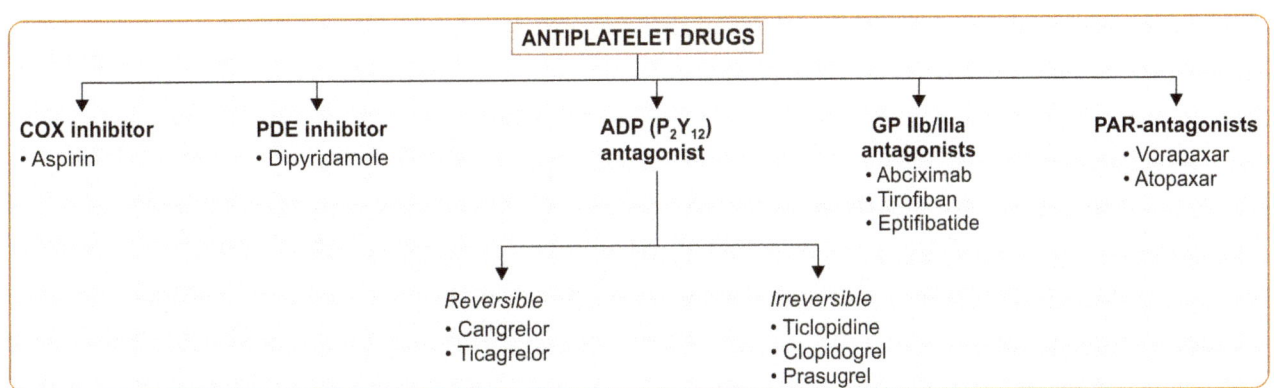

ANTIPLATELET DRUGS

- In arterial thrombi, platelets are the main constituents. Platelets first stick to damaged blood vessel wall and aggregation occurs which lead to release of ADP, TXA_2, serotonin and other substances that promote further aggregation by activating Gp IIb/IIIa receptors on the platelet surface. PGI_2 (prostacyclins) synthesized in vascular endothelium is a **potent inhibitor of aggregation of platelets**.
- Main drugs acting as **antiplatelet agents** are TXA_2 synthesis inhibitor (**aspirin**), ADP antagonists (**clopidogrel and ticlopidine**) and Gp IIb/IIIa antagonists (**abciximab, tirofiban, eptifibatide**).
- **Aspirin inhibits COX enzyme irreversibly** and thus results in decreased synthesis of TXA_2 as well as PGI_2. TXA_2 is produced by platelets and as platelets do not contain nuclei, TXA_2 is not synthesized till there is production of fresh platelets, whereas vessel wall contains nucleus and thus can resume the synthesis of enzymes required for the formation of prostacyclins. The net effect is inhibition of TXA_2 synthesis leading to anti-aggregatory effects.
- **Aspirin inhibits thromboxane synthesis but does not inhibit the enzyme thromboxane synthetase** (*dazoxiben is inhibitor of this enzyme*). **For antiplatelet action lowest doses of aspirin are required** (40-325 mg). It has no effect on platelet survival time and their adhesion to vessel wall.
- **Dipyridamole** is another drug that acts by **inhibiting phosphodiesterase** (which breaks down cAMP) resulting in increased cAMP that potentiates prostacyclins and thus **anti-aggregation**.
- **Ticlopidine, clopidogrel** and **prasugrel** act as **irreversible antagonists of P_2Y_{12} receptor of ADP**. These drugs interfere with the activation of platelets by ADP and fibrinogen. Like dipyridamole, these drugs also increase platelet survival time. *Ticlopidine and clopidogrel are prodrugs* and are converted to active metabolites in the liver by CYP_2C_{19}. *Genetic polymorphisms* in this enzyme can affect the antiplatelet action of these drugs. Further, *proton pump inhibitors* (like omeprazole) *inhibit CYP_2C_{19}* and thus prevent activation of these drugs resulting in decreased antiplatelet effect.
- **Ticlopidine causes severe neutropenia** (Absolute neutrophil count < 500/μL) and **thrombocytopenia** and thus less commonly used, whereas clopidogrel is better tolerated. **Most common side effects** of these drugs are **gastrointestinal**.

> - **Prasugrel** is *more potent antiplatelet drug* as compared to ticlopidine or clopidogrel. It is **faster acting than clopidogrel**. However, it also has higher risk of fatal bleeding and thus should be **avoided in elderly** patients (> 75 years old) and those with **history of stroke**.

- **Gp IIb/IIIa antagonists are strongest antiplatelet drugs** as they block aggregation induced by all agonists. **Abciximab** is a monoclonal antibody against this receptor and is not antigenic. **Eptifibatide** and **tirofiban** are other drugs in this category.
- **Cilostazol** is a *phosphodiesterase-3 inhibitors* and results in elevated cAMP levels. It reduces platelet aggregation and also possess peripheral vasodilatory action. It can be used for the *treatment of intermittent claudication*.
- **Bleeding** is the main problem with all antiplatelet drugs.
- Antiplatelet drugs are used for **prophylaxis of MI (aspirin is used most commonly), cerebrovascular disease and in artificial heart valves (dipyridamole + warfarin is preferred)**.

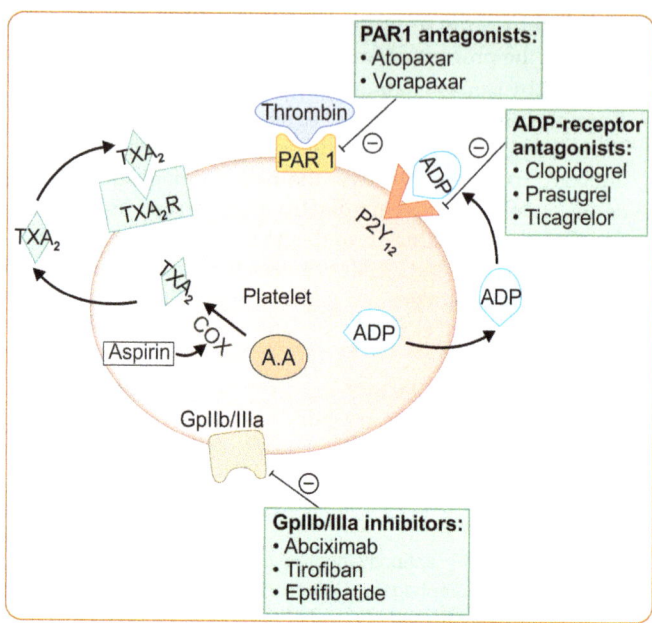

FIG. 9.2: Mechanism of action of antiplatelet drugs.

NEW ANTIPLATELET AGENTS

- Two groups of newer antiplatelet agents are in advanced stages of development.
- **Ticagrelor** and **cangrelor** are direct-acting **reversible** P_2Y_{12} receptor antagonists. *Ticagrelor is orally effective*.
  As compared to clopidogrel, it produces *greater and more predictable antiplatelet action*. It also has *more rapid onset and offset* of action as compared to clopidogrel. It is the first new antiplatelet drug to demonstrate a greater reduction in cardiovascular death than clopidogrel in patients with acute coronary syndromes. It has recently been approved by FDA. **Cangrelor** is *intravenous* reversible P_2Y_{12} receptor antagonist recently approved as an adjunct to PCI.
- **Vorapaxar** is an *orally active inhibitor of* thrombin receptors on platelets called *protease-activated receptor 1* (PAR-1). It has recently been approved as antiplatelet drug in patients with history of MI or peripheral artery disease.

COAGULANTS

Main coagulant in the body is vitamin K. It is of three types; K_1 (**phytonadione**), K_2 (**menaquinone**) and K_3 (**menadione**). *Vitamin K is involved in the activation of various clotting factors* (like II, VII, IX and X) *as well as anti-clotting proteins* (like protein C and S). It carries out the final step in activation of these factors, i.e. **gamma carboxylation of glutamate residues**. Main indications of using vitamin K are:

- Deficiency states like dietary deficiency, prolonged antimicrobial therapy, liver disease, etc.
- Newborns (because usually they have deficiency of this vitamin).
- Overdose of oral anticoagulants like warfarin.

For most of these indications, vitamin K_1 is used. **Menadione (K_3) is contraindicated in patient with G-6-PD deficiency** (causes hemolysis) and in **newborn** (more chances of **kernicterus** due to competitive inhibition of glucuronidation of bilirubin and its displacement from plasma protein binding sites).

ANTICOAGULANTS

Three major groups of anticoagulants are used; warfarin group, indirect thrombin inhibitors (heparin group) and direct thrombin inhibitors. Heparin can be used both in vivo as well as in vitro.

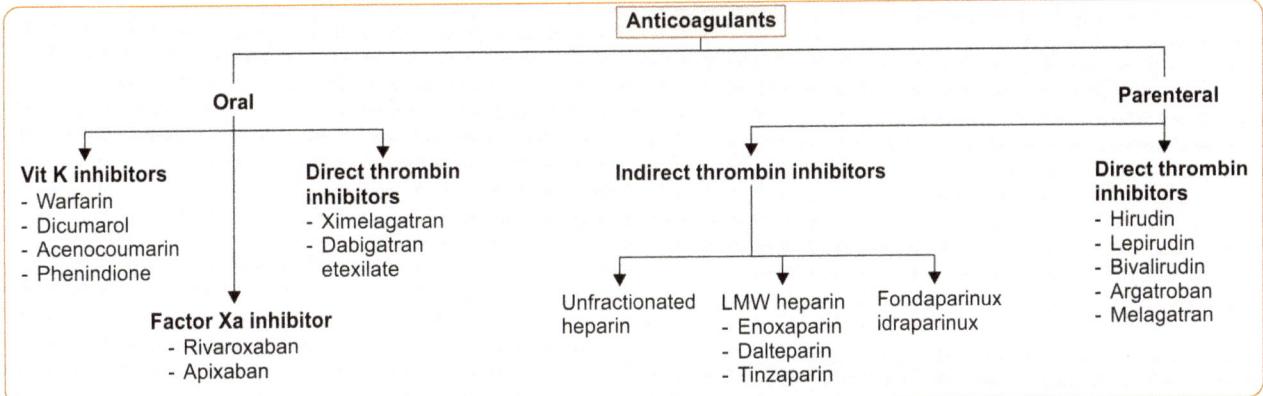

1. ORAL ANTICOAGULANTS

- Drugs in this group include **warfarin**, bishydroxycoumarin (**dicumarol**), **acenocoumarin, phenindione** etc. **Phenindione causes orange coloured urine** as well as liver and kidney damage.
- These drugs act by inhibiting the activation of vitamin K dependent clotting factors. These factors are synthesized by liver and activated by *gamma- carboxylation of glutamate residues* with the help of vitamin K. Hydroquinone form of vitamin K is converted to epoxide form in this reaction and regeneration of hydroquinone form by enzyme vitamin K epoxide reductase (VKOR) is required for this activity. Oral anticoagulants prevents this regeneration by inhibiting VKOR, thus **vitamin K dependent factors are not activated (Fig 9.3)**. These factors include clotting **factors II, VII, IX and X** as well as **anti-clotting proteins, protein C and protein S**. As already activated factors are not affected, the effects of these drugs depend on disappearance of already activated factors from the blood.

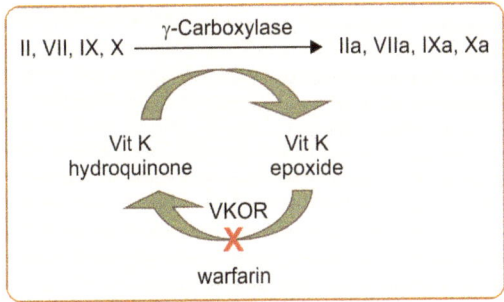

FIG. 9.3: Mechanism of action of warfarin.

- Warfarin is a racemic mixture of R and S isomers. S-warfarin is more active and is metabolized by CYP2C9. Polymorphisms in CYP2C9 may affect the activity of warfarin among different persons.
- **Protein C** has **shorter half life** than most clotting factors (8 hours) so it is the first factor to decline and its deficiency may lead to **dermal vascular necrosis and hypercoagulation** (protein C is anti-clotting) as early appearing (3-10 days after initiation of therapy) adverse effects of warfarin and other drugs of this group. Among **clotting factors, first to disappear is factor VII** ($t_{1/2}$ = 6 hours) and last to disappear is factor II ($t_{1/2}$ = 60 hours). Therefore, the effect of oral anticoagulants is always delayed (develops gradually over 1-3 days) and these are thus **used for maintenance** of anticoagulation rather than initiation of treatment.
- **Bleeding** is the most common **adverse effect** of all anticoagulants. If a patient develops **bleeding due to overdose** of warfarin, **four factor concentrate or fresh frozen plasma** (to supply clotting factors) is the **treatment of choice** but *specific antidote is vitamin K_1* (but the action will be delayed).
- Warfarin is absorbed well from GIT and it is highly plasma protein bound (99%). Its kinetics changes from first order to zero order within therapeutic concentrations.
- It crosses the placenta and can cause fetal warfarin syndrome; also known as Contradi syndrome (growth retardation, stippled epiphyses, hypoplasia of nose and hand bones etc.) if used during pregnancy (therefore contraindicated). However, it is not secreted in the breast milk and can be safely given to nursing mothers.
- Prothrombin time is used to adjust the dose of warfarin (*because it mainly affects the extrinsic pathway*). Better test for monitoring the effect of oral anticoagulants is INR (international normalized ratio). It has been developed by WHO and is based on human brain thromboplastin.

$$INR = (PT\ of\ patient/PT\ of\ reference)^{ISI}$$

- Where *ISI is international sensitivity index that depends on the sensitivity of reference thromboplastin to WHO standard thromboplastin.*
- **Management of warfarin overdose** is done as follows:

*INR < 5 but above therapeutic range	Discontinue warfarin temporarily and restart at low dose.
*INR 5-9	Vitamin K_1 (1 mg oral)
*INR > 9 but no bleeding	Vitamin K_1 (2 – 3 mg oral)
*INR ≥ 20 or bleeding	Four factor concentrate or Fresh frozen plasma.

- Warfarin shows a number of **drug interactions**, therefore requires dose adjustment with several medications.

- Drugs **increasing the effect of warfarin**, thus requiring dose reduction include **broad spectrum antibiotics, cephalosporins** like cefamandole, cefoperazone and moxalactam (cause hypoprothrombinemia), **aspirin, phenylbutazone** and various microsomal enzyme inhibitors (**isoniazid, amiodarone, erythromycin, cimetidine** etc.).
- On the other hand, **enzyme inducers** (like **rifampicin, carbamazepine, griseofulvin**, etc.) and **oral contraceptives** (increase clotting factors) **decrease the effect** and thus require increase in dose of warfarin.
- New **oral** anticoagulants include **dabigatran etexilate, rivaroxaban** and **apixaban**. These *do not require monitoring*. **Dabigatran etexilate** is a *prodrug* and its active metabolite is a *direct thrombin inhibitor* whereas **rivaroxaban and apixaban** are *factor Xa inhibitors*. Rivaroxaban has maximum (80%) whereas dabigatran etexilate has minimum (6%) oral bioavailability.

2. INDIRECT THROMBIN INHIBITORS

- This group **includes unfractionated heparin, low molecular weight heparin** (enoxaparin, dalteparin, tinzaparin, ardeparin, nadroparin and raviparin) and **fondaparinux and idraparinux.**
- **Heparin** is the **strongest organic acid** present in the body (in mast cells).
- Heparin is not physiologically active anticoagulant. Commercially it is produced from **ox lung** and **pig intestine**.
- This group of drugs act by **activating antithrombin III (AT III)** in plasma. Normally AT III inactivates several clotting factors, most importantly factor Xa and IIa (thrombin) but the reaction is very slow. Heparin accelerates this inactivation process by binding to ATIII and inducing the conformational change in it to expose the binding sites. Only conformational change is required for inactivation of factor Xa whereas inactivation of thrombin is also dependent on formation of scaffolding by heparin (that binds both ATIII and IIa). **Unfractionated heparin** provides this scaffolding and thus **inhibits both factor IIa and Xa** whereas **fondaparinux** only cause conformational change in ATIII and thus **inhibit only factor Xa (Fig 9.4)**.
- Only few molecules of LMWH are long enough to provide scaffolding for inhibition of factor IIa, thus **LMWH mainly inhibit factor Xa** (although some inhibition of factor IIa also occurs, but is unreliable)

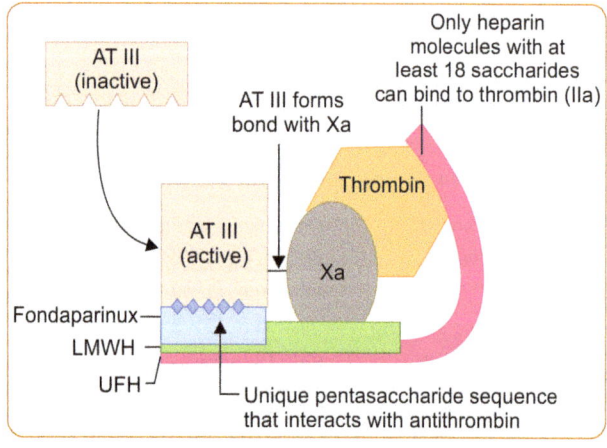

FIG. 9.4: Mechanism of action of anti-thrombin activators.

- Heparin also increases the release of tissue factor pathway inhibitor (TFPI) from the endothelium that may contribute to its anticoagulant activity.
- As heparin is inhibiting already activated factors, so there is no time lag between the administration and action of this drug, therefore it can be used for initiation of anticoagulant therapy.
- Heparin is not absorbed by oral route, therefore should be given either by SC or IV routes (IM route is contra-indicated due to more chances of hematoma formation).
- **Unfractionated heparin** is metabolized by *non-renal routes* whereas **LMW heparin and fondaparinux** are excreted *by kidney* and are contraindicated in renal failure.
- It does not cross the placenta and is thus **anticoagulant of choice during pregnancy.**
- At higher doses, heparin also exerts antiplatelet action.
- Bioavailability of unfractionated heparin is inconsistent after SC route and its effect is **monitored by** testing aPTT (at low doses it selectively affects the intrinsic pathway).
- **LMW heparin and fondaparinux** have long half lives and consistent SC absorption; therefore **do not require monitoring** and once daily SC doses are sufficient. Patients with **end stage renal failure and morbid obesity** may *require monitoring* with **anti-factor Xa assay.**

Feature	Heparin	LMWH
Bioavailability after SC administration.	90%	100%
Plasma $t_{1/2}$	4 hr	17 hr
Release of TFPI	Yes	No
Antidote	Protamine	No

- LMW heparins are preferred as initial parenteral anticoagulants over unfractionated heparin for most of the indications. Unfractionated heparin is preferred over LMW heparin in:

  - Patients with severe chronic kidney disease (creatinine clearance <30 mL/min.)
  - Concomitant thrombolysis is being considered (LMW heparins are contraindicated because of long $t_{1/2}$ and absence of antidote)
  - Patients with venous thromboembolism and a perceived higher risk of bleeding (e.g. post-surgery).
  - Patients with epidural catheters.

- The major **adverse effect** of these drugs also is **bleeding** which is **treated with fresh frozen plasma**. *Specific antidote of heparin is protamine* (highly basic drug that can cause release of histamine). It acts as **chemical antidote** and neutralizes heparin weight by weight. *Protamine sulfate partially neutralizes the effects of LMW heparins whereas it has no effect on fondaparinux's anticoagulant activity*. Other adverse effects include **thrombocytopenia, alopecia, osteoporosis, hyperkalemia, elevation in hepatic transaminases and hypersensitivity reactions.**

Advantages of LMWH over Heparin	
Advantage	*Consequence*
Better bioavailability and longer $t_{1/2}$ after SC injection	Can be given SC once or twice daily
Dose independent clearance	Simplified clearance
Predictable response	No need of monitoring
Lower risk of HIT-syndrome	Safer for long-term use
Lower risk of osteoporosis	Safer for long-term use

- **Pregnant females** receiving heparin therapy should be *supplemented with calcium* (to prevent osteoporosis).
- Thrombocytopenia (**HIT syndrome**; Heparin Induced Thrombocytopenia Syndrome) may occur due to formation of antibodies against complexes of heparin with platelet factor 4, that can result in *paradoxical thrombosis*. Most specific **diagnostic test** for HIT is *serotonin release assay*. Warfarin is contraindicated in such a case and LMW heparin should not be used. **Anticoagulant of choice for HIT syndrome is direct thrombin inhibitors** like **lepirudin** and **bivalirudin**. **Fondaparinux** *can be also used* for this condition.

> **Features of Heparin Induced Thrombocytopenia**
> - Platelet count < 100,000/μL or decreased by >50%.
> - Starts 5-10 days after starting heparin.
> - More common with unfractionated heparin (than LMW heparin), Surgical patients (than medical patients) and females (than males)
> - Venous thrombosis is more common than arterial.

Management of HIT
- Stop all forms of heparins and LMW heparins.
- Do not give platelet transfusions.
- Direct thrombin inhibitors (Lepirudin and Argatroban) are anticoagulants of choice.
- **L**epirudin is safe in **l**iver failure whereas **a**rgatroban can be safely administered in **a**nuria (renal failure).
- Initially, warfarin causes hypercoagulability, therefore should be avoided.
- Lepirudin is continued till platelet count reaches 1,00,000/μL.
- Now, warfarin should be started and direct thrombin inhibitors discontinued. Warfarin should be given for at least 30 days.
- Fondaparinux can also be used for HIT.

		Heparin	Oral Anticoagulants
1.	Route of administration	Parenteral (IV, SC)	Oral
2.	Onset of action	Rapid	Delayed (1-3 days)
3.	Activity	In vitro and in vivo	In vivo only
4.	MOA	Activates Antithrombin III	↓ Activation of II, VII, IX, X
5.	Monitoring by	aPTT	PT
6.	Antagonist	Protamine sulphate	Vit. K_1 (Phytonadione)
7.	Placental barrier	Does not cross placenta	Fetal warfarin syndrome
8.	Use	To initiate therapy	For maintenance

3. DIRECT THROMBIN INHIBITORS

This group includes **hirudin, lepirudin, bivalirudin, argatroban, dabigatran, melagatran** and **ximelagatran**. *Dabigatran and Ximelagatran (a prodrug of melagatran) can be given orally.* All other drugs are used parenterally. These drugs **directly inactivate factor IIa** (thrombin). These are the **anticoagulant of choice for heparin induced thrombocytopenia**. **Bleeding** is the major adverse effect of this group of drugs also. Effect of these drugs can be **monitored by aPTT**. All of these drugs (*except agratroban*) are *excreted by kidney*, therefore, should be avoided in renal failure. *Argatroban is secreted in bile and thus is safe in renal failure. Lepirudin can be used in liver disease.* **Idarucizumab** is a monoclonal antibody against dabigatran. It is approved for reversal of anticoagulant effect of dabigatran.

> **Note**
> - All can prolong aPTT whereas argatroban can prolong INR also.
> - Bivalirudin has shortest $t_{1/2}$ (25 min)

4. TARGET SPECIFIC ORAL ANTICOAGULANTS

Target specific (or direct) oral anticoagulants include dabigatran, rivaroxaban, edoxaban and apixaban. Dabigatran is a direct thrombin inhibitor. **Rivaroxaban, edoxaban, betrixaban** and **apixaban** are **new oral anticoagulants** that act by inhibiting factor Xa. These are **preferred over warfarin** in atrial fibrillation by European guidelines.

Key Points

Warfarin is preferred in patients with:
- Mechanical prosthetic valves
- Advanced kidney disease [CrCL < 30 mL/min]
- Moderate or severe mitral stenosis
- Cannot afford new drugs

Andexanet alpha is a new drug recently approved to reverse overdose of factor Xa inhibitors, like rivaroxaban and apixaban. When given intravenously, it binds to factor Xa inhibitors and reverse their action.

MNEMONIC

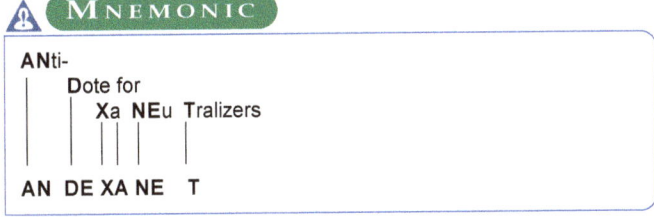

5. OTHER ANTICOAGULANTS

- **Danaparoid** (mixture of 84% heparan sulfate, 12% dermatan sulfate and 4% chondroitin sulfate) is approved for **prophylaxis of DVT**. It is also effective for **HIT syndrome**. It mainly promotes inhibition of factor Xa by antithrombin.
- **Rodenticides** *contain long acting anticoagulants* like *bromadiolone, brodifacoum, diphenadione, chlorphenacinone and pindone*. **Treatment is Vit. K.**
- **Drotrecogin alfa** is a recombinant form of **human activated protein C** that inhibits coagulation by proteolytic inactivation of factor Va and VIIIa. It also has anti-inflammatory activity. *It decreases mortality in patients with severe sepsis.*

Use of Anticoagulants

- These drugs are mainly used **for venous thrombosis** and are highly effective in the **treatment and prophylaxis of deep vein thrombosis**.
- **Warfarin** is the most commonly used drug in a patient with **chronic atrial fibrillation** (to prevent the thromboembolism).
- Aspirin and heparin in combination are recommended for unstable angina.
- **Heparin** can also be used in disseminated intravascular coagulation (**defibrination syndrome**).
- Anticoagulants are of little value in cerebral thrombosis once neurological deficit has occurred but these can be used to decrease the occurrence of **stroke** (**antiplatelet drugs are preferred** for this indication).

Contraindications of Anticoagulants

All anticoagulants are contraindicated in the conditions having increased risk of bleeding like *bleeding disorders, peptic ulcers, hemorrhoids, severe hypertension, subacute bacterial endocarditis, tuberculosis* and along *with aspirin and other antiplatelet drugs*.

FIBRINOLYTICS/THROMBOLYTICS

Insoluble fibrin molecules are broken down to soluble fragments with the help of plasmin, which is generated from plasminogen with the help of tissue plasminogen activator (tPA). tPA selectively activates plasminogen that is bound to fibrin (in the thrombus), whereas the excess plasmin generated is inactivated by circulating antiplasmins. **Fibrinolytics** are the drugs which **activate plasminogen to form plasmin** and thus help in lysis of thrombus (**Fig 9.5**). These drugs can cause bleeding as the major adverse effect due to lysis of physiological thrombi as well as due to excessive amount of plasmin generated in the circulation. Important fibrinolytic drugs are **streptokinase, anistreplase urokinase, alteplase, reteplase and tenecteplase**.

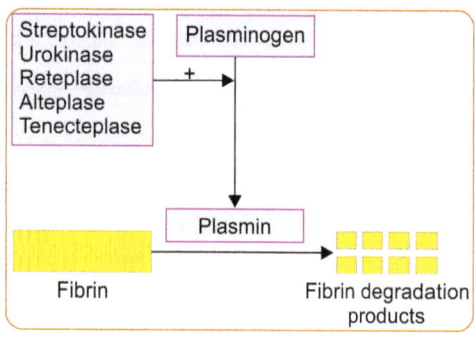

FIG. 9.5: Mechanism of fibrinolytics.

- **Streptokinase** is obtained from β **hemolytic streptococci**.
- Unlike other plasminogen activators, streptokinase does not directly convert plasminogen to plasmin. Instead, it forms a complex with plasminogen and exposes its active site. This altered plasminogen starts acting like tPA and activates other plasminogen molecules to plasmin.
- It **activates fibrin bound as well as circulating plasminogen**. This is **antigenic** and can lead to allergic reactions. It can also lead to formation of **neutralizing antibodies**, thus it is less effective if given repeatedly, however it is **least expensive**.

- **Anistreplase** is formed by *combining streptokinase with Lys-plasminogen*. The active site of plasminogen thus exposed is masked with anisoyl group. After IV infusion, the anisoyl group is slowly removed by deacylation, giving the complex a $t_½$ of approximately 100 minutes. This allows drug administration via a single bolus infusion. However, like streptokinase, anistreplase is *antigenic* and is *not specific for fibrin-bound plasminogen*.
- **Urokinase** is isolated from human **urine** and is not antigenic.
- It directly converts plasminogen to plasmin. Like streptokinase and anistreplase, it also does not discriminate between fibrin-bound and circulating plasminogen and can induce a systemic lytic state. It is often *used for catheter-directed lysis of thrombi in deep veins or peripheral arteries. Its availability is limited* due to production problems.
- **Alteplase, reteplase and tenecteplase are recombinant tPA**. These are not antigenic and are more efficacious than streptokinase but incidence of hemorrhage is similar to streptokinase and urokinase. *Reteplase and tenecteplase (longest acting) are known as bolus fibrinolytics* since administration do not require prolonged intravenous infusion.

Main indication of these drugs is treatment of **acute myocardial infarction (STEMI)**, for which these should be administered IV **within 12 hours** preferably within first 3-6 hours. These are **also indicated in severe, life threatening pulmonary embolism**. These drugs are also contraindicated in the conditions where risk of bleeding is more. Epsilon amino caproic acid **(EACA)** and tranexamic acid are specific antidotes for overdose of fibrinolytic agents.

Contraindications of Fibrinolytics

	Absolute		Relative
1.	Absolute of hemorrhagic stroke at any time	1.	Current use of anticoagulants (INR ≥ 2)
2.	History of non-hemorrhagic stroke within the past year	2.	Recent (> 2 weeks) invasive or surgical procedure.
3.	Marked hypertension (systolic > 180 and/or diastolic > 110 mm Hg).	3.	Prolonged (> 10 min.) cardiopulmonary resuscitation.
4.	Suspicion of aortic dissection	4.	Known bleeding diathesis
5.	Active internal bleeding (excluding menses)	5.	Pregnancy.
		6.	Hemorrhagic ophthalmic condition (e.g. hemorrhagic diabetic retinopathy.)
		7.	Active peptic ulcer disease.
		8.	History of severe hypertension that is currently adequately controlled.

PAROXYSMAL NOCTURNAL HEMOGLOBINURIA (PNH)

PNH is a condition characterized by **triad of hemolysis, pancytopenia and tendency to venous thrombosis**.

Normally, RBCs are protected from destruction by complement pathway due to presence of surface proteins like CD55 (also called DAF; Decay Accelerating Factor) and CD59

(Protectin). These proteins are attached to surface of RBC with the help of GPI (Glycosyl Phosphatidyl Inositol). PNH results due to deficiency of GPI because of mutations in the gene encoding enzymes (PIGA; Phosphatidyl Inositol Glycosyl A) required to form GPI. Mutations result in less formation of PIGA→ Less GPI→Less CD55 and CD59 on surface of RBC→Complement damage→Hemolysis.

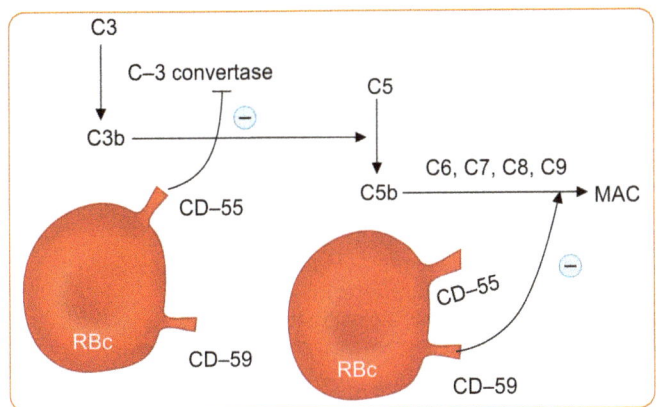

In complement cascade, C_3 convertase activates C_3 to C_{3b} (and C_{3a}). This C_{3b} helps in conversion of C_5 to C_{5b} that binds to C_6, C_7, C_8 and C_9 to form membrane attack complex (MAC).

Later (MAC) results in breakdown of cell (intravascular hemolysis). CD-55 protect the RBC from complement damage by inhibiting C_3 convertase whereas CD-59 inhibits the formation of MAC. In patients with PNH, these protective surface proteins (CD55 and CD-59) are deficient, therefore more risk of hemolysis.

Treatment of PNH:
- Bone marrow transplantation is the definitive treatment of PNH.
- Repeated blood transfusions are required for intravascular hemolytic episodes.
- **Monoclonal antibodies:**

Eculizumab and **Ravulizumab** are monoclonal antibodies against complement component C5. These bind to C5 and prevent the formation of MAC and thus intravascular hemolysis. These are given intravenously once in 14 days. However, these drugs do not inhibit the formation of C3b. MAC is not formed (because of inhibition of C5 by these antibodies) but C3b can opsonize the RBCs and promote extravascular hemolysis. So, these drugs **can prevent intravascular hemolysis but not extravascular hemolysis.**

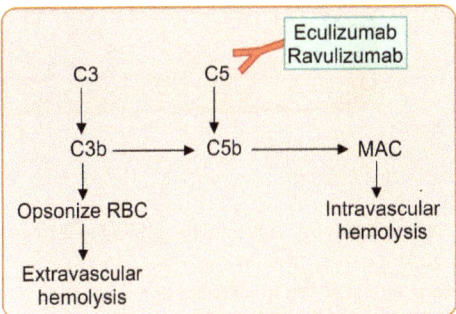

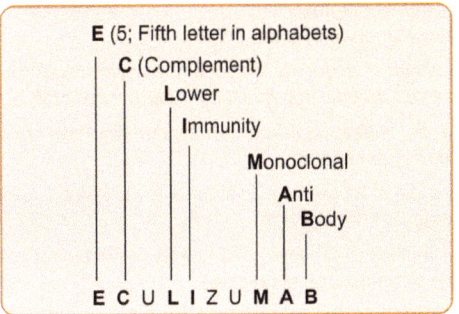

Pegcetacoplan is a complement C3 inhibitor and thus can prevent both intravascular (by decreasing formation of MAC) as well as extravascular (by decreasing opsonization of RBC due to less formation of C3b) hemolysis. It is pegylated and thus long acting.

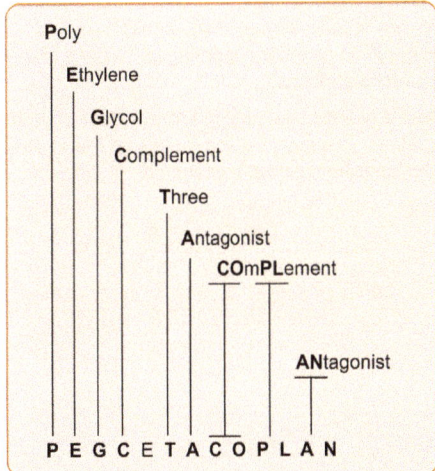

All three drugs, i.e. eculizumab, ravulizumab and pegcetacoplan are given IV and all three **increase the risk of infection by capsulated bacteria like meningococci.**

Golden Points

1. Iron is absorbed mostly in the duodenum in the ferrous form (Fe^{2+}).

2. Parenteral route (IV, IM) is indicated only when:
   - Oral iron is not tolerated
   - Oral iron is not absorbed
   - Along with erythropoietin.

3. The antidote of acute iron poisoning is desferrioxamine (IM) whereas for chronic iron overload, deferiprone (oral) is preferred.

4. Vitamin B_{12} is absorbed in terminal ileum whereas iron is absorbed in duodenum.

5. If the cause of megaloblastic anemia is not known, folic acid alone should not be given.

6. Aspirin inhibits thromboxane synthesis but does not inhibit the enzyme thromboxane synthetase.

7. **Ticlopidine, clopidogrel and prasugrel** act as **irreversible** antagonists of P_2Y_{12} receptor of ADP whereas **Ticagrelor and cangrelor** are direct-acting reversible P_2Y_{12} receptor antagonists.

8. Vitamin K is involved in the activation of various clotting factors (like II, VII, IX and X) as well as anti-clotting proteins (like protein C and S).

9. Warfarin may lead to dermal vascular necrosis and hypercoagulation as early appearing (3-10 days after initiation of therapy) adverse effects.

10. If a patient develops bleeding due to overdose of warfarin, fresh frozen plasma (to supply clotting factors) is the treatment of choice but specific antidote is vitamin K_1.

11. Unfractionated heparin provides this scaffolding and thus inhibits both factor IIa and Xa whereas LMW heparins and fondaparinux only cause conformational change in ATIII and thus inhibit only factor Xa.

12. Effect of unfractionated heparin is monitored by testing aPTT whereas effect of warfarin is monitored by PT or INR.

13. LMW heparin and fondaparinux have long half lives and consistent SC absorption; therefore do not require monitoring.

14. Pulmonary embolism (PE) is treated by anticoagulants. Indications of thrombolytics in PE are:
    - Massive PE, i.e with hemodynamic instability
    - PE without hemodynamic instability but right ventricular compromise.

15. Direct thrombin inhibitors (Lepirudin and Argatroban) are anticoagulants of choice for heparin induced thrombocytopenia.

16. **Idarucizumab** is a monoclonal antibody against dabigatran. It is approved for dabigatran toxicity.

17. **Rivaroxaban, Apixaban and Edoxaban** are new oral anti-coagulants that act by direct inhibition of factor Xa.

18. Reteplase and tenecteplase are known as bolus fibrinolytics.

19. Epsilon amino caproic acid (EACA) and tranexamic acid are specific antidotes for overdose of fibrinolytic agents.

20. Streptokinase, anistreplase and urokinase can activate fibrin bound as well as circulating plasminogen (can cause systemic lytic state) whereas reteplase, alteplase and tenecteplase are fibrin-specific.

Drug of Choice

Condition	Drug of choice
Anemia	
– Iron deficiency anemia	Ferrous sulphate
– Megaloblastic anemia	
- Folate deficiency	Folic acid
- B_{12} deficiency	Vitamin B_{12}
- Pernicious anemia	Vitamin B_{12}
- Chemotherapy induced anemia	Erythropoietin
– Anemia due to chronic kidney disease	Erythropoietin
Iron poisoning	
– Acute	Desferrioxamine
– Chronic	Deferiprone
Cyanide poisoning	Hydroxocobalamin/Amyl nitrite
Deep vein thrombosis	
– Prophylaxis	Warfarin
– Initiation of therapy	LMW heparin + warfarin
– With severe chronic kidney disease	Unfractionated heparin
Pulmonary embolism	
– Stable patient	LMW heparin
– Unstable patient	Thrombolytics (Reteplase)
Chronic Atrial fibrillation	
– Prophylaxis	Dabigatran or Rivaroxaban or Apixaban
– In mechanical prosthetic valves	Warfarin
– Advanced kidney disease	Warfarin
– Mitral stenosis	Warfarin
Myocardial Infarction	
– Acute STEMI	Thrombolytics (Reteplase)
– Prophylaxis	Aspirin
Heparin overdose	Protamine
Warfarin overdose	Vitamin K
Bleeding due to overdose of anticoagulants (heparins or warfarin)	Fresh frozen plasma
Fibrinolytic overdose	Tranexamic acid or Epsilon Amino Caproic Acid
Chemotherapy induced leukopenia	Sargramostim
Chemotherapy induced thrombocytopenia	Oprelvekin
Immune thrombocytopenic purpura	Corticosteroids
Heparin induced thrombocytopenia	Argatroban

Image Based Questions

1. Based on the mechanism shown in the below figure, Drug A is likely to be:

   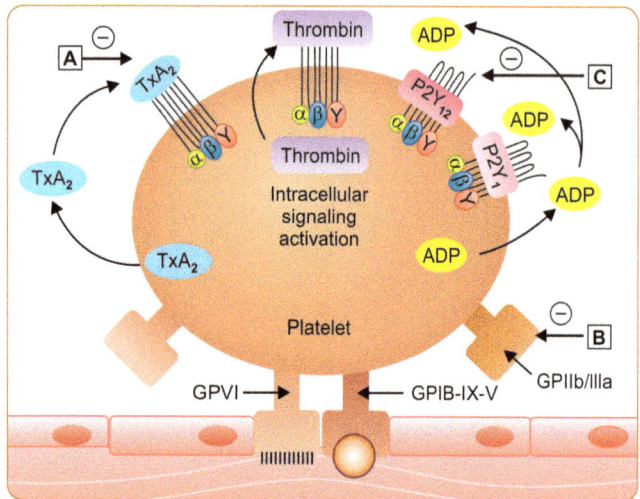

   (a) Aspirin (b) Clopidogrel
   (c) Abciximab (d) All of these

2. Based on the mechanism shown in the above figure, Drug B is likely to be:
   (a) Aspirin (b) Clopidogrel
   (c) Abciximab (d) All of these

3. Based on the mechanism shown in the above figure, Drug C is likely to be:
   (a) Aspirin (b) Clopidogrel
   (c) Abciximab (d) All of these

4. A patient was started on an anticoagulant therapy for DVT. Next day he presented with the features shown in the below figure. The implicated drug is:

   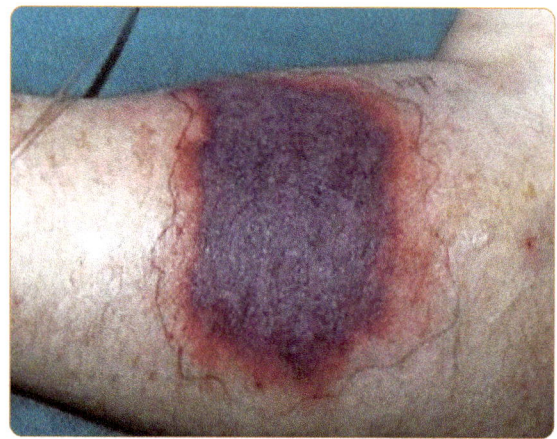

   (a) Warfarin (b) Heparin
   (c) Rivaroxaban (d) Dabigatran

5. A patient was started on an anticoagulant therapy for DVT. Next day he presented with the features shown in the below figure. The implicated drug is:

   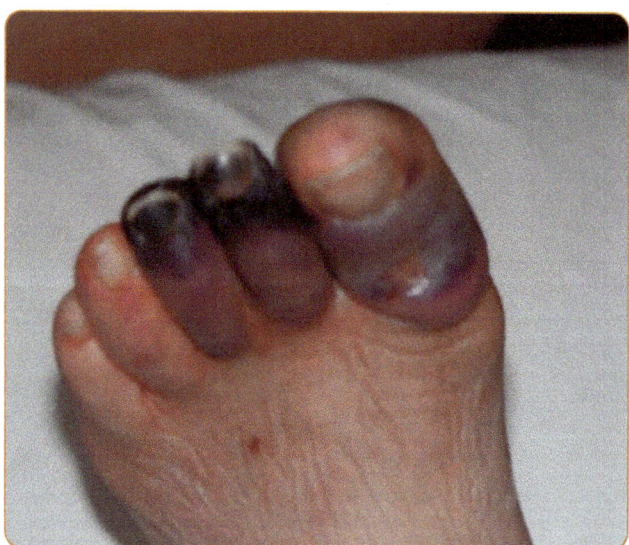

   (a) Warfarin (b) Heparin
   (c) Rivaroxaban (d) Dabigatran

Hematology

6. A 50-year-old male, Rajesh presented to OPD with fever and sore throat with mouth ulcers. He has a history of myocardial infarction and is taking several drugs. One month back he had an episode of transient ischemic attack. His complete blood count shows:

Hb 14.2 g/dL
WBC 900/mm³
Platelet 220000/mm³

If an antiplatelet drug is responsible for the above symptoms of the patients, Which of the following drugs is most likely mechanism of the drug as shown in below figure?

(a) A
(b) B
(c) C
(d) D

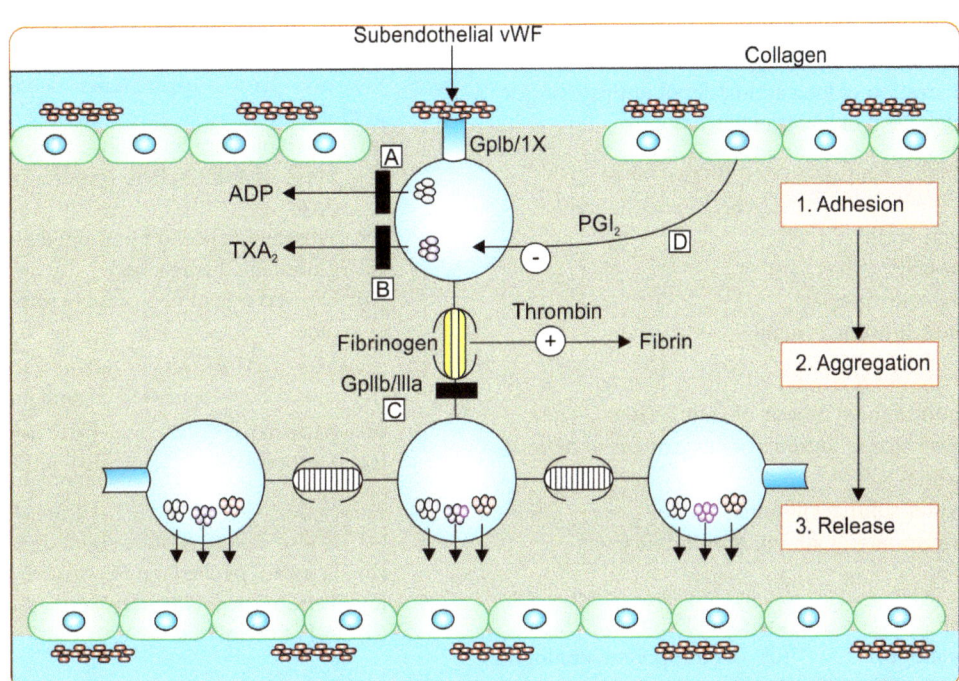

Explanations

1. **Ans. (a) Aspirin**
   Mechanism of action of anti-platelet drugs

Drug	Mechanism of action
Aspirin	Decrease formation of TXA2 by inhibiting COX
Clopidogrel Ticlopidine Prasugrel	Irreversible P2Y12 receptor antagonists of ADP
Cangrelor Ticagrelor	Reversible P2Y12 receptor antagonists of ADP
Abciximab Tirofiban Eptifibatide	GpIIb/IIIa antagonists
Dipyridamole	PDE inhibitor
Vorapaxar Atopaxar	Antagonists of protease activated receptors (PAR) of thrombin

2. **Ans. (c) Abciximab**

3. **Ans. (b) Clopidogrel**

4. **Ans. (a) Warfarin**
   The figure shows the dermal vascular necrosis which is an early adverse effect of warfarin. It is mainly seen in patients with genetic protein C deficiency.

5. **Ans. (a) Warfarin**
   This is also dermal vascular necrosis also known as 'purple toe syndrome'

6. **Ans. (a) A** *(Ref: Katzung 11/e p598)*
   The patient is having neutropenia and the drug most likely being discussed about is ticlopidine. Clopidogrel and ticlopidine act as ADP antagonists. Ticlopidine is rarely used due to the occurrence of serious side effects like neutropenia that typically presents with fever and mouth ulcers. Though this is rare, it is a serious complication and complete blood count should be monitored biweekly for the first three months.

Multiple Choice Questions

HEMATINICS AND GROWTH FACTORS

1. Z-track technique is used for: *(AIIMS Nov. 2019)*
   (a) Monitoring of lithium therapy
   (b) Monitoring of carbamazepine therapy
   (c) Administration of long acting depot antipsychotics
   (d) Administration of nicotine patches

2. True statement about pegylated filgrastim is: *(NEET Pattern Question 2019)*
   (a) It is given orally
   (b) It is GM-CSF
   (c) Reduces neutropenia
   (d) Has short duration of action

3. True about vitamin K is: *(NEET Pattern Question 2017-2018)*
   (a) It is required for synthesis of factor VII
   (b) Long term use of antimicrobials can cause deficiency of vitamin K
   (c) It is a water soluble vitamin
   (d) DVT is associated with vitamin K deficiency

4. Sargramostim is: *(NEET Pattern Question 2016-17)*
   (a) GM-CSF
   (b) G-CSF
   (c) IL-11 analogue
   (d) Erythropoietin analogue

5. Which of the following is true regarding iron replacement therapy in iron deficiency anemia? *(AIIMS Nov 2016)*
   (a) Oral iron should be given till hematocrit normalizes and discontinued later because of gastric adverse effects
   (b) Before giving parenteral iron, the dose should be diluted and checked for anaphylaxis
   (c) There is 50 percent absorption from 325 mg of ferrous sulphate by oral route
   (d) Because of adverse effects of oral iron, parenteral iron is the preferred treatment

6. Which of the following is given to treat thrombocytopenia secondary to anti-cancer therapy and is known to stimulate progenitor megakaryocytes? *(AI 2011)*
   (a) Filgrastim
   (b) Oprelvekin
   (c) Erythropoietin
   (d) Iron dextran

7. All of the following are characteristic features of treatment of iron deficiency anemia with oral iron supplements, *except*: *(Recent NEET Pattern Question)*
   (a) If 200-300 mg elemental iron is consumed, about 50 mg is absorbed
   (b) The proportion of iron absorbed reduces as hemoglobin improves
   (c) The reticulocyte count should begin to increase in two weeks and peak in 4 weeks — this suggests good response to treatment
   (d) The treatment should be discontinued immediately once hemoglobin normalizes to prevent side effects of iron.

8. Posterior column sensations in lower limbs are lost in: *(Recent NEET Pattern Question)*
   (a) Vitamin A deficiency
   (b) Vitamin B_{12} deficiency
   (c) Vitamin C deficiency
   (d) Vitamin D deficiency

9. For oral iron supplements used for iron deficiency anemia: *(Recent NEET Pattern Question)*
   (a) Tolerable dose will deliver 40 to 60 mg of iron per day
   (b) Mass of total salt is important in determining daily dose
   (c) Treatment should be stopped as soon as normal hemoglobin level is reached
   (d) Desired rate of hemoglobin improvement is 0.5 mg per day

10. Megaloblastic anemia is caused by all *except*: *(Recent NEET Pattern Question)*
    (a) Aspirin
    (b) Primidone
    (c) Methotrexate
    (d) N_2O

11. Folic acid: *(Recent NEET Pattern Question)*
    (a) Is also called as pteroylglutamic acid
    (b) Is useful in carriage of one carbon atom moiety
    (c) Tetrahydrofolate is the active form
    (d) All of the above

12. Filgrastim is a: *(Recent NEET Pattern Question)*
    (a) T-cell stimulating factor
    (b) GnRH analogue
    (c) G-CSF
    (d) GM-CSF

13. Erythropoietin is mainly produced in: *(Recent NEET Pattern Question)*
    (a) Liver
    (b) Kidney
    (c) Intestine
    (d) Bone

14. Indication for intramuscular iron therapy is: *(Recent NEET Pattern Question)*
    (a) Pregnancy
    (b) Postpartum period
    (c) Emergency surgery
    (d) Oral iron intolerance

15. Methotrexate should be given with which of the following to decrease its side effects? *(Recent NEET Pattern Question)*
    (a) Folic acid
    (b) Cyanocobalamin
    (c) Thiamine
    (d) Folinic acid

16. Macrocytic anemia is noted with all of the following *except*: *(Recent NEET Pattern Question)*
    (a) Phenytoin
    (b) Methotrexate
    (c) Pyrimethamine
    (d) Ciprofloxacin

17. Deficiency of this haemophilic factor during early pregnancy will result in neural tube defect: *(Recent NEET Pattern Question)*
    (a) Folic acid
    (b) Iron
    (c) Cyanocobalamine
    (d) Antioxidants

Hematology

18. Dose of vitamin K in case of serious bleeding is:
    (Recent NEET Pattern Question)
    (a) 2.5 mg   (b) 5 mg
    (c) 10 mg   (d) 20 mg

19. All are true about romiplostim except:
    (Recent NEET Pattern Question)
    (a) It is recombinant erythropoietin
    (b) It has a protein component in its structure
    (c) Its half life is variable
    (d) It is given subcutaneously

20. What is the formula for parenteral iron therapy?
    (Recent NEET Pattern Question)
    (a) $4.4 \times$ body weight (kg) $\times$ Hb deficit (g/dL)
    (b) $3.3 \times$ body weight (kg) $\times$ Hb deficit (g/dL)
    (c) $2.2 \times$ body weight (kg) $\times$ Hb deficit (g/dL)
    (d) $1.1 \times$ body weight (kg) $\times$ Hb deficit (g/dL)

21. Cyanide poisoning can be treated by:
    (Recent NEET Pattern Question)
    (a) Pyridoxine   (b) Vitamin B_{12}
    (c) Hyperbaric oxygen   (d) Flumazenil

22. Malonyl aciduria is seen in deficiency of:
    (Recent NEET Pattern Question)
    (a) Vitamin B_{12} (b) Vitamin B_2
    (c) Pyridoxine   (d) Folic acid

23. All of the following changes seen in megaloblastic anemia can be corrected by administration of folic acid except: *(Recent NEET Pattern Question)*
    (a) Megaloblastic hyperplasia of bone marrow
    (b) Macrocytic normochromic canges in RBC
    (c) Neurological changes
    (d) Loss of appetite and easy fatigue

24. Rate of iron uptake is regulated by which one of the following? *(Recent NEET Pattern Question)*
    (a) Mucosal cell iron stores
    (b) Route of administration
    (c) Preparation administered
    (d) Age of the patient

25. Which one of the following is ineffective in acute iron toxicity? *(Recent NEET Pattern Question)*
    (a) Desferrioxamine
    (b) BAL
    (c) Whole bowel irrigation
    (d) Deferasirox

ANTIPLATELETS

26. Which is an oral factor Xa inhibitor?
    (NEET Pattern Question 2019)
    (a) Rivaroxaban   (b) Dabigatran
    (c) Argatroban   (d) Fondaparinux

27. Which of the following statements about prasugrel is true as compared to clopidogrel?
    (NEET Pattern Question 2017-2018)
    (a) It is slower acting than clopidogrel
    (b) Due to higher risk of bleeding, prasugrel is contraindicated in stroke
    (c) It is reversible antagonist of ADP receptors
    (d) It is effective orally unlike clopidogrel

28. Which is not an antiplatelet drug?
    (NEET Pattern Question 2016-17)
    (a) Aspirin   (b) Streptokinase
    (c) Clopidogrel   (d) Ticlopidine

29. Which of the following drug is NOT a GpIIb/IIIa antagonist? *(AIIMS May 2016)*
    (a) Tirofiban   (b) Abciximab
    (c) Eptifibatide   (d) Prasugrel

30. Mechanism of action of aspirin as antiplatelet drug is its inhibitory action on: *(AIIMS Nov 2015)*
    (a) Prostacyclins   (b) PGF 2 alpha
    (c) Thromboxane A2   (d) Phospholipase C

31. Aspirin prolongs bleeding by inhibiting the synthesis of which of the following? *(Recent NEET Pattern Question)*
    (a) Adenosine receptors
    (b) Cyclic AMP
    (c) Prostacyclin
    (d) Thromboxane A_2

32. Glycoprotein IIb/IIIa receptor antagonist is:
    (Recent NEET Pattern Question)
    (a) Clopidogrel   (b) Abciximab
    (c) Tranexamic acid   (d) Ticlopidine

33. All are antiplatelet drugs except:
    (Recent NEET Pattern Question)
    (a) Aspirin   (b) Clopidogrel
    (c) Dipyridamole   (d) Warfarin

34. Clopidogrel is an antiplatelet agent that acts by:
    (Recent NEET Pattern Question)
    (a) Reducing myocardial oxygen requirements during exertion and stress
    (b) Reducing myocardial oxygen requirements and by inducing coronary artery vasodilatation
    (c) Inhibiting ADP-induced platelet aggregation
    (d) None of the above

35. Mechanism of action of aspirin is inhibition of:
    (Recent NEET Pattern Question)
    (a) Thromboxane A_2 synthesis
    (b) Phosphodiesterase
    (c) HMG-CoA reductase
    (d) Pancreatic lipase

36. Abciximab is: *(Recent NEET Pattern Question)*
    (a) Antibody against IIb/IIIa glycoprotein
    (b) Antibody against Ib/IX receptors
    (c) Topoisomerase inhibitor
    (d) Adenosine inhibitor

37. Tirofiban is a: *(Recent NEET Pattern Question)*
    (a) Monoclonal antibody
    (b) Antiplatelet drug
    (c) Anti-inflammatory drug
    (d) Antianginal drug

38. All are antiplatelet drugs except:
    (Recent NEET Pattern Question)
    (a) Clopidogrel   (b) Abciximab
    (c) Ticlopidine   (d) Aprotinin

39. Aspirin is not given in a patient who is already on heparin because aspirin causes: *(Recent NEET Pattern Question)*
    (a) Platelet dysfunction
    (b) Aspirin inhibits the action of heparin
    (c) Enhanced hypersensitivity of heparin
    (d) Therapy of heparin cannot be monitored

40. Which of the following is an antiplatelet drug? *(Recent NEET Pattern Question)*
    (a) Clopidogrel (b) Tranexamic acid
    (c) Streptokinase (d) Hirudin

41. Mechanism of action of clopidogrel is: *(Recent NEET Pattern Question)*
    (a) Thromboxane A_2 inhibition
    (b) Inhibit ADP mediated cAMP activation
    (c) GP IIb/IIIa inhibition
    (d) Phosphodiesterase inhibition

42. Ticlopidine act by: *(Recent NEET Pattern Question)*
    (a) Decreasing ADP mediated cAMP activation
    (b) Inhibiting COX enzyme irreversibly
    (c) GP IIb/IIIa antagonist
    (d) Phosphodiesterase inhibition

43. Action of aspirin is due to: *(Recent NEET Pattern Question)*
    (a) Decrease in thromboxane A_2
    (b) Inhibition of adenyl cyclase
    (c) GP IIb/IIIa inhibition
    (d) ADP antagonism

44. Aspirin is contraindicated in a patient who in on treatment with: *(Recent NEET Pattern Question)*
    (a) Prednisolone (b) Warfarin
    (c) Theophyline (d) Oral contraceptives

45. Mechanism of action of aspirin is: *(Recent NEET Pattern Question)*
    (a) Inhibits COX-2 preferentially
    (b) Inhibits COX-1 preferentially
    (c) Inhibits COX 1 and COX 2 reversibly
    (d) Inhibits COX 1 and COX 2 irreversibly

46. Clopidogrel inhibits platelet aggregation by: *(Recent NEET Pattern Question)*
    (a) Inhibits GpIIb/IIIa
    (b) Inhibits phosphodiesterase
    (c) Inhibits ADP
    (d) Inhibits cyclooxygenase

47. The most common adverse effect with ticlopidine is: *(Recent NEET Pattern Question)*
    (a) Neutropenia
    (b) Diarrhea
    (c) Hemorrhage
    (d) Thrombocytopenic purpura

48. Platelet aggregation is inhibited by all *except*: *(Recent NEET Pattern Question)*
    (a) Aspirin (b) Clopidogrel
    (c) Thromboxane A2 (d) Eptifibatide

49. Ticlopidine is an: *(Recent NEET Pattern Question)*
    (a) Antiplatelet drug
    (b) Antiarrhythmic drug
    (c) Anticoagulant drug
    (d) Antifibrinolytic drug

ANTICOAGULANTS

50. Most commonly used route of administration of heparin for postoperative thromboprophylaxis is: *(AIIMS Nov. 2019)*
    (a) Subcutaneous (b) Intravenous
    (c) Inhalational (d) Intramuscular

51. A patient is on warfarin therapy. All of the following drugs increase the risk of bleeding with warfarin *except*: *(AIIMS Nov. 2018)*
    (a) Isoniazid (b) Amiodarone
    (c) Carbamazepine (d) Cimetidine

52. Heparin acts via which of the following adjuvants? *(AIIMS May. 2018)*
    (a) Antithrombin 3 (b) Protein C
    (c) Protein S (d) Thrombomodulin

53. Which is an oral factor Xa inhibitor? *(NEET Pattern 2019)*
    (a) Rivaroxaban (b) Dabigatran
    (c) Argatroban (d) Fondaparinux

54. Drug monitoring is required for: *(NEET Pattern Question 2017-2018)*
    (a) Fondaparinux (b) Enoxaparin
    (c) Lepirudin (d) Dabigatran

55. Apixaban is: *(NEET Pattern Question 2017-2018)*
    (a) Direct thrombin inhibitor
    (b) Factor Xa inhibitor
    (c) Antithrombin 3 activator
    (d) Vitamin K antagonist

56. LMW heparin is preferred over unfractionated heparin because: *(AIIMS Nov 2013)*
    (a) LMW heparin directly inhibits thrombin whereas unfractionated heparin acts via activation of antithrombin
    (b) LMW heparins have lesser risk of causing bleeding
    (c) LMW heparin can be given subcutaneously as well as orally
    (d) LMW heparin has consistent bioavailability

57. Apixaban is a new drug that acts by: *(AI 2012)*
    (a) Inhibiting TNF alpha
    (b) Inhibiting coagulation factor Xa
    (c) Inhibiting platelet aggregation
    (d) Activating plasminogen

58. Recent oral direct thrombin inhibitor which can be used for prevention of stroke is: *(AIIMS Nov 2011)*
    (a) Dabigatran (b) Ximelagatran
    (c) Lepirudin (d) Saxagliptin

59. Vitamin K dependent clotting factors are: *(Recent NEET Pattern Question)*
    (a) Factor IX and X (b) Factor IV
    (c) Factor XII (d) Factor I

Hematology

60. **As compared to unfractionated heparin, low molecular weight heparins:** *(Recent NEET Pattern Question)*
    (a) Are absorbed more uniformly when given subcutaneously
    (b) Require more frequent laboratory monitoring
    (c) Can be given to patients with heparin induced thrombocytopenia
    (d) Predispose to a higher risk of osteopenia

61. **Heparin therapy should be monitored with intermittent estimation of:** *(Recent NEET Pattern Question)*
    (a) Bleeding time   (b) Prothrombin time
    (c) PTTK   (d) All of the above

62. **Heparin acts via activation of:** *(Recent NEET Pattern Question)*
    (a) Antithrombin III   (b) Factor VIII
    (c) Factor II and X   (d) Factor V

63. **The anticoagulant of choice in pregnancy is:** *(Recent NEET Pattern Question)*
    (a) Heparin   (b) Warfarin
    (c) Dicumarol   (d) Phenindione

64. **Which of the following drugs does not cross placenta?** *(Recent NEET Pattern Question)*
    (a) Heparin   (b) Warfarin
    (c) Dicumarol   (d) Nicoumalone

65. **All of the following are anticoagulants, except:** *(Recent NEET Pattern Question)*
    (a) Phytonadione   (b) Warfarin
    (c) LMW heparin   (d) Lepirudin

66. **Orally acting direct thrombin inhibitor is:** *(Recent NEET Pattern Question)*
    (a) Bivalirudin   (b) Ximelgatran
    (c) Melagatran   (d) Argatroban

67. **Heparin does not cause:** *(Recent NEET Pattern Question)*
    (a) Osteoporosis   (b) Factor V inhibition
    (c) Thrombocytopenia   (d) Prolongation of aPTT

68. **All of the following are seen with heparin therapy except:** *(Recent NEET Pattern Question)*
    (a) Skin necrosis
    (b) Thrombosis and thrombocytopenia
    (c) Osteoporosis
    (d) Alopecia

69. **Which of the following is NOT an adverse effect of heparin?** *(Recent NEET Pattern Question)*
    (a) Bleeding   (b) Thrombocytopenia
    (c) Hypokalemia   (d) Osteoporosis

70. **All of the following statements are true regarding warfarin toxicity (skin necrosis) except:** *(Recent NEET Pattern Question)*
    (a) Skin necrosis occurs during initiation of therapy
    (b) Most common sites are toes and tips of fingers
    (c) Decreased quantity of protein C
    (d) Decreased incidence of adverse effects if therapy with LMWH is started

71. **Oral anticoagulants are monitored by:**
    (a) Bleeding time (BT)   *(Recent NEET Pattern Question)*
    (b) Coagulation time (CT)
    (c) Prothrombin time (PT)
    (d) Partial thromboplastin time (PTT)

72. **Structurally, heparin is:** *(Recent NEET Pattern Question)*
    (a) Homopolysaccharide
    (b) Heteropolysaccharide
    (c) Glycoprotein
    (d) Mucoprotein

73. **Low molecular weight heparin inhibits clotting factor:** *(Recent NEET Pattern Question)*
    (a) IIa   (b) IXa
    (c) Xa   (d) Both (a) and (c)

74. **Low molecular weight heparin acts on factor:** *(Recent NEET Pattern Question)*
    (a) XIa   (b) Xa
    (c) IXa   (d) IIa

75. **All of the following have interaction with warfarin except:** *(Recent NEET Pattern Question)*
    (a) Barbiturates   (b) Oral contraceptives
    (c) Cephalosporins   (d) Benzodiazepines

76. **True about heparin induced thrombocytopenia are all except:** *(Recent NEET Pattern Question)*
    (a) Low molecular weight heparins should not be used for treatment
    (b) It causes both arterial and venous thrombosis
    (c) More common with fractionated heparin
    (d) Occurs after about a week of heparin therapy

77. **Protamine antagonism for heparin is:** *(Recent NEET Pattern Question)*
    (a) Competitive   (b) Chemical
    (c) Toxic   (d) Noncompetitive

78. **Low molecular weight heparin inhibits:** *(Recent NEET Pattern Question)*
    (a) Factor Xa   (b) Factors Xa and IIa
    (c) Factor IIa   (d) Factors II, VII, IX and X

79. **Warfarin anticoagulants inhibits following coagulation factors:** *(Recent NEET Pattern Question)*
    (a) II, V, VII, IX   (b) II, VII, IX, X
    (c) II, V, IX, X   (d) II, IX, X, XIII

80. **Which one of the following statement is incorrect regarding Heparin induced thrombocytopenia?** *(Recent NEET Pattern Question)*
    (a) Heparin should be discontinued immediately
    (b) Alternative anticoagulant such as lepirudin should be administered
    (c) Low molecular weight heparins should be avoided
    (d) Heparin should be replaced with Warfarin

81. **Decreased effect of warfarin is seen in case of:**
    (a) Nephrotic syndrome   *(Recent NEET Pattern Question)*
    (b) Acute intake of alcohol
    (c) Concurrent treatment with phenylbutazone
    (d) Congestive heart failure

82. **All of the following are true regarding LMWH (Low Molecular Weight Heparin) except:** *(Recent NEET Pattern Question)*
    (a) It has higher and predictable bioavailability
    (b) It inhibits both factor IIa and Xa
    (c) PT; aPTT monitoring is not required
    (d) It has more favorable pharmacokinetics

83. **Drug of choice for deep vein thrombosis prophylaxis in surgical patients is:** *(Recent NEET Pattern Question)*
    (a) Intravenous unfractionated heparin
    (b) Subcutaneous unfractionated heparin
    (c) Subcutaneous low molecular weight heparin
    (d) Warfarin

84. **Initial treatment for pulmonary embolism is:** *(Recent NEET Pattern Question)*
    (a) Fibrinolysis
    (b) Anticoagulation
    (c) Surgical embolectomy
    (d) Vena caval filter

85. **A patient diagnosed to have deep vein thrombosis is being treated with heparin. Which of the following test will you order to adjust its dosage?**
    (a) Platelet count *(Recent NEET Pattern Question)*
    (b) Prothrombin time
    (c) Bleeding time
    (d) Activated partial thromboplastin time

86. **Which of the following statements is not true for heparin?** *(Recent NEET Pattern Question)*
    (a) Acts by activating anti-thrombin III
    (b) Protamine sulphate antagonizes its action
    (c) Requires aPTT monitoring in patient
    (d) Has only in vivo anticoagulant action

87. **All of the following are vitamin K dependent coagulation factors except:** *(Recent NEET Pattern Question)*
    (a) Factor X
    (b) Factor VII
    (c) Factor II
    (d) Factor VIII

88. **Activity of extrinsic pathway of blood coagulation is measured by:** *(Recent NEET Pattern Question)*
    (a) Bleeding time
    (b) Prothrombin time/INR
    (c) aPTT
    (d) Thrombin time

89. **The biochemical role of vitamin K in the post translational modification of clotting factors is by:** *(Recent NEET Pattern Question)*
    (a) Glycosylation
    (b) Carboxylation
    (c) Acetylation
    (d) Phosphorylation

90. **Warfarin act by:** *(Recent NEET Pattern Question)*
    (a) Inhibiting the activation of vitamin K dependent factors
    (b) Inhibiting thrombin indirectly through antithrombin III
    (c) Directly inhibiting thrombin
    (d) Inhibiting Gp IIb/IIIa

91. **Anticoagulant not used in vitro is:** *(Recent NEET Pattern Question)*
    (a) Heparin
    (b) Warfarin
    (c) Oxalate
    (d) Citrate

92. **Antagonist of heparin is:** *(Recent NEET Pattern Question)*
    (a) Protamine
    (b) Vitamin K
    (c) Warfarin
    (d) Fresh frozen plasma

93. **All are true about heparin except:** *(Recent NEET Pattern Question)*
    (a) Antidote is protamine sulphate
    (b) Can be administered only in vivo
    (c) Cannot be given orally
    (d) Increases aPTT

FIBRINOLYTIS AND MISCELLANEOUS

94. **Antidote of fibrinolytic drugs is:** *(AIIMS May 2017)*
    (a) Heparin
    (b) Protamine
    (c) Epsilon amino caproic acid
    (d) Alteplase

95. **A young male patient presented with prolonged bleeding time. You take a detailed history and ask the patient for intake of NSAIDs as these can prolong the bleeding time. The patient refuses the intake of any form of NSAIDs. No other drug history was obtained. All of the following drugs can prolong bleeding time except:** *(AIIMS Nov 2016)*
    (a) Cephalosporins
    (b) Multivitamins containing Vitamin K
    (c) Methylxanthines
    (d) Anti-depressants

96. **Which of the following substance can be used as an antidote to fibrinolytics?** *(AIIMS Nov 2015)*
    (a) Epsilon amino caproic acid
    (b) Protamine
    (c) Alteplase
    (d) Dabigatran

97. **A substance has molecular weight 30,000. It exerts oncotic pressure similar to albumin and is non-antigenic. It does not interfere with blood grouping and cross-matching. It is:** *(AIIMS Nov 2014)*
    (a) Dextran 40
    (b) Dextran 70
    (c) Polygeline
    (d) Hetastarch

98. **Thrombolytics can provide relative mortality reduction in the treatment of acute myocardial infarction, if patient comes within:** *(AIIMS May 2012)*
    (a) 6 hours
    (b) 12 hours
    (c) 18 hours
    (d) 24 hours

99. **Which of the following drugs is not recommended in septic shock?** *(Recent NEET Pattern Question)*
    (a) Normal saline
    (b) Activated protein C
    (c) Steroids
    (d) Rituximab

100. **Dextran is a good plasma expanders, but it has disadvantage of:** *(Recent NEET Pattern Question)*
    (a) Interference with blood group matching
    (b) Causes thrombocytopenia
    (c) Decreases microcirculation
    (d) Promote roleaux formation

101. **Alteplase differs from streptokinase as it:**
    (a) Is longer acting *(Recent NEET Pattern Question)*
    (b) Is derived from human kidney
    (c) Is cheap
    (d) Activates plasminogen bound to fibrin

102. **Which of the following has proved antithrombotic property?** *(Recent NEET Pattern Question)*
    (a) Gelatin
    (b) Dextran 40
    (c) Dextran 100
    (d) Hetastarch

103. **Plasma expanders are used in:** *(Recent NEET Pattern Question)*
    (a) Severe anemia
    (b) Severe trauma
    (c) Pulmonary oedema
    (d) Cardiac failure

104. Thrombolytic therapy with streptokinase is contraindicated in all of the following *except*:
 (Recent NEET Pattern Question)
 (a) Supraventricular tachycardia
 (b) Recent trauma
 (c) Recent cerebral bleeding
 (d) Recent surgery

105. Activated protein C is used therapeutically in:
 (Recent NEET Pattern Question)
 (a) Abnormal PT/PTT (b) MI
 (c) Fungal infection (d) Sepsis

106. Absolute contraindication to thrombolytic therapy is:
 (Recent NEET Pattern Question)
 (a) Pregnancy
 (b) History of hemorrhagic stroke in past one year
 (c) Patients on nitrates
 (d) Hypertension

107. Which of the following plasminogen activator (fibrinolytic) can be given as bolus dose in patients with acute myocardial infarction? *(Recent NEET Pattern Question)*
 (a) Urokinase (b) Alteplase
 (c) Reteplase (d) None

108. A useful thrombolytic agent that leads to plasmin activation is: *(Recent NEET Pattern Question)*
 (a) Vitamin K (b) Heparin
 (c) Streptokinase (d) Aspirin

109. Relative contraindication to thrombolytic therapy includes all the following *except*:
 (Recent NEET Pattern Question)
 (a) Hypotension (b) Recent surgery
 (c) Active peptic ulcer (d) Pregnancy

110. Epsilon amino caproic acid is used to reduce bleeding due to: *(Recent NEET Pattern Question)*
 (a) Heparin
 (b) Warfarin
 (c) Thrombocytopenia
 (d) Hyperplasminemia

111. Epsilon amino caproic acid (EACA) can be used in the treatment of adverse effects caused by:
 (Recent NEET Pattern Question)
 (a) Streptokinase (b) Heparin
 (c) Warfarin (d) Any of the above

112. Which of the following drugs may cause thrombocytopenia? *(Recent NEET Pattern Question)*
 (a) Ticlopidine (b) Clopidogrel
 (c) Abciximab (d) Aspirin

113. Which one of the following preferentially activates plasminogen bound to fibrin and avoids the systemic lytic state? *(Recent NEET Pattern Question)*
 (a) Streptokinase (b) Amino caproic acid
 (c) Tranexamic acid (d) Alteplase

Explanations

1. **Ans. (c) Administration of long acting depot antipsychotics** *(Ref: KDT 8th/e p650)*
   Z track technique is a technique used for intramuscular injection.
   During Z track technique, skin is stretched to one side before injecting the needle so that the point of injection and point of deposition of drug are not in straight line. This decreases the risk of efflux back of drug
   Advantages of Z track technique:
   - It will not cause any pigmentation
     - Lithium and carbamazepine are oral drugs and monitoring is done by taking blood through veins.
     - Long acting depot antipsychotics are given by intramuscular route via Z-track technique.
     - Nicotine patches are applied on the skin.

2. **Ans. (c) Reduces neutropenia** *(Ref: Harrison 20/e p500)*
   - **Recombinant G-CSF is filgrastim** and recombinant **GM-CSF is sargramostim**.
   - Pegylation of filgrastim help in increasing the duration of action of the drug.
   - These are **used for leucopenia** induced by cancer chemotherapy and are also useful **for harvesting peripheral blood stem cells** (these substances result in mobilization of stem cells from bone marrow to peripheral blood, which can be utilized for transplantation).
   - These drugs are administered by subcutaneous route
   - Filgrastim is better tolerated although both can cause bone pain.
   - GM-CSF is associated with *capillary leak syndrome*.

3. **Ans. (b) Long-term use of antimicrobials can cause deficiency of vitamin K** *(Ref: KDT 8/e p661)*
   - Vitamin K is involved in activation of factor II, VII, IX and X (not synthesis)
   - It is a fat soluble vitamin like Vitamin A, D and E. Vitamin B and C are water soluble.
   - Warfarin (an inhibitor of vitamin K) is used for treatment of DVT.
   - Long term antimicrobial use can alter gut flora leading to deficiency of vitamin K.

4. **Ans. (a) GM-CSF** *(Ref: KDT 7/e p936)*

5. **Ans. (b) Before giving parenteral iron, the dose should be diluted and checked for anaphylaxis** *(Ref: KDT 8/e p649)*
   - Parenteral iron can lead to allergic reactions, therefore skin testing must be done
   - Oral iron should be continued for 2 to 3 months after the hemoglobin normalizes, to replenish the stores.
   - Ferrous sulphate has only 20 percent absorption.
   - Oral iron is the preferred treatment of iron deficiency anemia. Parenteral iron is indicated only when oral iron is not tolerated or not absorbed.

6. **Ans (b) Oprelvekin** *(Ref: Katzung's 11/e p580-581)*
   Oprelvekin (IL-11) is used to prevent and treat thrombocytopenia.

7. **Ans. (d) The treatment should be discontinued immediately once hemoglobin normalizes to prevent side effects of iron** *(Ref: Katzung 11/e p571-572)*
   - A normal individual without iron deficiency absorbs 5–10% of iron, or about 0.5–1 mg daily. Iron absorption increases in response to low iron stores or increased iron requirements
   - In an iron deficient individual, about 50–100 mg of iron can be incorporated into hemoglobin daily, and about 25% of oral iron given as ferrous salt can be absorbed. Therefore, 200–400 mg of elemental iron should be given daily to correct iron deficiency most rapidly.
   - The reticulocyte count should begin to increase in two weeks and peak in 4 weeks. This suggests good response to treatment
   - Treatment with oral iron should be continued for 3–6 months. This will correct the anemia and replenish iron stores.

8. **Ans. (b) Vitamin B_{12} deficiency** *(Ref: KDT 8/e p654)*
   - Deficiency of vitamin B_{12} leads to megaloblastic anemia which is indistinguishable from folic acid deficiency.
   - Deficiency also have manifestations related to loss of myelin like subacute combined degeneration of spinal cord (symptoms of lesions of posterior column like loss of vibration and proprioception, paraesthesia, depressed stretch reflexes and mental changes like poor memory and hallucinations etc.)

9. **Ans. (a) Tolerable dose will deliver 40 to 60 mg of iron per day** *(Ref: Katzung 10/e p530; KDT 8/e p649)*

   - Tolerable dose of elemental iron is 200 mg per day in three divided doses i.e. app. 60 mg per dose.
   - Mass of elemental iron is more important in determining daily dose rather than mass of total salt, because different salts provide different amount of elemental iron.
   - Treatment with oral iron should be continued even after reaching the desired hemoglobin level to replenish the stores.
   - Desired rate of hemoglobin improvement is 0.5 to 1 mg per week (not day).

10. **Ans. (a) Aspirin** *(Ref: Harrison's 17/e p647,649; KDT 8/e p656,657)*

11. **Ans. (d) All of the above** *(Ref: KDT 8/e p655,656)*

12. **Ans. (c) G-CSF** *(Ref: Katzung 11/e p581, KDT 8/e p936)*

13. **Ans. (b) Kidney** *(Ref: KDT 8/e p657)*

14. **Ans. (d) Oral iron intolerance** *(Ref: KDT 8/e p649)*

15. **Ans. (d) Folinic acid** *(Ref: KDT 8/e p921)*

16. **Ans. (d) Ciprofloxacin** *(Ref: KDT 8/e p441, 884,921)*

17. **Ans. (a) Folic acid** *(Ref: KDT 8/e p657)*

18. **Ans. (c) 10 mg** *(Ref: KDT 8/e p661)*

19. **Ans. (a) It is recombinant erythropoietin** *(Ref. CMDT 2015/540)*

20. Ans. (a) 4.4. × body weight (kg) × Hb deficit (g/dL)
    (Ref: KDT 8/e p649)
21. Ans. (b) Vitamin B_{12} *(Ref: KDT 8/e p655)*
22. Ans. (a) Vitamin B_{12} *(Ref: KDT 8/e p653)*
23. Ans. (c) Neurological changes *(Ref: KDT 8/e p656)*
24. Ans. (a) Mucosal cell iron stores *(Ref: KDT 8/e p652)*
25. Ans. (b) BAL *(Ref: KDT 7/e p906)*
26. Ans. (a) Rivaroxaban *(Ref: Harrison 20/e p854)*
    - New **oral** anticoagulants include **dabigatran etexilate, rivaroxaban, apixaban, edoxaban and betrixaban.**
    - These *do not require monitoring*.
    - **Dabigatran etexilate** is a *prodrug* and its active metabolite is a *direct thrombin inhibitor*.
    - **Rivaroxaban, betrixaban, edoxaban and apixaban** are *factor Xa inhibitors*.
    - Argatroban is an injectable thrombin inhibitor
    - Fondaparinux is a pentasaccharide portion of heparin and acts by activating anti-thrombin 3
27. Ans. (b) Due to higher risk of bleeding, prasugrel is contraindicated in stroke *(Ref: CMDT 2018/e p374, KDT 8/e p679)*
    - Prasugrel is irreversible antagonist of ADP receptors like clopidogrel.
    - Prasugrel is more potent and faster acting than clopidogrel
    - Both clopidogrel and prasugrel are given orally.
    - Prasugrel has higher risk of intracranial bleeding in patients with TIA and stroke and is thus contraindicated.
28. Ans. (b) Streptokinase *(Ref: KDT's 8/e p674)*
29. Ans. (d) Prasugrel *(Ref: Katzung 13/e p596, KDT 8/e p677)*
    Prasugrel is an antagonist of P_2Y_{12} receptors of ADP like clopidogrel.

GpIIb/IIIa antagonists include
• Abciximab
• Tirofiban
• Eptifibatide

30. Ans. (c) Thromboxane A2 *(Ref: KDT 8/e p677)*
    By inhibiting cyclooxygenase enzyme, aspirin initially decreases the level of both prostacyclins (in endothelium) and TXA2 (in platelets). However after some time prostacyclin synthesis resumes due to presence of nucleus in endothelium whereas TXA2 remain depressed because platelets are enucleated. Thus final effects of aspirin are due to decrease in TXA2 synthesis.
31. Ans. (d) Thromboxane A_2 *(Ref: KDT 8/e p677)*
32. Ans. (b) Abciximab *(Ref: Katzung 11/e p599, KDT 8/e p679)*
33. Ans. (d) Warfarin *(Ref: Katzung 11/e p598-599)*
34. Ans. (c) Inhibiting ADP-induced platelet aggregation
    (Ref: KDT 8/e p678)
35. Ans. (a) Thromboxane A_2 synthesis *(Ref: KDT 8/e p677)*
36. Ans. (a) Antibody against IIb/IIIa glycoprotein
    (Ref: KDT 8/e p679)
37. Ans. (b) Antiplatelet drug *(Ref: KDT 8/e p680)*
38. Ans. (d) Aprotinin *(Ref: KDT 8/e p677)*
    Aprotinin is a natural proteinase inhibitor identical to pancreatic trypsin inhibitor. It inhibits mediators of inflammatory response, fibrinolysis and thrombin generation. Aprotonin decreases the requirement of blood transfusions in patients undergoing CABG. It has been withdrawn because of high mortality and renal morbidity.
39. Ans. (a) Platelet dysfunction *(Ref: KDT 8/e p655)*
40. Ans. (a) Clopidogrel *(Ref: KDT 8/e p677)*
41. Ans. (b) Inhibit ADP mediated cAMP activation
    (Ref: KDT 8/e 678)
42. Ans (a) Decreasing ADP mediated cAMP activation
    (Ref: KDT 8/e p678)
43. Ans (a) Decrease in thromoboxane A_2 *(Ref: KDT 8/e p677)*
44. Ans. (b) Warfarin *(Ref: KDT 8/e p670)*
45. Ans. (d) Inhibits COX 1 and COX 2 irreversibly
    (Ref: KDT 8/e p677)
46. Ans. (c) Inhibits ADP *(Ref: KDT 8/e p678)*
47. Ans. (b) Diarrhea *(Ref: KDT 7/e p630)*
48. Ans. (c) Thromboxane A2 *(Ref: KDT 8/e p677)*
49. Ans. (a) Antiplatelet drug *(Ref: KDT 8/e p677)*
50. Ans. (a) Subcutaneous *(Ref: KDT 8th/e p665)*
    Unfractionated heparin is injected subcutaneously every 8–12 hours, started before surgery and continued for 7–10 day, or till the patient starts moving about. This regimen has been found to prevent postoperative deep vein thrombosis (postoperative thromboprophylaxis) without increasing the risk of surgical bleeding.
51. Ans. (c) Carbamazepine *(Ref: KDT 8th/e p670)*
    Warfarin shows a number of **drug interactions**, therefore requires dose adjustment with several medications.
    - Drugs **increasing the effect of warfarin**, thus requiring dose reduction include:
      - **Broad spectrum antibiotics**
      - **Cephalosporins** like cefamandole, cefoperazone and moxalactam (cause hypoprothrombinemia)
      - **Aspirin**
      - Drugs displacing warfarin from PPB sites like **sulfonamides, phenytoin, probenecid, indomethacin**
      - Enzyme inhibitors like **isoniazid, amiodarone, erythromycin, cimetidine**, etc.
    - Drugs reducing the effect of warfarin include:
      - **Enzyme inducers** like **rifampicin, barbiturates, carbamazepine, griseofulvin**, etc.
      - **Oral contraceptives** (increase clotting factors)
52. Ans. (a) Antithrombin 3 *(Ref: KDT 8th/e p663)*
    - Heparins act by **activating antithrombin III** (AT III) in plasma.
    - Normally AT III inactivates several clotting factors, most importantly factor Xa and IIa (thrombin) but the reaction is very slow.

- Heparin accelerates this inactivation process by binding to ATIII and inducing the conformational change in it to expose the binding sites. Only conformational change is required for inactivation of factor Xa whereas inactivation of thrombin is also dependent on formation of scaffolding by heparin (that binds both ATIII and IIa). **Unfractionated heparin** provides this scaffolding and thus **inhibits both factor IIa and Xa.**

53. **Ans. (a) Rivaroxaban** *(Ref: Harrison 20th/e p854)*
    - New **oral** anticoagulants include **dabigatran etexilate, rivaroxaban, apixaban, edoxaban and betrixaban.**
    - These *do not require monitoring.*
    - **Dabigatran etexilate** is a *prodrug* and its active metabolite is a *direct thrombin inhibitor.*
    - **Rivaroxaban, betrixaban, edoxaban and apixaban** are *factor Xa inhibitors.*
    - Argatroban is an injectable thrombin inhibitor
    - Fondaparinux is a pentasaccharide portion of heparin and acts by activating anti-thrombin 3

54. **Ans. (c) Lepirudin** *(Ref: Harrison 19/e p754)*
    Low molecular weight heparins (like enoxaparin) and Fondaprinux does not require monitoring. Similarly oral direct acting anticoagulants like dabigatran, rivaroxaban etc also does not require monitoring. Direct thrombin inhibitors like lepirudin can be monitored by measuring the aPTT.

55. **Ans. (b) Factor Xa inhibitor**
    (Ref: CMDT 2018/e p671, KDT 8/e p671)

56. **Ans. (d) LMW heparin has consistent bioavailability** *(Ref: KDT 8/e p665)*
    - Major advantage of LMW heparins over unfractionated heparin is that it does not require monitoring as it has consistent subcutaneous bioavailability
    - Both of these work by activating antithrombin. Unfractionated heparin act by inhibiting both factor X and factor II whereas low molecular weight heparin can inhibit only factor X
    - Risk of bleeding is present with both LMW as well as unfractionated heparin
    - None of these is effective orally. These are administered either by IV or by subcutaneous route.

57. **Ans. (b) Inhibiting coagulation factor Xa**
    (Ref: Harrison 18/e p1000, KDT 8/e p671)
    Rivaroxaban and Apixaban are newer oral anticoagulants that act by inhibiting factor Xa.

    > **Newer oral anticoagulants that are currently being asked in the exams are:**
    > - Dabigatran (Direct thrombin inhibitor)
    > - Rivaroxaban
    > - Apixaban

58. **Ans. (a) Dabigatran**
    (Ref: Katzung 11/e p594, CMDT 2012/537, KDT 8/e p671,672)
    Ximelagatran was the first oral direct thrombin inhibitor approved; however it was later withdrawn because of **hepatotoxicity.** Recently a new direct thrombin inhibitor dabigatran has been approved for the prophylaxis of stroke and systemic embolism in nonvalvular atrial fibrillation. It is administered as a prodrug; dabigatran etexilate. It is not metabolized by CYP enzymes however dose adjustment is required in renal failure.

59. **Ans. (a) Factor IX and X** *(Ref: Katzung 11/e p595)*

60. **Ans. (a) Are absorbed more uniformly when given subcutaneously** *(Ref: Katzung 10/e p546; KDT 8/e p665)*
    - Unlike unfractionated heparin, LMW heparins have more consistent SC bioavailability and thus do not require monitoring.
    - Adverse effects of both type of heparins are similar.
    - Both are contraindicated in heparin induced thrombocytopenia where the agent of choice is direct thrombin inhibitors like lepirudin.

61. **Ans. (c) PTTK** *(Ref: KDT 8/e p663)*
62. **Ans. (a) Antithrombin III** *(Ref: KDT 8/e p663)*
63. **Ans. (a) Heparin** *(Ref: KDT 8/e p664)*
64. **Ans. (a) Heparin** *(Ref: KDT 8/e p664)*
65. **Ans. (a) Phytonadione** *(Ref: KDT 8/e p660,663)*
66. **Ans. (b) Ximelgatran** *(Ref: Katzung 11/e p514)*
67. **Ans. (b) Factor V inhibition** *(Ref: KDT 8/e p665)*
68. **Ans. (a) Skin necrosis** *(Ref: KDT 8/e p665)*
69. **Ans. (c) Hypokalemia** *(Ref: KDT 8/e p665)*
70. **Ans. (b) Most common sites are toes and tips of fingers** *(Ref: Harrison 18/e p433)*
    Common sites of warfarin-induced skin necrosis are breasts, thighs and buttocks.

71. **Ans. (c) Prothrombin time (PT)** *(Ref: KDT 8/e p668)*
72. **Ans. (b) Heteropolysaccharide** *(Ref: Katzung 11/e p591)*
73. **Ans. (c) Xa** *(Ref: KDT 8/e p665)*
74. **Ans. (b) Xa** *(Ref: KDT 8/e p665)*
75. **Ans. (d) Benzodiazepines** *(Ref: KDT 8/e p670)*
76. **Ans. (c) More common with fractionated heparin** *(Ref: CMDT p526-527)*
77. **Ans. (b) Chemical** *(Ref: KDT 8/e p666)*
78. **Ans. (a) Factor Xa** *(Ref: KDT 8/e p665)*
79. **Ans. (b) II, VII, IX, X** *(Ref: KDT 8/e p667)*
80. **Ans. (d) Heparin should be replaced with Warfarin** *(Ref: KDT 8/e p665)*
81. **Ans. (a) Nephrotic syndrome** *(Ref: KDT 8/e p669)*
82. **Ans. (b) It inhibits both factor IIa and Xa** *(Ref: KDT 8/e p665)*
83. **Ans. (d) Warfarin** *(Ref: KDT 8/e p672)*
84. **Ans. (b) Anticoagulation** *(Ref: CMDT 2014/e p291)*
85. **Ans. (d) Activated partial thromboplastin time** *(Ref: KDT 8/e p664)*
86. **Ans. (d) Has only in vivo anticoagulant action** *(Ref: KDT 8/e p663)*
87. **Ans. (d) Factor VIII** *(Ref: KDT 8/e p667)*
88. **Ans. (b) Prothrombin time/INR** *(Ref: KDT 8/e p669)*

89. Ans. (b) Carboxylation (Ref: KDT 8/e p661)
90. Ans. (a) Inhibiting the activation of vitamin K dependent factors (Ref: KDT 8/e p667)
91. Ans. (b) Warfarin (Ref: KDT 8/e p667)
92. Ans. (a) Protamine (Ref: KDT 8/e p666)
93. Ans. (b) Can be administered only in vivo (Ref: KDT 8/e p663-664)
94. Ans. (c) Epsilon amino caproic acid (Ref: KDT 7/e p628)
    EACA and tranexamic acid act as antidote for fibrinolytic drugs.
95. Ans. (b) Multivitamins containing Vitamin K (Ref: Goodman and Gilman 12/e p1806)
    Vitamin K is involved in activation of clotting factors II, VII, IX and X. It thus, decreases the risk of bleeding.
96. Ans. (a) Epsilon amino caproic acid (Ref: KDT 8/e p676)
    Epsilon amino caproic acid (EACA) and tranexamic acid are used as antidote to fibrinolytic drugs like streptokinase.
97. Ans. (c) Polygeline (Ref: KDT 7/e p645)
98. Ans. (b) 12 hours (Ref: Harrison 18/e p2027)
    Thrombolytic drugs should be given within 12 hours after onset of acute MI and within 3 hours of acute stroke.
99. Ans. (d) Rituximab (Ref: Harrison 17/e p1700-1701)
    - Septic shock is managed by maintaining the cardiovascular system with the help of i.v. fluids particularly normal saline along with antibiotics.
    - Adrenal insufficiency has been noted in many cases of septic shock that can be treated by steroids.
    - Activated protein C available as drotrecogin alpha is also approved for septic shock.
    - Rituximab has no role in treatment of septic shock.
100. Ans. (a) Interference with blood group matching (Ref: KDT 7/e p645)
    Dextran is a polysaccharide obtained from sugar beat. It is a plasma expander and have all properties of an ideal plasma expander *except*:

- May interfere with **blood grouping** and **cross matching.**
- Some polysaccharide reacting antibodies if present in patients may cross-react with dextran and trigger an **anaphylactoid reaction.**
- They coat the platelets and coagulation factors and may interfere with **coagulation** and **platelet function,** thus prolong bleeding time. It is not used when hypofibrinogenemia, thrombocytopenia or bleeding is present.
- Dextran prevent roleaux formation of RBCs and have anti-sludging effects, thereby increases microcirculation. [Satoskar 18/e p453].

101. Ans. (d) Activates plasminogen bound to fibrin (Ref: KDT 8/e p674)
    Fibrinolytics are the drugs which activate plasminogen to form plasmin and thus help in lysis of thrombus. These drugs can cause bleeding as the major adverse effect due to lysis of physiological thrombi as well as due to excessive amount of plasmin generated in the circulation.
102. Ans. (b) Dextran 40 (Ref: KDT 7/e p645)
    Dextran 40 and 70 interferes with coagulation and platelet function and thus prolong bleeding time and so is not used in hypofibrinogenemia, thrombocytopenia or in presence of bleeding.
103. Ans. (b) Severe trauma (Ref: KDT 7/e p645)
104. Ans. (a) Supraventricular tachycardia (Ref: KDT 8/e p675)
105. Ans. (d) Sepsis (Ref: CMDT/2010, 437)
106. Ans. (b) History of hemorrhagic stroke in past one year (Ref: KDT 8/e p675)
107. Ans. (c) Reteplase (Ref: KDT 8/e p674)
108. Ans. (c) Streptokinase (Ref: KDT 8/e p674)
109. Ans. (a) Hypotension (Ref: KDT 8/e p675)
110. Ans. (d) Hyperplasminemia (Ref: KDT 8/e p676)
111. Ans. (a) Streptokinase (Ref: KDT 8/e p676)
112. Ans. (a) Ticlopidine (Ref: KDT 8/e p678)
113. Ans. (d) Alteplase (Ref: KDT 8/e p674)

Respiratory System

CHAPTER 10

COUGH

It may be productive (with expectoration) or non productive (dry cough). Dry cough is useless and should be suppressed by using an anti-tussive agent. On the other hand, productive cough should be allowed but made easier by the use of expectorants or mucolytics.

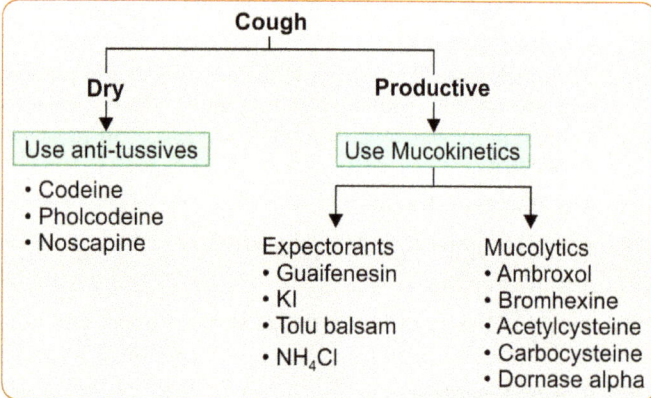

Mucokinetics

These are the drugs which help in clearance of mucus from airways. These may be expectorants or mucolytics.

- **Expectorants**: These increase the amount and hydration of secretions. These include guaifenesin, sodium citrate, potassium citrate, potassium iodide, tolu balsam, vasaka and ammonium chloride etc.
  - **Guaifenesin** is commonly added expectorant in cough syrups
  - **Potassium iodide** acts directly (by irritating bronchial glands) as well as indirectly (by gastric irritation) to increase bronchial secretions. However, it interferes with thyroid function tests and on prolonged use, can also lead to hypothyroidism. It **may** also **lead to flaring up of acne** in adolescents. It should not be used in pregnancy (risk of fetal hypothyroidism) and in patients sensitive to iodine.
- **Mucolytics**: These agents dissolve thick mucus and help to relieve respiratory difficulties. Mucolytics dissolve various chemical bonds within secretions that help in lowering the viscosity of secretions. These include acetylcysteine, carbocysteine, ambroxol, bromhexine and dornase alpha etc.
  - **Dornase alpha** is an enzyme that acts as a mucolytic agent
  - **Acetylcysteine** and **carbocysteine** also help in decreasing viscosity of secretions
  - **Bromhexine** causes depolymerization of mucopolysaccharides and thus results in making the mucus less viscid (mucolytic).
  - **Ambroxol** (metabolite of bromhexine) is also a mucolytic drug.

Anti-tussives

These drugs suppress cough, either by acting directly in the CNS or by inhibiting cough impulses in the respiratory tract. These drugs should be used **only for dry** (non productive) **cough**. Anti-tussives include **codeine, pholcodeine, noscapine** and **dextromethorphan**.

BRONCHIAL ASTHMA

It is a condition of bronchial hyperreactivity associated with inflammation. IgE binds to mast cells on first exposure to antigen. On subsequent exposure, the antigen binds to this IgE (bound to mast cells) and its activation leads to degranulation of mast cells, resulting in the release of mediators. Important mediators include leukotrienes (LTs), prostaglandins (PGs), platelet activating factor (PAF), histamine and protease enzymes. These mediators can lead to bronchoconstriction (and thus acute attack of asthma) as well as inflammation leading to hyperreactivity. **The only drugs effective for the treatment of acute attack of bronchial asthma are bronchodilators** (sympathomimetics, parasympatholytics and methyl xanthines). Other drugs used in asthma include those inhibiting IgE (omalizumab), stabilizing mast cells (sodium cromoglycate), decreasing production of mediators (corticosteroids and zileuton) and those inhibiting the actions of mediators (zafirlukast, montelukast) **(Fig. 10.1)**.

 Key Points

The only drugs effective for the treatment of acute attack of bronchial asthma are bronchodilators.

1. BRONCHODILATORS (FIG. 10.2)

These are the only drugs useful in terminating acute attack of bronchial asthma. Three group of drugs may act as bronchodilators:

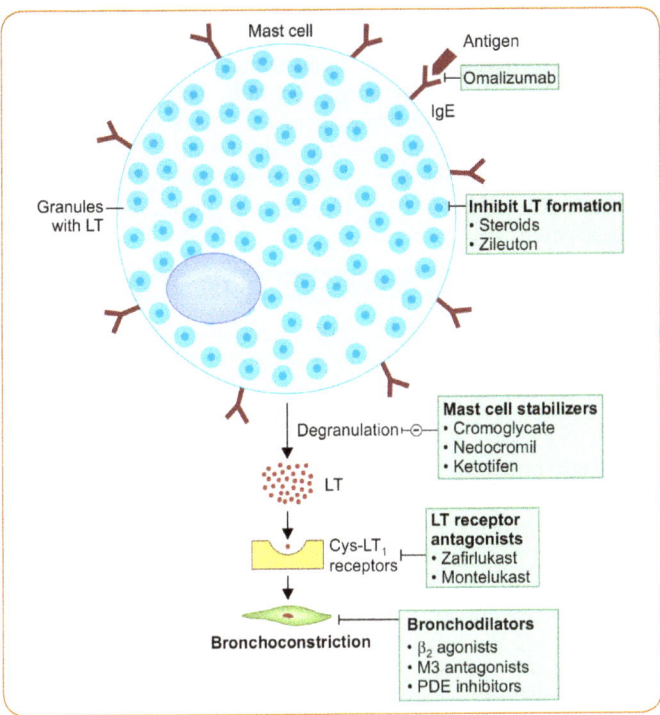

FIG. 10.1: Targets for treatment and prophylaxis of bronchial asthma.

Sympathomimetics

- Adrenergic drugs (β_2 agonists) act by:
  - Stimulating GPCRs that result in the activation of adenylyl cyclase and finally increase in cAMP, which cause smooth muscle relaxation (*bronchodilation*).
  - cAMP also *decreases the mediator release from mast cells.*
  - These drugs *also inhibit microvascular leakage and increase mucociliary transport* by increasing ciliary activity.
- By inhalational route, these are the **fastest acting drugs**. Adrenaline and isoprenaline produce bronchodilation quickly whereas ephedrine has slower onset of action. Above mentioned drugs are non selective and thus are not preferred (tachycardia and increase in the BP are their side effects). Selective β_2 agonists are preferred agents for bronchial asthma. *Salbutamol, Levalbuterol, pirbuterol, terbutaline, isoetharine, bitolterol, fenoterol and procaterol are short acting whereas salmeterol, formoterol, arformoterol, carmoterol, olodaterol and indacterol are long acting β_2 agonists.*
- **Salbutamol (albuterol), metaproternol, pirbuterol and terbutaline** are fast acting drugs by inhalational route (*optimal particle size: 2-5 µm, deposition can be increased by holding the breath in inspiration*), so they are used for aborting an attack of acute asthma. These drugs are **not suitable for prophylaxis** because of shorter duration of action.
- Chronic use of long acting β_2 agonists may lead to tolerance due to down regulation of β_2 receptors. **Salmeterol, bambuterol (prodrug of terbutaline) and formoterol are long acting β_2 selective agonists.**
- **Salmeterol** is **delayed acting**, therefore useful only for prophylaxis whereas **formoterol** is **fast acting also**, so it is useful in aborting acute attack of bronchial asthma as well as for prophylaxis.
- *Bitolterol is a prodrug and is activated to form colterol by esterases in lung.*

- **Muscle tremor** and tachycardia are the major side effect of β_2 agonists.
- Salbutamol causes intracellular movement of potassium from blood and result in hypokalmia

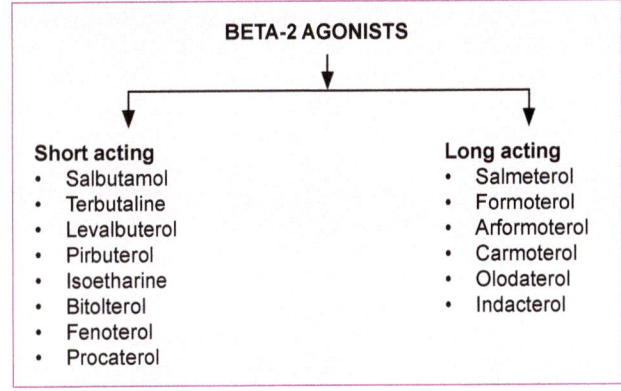

MNEMONIC

SalMETEROl and ForMOTEROl contains metro in name. Metro runs long distances, so these are long acting.
Salmeterol contains S, i.e. slow acting (not for acute attack) whereas Formoterol starts with F, i.e. fast acting (so, can be used for acute attack).

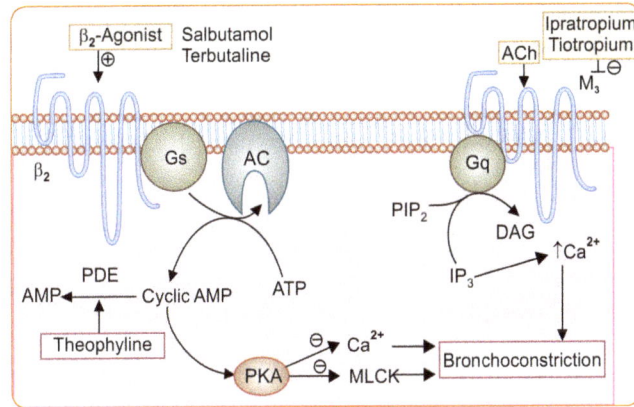

FIG. 10.2: Mechanism of action of bronchodilators.

Anticholinergics

These drugs cause dilation of mainly **large airways** (β_2 agonists cause bronchiolar dilation). These are **less efficacious and slower acting** bronchodilators than sympathomimetics. These drugs are **more effective for COPD** than bronchial asthma. **Ipratropium, tiotropium and umiclidinium** are anticholinergic drugs (M_3 antagonists) that can be used only by inhalational route. **Tiotropium and umiclidinium are longer acting** than ipratropium. Titropium is used in long-term prophylaxis of bronchial asthma (only in combination with corticosteroids) whereas umeclidinium is used for maintenance treatment of airflow obstruction in COPD. These drugs are **bronchodilators of choice in patients** of bronchial asthma **on β blocker therapy** (β_2 agonists will be ineffective).

Revefenacin is a new anticholinergic drug. It has recently been approved for COPD by inhalational route.

Methylxanthines

This group includes caffeine, theophylline and theobromine. Methylxanthines *act by blockade of adenosine receptors* (adenosine is a bronchoconstrictor) and by *inhibition of enzyme phosphodiesterase* (involved in the breakdown of cAMP). At high dose, these drugs can result in *release of Ca^{++}* from sarcoplasmic reticulum in skeletal and cardiac muscles. These drugs are *CNS stimulant drugs* and at toxic dose can result in tremors, delirium and convulsions. These can lead to vomiting due to gastric irritation and CTZ stimulation. **Theophylline** is a potent vasodilator (due to increase in cAMP) and can cause hypotension which leads to reflex tachycardia. *Positive chronotropic and inotropic effects* may be produced even at low doses due to inhibition of presynaptic adenosine receptors (heteroceptors at sympathetic nerve endings). At toxic doses, arrhythmias can be produced. Caffeine can cause *vasoconstriction of cranial vessels* (so useful in migraine) whereas *dilation of other blood vessels* takes place with methylxanthines. Therapeutic effect of methylxanthines in bronchial asthma is due to *bronchodilation, which is slow but sustained.* Theophylline is given by oral route and **aminophylline** is administered by **slow IV infusion**. Kinetics of **theophylline** changes from first order to **zero order** within therapeutic dose range. It has **narrow therapeutic index**. Toxic symptoms are related to GIT, CNS and CVS as described above. *Smoking* and enzyme inducers (phenytoin, phenobarbitone, rifampicin etc.) decrease the plasma levels of theophylline, therefore *require increase in dose*. On the other hand, drugs like *ciprofloxacin, erythromycin and cimetidine* are powerful microsomal enzyme inhibitors, *predisposing to toxicity of theophylline*. **Children clear theophylline faster than adults** (require high dose) whereas clearance of theophylline is **slower in elderly, premature infants and neonates** (require less dose). Further, children are more liable to develop CNS toxicity.

Interactions of Theophylline

Dose reduction is required in	Dose should be increased in
• Elderly	• Smokers
• Patients with CHF	• Children
• Patients of pneumonia	• With enzyme inducers like rifampicin and phenobarbitone
• Hepatic insufficiency	
• With enzyme inhibitors like ciprofloxacin, cimetidine and erythromycin	

Apart from bronchial asthma, theophylline can also be used to **reduce** the frequency of **episodes of apnea in premature infants** because methylxanthines improve contractility and reverse fatigue of diaphragam. **Roflumilast, cilomilast and tofimilast** are *PDE-4 inhibitors* being tried for bronchial asthma.

> **Note**
> Recently, it has been found that theophylline at low doses exert anti-inflammatory action by activating a nuclear enzyme; histone deacetylase-2.

2. DRUG INHIBITING IGE ACTION

Omalizumab is a monoclonal antibody against circulating IgE and is indicated to prevent the attack of bronchial asthma in patients not responding to combination of long acting β_2 agonist and a high dose of inhalational steroid. It is administered by subcutaneous route.

3. MAST CELL STABILIZERS

Sodium cromoglycate and **nedocromil** prevent the degranulation of mast cells by trigger stimuli. These are indicated only for prophylaxis of bronchial asthma. These are given by inhalational route. **Ketotifen** has antihistaminic action apart from mast cell stabilizing property and is specially indicated for patients with multiple disorders (atopic dermatitis, perennial rhinitis, conjunctivitis, etc.).

4. DRUGS DECREASING THE ACTION OF LTS

This group includes the drugs that interfere with generation of LTs (corticosteroids and lipoxygenase inhibitors) and also that interfere with the action of LTs (leukotriene receptor antagonists).

Corticosteroids

These are potent anti-inflammatory drugs and also decrease bronchial hyperreactivity and mucosal edema. Anti-inflammatory action is due to decreased recruitment of inflammatory cells as well as decreased production of PGs and LTs. Arachidonic acid (AA) is released from the membrane phospholipids with the help of enzyme phospholipase A_2 that is inhibited by corticosteroids. AA is converted to PG and TX by cyclooxygenase and to LT with the help of enzyme 5-lipooxygenase (5 LOX). Thus, these mediators are not generated when corticosteroid therapy is initiated. Systemic steroids have a lot of adverse effects, therefore are reserved for resistant severe chronic asthma and in status asthmaticus. These are not bronchodilators but increase the sensitivity to β_2 agonists. **Inhaled steroids** include **beclomethasone, budesonide, mometasone, fluticasone, flunisolide** and **triamcinolone**. These have very little oral absorption and thus little systemic activity after inhalation (>90% reaches GIT after inhalational route, only 4-5% is retained in lungs). **Hoarseness of voice** and **oropharyngeal candidiasis** are very common adverse effects. Candidiasis can be prevented by gargling after each dose and topical nystatin (can be used for treatment also). *Systemic corticosteroids should be avoided in pregnancy but inhaled steroids are safe.* **Ciclesonide** is an inhaled corticosteroid which is metabolized by enzymes in the lungs. Thus, it has least risk of toxicity from systemic absorption when given inhalationally. It is known as soft steroid.

Intramuscular triamcinolone acetonide is a depot preparation but proximal myopathy is a major problem with this therapy.

Lipoxygenase Inhibitors

Zileuton inhibits synthesis of LTB_4 (chemotactic) and LTC_4 and LTD_4 (bronchoconstrictor). Limiting features of this drug are short duration of action and **hepatotoxicity**.

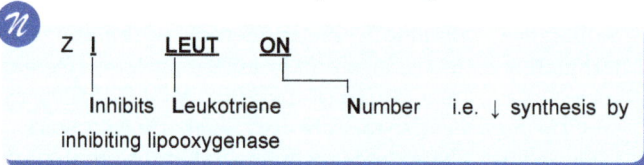

LT Receptor Antagonists

Montelukast and **zafirlukast** inhibit the bronchoconstrictor action of LTs at cys LT_1 receptor. These are used as prophylactic agents for bronchial asthma. These are very safe drugs but few cases of **Churg Strauss syndrome** (vasculitis with eosinophilia) have been associated with their use.

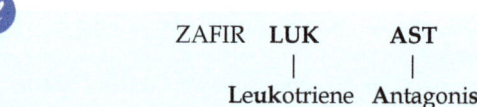

5. MONOCLONAL ANTIBODIES AGAINST IL-4 AND IL-5

- *Mepolizumab* and *reslizumab* are monoclonal antibodies against IL-5. These act by inhibiting the recruitment of eosinophils.
- **Dupilumab** is a monoclonal antibody against IL-4.

SPECIAL TYPES OF ASTHMA

- **Exercise-Induced Asthma:** It typically begins after the end of exercise and recovers spontaneously within 30 minutes. Treatment is usually not required but can be done by SABA. Best method to prevent exercise-induced asthma is regular treatment with **inhaled corticosteroids** (Ref. Harrison 17th/1601) which reduces mast cells. Anti-leukotrienes, mast cell stabilizers and β_2 agonists can also be used for this function.
- **Aspirin Induced Asthma:** Recently, it has been found that aspirin acetytelated COX-2 enzyme can convert arachidonic acid to 15-HETE (15-hydroxyeicosatetraenoic acid). In WBCs, 15-HETE is converted to epi-lipoxins (15-epi-LXA_4 or 15-epi LXB_4). These are called **aspirin-triggered lipoxins** and have powerful bronchoconstrictor action. This finding can explain induction of asthma with aspirin but not by other COX-inhibitors.
- **Brittle asthma** is very severe form of asthma resistant to inhalational beta 2 agonists. DOC for Type 1 brittle asthma is subcutaneous terbutaline and for type 2 brittle asthma, it is subcutaneous adrenaline.

Note
- *LABA should not be given in the absence of ICS therapy* as they do not control the underlying inflammation. Recently, FDA has issued a black box warning for this combination due to slightly increased risk of mortality from asthma attacks.
- In pregnancy; *SABA, ICS and theophylline are considered safe.* If oral corticosteroids are required prednisone should be used. Because, for action it needs to be converted to prednisolone and fetal liver cannot carry out this reaction. Fetus is thus protected from the systemic effects of corticosteroids.

AEROSOL DELIVERY OF DRUGS

Four classes of anti-asthma drugs (β_2 **agonists, anticholinergics, sodium cromoglycate and steroids**) can be administered by inhalational route. This route is aimed to decrease systemic side effects of these drugs. Two types of aerosols can be used.

- *Aerosols using drug in solution:* These include *metered dose inhaler* (MDI) and *nebulizer*.

  - **MDI** use chlorofluorocarbons (less preferred due to their effect on ozone layer) or hydrofluoroalkane propellants. These deliver the drug in spray form. Disadvantage of these devices is that they *require proper co-ordination* between deep inspiration and inhaler activation which many patients (especially children and elderly) are unable to do. Use of a spacer decrease the requirement of this co-ordination
  - **Nebulizers** produce a mist of drug solution generated by pressurized air. These *do not require hand-inspiration co-ordination* and are therefore preferred in children, elderly and very severe episodes of asthma.

- *Aerosols using drugs as dry powder:* These include **spinhaler and rotahaler**. Disadvantage of these devices is that they *require high velocity inspiration* (not suitable for children, elderly and very sick patients) and these can cause *irritation of the air passage* (leading to cough and bronchoconstriction).

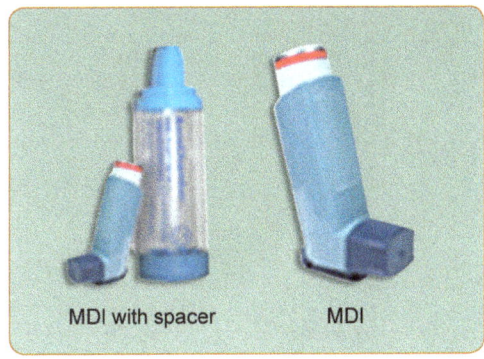

MDI with spacer — MDI

GLOBAL INITIATIVE OF ASTHMA (GINA)–2021 GUIDELINES

- According to GINA-2021 guidelines, short acting beta 2 agonists (SABA) alone are not recommended for treatment of asthma. Patients should receive Inhaled corticosteroids (ICS) containing controller regimen to reduce the risk of serious exacerbations and to control symptoms.
- Treatment figures for adult and adolescents have two tracks based on choice of reliever medication:
  - **Track 1:** It is *preferred approach*. The reliever is low dose ICS—Formoterol combination
  - **Track 2:** It is *alternative* approach. SABA is reliever

Presenting symptoms	Step	Track 1 (Preferred initial treatment)	Track 2 (Alternative initial treatment)
• Asthma symptoms less than twice a month • No risk factors for exacerbations	Step 1	As-needed Low dose ICS + Formoterol	Take ICS with or just after SABA (whenever needed)
Symptoms twice a month or more but less than 4-5 days a week	Step 2	As-needed Low dose ICS + Formoterol	Low dose ICS maintenance daily + As-needed SABA
Symptoms most days or waking due to asthma once a week or more	Step 3	Low dose ICS + Formoterol maintenance + As-needed low dose ICS + formoterol (MART: maintenance and reliever therapy)	Low dose ICS + LABA maintenance + As-needed SABA
Daily symptoms or waking with asthma once a week or more and low lung function	Step 4	Medium dose ICS + formoterol maintenance + As-needed low dose ICS + formoterol	Medium dose ICS + LABA maintenance + As-needed SABA
Severely uncontrolled symptoms	Step 5	High dose ICS + formoterol (OCS may be required) + Add on LAMA ± Biological drugs	High dose ICS + LABA (OCS may be needed) + Add on LAMA ± Biological agents

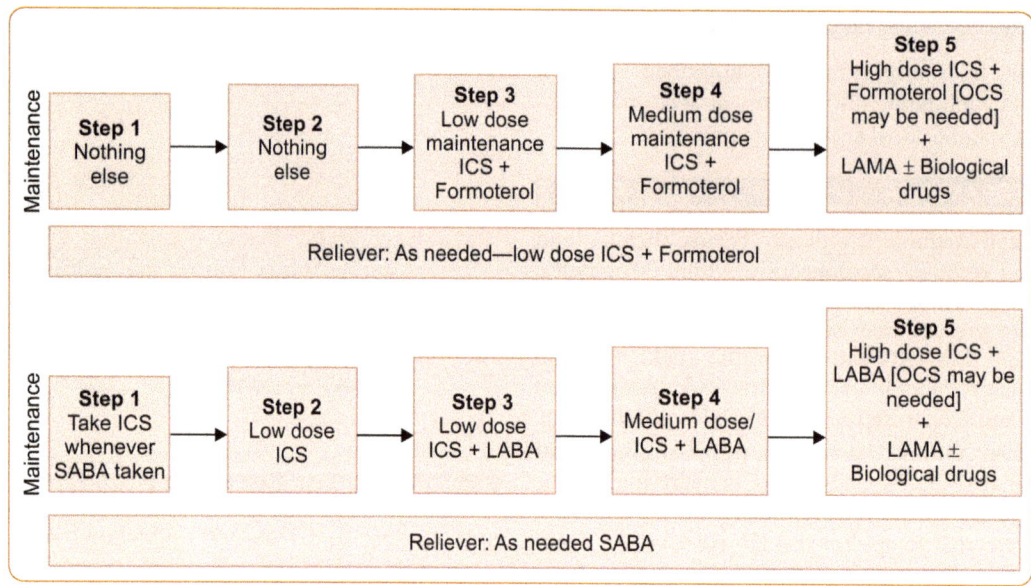

Note :

1. SABA is short acting β_2 agonists (like salbutamol and terbutaline) whereas LABA is long acting β_2 agonists (like salmeterol and Formoterol).
2. ICS means inhaled corticosteroids and OCS means oral corticosteroids
3. LAMA is long acting muscarinic antagonists like tiotropium
4. Biological drugs may be anti-IgE (Omalizumab), anti IL-5 (Reslizumab, Mepolizumab) and anti IL-4R (dupilumab)
5. Azithromycin may be added in Step 5 after specialist referal.

Golden Points

1. Potassium iodide acts directly (by irritating bronchial glands) as well as indirectly (by gastric irritation) to increase bronchial secretions.
2. **Umeclidinium** (anticholinergic) plus **vilanterol** (LABA) combination is recently approved for maintenance treatment of COPD.
3. Anticholinergics are more effective for COPD than bronchial asthma.
4. Anticholinergic drugs are bronchodilators of choice in patients of bronchial asthma on β blocker therapy.
5. Theophylline is a potent vasodilator and can cause hypotension which leads to reflex tachycardia.
6. Children clear theophylline faster than adults (require high dose) whereas clearance of theophylline is slower in eldery, premature infants and neonates (require less dose).
7. Roflumilast, cilomilast and tofimilast are PDE-4 inhibitors being tried for bronchial asthma.
8. Ketotifen has antihistaminic action apart from mast cell stabilizing property.
9. **Mepolizumab** is an IL-5 antagonist indicated for add-on therapy in severe asthma
10. **Ciclesonide** is an inhaled corticosteroid which is metabolized by enzymes in the lungs. Thus, it has least risk of toxicity from systemic absorption when given inhalationally. It is known as **soft steroid**.
11. Recently $MgSO_4$ by intravenous and inhalational route has been tried for acute severe asthma.

Drug of Choice

Condition	Drug of choice
• Bronchial Asthma	
– Acute attack	Low dose ICS + formoterol
– Acute attack during labour	Ipratropium
– Acute attack in patients on beta blocker therapy	Ipratropium
– Prophylaxis	Corticosteroids
• Exercise-induced asthma	
– Acute attack	Low dose ICS + formoterol
– Prophylaxis	Corticosteroids
• Aspirin-induced asthma	
– Acute attack	Low dose ICS + formoterol
– Prophylaxis	Corticosteroids
• Brittle asthma	
– Type 1	SC Terbutaline infusion
– Type 2	SC Adrenaline

Image Based Questions

1. A 20-year-old male, Chintu is being treated with zafirlukast for bronchial asthma. The most likely site of action of this drug from the below Figure can be deciphered as:
   (a) A
   (b) B
   (c) C
   (d) D

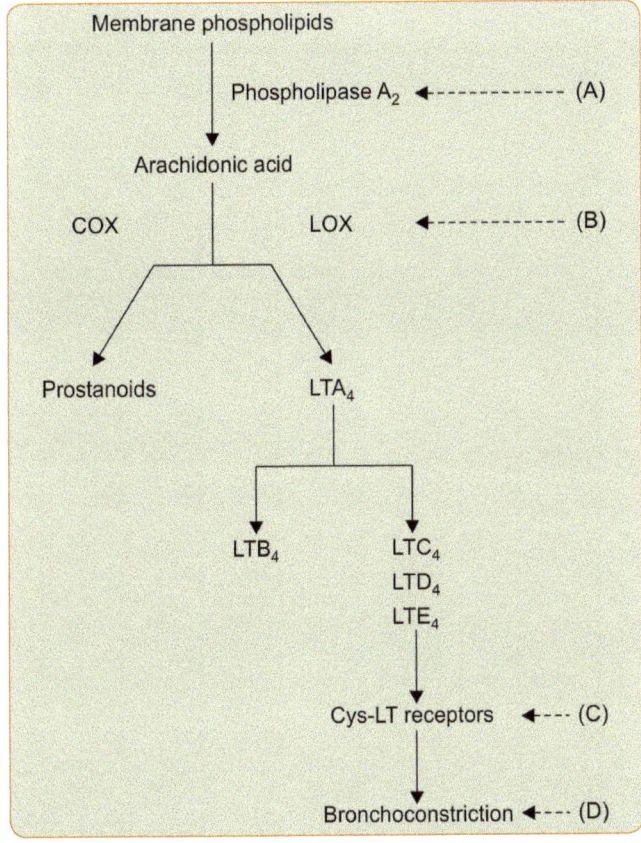

2. Which of the following drug cannot be given by the route shown in the figure?

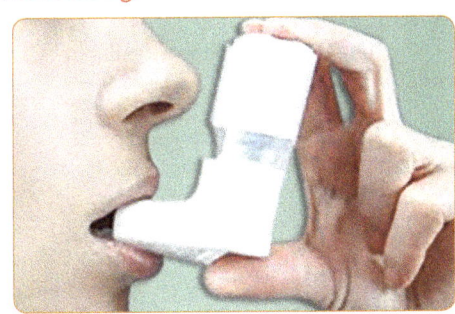

   (a) Salbutamol   (b) Budesonide
   (c) Cromoglycate   (d) Montelukast

3. For which of the following type of patients, the device shown in image should be used for delivering the drug?

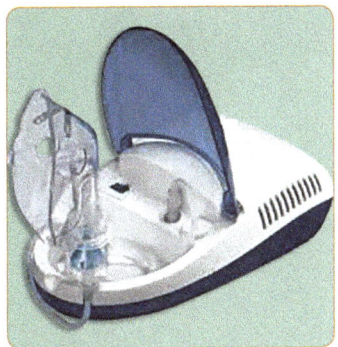

   a. An elderly patient presenting in emergency with exacerbation of acute attack of asthma
   b. Routine use for prophylaxis of asthma in 40 years old male with frequent travelling job
   c. A 5-year-old child with asthma
   d. Both a and c

Explanations

1. **Ans. (c) C** *(Ref: Katzung 11th/e p349)*
   The drug zafirlukast is a cys-LT receptor antagonist.

2. **Ans (d) Montelukast**
   The anti-asthma drugs which are available by inhalational route are:

   - Beta 2 agonists like salbutamol, terbutaline
   - Anticholinergics like ipratropium
   - Steroids like budesonide
   - Mast cell stabilizer like cromoglycate

3. **Ans. (d) Both a and c**
   The device shown in the figure is a nebulizer. It is used to deliver inhalational drugs (mostly bronchodilators) for:

   - Acute severe asthma
   - Elderly patients and patients who are unable to take deep inspiration
   - Children

Multiple Choice Questions

1. Theophylline causes diuresis because of:
   (NEET Pattern 2020)
   (a) PDE4 inhibition
   (b) Adenosine A1 receptor antagonism
   (c) Beta 2 agonism
   (d) PDE 3 inhibition

2. Which of the following antimicrobials should not be given to a chronic asthmatic patient managed on theophylline therapy? *(NEET Pattern 2020)*
   (a) Erythromycin (b) Cefotaxime
   (c) Cotrimoxazole (d) Amoxicillin

3. Which of the following is not an adverse effect of salbutamol? *(AIIMS May 2018)*
   (a) Hypoglycemia (b) Hypokalemia
   (c) Tremors (d) Tachycardia

4. A patient presented with acute exacerbation of bronchial asthma. Salbutamol inhalation did not improve the condition of the patient. So, intravenous corticosteroids and aminophylline were added and the condition improved. What is the mechanism of action of corticosteroids in this condition? *(AIIMS Nov 2017)*
   (a) They cause bronchodilation when given with xanthines
   (b) They increase bronchial responsiveness to salbutamol
   (c) They increase the action of aminophylline on adenosine receptors
   (d) They increase the mucociliary clearance

5. A patient of bronchial asthma was prescribed 2 puffs from a metered dose inhaler of budesonide. Which of the following should NOT be done? *(AIIMS Nov 2016)*
   (a) Shake the inhaler well before use
   (b) Clean the inhaler after every use
   (c) Wait for 1 minute in between puffs
   (d) Rinse mouth after every use

6. Which of the following drugs can be administered by subcutaneous route? *(AIIMS May 2013)*
   (a) Albuterol (b) Terbutaline
   (c) Metaproterenol (d) Pirbuterol

7. Mechanism of action of theophylline in bronchial asthma is: *(AI 2010)*
   (a) Phosphodiesterase 4 inhibition
   (b) Beta2 agonism
   (c) Anticholinergic action
   (d) Inhibition of mucociliary clearance

8. To prevent exercise induced bronchial asthma drug used is: *(Recent NEET Pattern Question)*
   (a) Sodium cromoglycate
   (b) Ipratropium bromide
   (c) Terbutaline
   (d) Epinephrine

9. Which of the following drugs has been found to be useful in acute severe asthma? *(Recent NEET Pattern Question)*
   (a) Magnesium Sulphate (b) Anti-leukotrine
   (c) Cromolyn Sodium (d) Cyclosporine

10. The following drug is NOT useful during acute attack of bronchial asthma: *(Recent NEET Pattern Question)*
    (a) Salbutamol (b) Hydrocortisone
    (c) Cromolyn sodium (d) Theophylline

11. All of the following drugs useful in bronchial asthma are bronchodilators *except*: *(Recent NEET Pattern Question)*
    (a) Theophylline (b) Salmeterol
    (c) Beclomethasone (d) Ipratropium

12. All of the following are the adverse effects seen with the use of salbutamol *except*: *(Recent NEET Pattern Question)*
    (a) Tremors (b) Palpitation
    (c) Hypotension (d) Hypokalemia

13. Which of the following is a bronchodilator? *(Recent NEET Pattern Question)*
    (a) Corticosteroids (b) Salmeterol
    (c) Ketotifen (d) Sodium cromoglycate

14. The drug that does not result in theophylline toxicity is: *(Recent NEET Pattern Question)*
    (a) Ciprofloxacin (b) Amoxicillin
    (c) Erythromycin (d) Cimetidine

15. All of the following drugs can precipitate acute attack of asthma *except*: *(Recent NEET Pattern Question)*
    (a) Phenylbutazone (b) Naproxen
    (c) Glucocorticoids (d) Aspirin

16. Ipratropium bromide used in bronchial asthma, is: *(Recent NEET Pattern Question)*
    (a) β-Sympathomimetics (b) Methylxanthines
    (c) Anticholinergics (d) Mast cell stabilizers

17. Which of the following is long acting sympathomimetics used in bronchial asthma? *(Recent NEET Pattern Question)*
    (a) Salbutamol (b) Terbutaline
    (c) Bambuterol (d) Salmeterol

18. Dextromethorphan is an: *(Recent NEET Pattern Question)*
    (a) Antihistaminic (b) Antitussive
    (c) Expectorant (d) Antiallergic

19. Disodium cromoglycate is used by which of the following routes? *(Recent NEET Pattern Question)*
    (a) Inhalation (b) Oral
    (c) IV (d) IM

20. Which is a "Soft steroid" used in bronchial asthma? *(Recent NEET Pattern Question)*
    (a) Budesonide (b) Dexamethasone
    (c) Ciclesonide (d) Flunisolide

21. Omalizumab is administered in bronchial asthma by which route? *(Recent NEET Pattern Question)*
    (a) Oral
    (b) Intravenous
    (c) Subcutaneous
    (d) Aerosol

22. Directly acting cough suppressant is: *(Recent NEET Pattern Question)*
    (a) Dextromethorphan
    (b) Bromhexine
    (c) Actyl cysteine
    (d) Carbapentate

23. In a patient of chronic asthma on treatment with theophyline, which of the following should not be used to treat his upper respiratory tract infection? *(Recent NEET Pattern Question)*
    (a) Ampicillin
    (b) Cephalexin
    (c) Erythromycin
    (d) All

24. Which of the following inhibits theophylline metabolism? *(Recent NEET Pattern Question)*
    (a) INH
    (b) Griseofulvin
    (c) Prednisolone
    (d) Ciprofloxacin

25. Longest acting β-agonist is: *(Recent NEET Pattern Question)*
    (a) Salbutamol
    (b) Terbutaline
    (c) Salmeterol
    (d) Theophylline

26. Common complication of aerosol steroids use include: *(Recent NEET Pattern Question)*
    (a) Oral candidiasis
    (b) Cushing's syndrome
    (c) Decreased ACTH
    (d) Systemic complications

27. The following drug is contraindicated in bronchial asthma: *(Recent NEET Pattern Question)*
    (a) Propranolol
    (b) Ipratropium bromide
    (c) Theophylline
    (d) Ketotifen

28. Release of histamine and leukotrienes from mast cells is prevented by: *(Recent NEET Pattern Question)*
    (a) Zileuton
    (b) Nedocromil sodium
    (c) Zafirlukast
    (d) Fexofenadine

29. Advantage of salmeterol over salbutamol is its: *(Recent NEET Pattern Question)*
    (a) Shorter duration of action
    (b) More potency
    (c) Longer duration of action
    (d) Lesser cardiac effects

30. Interaction of theophylline with ciprofloxacin is: *(Recent NEET Pattern Question)*
    (a) Ciprofloxacin increases theophylline metabolism
    (b) Ciprofloxacin decreases theophylline metabolism
    (c) Theophylline increases ciprofloxacin metabolism
    (d) Theophylline decreases ciprofloxacin metabolism

31. Theophylline overdose causes: *(Recent NEET Pattern Question)*
    (a) Bradycardia
    (b) Seizures
    (c) Drowsiness
    (d) Bronchospasm

32. Therapeutic blood range of theophylline in microgram per mililitre is: *(Recent NEET Pattern Question)*
    (a) 0-5
    (b) 5-10
    (c) 5-15
    (d) 5-20

33. In theophylline metabolism, drug interactions occurs with all *except*: *(Recent NEET Pattern Question)*
    (a) Cimetidine
    (b) Phenobarbitone
    (c) Rifamipine
    (d) Tetracyclines

34. Mechanism of action of theophylline in bronchial asthma include all of the following *except*: *(Recent NEET Pattern Question)*
    (a) Phosphodiesterase inhibition
    (b) Adenosine receptor antagonism
    (c) Increased histone deacetylation
    (d) Beta -2 receptor stimulation

35. Which of the following is a long acting beta 2 agonist? *(Recent NEET Pattern Question)*
    (a) Salmeterol
    (b) Orciprenaline
    (c) Penoterol
    (d) Pexbaterol

36. Efficacy of salmeterol is increased if it is given along with: *(Recent NEET Pattern Question)*
    (a) Theophylline
    (b) Corticosteroid
    (c) Ipratropium
    (d) Sodium cromoglycate

37. Omalizumab is indicated for which of the following conditions? *(Recent NEET Pattern Question)*
    (a) Multiple myeloma
    (b) Psoriasis
    (c) Bronchial asthma
    (d) Rheumatoid arthritis

38. Most common dose related side effects of salbutamol is: *(Recent NEET Pattern Question)*
    (a) Nervousness
    (b) Palpitations
    (c) Restlessness
    (d) Tremors

39. Which of the following is a long acting beta 2 agonist? *(Recent NEET Pattern Question)*
    (a) Salbutamol
    (b) Salmeterol
    (c) Terbutaline
    (d) Levalbuterol

40. Mechanism of actions of montelukast is: *(Recent NEET Pattern Question)*
    (a) Competitive antagonist of leukotriene receptors
    (b) Inhibits alpha receptor
    (c) Beta receptor agonist
    (d) Non-competitive inhibitor of leukotriene synthesis

41. Mechanism of action of zileuton is: *(Recent NEET Pattern Question)*
    (a) Inhibits production of IgE
    (b) Inhibits Lipoxygenase
    (c) Inhibits Cyclooxygenase
    (d) Inhibits activity of mast cells

42. Which of the following does not have a role in acute attack of asthma? *(Recent NEET Pattern Question)*
    (a) Cromolyn sodium
    (b) Ipratropium
    (c) Steroids
    (d) Salbutamol

43. Which of the following is not a bronchodilator?
    (a) Beta 2 agonists *(Recent NEET Pattern Question)*
    (b) Methylaxanthines
    (c) Steroids
    (d) Anticholinergic

44. Drug of choice for treatment of acute asthmatic attacks is: *(Recent NEET Pattern Question)*
    (a) Leukotriene antagonists
    (b) Lipoxygenase inhibitors
    (c) Beta 2 agonists
    (d) Anticholinergics

45. Which of the following class of drugs is a precipitant of acute asthma? *(Recent NEET Pattern Question)*
    (a) Beta-adrenergic receptor agonists
    (b) NSAIDs
    (c) Calcium channel blockers
    (d) H_1 blockers

46. Adverse effects of salmeterol include:
    (a) Hyperkalemia *(Recent NEET Pattern Question)*
    (b) Seizures
    (c) Tremors
    (d) Interstitial nephritis

47. A 34-year-old man with a long history of asthma is referred to pulmonologist. The physician decides to prescribe zileuton. The mechanism of action of this drug is to: *(Recent NEET Pattern Question)*
    (a) Antagonize leukotriene D4 receptor
    (b) Inhibits 5-lipoxygenase
    (c) Inhibit phosphodiesterases
    (d) Stimulate beta2 receptors

48. Select the correct statement regarding use of inhaled glucocorticoids in bronchial asthma: *(Recent NEET Pattern Question)*
    (a) They are used for acute attacks of asthma
    (b) They have high systemic activity
    (c) They are superior to β_2 agonists in symptom control
    (d) Oral candidiasis can occur as a side effect

49. Which of the following drug is not used in the treatment of bronchial asthma? *(Recent NEET Pattern Question)*
    (a) β_2 agonists
    (b) Corticosteroids
    (c) Cholinesterase inhibitors
    (d) Phosphodiesterase inhibitors

50. All of the following are useful in the management of acute asthma *except*: *(Recent NEET Pattern Question)*
    (a) Hydrocortisone intravenously
    (b) Salbutamol inhalation
    (c) Salmeterol inhalation
    (d) Terbutaline inhalation

51. Which of the following drugs prevents the release of leukotrienes and histamine from mast cells? *(Recent NEET Pattern Question)*
    (a) Zileuton
    (b) Fexofenadine
    (c) Nedocromil
    (d) Tiotropium

52. Which of the following is a long acting β2 selective agonist? *(Recent NEET Pattern Question)*
    (a) Formoterol
    (b) Isoprenaline
    (c) Salbutamol
    (d) Ephedrine

53. In bronchial asthma the mechanism of action of corticosteroids is: *(Recent NEET Pattern Question)*
    (a) Relax airway smooth muscle directly
    (b) Inhibits mast cell deregulation
    (c) Inhibits adenosine receptors
    (d) Inhibits lymphocytic eosinophilic mucosal inflammation

54. Leukotrienes inhibitors are very effective in which one of the following conditions? *(Recent NEET Pattern Question)*
    (a) Exercise induced asthma
    (b) Antigen induced asthma
    (c) Aspirin induced asthma
    (d) Occupational asthma

55. Inhaled sodium cromoglycate: *(Recent NEET Pattern Question)*
    (a) Prevents the antigen antibody combination
    (b) May cause cardiac arrhythmias
    (c) Is of benefit in preventing exercise induced bronchial spasm
    (d) Is effective in alleviating an acute episode of allergic asthma

56. Most common side effect of inhalational beclomethasone is: *(Recent NEET Pattern Question)*
    (a) Adrenal suppression
    (b) Oropharyngeal candidiasis
    (c) Bronchoconstriction
    (d) Hepatitis

57. Efficacy of inhaled steroids is maximum when particle size is: *(Recent NEET Pattern Question)*
    (a) 1-5 μm
    (b) 5-10 μm
    (c) 10-15 μm
    (d) 15-20 μm

58. Zileuton is: *(Recent NEET Pattern Question)*
    (a) 5 lipoxygenase inhibitor
    (b) TX A_2 inhibitor
    (c) Leukotriene receptor antagonist
    (d) Prostaglandin synthesis inhibitor

Explanations

1. **Ans. (b) Adenosine A1 receptor antagonism**
   (Ref: KDT 8th/e p246)
   - Theophylline causes bronchodilation by two major mechanisms
     - Phosphodiesterase inhibition
     - Adenosine A1 antagonism
   - Adverse effects of theophylline are also attributed to these two mechanisms

Adverse effect	Mechanism
Nausea and vomiting	PDE inhibition
Headache	PDE inhibition
Gastric discomfort	PDE inhibition
Diuresis	Adenosine A1 antagonism
Arrhythmias	PDE inhibition, Adenosine A1 antagonism
Seizures	Adenosine A1 antagonism

2. **Ans. (a) Erythromycin** *(Ref: KDT 8th/e p246)*
   Erythromycin is a microsomal enzyme inhibitor. If given along with theophylline, enzyme inhibitors like erythromycin increase the risk of theophylline toxicity.
   Drugs which inhibit theophylline metabolism and increase its plasma level are:
   - Erythromycin
   - Ciprofloxacin
   - Cimetidine
   - Oral contraceptives
   - Allopurinol

3. **Ans. (a) Hypoglycemia** *(Ref: KDT 8th/e p242)*
   Major adverse effects of beta 2 agonists include:
   - Tremors (most common)
   - Tachycardia (mainly at high doses)
   - Tolerance (seen with long acting beta 2 agonists)
   - Hypokalemia.

4. **Ans. (b) They increase bronchial responsiveness to salbutamol** *(Ref: KDT 7th/e p229)*
   Mechanism of action of steroids in acute attack of bronchial asthma is to increase the bronchodilatory effect of beta 2 agonists whereas in prophylaxis their major mechanism is anti-inflammatory.

5. **Ans. (b) Clean the inhaler after every use** *(Ref: Practical Manual of Pharmacology by Dinesh Badyal 1st ed/63-64)*
   Steps to use metered dose inhaler (MDI):
   - Take off the cap and hold inhaler upright.
   - Shake the inhaler.
   - Tilt the head back slightly and slowly breathe out completely for 3-5 seconds.
   - Simultaneously breathe in slowly through the mouth and press down on the inhaler 1 time to release the medication.
   - Keep breathing in slowly, as deeply and evenly as possible.
   - If possible, hold the breath while counting to 10 slowly; this allows the medicine to reach deep into the lungs
   - Breathe out through nose.
   - Repeat the above process if more than 1 puff (actuation) is prescribed.
   - Wait 1 minute between actuations; this may improve penetration of the second actuation into lung airways.
   - Rinse the mouth with warm water.
   - For steroid inhalers, rinse mouth and gargle after every use to remove deposited drug.

6. **Ans. (b) Terbutaline**
   (Ref: Katzung 12th/e p344, KDT 8th/e p243)
   All four drugs i.e. albuterol (salbutamol), terbutaline, metaproterenol and pirbuterol are available as metered dose inhaler
   Salbutamol and terbutaline are also available in tablet forms
   Only terbutaline is available as subcutaneous injection. This route is indicated only for severe asthma requiring emergency treatment when aerosolized therapy is not available or has been ineffective.

7. **Ans. (a) Phosphodiesterase 4 inhibition**
   (Ref: Katzung 11th/e p345; KDT 8th/e p245)
   Theophylline is used in bronchial asthma. Its mechanism of action is:
   - Inhibition of phosphodiesterases particularly PDE-4.
   - Antagonism of adenosine receptors.
   - Enhancement of histone deacetylation. Acetylation of histone is required for activation of inflammatory gene transcription. By inhibiting this process, low-dose theophylline may restore responsiveness to corticosteroids.

8. **Ans. (a) Sodium cromoglycate**
   (Ref: Katzung 10th/e p325; KDT 8th/e p249)
   Mast cell stabilizers like cromoglycate and nedocromil are used to prevent exercise induced asthma. However, corticosteroids are preferred for this indication.

9. **Ans. (a) Magnesium sulphate** *(Ref: Harrison 17th/e p1605)*
   Magnesium sulphate by i.v. or inhalational route has been used for the treatment of acute severe asthma. All other drugs mentioned in the options are used for prophylaxis of asthma.

10. **Ans. (c) Cromolyn sodium** *(Ref: KDT 8th/e p249)*
11. **Ans. (c) Beclomethasone** *(Ref: KDT 8th/e p251)*
12. **Ans. (c) Hypotension** *(Ref: KDT 8th/e p242)*
13. **Ans. (b) Salmeterol** *(Ref: KDT 8th/e p242)*
14. **Ans. (b) Amoxicillin** *(Ref: KDT 8th/e p246)*
15. **Ans. (c) Glucocorticoids** *(Ref: KDT 8th/e p250)*

- COX inhibitors like aspirin, indomethacin, naproxen and phenylbutazone etc. inhibit the formation of PGs from arachidonic acid. This results in diversion of metabolism of arachidonic acid to produce LTs. Large excess of LTs are therefore produced with the use of NSAIDs. These drugs therefore, can result in precipitation of acute attack of asthma (because LTs are bronchoconstrictors).
- Glucocorticoids are useful in the treatment and prophylaxis of bronchial asthma.

16. Ans. (c) Anticholinergics *(Ref: KDT 8th/e p247,248)*
17. Ans. (d) Salmeterol *(Ref: KDT 8th/e p243)*
18. Ans. (b) Antitussive *(Ref: KDT 8th/e p237)*
19. Ans. (a) Inhalation *(Ref: KDT 8th/e p249)*
20. Ans. (c) Ciclesonide *(Ref: Katzung 11/e p348)*

    Ciclesonide has got high topical: systemic activity ratio.

21. Ans. (c) Subcutaneous
    (Ref: Katzung 11th/e p355, KDT 8th/e p251)
22. Ans. (a) Dextromethorphan *(Ref: KDT 8th/e p239)*
23. Ans. (c) Erythromycin *(Ref: KDT 8th/e p246)*
24. Ans. (d) Ciprofloxacin *(Ref: KDT 8th/e p246)*
25. Ans. (c) Salmeterol *(Ref: KDT 8th/e p243)*
26. Ans. (a) Oral candidiasis *(Ref: KDT 8th/e p250)*
27. Ans. (a) Propranolol *(Ref: KDT 8th/e p160)*
28. Ans. (b) Nedocromil sodium *(Ref: KDT 8th/e p249)*
29. Ans. (c) Longer duration of action *(Ref: KDT 8th/e p243)*
30. Ans. (b) Ciprofloxacin decreases theophylline metabolism *(Ref: KDT 8th/e p246)*
31. Ans. (b) Seizures *(Ref: KDT 8th/e p246)*
32. Ans. (d) 5-20 *(Ref: KDT 8th/e p246)*
33. Ans. (d) Tetracyclines *(Ref: KDT 8th/e p246)*
34. Ans (d) Beta 2 receptor stimulation *(Ref: KDT 8th/e p245)*
35. Ans (a) Salmeterol *(Ref: KDT 8th/e p242)*
36. Ans (b) Corticosteroid *(Ref: KDT 8th/e p250)*
37. Ans. (c) Bronchial asthma *(Ref: KDT 8th/e p251)*
38. Ans. (d) Tremors *(Ref: KDT 8th/e p243)*
39. Ans. (b) Salmeterol *(Ref: KDT 8th/e p243)*
40. Ans. (a) Competitive antagonist of leukotriene receptors *(Ref: KDT 8th/e p248)*
41. Ans. (b) Inhibits Lipoxygenase *(Ref: KDT 8th/e p249)*
42. Ans. (a) Cromolyn sodium *(Ref: KDT 8th/e p249)*
43. Ans. (c) Steroids *(Ref: KDT 8th/e p249)*
44. Ans. (c) Beta 2 agonists *(Ref: KDT 8th/e p253)*
45. Ans. (b) NSAIDs *(Ref: KDT 8th/e p214)*
46. Ans. (c) Tremors *(Ref: KDT 8th/e p242)*
47. Ans. (b) Inhibits 5-lipoxygenase *(Ref: KDT 8th/e p249)*
48. Ans. (d) Oral candidiasis can occur as a side effect *(Ref: KDT 8th/e p250)*
49. Ans. (c) Cholinesterase inhibitors *(Ref: KDT 8th/e p242)*
50. Ans. (c) Salmeterol inhalation *(Ref: KDT 8th/e p242)*
51. Ans. (c) Nedocromil *(Ref: KDT 8th/e p249)*
52. Ans. (a) Formoterol *(Ref: KDT 8th/e p242)*
53. Ans. (d) Inhibits lymphocytic eosinophilic mucosal inflammation *(Ref: KDT 8th/e p249)*
54. Ans. (c) Aspirin induced asthma *(Ref: KDT 8th/e p214)*
55. Ans. (c) Is of benefit in preventing exercise induced bronchial spasm *(Ref: KDT 8th/e p249)*
56. Ans. (b) Oropharyngeal candidiasis *(Ref: KDT 8th/e p250)*
57. Ans. (a) 1–5 μm *(Ref: KDT 8th/e p252)*
58. Ans. (a) 5 lipoxygenase inhibitor *(Ref: KDT 8th/e p249)*

Gastrointestinal Tract

CHAPTER 11

PEPTIC ULCER DISEASE

Peptic ulcer disease arises from the *imbalance between defensive factors* (mucus, bicarbonate and mucosal blood flow) *and aggressive factors* (acid, pepsin, NSAIDs and *Helicobacter pylori*).

Hydrochloric acid is secreted by gastric parietal cells due to stimulation of H^+K^+ ATPase (proton pump). Histamine (through H_2 receptors), acetylcholine (through M_1 and M_3 receptors) and gastrin (through CCK receptors) are important stimulators of proton pump. *ACh and gastrin exert their action directly as well as through release of histamine.*

Antral G-cells produce gastrin on stimulation by dietary peptides. Gastrin mainly stimulates release of histamine from entero-chromaffin like (ECL) cell and weakly stimulates proton pump itself. Parietal cells secrete H^+ in the lumen through $H^+ - K^+ -$ ATPase (proton pump). Vagus nerve (via ACh) help in increasing acid by three mechanisms:

- Direct stimulation of proton pump
- Stimulation of ECL-cells to release histamine
- Direct release of gastrin (by action of G-cells) and inhibition of somatostatin by action on D-cells (later inhibits release of gastrin).

The main strategies employed for the treatment of peptic ulcer disease and gastritis are to:

1. Neutralize gastric acid by *antacids*.
2. *Decrease secretion of acid* in stomach.
3. *Increase* protective factors like *mucus and bicarbonate*.
4. *Protect the ulcer* by forming a layer over it.
5. *Stimulate the healing* of ulcer.
6. *Kill H. pylori* associated with peptic ulcer disease.

ANTACIDS

These drugs are weak bases that neutralize gastric acid (do not decrease the volume of acid secreted). Their **major role** in peptic ulcer is to provide **prompt relief from ulcer pain**. Antacids may be systemic (absorbed from the GIT) or local (poorly absorbed). **Sodium bicarbonate** is rapidly acting **systemic antacid**. It is not indicated for long term use because:

- It releases CO_2 that can cause belching and gastric distension (ulcer perforation can occur).
- Sodium chloride formed in the neutralization reaction can be absorbed that can exacerbate fluid retention in patients of CHF and hypertension.
- Systemic and urinary alkalosis may occur.
- Rebound hyperacidity can occur.

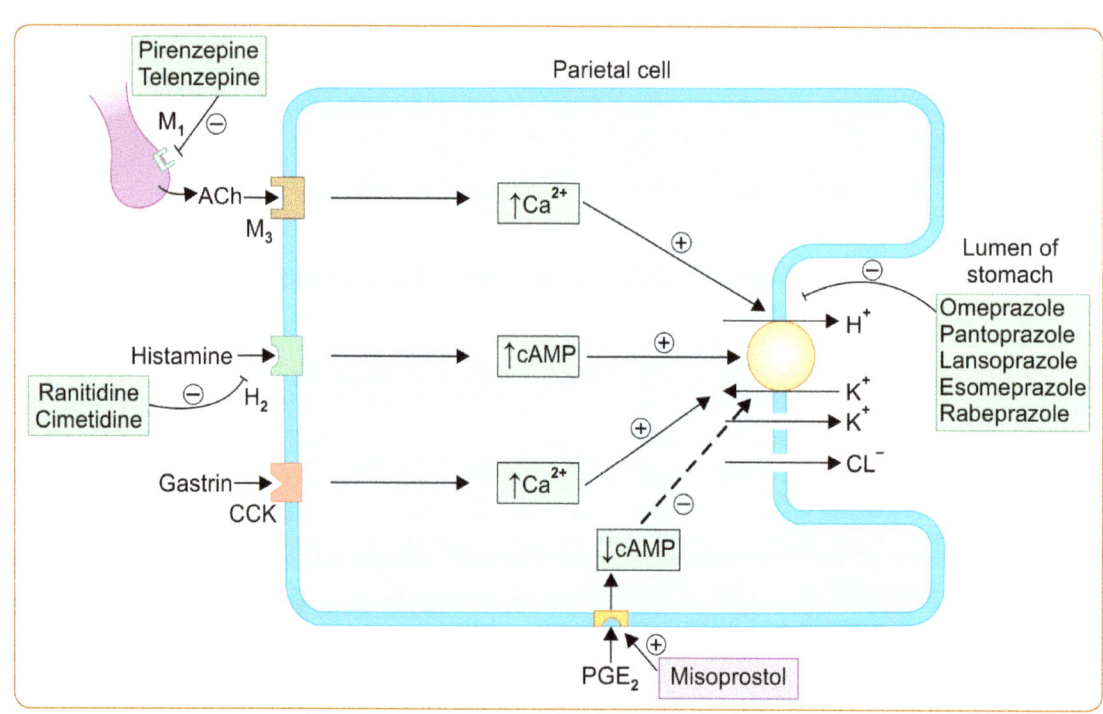

- **Aluminium hydroxide** [Al(OH)$_3$], **magnesium trisilicate, megaldrate** and **magnesium hydroxide** [Mg(OH)$_2$] are **non systemic antacids**. These are slower but longer acting drugs. Rebound acidity does not occur. **Al(OH)$_3$ causes constipation** whereas **magnesium** salts are responsible for **diarrhea**. Most of the market preparations contain these agents in combination to minimize the impact on bowel movements.
- **Simethicone** is a water repellant, pharmacologically inert **anti-foaming agent**. It reduces flatulence and can also be used to prevent bed sores.
- Antacids decrease the absorption of acidic drugs (acidic drugs are ionized in alkaline medium) and tetracyclines (by forming complexes).
- **Milk alkali syndrome** (*hypercalcemia, renal insufficiency and metabolic alkalosis*) may be caused by excessive doses of Na$_2$CO$_3$ or CaCO$_3$ with calcium containing foods (like milk).

DRUGS DECREASING ACID SECRETION

Proton Pump Inhibitors (PPIs)

- These are **prodrugs** (active moiety is sulfenamide) and act **by irreversibly inhibiting H$^+$ K$^+$ ATPase** in gastric parietal cells. The drugs in this group include **omeprazole, pantoprazole, esomeprazole, lansoprazole, rabeprazole, tenatoprazole** (approved in Japan) and **ilaprazole** (approved in Korea). These drugs are weak bases and can be destroyed by gastric acid. To protect them from gastric acid, these are given as enteric coated tablets. This coating dissolves in alkaline medium (intestinal juice) and prodrugs are absorbed. On reaching parietal cells, active moiety (sulfenamide) is formed and gets trapped. These can *inhibit both basal acid output* (nocturnal acid secretion) as well as *meal stimulated acid output* (maximal acid output).
- **Tenatoprazole** is a very long acting PPI and can effectively suppress nocturnal acid secretion.
- PPIs are given orally in early morning empty stomach (just before breakfast). **Pantoprazole, esomeprazole** and lansoprazole **can be given IV**. These drugs have short $t_{1/2}$ but can inhibit acid secretion for more than 24 hours (**hit and run drugs**, inhibit proton pump irreversibly).
- PPIs are the drugs of choice for **peptic ulcer disease (PUD) due to any etiology (even NSAID induced)**. These are **also** the agents of choice **for gastroesophageal reflux disease (GERD) and** Zollinger Ellison Syndrome **(ZES)**. *For prevention of stress induced gastric bleeding, H$_2$ blockers (IV infusion) are preferred over PPIs*. In patients with nasoenteric tube, immediate release omeprazole (by nasogastric tube) is currently preferred.
- PPIs are quite safe drugs and have diarrhea, headache and abdominal pain as adverse effects. These have been shown to be **carcinogenic in rodents** but no such case has been reported in humans.
- All PPIs are substrates of CYP2C19 and CYP3A4 **except rabeprazole**. PPIs can also inhibit these microsomal enzymes leading to drug interactions. Particularly important is their interaction with clopidogrel. Later is a prodrug which is activated by CYP2C19. Omeprazole and other PPIs inhibit this enzyme and result in decreased activity of clopidogrel.

Rabeprazole followed by pantoprazole has **minimum** risk of **drug interactions**.

Long-term use of PPI is associated with:
- Subnormal vitamin B$_{12}$ levels (reduced absorption)
- Increase in risk of hip fractures (reduced Ca^{2+} absorption)
- Increased risk of enteric bacterial infections
  - *C. difficile* infections
  - Bacterial gastroenteritis
- Pneumonia

> **Note**
> - **Lanoprazole is most potent** PPI.
> - Lansoprazole is safest PPI in **pregnancy**.
> - **Rabeprazole** is **fastest** acting PPI.
> - **Rabeprazole has minimum inhibitory effect on CYP**.

Potassium Competitive Acid Blockers

These are the drugs that inhibit proton pump by **competitive** binding to potassium site of proton pump. These are reversible drugs and duration of action of these drugs depends upon their half lives. **Vonoprazan** (approved in Japan) and **Revaprazan** (approved in Korea) are the important drugs in this group. Major advantage of these drugs over irreversible proton pump inhibitors is that these **cause very fast acid suppression**.

H$_2$ Receptor Antagonists

- These drugs competitively inhibit H$_2$ receptors in parietal cells, thus inhibiting the acid secretion. ACh and gastrin act partly by causing the release of histamine, therefore acid secreting capacity of these agents also is decreased by H$_2$ blockers. Drugs in this group are **cimetidine, ranitidine, famotidine, roxatidine, nizatidine and loxatidine**.
- These drugs are *more effective for reducing basal (nocturnal) acid secretion (histamine mediated) than stimulated acid secretion* (stimulated by gastrin, ACh, as well as histamine). These drugs can be used for GERD, PUD, ZES and prevention of stress induced ulcers. **Cimetidine is not used routinely** because:
  - It can cross blood brain barrier and result in **mental state changes**.
  - It inhibits binding of dihydrotestosterone to androgen receptors that can manifest as **impotence** in males.
  - It inhibits metabolism of estradiol and increases serum prolactin levels on long term use, thus can cause gynaecomastia (in males) and galactorrhoea (in females).
  - **It is a potent inhibitor of CYP enzymes** and can increase plasma concentration of warfarin, theophylline and many other drugs.
  - It is the **least potent H$_2$ blocker**.

> **Note**
> - **Famotidine is most potent** H$_2$ blocker.
> - All H$_2$ blockers except famotidine inhibits the gastric first pass metabolism of ethanol
> - **Loxatidine is a non-competitive blocker** of H$_2$ receptors.
> - **Nizatidine also possess anti-AChE activity** and can cause bradycardia and enhanced gastric emptying.
> - **Nizatidine** is having negligible first pass metabolism (**~100% bioavailability**).

Anticholinergics

- Non-selective anti-muscarinic drugs like propantheline and oxyphenonium can be used for decreasing gastric acid secretion. However, by increasing gastric emptying time, these drugs prolong the exposure of ulcer bed to gastric acid. Further anticholinergic adverse effects like dry mouth, blurred vision, constipation and urinary retention are commonly seen with these drugs. **Pirenzepine and telenzepine** are **selective M_1 blockers** that are preferred antimuscarinic agents for peptic ulcer disease as these are devoid of anticholinergic adverse effects.

DRUGS INCREASING PROTECTIVE FACTORS

PGE_1, PGE_2 and PGI_2 act as anti-ulcer drugs by increasing the release of mucus and bicarbonate and by increasing the mucosal blood flow. PGs also inhibit $H^+ K^+$ ATPase and decrease the acid production. **Misoprostol** (PGE$_1$ analogue) is the **MOST SPECIFIC drug for** treatment and prevention of **NSAID induced peptic ulcer** *(DOC is PPI)*. **Enprostil** and **rioprostil** (PGE$_2$ analogue) are other drugs in this group. Commonest side effect of PG analogues is diarrhea and colicky abdominal pain.

ULCER PROTECTIVE AGENTS

These drugs form a covering over the ulcer bed that prevents its exposure to gastric acid. **Sucralfate and colloidal bismuth subcitrate** are two important ulcer protective drugs.

- **Sucralfate:** It is aluminium salt of sulfated sucrose. At pH below 4, its molecules polymerize to form a sticky layer that covers the ulcer base and acts as a physical barrier to prevent acid exposure. It can bind phosphates also and **can result in hypophosphatemia**. It **should not be given with antacids** because it acts only in acidic medium (antacids raise the pH by neutralizing the gastric acid). *Most common side effect of sucralfate is constipation.*
- **Colloidal bismuth subcitrate:** It also forms an acid resistant coating over the ulcer. It **also dislodges** *H. pylori* from the surface of gastric mucosa and kills it. Adverse effects include blackening of tongue and bismuth toxicity (osteodystrophy and encephalopathy).
- **Rebamipide** and **Ecabet** are *cytoprotective drugs* acting by increase in PG generation and by scavenging reactive oxygen species.

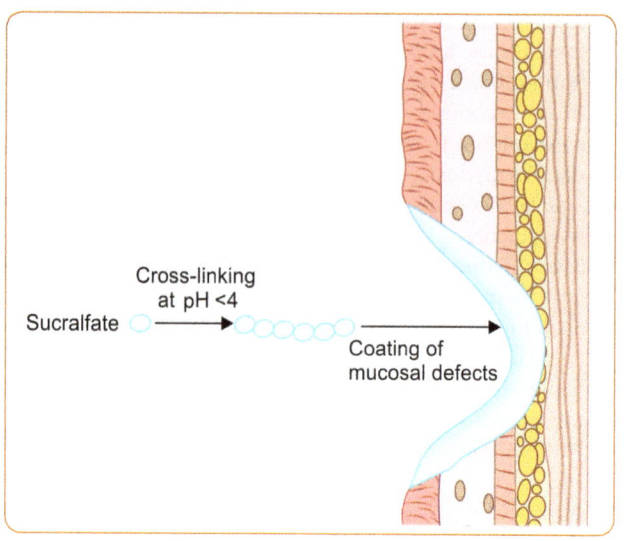

ULCER HEALING DRUGS

Carbenoloxone is obtained from the roots of licorice. It causes epithelisation of ulcer without decreasing acid production. It can displace aldosterone from plasma protein binding sites and result in hypertension, sodium and water retention and hypokalemia.

ANTI-HELICOBACTER PYLORI DRUGS

H. pylori infection can be detected by *"urea breath test"*. It is responsible for relapse of PUD. Drugs used for the treatment of *H. pylori* include:

- *Metronidazole/tinidazole*
- Amoxicillin
- Clarithromycin
- Tetracycline
- Colloidal bismuth subcitrate
- *Omeprazole/lansoprazole*

Triple drug therapy for H. Pylori
C–Clarithromycin
A–Amoxycillin
P–Proton pump inhibitor

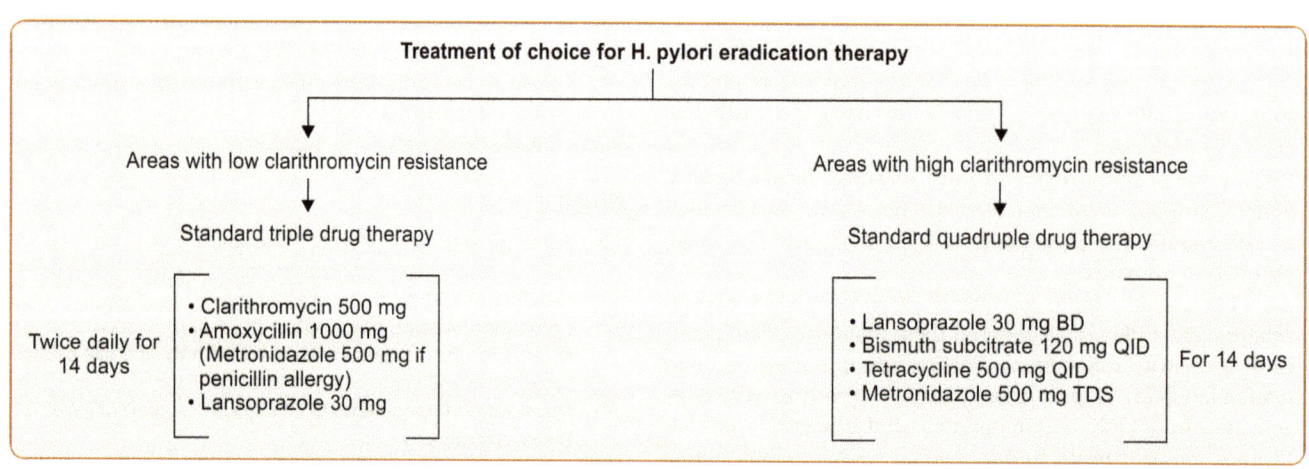

ANTI-EMETIC DRUGS

Vomiting (emesis) occurs due to stimulation of vomiting centre (VC) in lateral medullary reticular formation. It receives input from GI mucosa, chemoreceptor trigger zone (CTZ) and vestibular apparatus.

- Irritation of GI mucosa by drugs or irritants leads to release of serotonin that stimulates VC via $5HT_3$ receptors.
- CTZ is rich in dopamine (D_2) and serotonin ($5HT_3$) and neurokinin (NK_1) receptor.
- Motion sickness occurs due to stimulation of vestibular apparatus and cerebellum. These structures result in stimulation of VC by activating M_1 and H_1 receptors.
- By stimulation of H_1 receptors, histamine plays a permissive role in all types of vomiting.

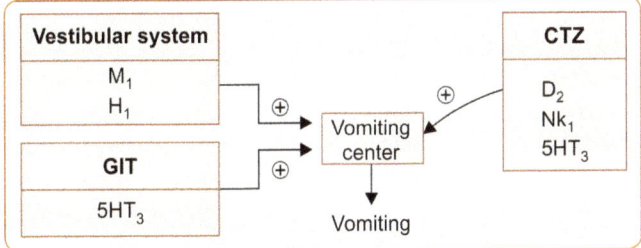

DRUGS FOR MOTION SICKNESS

- **Hyoscine** is used as IM injection or transdermal patch (applied behind pinna) for **prophylaxis of motion sickness**. It has **no role in treatment**, once the vomiting starts.
- **Antihistaminics** like promethazine, diphenhydramine, cyclizine or meclizine can also be used for prophylaxis.
- **Cinnarizine** (antihistaminic with anticholinergic and antiserotonergic properties) is used **for** treatment of **vertigo**.

DRUGS FOR MORNING SICKNESS

- Combination of **doxylamine** (antihistaminic) **with pyridoxine** (Vit B_6) in high dose is **safest anti-emetic drug in pregnancy**
- D_2 **blockers** although effective should not be used due to their **teratogenic** potential.

DRUGS FOR CHEMOTHERAPY AND RADIATION THERAPY INDUCED VOMITING

- **5 HT_3 blockers** like ondansetron, granisetron, dolasetron, palonosetron and ramosetron are DOC for this condition.
- **Palonosetron** is **most potent** 5 HT_3 blocker. **Dolasetron may prolong QT interval.**
- **Palonosetron** has *longest $t_{1/2}$* whereas *ondansetron has shortest $t_{1/2}$*.
- Efficacy of these drugs increases if used along with antihistaminics, D_2 blockers or dexamethasone.
- These drugs are also effective in *hyperemesis of pregnancy and postoperative nausea*.
- D_2 blockers like metoclopramide and domperidone can also be used.
- Vomiting due to **cisplatin (most emetogenic anti cancer drug)** can occur *within 24 hours* or it may be **delayed (after 2 days)**. DOC for the former condition is *$5HT_3$ blocker* whereas for the latter condition, DOC is **aprepitant** (substance P antagonist). *Palonosetron may also be effective in delayed emesis.*
- **Aprepitant** is a *highly selective NK1 receptor antagonist*, **orally active**, and enter the brain. It is *metabolized by CYP3A4 enzymes* and can also inhibit the metabolism of drugs metabolized by this enzyme, e.g. warfarin.
- **Fosaprepitant** is an *intravenous prodrug of aprepitant*.
- **Netupitant** is a newer NK1 antagonist approved for chemotherapy induced vomiting (both acute and delayed in combination with palonosetron).
- **Rolapitant** is recently approved NK 1 antagonist for delayed vomiting.
- **Dronabinol** can be used in patients not responding to other drugs.

DRUGS FOR POSTOPERATIVE VOMITING

- **5 HT_3 antagonists** are preferred over other drugs.
- **Amisulpiride** (D_2 antagonist) can also be used for this indication.

OTHER DRUGS FOR VOMITING

- **Steroids** like dexamethasone can be used as anti-emetic agents in chemotherapy induced vomiting.
- **Benzodiazepines** like lorazepam and alprazolam may be useful for anticipatory component of nausea and vomiting before surgery.
- **Dronabinol (a cannabinoid)** possesses anti-emetic properties and acts by stimulating CB_1 receptors. It can also **stimulate appetite** (*used for AIDS with anorexia*). *Central sympathomimetic (tachycardia, palpitations etc.) effects, paranoid reactions and thinking abnormalities* may appear as adverse effects. It is also approved for chemotherapy-induced vomiting that fails to respond to conventional anti-emetic drugs.

EMETIC DRUGS

Apomorphine and ipecacuanha can be used to produce vomiting for treatment of poisonings. *Emetics should not be used for kerosene and corrosive (acid and alkali) poisonings.*

GASTROESOPHAGEAL REFLUX DISEASE (GERD)

It is a condition in which acid in the stomach reaches the esophagus and causes mucosal inflammation. *Two strategies for the management of this condition are either to decrease the acid production* (by PPIs) *or to increase the forward movement of GIT* (so that the contents do not reflux upwards). The drugs used for increasing the GI motility are known as prokinetic drugs. These drugs can also be used for the treatment of gastroparesis, postoperative paralytic ileus and constipation.

PROKINETIC DRUGS

- ACh is the main excitatory neurotransmitter in the GIT. Cholinergic neurons contain excitatory ($5-HT_4$) as well as inhibitory ($5HT_3$, D_2) presynaptic receptors.
- Thus D_2 and $5HT_3$ antagonists and 5 HT_4 agonists will increase the release of ACh and stimulate the GI motility.

Metoclopramide

It possesses *central as well as peripheral D2 blocking action*. Central D_2 blocking action is responsible for its antiemetic effects.

> - It is also a prokinetic drug due to **agonistic** action at **$5HT_4$ receptors** (main mechanism) and **antagonistic action** at **$5HT_3$** receptors.
> - **Prokinetic action** is due to release of ACh and thus *can be antagonized by atropine*. It *increases gastric peristalsis (enhances gastric emptying) and LES tone but has no effect on colonic motility*.
> - Metoclopramide is mainly used as an **antiemetic** agent. It can also be used in **GERD** and for the treatment of **gastroparesis** (in diabetic patients). Another indication of this drug is to **enhance gastric emptying** for emergency general anaesthesia (if the patient has taken food within 4 hrs.)
> - D2 blocking action can result in extrapyramidal side effects (muscle dystonia, Parkinsonism, etc.) and *hyperprolactinemia* (leading to **galactorrhoea**).

Domperidone

It is a D_2 receptor antagonist and **cannot cross blood brain barrier**. It is mainly used as an antiemetic (less efficacious than metoclopramide) drug and is devoid of extrapyramidal and hyperprolactinemic adverse effects. *It decreases l-dopa induced vomiting without interfering with its efficacy*.

$5HT_4$ Agonists

Cisapride, mosapride, renzapride, prucalopride and tegaserod are $5-HT_4$ agonistic drugs with no action on D_2 receptors (no antiemetic property). These drugs *increase whole GI motility including colon*.

- **Cisapride** was previously used for the treatment of GERD but it has been withdrawn in some countries due to its **QT prolonging action**. It is metabolized by CYP 3A4 and therefore **should not be administered with** microsomal enzyme inhibitors like **ketoconazole and erythromycin** (increased chances of torsades de pointes, an arrhythmia with QT prolongation). *Mosapride and renzapride do not prolong QT interval*. **Tegaserod** can be used for constipation dominant irritable bowel syndrome. However, recently it has also been **withdrawn** from India due to increased incidence of *myocardial infarction and stroke*.

Other Prokinetic Drugs

- *Levosulpiride* (l-isomer of sulpiride; an antipsychotic drug) is a newer D_2 blocker having prokinetic activity.
- *Loxiglumide* is a CCK1 receptor antagonist indicated for constipation dominant IBS.
- *Macrolides* (like erythromycin) are *motilin agonists*. Erythromycin is indicated in diabetic gastroparesis. Rapid development of tolerance limits this use.

IRRITABLE BOWEL SYNDROME (IBS)

- It is a condition characterized by abdominal pain, bloating and altered bowel habits (diarrhea or constipation)
- **For relieving pain**, the drugs used are **TCAs** (fluoxetine is less effective) **and anticholinergics** like dicyclomine and hyoscine. **Mebeverine** is an antispasmodic agent that exerts direct action on GI smooth muscle without affecting motility.
- **Diarrhea-dominant IBS** can be managed by opioids like **loperamide**. Newer opioids like **fedotozine** (k receptor agonist) and **eluxadoline** (μ and k agonist, δ-antagonist) can also be used. $5HT_3$ antagonists like **alosetron** and **cilansetron** are indicated in selected cases. Major adverse effect of $5HT_3$ antagonists is development of **ischemic colitis**.
- **Constipation** in IBS patients can be managed by dietary fibres and laxatives like methylcellulose and polyethylene glycol. **Lubipristone** (a chloride channel activator) and **linaclotide** (a guanylate cyclase-C agonist) stimulate chloride secretion in GIT that induces passive movement of sodium and water into the bowel lumen.
- **Tenapanor** is an inhibitor of sodium hydrogen exchanger-3 (NHE-3) in intestine. NHE-3 helps in absorption of Na^+ in GIT. By inhibiting this transporter, tenapanor prevents absorption of Na^+ in the intestine. Elevated sodium leads to water secretion and makes stool soft. It is approved for IBS with constipation. It is **contraindicated in children less than 6 years** of age due to risk of **severe dehydration**.

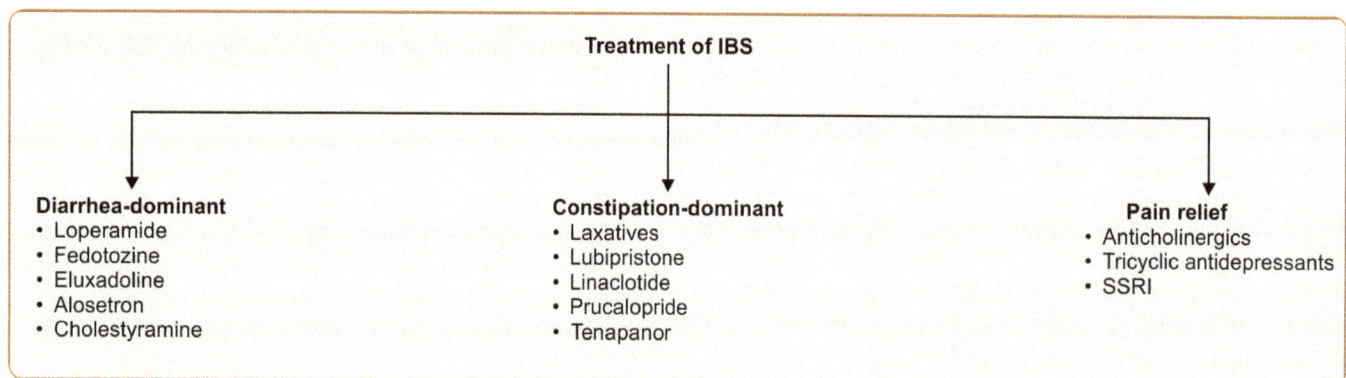

Treatment of IBS

Diarrhea-dominant
- Loperamide
- Fedotozine
- Eluxadoline
- Alosetron
- Cholestyramine

Constipation-dominant
- Laxatives
- Lubipristone
- Linaclotide
- Prucalopride
- Tenapanor

Pain relief
- Anticholinergics
- Tricyclic antidepressants
- SSRI

CONSTIPATION

High fibre diet, adequate fluid intake and regular exercise are best measures to prevent constipation. Patients not responding to these measures may require laxatives. These can be classified as:

Gastrointestinal Tract

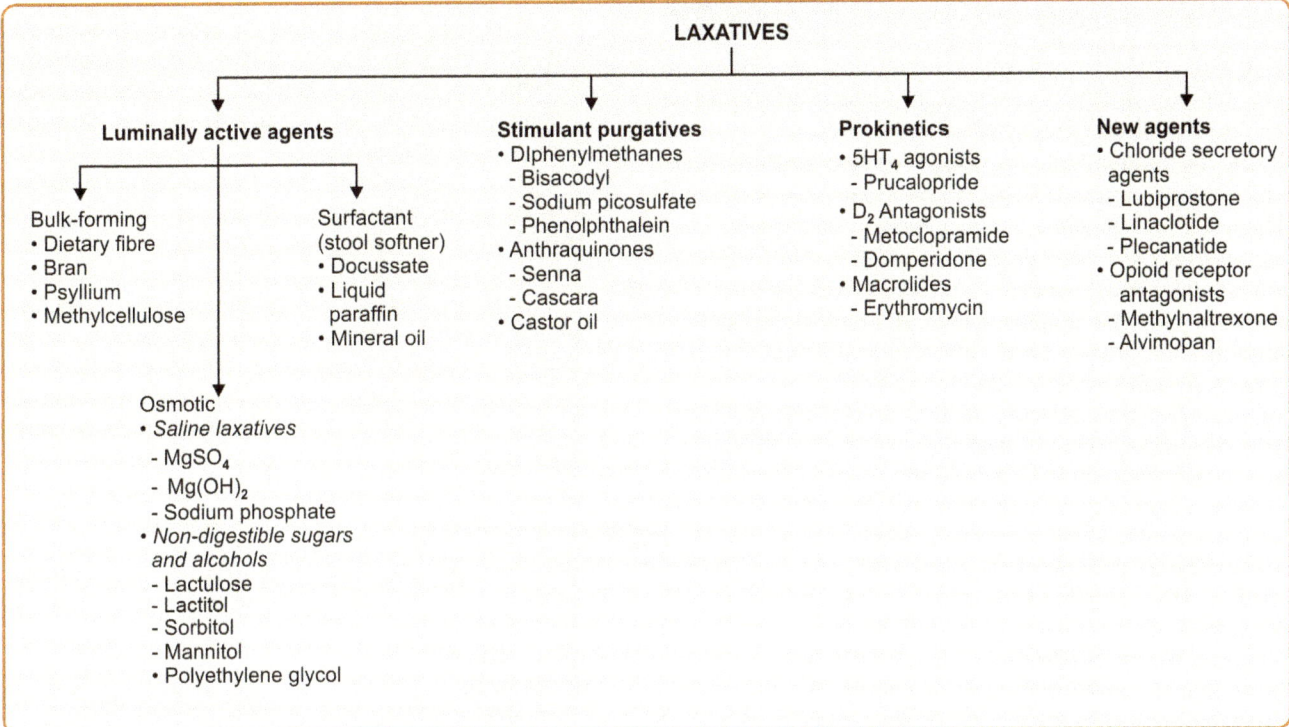

- Bulk-forming agents are contraindicated in presence of megacolon.
- Saline purgatives should not be given in chronic renal failure.
- Stimulant purgatives are contraindicated in presence of intestinal obstruction.
- *Chronic use of anthraquinone derivatives (like senna and cascara) may lead to melanosis coli* (brown pigmentation of colon)
- *Phenolphthalein* is not used now due to risk of *potential carcinogenicity.*
- *Prucalopride* is a 5HT$_4$ agonist and is recently approved for oral treatment of chronic idiopathic constipation.
- *Lubiprostone and Linaclotide:* These stimulate Cl⁻ channel opening in the intestine, increase liquid secretion in gut and decrease transit time, therefore used for chronic constipation.

Plecanatide is a guanylate cyclase C agonist. It activates CFTR leading to increased flow of chloride and water into the lumen of GIT. It is recently approved for **chronic idiopathic constipation**.

- **Methylnaltrexone, naldemedine and naloxegol** are peripheral opioid antagonists and are used for opioid induced constipation.

Key Points

Lubiprostone is used for chronic constipation. It acts by
- Stimulating Cl⁻ channel opening in the intestine,
- Increasing liquid secretion in gut
- Decreasing transit time.

DIARRHEA

Diarrhea can be treated by antibiotics effective against the causative organism. In non-infective diarrhea, drugs useful are:

Opioids

Loperamide is a non-addictive over the counter anti-diarrheal drug. **Diphenoxylate** is another opioid but has addictive potential if used for prolonged periods. It is always given in combination **with atropine to prevent the abuse** (atropine will produce dry mouth and other anticholinergic side effects). These drugs are **contraindicated in infective diarrhea**.

Octreotide

This long acting **somatostatin analog** can be used to decrease **secretory diarrhea** and other symptoms of carcinoid syndrome and VIPoma. *In low doses* (50 μg, SC), *it stimulates motility, whereas at high doses* (100-250 μg, SC), *it inhibits motility*. In higher doses, it is also useful for the treatment of diarrhea due to vagotomy, short bowel syndrome and AIDS. It can also be used for treatment and prophylaxis of **acute pancreatitis.**

Other Drugs

- **Racecadrotil** is *enkephalinase inhibitor* (inhibits breakdown of enkephalins; endogenous opioids) having antidiarrheal effect.
- **Clonidine** is indicated for diabetics with chronic diarrhea.
- **Crofelemer** is a new drug approved for relieving symptoms of diarrhea in AIDS patients taking anti-retroviral therapy. It acts by blocking two chloride channels; CFTR and anoctamin-1.
- **Bezlotoxumab** is a monoclonal antibody that binds to C. difficile toxin B and neutralizes its effect. It is used to reduce recurrence of C. difficile infection.
- **Telotristat ethyl** is a tryptophan hydroxylase inhibitor. It decreases the formation of serotonin. It is approved for diarrhea due to carcinoid syndrome.

ORAL REHYDRATION SOLUTION (ORS)

- Hydration must be maintained in all cases of diarrhea to prevent fluid depletion and shock. It is mostly accomplished by the institution of oral rehydration solution.
- It contains sodium and potassium chloride, trisodium citrate and glucose. Glucose helps in the absorption of sodium because *glucose facilitated sodium reabsorption remains intact even in severe diarrhea*. Trisodium citrate is added to prevent acidosis. Previously sodium bicarbonate was used for this function but now sodium citrate is preferred because it imparts a longer shelf life to ORS. Composition of ORS used previously and now is as follows:

	Standard formula ORS	New formula WHO-ORS
NaCl	3.5 g	2.6 g
KCl	1.5 g	1.5 g
Trisodium citrate	2.9 g	2.9 g
Glucose	20 g	13.5 g
Water	1 L	1 L
Na^+	90 mmol/L	75 mmol/L
K^+	20 mmol/L	20 mmol/L
Cl^-	80 mmol/L	65 mmol/L
Citrate	10 mmol/L	10 mmol/L
Glucose	111 mmol/L	75 mmol/L
Total osmolality	311 mosm/L	245 mosm/L

In new formula WHO-ORS, concentration of NaCl and glucose as well as total osmolarity is decreased because

- WHO standard formula was based on *cholera stools* in which loss of Na^+ was more. There is a significant decrease in cholera cases and major cause of diarrhea now-a-days is rota virus. New composition ORS is based on stool composition of rota virus patients.
- Use of *standard formula* ORS has *lead to* development of *edema* (excess of sodium) *and increased stool frequency* (unabsorbed glucose acts as laxative) in some patients.

INFLAMMATORY BOWEL DISEASE

Ulcerative colitis and Crohn's disease are two distinct disorders classified under inflammatory bowel disease (IBD).

Aminosalicylates

- **5-aminosalicylic acid** (5-ASA) is the main anti-inflammatory compound that acts locally in the colon. When given alone by oral route, more than 80% is absorbed in proximal intestine and very little reaches the diseased site i.e. colon. To decrease the absorption it may be associated with some inert compound. **Sulfasalazine** (5-ASA + sulfapyridine), **olsalazine** (5-ASA + 5-ASA) and **balsalazide** (5-ASA + amino benzoyl alanine) are effective for the treatment of ulcerative colitis.

The inert compound prevents the absorption in proximal GIT and the combination reaches the colon where the bacteria cleaves the azo bond to free 5-ASA for action. Approximately 85% sulfapyridine is absorbed from colon leading to adverse effects.

- **Different formulations** (like **time release tablets** and **coating in pH sensitive resins** that dissolve at pH 7) of 5-ASA have been developed to deliver it to colon. These formulations are known as **mesalamine**.
- **5-ASA is the first line treatment for mild to moderate ulcerative colitis**. Efficacy in Crohn's disease has not been established. Absorption of sulfapyridine (in sulfasalazine) lead to nausea, vomiting, GI upset, bone marrow suppression, hypersensitivity and oligospermia. Olsalazine may result in secretory diarrhea.

Glucocorticoids

- **Prednisone, prednisolone, hydrocortisone and budesonide** are used in the treatment of moderate to severe ulcerative colitis and Crohn's disease.
- Purine analogs.
- **Azathioprine and 6-MP** are important agents for the induction and maintenance of remission of ulcerative colitis and Crohn's disease.

Methotrexate

- It is used for the induction and maintenance of remission of Crohn's disease but not ulcerative colitis.

Anti TNF-α Therapy

- **Infliximab, adalimumab and certolizumab** are useful in Crohn's disease. Efficacy in ulcerative colitis is doubtful. **Infliximab** is given by **IV** route whereas other two are administered SC **Certolizumab** is a pegylated anti-TNF-α indicated for Crohn's disease.

Anti-integrin Therapy

- **Natalizumab** is recently approved for moderate to severe Crohn's disease not responding to other therapies. It is targeted against $α_4$ **subunit of integrins**. The patient on natalizumab therapy should not be on other immunosuppressants due to risk of **progressive multifocal leukoencephalopathy (PML)**.
- **Vedolizumab** is a new anti-integrin that block α4 β7 in GIT but not in brain. It is, thus, less likely to cause PML.

 Key Points

Monoclonal Antibodies for Crohn's Disease
- Infliximab
- Adalimumab
- Certolizumab
- Natalizumab
- Vedolizumab

Golden Points

1. **Proton pump is stimulated by**
   - Histamine (H_1 receptors)
   - Acetylcholine (M_1 and M_3 receptors)
   - Gastrin (CCK receptors)

2. Major role of antacids in peptic ulcer is to provide prompt relief from ulcer pain.

3. $Al(OH)_3$ causes constipation whereas magnesium salts are responsible for diarrhea.

4. Recent studies have suggested an increase in risk of hip fracture in patients taking PPI on long term.

5. Anti-histaminics (H_2 blockers) are more effective for reducing basal (nocturnal) acid secretion (histamine mediated) than stimulated acid secretion (stimulated by gastrin, ACh, as well as histamine).

6. Acid suppressing agents (like PPIs, H_2 blockers etc.) can result in tolerance and rebound hyperacidity due to secondary hyper-gastrinemia.

7. Misoprostol (PGE_1 analogue) is the MOST SPECIFIC drug for treatment and prevention of NSAID induced peptic ulcer whereas drug of choice is proton pump inhibitor.

8. Sucralfate should not be given with antacids as it polymerises only in acidic medium.

9. Combination of doxylamine (antihistaminic) with pyridoxine (Vit B_6) in high dose is safest anti-emetic drug in pregnancy.

10. $5HT_3$ blockers like ondansetron, granisetron, dolasetron, palonosetron and ramosetron are DOC for chemotherapy induced vomiting.

11. Domperidone decreases l-dopa induced vomiting without interfering with its efficacy.

12. Cisapride has been withdrawn in some countries due to its QT prolonging action whereas Tegaserod has been withdrawn from India due to increased incidence of myocardial infarction and stroke.

13. **Linaclotide** is a guanylate cyclase agonist indicated for oral treatment of idiopathic constipation and IBS with constipation.

14. Atropine is added to lopermide to decrease its addictive potential.

15. In new formula WHO-ORS, concentration of NaCl and glucose as well as total osmolarity is decreased.

16. 5-ASA is the first line treatment for mild to moderate ulcerative colitis.

17. **PPIs are drugs of choice for**
    - Peptic ulcer disease (PUD) due to any etiology (even NSAID induced).
    - Gastroesophageal reflux disease (GERD).
    - Zollinger-Ellison syndrome (ZES).

Drug of Choice

Condition	Drug of choice
• Peptic ulcer	
– Gastric ulcer	Proton pump inhibitors (PPI)
– Duodenal ulcer	PPI
– Stress ulcer	PPI
– NSAID-induced	PPI
– H. pylori associated	Lansoprazole + Amoxycillin + Clarithromycin
– Zollinger Ellison syndrome	PPI
– Gastro esophageal Reflux Disease	PPI
• Vomiting	
– Chemotherapy induced	5-HT_3 antagonists like palonosetron
– Levo-dopa induced	Domperidone
– Migraine associated	Metoclopramide
– Drug or disease associated	Metoclopramide
– Postoperative	Ondansetron
– Radiation induced	Ondansetron
– Cisplatin - induced	
- Early	5-HT_3 antagonists
- Delayed	Aprepitant
• Prophylaxis of motion sickness	Hyoscine
• Pregnancy (Morning sickness)	Doxylamine + Pyridoxine
• Opioid induced constipation	Methylnaltrexone
• Diarrhea in carcinoid syndrome	Octreotide
• To prevent dehydration in diarrhea	ORS
• Crohn's disease	Corticosteroids
• Ulcerative colitis	5-ASA derivatives
• Hepatic encephalopathy	Lactulose

Image Based Questions

1. A new drug L has been approved for constipation-dominant irritable bowel syndrome. Its mechanism of action is shown in the image. Drug L is likely to be:

   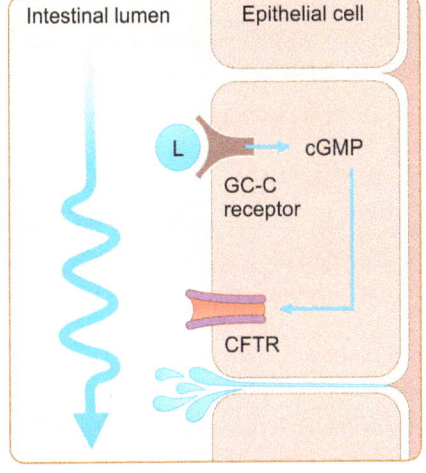

   (a) Prucalopride (b) Alvimopan
   (c) Plecanatide   (d) Ivacaftor

2. A patient was taking laxatives since many years. His colonoscopy revealed the following features. The likely laxative responsible for these features is:

   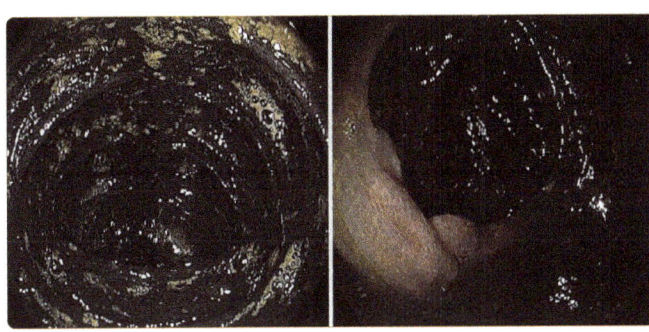

   (a) Senna
   (b) Bisacodyl
   (c) Dietary fibre
   (d) Lactulose

Explanations

1. **Ans. (c) Plecanatide**
   Plecanatide is a new drug which acts as an agonist of guanylate cyclase C receptors. It increases chloride secretion by activating the CFTR via this mechanism.

2. **Ans. (a) Senna**
   Anthraquinone laxatives like senna and cascara can result in melanosis coli (as shown in the image).

Multiple Choice Questions

PEPTIC ULCER DISEASE

1. Pirenzepine is used for:
   (NEET Pattern Question 2017-2018)
   - (a) Peptic ulcer
   - (b) Motion sickness
   - (c) Constipation
   - (d) Bronchial asthma

2. Which of the following drugs have least affinity for CYP3A4? *(AIIMS May 2016)*
   - (a) Omeprazole
   - (b) Lansoprazole
   - (c) Esomeprazole
   - (d) Rabeprazole

3. All of the following adverse effects are associated with the use of proton pump inhibitors *except*:
   - (a) Community acquired pneumonia *(AIIMS Nov 2015)*
   - (b) *Clostridium difficile* infection
   - (c) Osteoporosis leading to hip fracture
   - (d) Hypothyroidism

4. Despite their short half-lives (2 hrs), proton pump inhibitors (PPIs) cause a prolonged suppression of acid secretion (up to 48 h) because: *(AIIMS May 2012)*
   - (a) They are prodrugs and undergo activation gradually
   - (b) They exit from the plasma and enter acid secretory canaliculi and stay there, blocking the secretion of acid for a long time
   - (c) They irreversibly inhibit the proton pump molecule and hence, acid secretion requires synthesis of new proton pumps
   - (d) They are available as enteric coated capsules, from which drug is gradually released

5. Cimetidine inhibits the metabolism of all of the following drugs *except*: *(Recent NEET Pattern Question)*
   - (a) Phenytoin
   - (b) Warfarin
   - (c) Ketoconazole
   - (d) Diazepam

6. Drug used in the treatment of gastric ulcer due to *H. pylori* is: *(Recent NEET Pattern Question)*
   - (a) Anticholinergics
   - (b) Carbenoxolone sodium
   - (c) Bismuth subcitrate
   - (d) Corticosteroid

7. Which one of the following is not an antacid?
   - (a) Magnesium sulfate *(Recent NEET Pattern Question)*
   - (b) Magaldrate
   - (c) Magnesium carbonate
   - (d) Magnesium phosphate

8. NSAID induced ulcer are treated by:
   - (a) Antacids *(Recent NEET Pattern Question)*
   - (b) H_2 blockers
   - (c) Misoprostol
   - (d) PPI (proton pump inhibitors)

9. Which of the following is not the effect of ranitidine as compared to cimetidine? *(Recent NEET Pattern Question)*
   - (a) Action on H_2 receptors
   - (b) Given orally
   - (c) Used with proton pump blockers
   - (d) Anti-androgenic action

10. Esomeprazole acts by inhibiting:
    (Recent NEET Pattern Question)
    - (a) H^+K^+ ATPase pump
    - (b) H^+Na^+ ATPase pump
    - (c) H^+ pump
    - (d) Any of the above

11. Antacid drug that typically causes diarrhea:
    - (a) Sodium bicarbonate *(Recent NEET Pattern Question)*
    - (b) Magnesium hydroxide
    - (c) Calcium bicarbonate
    - (d) Aluminium hydroxide

12. The inhibition of hydrochloric acid (HCl) secretion by omeprazole occurs within an hour, reaches a peak at 2 hours, and plateaus by 4th day. After how many days will the secretion gradually normalize?
    (Recent NEET Pattern Question)
    - (a) < 24 hours
    - (b) 1-2 days
    - (c) 3-5 days
    - (d) 6-10 days

13. All are H_2 blocker *except*: *(Recent NEET Pattern Question)*
    - (a) Omeprazole
    - (b) Cimetidine
    - (c) Famatodine
    - (d) Ranitidine

14. The following appears to affect the integrity of the adherent gel of sucralfate interfering with its action:
    (Recent NEET Pattern Question)
    - (a) Antacids
    - (b) Food
    - (c) Mucin
    - (d) Proteins in foodstuffs

15. A patient presents with Zollinger-Ellison syndrome due to gastrinoma. He has two bleeding ulcers and diarrhoea. A drug that irreversibly inhibits the H^+/K^+ ATPase in gastric parietal cells is:
    (Recent NEET Pattern Question)
    - (a) Cimetidine
    - (b) Cisapride
    - (c) Glycopyrrolate
    - (d) Omeprazole

16. Which is not an adverse effect of cimetidine?
    (Recent NEET Pattern Question)
    - (a) Impotence
    - (b) Gynaecomastia
    - (c) Atrophic gastritis
    - (d) Galactorrhea

17. Primary role of antacids in peptic ulcer is:
    (Recent NEET Pattern Question)
    - (a) Pain relief
    - (b) Ulcer healing
    - (c) H. pylori eradication
    - (d) All of the above

18. Drug not used in the treatment of *H. pylori* is:
    (Recent NEET Pattern Question)
    - (a) Cisapride
    - (b) Clarithromycin
    - (c) Metronidazole
    - (d) Omeprazole

Gastrointestinal Tract

19. All of the following antibiotics have been used in treatment of *H. pylori* infection, *except*:
    (Recent NEET Pattern Question)
    (a) Clarithromycin (b) Amoxicillin
    (c) Metronidazole (d) Ciprofloxacin

20. Which group of drugs is most effective for the healing of Nonsteroidal AntiInflammatory Drug (NSAID) induced gastric ulcer? *(Recent NEET Pattern Question)*
    (a) Prostaglandin analogues
    (b) H_2-receptor antagonists
    (c) Proton pump inhibitors
    (d) Antacids

21. Effective ulcer treatment that works by inhibitory action on gastric acid secretion is:
    (Recent NEET Pattern Question)
    (a) Lactulose (b) Aluminium hydroxide
    (c) Sucralfate (d) Ranitidine

22. Which of the following is the drug of choice for treatment of peptic ulcer disease?
    (Recent NEET Pattern Question)
    (a) Omeprazole (b) Pirenzepine
    (c) Ranitidine (d) Sucralfate

23. On chronic use which of the following drugs may cause reversible gynaecomastia? *(Recent NEET Pattern Question)*
    (a) Cimetidine (b) Omeprazole
    (c) Pirenzepine (d) Sucralfate

24. A 30 years old pregnant woman has a history of rheumatoid arthritis which has been managed successfully with NSAIDs. However, she has recently visited her general practitioner complaining of burning epigastric pain worsened by food intake. Which of the following ulcer medication is most likely contraindicated in this patient? *(Recent NEET Pattern Question)*
    (a) Famotidine (b) Omeprazole
    (c) Misoprostol (d) Ranitidine

25. Omeprazole acts by inhibiting:
    (Recent NEET Pattern Question)
    (a) $Na^+H^+ATPase$ (b) $Na^+K^+ATPase$
    (c) Calcium channels (d) $H^+K^+ATPase$

ANTI-EMETICS AND GERD

26. A patient presented with history of few episodes of vomiting and was given an anti-emetic drug by the intern. Few hours later, the patient developed an abnormal posture. Which of the following is likely drug administered to him? *(AIIMS May 2018)*
    (a) Metoclopramide
    (b) Ondansetron
    (c) Domperidone
    (d) Dexamethasone

27. Most specific antiemetic for chemotherapy induced vomiting is: *(NEET Pattern Question 2019)*
    (a) Granisetron (b) Tegaserod
    (c) Domperidone (d) Doxylamine

28. Which of the following drugs has both $5HT_4$ agonist and D_2 antagonist property? *(NEET Pattern Question 2016-17)*
    (a) Ondansetron
    (b) Metoclopramide
    (c) Benzhexol
    (d) Ibutilide

29. A person has to go to Shimla next morning. What drug should be given to prevent motion sickness in this person? *(AIIMS Nov 2017)*
    (a) Scopolamine patch a night before
    (b) Ranitidine one night before and then before the trip
    (c) Dimenhydrinate 1 hour before journey
    (d) Omeprazole half an hour before the trip

30. Antiemetic effect of metoclopramide is mainly due to its action as: *(AIIMS May 2016)*
    (a) 5HT3 antagonist (b) D2 antagonist
    (c) M3 antagonist (d) 5HT4 agonist

31. Which of the following is an antagonist of a peptide and is used to reduce chemotherapy induced nausea and vomiting? *(AIIMS May 2013)*
    (a) Atrial natriuretic peptide
    (b) Aprepitant
    (c) Bradykinin
    (d) Enalapril

32. Drug given for metoclopramide induced dystonic reaction is: *(Recent NEET Pattern Question)*
    (a) Pheniramine
    (b) Promethazine
    (c) Chlorpromazine
    (d) Prochlorperazine

33. Metoclopramide: *(Recent NEET Pattern Question)*
    (a) Inhibit cholinergic smooth muscle stimulation in the gastrointestinal tract
    (b) Decrease lower esophageal sphincter pressure
    (c) Stimulate D_2 receptor
    (d) Enhance colonic motility

34. Drug implicated in prolonging QT interval is:
    (Recent NEET Pattern Question)
    (a) Domperidone
    (b) Metoclopramide
    (c) Cisapride
    (d) Omeprazole

35. Ondansetron acts by inhibiting which of the following receptors? *(Recent NEET Pattern Question)*
    (a) $5-HT_1$ (b) $5-HT_2$
    (c) $5-HT_3$ (d) $5-HT_4$

36. Drug stimulating 5HT4 receptors to act as prokinetic agents are all of the following *except*:
    (Recent NEET Pattern Question)
    (a) Renzapride (b) Metoclopramide
    (c) Domperidone (d) Cisapride

37. Which of the following drugs is not used for motion sickness? *(Recent NEET Pattern Question)*
    (a) Metoclopramide (b) Cyclizine
    (c) Cinnarizine (d) Scopolamine

38. All of the following are true about ondansetron *except*:
    (Recent NEET Pattern Question)
    (a) Drug of choice for chemotherapy induced vomiting
    (b) Dopamine antagonist
    (c) 5HT$_3$ antagonist
    (d) Used to prevent relapse in alcohol dependence

39. Which of the following is the most potent 5HT$_3$ antagonist? *(Recent NEET Pattern Question)*
    (a) Ondansetron
    (b) Granisetron
    (c) Dolasetron
    (d) Palonosetron

40. Which drug is given in delayed vomitting after chemotherapy? *(Recent NEET Pattern Question)*
    (a) Metoclopramide (b) Hyoscine
    (c) Domperiodone (d) Aprepitant

41. Antiemetic used in vomiting induced by anticancer drugs is: *(Recent NEET Pattern Question)*
    (a) Ondansetron (b) Cisapride
    (c) Metoclopramide (d) Trifluopromazine

42. Drug used in cancer chemotherapy induced vomiting is:
    (Recent NEET Pattern Question)
    (a) Aprepitant (b) Dexamethasone
    (c) Ondansetron (d) All of the above

43. All of the following are true for metoclopramide *except*:
    (Recent NEET Pattern Question)
    (a) Chemically related to procainamide
    (b) Speeds gastric emptying
    (c) Stimulates chemoreceptor trigger zone
    (d) Blocks D$_2$ receptors

44. Which of the following 5-HT receptors play an important role in causing emesis?
    (Recent NEET Pattern Question)
    (a) 5HT$_1$ (b) 5HT$_{2A/2C}$
    (c) 5HT$_3$ (d) 5HT$_4$

45. A prokinetic drug which lacks D$_2$ receptor antagonistic action is which one of the following?
    (Recent NEET Pattern Question)
    (a) Metoclopramide
    (b) Domperidone
    (c) Cisapride
    (d) Chlorpromazine

46. All of the following are effective against cytotoxic drug induced emesis *except*: *(Recent NEET Pattern Question)*
    (a) Dronabinol (b) Hyoscine
    (c) Metoclopramide (d) Ondansetron

DIARRHEA, CONSTIPATION, IBS

47. Which of the following is not a prokinetic?
    (NEET Pattern 2020)
    (a) 5HT$_4$ agonist (b) D$_2$ blocker
    (c) Motilide (d) Diphenoxymethane

48. Prucalopride is a: *(AIIMS Nov. 2019)*
    (a) 5HT$_4$ agonist (b) 5HT$_{2b}$ agonist
    (c) 5HT$_{2b}$ antagonist (d) 5HT$_{1a}$ partial agonist

49. Melanosis coli is caused by:
    (NEET Pattern Question 2017-2018)
    (a) Bisacodyl (b) Senna
    (c) Magnesium sulfate (d) Lactulos

50. False statement about rececadotril is:
    (NEET Pattern Question 2016-17)
    (a) It is a prodrug that is converted to peripherally acting enkephalinase inhibitor
    (b) It is a drug used in constipation
    (c) It is metabolised by liver
    (d) It has anti-secretory action in GIT

51. Drug use in treatment of steroid-resistant ulcerative colitis is: *(NEET Pattern Question 2016-17)*
    (a) Cyclosporine (b) 5-ASA
    (c) Azathioprine (d) Racecadotril

52. Laxative abuse is associated with: *(AIIMS May. 2014)*
    (a) Hypokalemia (b) Hypomagnesemia
    (c) Hypoglycemia (d) Colonic spacticity

53. Drug used in irritable bowel syndrome with constipation is: *(AI 2012)*
    (a) Lubiprostone (b) Loperamide
    (c) Alosetron (d) Clonidine

54. Bisacodyl is: *(Recent NEET Pattern Question)*
    (a) Bulk forming
    (b) Stool softner
    (c) Stimulant purgative
    (d) Osmotic purgative

55. Sulfa drug used in inflammatory bowel disease includes:
    (a) Sulfasalazine *(Recent NEET Pattern Question)*
    (b) Sulfamethoxazole
    (c) Sulfinpyrazone
    (d) Sulphadoxine

56. Best for treatment of irritable bowel syndrome with spastic colon is: *(Recent NEET Pattern Question)*
    (a) Liquid parafin (b) Senna
    (c) Bisacodyl (d) Dietary fibers

57. Diarrhea (loose stools) is side effect of:
    (Recent NEET Pattern Question)
    (a) Omeprazole (b) Sucralfate
    (c) Metoclopramide (d) Misoprostol

58. Not true about the composition of ORS:
    (Recent NEET Pattern Question)
    (a) NaCl -3.5 g (b) KCl -1.5 g
    (c) Bicarbonate -2 g (d) Glucose -20 g

59. Which one of the drugs is useful in treating Crohn's disease? *(Recent NEET Pattern Question)*
    (a) Infliximab
    (b) Azathioprine
    (c) Tacrolimus
    (d) Cyclosporine

60. Drug useful in hepatic encephalopathy is:
    (Recent NEET Pattern Question)
    (a) Magnesium sulphate
    (b) Lactulose
    (c) Bisacodyl
    (d) Biphosphonates

Gastrointestinal Tract

61. Which of the following stool softeners does not interfere with fat absorption? *(Recent NEET Pattern Question)*
    (a) Docussates
    (b) Phenolphthalein
    (c) Liquid paraffin
    (d) Castor oil

62. Which of the following is not used in Crohn's disease? *(Recent NEET Pattern Question)*
    (a) Infliximab
    (b) Adalimumab
    (c) Ustekinumab
    (d) Natalizumab

63. Which laxative acts by opening of chloride channels? *(Recent NEET Pattern Question)*
    (a) Docusate
    (b) Anthraquinone
    (c) Lubiprostone
    (d) Bisacodyl

64. Which of the following purgative increases the fecal bulk due to their water absorbing and retaining capacity?
    (a) Methyl cellulose *(Recent NEET Pattern Question)*
    (b) Lactulose
    (c) Liquid paraffin
    (d) Dioctyl sodium sulfosuccinate

65. All of the following statements about treatment of diarrhea are correct *except*: *(Recent NEET Pattern Question)*
    (a) Opioids delay passage of gut contents by reducing peristalsis
    (b) Loperamide is an opioid with anti motility action
    (c) Antimotility drugs are best drugs for infective diarrhea
    (d) Diphenoxylate overlose can cause respiratory depression

66. Sulfasalazine is used in: *(Recent NEET Pattern Question)*
    (a) Ulcerative colitis
    (b) Osteoarthritis
    (c) Gouty arthritis
    (d) Irritable bowel syndrome

67. Glucose is added in ORS to:
    (a) Improve taste *(Recent NEET Pattern Question)*
    (b) Decrease bacterial colonization of GIT
    (c) Increase the stability
    (d) Increase the absorption of sodium

Explanations

1. **Ans. (a) Peptic ulcer** *(Ref: KDT 8th/e p702)*

2. **Ans. (d) Rabeprazole** *(Ref: Katzung 13th/1060, KDT 8th/e p701)*
   Proton pump inhibitors are metabolized by CYP3A4 and CYP2C19. They are also inhibitors of these enzymes. Rabeprazole and pantoprazole has less affinity for these enzymes.

3. **Ans. (d) Hypothyroidism**
   (Ref: CMDT 2015/609-610, KDT 8th/e p701.)
   - Long-term use of proton pump inhibitors may lead to
     - Mild to moderate decrease in vitamin B_{12}, iron and calcium absorption.
     - Increased risk of enteric infections including *C. difficile* and bacterial gastroenteritis.
     - Modest increase in risk of hip fractures.
     - Modest increase in risk of pneumonia.

4. **Ans. (c) They irreversibly inhibit the proton pump molecule and hence, acid secretion requires synthesis of new proton pumps** *(Ref: Rang and Dale 5th/e p370-371, Goodman Gilman 12th/e p1311-1312, KDT 8th/e p700)*

   - The activated form of PPIs binds covalently with sulfhydryl groups of cysteines in the H^+, K^+-ATPase, irreversibly inactivating the pump molecule. Acid secretion resumes only after new pump molecules are synthesized and inserted into the luminal membrane, providing a prolonged (up to 24- to 48-hour) suppression of acid secretion, despite the much shorter plasma half-lives (0.5-2 hours) of the parent compounds.
   - Because not all pumps or all parietal cells are active simultaneously, maximal suppression of acid secretion requires several doses of the proton pump inhibitors. For example, it may take 2-5 days of therapy with once-daily dosing to achieve the 70% inhibition of proton pumps that is seen at steady state.

5. **Ans. (c) Ketoconazole** *(Ref: KDT 8th/e p698)*
   Cimetidine is a potent inhibitor of microsomal enzymes. It prolongs the half lives of warfarin, theophylline, phenytoin, oral hypoglycemic agents, alcohol and benzodiazepines.

6. **Ans. (c) Bismuth subcitrate** *(Ref: KDT 8th/e p705)*

7. **Ans. (a) Magnesium sulfate** *(Ref: KDT 8th/e p703)*

8. **Ans. (d) PPI** *(Ref: KDT 8th/e p701)*

9. **Ans. (d) Anti-androgenic action** *(Ref: KDT 8th/e p698)*

10. **Ans. (a) H^+K^+ ATPase pump** *(Ref: KDT 8th/e p701, 702)*

11. **Ans. (b) Magnesium hydroxide** *(Ref: KDT 8th/e p703)*

12. **Ans. (c) 3-5 days** *(Ref: KDT 8th/e p700)*

13. **Ans. (a) Omeprazole** *(Ref: KDT 8th/e p700)*

14. **Ans. (a) Antacids** *(Ref: KDT 8th/e p705)*

15. **Ans. (d) Omeprazole** *(Ref: KDT 8th/e p700)*

16. **Ans. (c) Atrophic gastritis** *(Ref: KDT 8th/e p698)*

17. **Ans. (a) Pain relief** *(Ref: KDT 8th/e p703)*

18. **Ans. (a) Cisapride** *(Ref: KDT 8th/e p705)*

19. **Ans. (d) Ciprofloxacin** *(Ref: KDT 8th/e p705, 706)*

20. **Ans. (c) Proton pump inhibitors** *(Ref: KDT 8th/e p701)*

21. **Ans. (d) Ranitidine** *(Ref: KDT 8th/e p697)*

22. **Ans. (a) Omeprazole** *(Ref: KDT 8th/e p701)*

23. **Ans. (a) Cimetidine** *(Ref: KDT 8th/e p698)*

24. **Ans. (c) Misoprostol** *(Ref: KDT 8th/e p702)*

25. **Ans. (d) $H^+ - K^+$ ATPase** *(Ref: KDT 8th/e p700)*

26. **Ans. (a) Metoclopramide** *(Ref: KDT 8th/e p714)*
    - The abnormal posture is likely to be muscular dystonia. Metoclopramide can result in dystonias due to its D_2 receptor blocking property in the CNS.
    - Domperidone also blocks D_2 receptors but does not cross the blood brain barrier.

27. **Ans. (a) Granisetron** *(Ref: Harrison 20th/e p 501)*
    Drugs for chemotherapy induced vomiting
    - 5 HT_3 blockers like ondansetron, granisetron, dolasetron, palonosetron and ramosetron are DOC for this condition.
    - Palonosetron is most potent 5 HT_3 blocker. Dolasetron may prolong QT interval.
    - Palonosetron has longest $t_{1/2}$ whereas ondansetron has shortest $t_{1/2}$.
    - Efficacy of these drugs increases if used along with antihistaminics, D_2 blockers or dexamethasone.

28. **Ans. (b) Metoclopramide** *(Ref: KDT's 8th/e p713)*

29. **Ans. (a) Scopolamine patch a night before**
    (Ref: KDT 7/e p120)
    Scopolamine (hyoscine) is drug of choice for motion sickness. It should be given as transdermal patch (a night before) or orally (half an hour before journey).

30. **Ans. (b) D_2 antagonist**
    (Ref: Katzung 13th/1070, KDT 8th/e p713)
    Metoclopramide has action on several receptors.
    - Main action as anti-emetic is because of D_2 receptor antagonism.
    - Main action as prokinetic is because of $5HT_4$ agonism.

Mechanism of actions of metoclopramide

Receptor	Action	Clinical effect
D_2	Antagonism	Anti-emetic
$5HT_3$	Antagonism	Anti-emetic Prokinetic
$5HT_4$	Agonism	Prokinetic

31. Ans. (b) Aprepitant *(Ref: Goodman & Gilman 11/e p1005)*
This drug is an antagonist of substance P. It is particularly useful in delayed phase of chemotherapy induced vomiting.

32. Ans. (b) Promethazine *(Ref: KDT 8th/e p180)*
- "Acute muscle dystonia caused by antiemetic-antipsychotic drugs is promptly relieved by parenteral promethazine or hydroxyzine." This is based on central anti-cholinergic action of the drugs.
- Promethazine is a first generation anti-histaminic which has maximum penetration of blood brain barrier and maximum anticholinergic activity.

33. Ans. (d) Enhances colonic motility
(Ref: Katzung 10/e p1021; KDT 8th/e p713)

- Metoclopramide is a D_2 receptor antagonist that increases cholinergic activity by inhibiting pre-synpatic D_2 receptors in GIT (D_2 receptor stimulation inhibits the release of ACh).
- It increase LES tone that is also responsible for anti-emetic action.
- It does not significantly increase colonic motility.
- But out of the four options, this is the best answer, because although not significantly but it can increase colonic motility, whereas other options are definitely wrong.

34. Ans. (c) Cisapride *(Ref: KDT 8th/e p715)*
Cisapride is a $5HT_4$ agonist that is useful as a prokinetic agent. At high plasma concentration, it can block cardiac K^+ channels leading to polymorphic ventricular tachycardia (torsades de pointes). It is manifested in the ECG as QT prolongation. Therefore, cisapride should not be combined with microsomal enzyme inhibitors like erythromycin and ketoconazole. Other important drugs causing QT prolongation are:
- Terfenadine
- Astemizole
- Ziprasidone

35. Ans. (c) 5HT3 *(Ref: KDT 8th/e p711)*

36. Ans. (c) Domperidone *(Ref: KDT 8th/e p715)*

37. Ans. (a) Metoclopramide *(Ref: KDT 8th/e p711-713)*

38. Ans. (b) Dopamine antagonist *(Ref: KDT 8th/e p716-717)*

39. Ans. (d) Palonosetron *(Ref: KDT 8th/e p717)*

40. Ans. (d) Aprepitant *(Ref: KDT 8th/e p718)*

41. Ans. (a) Ondansetron *(Ref: KDT 8th/e p717)*

42. Ans. (d) All of the above *(Ref: KDT 8th/e p717, 935)*
- Ondansetron is drug of choice for chemotherapy induced vomiting
- Dexamethasone, lorazepam and aprepitant are also used for chemotherapy induced vomiting.

43. Ans. (c) Stimulates chemoreceptor trigger zone
(Ref: KDT 8th/e p713-714)

44. Ans. (c) 5HT3 *(Ref: KDT 8th/e p709)*

45. Ans. (c) Cisapride *(Ref: KDT 8th/e p715)*

46. Ans. (b) Hyoscine *(Ref: KDT 8th/e p714, 717, 719)*

47. Ans. (d) Diphenoxymethane *(Ref: KDT 8th/e p713)*
- Prokinetics are the drugs which promote gastrointestinal transit and speed gastric emptying by increasing propulsive motility of GIT.
- These include:
  - D_2 blockers e.g. domperidone, metoclopramide
  - $5HT_4$ agonists like cisapride.
  - Motilin receptor agonsits (motilides) like macrolides e.g. erythromycin. Name motilide is a combination of motilin receptor agonist and macrolide.
- Diphenoxymethane derivative like hydroxyzine is used for anti-allergic purpose.

48. Ans. (a) $5HT_4$ agonist *(Ref: KDT 8th/e p724)*
Prucalopride
- It is a selective **5-HT_4 receptor agonist** approved recently for the treatment of chronic constipation, when other laxatives fail to provide adequate relief.
- It activates pre-junctional 5-HT_4 receptors on intrinsic enteric neurons to enhance release of the excitatory transmitter ACh. It, thereby promotes the propulsive contractions in ileum and more prominently in colon.
- Prucalopride is shown to have negligible affinity for cardiac K^+ channels. It is therefore, believed to be free of cardiovascular risk. No Q-T prolongation has been noted during clinical trial.

49. Ans. (b) Senna *(Ref: KDT 8th/e p724)*
Anthraquinones like Senna and Cascara can cause melanosis coli.

50. Ans. (b) It is a drug used in constipation
(Ref: KDT's 8th/e p733)

51. Ans. (a) Cyclosporine *(Ref: KDT 8th/e p737)*

52. Ans. (a) Hypokalemia *(Ref: Harrison 18th/351)*
Laxative abuse is associated with hypokalemia.

53. Ans. (a) Lubiprostone *(Ref: Katzung 11/e p1080)*
Lubiprostone acts by stimulating Cl^- channel opening in the intestine, increasing liquid secretion in gut and decreasing transit time, therefore used for chronic constipation. It has also been approved for constipation dominant irritable bowel syndrome in women.

54. Ans. (c) Stimulant purgative *(Ref: KDT 8th/e p723)*

55. Ans. (a) Sulfasalazine *(Ref: KDT 8th/e p734)*

56. Ans. (d) Dietary fibers *(Ref: KDT 8th/e p722)*

57. Ans. (d) Misoprostol *(Ref: KDT 8th/e p207)*

58. Ans. (c) Bicarbonate -2 g *(Ref: KDT 8th/e p729)*

59. Ans. (a) Infliximab *(Ref: KDT 8th/e p737)*

60. **Ans. (b) Lactulose** *(Ref: KDT 8th/e p725)*
    - Lactulose is a laxative that acts by conversion to short chain fatty acids in the colon.
    - These fatty acids result in decrease in pH of intestinal juice.
    - At low pH, ammonia becomes ionized (NH4+) and thus cannot be absorbed.

61. **Ans. (a) Docussates** *(Ref: KDT 8th/e p723)*
    Phenolphthalein and castor oil are stimulant purgatives whereas docussates (DOSS) and liquid paraffin are stool softners. Liquid paraffin may cause deficiency of fat soluble vitamins.

62. **Ans. (c) Ustekinumab** *(Ref: CMDT 2014 p620)*

63. **Ans. (c) Lubiprostone** *(Ref: KDT 8th/e p724)*

64. **Ans. (a) Methyl cellulose** *(Ref: KDT 8th/e p722)*

65. **Ans. (c) Antimotility drugs are best drugs for infective diarrhea** *(Ref: KDT 8th/e p733)*

66. **Ans. (a) Ulcerative colitis** *(Ref: KDT 8th/e p734)*

67. **Ans. (d) Increase the absorption of sodium** *(Ref: KDT 8th/e p727)*

Chemotherapy A: General Considerations and Non-specific Antimicrobial Agents

CHAPTER 12

Antibiotics are the substances produced by microorganisms, which suppress the growth of or kill other microorganisms at very low concentrations.

GENERAL CONSIDERATIONS

DRUG RESISTANCE

Drug resistance in bacteria may be natural or acquired. Development of acquired resistance may be due to **single step mutation** (as seen with *streptomycin and rifampicin*) or **multi step mutation** (*erythromycin, tetracycline and chloramphenicol*).

Drug resistance can be transferred from one microorganism to other by gene transfer (also called infectious resistance) via conjugation, transduction or transformation.

- **Conjugation:** It is due to the physical contact between bacteria and is responsible for multidrug resistance. This is a very important mechanism for the development of resistance against *chloramphenicol and streptomycin*.
- **Transduction:** It is the transfer of resistance gene through bacteriophage e.g. *penicillin, erythromycin and chloramphenicol*.
- **Transformation:** It is the transfer of resistance gene through environment and is *not significant* clinically e.g. penicillin G.

Resistance once acquired becomes prevalent due to *selection pressure* of a widely used antimicrobial agent i.e. antimicrobials allow resistant organisms to grow preferentially.

Mechanism of Resistance

Microorganism may develop resistance due to

- **Decreased affinity for the target** e.g. pneumococci and staphylococci may develop altered penicillin binding proteins.
- Development of **alternative metabolic pathway** e.g. sulfonamide resistant organisms start utilizing preformed folic acid in place of synthesizing it from PABA.
- Elaboration of the **enzymes which inactivate the drug** e.g. β-lactamases (penicillins and cephalosporins), chloramphenicol acetyl transferase (chloramphenicol) and aminoglycoside inactivating enzymes (aminoglycosides).

> **MNEMONIC**
> Drug resistance by Inactivating enzymes
> A – **A**minoglycosides
> B – **B**eta lactams
> C – **C**hloramphenicol

- **Decreased drug permeability** due to the loss of specific channels e.g. *aminoglycosides and tetracyclines* attain much lower drug concentration in the resistant organisms than in the sensitive organisms.
- Development of **efflux pumps** (*tetracyclines, erythromycin and fluoroquinolones*) results in active extrusion of the drug from the resistant microorganisms.

Mechanism of resistance	Drug
↓ Affinity for target	MRSA
	Vancomycin
Alternative metabolic pathway	Sulfonamides
Inactivating enzymes	Aminoglycosides
	Beta lactams
	Chloramphenicol
↓ Permeability	Aminoglycosides
	Tetracyclines
Efflux pumps	Tetracyclines
	Erythromycin
	Fluoroquinolones

SUPERINFECTION

It refers to the appearance of a new infection as a result of antimicrobial therapy. Normal microbial flora contributes to host defense by development of bacteriocins. Pathogens also have to compete with the normal flora for nutrients. **Broad spectrum antibiotics** (*tetracyclines, chloramphenicol, clindamycin, aminoglycosides and ampicillin*) may kill the normal flora and result in the development of new infection. Superinfection is more commonly seen in immunocompromised patients. Oropharynx, intestine, respiratory and genitourinary tracts are common sites for the development of new infection. The organisms frequently involved are *Candida albicans, Clostridium difficile*, staphylococci, proteus and pseudomonas. *Clostridium difficile* superinfection may result in **pseudomembranous colitis** (most commonly due to third generation cephalosporins). **Fidaxomicin** and **Oral vancomycin** are the first line drugs for **pseudomembranous colitis** (*alternative drug is metronidazole*). Recently, a monoclonal antibody against *C. difficile* toxin B (**Bezlotoxumab**) has been approved to reduce the recurrence of *C. difficile* infection. Further, due to the loss of commensal flora, there may be decreased formation of vitamin K leading to enhanced anticoagulant effects of warfarin.

> **Note**
> According to latest IDCS guidelines, fidaxomicin is the first choice drug for treatment of pseudomembranous colitis due to its relapse preventing action.

Pseudomembranous colitis

Most common bacteria involved:	Clostridium difficile
Most common cause:	Cephalosporins > Clindamycin
Drug of choice:	Fidaxomicin
Drug having maximum relapse preventing action	Fidaxomicin

CONCENTRATION-DEPENDENT KILLING (CDK) AND TIME-DEPENDENT KILLING (TDK)

(Ref. Katzung 13th/e p879)

Bactericidal agents can be divided into two groups: agents that exhibit **concentration-dependent killing** and agents that exhibit **time-dependent killing**.

- **CDK** means that killing effect of a drug is high when ratio of peak concentration to MIC is more. This type of killing behaviour is exhibited by **aminoglycosides and fluoroquinolones**. These drugs produces better action when **used as a large single dose** as compared to same daily dose divided into 2-3 portions.
- **TDK** means antimicrobial action depends on the length of time the concentration remains above the MIC. This is exhibited by **β-lactams and vancomycin**. For these drugs **multiple daily doses** are preferred over single dose. Macrolides and clindamycin also possess time dependent activity. However, as these are static drugs, we cannot use the term TDK.
- **Post-antibiotic effect (PAE):** After exposure of an organism to the antibiotic, its growth stops. When it is placed in the antibiotic free medium, the growth resumes but only after a lag period. This signifies that inhibitory effect of antibiotics is present even when their concentration is below MIC. This period is known as PAE. *Most of the antimicrobials have long PAE (≥ 1.5 hours) against gram postive bacteria.* **Carbapenems and drug affecting protein synthesis (aminoglycosides, chloramphenicol, tetracyclines) or DNA synthesis (quinolones, rifampicin) have long PAE against gram negative bacteria also.** *Rifampicin prolongs the PAE of isoniazid.* Due to this reason isoniazid can be given thrice weekly when given in combination with rifampicin in short course chemotherapy of tuberculosis (it needs to be administered daily if used alone).

Antimicrobials with long PAE *(Ref. Katzung 13th/e p879)*

Against gram-positive cocci
- Beta lactams
  - Penicillins
  - Cephalosporins
  - Carbapenems
- Glycopeptides
  - Vancomycin
- Protein synthesis inhibitors
  - Tetracyclines
  - Tigecycline
  - Chloramphenicol
  - Macrolides

Against gram-negative bacilli
- Bactericidal
  - Aminoglycosides
  - Carbapenems
  - Quinolones
  - Rifampicin
- Bacteriostatic
  - Chloramphenicol
  - Tetracyclines
  - Tigecycline

Contd...

Contd...
  - Ketolides
  - Clindamycin
  - Streptogramins
  - Linezolide
  - Aminoglycosides
- Metabolism inhibitors
  - Sulfonamides
  - Trimethoprim
- Nucleic acid inhibitors
  - Fluoroquinolones
  - Rifampicin
- Daptomycin

COMBINED USE OF ANTIBIOTICS

Though every combination is unique but the general guidelines are that:

- *Two bacteriostatic* agents often show *additive* effect.
- *Two bactericidal* agents are *additive if the organism is sensitive to both* e.g. isoniazid and rifampicin in tuberculosis.
- Combination of a *bactericidal with a bacteriostatic* drug is *additive if* the organism has *low sensitivity to the cidal drug* e.g. streptomycin + tetracycline for brucellosis.
- Combination of *bactericidal with bacteriostatic* agent is *antagonistic if the organism has high sensitivity to cidal drug* e.g. penicillin + tetracycline (or chloramphenicol) for pneumococci.

FACTORS AFFECTING THE CHOICE OF AN ANTIMICROBIAL AGENT

1. Age

- *Chloramphenicol* in new born may cause *grey baby syndrome*.
- *Sulfonamides* in new born may cause *kernicterus*.
- Half life of aminoglycosides is prolonged in the elderly.
- *Tetracyclines* are contra-indicated in children below 6 years because it accumulates in the developing *teeth and bone*.

2. Pregnancy

All antibiotics pose risk to the fetus when used in pregnancy. *Penicillins, most cephalosporins and macrolides (PCM) appear safe*.

3. Impaired Host Defenses

Bactericidal drugs are must in immunocompromised patients.

4. Renal Function

Drugs contraindicated in renal disease	Dose reduction required in renal failure
Cephalothin	Aminoglycosides
Cephaloridine	Amphotericin B
Nitrofurantoin	Vancomycin
Nalidixic acid	Ethambutol
Tetracyclines (except doxycycline)	

> **Note**
> Penicillins and rifampicin do not require dose adjustment in renal disease.

5. Liver Function

Drugs contra-indicated in liver disease	Dose reduction required in liver failure
Erythromycin estolate	Chloramphenicol
Tetracyclines	Isoniazid
Pyrazinamide	Rifampicin
Pefloxacin	Clindamycin

6. Secreted in Bile

Antimicrobials that are secreted in bile, can be excreted in faeces. Therefore, these do not require dose reduction in renal failure. Important drugs secreted in bile are:

Safe (**Cef**)	- Ceftriaxone	**N**	- Nafcillin
	- Cefoperazone	**A**	- Ampicillin
in		**L**	- Lincosamides
The	- **T**igecycline		(Clindamycin)
R	- **R**ifampicin	**Disease**	- **D**oxycycline
E	- **E**rythromycin		

7. Genetic Factors

Antimicrobials producing **hemolysis in glucose-6-phosphate dehydrogenase (G-6PD) deficient patients** are *primaquine, chloroquine, quinine, chloramphenicol, nitrofurantoin, fluoroquinolones, dapsone and sulfonamides*, etc.

CLASSIFICATION OF ANTIMICROBIAL AGENTS

Antimicrobials can be classified according to several characteristics:

BASED ON THE MECHANISM OF ACTION

Antimicrobials may act on different parts of the bacterial cell like on cell wall or plasma membranes. These may also act by inhibiting nucleic acids, protein synthesis or metabolism (**Fig. 12.1**).

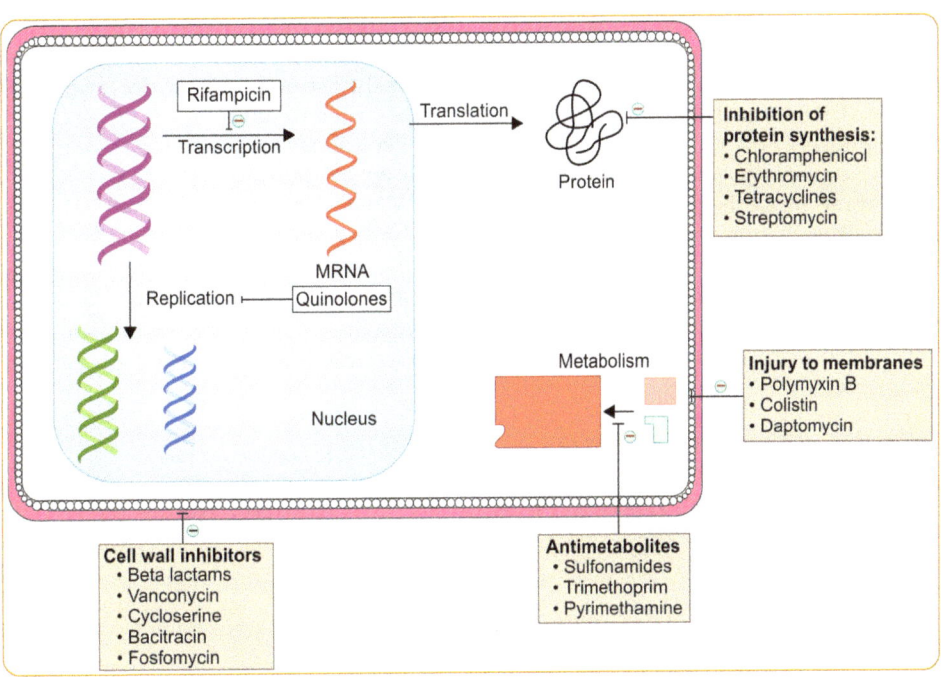

FIG. 12.1: Mechanism of action of different antimicrobials

BASED ON THE TYPE OF ACTION

According to this classification, drugs may be bacteriostatic or bactericidal (*see* **Table 12.1**).

TABLE 12.1: Classification of antibiotics according to the type of action

Bacteriostatic	Bactericidal
Protein synthesis inhibitors	**Protein synthesis inhibitors**
Tetracyclines	Aminoglycosides
Tigecycline	Streptogramins
Chloramphenicol	
Macrolides	
Lincosamides	
Linezolid	
Drugs affecting DNA	**Drugs affecting DNA**
Nitrofurantoin	Quinolones
Novobiocin	Metronidazole
Drugs affecting metabolism	**Polypeptide antibiotics**
Sulfonamides	Polymixin B
Dapsone	Colistin
PAS	Amphotericin B
Trimethoprim	
Ethambutol	
	Cell wall synthesis inhibitors
	Fosfomycin
	Cycloserine
	Bacitracin
	Vancomycin
	Penicillins
	Cephalosporins

Minimum bactericidal concentration (**MBC**) of an antibiotic is the concentration which **kills 99.9%** of the bacteria whereas minimum inhibitory concentration (**MIC**) of the antibiotic is the concentration which **prevents visible growth** of bacteria in culture plates using serial dilutions. A *small difference between MIC and MBC indicates* that the antibiotic is primarily *bactericidal, whereas* a *large difference* indicates *bacteriostatic action*. In immunocompromised patients (patients with HIV, on steroid therapy, neutropenic etc.), only bactericidal drugs should be used.

BASED ON THE THERAPEUTIC INDEX (TI)

High TI	Low TI	Very low TI
Penicillins	Chloramphenicol	Polymixin B
Cephalosporins	Aminoglycosides	Vancomycin
Macrolides	Tetracyclines	Ampho tericin B

DRUGS INHIBITING CELL WALL SYNTHESIS

Bacterial cell wall **(Fig. 12.2)** is composed of peptidoglycan that contains N-acetylmuramic acid and N-acetylglucosamine. It also contains a pentapeptide unit which is attached to N-acetylmuramic acid. Cell wall synthesis starts by conversion of UDP-N-acetylglucosamine (**UDP-G**) to UDP-N-acetylmuramic acid (**UDP-M**) in the presence of enzyme **enolpyruvate transferase**. UDP-M then acquires the pentapeptide. **Alanine racemase and alanine-alanine ligase helps in the formation of pentapeptide unit**. UDP is then removed from UDP-M-pentapeptide by bactoprenol (membrane lipid carrier) and N-acetylglucosamine is added to it (which is carried by UDP-G). These all reactions occur in the cytoplasm. The resulting molecule formed is **transported across the plasma membrane by bactoprenol. Elongation** of the peptidoglycan chain occurs with the help of enzyme **transglycosylase**. Strength to peptidoglycan chain is provided by **cross linking** of elongated chains with the help of **transpeptidase**.

Various antibiotics can act by inhibiting one of these steps in cell wall synthesis as shown in **Table 12.2** below. All of these are **bactericidal drugs**.

TABLE 12.2: Mechanism of action of cell wall synthesis inhibiting antimicrobial drugs

	Drug	Step in cell wall synthesis inhibited
Firmly Bind to Bacterial Cell Vall	Fosfomycin	Enolpyruvate transferase
	Beta lactam antibiotics	Transpeptidase
	Bacitracin	Dephosphorylation of bactoprenol
	Cycloserine	Alanine racemase and alanine ligase
	Vancomycin	Transglycosylase

BETA – LACTAM ANTIBIOTICS

Beta lactam antibiotics are those drugs that contain β-**lactam ring** in their structure. These drugs act by inhibiting the cell wall synthesis and include
- Penicillins
- Cephalosporins
- Monobactams e.g. aztreonam
- Carbapenems e.g. imipenem

All β-lactam antibiotics **are bactericidal** drugs. These bind to specific receptors (penicillin binding proteins; PBPs) on bacterial cell membrane and **inhibit transpeptidase** enzyme responsible for the cross linking of peptidoglycan chains. Bacteria formed

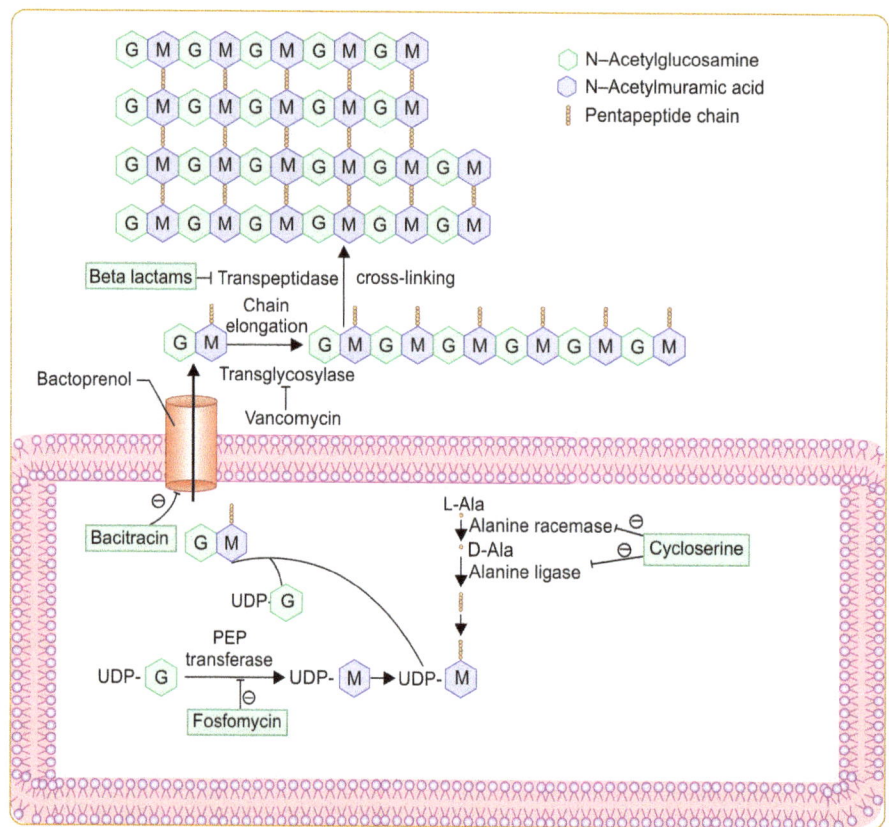

FIG.12.2: Bacterial cell wall synthesis and drugs inhibiting various steps

Chemotherapy A: General Considerations and Non-specific Antimicrobial Agents

in the presence of these drugs are without cell wall and die due to imbibition of water (cell wall provides turgidity). Bacteria like **mycoplasma** are *intrinsically resistant to beta-lactams and vancomycin* because they lack cell-wall.

Penicillins

Penicillin G is commercially obtained from *Penicillium chrysogenum*. It is the **only naturally occurring penicillin** (all others are semi-synthetic penicillins). It had a lot of limitations in its clinical use. Important among these are:

- It is **not effective orally** because of breakdown by acid in the stomach.
- It has **short duration of action** due to its rapid excretion from kidney through tubular secretion.
- It has **narrow spectrum** of activity covering mainly gram positive bacteria.
- Even, gram positive bacteria have now become **resistant** to penicillin G mainly due to development of penicillinase (β-lactamase) or altered penicillin binding proteins (PBPs).
- It can cause hypersensitivity reactions.

Newer Penicillins have been Designed to Overcome These Shortcomings

1. Penicillin G is not effective orally due to acid lability. New penicillins have been developed that are acid-resistant and can be given orally. These include: penicillin V, oxacillin, dicloxacillin, cloxacillin, amoxycillin and ampicillin.

MNEMONIC

Acid-resistant penicillins
V – Penicillin V
O – Oxacillin
D – Dicloxacillin
K – Cloxacillin
A – Amoxycillin and Ampicillin

2. Penicillin G is short acting. To overcome this problem:
   (a) Benzathine and procaine group can be added to penicillin G to make it long acting. Benzathine penicillin G is longest acting penicillin.
   (b) Probenecid can be administered with penicillins. Former inhibits the tubular secretion.
   (c) Penicillins have wide therapeutic index. A high initial dose can be used.
3. Penicillin G has narrow spectrum of antibacterial activity. Several new penicillins with extended spectrum have been developed.

MNEMONIC

Extended spectrum penicillins:
Aminopenicillins: Ampicillin
 Amoxycillin
Carboxypenicillins: Carbenicillin
 Ticarcillin
Ureidopenicillins: Mezlocillin
 Azlocillin
 Piperacillin

Mnemonic: A CT MAP
  - All of these are effective against gram negative bacteria like E. coli, salmonella, shigella (except amoxycilin) etc.
  - Last five penicillins (CT MAP) are effective against Pseudomonas.
  - Last three (MAP) are effective against Klebsiella also.

4. Problem of resistance can be tackled by:
   (a) Adding β-lactamase inhibitors to penicilins. These inhibit the bacterial enzyme and penicillins escape degradation.
   (b) By administering penicillinase resistant penicillins like cloxacillin, oxacillin, nafcillin, dicloxacillin or methicillin.

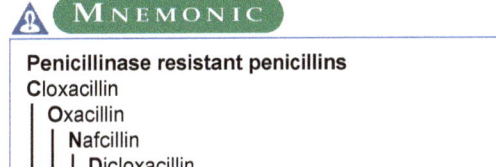

Penicillinase resistant penicillins
Cloxacillin
 Oxacillin
  Nafcillin
   Dicloxacillin
    Methicillin
C O N D O M

5. **Hypersensitivity reactions** can occur with any penicillin. Infact, penicillins are the most common drugs responsible for anaphylactic shock. If a person is severely allergic to any penicillin, no β-lactam (except monobactams) should be administered to that person. Intra-dermal skin testing can be used to prevent severe allergic reactions.

Pharmacokinetics

- *One gram of penicillin is equivalent to 1.6 million units.*
- *Gastric acid breaks down penicillins and results in decreased oral bioavailability.* Penicillin G can be used orally only for infections in which clinical experience has proven efficacy.
- *Ampicillin and nafcillin are excreted partly in the bile.*
- Benzyl penicillin (Penicillin G) is given by i.m. injection. It has short $t_{1/2}$ so given 6-12 hourly whereas procaine penicillin (12-24 hourly) and **benzathine penicillin (longest acting)** are long acting due to slow release. **Procaine** helps to **prolong the duration** of action.

Clinical Uses

- **Penicillin G:** It is the *drug of choice for syphilis*. Benzathine penicillin G is used for primary, secondary and early latent syphilis (**2.4 million units i.m.**) as single dose and late latent and tertiary syphilis for 3 weeks (once weekly). **Aqueous penicillin G is DOC for neurosyphilis** (benzathine penicillin has little entry in brain). It can also be used for gram positive bacteria like streptococci and meningococci. **Penicillin G** is also the *drug of choice for meningococcus, actinomycosis, tetanus, gas gangrene, rat bite fever, yaws, leptospirosis, group A and B streptococcal infections and viridan streptococcal endocarditis*. Most staphylococci and gonococci are now resistant. It is effective against *anaerobic bacteria except bacteroides*.

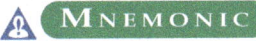
MNEMONIC

Penicillin G is drug of choice for:
L - Leptospira
A - Actinomyces
S - Streptococcus
  Staphylococcus (non-penicillinase-producing)
T - Treponema
   * Syphilis (see details on next page)
   * Yaws
  - Tetanus (and Gas gangrene)
M - Meningococcus
A]
N] - ANthrax (Ciprofloxacin is also first-line drug)

- **Methicillin, nafcillin, oxacillin and cloxacillin:** Main use of these drugs is for the treatment of *Staphylococcus aureus* infections although organisms resistant to these drugs also have been isolated. Methicillin resistance is developed due to the formation of alternative penicillin binding proteins that have less affinity for the drugs. *Organisms resistant to methicillin (MRSA) are resistant to all other beta lactam drugs*. These resistant organisms are *treated by vancomycin or teicoplanin*. Vancomycin resistant staphylococcus (VRSA) *can be treated by linezolid or streptogramins*.
- **Ampicillin, amoxicillin:** These are wide spectrum penicillinase sensitive antibiotics. In addition to gram positive organisms, these are also effective against *enterococci, listeria and haemophilus* organisms. The activity of these drugs is enhanced when used with beta lactamase inhibitors like sulbactam or clavulanic acid. **Ampicillin** is *drug of choice for listeria meningitis (cephalosporins are not effective) and UTI caused by E. faecalis*.
- **Piperacillin, ticarcillin, carbenicillin, azlocillin and mezlocillin:** These possess activity against gram negative rods including Pseudomonas. These are used with beta lactamase inhibitors and with aminoglycosides. Ureido-penicillins (piperacillin, azlocillin and mezlocillin) are also highly effective against klebsiella species.

> **MNEMONIC**
>
> **Anti-pseudomonal penicillins**
> C – Carbenicillin
> T – Ticarcillin
> M – Mezlocillin
> A – Azlocillin
> P – Piperacillin

- MRSA is not susceptible to β-lactam antibiotics.

Recommended Treatment of Syphilis

Stage of syphilis	Treatment
Primary, secondary, or early latent	Benzathine penicillin G 2.4 million units IM once
Late latent or uncertain duration	Benzathine penicillin G 2.4 million units IM weekly for 3 weeks
Tertiary without neurosyphilis	Benzathine penicillin G 2.4 million units IM weekly for 3 weeks
Neurosyphilis	Aqueous penicillin G 18-24 million units IV daily, given every 3-4 hours or as continuous infusion for 10-14 days

> **Note**
> Penicillin is the only documented effective treatment in pregnancy, so pregnant patients with true allergy should be desensitized and treated with penicillin according to stage of disease as above.

Toxicity

- Main toxicity is hypersensitivity including serum sickness. **Anaphylaxis** is most commonly associated with these drugs; therefore intra-dermal sensitivity testing is must before administration of penicillins. *If a patient develops severe hypersensitivity reaction to a penicillin, all other beta lactam antibiotic are contra-indicated* **except aztreonam** (cross sensitivity is not present).
- *Ampicillin* is involved in causing maculopapular skin *rash in* the patients with *viral diseases* like infectious mononucleosis.
- *Methicillin* is the most common antibiotic implicated in causing *interstitial nephritis*.
- Nausea and diarrhea may be caused by oral drugs like amoxicillin and ampicillin. *Ampicillin causes diarrhea* more frequently, because it is incompletely absorbed and causes more suppression of normal microbial flora. It can also cause pseudomembranous colitis.
- *Procaine penicillin* in high doses can result in *seizures* and CNS abnormalities (*due to procaine*).
- *Oxacillin* can cause *hepatitis* and *nafcillin* is involved in causing *neutropenia*.

> **MNEMONIC**
>
> Nafcillin can cause Neutropenia

- *Carbenicillin* in high dose can result in *bleeding*.

Cephalosporins

These are β-lactam antibiotics having 7-aminocephalosporanic acid nucleus. These are classified into four generations.

First generation		Second generation		Third generation		Fourth generation	Fifth generation
Oral	Parenteral	Oral	Parenteral	Oral	Parenteral	Parenteral	Parenteral
Cephalexin	Cefazolin	Cefaclor	Cefuroxime	Cefixime	Cefotaxime	Cefepime	Ceftaroline
Cefadroxil		Cefuroxime axetil	Cefotetan	Cefpodoxime	Ceftizoxime	Cefpirome	Ceftobiprole
Cepharadine			Cefoxitin	Ceftibuten	Ceftriaxone		
		Loracarbef	Cefmetazole	Cefditoren	Ceftazidime		
		Cefprozil		Cefdinir	Cefoperazone		
					Moxalactam		

Chemotherapy A: General Considerations and Non-specific Antimicrobial Agents

> **MNEMONIC**
>
> 1. **Which generation?**
>   - All drugs having 'a' after cef are 1st generation except cefaclor [e.g. cefazolin, cefadroxil]
>   - Drugs with 'PI' in the name are 4th generation (cefePIme and cefPIrome)
>   - Drugs with 'ROL' in the name are 5th generation [CeftibipROLe, ceftaROLine]
>   - Drugs ending with ME except cefuroxime (CefixiME, CefpodoxiME, CeftazidiME, CefotaxiME, CeftizoxiME), ONE (ceftriaxONE, CefoperazONE) or TEN (ceftibutTEN, CefditorEN) are 3rd generation.
>   - Rest of the drugs (except cefdinir and moxalactam) are 2nd generation.
> 2. **Whether oral or parenteral?**
>   - Drugs with OR in the name are ORal (e.g. CefaclOR, CefditOREn, LORarcarbef)
>   - Apart from these, drugs having 't' in the name are injectable except ceftibuten (CefoTetan, CefTazidime, CefoTaxime, CefTizoxime, CefTriaxone, moxalacTam, CefTaroline, CefTobiprole)

Pharmacokinetics

- Most cephalosporins are excreted via kidney *through tubular secretion*.
- **Ceftriaxone and cefoperazone** are secreted in the **bile**.
- *Nephrotoxicity* of these drugs is *increased with loop diuretics*.

Antibacterial Spectrum

	Useful spectrum of cephalosporins	
Generation	**Organism**	**Remarks**
First	**Gram +ve Cocci** Streptococci Staphylococci	Not active against penicillin resistant strains
Second	**Gram –ve bacilli** E. coli Klebsiella Proteus H. influenza M. catarrhalis Bacteroides	Only cefoxitin, cefmetazole and cefotetan are effective against *Bacteroides*
Third	**Gram +ve cocci** Streptococci Staphylococci **Gram –ve cocci** Gonococci **Gram –ve bacilli** Enterobacteriaceae Serratia Pseudomonas **Anaerobes** Bacteroides	Only ceftazidime and cefoperazone are effective against *Pseudomonas* Activity against gram +ve cocci is same as 1st generation agents Activity against *Bacteroides* is less than cefoxitin
Fourth	Same as 3rd Generation	More resistant to β-lactamases

Clinical Uses

First Generation

These are active *against gram positive cocci* including staphylococci. *MRSA is resistant to cephalosporins also*. **Cefazolin is the drug of choice for surgical prophylaxis.**

Second Generation

This group of drugs is less active against gram positive organisms than first generation agents but has extended gram negative coverage. **Cefotetan, cefmetazole and cefoxitin are active against anaerobes like *Bacteroides fragilis*.** *Cefuroxime attains higher CSF levels as compared to other second generation cephalosporins. It can be used for bacterial meningitis. However, ceftriaxone is preferred.*

Third Generation

- These are active against gram negative organisms resistant to other beta lactam antibiotics.
- These can also *penetrate the blood brain barrier (except cefoperazone and cefixime)*.
- **Ceftazidime (maximum), ceftolozane and cefoperazone** are active **against Pseudomonas.**
- **Ceftazidime** is *drug of choice for melioidiosis (caused by Burkholderia pseudomallei)*.
- *Ceftizoxime* has maximum activity against *Bacteroides*.
- **Ceftriaxone** is the *first choice drug for gonorrhoea, salmonellosis (including typhoid), E. coli sepsis, Proteus, Serratia, Haemophilus and empirical therapy for bacterial meningitis*.
- Long term use of > 2g/d of **ceftriaxone** is associated with **biliary sludging syndrome** and cholelithiasis due to precipitation in bile.
- Most of these drugs are reserved for serious infections.
- Ceftriaxone has long plasma half life.
- Cefotaxime is metabolized to an active metabolite (desacetyl-cefotaxime).

Fourth Generation

These drugs possess activity against gram negative organisms (including Pseudomonas) resistant to 3rd generation cephalosporins. Their efficacy against gram positive cocci is similiar to 3rd generation compounds. However, these are not active against anaerobes.

Fifth Generation

Ceftaroline and **ceftobiprole** are fifth generation cephalosporins approved for treatment of community acquired pneumonia and MRSA infections. Ceftobiprole is also effective against MRSA and Pseudomonas.

> **Note**
> - No cephalosporin is active against Enterococcus fecalis, MRSA and Listeria monocytogenes.
> - **Ceftazidime plus aminoglycoside is the treatment of choice for pseudomonas infections.**

Cefiderocol is a cephalosporin that is approved for complicated UTI by intravenous route. Unlike other cephalosporins, it is a **siderophore**. It can undergo active transport in the bacterial cell through iron channels. It is effective against wide range of gram negative bacteria including Pseudomonas.

Toxicity

- Cephalosporins can cause *hypersensitivity* reactions. There is complete cross reactivity between different cephalosporins and also 5–10% cross-reactivity with penicillins.

- Drugs containing a methylthiotetrazole group like *cefamandole, cefoperazone, moxalactam and cefotetan* may cause *hypoprothrombinemia (bleeding) and disulfiram like reaction* with alcohol.
- *Ceftazidime* is implicated in causing *neutropenia*.

 Key Points

Meningococcal meningitis	
Empirical treatment of choice:	Ceftriaxone
Definitive treatment of choice:	Penicillin G
Drugs used for chemoprophylaxis:	Ciprofloxacin
	Ceftriaxone
	Rifampicin
Drugs of choice for mass chemoprophylaxis:	Ciprofloxacin > Rifampicin
Most effective drug for chemoprophylaxis:	Ceftriaxone

Other Beta Lactam Antibiotics

Monobactams

This group includes **aztreonam**. This is active against β-lactamase producing *gram negative rods* including pseudomonas but has no activity against gram positive organisms or anaerobes. It is administered i.v. and its half life is prolonged in renal failure. **It is the only beta lactam antibiotic that can be used in patients having severe allergy to penicillins or cephalosporins** (as it is not cross allergenic).

Carbapenems

These include *imipenem, doripenem, meropenem, faropenem and ertapenem*. These have *wide spectrum* of activity including gram positive cocci, gram negative rods as well as anaerobes. For the treatment of pseudomonas (meropenem is most active whereas ertapenem is least) infections, these drugs should be combined with aminoglycosides. Carbapenems are β-lactamase resistant and are *drugs of choice for Enterobacter, Klebsiella and acinetobacter species*. These are the **only β-lactams which are reliably efficacious against ESBL** (extended spectrum β-lactamase) producing organisms and are thus **drug of choice** for ESBL- producing bacteria. **Imipenem is rapidly inactivated by renal dehydropeptidase I, so it is combined with cilastatin**, an inhibitor of this enzyme. *Cilastatin increases the half life of imipenem and also inhibits the formation of nephrotoxic metabolite*. Main adverse effects of imipenem-cilastatin combination include **seizures** and gastrointestinal distress. *Meropenem, doripenem and ertapenem are not metabolized by renal dehydropeptidase and are less likely to cause seizures*. **Ertapenem is very long acting and is inactive against Pseudomonas.**

 Key Points

- Imipenem is given with cilastatin
- Imipenem has highest risk of seizures among carbapenems.
- Ertapenem is not effective against Pseudomonas
- Faropenem is only carbapenem effective orally.

Loracarbef: It is chemically *similar to cefaclor*. It can be administered orally and its uses and spectrum resembles second generation cephalosporins. *Its overdose can cause seizures.*

Beta Lactamase Inhibitors

- These include *clavulanic acid, sulbactam, tazobactam and avibactam*. These are more active against plasmid encoded beta-lactamases (produced by gonococci and E. coli) than against inducible chromosomal beta-lactamases (produced by pseudomonas and enterobacter)

  - *Amoxicillin* is combined with *clavulanic acid* (Co-amoxy-clav).
  - *Ampicillin* is combined with *sulbactam* (Sultamicin).
  - *Piperacillin* is combined with *tazobactam*.
  - **Ceftazidime-avibactam combination** is approved for complicated UTI (including pyelonephritis) and complicated intra-abdominal infections.
  - **Meropenem-vaborbactam** is a new combination approved for complicated UTI.
  - **Relebactam** has been approved in combination with imipenem-cilastatin for treatment of intra-abdominal infections and UTI.

Extended Spectrum Beta Lactamases (ESBL)

These are the enzymes that confer resistance to most beta lactams antibiotics including penicillins, cephalosporins and monobactams. ESBL have been found exclusively in gram negative organisms primarily in Klebsiella and E. coli. The important characteristics of ESBL are:

- These belong to functional (Bush) group 2be and molecular (Amber) group A.
- These **can be inhibited by clavulanic acid or tazobactam.**
- These can hydrolyze penicillins, cephalosporins (including cefotaxime, ceftazidime, ceftriazone, cefepime) as well monobactams (aztreonam).
- These cannot hydrolyze cephamycins (cefoxitin, cefotetan and cefmetazole).
- These **cannot hydrolyze carbapenems** (imipenem, meropenem etc.)
- **Carbapenems are drug of choice for treatment of infections caused by a bacteria producing ESBL.**

OTHER CELL WALL SYNTHESIS INHIBITORS

Glycopeptides

- **Vancomycin** is a bactericidal *glycopeptide antibiotic* that inhibits cell wall synthesis by *inhibiting transglycosylase* enzyme (involved in chain elongation).
- It has narrow spectrum and is effective against **gram positive organisms** including MRSA, penicillin resistant pneumococci and *Clostridium difficile*. It is *drug of choice for MRSA, Corynebacterium jeikeium and for serious infections in penicillin allergic patients.*

 Key Points

Vancomycin is drug of choice for
- MRSA
- Corynebacterium jeikeium
- Serious infections in penicillin allergic patients.

- **Teicoplanin** is another glycopeptide with similar characteristics but can be given once daily due to **long $t_{1/2}$** (45-70 hours).
- These are administered parenterally *(vancomycin by IV route and teicoplanin by IV or IM route)* and are excreted unchanged in urine.

- Rapid IV infusion of high doses of vancomycin can cause *RED MAN SYNDROME* (diffuse flushing due to histamine release). It is the **most common adverse reaction** to vancomycin.
- Other toxic effects of vancomycin are *chills, ototoxicity and nephrotoxicity*. Its dose should be decreased in renal failure. Teicoplanin does not cause red man syndrome or nephrotoxicity.
- Vancomycin is used *ORALLY to treat pseudomembranous colitis* by *Clostridium difficile* because it is not absorbed from the gastrointestinal tract and higher concentration reaches the colon.

> **Key Points**
>
> **Vancomycin resistance** to Enterococci and Staphylococcus aureus develops because of **replacement of terminal Alanine-Alanine by Alanine-Lactate of** peptidoglycan. This decreases its affinity for transglycosylase

- **Oritavancin** is a newer glycopeptide antibiotic that is being developed for the treatment of MRSA infections.
- **Telavancin** has been approved for complicated skin and skin structure infections. It is effective against MRSA. Apart from vancomycin like mechanism, it also disrupts membrane potential.
- **Dalbavancin** is **once-weekly** drug being developed for MRSA and VRSA acting by same mechanism as vancomycin.

Fosfomycin

It inhibits cell wall synthesis by *inhibiting enolpyruvate transferase*. Diarrhea is quite common with its use. It is drug of choice (along with nitrofurantoin), for uncomplicated urinary tract infections.

Bacitracin

It also inhibits cell wall synthesis but because of *marked nephrotoxicity*, it is indicated *only for topical use*. It is selectively active against gram positive bacteria.

Cycloserine

It also inhibits cell wall synthesis. It has potential neurotoxic effects (tremors and seizures). It also causes **neuropsychiatric symptoms**. It is one of the **second line drugs for the treatment of tuberculosis**.

DRUGS INHIBITING PROTEIN SYNTHESIS

Protein synthesis in the bacteria is accomplished with the use of 70S ribosome, mRNA and tRNA. 70S ribosome consists of two subunits 30S and 50S. Latter (50S subunit) contains two sites; *A site (acceptor)* and *P site (peptidyl)*. Nascent (already formed) peptide chain is attached to P site. Next amino acid is transported to the A site by tRNA having complementary base pairs (anticodons). Peptide bond forms between the peptide chain and the newly attached amino acid with the help of enzyme *peptidyl transferase*. The nascent peptide chain is thus shifted from P site to A site. For further elongation of the peptide chain, A site must be free because the next amino acid attaches to A site only. This is carried out by *translocation* of the peptide chain from A site to P site. Ribosome moves forward along the mRNA to expose the next codon **(Fig. 12.3)**. All of these steps keep on repeating till there is a termination codon on the mRNA (at this point protein synthesis stops). *All drugs inhibiting protein synthesis are bacteriostatic except aminoglycosides and streptogramins.*

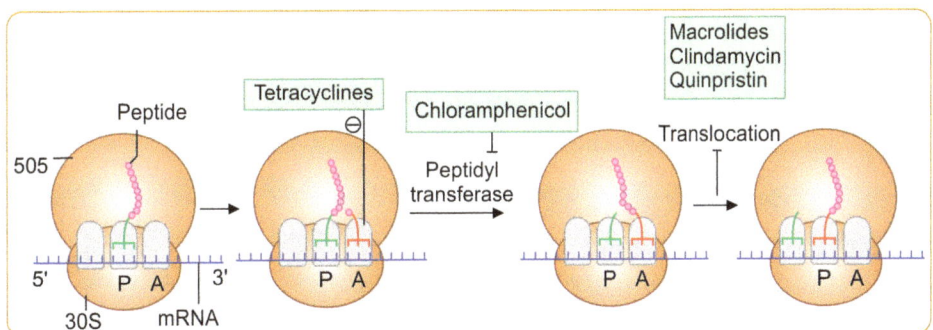

FIG. 12.3: Steps of protein synthesis and the mechanism of action of drugs

TABLE 12.3: Mechanism of action of protein synthesis inhibiting antimicrobial drugs

	Drugs	Binds to	Mechanism of action
1.	Aminoglycosides	Several sites at 30 S and 50 S subunits as well as to their interface	• Freezing of initiation • Interference with polysome formation • Misreading of mRNA code
2.	Tetracyclines and Glycylcyclines	30S ribosome	• Inhibit aminoacyl-tRNA attachment to A Site
3.	Chloramphenicol	50S ribosome	• Inhibits peptidyl transferase that results in the inhibition of peptide bond formation and transfer of peptide chain from P to A site
4.	Macrolides Lincosamides Streptogramins	50S ribosome	• Inhibit translocation of peptide chain from A site to P site
5.	Linezolid	23S fraction of 50S ribosome	• Inhibits initiation

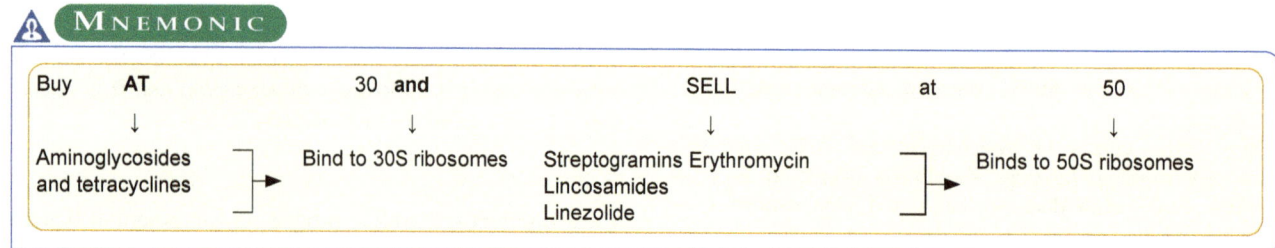

According to spectrum of activity, these may be classified as:
- **Broad spectrum:** Chloramphenicol and tetracyclines
- **Moderate spectrum:** Macrolides and ketolides
- **Narrow spectrum:** Lincosamides, streptogramins and oxazolidinones

CHLORAMPHENICOL

It inhibits protein synthesis by binding to 50S ribosomal subunit and causing the *inhibition of peptidyl transferase*. Chloramphenicol **undergoes enterohepatic circulation** and is mainly inactivated by hepatic glucuronidation. It is a *bacteriostatic* drug with wide spectrum of antimicrobial activity. *Resistance* develops to this drug due to the formation of *inactivating enzyme* acetyl transferase. Because of the rapid development of resistance and high toxicity, this drug has very few systemic uses. Earlier, it was the drug of choice for typhoid fever (enteric fever) but due to the development of resistance, ceftriaxone or ciprofloxacin are now the preferred drugs. It is also *active against anaerobes*. Due to its wide spectrum, it may cause superinfection diarrhea. It can also cause dose dependent and **reversible bone marrow suppression** as well as idiosyncratic, **irreversible myelosuppression** (can occur even after ocular administration). Neonates and premature infants are deficient in hepatic glucuronyl transferase and because it is excreted in the kidney after glucuronidation, these are very sensitive to its toxicity. In such patients, it may lead to **grey baby syndrome** characterized by decreased RBCs, cyanosis and cardiovascular collapse.

TETRACYCLINES

Tetracyclines bind to 30S ribosomal subunit and *inhibit the binding of aminoacyl-tRNA to the A site*. These are classified as:
- **Group I:** Tetracycline, chlortetracycline, oxytetracycline
- **Group II:** Demeclocycline, lymecycline
- **Group III:** Doxycycline, minocycline
- **New drugs:** Eravacycline, omadacycline, sarecycline

Pharmacokinetics

- Oral *absorption* of tetracyclines is *impaired by food and multivalent cations* (calcium, iron, aluminium etc.). Yoghurt decreases the absorption of tetracyclines because it contains cations like calcium and magnesium.
- Tetracyclines *cross the placenta* and affect the fetus, if administered to a pregnant female.
- All tetracyclines undergo *enterohepatic circulation*.
- All tetracyclines are excreted primarily in the urine except doxycycline. **Doxycycline is excreted in the feces and thus can be used in the presence of renal failure.**
- Half life of doxycycline and minocycline is longer than other tetracyclines.

Clinical Uses

Tetracyclines are broad spectrum *bacteriostatic* drugs. Development of **resistance** to tetracyclines is mainly due to the development of **efflux pumps. Tetracyclines are first choice drugs for**

- Lymphogranuloma venereum (LGV)
- Granuloma inguinale
- Atypical pneumonia due to chlamydia (Now preferred drug is azithromycin)
- Cholera
- Brucellosis (with rifampicin)
- Plague prophylaxis (Drug of choice for treatment is streptomycin)
- Relapsing fever (Doxycycline)
- Lyme's disease (Doxycycline)
- Rickettsial infections (Doxycycline)
- Chlamydial infections (Doxycycline)

Other Uses of Individual Tetracyclines include

- Meningococcal carrier state (Minocycline)
- Malaria prophylaxis (Doxycycline)
- Amoebiasis (Doxycycline)
- Syndrome of inappropriate ADH secretion (Demeclocycline)
- As secondary drugs for gonorrhoea, syphilis and chlamydial infections
- For pleurodesmosis in malignant pleural effusion.
- Leprosy (minocycline)
- Peptic ulcer by *H. pylori* (tetracycline)

New Tetracyclines

Drug	Route	Indication
Eravacycline	IV	Complicated intra-abdominal infections
Omadacycline	Oral, IV	Community acquired pneumonia Acute skin and skin structure infections
Sarecycline	Oral	Inflammatory lesions of non-nodular acne

MNEMONIC

Uses of tetracyclines
- R–Rickettsia, Relapsing fever
- B–Brucellosis
- C–Cholera, Chlamydia
- IN–Inguinale (Granuloma)
- P–Plague, Peptic ulcer, Pleurodesmosis
- L–LGV, Lyme, Leprosy
- A–Atypical pneumonia
- S–SIADH
- M–Malaria
- A–Amoebiasis

Toxicity

- Tetracyclines may cause *superinfection diarrhea and pseudomembranous colitis. Gastrointestinal side effects* are *most common* adverse effects.

- These are contra-indicated in pregnancy due to the risk of *fetal tooth enamel dysplasia and irregularities in the fetal bone growth*.
- Treatment of *young children (<8 years)* with tetracyclines may *cause dentition abnormalities*. Doxycycline is less likely to cause this adverse effect.
- High dose of tetracyclines may lead to *hepatic necrosis* especially in pregnant females.
- *Outdated* tetracycline use may lead to *Fanconi's syndrome* (a type of renal tubular acidosis).
- Tetracyclines may *exacerbate pre-existing renal dysfunction* although these are not directly nephrotoxic.
- *Demeclocycline (maximum)* and doxycycline can result in *photosensitivity*.
- **Minocycline** may lead to dose dependent **vestibular toxicity** (more in women).
- **Diabetes insipidus** may be precipitated *by* ADH antagonistic action of **demeclocycline**.
- Tetracyclines also possess anti-anabolic effects.

MNEMONIC

- K – Kidney Failure (All are contra-indicated except doxycycline)
- A – Antianabolic effect
- P – Photosensitivity (Maximum with demeclocycline)
- I – Insipidus (diabetes insipidus; maximum with demeclocycline)
- L – Liver Toxicity (hepatic necrosis)
- D – Dentition and Bone defects (contra-indicated in pregnancy and children)
- E – Expired drugs can cause Fanconi's syndrome
- V – Vestibular dysfunction (maximum with minocycline)

Tigecycline

- It belongs to a new group of antibiotics called glycylcyclines, which act by inhibiting protein synthesis via a mechanism *similar to tetracyclines*. But it is *more resistant* than tetracyclines *to efflux pumps* developed by the microorganisms.
- Its main indication is *serious complicated skin and skin structures infections* and intra-abdominal infections.
- It has a **broad spectrum** including MRSA, VRSA, streptococci, enterococci, anaerobes, rickettsia, chlamydia, legionella and rapidly growing mycobacteria.
- However, tigecycline is **ineffective against Proteus and Pseudomonas**.
- *Tigecycline is administered* **intravenously**.
- *It is mainly excreted in bile, so* **does not require dose adjustment in renal failure**.

SYNDROMIC MANAGEMENT OF STDS

Syndrome	Likely organism	Kit No.	Color	Content & Treatment
Urethral discharge or Cervicitis	N. gonorrhoea C. trachomatis	1	Grey	Tab. Azithromycin* 1 g single dose Tab. Cefixime 400 mg single dose
Vaginitis	Trichomonas Gardernella Candida	2	Green	Tab. Secnidazole 1g single dose Tab. Fluconazole 150 mg single dose
Genital ulcer (Non-herpetic)	Syphilis Chancroid	3	White	Inj. Benzathine penicillin 2.4 MU i.m. once Tab. Azithromycin 1 g once
Genital ulcer (Non-herpetic) allergic to penicillins	Syphilis Chancroid	4	Blue	Tab. Doxycycline 100 mg BD for 14 days Tab. Azithromycin 1 g once
Genital ulcer (Herpetic)	H. simplex	5	Red	Tab. Acyclovir 400 mg TDS for 7 days
Lower abdominal pain (PID)	N. gonorrhoea C. trachomatis Anaerobes	6	Yellow	Tab. Cefixime 400 mg once Tab. Metronidazole 400 mg BD x 14 days Tab. Doxycycline 100 mg BD x 14 days
Inguinal bubo	LGV	7	Black	Tab. Doxycycline 100 mg BD x 21 days Tab. Azithromycin 1 g once

*Azithromycin (2 g) is effective against both gonococcal and non-gonococcal urethritis.

MACROLIDES

These antibiotics have large cyclic lactone ring structure with attached sugars. The drugs included in this group are *erythromycin, azithromycin, roxithromycin and clarithromycin*. An immunosuppressant drug, **tacrolimus is also a macrolide** antibiotic. These drugs bind to 50S ribosome and **block the translocation** of peptide chain from A to P site. *Ketolides and lincosamides have similar mechanism* of action.

Pharmacokinetics

These drugs are well absorbed orally. **Erythromycin is excreted by biliary route** and clarithromycin by both renal and biliary routes. Excretion of **azithromycin** is quite slow (**longest half life**) and mainly in the urine. Erythromycin is administered four times a day whereas azithromycin is administered as a single daily dose.

Clinical Uses

Macrolides are the **drug of choice** for (remembered as **CLAW**)

MNEMONIC

- **C**hancroid by *Haemophilus ducreyi* (Azithromycin single dose), **C**orynebacterium (diptheria), **C**ampylobacter
- **L**egionella infections
- **A**typical pneumonia
- **W**hooping cough by *Bordetella pertussis*

It can also be used for diphtheria and the infections caused by chlamydia and gram positive organisms (as second choice drugs to penicillins).

- Azithromycin has similar spectrum but is more active against *H. influenza and Neisseria*. Because of its long t1/2, **a single dose** is effective in the treatment of urogenital infections and trachoma caused by **chlamydia**. It can be used once weekly in the prophylaxis of MAC infections.
- Roxithromycin has similar spectrum as that of azithromycin.
- *Clarithromycin* is approved for the prophylaxis and treatment of *Mycobacterium avium complex* and in the treatment of peptic ulcer caused by *H. pylori*.

- Macrolides have **anti-inflammatory** action due to their effect on neutrophils and inflammatory cytokines. This action is responsible for the use of macrolides in the prevention of cystic fibrosis exacerbation.
- **Spiramycin** is another macrolide antibiotic that is the **drug of choice for the treatment of toxoplasmosis in pregnancy**.
- **Fidaxomycin** is a non-absorbed macrolide approved for treatment of *C. difficile* infection.

> **MNEMONIC**
>
> **Clinical uses of Azithromycin and Clarithromycin**
> C – Chlamydia
> H – H.influezae
> A – MAC
> T – Toxoplasma

Toxicity

- Erythromycin can cause *diarrhea* by the stimulation of **motilin receptors**. *Gastrointestinal effects* are *most common* side effects of all macrolides.
- **Erythromycin estolate** is implicated in the causation of **acute cholestatic hepatitis** especially in pregnant females. Other salts of erythromycin are safe.
- Use of **erythromycin** in infants < 6 weeks of age increases the **risk of** developing **infantile hypertrophic pyloric stenosis**.
- *Erythromycin, roxithromycin and clarithromycin inhibit CYP3A4*. If administered to patients receiving *terfenadine, astemizole or cisapride* (substrates of CYP3A4), these drugs may lead to prolongation of QT interval and serious polymorphic ventricular tachycardia (*torsades de pointes*). **Azithromycin is not an enzyme inhibitor** and is free from these drugs interactions.
- *Intravenous erythromycin* (not oral) can cause dose dependent reversible ototoxicity.
- *Erythromycin also increases the plasma concentration of theophylline* by inhibiting CYP1A2.

> **MNEMONIC**
>
> **Adverse Effect of Macrolides**
> M – Motilin receptor agonists
> A – Allergy
> C – Cholestasis
> R – Reversible
> O – Ototoxicity

KETOLIDES

This group includes *telithromycin*. It has the same mechanism of action and indications as macrolides. It is excreted in the bile and urine and is a potent inhibitor of CYP3A4.

LINCOSAMIDES

This group includes *clindamycin and lincomycin*. These have same mechanism of action as macrolides. Main use of clindamycin is against *anaerobes like bacteroides* and propionbacterium (responsible for acne). It is also a *drug of choice* for treatment of *severe, invasive group A streptococcal infections along with penicillin*.

It was also active against *Pneumocystis jiroveci* (previously called *P. carnii*) and *Toxoplasma gondii. It is used as an alternative to amoxycillin or ampicilin for prophylaxis against endocarditis following dental procedures*. It was the **most common antibiotic implicated in causing pseudomembranous colitis but now second and third generation cephalosporins (particularly cefotaxime, cefuroxime, ceftriaxone and ceftazidime) are most frequently responsible**. It can also cause hepatic dysfunction.

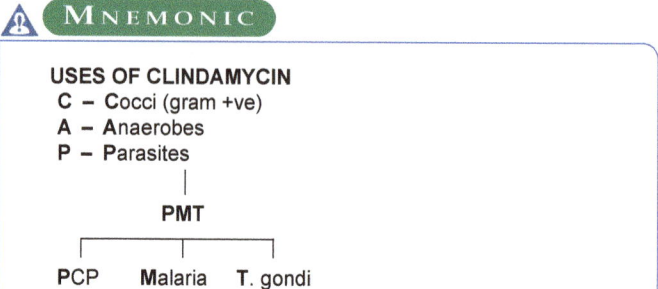

STREPTOGRAMINS

These are **bactericidal** for most susceptible organisms. These drugs bind to 50S ribosomal subunit and constrict the exit channel on the ribosome through which nascent polypeptides are extruded. These drugs also inhibit tRNA synthetase activity. **Quinpristin – dalfopristin** is a bactericidal combination of two streptogramins with prolonged PAE. Resistance to macrolides, lincosamides and streptogramins may be inherited together (**MLS-B resistance**). Quinpristin- dalfopristin combination is **effective against gram positive bacteria including penicillin-resistant pneumococci, Methicillin resistant Enterococcus faecium (not faecalis), MRSA as well as VRSA**. It is also effective against **Legionella and Mycoplasma**. These drugs are potent inhibitors of CYP3A4, therefore drug interactions are possible. *Venous irritation* is very common side effect (mostly required to be given by central line). Other adverse effects include *arthralgia myalgia syndrome*.

OXAZOLIDINONES

This group includes the drugs **linezolid and tedizolide**. These act by *binding to 23S part of 50S ribosomal subunit* and inhibits the initiation of protein synthesis. These have *no cross resistance with other protein synthesis inhibiting drugs*. These are **active against MRSA, VRSA and vancomycin resistant Enterococcus faecium as well as faecalis**. Major adverse effect of linezolid is *thrombocytopenia and neutropenia*. Blood counts should be monitored if duration of therapy exceeds one week. It also possesses MAO inhibitory activity and can cause **serotonin syndrome** if administered with SSRI or other serotonergic drugs. Optic neuritis, peripheral neuropathy and lactic acidosis have also been reported with this drug.

AMINOGLYCOSIDES

These include *streptomycin, gentamicin, kanamycin, tobramycin, amikacin, sisomicin, netilmicin, neomycin and framycetin*. These drugs **exhibit CDK** and have **prolonged PAE**, therefore are administered as *single daily dose*. Aminoglycosides are

bactericidal inhibitors of protein synthesis. *Their penetration across the cell wall is dependent on the oxygen dependent transport,* therefore these drugs are **inactive against anaerobes**. Their transport is enhanced if used along with cell wall synthesis inhibitors like penicillins. These bind to 30S and 50S ribosomes and *freeze initiation, interfere with polysome formation and cause misreading of mRNA code.*

Pharmacokinetics

These are *not absorbed orally* and do not cross blood brain barrier. These are *excreted primarily by glomerular filtration* and the dose should be decreased in renal insufficiency.

Resistance to these drugs develops due to the formation of **inactivating enzymes** which acetylate, phosphorylate or adenylate the aminoglycosides. All aminoglycosides except amikacin and netilmicin are susceptible to these enzymes. Thus *amikacin and netilmicin may be effective against organisms resistant to other aminoglycosides.*

Clinical Uses

- Gentamicin, tobramycin and amikacin are effective against *gram negative organisms* including pseudomonas (except salmonella). However these are not reliable for gram positive organisms if used alone.
- Aminoglycosides produce synergistic effects against gram positive bacteria when combined with β-lactams or vancomycin.
- *Streptomycin is the first line drug for the treatment of tuberculosis, plague and tularemia.*
- Amikacin is a second line drug for the treatment of tuberculosis and is also used for *MDR tuberculosis*.
- Netilmicin is used for serious infections only.
- Neomycin and framycetin are used only topically because of their high toxic potential.
- *Neomycin can also be used orally for gut sterilization in hepatic encephalopathy.*
- **Spectinomycin** is a drug related to aminoglycosides, which is used as a **single dose treatment for** penicillinase producing *Neisseria gonorrhoea* (**PPNG**) and for gonorrhea in penicillin-allergic patients.

> **Note**
> Tobramycin is much less active against enterococcal endocarditis than gentamicin or streptomycin.

Toxicity

- **Ototoxicity:** It can occur due to damage to hair cells. This adverse effect is more likely with prolonged use, high serum concentrations (especially with renal impairment), hypovolemia and other ototoxic medications (like ethacrynic acid). *Amikacin, kanamycin and neomycin are more likely to cause hearing loss whereas streptomycin and gentamicin cause predominantly vestibular dysfunction.* Tobramycin cause both abnormalities equally. Ototoxicity is largely **irreversible** and progress from base of cochlea (high frequency) to the apex (low frequencies). Very early changes can be reversed by Ca^{2+}. Amikacin cause maximum hearing loss whereas streptomycin is most vestibulotoxic. Netilmicin is least ototoxic aminoglycoside.
- **Nephrotoxicity:** It results from toxicity to proximal tubular cells and is almost always **reversible**. Risk factors for nephrotoxicity include *hypokalemia, pre-existing renal disease and concomitant nephrotoxic medications* (like AMB, vancomycin etc.). Neomycin is most nephrototoxic and is not indicated for systemic use. Among the systemically used aminoglycosides, gentamicin is most nephrotoxic followed by tobramycin. Streptomycin is least nephrotoxic.
- **Neuromuscular blockade:** This adverse effect can lead to rare but severe respiratory depression. It can occur due to *inhibition of pre-synaptic release of ACh* and partly by *decreased sensitivity of post-synaptic receptors.* **Hypocalcemia, peritoneal administration, use of neuromuscular blockers and pre-existing respiratory depression** constitutes risk factors. This complication can be avoided by slow i.v. infusion (over 30 min.) or by i.m. route. If *respiratory depression occurs, it is reversed by i.v. administration of calcium.* Neomycin (not used) and streptomycin have maximum potency of causing neuromuscular block whereas tobramycin is least potent in this regard. These drugs are therefore contra-indicated in mysthenia gravis.

	Maximum	**Minimum**
Nephrotoxicity	Neomycin > Gentamicin	Streptomycin
Ototoxicity	Amikacin (Auditory) Streptomycin (vestibular)	Netilmicin
Neuromuscular blockade	Neomycin > Streptomycin	Tobramycin

- **Intra-vitreal injection of gentamicin** can result in **macular infarction**.

> Plazomicin is a recently approved aminoglycosides. It is given intravenously for complicated UTI.

PLEUROMUTILINS

Retapamulin is a new drug of this class approved for *topical treatment of impetigo due to methicillin-sensitive Staphylococcus aureus or Streptococcus pyogenes.* It acts by inhibiting protein synthesis after binding to 50S ribosomes. **Lefamulin** is a new drug in this group which is approved for treatment of community acquired pneumonia.

MUPIROCIN (PSEUDOMONIC ACID)

It acts on gram positive organisms by inhibiting protein synthesis due to binding with isoleucyl-tRNA. It is active against most gram positive cocci including MRSA (but not enterococci). It is *used topically* or nasally **for eliminating staphylococcal nasal carriage**.

FUSIDIC ACID

It acts by blocking protein synthesis and is used *topically* for staphylococcal infections.

ANTIMETABOLITES

The drugs that are able to interfere with the role of an endogenous compound in the cellular metabolism are called antimetabolites e.g. *sulfonamides, trimethoprim, pyrimethamine, proguanil and methotrexate.* Most important metabolic step amenable to inhibition by the drugs is folic acid synthesis.

- **Drugs inhibiting folic acid synthesis:** Folic acid synthase (dihydropteroate synthase) results in the formation of folic acid by incorporation of PABA. *Sulfonamides, dapsone and paraaminosalicylic acid (PAS)* are structural analogues of paraaminobenzoic acid (PABA). There drugs act as competitive inhibitors of folic acid synthase.
- **Dihydrofolate reductase (DHFRase) inhibitors:** DHF-Rase is the enzyme responsible for conversion of dihydrofolic acid to tetrahydrofolic acid. Latter is the active form required for the transfer of one carbon units. Drugs inhibiting this enzyme are *trimethoprim, pyrimethamine, proguanil and methotrexate.*

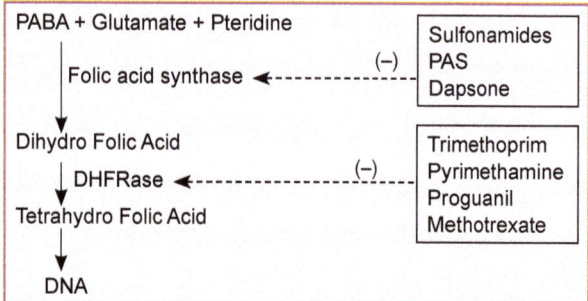

- **Arabinogalactan synthesis inhibitors:** Ethambutol inhibits arabinogalactan synthesis and thus incorporation of mycolic acid in the cell wall of mycobacteria.

SULFONAMIDES

- These drugs are *bacteriostatic* agents and act by *inhibiting folate synthase competitively*.
- The selective toxicity to bacteria is due to the reason that mammalian cells do not synthesize folic acid and utilize preformed folic acid in the diet.
- Sulfonamides are **not effective in the presence of pus** because it contains large amount of PABA.
- These drugs undergo hepatic metabolism by **ACETYLATION** (Drugs undergoing acetylation are **SHIP:** Sulfonamides including dapsone, Hydralazine, Isoniazid and Procainamide) and can cause SLE.
- The solubility of sulfonamides decrease in the acidic urine, which may result in precipitation of the drug causing **crystalluria**. Risk is **minimum with** soluble drugs like **sulfisoxazole**.
- **Sulfadoxine** is **longest acting** whereas **sulfacytine** is **shortest** acting sulfonamide.

Classification

- For systemic use as oral agents
  - Short acting: Sulfisoxazole, sulfamethiazole, Sulfacytine
  - Intermediate acting: Sulfamethoxazole, Sulfadiazine
  - Long acting: Sulfadoxine
- **For use in GIT:** Sulfasalazine, olsalazine
- **For topical use:** Sulfacetamide, silver sulfadiazine, mafenide

Clinical Uses

- *Sulfacetamide* is used for *ocular infections* whereas *mafenide and silver sulfadiazine* are used in *burn patients* as topical agents.
- *Sulfadiazine* can be used for *nocardiosis* and *sulfisoxazole* for *urinary tract infections.*
- *Sulfasalazine and olsalazine* are used for the treatment of *ulcerative colitis.*
- *Sulfadoxine plus pyrimethamine* is used for *malaria.*
- *Sulfadiazine and pyrimethamine* combination can be used for the *treatment of toxoplasmosis* and *prophylaxis of Pneumocystis jiroveci* pneumonia in AIDS patients.
- **Silver sulfadiazine** is also used for **fungal keratomycosis.**

Toxicity

- *Skin rash* due to hypersensitivity is the *most common* adverse effect.
- These can also cause *granulocytopenia, thrombocytopenia and aplastic anemia* (more common in HIV infected patients).
- Sulfonamides can cause acute *hemolysis* in patients with G-6 PD deficiency.
- These can precipitate in the urine at acidic pH and may result in *crystalluria* and hematuria.
- These can displace bilirubin from plasma protein binding sites and may result in *kernicterus in the new born* (if given in third trimester of pregnancy).

MNEMONIC

Sulfonamides commonly cause rash, so to remember adverse effects of sulfonamides, one must know ABC of RASH.
- A – Aplastic anemia
- B – Bilirubin displacement (kernicterus)
- C – Crystalluria
- R – Rash (MC side effect)
- A – Acetylation
- S – SLE
- H – Hemolysis in G-6-PD deficiency

TRIMETHOPRIM

It is a **bacteriostatic antimetabolite** that *inhibits dihydrofolate reductase. It attains high concentrations in the prostate and vaginal fluids.* For most of the indications, it is combined with sulfonamides; however it *can be used alone in prostatitis and UTI.* It can cause *megaloblastic anemia* (can be ameliorated by folinic acid), leucopenia and pancytopenia. It can also result in *hyperkalemia* (due to amiloride like action i.e., inhibition of epithelial Na⁺ channels in CD).

Note
- Other DHFRase inhibitors are pyrimethamine, methotrexate, proguanil and pentamidine.
- All DHFRase inhibitors can cause megaloblastic anemia.

COTRIMOXAZOLE

This is a fixed dose *combination of sulfamethoxazole and trimethoprim in a ratio of 5:1.* Commercially available double strength septran contains 800 mg sulfamethoxazole and 160 mg trimethoprim. Both drugs have similar half life and the combination is **bactericidal** to most pathogens. Due to different bioavailability (more for sulfamethoxazole), *plasma concentration* of the two drugs *attained is 20:1.* The bactericidal activity is due to **sequential blockade** at two steps in the DNA synthesis (sulfamethoxazole inhibits folate synthase and trimethoprim inhibits DHFRase). Cotrimoxazole is effective in UTI, respiratory tract infections, MRSA, middle ear and sinus infections caused by hemophilus and moraxella. It is the *drug* of choice for pneumocystosis, nocardiosis and infections caused by *Burkholderia cepacia*. Adverse effects are similar to sulfonamides and trimethoprim.

> **MNEMONIC**
>
> Cotrimoxazole is drug of choice for:
> Punjab: Pneumocystis
> National: Nocardia
> Bank: Burkholderia cepacia

DRUGS AFFECTING NUCLEIC ACIDS

These drugs include:

- **DNA gyrase inhibitors:** DNA replication occurs on the straight strands of DNA and in this process positive supercoils are introduced. DNA gyrase *nicks* the double stranded DNA, *introduces negative supercoils* and then *reseals* the nicked ends. This prevents excessive supercoiling. In gram positive bacteria, same function is carried out by a similar enzyme topoisomerase IV. The drugs inhibiting DNA gyrase or topoisomerase are *quinolones (nalidixic acid and fluoroquinolones) and novobiocin*.
- **RNA polymerase inhibitors:** *Rifampicin* inhibits transcription by inhibiting DNA dependent RNA polymerase.
- **Drugs destroying DNA:** *Metronidazole* generates reactive nitro radicals (in anaerobic conditions) that results in DNA helix destabilization and strand breakage. *Nitrofurantoin* is also considered to be acting by the destruction of DNA.
- **Nucleotide/Nucleoside analogues:** Drugs that are structurally similar to nucleosides (nitrogen base plus sugar) or nucleotides (nitrogen base plus sugar plus phosphate) gets incorporated in the DNA or RNA. This results in the formation of faulty nucleic acids that may be non-functional or unstable (degrade easily). *Idoxuridine, acyclovir, NRTI* etc. are analogues of nucleosides/nucleotides.

FLUOROQUINOLONES

These drugs act by **inhibiting DNA gyrase** (topoisomerase II) and topoisomerase IV resulting in the inhibition of DNA replication. These drugs have *long PAE*. Important drugs in this group include *norfloxacin, lomefloxacin, ciprofloxacin, ofloxacin, levofloxacin, gatifloxacin, pefloxacin, sparfloxacin, moxifloxacin, fleroxacin, garenoxacin, gemifloxacin, delafloxacin and trovafloxacin*.

Pharmacokinetics

- These have *good oral bioavailability* (except norfloxacin) but like tetracycline multivalent cations interfere with absorption.
- **Norfloxacin** has *minimum oral bioavailability* whereas **levofloxacin** has *maximum*.
- Excretion of *moxifloxacin and trovafloxacin* is by *hepatic metabolism and biliary excretion*. *Sparfloxacin* and *pefloxacin* are excreted by *both* renal and hepatic route. All *other drugs* (ciprofloxacin, gatifloxacin, levofloxacin, lomefloxacin, norfloxacin and ofloxacin) are excreted by *tubular secretion in the kidneys*. Probenecid inhibits tubular secretion of these drugs. *Dose adjustment is required in renal disease for all fluoroquinolones except pefloxacin, moxifloxacin and trovafloxacin* (remembered as PMT).
- *Sparfloxacin, moxifloxacin and trovafloxacin* have **long half-lives** and can be administered once daily. **Sparfloxacin** (followed by moxifloxacin) has *longest* half-life among fluoroquinolones.

Clinical Uses

- Quinolones are the oral agents with greatest activity against pseudomonas (maximum with ciprofloxacin).
- First generation drugs like *norfloxacin have narrow spectrum*. The concentration of norfloxacin reached in urine is bactericidal, thus it can be used for *UTI* but it is not effective for systemic use.
- Second generation drugs like ciprofloxacin and ofloxacin are effective against gonorrhoea and other gram negative organisms including pseudomonas. **Ciprofloxacin** is the *drug of choice for prophylaxis and treatment of anthrax and for prophylaxis of meningococcal meningitis*.
- **Ciprofloxacin and levofloxacin are the only fluoroquinolones effective against *Pseudomonas*.**
- Levofloxacin is l-isomer of ofloxacin and is effective against infections caused by atypical microorganisms like mycoplasma. Sparfloxacin has greater activity against gram positive organisms but is not effective against pseudomonas.
- *Levofloxacin, gatifloxacin, gemifloxacin and moxifloxacin* are called **respiratory fluoroquinolones** due to their enhanced activity against gram positive and atypical organisms (like chlamydia, mycoplasma and legionella).
- Moxifloxacin and trovafloxacin have widest spectrum including gram negative and gram positive microorganisms as well as anaerobes.
- *Fluoroquinolones (ciprofloxacin, levofloxacin and moxifloxacin) are also effective in tuberculosis* and can be used for the *prophylaxis of neutropenic patients*.
- Finafloxacin is a fluoroquinolone that has been approved recently for topical treatment of acute otitis externa caused by *Pseudomonas* and *Staphylococcus*.
- **T. Pallidum and Nocardia are resistant to all fluoroquinolones.**

Toxicity

- *GI distress* is the *most common* side effect followed by CNS side effects (headache and dizziness; rarely seizures also).
- These may also cause *cartilage problems*, thus are not advocated in *children* less than 18 years old and in pregnancy. However when benefits outweighs risks, these can be indicated e.g. in *adolescent patients with cystic fibrosis who have pulmonary exacerbations*.
- *Tendinitis* resulting in tendon rupture can be seen rarely in adults.
- These drugs can also cause *phototoxicity*, the incidence of which is *maximum with lomefloxacin and sparfloxacin*.
- Gatifloxacin has recently been with drawn from India due to its dysglycemic effects. Moxifloxacin can also cause hypoglycemia.
- *Sparfloxacin and gatifloxacin prolong QTc interval (grepafloxacin was withdrawn because of arrhythmias caused due to prolongation of QT interval). Gatifloxacin can also result in hypo or hyperglycemia*.
- *Trovafloxacin* has *hepatotoxic* potential.
- Fluoroquinolones particularly ciprofloxacin or pefloxacin *increase the plasma concentration of methylxanthines* like theophylline and thus enhance their toxicity.

- NSAIDs increase CNS toxicity (seizures) of these drugs. Fluoroquinolones are *contra-indicated in epilepsy*.
- Several fluoroquinolones have been **withdrawn** from the market like **temafloxacin** (*immune hemolytic anemia*), **trovafloxacin** (*hepatotoxicity*), **grepafloxacin** (*cardiotoxicity; increase QT interval*) and **clinafloxacin** (*phototoxicity*).
- Recently, FDA has issued warning regarding **Peripheral Neuropathy** caused by fluoroquinolones.

URINARY ANTISEPTICS

These are oral drugs that are rapidly excreted in the urine and suppress the bacterial growth in urinary tract. These are *more effective in acidic urine because low pH is an independent inhibitor of bacterial growth*. Nitrofurantoin, methanamine mandelate and nalidixic acid are three important urinary antiseptic drugs.

Nitrofurantoin

After reduction by bacterial enzymes, nitrofurantoin result in DNA damage. It is active against most urinary pathogens *except pseudomonas and proteus*. Resistance against it develops slowly. Now it is used infrequently. Adverse effects include diarrhea, phototoxicity, neurotoxicity and *hemolysis in G-6-PD deficient* patients.

Methanamine Mandelate

Methanamine *release formaldehyde at low pH* (below 5.5), which is the major compound having antibacterial activity. *Mandelate salt is used because it itself is urine acidifying* agent. This drug is *not effective against proteus* because it releases NH_3 and alkalinizes the urine. Insoluble complex forms between formaldehyde and sulfonamides, so methanamine *should not be used with sulfonamides*.

Nalidixic Acid

This is a **quinolone** drug and acts by *inhibiting DNA gyrase*. This too is not effective against pseudomonas and proteus. Resistance emerges rapidly and *main adverse effect is neurotoxicity*.

Phenazopyridine

It is not a urinary antiseptic but possesses analgesic action and alleviates symptoms of dysuria, frequency, burning and urgency.

DRUGS AFFECTING CELL MEMBRANE

These drugs act by causing disruption of cell membrane and leakage of ions and molecules from the cell. The drugs include
- **Polypeptide antibiotics:** *Polymixin B, colistin and tyrothricin* (bacitracin is also a polypeptide but acts by inhibiting cell wall synthesis)
- **Polyene antibiotics:** *Amphotericin B, nystatin, hamycin, natamycin*
- **Azoles:** *Ketoconazole, fluconazole, itraconazole*

DAPTOMYCIN

It is a **lipopeptide** bactericidal drug that acts *by causing depolarization of bacterial cell membranes* with K^+ efflux and rapid cell death. It is used for serious gram positive infections including *penicillin resistant pneumococci, MRSA and VRSA*. **Daptomycin is now drug of choice for VRSA.** It is also effective against organisms resistant to linezolid and streptogramins. *Myopathy* is the dose limiting toxicity of this drug. **Pulmonary surfactant** *antagonizes daptomycin*, therefore, the latter should not be used to treat pneumonia.

POLYPEPTIDE ANTIBIOTICS

These include *polymyxin B, bacitracin, colistin and tyrothricin*. **All of these except bacitracin affect cell membrane**. Bacitracin inhibits cell wall synthesis. *Because of neurotoxicity and renal damage, these antibiotics are used only topically*.

IMPORTANT POINTS ABOUT ANTIMICROBIALS

1. **Drugs Effective Against Anaerobic Organisms**

   - Clindamycin
   - Cefotetan
   - Moxifloxacin
   - Cefmetazole
   - Trovafloxacin
   - Cefoxitin
   - Metronidazole
   - Chloramphenicol
   - Vancomycin

   > **Note**
   > **Aminoglycosides** are NOT EFFECTIVE against **anaerobic** microorganisms.

2. **Drugs Effective Against Pseudomonas**

   Beta lactam antibiotics
   - Carboxypenicillins (*Carbenicillin, ticarcillin*)
   - Ureidopenicillin (*Piperacillin, azlocillin and mezlocillin*)
   - Carbapenems (*Imipenem, doripenem, meropenem*)
   - Monobactams (*Aztreonam*)
   - Cephalosporins (*Ceftazidime, cefoperazone, moxalactam, cefepime, cefpirome*).

   Fluoroquinolones
   - Ciprofloxacin, Levofloxacin

   Polypeptide Antibiotics
   - Colistin, Polymixin B.

   Aminoglycosides

   > **Note**
   > - **Vancomycin** is NOT ACTIVE against **Pseudomonas**.
   > - Ceftazidime plus aminoglycoside is the treatment of choice for pseudomonas infections.

3. **Drugs Effecive Against MRSA**

   - Vancomycin
   - Teicoplanin
   - Oritavancin
   - Telavancin
   - Dalbavancin
   - Streptogramins
   - Linezolide
   - Daptomycin
   - Cotrimoxazole
   - Rifampicin
   - Tetracyclines

   > **Note**
   > No β-lactam is effective against MRSA except 5th generation cephalosporins.

Chemotherapy A: General Considerations and Non-specific Antimicrobial Agents

4. Antimicrobials of Choice for Prophylaxis
(Ref: Katzung 13th/884)

Cholera	Tetracycline
Rheumatic fever	Benzathine penicillin
Tuberculosis	Isoniazid alone or with rifampicin
Meningococcal meningitis	Rifampicin/Ciprofloxacin/Ceftriaxone
Malaria	Chloroquine/Mefloquine/Doxycycline
Influenza A and B	Osetamivir
Surgical prophylaxis	Cefazolin
Anthrax	Ciprofloxacin/Doxycycline
Diphtheria	Penicillin/Erythromycin
Endocarditis	Amoxycillin/Clindamycin
Herpes Simplex	Acyclovir
Group B streptococcal infection	Ampicillin
Hemophilus influenza type B	Rifampicin
Mycobacterium avium complex (MAC)	Azithromycin/Clarithromycin/Rifabutin
Otitis media	Amoxicillin
Pertussis	Azithromycin
Plague	Tetracycline
Pneumocystis jiroveci	Cotrimoxazole/Dapsone/Atovaquone
Toxoplasmosis	Cotrimoxazole
Urinary tract infections	Cotrimoxazole

5. Most Important Mechanism of Drug Resistance

Beta lactams	Inactivating enzyme (beta lactamase)
Tetracyclines	Efflux pump (decreased concentration in the cell)
Chloramphenicol	Inactivating enzyme (acetyl transferase)
Aminoglycosides	Inactivating enzyme
Macrolides	Decreased permeability or efflux pumps
Sulfonamides	Form large amount of PABA
	Decreased activity of folate synthase
Fluoroquinolones	*Altered DNA gyrase* with reduced affinity

Note
Transfer of resistance against all antibiotics is plasmid mediated except fluoroquinolones (due to chromosomal mutation).

6. Drugs of Choice for Suspected or Proved Microbial Pathogens
(Ref: CMDT, 2019)

Organism	Drug of Choice
Gram-positive cocci	
Streptococcus	
• S. pneumoniae	• Penicillin G[1]
• Hemolytic, groups A, B, C, G	• Penicillin G[1]
• S. viridans	• Penicillin G[1,2]
Staphylococcus	
• Non penicillinase producing	• Penicillin G[1]
• Penicillinase producing	• Penicillinase resistant penicillin (cloxa, oxa, naf or dicloxacillin)
• Methicillin resistant (MRSA)	• Vancomycin
• Coagulase negative	• Vancomycin
Enterococcus	
• Faecalis	• Ampiillin[3]
• Faecium	• Vancomycin[3]
Gram-positive bacilli	
• Actinomyces	• Penicillin G
• Bacillus including anthrax	• Penicilling G
• Clostridium	• Pencillin G
• Corynebacterium	• Erythromycin[4]
• Listeria	• Ampicillin[5]
Gram-negative cocci	
• Neisseria	
– Meningitidis	• Penicillin G
– Gonorrhae	• Ceftriaxone + Azithromycin/Doxycycline
• Moraxella	• Cefuroxime
Gram-negative bacilli	
• Campylobacter	• Macrolides
• Legionella	• Macrolides
• Bordetella	• Macrolides
• Brucella	• Doxycyline + Rifampicin
• Acinetobacter	• Carbapenems
• Hemophilus	
– Serious infections like meningitis	• Ceftriaxone
– Respiratory infections, otitis	• Ampicillin-sulbactam
– Ducreyi (chancroid)	• Azithromycin
• Prevotella	• Clindamycin
• Bacteroides	• Metronidazole
• Pseudomonas	• Anti-Pseudomonal β-lactam (piperacillin or ceftazidime or cefepime or imipenem) + Gentamicin
• Burkholderia	
– Mallei (glanders)	• Streptomycin + Tetracycline
– Pseudomallei (melioidosis)	• Ceftazidime
– Cepacia	• Cotrimoxazole
• Helicobacter pylori	• Clarithromycin + Amoxycillin + Proton pump inhibitor
• Vibrio (cholera, sepsis)	• Tetracyclines
• Enterobactericiae	
– Salmonella	• Ceftriaxone
– E. coli UTI	• Nitrofurantoin/Fosfomycin
– E. coli sepsis	• Ceftriaxone[6]
– Klebsiella	• Ceftriaxone[7]
– Proteus vulgaris	• Ceftriaxone[8]
– Proteus mirabilis	• Ampicillin
– Enterobacter	• Carbapenems
– Serratia	• Carbapenems
– Shigella	• Fluoroquinolones
– Yersinia (plague)	• Streptomycin ± Tetracycline

Organism	Drug of Choice
Spirochetes	
• Treponema	
– Pallidum (syphilis)	• Penicillin G
– Pertenue (yaws)	• Penicillin G
• Leptospira	• Penicillin G
• Borrelia	
– Burgdorferi (Lyme's)	• Doxycycline
– Recurrentis (Relapsing fever)	• Doxycycline
Chlamydiae	
• C. psittaci	• Doxycycline
• C. trachomatis	• Doxycycline or azithromycin
• C. pneumoniae	• Doxycycline
Rickettsiae	
• R. prowazekii (Epidemic typhus)	• Doxycycline
• R. typhi (Endemic typhus)	• Doxycycline
• Orientia tsutsugamushi (scrub typhus)	• Doxycycline
• R. rickettssi (Rocky mounted spotted fever)	• Doxycycline
• R. akari (Rickettsial pox)	• Doxycycline
• Rickettsia fever	• Doxycycline
• Ehrlichia	• Doxycycline
• Coxiella burnetii (Q fever)	• Doxycycline
Mycoplasma	• Azithromycin
Nocardia	• Cotrimoxazole

1. Oral penicillin V can be used for mild cases
2. Addition of gentamicin decreases the duration of treatment
3. Gentamicin is added for meningitis or endocarditis
4. For C. jeikium, vancomycin is drug of choice
5. Gentamicin is added for first few days
6. For UTI by E.coli, nitrofurantion or fosfomycin are used
7. For ESBL producing strains, carbapenems are drug of choice
8. For P. mirabilis, ampicillin is drug of choice

7. Examples of Initial Antimicrobial Therapy for Acutely ill, Hospitalized Adults Pending Identification of Causative Organism (Ref: CMDT 2019)

Clinical diagnosis	Empirical antimicrobial of choice
• **Bacteral Meningitis**	
– Age 18-50 years	• Vancomycin + ceftriaxone
– >50 years	• Vacomycin + ceftriaxone + ampicillin (to cover Listeria)
– Post-operative or post-traumatic	• Vancomycin + cefepime
• **Brain Abcess**	• Vancomycin + ceftriaxone + metronidazole
• **Pneumonia**	
– Community acquired	• Respiratory fluoroquinolone[1,2]
– Nosocomial	
*Low risk of MDR organisms	• Respiratory fluoroquinolone[1]
*High risk of MDR organisms	• [Ceftazidime + gentamicin] to cover Pseudomonas + Vancomycin for MRSA
• **Endocarditis**	• Vancomycin + gentamicin
• **Septic thrombophlebitis**	• Vancomycin + ceftriaxone
• **Osteomyelitis**	• Nafcilin[3]
• **Septic Arthritis**	• Ceftriaxone
• **Pyelonephritis**	• Ceftriaxone
• **Febrile neutropenia**	• Cefepime
• **Intra-abdominal sepsis**	• Ertapenem

1. Respiratory fluoroquinolones include levofloxacin, moxifloxacin and gemifloxacin.
2. Azithromycin plus ceftriaxone is also first line treatment.
3. Cefazolin can also be used as first line drug.

8. Example of Empiric Choices of Antimicrobials for Adult Outpatient Infections (Ref. CMDT 2019)

Clinical diagnosis	Likely etiologic diagnosis
• **Streptococcal skin infections**	
– Erysipelas	Penicillin V
– Impetigo	
– Cellulitis	
– Lymphangitis	
• **Staphylococcal skin infection**	
– Furuncle (Methicillin-sensitive)	• Dicloxacillin
– Furuncle (MRSA)	• Cotrimoxazole or Clindamycin
• **Pharyngitis**	• Penicillin V
• **Otitis media**	• Amoxycillin
• **Malignant otitis externa**	• Ciprofloxacin
• **Acute sinusitis**	• Amoxycilin + clavulanic acid
• **Pneumonia**	
– Aspiration	• Clindamycin
– Community acquired	• Doxycycline
• **Urinary tract infections**	
– Cystitis	• Nitrofurantoin or Fosfomycin
– Pyelonephritis	• Fluoroquinolone
• **Gastroenteritis**	
– Salmonella	• No treatment
– Shigella	• Ciprofloxacin
– Campylobacter	• Ciprofloxacin
– Entameoba	• Metronidazole
• **Urethritis or epididymitis**	
– Gonococcal	• Ceftriaxone + Azithromycin
– Chlamydial	• Azithromycin
Pelvic inflammatory Disease (PID)	• Ceftriaxone + Doxycycline ± Metronidazole
• **Syphilis**	
– Early (Primary, secondary, latent < 1 year)	• Benzathine Penicillin G once
– Latent > 1 year	• Benzathine Pencillin G × 3 weeks
– Cardiovacuar	• Benzathine Pencillin G × 3 weeks
– Neurosyphilis	• Aqueous pencillin G × 10-14 days

Golden Points

1. **Pseudomembranous Colitis**
   - Most common organism implicated: Clostridium difficile
   - Most common antimicrobial implicated: Third generation cephalosporins > Clindamycin
   - Treatment of choice: Vancomycin
2. **Drugs having**
   - **CDK**
     - Aminoglycosides
     - Fluoroquinolones
   - **TDK**
     - Beta lactams
     - Vancomycin
   - **Time dependent inhibitory activity**
     - Macrolides
     - Clindamycin
   - **Prolonged PAE against gram negative bacteria**
     - Carbapenems
     - Tetracyclines
     - Chloramphenicol
     - Aminoglycosides
     - Fluoroquinolones
     - Rifampicin
3. **Puromycin** resembles 3'-end of aminoacyl-tRNA. It enters the A-site and transfers to growing chain (forming covalent bond) and causes premature chain termination. It inhibits protein synthesis in both prokaryotes as well as eukaryotes.
4. Methicillin resistance occurs due to altered PBPs, thus no penicillin, (infact no β-lactam antibiotic) is useful against methicillin-resistant Staphylococcus aureus (MRSA) infections.
5. Ampicillin should be avoided in patients with viral illness particularly EBV because it can cause rash in these patients.
6. Ceftriaxone and cefoperazone are secreted in the bile.
7. Cefazolin is the drug of choice for surgical prophylaxis.
8. Cefotetan, cefmetazole and cefoxitin are active against anaerobes like Bacteroides fragilis.
9. Aztreonam is the only beta lactam antibiotic that can be used in patients having severe allergy to penicillins or cephalosporins.
10. Carbapenems are the only β-lactams which are reliably efficacious against ESBL (extended spectrum β-lactamase) producing organisms.
11. Cycloserine has potential neurotoxic effects (tremors and seizures). It also causes **neuropsychiatric symptoms**.
12. Chloramphenicol may lead to grey baby syndrome and bone marrow suppression.
13. All tetracyclines are excreted primarily in the urine except doxycycline. Doxycycline is excreted in the feces and thus can be used in the presence of renal failure.
14. Aminoglycosides exhibit CDK and have prolonged PAE, therefore are administered as single daily dose.
15. Sulfisoxazole is most water-soluble sulfonamide. Thus it has minimum risk of causing crystalluria.
16. Cotrimoxazole is the drug of choice for pneumocystosis and nocardiosis.
17. Gatifloxacin has recently been withdrawn from India due to its dysglycemic effects.
18. NSAIDs increase CNS toxicity (seizures) of fluoroquinolones.
19. Recently, FDA has issued warning regarding peripheral neuropathy caused by fluoroquinolones.

Image Based Questions

1. In the given below figure at which site does penicillinase work?

   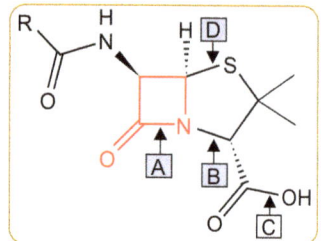

   (a) Site A (b) Site B
   (c) Site C (d) Site D

2. The drug shown in the figure is treatment of choice for:

   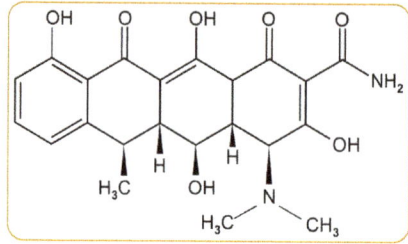

   (a) Enteric fever (b) Q Fever
   (c) MRSA (d) Gonorrhea

3. Identify drug A by its mechanism of action as shown in the figure:

   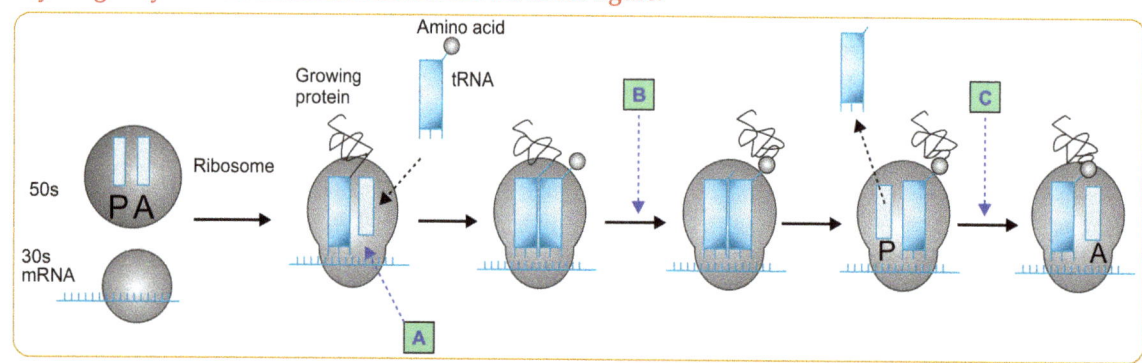

   (a) Doxycycline (b) Chloramphenicol (c) Azithromycin (d) Penicillin G

4. Identify drug B by its mechanism of action as shown in the above figure:
   (a) Doxycycline
   (b) Chloramphenicol
   (c) Azithromycin
   (d) Penicillin G

5. Identify drug C by its mechanism of action as shown in the above figure:
   (a) Doxycycline (b) Chloramphenicol
   (c) Azithromycin (d) Penicillin G

6. Mechanism of transfer of drug resistance shown in the given below figure:

   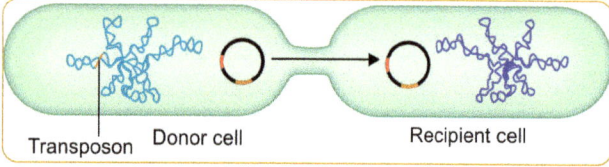

   (a) Conjugation
   (b) Transformation
   (c) Transduction
   (d) Mutation

7. Mechanism of transfer of drug resistance shown in the given below figure:

   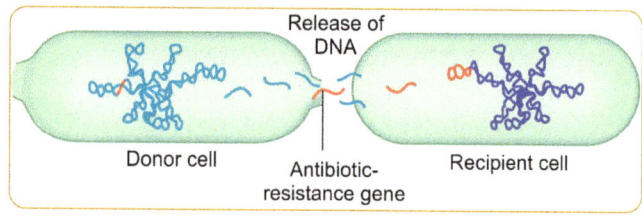

   (a) Conjugation (b) Transformation
   (c) Transduction (d) Mutation

8. Mechanism of transfer of drug resistance shown in the given below figure:

   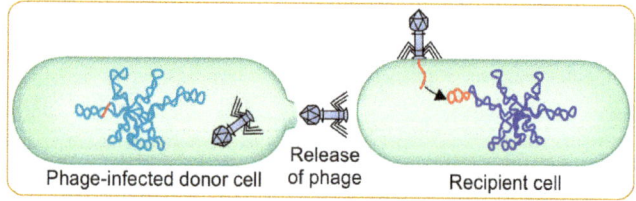

   (a) Conjugation (b) Transformation
   (c) Transduction (d) Mutation

9. Biochemical mechanisms of drug resistance are shown in the given below figure. Most important mode of resistance in MRSA is:

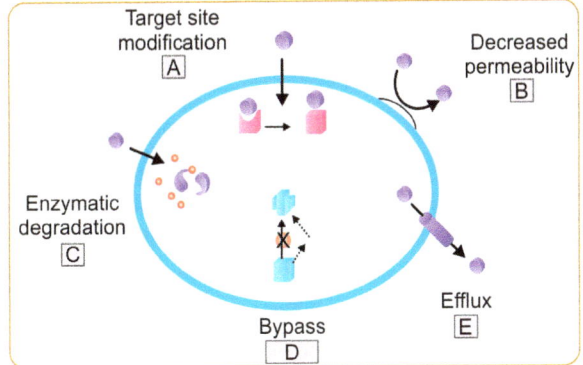

(a) A
(b) B
(c) C
(d) D

10. Vancomycin develops resistance to Enterococcus by which mechanism (as shown in figure in question 9)?
(a) A
(b) B
(c) C
(d) D

11. C is the major mechanism of resistance (according to figure in question 9) against:
(a) Fluoroquinolones
(b) Aminoglycosides
(c) Tetracyclines
(d) Sufonamides

12. Major mechanism of development of resistance against cotrimoxazole (in figure in question 9) is:
(a) B
(b) C
(c) D
(d) E

13. E is the major mode of resistance against (as shown in figure in question 9):
(a) Tetracyclines
(b) Chloramphenicol
(c) Ampicillin
(d) Ciprofloxacin

1. **Ans. (a) Site A**
   The four member ring is beta lactam ring and its integrity is required for antibacterial activity. Beta lactamase break this ring between N and C=O group and can result in resistance.

2. **Ans. (b) Q fever**
   The structure shows that the drug contains four cycles, therefore it is a drug in the group 'tetracyclines'. This is the chemical structure of doxycycline. Doxycycline is DOC for Q fever.

3. **Ans. (a) Doxycycline**
   Mechanism of action of protein synthesis inhibitors

Drug	Bind to which ribosome	Mechanism of action by inhibiting
Tetracyclines	30S	Attachment of tRNA to A site
Chloramphenicol	50S	Peptidyl transferase and transfer of peptide chain from A to P site
Macrolides	50S	Translocation (transfer of peptide chain from P to A site)
Clindamycin	50S	Translocation
Quinpristin-Dalfopristin	50S	Translocation
Linezolide	50S	Initiation
Aminoglycosides	30S and 50S	Initiation and cause misreading of mRNA code

4. **Ans. (b) Chloramphenicol**
5. **Ans. (c) Azithromycin**
6. **Ans. (a) Conjugation**

   Methods of horizontal transfer of drug resistance

Mechanism	Procedure
Conjugation	By forming sex pili between to bacteria through physical contact
Transformation	Through environment
Transduction	Through bacteriophage

7. **Ans. (b) Transformation**
8. **Ans. (c) Transduction**
9. **Ans. (a) A**
   Resistance in MRSA occurs mainly because of altered penicillin binding proteins
   Biochemical mode of transfer of drug resistance

Mechanism	Main drugs
Enzymatic breakdown	A: Aminoglycosides B: Beta lactams C: Chloramphenicol
Decreased permeability	Aminoglycosides
Efflux pumps	Tetracyclines
Altered metabolic pathway	Sulfonamides
Altered target	MRSA Vancomycin Fluoroquinolones

10. **Ans. (a) A**
    Vancomycin resistance occurs due to altered binding site whose structure changes from Alanine-Alanine to Alanine-Lactate

11. **Ans. (b) Aminoglycosides**

12. **Ans. (c) D**
    Cotrimoxazole contains sulfamethoxazole (a sulfonamide) and trimethoprim. Resistance to sulfonamides and thus cotrimoxazole occurs due to alternative metabolic pathway ie bacteria start utilizing preformed folic acid.

13. **(a) Tetracyclines**

Chemotherapy A: General Considerations and Non-specific Antimicrobial Agents

Multiple Choice Questions

GENERAL AND CLASSIFICATION

1. Which of the following drugs act by inhibiting DNA replication? *(NEET Pattern 2020)*
   - (a) 6-Mercaptopurine
   - (b) Actinomycin D
   - (c) Mitomycin C
   - (d) Asparaginase

2. Which of the following drug acts by inhibiting RNA synthesis? *(NEET Pattern 2020)*
   - (a) Rifampicin
   - (b) Nitrofurantoin
   - (c) Ciprofloxacin
   - (d) Novobiocin

3. All of the following drugs require dose reduction in renal failure *except*: *(AIIMS Nov. 2018)*
   - (a) Amphotericin B
   - (b) Vancomycin
   - (c) Gentamicin
   - (d) Doxycycline

4. Which of the following drugs is not used in typhoid fever? *(AIIMS May. 2018)*
   - (a) Amikacin
   - (b) Cefixime
   - (c) Azithromycin
   - (d) Ciprofloxacin

5. All of the following drugs are bacteriostatic *except*: *(Recent NEET Pattern Question 2017-2018)*
   - (a) Vancomycin
   - (b) Clindamycin
   - (c) Linezolide
   - (d) Tigecycline

6. Anaerobic bacteria are intrinsically resistant to: *(Recent NEET Pattern Question 2017-2018)*
   - (a) Beta lactams
   - (b) Aminoglycosides
   - (c) Chloramphenicol
   - (d) Metronidazole

7. Mycoplasma is resistant to: *(Recent NEET Pattern Question 2017-2018)*
   - (a) Vancomycin
   - (b) Doxycycline
   - (c) Moxifloxacin
   - (d) Azithromycin

8. Which of the following drug is used for mass prophylaxis for prevention of meningococcal meningtitis? *(Recent NEET Pattern Question 2017-2018)*
   - (a) Ciprofloxacin
   - (b) Rifampicin
   - (c) Ceftriaxone
   - (d) Minocycline

9. Which of the following is a beta-lactam antibiotic? *(Recent NEET Pattern Question 2016-17)*
   - (a) Vancomycin
   - (b) Dactinomycin
   - (c) Quinupristin
   - (d) Imipenem

10. Mechanism of action of vancomycin is:
    - (a) Cell wall synthesis inhibition *(AIIMS Nov 2017)*
    - (b) Protein synthesis inhibition
    - (c) Increase in membrane permeability
    - (d) Inhibition of folic acid metabolism

11. All of the following drugs act on nucleic acids *except*:
    - (a) Fluoroquinolones *(AIIMS Nov. 2015)*
    - (b) Linezolide
    - (c) Rifampicin
    - (d) Nalidixic acid

12. Tim- dependent killing and prolonged post-antibiotic effect is seen with: *(AIIMS Nov. 2014, May 2013, 2014)*
    - (a) Fluoroquinolones
    - (b) Beta-lactams
    - (c) Clindamycin
    - (d) Erythromycin

13. All of the following drugs are bactericidal *except*:
    - (a) Isoniazid *(AI 2012)*
    - (b) Tigecycline
    - (c) Daptomycin
    - (d) Ciprofloxacin

14. Drug resistance transmitting factor present in bacteria is: *(AI 2012)*
    - (a) Plasmid
    - (b) Chromosome
    - (c) Introns
    - (d) Centromere

15. Enzyme inactivation is the main mode of resistance to:
    - (a) Aminoglycosides *(Recent NEET Pattern Question)*
    - (b) Quinolones
    - (c) Rifamycins
    - (d) Glycopeptides

16. All of the following drug combinations shows antimicrobial synergism *except*: *(Recent Neet Pattern Question)*
    - (a) Penicillin + streptomycin in SABE
    - (b) Ampicillin + tetracycline in endocarditis
    - (c) Sulfamethoxazole + trimethoprim in UTI
    - (d) Amphotericin B + flucytosine in cryptococcal meningitis

17. Multiple drug resistance is transferred through:
    - (a) Transduction *(Recent NEET Pattern Question)*
    - (b) Transformation
    - (c) Conjugation
    - (d) Mutation

18. Most common mechanism for transfer of resistance in *Staphylococcus aureus* is: *(Recent NEET Pattern Question)*
    - (a) Conjugation
    - (b) Transduction
    - (c) Transformation
    - (d) Mutation

19. Elaboration of inactivating enzymes are the important mechanism of drug resistance among all of these antibiotics *except*: *(Recent NEET Pattern Question)*
    - (a) Quinolones
    - (b) Penicillin
    - (c) Chloramphenicol
    - (d) Aminoglycosides

20. Pneumococcal resistance to penicillin G is mainly acquired by: *(Recent NEET Pattern Question)*
    - (a) Conjugation
    - (b) Transduction
    - (c) Transformation
    - (d) All of the above

21. A bactericidal drug would be preferred over a bacteriostatic drug in a patient with:
    (Recent NEET Pattern Question)
    (a) Neutropenia (b) Cirrhosis
    (c) Pneumonia (d) Heart disease

22. Which of the following antibiotic acts by inhibiting cell wall synthesis? *(Recent NEET Pattern Question)*
    (a) Chloramphenicol (b) Gentamicin
    (c) Erythromycin (d) Penicillin

23. Which of the following drugs acts by inhibiting cell wall synthesis? *(Recent NEET Pattern Question)*
    (a) Erythromycin (b) Cephalosporins
    (c) Chloramphenicol (d) Sulfonamides

24. In Staphylococci, plasmids encoding beta-lactamase are transmitted by: *(Recent NEET Pattern Question)*
    (a) Conjugation (b) Transduction
    (c) Transposon (d) Transformation

25. Which of the following drug is bactericidal?
    (a) Sulfonamides *(Recent NEET Pattern Question)*
    (b) Erythromycin
    (c) Chloramphenicol
    (d) Cotrimoxazole

26. Superinfection is common in:
    (Recent NEET Pattern Question)
    (a) Narrow spectrum antibiotics
    (b) Immunocompromised host
    (c) Low spectrum antibiotics
    (d) Nutritional deficiency

27. Which of the following is a broad spectrum antibiotic?
    (a) Erythromycin *(Recent NEET Pattern Question)*
    (b) Streptomycin
    (c) Tetracycline
    (d) All

28. Which of the following antibiotic does not act by inhibiting protein synthesis?
    (a) Vancomycin *(Recent NEET Pattern Question)*
    (b) Tetracycline
    (c) Streptomycin
    (d) Azithromycin

29. Drug that inhibits cell wall synthesis is:
    (a) Tetracyclines *(Recent NEET Pattern Question)*
    (b) Penicillins
    (c) Aminoglycosides
    (d) Chloramphenicol

30. Which of the following is responsible for antibiotic associated colitis? *(Recent NEET Pattern Question)*
    (a) Clostridium botulinum
    (b) Clostridium perfringens
    (c) Clostridium difficile
    (d) Actinomyces species

31. Which amongst the following antimicrobials exhibits a long post antibiotic effect? *(Recent NEET Pattern Question)*
    (a) Quinolones (b) Macrolides
    (c) Beta-lactams (d) Oxazolidinones

32. The persistent suppression of bacterial growth that may occur after limited exposure to some antimicrobial drug is called: *(Recent NEET Pattern Question)*
    (a) Time dependent killing
    (b) Concentration dependent killing
    (c) Post-antibiotic effect
    (d) Sequential blockade

33. Which of the following antimicrobial agents act solely on the gram positive bacterial cell wall?
    (Recent NEET Pattern Question)
    (a) Ciprofloxacin (b) Gentamicin
    (c) Tetracycline (d) Vancomycin

34. Dosage of benzathine penicillin G in treatment of primary syphilis is: *(Recent NEET Pattern Question)*
    (a) 1.2 MU single i.m. (b) 1.2 MU single i.v.
    (c) 2.4 MU single i.m. (d) 4.8 MU single i.m.

CELL WALL SYNTHESIS INHIBITORS

35. Mechanism of resistance to penicillins via beta lactamase is: *(NEET Pattern 2020)*
    (a) Altered penicillin binding proteins
    (b) Drug efflux
    (c) Breaks drug structure
    (d) Alteration in 50S ribosome structure

36. There was outbreak of MRSA in the hospital and it was found that a nurse of NICU had MRSA colonization of anterior nares. What is the best treatment?
    (AIIMS Nov. 2019)
    (a) Topical mupirocin (b) Oral vancomycin
    (c) Inhaled colistin (d) IV cefazolin

37. Treatment of choice for late cardiovascular syphilis is:
    (AIIMS May 2018)
    (a) Benzathine penicillin 7.2 million units in three divided doses
    (b) Benzathine penicillin 2.4 million units single dose
    (c) Benzyl penicillin 12–24 million units for 21 days
    (d) Tetracycline 2 g daily

38. Imipenem is combined with cilastatin to:
    (Recent NEET Pattern Question 2019)
    (a) Cilastatin prevents degradation of imipenem in kidney
    (b) Cilastatin inreases intestinal absorption of imipenem
    (c) Cilastatin inhibits beta lactamase activity
    (d) Both have synergistic activity against Pseudomonas

39. Carbapenem with maximum risk of seizures is:
    (Recent NEET Pattern Question 2019)
    (a) Imipenem (b) Meropenem
    (c) Ertapenem (d) Doripenem

40. Antimicrobial agent effective against ESBL producing microorgansims is: *(Recent NEET Pattern Question 2017-2018)*
    (a) Beta lactam plus beta lactamase inhibitor
    (b) Ampicillin
    (c) Ceftriaxone
    (d) Aztreonam

41. Red man syndrome is caused by which drug?
    (Recent Question 2016-17)
    (a) Linezolid (b) Clindamycin
    (c) Vancomycin (d) Teicoplanin

42. Some gram-negative bacteria produce an enzyme that blocks the action of beta lactam antibiotics in periplasmic space. Which arrow in the structural diagram of Penicillin G denotes the site of action of this enzyme? *(AIIMS Nov. 2015)*

    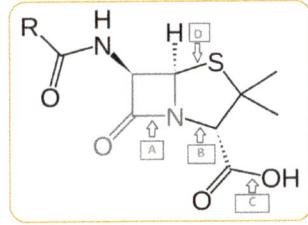

    (a) A (b) B
    (c) C (d) D

43. A child was admitted to the hospital with H. influenza meningitis. Cefotaxime is preferred over ampicillin because: *(AIIMS May. 2015)*
    (a) Cefotaxime has more oral bioavailability
    (b) Cefotaxime is more active against H influenza having altered penicillin binding proteins
    (c) Cefotaxime is cidal drug whereas ampicillin is bacterostatic
    (d) Cefotaxime is more active against beta-lactamase producing strains

44. Which of the following statements about cefepime is true? *(Recent NEET Pattern Question)*
    (a) It is a 4th generation cephalosporin
    (b) Once a day dosing is given
    (c) It is not active against Pseudomonas
    (d) It is a prodrug

45. Therapeutic uses of penicillin G include all *except*:
    (a) Bacterial meningitis *(Recent NEET Pattern Question)*
    (b) Syphilis
    (c) Rickettsial infections
    (d) Anthrax

46. Combination of amoxycillin with clavulanic acid is active against all of the following organisms *except*:
    (a) MRSA *(Recent NEET Pattern Question)*
    (b) Penicillinase producing *Staph. aureus*
    (c) Penicillinase producing *N. gonorrhoea*
    (d) Beta lactamase producing *E. coli*

47. Which of the following statements about cefuroxime is true? *(Recent NEET Pattern Question)*
    (a) It is active against bacteroides
    (b) It is superior to ceftriaxone for treatment of meningitis
    (c) It has poor CSF penetration
    (d) It is rapidly excreted by kidneys

48. Which of the following is not a semi-synthetic penicillin? *(Recent NEET Pattern Question)*
    (a) Penicillin V (b) Penicillin G
    (c) Methicillin   (d) Amoxycillin

49. Regarding vancomycin resistant enterococci, true statement is: *(Recent NEET Pattern Question)*
    (a) Resistance is plasmid-mediated
    (b) Resistance is due to development of inactivating enzyme
    (c) Third-generation cephalosporins can be used for treatment
    (d) VRE can cause epidemics throughout the world

50. Which of the following cephalosporin has activity against methicillin resistant Staphylococcus aureus? *(AIIMS Nov 2014)*
    (a) Ceftriaxone   (b) Ceftazidime
    (c) Cefuroxime   (d) Ceftobiprole

51. TRUE statement about penicillin G is:
    (a) It is administered orally *(AIIMS Nov 2014)*
    (b) It has a wide spectrum
    (c) It can be used for rat bite fever
    (d) Co-administration of probenecid decreases its duration of action

52. Which of the following drugs is active against Pseudomonas? *(AIIMS Nov 2014)*
    (a) Ceftriaxone
    (b) Piperacillin-tazobactam
    (c) Ampicillin
    (d) Cefalexin

53. Which of the following antimicrobial is effective against an organism producing extended spectrum beta lactamase? *(AIIMS Nov 2012)*
    (a) Amoxicillin–Clavulinic acid
    (b) Cefepime
    (c) Piperacillin-Tazobactam
    (d) Ceftriaxone

54. Which of the following statement about Penicillin G is true? *(AIIMS Nov 2012)*
    (a) It is commonly administered orally
    (b) It has a broad spectrum of antibacterial activity
    (c) It can be used for the treatment of rat bite fever
    (d) Concomitant probenecid decreases its duration of action

55. Which of the following beta-lactam antibiotics can be safely used in a patient with a history of allergy to penicillins? *(Recent NEET Pattern Question)*
    (a) Aztreonam   (b) Cefepime
    (c) Loracarbef (d) Ceftriaxone

56. Extended spectrum beta lactamases (ESBLs) are characterized by activity against all *except*: *(Recent NEET Pattern Question)*
    (a) Penicillinases
    (b) Cephalosporinases
    (c) Oxyimino-cephalosporinases
    (d) Carbapenems

57. Not true about cefepime is: *(Recent NEET Pattern Question)*
    (a) 4th generation cephalosporin
    (b) Useful in hospital acquired infection
    (c) Inhibits transpeptidase
    (d) Given twice daily orally

58. Antipseudomonals are all, *except*: *(Recent NEET Pattern Question)*
    (a) Cephalexin (b) Carbenicillin
    (c) Piperacillin (d) Ceftazidime

59. Cilastatin is given along with: *(Recent NEET Pattern Question)*
    (a) Imipenem   (b) Amoxicillin
    (c) Erythromycin (d) Ampicillin

60. Which of the following cephalosporins is active against Pseudomonas aeruginosa? *(Recent NEET Pattern Question)*
    (a) Ceftriaxone (b) Cephalothin
    (c) Ceftazidime (d) Cefotaxime

61. Which of the following is not true about penicillins? *(Recent NEET Pattern Question)*
    (a) Penicillin V is absorbed orally
    (b) Benzathine penicillin is short-acting penicillin
    (c) Cloxacillin is b-lactamase and acid resistant
    (d) Ampicillin is not resistant to b-lactamases

62. Mechanism of action of vancomycin is: *(Recent NEET Pattern Question)*
    (a) Inhibition of cell wall synthesis
    (b) Inhibition of protein synthesis
    (c) Leakage from cell membrane
    (d) Inhibition of DNA gyrase

63. Carbenicillin: *(Recent NEET Pattern Question)*
    (a) Is effective in pseudomonas infection
    (b) Has no effect in Proteus infection
    (c) Is a macrolide antibiotic
    (d) Is administered orally

64. A potent inhibitor of beta-lactamase is: *(Recent NEET Pattern Question)*
    (a) Carbenicillin
    (b) Clavulanic acid
    (c) Cefamandole
    (d) Idoxuridine

65. All are true about cefuroxime *except*: *(Recent NEET Pattern Question)*
    (a) Inhibit cell wall synthesis
    (b) Third-generation cephalosporin
    (c) Some acquired resistance with penicillin
    (d) More active against gram negative organisms

66. Amoxycillin is better than ampicillin due to: *(Recent NEET Pattern Question)*
    (a) Better bioavailability if taken with food
    (b) Lesser bioavailability if taken with food
    (c) Incidence of diarrhea is higher
    (d) More active against Shigella and H. influenza

67. Mechanism of action of penicillins and cephalosporins is to inhibit: *(Recent NEET Pattern Question)*
    (a) Cell wall synthesis
    (b) Leakage from cell membrane
    (c) Protein synthesis
    (d) DNA gyrase

68. The following organisms are known to develop resistance to Penicillin *except*: *(Recent NEET Pattern Question)*
    (a) Staphylococcus (b) Streptococcus
    (c) Pneumococcus (d) Treponema

69. Ceftriaxone is: *(Recent NEET Pattern Question)*
    (a) IInd generation short Acting cephalosporin
    (b) Has activity against beta lactamase Producing bacteria
    (c) IVth generation long Acting cephalosporin
    (d) IIIrd generation long Acting cephalosporin

70. Acid-susceptible penicillin is: *(Recent NEET Pattern Question)*
    (a) Methicillin (b) Ampicillin
    (c) Amoxicillin (d) Cloxacillin

71. All are first generation cephalosporins *except*: *(Recent NEET Pattern Question)*
    (a) Cefadroxil (b) Cefazolin
    (c) Cephalexin (d) Cefaclor

72. Which is not a beta lactum antibiotic? *(Recent NEET Pattern Question)*
    (a) Penicillin (b) Carbepenem
    (c) Monobactum (d) Azithromycin

73. Second generation cephalosporin that can be used orally is: *(Recent NEET Pattern Question)*
    (a) Cefepime (b) Cefalothin
    (c) Cefaclor (d) Cefadroxil

74. Third generation cephalosporin that can be given orally is: *(Recent NEET Pattern Question)*
    (a) Cefixime (b) Cefpirome
    (c) Cefaclor (d) Cefadroxil

75. Ampicillin is not given in EB virus infection due to: *(Recent NEET Pattern Question)*
    (a) Due to increased toxicity
    (b) Skin rash
    (c) Blindness
    (d) Convulsions

76. Which among the following is not a beta lactamase inhibitor? *(Recent NEET Pattern Question)*
    (a) Sulbactam (b) Calvulanic acid
    (c) Piperacillin (d) None

77. Oral cephalosporin among these is: *(Recent NEET Pattern Question)*
    (a) Cefatoxime (b) Ceftriaxone
    (c) Cefaclor (d) Ceftazidime

78. Beta lactam antibiotics act by inhibiting: *(Recent NEET Pattern Question)*
    (a) Cell wall synthesis (b) Protein synthesis
    (c) RNA synthesis (d) DNA synthesis

79. Which one of the following is a fourth generation cephalosporin? *(Recent NEET Pattern Question)*
    (a) Cefuroxime (b) Ceftazidime
    (c) Cefepime (d) Cefamandole

80. Neutropenia is associated with: *(Recent NEET Pattern Question)*
    (a) Nafcillin (b) Methicillin
    (c) Carbencillin (d) Ampicillin

81. Third-generation cephalosporins include all of the following *except*: *(Recent NEET Pattern Question)*
    (a) Ceftizoxime (b) Cefoperazone
    (c) Cefoxitin (d) Cefixime

82. Which one of the following statement about imipenem is most accurate? *(Recent NEET Pattern Question)*
    (a) The drug has a narrow spectrum of anti-bacterial action
    (b) It is used in fixed combination with sulbactam
    (c) Imipenem is highly susceptible to beta lactamase produced by enterobacteriaciae
    (d) In renal dysfunction, dosage reduction is necessary to avoid seizures

83. Which of the following is fourth generation cephalosporin? *(Recent NEET Pattern Question)*
    (a) Cefamandole (b) Cefpirome
    (c) Cephalexin (d) Cefuroxine

84. Penicillinase resistant penicillins include all of the following drugs *except*: *(Recent NEET Pattern Question)*
    (a) Cloxacillin (b) Nafcillin
    (c) Oxacillin (d) Carbenicillin

85. Ampicillin is used in: *(Recent NEET Pattern Question)*
    (a) Listeria (b) Pertussis
    (c) Atypical pneumonia (d) Gonococci

86. Red man syndrome is due to: *(Recent NEET Pattern Question)*
    (a) Vancomycin (b) Polymyxin
    (c) Rifampicin (d) Teicoplanin

87. Bleeding is a risk with the use of: *(Recent NEET Pattern Question)*
    (a) Cefaloridine (b) Cefazolin
    (c) Moxalactam (d) Ceftazidime

88. True about imipenem is: *(Recent NEET Pattern Question)*
    (a) It is narrow spectrum antibiotic
    (b) It is easily broken by beta lactamases
    (c) It should be used with cilastatin
    (d) It is used with sulbactam

89. Which among the following is not a beta lactamase resistant Penicillin? *(Recent NEET Pattern Question)*
    (a) Methicillin (b) Carbenicillin
    (c) Nafcillin (d) Oxacillin

90. All are third-generation Cephalosporins *except*: *(Recent NEET Pattern Question)*
    (a) Ceftriaxone (b) Ceftazidime
    (c) Cefuroxime (d) Cefoperazone

91. All of the following have beta lactam ring *except*: *(Recent NEET Pattern Question)*
    (a) Penicillin (b) Linezolid
    (c) Cefotaxime (d) Imipenem

92. All of the following beta-lactam antibiotics possess anti-pseudomonal action *except*: *(Recent NEET Pattern Question)*
    (a) Piperacillin (b) Ceftriaxone
    (c) Ceftazidime (d) Cefoperazone

93. All of the following are beta lactamase inhibitors *except*: *(Recent NEET Pattern Question)*
    (a) Clavulanic acid (b) Sulbactam
    (c) Tazobactam (d) Aztreonam

94. Which one of the following is true about the beta lactam antibiotics? *(Recent NEET Pattern Question)*
    (a) All are based on the 6-amino-penicillanic acid structure
    (b) Include amikacin
    (c) Are safe in pregnancy
    (d) Are uniformly ineffective against pseudomonas aeruginosa

95. The preferred treatment option for primary syphilis is: *(Recent NEET Pattern Question)*
    (a) Injection Benzathine pencillin 2.4 million units IM single dose
    (b) Injection Benzathine penicillin 2.4 million units IM once a week for 3 weeks
    (c) Cap. Doxycycline 100 mg orally twice a day for 2 weeks
    (d) Tab. Azithromycin 2 gm single dose

96. Oral vancomycin can be used for treatment of: *(Recent NEET Pattern Question)*
    (a) Hepatic encephalopathy
    (b) Pseudomembranous colitis
    (c) Staphylococcal food poisoning
    (d) None of the above

97. Which of the following drugs is an anti-Pseudomonal penicillin? *(Recent NEET Pattern Question)*
    (a) Cephalexin (b) Dicloxacillin
    (c) Piperacillin (d) Cloxacillin

98. Which of the following drugs is a 4th generation cephalosporin? *(Recent NEET Pattern Question)*
    (a) Cefixime (b) Ceftriaxone
    (c) Cefpirome (d) Cefazolin

99. Beta lactam antibiotics are all *except*: *(Recent NEET Pattern Question)*
    (a) Amoxicillin (b) Aztreonam
    (c) Ceftriaxone (d) Vancomycin

100. Not true about vancomycin is: *(Recent NEET Pattern Question)*
    (a) 95% oral bioavailability
    (b) Inhibits cells wall synthesis
    (c) Can be used parenterally as well as orally
    (d) Indicated for MRSA infections

101. Route of administration of vancomycin in pseudomembranous colitis is: *(Recent NEET Pattern Question)*
    (a) i.m. (b) oral
    (c) i.v. (d) s.c.

102. In treatment of Pseudomonas infections, carbenicillin is frequently combined with: *(Recent NEET Pattern Question)*
    (a) Penicillin
    (b) Gentamicin
    (c) Ciprofloxacin
    (d) Amoxycillin

103. All of the following are true regarding cephalosporins *except*: *(Recent NEET Pattern Question)*
    (a) Bactericidal agents
    (b) Active against only gram negative bacteria
    (c) IIIrd Generation are resistant to b-lactamases from gram negative bacteria
    (d) ceftriaxone is administered parenterally

104. Penicillinase-resistant penicillin is: *(Recent NEET Pattern Question)*
    (a) Methicillin (b) Ampicillin
    (c) Carbenecillin (d) Ticarcillin

PROTEIN SYNTHESIS INHIBITORS

105. Which of the following statements about tedizolide is true? *(AIIMS Nov. 2019)*
    (a) Peripheral neuropathy is a common adverse effect
    (b) It is active against gram positive organisms
    (c) It has poor oral bioavailability
    (d) Major mode of elimination is renal excretion

106. Drug of choice for prophylaxis of diphtheria is:
 (Recent Question 2019)
    (a) Erythromycin (b) Rifampicin
    (c) Cloxacillin (d) Doxycycline

107. Which of the following statements regarding tigecycline is true? *(Recent Question 2017-2018)*
    (a) It is a bactericidal drug
    (b) It does not require dose adjustment in renal failure
    (c) Approximately 95% of Pseudomonas are susceptible to tigecycline
    (d) It has narrow spectrum antibacterial action

108. Mechanism of action of tetracycline is:
 (Recent Question 2016-17)
    (a) Block translocation
    (b) Block cell wall synthesis
    (c) Block DNA synthesis
    (d) Inhibits binding of amino acyl t-RNA to A site

109. Mechanism of action of Linezolid is:
    (a) Binds to 30S ribosome and inhibits t-RNAfMet initiation complex *(Recent Question 2016-17)*
    (b) Binds to 50S ribosome and inhibits t-RNAfMet initiation complex
    (c) Inhibits attachment of aminoacyl tRNA to A-site
    (d) Inhibits peptidyltransferase

110. Which of the following mechanism is mainly responsible for gentamicin induced ototoxicity?
    (a) Direct hair cell toxicity *(AIIMS Nov 2012)*
    (b) Binding to and inhibition of hair cell Na^+ K^+ ATPase
    (c) Non-cumulative toxicity
    (d) Bind to Ca^{2+} channels

111. The antibiotic that inhibits protein synthesis by premature termination and which structurally resembles amino acyl t-RNA is: *(Recent NEET Pattern Question)*
    (a) Tetracycline (b) Chloramphenicol
    (c) Puromycin (d) Erythromycin

112. Which of the following drugs act by inhibiting bacterial protein synthesis? *(Recent NEET Pattern Question)*
    (a) Bacitracin (b) Dapsone
    (c) Ethambutol (d) Streptomycin

113. Tetracyclines are not useful for:
 (Recent NEET Pattern Question)
    (a) Trichomonas (b) Chlamydia
    (c) Syphilis (d) Rickettsia

114. The following drug interferes with translocation of protein synthesis: *(Recent NEET Pattern Question)*
    (a) Erythromycin (b) Tetracycline
    (c) Chloramphenicol (d) Penicillins

115. Chloramphenicol act through action on:
 (Recent NEET Pattern Question)
    (a) 50S ribosome (b) 30S ribosome
    (c) Nucleus (d) Mitochondria

116. Tetracyclines can be given in all forms *except*:
 (Recent NEET Pattern Question)
    (a) Oral (b) Intravenous
    (c) Topical in eye (d) Topical in open wound

117. All are aminoglycosides *except*:
 (Recent NEET Pattern Question)
    (a) Netilmycin (b) Streptomycin
    (c) Kanamycin (d) Azithromycin

118. Which of the following aminoglycosides has highest nephrotoxicity? *(Recent NEET Pattern Question)*
    (a) Paramomycin (b) Streptomycin
    (c) Amikacin (d) Neomycin

119. Auditory toxicity is maximum with:
 (Recent NEET Pattern Question)
    (a) Streptomycin (b) Kanamycin
    (c) Tobramycin (d) Amikacin

120. Erythromycin acts by interfering with:
 (Recent NEET Pattern Question)
    (a) Translocation of 50S ribosome
    (b) Translocation of 50S ribosome
    (c) Transcription of 50S ribosome
    (d) Signal transduction of 50S ribosome

121. Single dose aminoglycoside administration is more preferable than 8 hourly dose because of:
    (a) MIC *(Recent NEET Pattern Question)*
    (b) Increase perfusion of renal cortex
    (c) Post-antibiotic effect
    (d) None

122. Linezolid is best used for: *(Recent NEET Pattern Question)*
    (a) MRSA (b) VRSA
    (c) K.pneumoniae (d) E.coli

123. Doxycycline is used in the treatment of following diseases *except*: *(Recent NEET Pattern Question)*
    (a) Leptospirosis (b) Q fever
    (c) Borrelliosis (d) All of the above

124. This bacterial protein synthesis inhibitor is used for management of abdominal abcess caused by Bacteroides fragilis. Antibiotic associated colitis commonly occurs with use of this drug. Which of the following drug is being described? *(Recent NEET Pattern Question)*
    (a) Clarithromycin (b) Clindamycin
    (c) Minocycline (d) Ticarcillin

125. Ketolide antimicrobial among the following is:
    (a) Erythromycin *(Recent NEET Pattern Question)*
    (b) Azithromycin
    (c) Telithromycin
    (d) Clarithromycin

126. Streptogramins are not effective against:
 (Recent NEET Pattern Question)
    (a) E. coli (b) Staph. aureus
    (c) Legionella (d) Mycoplasma

127. Drug causing macular infraction on intravitreal use is:
 (Recent NEET Pattern Question)
    (a) Penicillin (b) Gentamicin
    (c) Amoxycillin (d) Metronidazole

128. Erythromycin is drug of choice for treatment of diarrhea in children caused by: *(Recent NEET Pattern Question)*
    (a) Giardia lamblia
    (b) Vibrio cholerae
    (c) Staph. aureus
    (d) Campylobacter jejuni

Chemotherapy A: General Considerations and Non-specific Antimicrobial Agents

129. Ototoxicity caused by aminoglycosides first involves:
     (Recent NEET Pattern Question)
     (a) Outer hair cells and base of cochlea
     (b) Apex of cochlea
     (c) Vestibular nerve
     (d) Cochlear nerve

ANTIMETABOLITES, FLUOROQUINOLONES AND MISCELLANEOUS ANTIMICROBIALS

130. Fluoroquinolone contraindicated in liver disease is:
     (NEET Pattern 2020)
     (a) Levofloxacin   (b) Pefloxacin
     (c) Ofloxacin   (d) Lomefloxacin

131. Fluoroquinolone with highest oral bioavailability is:
     (Recent NEET Pattern Question 2019)
     (a) Levofloxacin
     (b) Gemifloxacin
     (c) Ciprofloxacin
     (d) Norfloxacin

132. Fluoroquinolone having longest half-life is: *(AI 2012)*
     (a) Levofloxacin   (b) Lomefloxacin
     (c) Ciprofloxacin   (d) Moxifloxacin

133. Ciprofloxacin should not be given to an asthmatic using theophylline because: *(Recent NEET Pattern Question)*
     (a) Ciprofloxacin inhibits theophylline metabolism
     (b) Theophylline inhibits ciprofloxacin metabolism
     (c) Ciprofloxacin decreases effect of theophylline
     (d) Theophylline induces metabolism of ciprofloxacin

134. Mechanism of action of fluoroquinolones is:
     (Recent NEET Pattern Question)
     (a) Inhibits cell wall synthesis
     (b) Inhibits DNA gyrase
     (c) Interferes with intermediary metabolism

135. Eye drops of which sulphonamide is used clinically?
     (Recent NEET Pattern Question)
     (a) Sulfacetamide   (b) Sulfamethoxazole
     (c) Sulfinpyrazone   (d) All

136. Which is of the following can be used safely in renal failure? *(Recent NEET Pattern Question)*
     (a) Ciprofloxacin   (b) Ofloxacin
     (c) Lomefloxacin   (d) Pefloxacin

137. Mechanism of action of quinolones is by:
     (Recent NEET Pattern Question)
     (a) Inhibiting DHFRase
     (b) Inhibiting DNA gyrase
     (c) Inhibiting protein synthesis
     (d) Inhibiting cell wall synthesis

138. Longest acting sulphonamide is:
     (Recent NEET Pattern Question)
     (a) Sulfadiazine   (b) Sulfadoxine
     (c) Sulfamethoxazole (d) Sulfamethiazole

139. All are true about ciprofloxacin *except*:
     (Recent NEET Pattern Question)
     (a) Contra-indicated in pregnancy
     (b) DNA inhibition
     (c) Most potent first generation fluoroquinolone
     (d) More active at acidic pH

140. Sulfonamides inhibit bacterial synthesis of folic acid by:
     (Recent NEET Pattern Question)
     (a) Uncompetitive inhibition
     (b) Allosteric inhibition
     (c) Competitive inhibition
     (d) Non competitive inhibition

141. Highest photosensitivity is seen with:
     (Recent NEET Pattern Question)
     (a) Pefloxacin   (b) Gatifloxacin
     (c) Levofloxacin   (d) Sprafloxacin

142. Fluoroquinoline with least oral bioavailability is:
     (Recent NEET Pattern Question)
     (a) Norfloxacin   (b) Ofloxacin
     (c) Ciprofloxacin   (d) Levofloxacin

143. Drug used for treatment of impetigo is:
     (Recent NEET Pattern Question)
     (a) Dicloxacillin   (b) Ciprofloxacin
     (c) Gentamicin   (d) Amoxycillin

144. Fluoroquinolone with longest half-life is:
     (Recent NEET Pattern Question)
     (a) Levofloxacin   (b) Lomefloxacin
     (c) Ciprofloxacin   (d) Moxifloxacin

145. Drug used to prevent staphylococcal colonization of nose in patients of recurrent pyoderma is:
     (Recent NEET Pattern Question)
     (a) Rifampicin   (b) Amoxycillin
     (c) Tetracycline   (d) Mupirocin

CLINICAL USES OF ANTIMICROBIALS

146. **Assertion**: In a patient admitted in hospital for community acquired pneumonia, combination therapy of beta lactams and azithromycin is given.
     Reason: The combination covers gram positive organisms as well as anaerobes. *(AIIMS Nov. 2019)*
     (a) Both A and R are correct and R is correct explanation of A
     (b) Both A and R are correct and R is not the correct explanation of A
     (c) A is true and R is false
     (d) A is false and R is true
     (e) Both A and R are false statements

147. Clostridium difficile diarrhea is most commonly associated with: *(AIIMS Nov. 2019)*
     (a) Aminopenicillins (b) Fluoroquinolones
     (c) Macrolides   (d) Carbapenems

148. Pediatrician was called for attending a new born baby. The serum unconjugated bilirubin of this baby was 33 mg/dL. Which of the following drug taken by mother in late 3rd trimester might have resulted in this problem?
     (AIIMS Nov. 2018)
     (a) Cotrimoxazole   (b) Azithromycin
     (c) Ampicillin   (d) Chloroquine

149. Drug of choice for scrub typhus is: *(AIIMS May 2018)*
     (a) Doxycycline   (b) Metronidazole
     (c) Sulfonamides   (d) Erythromycin

150. Which of the following drug is commonly used for community acquired pneumonia caused by S. aureus?
    (AIIMS May 2018)
    (a) Vancomycin (b) Ceftriaxone
    (c) Azithromycin (d) Streptomycin

151. Drug of choice for prophylaxis of diphtheria is:
    (NEET Pattern 2019)
    (a) Erythromycin (b) Rifampicin
    (c) Cloxacillin (d) Doxycycline

152. Drug of choice for mastitis is:
    (Recent NEET Pattern Question 2019)
    (a) Cloxacillin (b) Metronidazole
    (c) Amoxicillin (d) Cefazolin

153. Burkholderia cepacia is intrinsically resistant to:
    (Recent NEET Pattern Question 2017-2018)
    (a) Doxycycline (b) Polymyxin B
    (c) Cotrimoxazole (d) Ceftazidime

154. Drug of choice for confirmed case of gonococcal urethritis is: *(Recent Question 2016-17)*
    (a) Cefixime 400 mg + Azithromycin 1g
    (b) Ceftriaxone 250 mg i/m single dose + Azithromycin 400 mg
    (c) Doxycycline 100 mg + Probenecid 1 g oral
    (d) Ceftriaxone 250 mg i/m single dose + Azithromycin 1 g oral

155. Which of the following drug should be avoided in a 7-year-old child? *(Recent NEET Pattern Question 2016-17)*
    (a) Cefixime (b) Erythromycin
    (c) Ofloxacin (d) Amoxicillin

156. Drug of choice for scrub typhus is: *(AIIMS Nov 2017)*
    (a) Azithromycin
    (b) Ciprofloxacin
    (c) Doxycycline
    (d) Chloramphenicol

157. Treatment of choice for a patient with gonococcal as well as non-gonococcal urethritis is: *(AIIMS Nov 2017)*
    (a) Ceftriaxone 250 mg im single dose
    (b) Cefixime 400 mg oral single dose
    (c) Ciprofloxacin 500 mg oral single dose
    (d) Azithromycin 2 g oral single dose

158. Drug of choice for prophylaxis of Pneumocystis jiroveci pneumonia in immunocompromised patients is:
    (a) Cotrimoxazole *(AIIMS May 2017)*
    (b) Amoxycillin
    (c) Dexamethasone
    (d) Cefotetan

159. Drug of choice for Burkholderia cepacia pneumonia is:
    (a) Cotrimoxazole *(AIIMS May 2017)*
    (b) Carbapenem
    (c) Cefepime
    (d) Colistin

160. Empirical treatment for meningococcal meningitis is:
    (AIIMS May 2017)
    (a) Ceftriaxone
    (b) Cefotetan
    (c) Gentamicin
    (d) Cefoxitin

161. Drug of choice for antibiotic associated pseudomembranous colitis is: *(AIIMS Nov 2014)*
    (a) Oral vancomycin (b) Metronidazole
    (c) Clindamycin (d) Penicillin G

162. Which of the following drugs is used in the treatment of acute bacterial meningitis? *(AIIMS May 2014)*
    (a) Erythromycin (b) Sulfamethoxazole
    (c) Ceftriaxone (d) Streptomycin

163. Drug-induced colitis is most frequently associated with:
    (AIIMS May 2012)
    (a) Neomycin (b) Vancomycin
    (c) Clindamycin (d) Chloramphenicol

164. A 26-year-old patient presents with suspected pneumococcal meningitis. CSF culture is sent for antibiotic sensitivity. Which empirical antibiotic should be given till culture sensitivity result come? *(AIIMS May 2012)*
    (a) Penicillin G
    (b) Ceftriaxone + metronidazole
    (c) Doxycycline
    (d) Cefotaxime + vancomycin

165. A patient develops an infection of methicillin resistant Staphylococcus aureus. All of the following can be used to treat this infection *except*: *(AI 2012)*
    (a) Cotrimoxazole *(AIIMS Nov. 2011)*
    (b) Cefaclor
    (c) Ciprofloxacin
    (d) Vancomycin

166. Drug of choice for syphilis in a pregnant lady is:
    (a) Penicillin *(AI 2012)*
    (b) Azithromycin
    (c) Tetracycline
    (d) Ceftriaxone

167. Which of the following antibiotic is used in the treatment of Clostridium difficile associated diarrhea?
    (a) Ciprofloxacin *(Recent NEET Pattern Question)*
    (b) Metronidazole
    (c) Piperacillin
    (d) Clindamycin

168. Which of the following drug should not be used to treat Klebsiella infection? *(Recent NEET Pattern Question)*
    (a) Ampicillin (b) Amikacin
    (c) Imipenem (d) Tigecycline

169. Which of the following drugs is effective against Pseudomonas infection? *(Recent NEET Pattern Question)*
    (a) Ampicillin (b) Ceftriaxone
    (c) Colistin (d) Cefixime

170. Drug of choice for treatment of infection caused by methicillin resistant Staphylococcus aureus is:
    (a) Macrolides *(Recent NEET Pattern Question)*
    (b) Third generation cephalosporins
    (c) Carbapenems
    (d) Glycopeptides

171. Methicillin resistant Staphylococcus aureus is not expected to respond to: *(Recent NEET Pattern Question)*
    (a) Aminoglycoside
    (b) Lincosamide
    (c) Oxazolidinone
    (d) Carbapenem

Chemotherapy A: General Considerations and Non-specific Antimicrobial Agents

172. Fixed drug eruptions can be seen more frequently with:
(Recent NEET Pattern Question)
(a) Penicillin (b) Sulfonamide
(c) Cetrizine (d) Roxithromycin

173. Red man syndrome occurs with:
(Recent NEET Pattern Question)
(a) Clindamycin (b) Teicoplanin
(c) Vancomycin (d) Polymyxin

174. Which of the following antimicrobials needs dose reduction even in mild renal failure?
(Recent NEET Pattern Question)
(a) Ciprofloxacin (b) Carbenicillin
(c) Cefotaxime (d) Ethambutol

175. Which of the following drug can cause cartilage damage in children? *(Recent NEET Pattern Question)*
(a) Cotrimoxazole (b) Penicillin
(c) Ciprofloxacin (d) Metronidazole

176. Gray baby syndrome is caused by:
(Recent NEET Pattern Question)
(a) Chlorpromazine (b) Chloramphenicol
(c) Phenytoin (d) Gentamycin

177. Macrocytic anaemia is caused by all *except*:
(Recent NEET Pattern Question)
(a) Pyrimethamine (b) Methotrexate
(c) Pentamidine (d) Trimethoprim

178. Which of the following drugs is most commonly associated with Clostridium difficile colitis?
(Recent NEET Pattern Question)
(a) Vancomycin (b) Metronidazole
(c) Clindamycin (d) Erythromycin

179. Which of the following is not nephrotoxic?
(Recent NEET Pattern Question)
(a) Tobramycin (b) Kanamycin
(c) Ampicillin (d) Amphotericin B

180. Dose of which of the following antibiotic does not require alteration in renal failure?
(Recent NEET Pattern Question)
(a) Vancomycin (b) Ethambutol
(c) Erythromycin (d) Metronidazole

181. Drug of choice for sore throat caused by Group A beta hemolytic streptococcus is:
(Recent NEET Pattern Question)
(a) Erythromycin (b) Penicillin
(c) Ceftriaxone (d) Sulfonamides

182. Nephrotoxicity is seen with:
(Recent NEET Pattern Question)
(a) Doxycycline (b) Aminoglycosides
(c) Erythromycin (d) Rifampicin

183. Drug which should not be given in renal disease is:
(Recent NEET Pattern Question)
(a) Gentamicin (b) Nitroprusside
(c) Doxycycline (d) Ceftriaxone

184. Drug causing megaloblastic anemia is:
(Recent NEET Pattern Question)
(a) INH (b) Chloramphenicol
(c) Pyrimethamine (d) Methyldopa

185. All are hepatotoxic drugs *except*:
(Recent NEET Pattern Question)
(a) Erythromycin estolate
(b) Rifampicin
(c) Tetracycline
(d) None

186. Jarisch-Herxheimer reaction is seen in syphilis with:
(Recent NEET Pattern Question)
(a) Tetracyclines (b) Penicillins
(c) Co-trimoxazole (d) Sulfonamides

187. Which of the following drug is not used against Pseudomonas? *(Recent NEET Pattern Question)*
(a) Piperacillin (b) Carbenicillin
(c) Ticarcillin (d) Oxacillin

188. Red cell aplasia can be caused by:
(Recent NEET Pattern Question)
(a) Aminoglycosides (b) Chloramphenicol
(c) Penicillins (d) Ciprofloxacin

189. Which of the following drug is safe during pregnancy?
(Recent NEET Pattern Question)
(a) Aminoglycoside (b) Ampicillin
(c) Chloramphenicol (d) Cotrimoxazole

190. Which one of the following is used in the prophylaxis of streptococcal sore throat? *(Recent NEET Pattern Question)*
(a) Phenoxy methyl penicillin
(b) Inj. Benzathine Penicillin
(c) Crystalline penicillin
(d) Both A and B are true

191. Drug of choice for plague is:
(Recent NEET Pattern Question)
(a) Erythromycin (b) Tetracyclines
(c) Ampicillin (d) Cotrimoxazole

192. Which one of the following is primarily bacteriostatic?
(Recent NEET Pattern Question)
(a) Ciprofloxacin (b) Chloramphenicol
(c) Vancomycin (d) Rifampicin

193. Drug of choice for prophylaxis of meningococcal meningitis is: *(Recent NEET Pattern Question)*
(a) Penicillin (b) Erythromycin
(c) Septran (d) Rifampicin

194. Drug with high degree of photosensitivity is:
(Recent NEET Pattern Question)
(a) Tetracycline (b) Doxycycline
(c) Minocycline (d) Methacycline

195. Drug used for treatment of methicillin resistant staphylococcus aureus is: *(Recent NEET Pattern Question)*
(a) Teicoplanin (b) Vancomycin
(c) Both (d) None

196. Drug of choice in pertussis is:
(Recent NEET Pattern Question)
(a) Penicillin (b) Doxycycline
(c) Erythromycin (d) Ciprofloxacin

197. Drug effective against pseudomonas is:
(Recent NEET Pattern Question)
(a) Penicillin G (b) Gentamicin
(c) Tetracycline (d) Chloramphenicol

198. Treatment of choice for chancroid is: *(Recent NEET Pattern Question)*
    (a) Penicillin (b) Chloramphenicol
    (c) Tetracyclines (d) Erythromycin

199. Pseudomembranous colitis is associated mostly with which drug? *(Recent NEET Pattern Question)*
    (a) Erythromycin (b) Ampicillin
    (c) Vancomycin (d) Ciprofloxacin

200. Drug of choice for primary syphilis is: *(Recent NEET Pattern Question)*
    (a) Ampicillin (b) Benzathine penicillin
    (c) Erythromycin (d) Tetracycline

201. Drug of choice for syphilis during pregnancy is: *(Recent NEET Pattern Question)*
    (a) Ampicillin (b) Erythromycin
    (c) Benzathine penicillin (d) Tetracyclines

202. Drug that is not contraindicated in G-6 PD deficiency is: *(Recent NEET Pattern Question)*
    (a) Primaquine (b) Nitrofurantoin
    (c) Dapsone (d) INH

203. Which of the following drug is contraindicated in pregnancy? *(Recent NEET Pattern Question)*
    (a) Chloroquine (b) Erythromycin
    (c) Ampicillin (d) Primaquine

204. Absorption of which of the following drug increases with food intake? *(Recent NEET Pattern Question)*
    (a) Tetracycline (b) Diazepam
    (c) Griseofulvin (d) Ampicilin

205. Which of the following prokinetic drug acts on motilin receptors? *(Recent NEET Pattern Question)*
    (a) Erythromycin (b) Metoclopramide
    (c) Loxiglumide (d) Cisapride

206. The antibiotic which can be given safely in a pregnant women is: *(Recent NEET Pattern Question)*
    (a) Ciprofloxacin (b) Cefuroxime
    (c) Metronidazole (d) Chloramphenicol

207. Drug of choice for Mycoplasma pneumoniae infection is: *(Recent NEET Pattern Question)*
    (a) Gentamicin (b) Amoxyclillin
    (c) Azithromycin (d) Cefotaxime

208. Drug of choice for acute (pneumococcal) lobar pneumonia is: *(Recent NEET Pattern Question)*
    (a) Amoxicillin clavulanic acid combination
    (b) Ciprofloxacin
    (c) Co-trimoxazole
    (d) Crystalline penicillin (Pen. G)

209. Drug of choice for acute meningococcal pyogenic meningitis is: *(Recent NEET Pattern Question)*
    (a) Crystalline penicillin (Pen. G)
    (b) Sulphonamides
    (c) Chloramphenicol
    (d) Amoxycillin

210. Which of the following is not given in myasthenia gravis? *(Recent NEET Pattern Question)*
    (a) Clofibrate (b) Polymixin B
    (c) Penicillin (d) All

211. Which of following drug's absorption is increased in gastric achlorhydria? *(Recent NEET Pattern Question)*
    (a) Ketoconazole (b) Penicillin G
    (c) Chloramphenicol (d) Ciprofloxacin

212. Which does not cause pseudomembranous enterocolitis? *(Recent NEET Pattern Question)*
    (a) Vancomycin (b) Levofloxacin
    (c) Clindamycin (d) Ceftazidime

213. Single dose treatment for chlamydia is: *(Recent NEET Pattern Question)*
    (a) Doxycycline (b) Tetracycline
    (c) Azithromycin (d) Erythromycin

214. Widest spectrum aminoglycoside is: *(Recent NEET Pattern Question)*
    (a) Streptomycin (b) Amikacin
    (c) Framycetin (d) Netilmicin

215. Pseudomonas is resistant to: *(Recent NEET Pattern Question)*
    (a) Vancomycin (b) Aztreonam
    (c) Ciprofloxacin (d) Polymyxin B

216. Which of the following is contra indicated in pregnancy? *(Recent NEET Pattern Question)*
    (a) Tetracycline (b) Erythromycin
    (c) Ampicillin (d) Chloroquine

217. Drug of choice for syphilis is: *(Recent NEET Pattern Question)*
    (a) Penicillin (b) Rifampicin
    (c) Tetracycline (d) Erythromycin

218. Actinomycete is the source of which of the following anti microbials? *(Recent NEET Pattern Question)*
    (a) Tetracycline (b) Polyene
    (c) Aztreonam (d) Colistin

219. Drug that can cause hypertrophic pyloric stenosis is: *(Recent NEET Pattern Question)*
    (a) Tertacycline (b) Erythromycin
    (c) Ampicillin (d) Rifampicin

220. Which of the following tetracycline can be used in renal failure without dose adjustment? *(Recent NEET Pattern Question)*
    (a) Oxytetracycline (b) Doxycycline
    (c) Demeclocycline (d) Tetracycline

221. Drug of choice in pregnant women with secondary syphills is: *(Recent NEET Pattern Question)*
    (a) Doxycycline (b) Benzathine Penicillin
    (c) Ceftriaxone (d) Cotrimoxazole

222. Drug of choice for Treponema pallidum is: *(Recent NEET Pattern Question)*
    (a) Penicillin G (b) Tetracycline
    (c) Azithromycin (d) Doxycycline

223. Treatment for clostridial myonecrosis is: *(Recent NEET Pattern Question)*
    (a) Amikacin (b) Penicillin
    (c) Ampicillin (d) Gentamicin

Chemotherapy A: General Considerations and Non-specific Antimicrobial Agents

224. Drug of choice for treatment of infections caused by MRSA is: *(Recent NEET Pattern Question)*
    (a) Metronidazole (b) Vancomycin
    (c) Imipenem (d) Clindamycin

225. All of the following are common antimicrobial agents used in treatment of typhoid fever except: *(Recent NEET Pattern Question)*
    (a) Ceftriaxone (b) Quinolones
    (c) Clindamycin (d) Azithromycin

226. The drug of choice in lymphogranuloma venereum is:
    (a) Penicillin *(Recent NEET Pattern Question)*
    (b) Ciprofloxacin
    (c) Tetracycline
    (d) Erythromycin

227. Antacid interfere with absorption of all of the following except: *(Recent NEET Pattern Question)*
    (a) Ketoconazole (b) Azithromycin
    (c) Oxytetracycline (d) Ofloxacin

228. Antibiotic which is effective as a single dose therapy for trachoma is: *(Recent NEET Pattern Question)*
    (a) Doxycycline
    (b) Clarithromycin
    (c) Azithromycin
    (d) Erythromycin

229. The prophylactic antibiotic indicated to prevent infection in lymphoedema is: *(Recent NEET Pattern Question)*
    (a) Vancomycin (b) Penicillin
    (c) Amikacin (d) Quinolones

230. Which of the following antibacterial causes both ototoxicity and nephrotoxicity? *(Recent NEET Pattern Question)*
    (a) Methicillin (b) Vancomycin
    (c) Clindamycin (d) Azithromycin

231. All of the following drugs can cause cholestatic jaundice except: *(Recent NEET Pattern Question)*
    (a) Ethambutol
    (b) Chlorpromazine
    (c) Erythromycin estolate
    (d) Estrogens

232. Which of the following antibiotics class is not safe in pregnancy? *(Recent NEET Pattern Question)*
    (a) Quinolones (b) Cephalosporins
    (c) Penicillins (d) Macrolides

233. Which of the following drugs is avoided in a patient with high serum creatinine (> 3 mg/dL)? *(Recent NEET Pattern Question)*
    (a) Gentamicin (b) Azithromycin
    (c) Moxifloxacin (d) Amlodipine

234. Which of the following is used in the prophylactic treatment of rheumatic heart disease?
    (a) Ampicillin *(Recent NEET Pattern Question)*
    (b) Penicillin-G
    (c) Benzathine penicillin
    (d) Phenoxy-methyl penicillin

235. Prophylactic antibiotics to prevent surgical site infection are best administered: *(Recent NEET Pattern Question)*
    (a) After commencement of surgery
    (b) 30 minutes before incision
    (c) At the end of surgery
    (d) With pre medication

236. Which can be given safely in renal failure? *(Recent NEET Pattern Question)*
    (a) Tetracycline (b) Gentamicin
    (c) Amphotericin B (d) Doxycycline

237. Drug of choice in pneumonia caused by P carnii is: *(Recent NEET Pattern Question)*
    (a) Penicillin (b) Cotrimoxazole
    (c) Kanamycin (d) Levofloxacin

238. Which of the following drugs should not be given in renal failure? *(Recent NEET Pattern Question)*
    (a) Clindamycin (b) Methicillin
    (c) Amoxicillin (d) Rifampicin

239. All of the following drugs are administered orally except: *(Recent NEET Pattern Question)*
    (a) Ciprofloxacin (b) Cotrimoxazole
    (c) Gentamicin (d) Amoxicillin

240. Aplastic anemia is the adverse effect of: *(Recent NEET Pattern Question)*
    (a) Chloramphenicol (b) Ciprofloxacin
    (c) Penicillin (d) Gentamicin

241. Dosage of topical tobramycin eye drops: *(Recent NEET Pattern Question)*
    (a) 1 mg/mL (b) 2 mg/mL
    (c) 3 mg/mL (d) 4 mg/mL

242. Treatment of non-specific urethritis is: *(Recent NEET Pattern Question)*
    (a) Erythromycin (b) Sulphonamides
    (c) Tetracycline (d) Ampicillin

243. Hemolysis in G-6 deficiency is precipitated by all of the following except: *(Recent NEET Pattern Question)*
    (a) Dapsone (b) Cotrimoxazole
    (c) Quinine (d) Penicillin

244. Drug used in the treatment of resistant gonorrhoea is: *(Recent NEET Pattern Question)*
    (a) Penicillin (b) Cotrimoxazone
    (c) Spectinomycin (d) Erythromycin

Explanations

1. **Ans. (a) 6-Mercaptopurine** *(Ref: KDT 8th/e p922)*
   - 6-Mercaptopurine is a purine antimetabolite. It acts as a competitive inhibitor of DNA polymerase and therefore it prevents DNA replication.
   - Mitomycin C is an antitumor antibiotic that inhibits DNA synthesis by producing DNA cross-links which halt cell replication and eventually cause cell death.
   - Actinomycin D acts by inhibiting DNA dependent RNA synthesis.
   - L-Asparginase is an enzyme that catalyzes the hydrolysis of l-asparagine to l-aspartic acid and ammonia. It inhibits protein synthesis in tumor cells by depriving them of the amino acid asparagine.

2. **Ans. (a) Rifampicin** *(Ref: KDT 8th/e p818)*
   - Rifampin interrupts RNA synthesis by binding to sub-unit of mycobacterial DNA-dependent RNA polymerase (encoded by rpo B gene) and blocking its polymerizing function.
   - Nitrofurantoin is a urinary antiseptic and after reduction by bacterial enzymes, it results in DNA damage.
   - Ciprofloxacin is a fluoroquinolone that acts by inhibiting DNA gyrase (topoisomerase II) and topoisomerase IV resulting in the inhibition of DNA replication.
   - Novobiocin binds to DNA gyrase, and blocks adenosine triphosphatase (ATPase) activity.

3. **Ans. (d) Doxycycline** *(Ref: KDT 8th/e p786)*
   Antimicrobials that are secreted in bile, can be excreted in feces. Therefore, these do not require dose reduction in renal failure. Important drugs secreted in bile are:

Safe (Cef) - **Cef**triaxone
- **Cef**operazone in
The - **T**igecycline
R - **R**ifampicin
E - **E**rythromycin
N - **N**afcillin
A - **A**mpicillin
L - **L**incosamides (Clindamycin)
Disease - **D**oxycycline

4. **Ans. (a) Amikacin** *(Ref: KDT 8th/e p762)*
   Normally we need to remember which antimicrobials are effective against which bacteria. However, many questions can be answered if we know some antimicrobials are not effective against certain bacteria. The important among these are:

Organism	Does not respond to	Special point
MRSA	Beta lactams except 5th generation cephalosporins	DOC is vancomycin
Pseudomonas (most gram negative bacteria)	Vancomycin	Aminoglycoside + ceftazidime
Anaerobes	Aminoglycosides	Metronidazole
Salmonella (enteric fever)	Aminoglycosides	Ceftriaxone
Mycoplasma	Cell wall synthesis inhibitors (beta lactams and vancomycin)	Azithromycin
Burkholderia cepacia	Polymyxins	Cotrimoxazole

5. **Ans. (a) Vancomycin** *(Ref: KK Sharma 2nd/699, KDT 8/e p806)*

6. **Ans. (b) Aminoglycosides** *(Ref: Goodman and Gilman 13th/1040, KDT 8/e p794)*

7. **Ans. (a) Vancomycin** *(Ref: Harrison 19th/e p1164)*
   Mycoplasma lacks cell wall. Thus any drug acting by inhibition of cell wall synthesis (like vancomycin and beta lactams) is likely to be ineffective.

8. **Ans. (a) Ciprofloxacin** *(Ref: Park 24th/176)*
   All the drugs mentioned in the options can be used for prophylaxis of meningococcal meningitis. Earlier rifampicin was used as drug of choice but now many species resistant to rifampicin have been isolated. Ciprofloxacin is preferred for mass prophylaxis now.

9. **Ans. (d) Imipenem** *(Ref: KDT's 8/e p782)*

10. **Ans. (a) Cell wall synthesis inhibition** *(Ref: KDT 7/e p757)*
    - Vancomycin acts by inhibiting transglycosylase enzyme which is involved in cell wall synthesis.
    - Beta lactams also inhibit cell wall synthesis but by inhibiting the enzyme transpeptidase.

11. **Ans. (b) Linezolide** *(Ref: KDT 8th/e p741)*
    Linezolide act by inhibiting cell wall synthesis whereas quinolones (nalidixic acid and fluoroquinolones) inhibit DNA gyrase and rifampicin inhibit RNA polymerase.

12. **Ans. (b) Beta-lactams** *(Ref: Katzung 13th/e p879)*
    Friends, this question has been unnecessarily made controversial by giving different answers in different books for competitive exams. Please try to search for the references provided in those books. Now coming to explanation:
    - The terms time dependent killing (TDK) and concentration dependent killing (CDK) are applicable only for cidal drugs. Beta lactams and vancomycin follow TDK whereas aminoglycosides and fluoroquinolones follow CDK.
    - Long post-antibiotic effect is shown by most of the drugs against gram positive bacteria (including aminoglycosides, beta lactams, clindamycin and macrolides) but few drugs have long PAE against gram negative bacteria. The table given in katzung is modified as:

Long PAE against	
Gram +ve cocci	Gram –ve bacilli
• Aminoglycosides	• Aminoglycosides
• Beta lactams	• Carbapenems
• Chloramphenicol	• Fluoroquinolones
• Clindamycin	• Chloramphenicol
• Daptomycin	• Rifampicin
• Vancomycin	• Tetracyclines
• Macrolides	
• Linezolide	
• Fluoroquinolones	
• Rifampicin	
• Sulfonamides	
• Tetracyclines	
• Streptogramins	

Chemotherapy A: General Considerations and Non-specific Antimicrobial Agents

- Clindamycin and erythromycin are static drugs that exhibit time dependent inhibitory activity. As these are bacteriostatic, so these can be easily excluded
- Fluoroquinolones follow CDK.
- So, answer is beta lactams as these follows TDK, have long PAE against gram positive cocci and some (carbapenems) have long PAE against gram negative bacilli also.

13. **Ans. (b) Tigecycline**
    (Ref: KK Sharma 2/e p733,750, KDT 8th/e p741,789)
    Tigecycline is a newer drug in the class 'Glycylcyclines.' Its mechanism of action and most properties are similar to tetracyclines. However, it is resistant to efflux pump (major mechanism of resistance against tetracyclines). Most protein synthesis inhibiting drugs (including tetracyclines and tigecycline) are bacteriostatic except aminoglycosides. Isoniazid, ciprofloxacin and daptomycin are bactericidal.

14. **Ans. (a) Plasmid** *(Ref: KDT 8/e p743)*
    Plasmids contain extra-chromosomal DNAs that help in transferring the genes responsible for multiple drug resistance among bacteria. These are therefore involved in horizontal transfer of resistance.
    As it is not due to penicillinase, beta lactamase inhibitors like clavulanic acid cannot reverse this resistance.

15. **Ans. (a) Aminoglycosides** *(Ref: KDT 8/e p743)*
    Resistance to quinolones is due to altered DNA gyrase, to rifamycin is due to mutation in gene rpo B reducing its ability for the target and for glycopeptides like vancomycin due to reduced affinity for target site.

16. **Ans. (b) Ampicillin + tetracycline in endocardites** *(Ref: KDT 8/e p749)*

    > **Antimicrobial drugs showing synergism are:**
    > - Penicillin/ampicillin + streptomycin/gentamicin for enterococcal SABE
    > - Carbenicillin/ticarcillin + gentamicin for pseudomonas infection, specially neutropenic patients.
    > - Ceftazidime + ciprofloxacin for pseudomonas infected orthopedic prosthesis.
    > - Rifampicin + INH in tubercular infection.
    > - Flucytosine has supra additive action with amphotericin-B in cryptococcal meningitis.
    > - Sufamethoxazole + trimethoprim in UTI.

17. **Ans. (c) Conjugation** *(Ref: KDT 8/e p743)*
    Multiple drug resistance is transferred through plasmids, mostly by conjugation.

18. **Ans. (b) Transduction**
    (Ref: Goodman & Gilman 11/e p1098; KDT 8/e p743)
    - Transduction is particularly important in transfer of resistance among staphylococci.
    - Multidrug resistance is transferred by conjugation.

19. **Ans. (a) Quinolones** *(Ref: KDT 8/e p760)*
    Resistance to fluoroquinolones is mediated by mutation in DNA gyrase.

20. **Ans. (c) Transformation** *(Ref: KDT 8/e p743)*
    - Acquisition of antibiotic resistance by Transduction is common in Staphylococcal and that of by Transformation in Pneumococcus and Neisseria.
    - Vancomycin resistance in enterococci and staphylococcus is mediated by conjugative plasmid.

21. **Ans. (a) Neutropenia**
    (Ref: Robbins 7th/640; KDT 8/e p686,806)
    Bactericidal drugs kill the bacteria whereas bacteriostatic drugs only inhibits bacterial growth. Bacteriostatic activity is adequate for the treatment of most infections, **bactericidal activity may be necessary for cure in patients with altered immune systems like: neutropenias, HIV and other immunosuppressive conditions.**

22. **Ans. (d) Penicillin** *(Ref: KDT 8/e p741)*
23. **Ans. (b) Cephalosporins** *(Ref: KDT 8/e p741)*
24. **Ans. (b) Transduction**
    (Ref: Goodman & Gilman 11/e p1133)
    Beta lactamases are encoded by plasmids that can be transferred with the help of bacteriophage (transduction) in staphylococci and by transformation in Pneumococci.

25. **Ans. (d) Cotrimoxazole** *(Ref: Katzung 11/e p817)*
26. **Ans. (b) Immunocompromised host**
    (Ref: K.D. Tripathi 6/e p672)
27. **Ans. (c) Tetracycline** *(Ref: KDT 8/e p784)*
28. **Ans. (a) Vancomycin** *(Ref: KDT 8/e p741)*
29. **Ans. (b) Penicillins** *(Ref: KDT 8/e p741)*
30. **Ans. (c) Clostridium difficile** *(Ref: KDT 8/e p745)*
31. **Ans. (a) Quinolones** *(Ref: KDT 8/e p748)*
32. **Ans. (c) Post-antibiotic effect** *(Ref: KDT 8/e p748)*
33. **Ans. (d) Vancomycin** *(Ref: KDT 8/e p806)*
34. **Ans. (c) 2.4 MU single i.m.** *(Ref: KDT 8/e p813)*
35. **Ans. (c) Break drug structure** *(Ref: KDT 8th/e p768)*
    - Beta lactamases (e.g. penicillinase) break down the beta lactam ring of drugs like penicillin. Therefore, the mechanism of resistance to penicillins via beta lactamase is Breaking drug structure.
    - Altered penicillin binding proteins cause resistance to methicillin.
    - Development of efflux pumps is important method of drug resistance in tetracyclines.
    - Alteration in 50S ribosome structure produces resistance to aminoglycosides.

36. **Ans. (a) Topical mupirocin** *(Ref: KDT 8th/e p809)*
    - Anterior nares is the most common site of colonization in carrier state of MRSA.
    - **Mupirocin** (2% topical cream) is DOC for MRSA carriers. Other drug that can be used is topical Bacitracin.
    - Vancomycin is intravenous DOC for treatment of severe infections caused by MRSA.
    - Colistin (cell membrane inhibitor) is DOC for Superbug [bacteria (mostly Klebsiella) producing New Delhi Metallo-beta-lactamase].
    - Cefazolin is first generation cephalosporin.

37. **Ans. (a) Benzathine penicillin 7.2 million units in three divided doses**

Syphilis	Drug of choice	Route	Dose	Frequency	Duration
Primary	Benzathine Penicillin G	Intramuscular	2.4 MU	Single dose	Single dose
Secondary	Benzathine Penicillin G	Intramuscular	2.4 MU	Single dose	Single dose
Early latent	Benzathine Penicillin G	Intramuscular	2.4 MU	Single dose	Single dose
Late latent	Benzathine Penicillin G	Intramuscular	2.4 MU	Weekly	3 weeks
Tertiary except neurosyphilis	Benzathine Penicillin G	Intramuscular	2.4 MU	Weekly	3 weeks
Neurosyphilis	Penicillin G	Intramuscular	5 MU	6 hourly	10–14 days

38. **Ans (a) Cilastatin prevents degradation of imipenem in kidney** *(Ref: Goodman and Gilman 13th/e p1035)*
    - Imipenem is rapidly inactivated by renal dehydropeptidase I, so it is combined with cilastatin, an inhibitor of this enzyme.
    - Cilastatin *increases the half life* of imipenem and also *inhibits the formation of nephrotoxic metabolite*.
    - *Meropenem, doripenem and ertapenem* are *not metabolized by renal dehydropeptidase*

39. **Ans. (a) Imipenem** *(Ref: Goodman and Gilman 13th/e p1035)*

    Carbapenems
    - These include *imipenem, doripenem, meropenem and ertapenem*.
    - These have *wide spectrum* of activity including gram positive cocci, gram negative rods as well as anaerobes.
    - For the treatment of pseudomonas (meropenem is most active whereas ertapenem is least) infections, these drugs should be combined with aminoglycosides.
    - Carbapenems are β-lactamase resistant and are *drugs of choice for Enterobacter, Klebsiella and acinetobacter species*.
    - These are the only β-lactams which are reliably efficacious against ESBL (extended spectrum β-lactamase) producing organisms and are thus drug of choice for ESBL- producing bacteria.
    - Main adverse effects of imipenem-cilastatin combination include seizures.
    - *Meropenem, doripenem and ertapenem* are *less likely to cause seizures*.
    - Ertapenem is very long acting and is inactive against Pseudomonas.

40. **Ans. (a) Beta lactam plus beta lactamase inhibitor** *(Ref: Harrison 19th/e p933)*
    ESBL is resistant to most of the beta lactam antibiotics except carbapenems. However, beta lactamase inhibitors can inhibit its activity. Piperacillin-tazobactam combination can be used for ESBL producing bacteria.

41. **Ans. (c) Vancomycin** *(Ref: KDT's 8/e p806)*

42. **Ans. (a) A** *(Ref: Goodman Gilman 12th/e p1478; Katzung 12th/e p791; KDT 8th/e p766)*
    Beta lactamase inhibitors work on beta lactam ring between N and C = O. All other options given are the sites at the other ring.

43. **Ans. (d) Cefotaxime is more active against beta-lactamase producing strains** *(Ref: Harrison 19th/e p1011)*
    - Cefotaxime is injectable 3rd generation dcephalosporin whereas ampicillin is oral penicillin. therefore, ampicillin must be having higher oral bioavailability as compared to cefotaxime.
    - All beta lactams (including cefotaxime and ampicillin) are bactericidal drugs
    - Resistance to most strains of H influenza occurs due to production of beta lactamases. Therefore ampicillin (whih was drug of choice earlier) is not effective in many patients. Now, a third generation cephalosporin like cefotaxime or amoxicillin-clavulanic acid combination is preferred among beta lactams. Another highly effective drug for H. influenza is azithromycin.

44. **Ans. (a) It is a 4th generation cephalosporin.** *(Ref: Goodman Gilman 12th/e p1498, KDT 8/e p779)*
    - Cefepime is 4th generation cephalosporin with good activity against Pseudomonas
    - It is given 8-12 hourly

45. **Ans. (c) Rickettsial infections** *(Ref: GG-1484-1485)*

46. **Ans. (a) MRSA** *(Ref: GG 1479)*
    Methicillin resistance occurs due to altered penicillin binding proteins, there fore cannot be reversed by β-lactamase inhibitor like clavulanic acid

47. **Ans. (d) It is rapidly excreted by kidneys** *(Ref: GG 1497)*
    - Cefuroxime has good CSF penetration. It can be used for meningitis, however ceftriaxone is superior
    - Cefuroxime is not effective against anaerobes

48. **Ans. (b) Penicillin G** *(Ref: GG 1477, KDT 8/e p768)*
    Penicillin G is natural penicillin, all other are semi-synthetic.

49. **Ans. (a) Resistance is plasmid-mediated** *(Ref: GG 1541, KDT 8/e p806)*

50. **Ans. (d) Ceftobiprole** *(Ref: Harrison 18th/e p1247-1248, KDT 8/e p780)*
    Fifth generation cephalosporins (ceftobiprole and ceftaroline) are the only beta-lactams active against MRSA.

51. **Ans. (c) It can be used for rat bite fever** *(Ref: KDT 8th/e p768-770)*

    Penicillin G
    - It is acid labile, thus not effective orally.
    - Penicillin G has short duration of action. Probenecid inhibits tubular secretion and prolongs its duration of action.
    - It has narrow antibacterial spectrum, mainly for gram positive bacteria.

Chemotherapy A: General Considerations and Non-specific Antimicrobial Agents

- Penicillin G is drug of choice for infections caused by Treponema like syphilis (*T. pallidum*) and Rat bite fever (*Spirillum minus*).

52. Ans. (b) Piperacillin-tazobactam *(Ref: KDT 8th/e p774)*

53. Ans. (c) Piperacillin-Tazobactam
(Ref: Harrison 18th/e p1247)

- Organisms producing ESBL-like Klebsiella are resistant to most beta-lactams except carbapenems.
- ESBL can be inhibited by beta lactamase inhibitors.
- Amoxicillin is not effective against Klebsiella whereas piperacillin has wide spectrum including Klesiella.

54. Ans. (c) It can be used for the treatment of rat bite fever
(Ref: H-18/e p24, 3, Katzung 10/e p726-731: KDT 8/e p770)
- It is **not effective orall**y because of breakdown by acid in the stomach.
- It has **short duration of action** due to its rapid excretion from kidney through tubular secretion. Probenecid decreases its tubular secretion, thus can be used **to prolong its action**.
- It has **narrow spectrum** of activity covering mainly gram positive bacteria.
- It is drug of choice for rat bite fever

55. Ans. (a) Aztreonam *(Ref: KDT 8/e p781)*
Aztreonam is the only beta lactam antibiotic that can be used in patients having severe allergy to penicillins or cephalosporins (as it is not cross allergenic).

56. Ans. (d) Carbapenems *(Ref: Katzung 10/e p739)*
Carbapenems like imipenem are the only beta lactams reliably efficacious against ESBL producing bacteria.

57. Ans. (d) Given twice daily orally *(Ref: KDT 8/e p779)*
- Cefepime is a a 4th generation cephalosporin.
- Due to high potency and extended spectrum, it is effective in many serious infections like hospital acquired pneumonia, febrile neutropenia, bacteremia, septicemia etc.
- All β-lactam antibiotics act by inhibiting the enzyme transpeptidase.
- Cefepime is given by i.v. route as it is not effctive orally.

58. Ans. (a) Cephalexin
(Ref: KDT 8/e p773,774,776; Goodman & Gilman 10/e p1209)
Cephalexin is an orally effective first generation cephalosporin active against gram positive but not against gram negative organisms like pseudomonas.

59. Ans. (a) Imipenem *(Ref: KDT 8/e p782)*

60. Ans. (c) Ceftazidime *(Ref: KDT 8/e p778)*

61. Ans. (b) Benzathine penicillin is short-acting penicillin
(Ref: KDT 8/e p770)
Benzathine penicillin is the longest acting penicillin.

62. Ans. (a) Inhibition of cell wall synthesis
(Ref: KDT 8/e p806)

63. Ans. (a) Is effective in pseudomonas infection
(Ref: KDT 8/e p773)
- Carbenicillin is a penicillin congener effective against pseudomonas and indole positive proteus which are not inhibited by penicillin G or ampicillin/amoxicillin.
- It is inactive orally and excreted rapidly in urine. It is sensitive to penicillinase and acid, so administered parenterally as sodium salt.

64. Ans. (b) Clavulanic acid *(Ref: KDT 8/e p774)*

65. Ans. (b) Third-generation cephalosporin
(Ref: KDT 8/e p774)

66. Ans. (a) Better bioavailability if taken with food
(Ref: KDT 8/e p773)

67. Ans. (a) Cell wall synthesis *(Ref: Katzung 11/e p775)*

68. Ans. (d) Treponema *(Ref: KDT 8/e p770)*

69. Ans. (d) IIIrd generation long-acting cephalosporin
(Ref: KDT 8/e p778)

70. Ans. (a) Methicillin *(Ref: KDT 8/e p771)*

71. Ans. (d) Cefaclor *(Ref: KDT 8/e p776)*

72. Ans. (d) Azithromycin *(Ref: KDT 8/e p804)*

73. Ans. (c) Cefaclor *(Ref: KDT 8/e p777)*

74. Ans. (a) Cefixime *(Ref: KDT 8/e p778)*

75. Ans. (b) Skin rash *(Ref: KDT 8/e p773)*

76. Ans. (c) Piperacillin *(Ref: KDT 8/e p774,775)*

77. Ans. (c) Cefaclor *(Ref: KDT 8/e p777)*

78. Ans. (a) Cell wall synthesis *(Ref: KDT 8/e p767)*

79. Ans. (c) Cefepime *(Ref : KDT 8/e p779)*

80. Ans. (a) Nafcillin *(Ref: KDT 8/e p772-773)*

81. Ans. (c) Cefoxitin *(Ref: KDT 8/e p776)*

82. Ans. (d) In renal dysfunction, dosage reduction is necessary to avoid seizures *(Ref: KDT 8/e p708,709)*

83. Ans. (b) Cefpirome *(Ref: K.D. Tripathi 8/e p776)*

84. Ans. (d) Carbenicillin *(Ref: KDT 8th/e p771)*

85. Ans. (a) Listeria *(Ref: KDT 8th/e p772)*

86. Ans. (a) Vancomycin *(Ref: KDT 8th/e p806)*

87. Ans. (c) Moxalactam *(Ref: CMDT 2015/547)*

88. Ans. (c) It should be used with cilastatin *(Ref: KDT 8/e p782)*

89. Ans. (b) Carbenicillin *(Ref: KDT 8/e p771)*

90. Ans. (c) Cefuroxime *(Ref: KDT 8/e p776)*

91. Ans. (b) Linezolid *(Ref: KDT 8/e p767)*

92. Ans. (b) Ceftriaxone *(Ref: KDT 8/e p774,778)*

93. Ans. (d) Aztreonam *(Ref: KDT 8/e p781)*

94. Ans. (c) Are safe in pregnancy *(Ref: KDT 8/e 746)*

95. Ans. (a) Injection Benzathine pencillin 2.4 million units IM single dose *(Ref: CMDT 2014/ p1258)*

96. Ans. (b) Pseudomembranous colitis *(Ref: KDT 8/e p806)*

97. Ans. (c) Piperacillin *(Ref: KDT 8/e p774)*

98. Ans. (c) Cefpirome *(Ref: KDT 8/e p776)*

99. Ans. (d) Vancomycin *(Ref: KDT 8/e p766,778)*

100. Ans. (a) 95% oral bioavailability *(Ref: KDT 8/e p806)*

101. Ans. (b) oral (Ref: KDT 8/e p806)

102. Ans. (b) Gentamicin (Ref: KDT 8/e p797)

103. Ans. (b) Active against only gram negative bacteria (Ref: KDT 8/e p775,778)

104. Ans. (a) Methicillin (Ref: KDT 8/e p771)

105. Ans. (b) It is active against gram positive organisms (Ref: KDT 8th/e p808)

    Tedizolide is a drug similar to linezolide.
    - Tedizolide is a protein synthesis inhibitor. It binds to 50S ribosome and inhibits the protein synthesis.
    - It is mainly used for gram positive organisms e.g. vancomycin resistant Staphylococcus aureus (VRSA).
    - Peripheral neuropathy and lactic acidosis are the adverse effects of tedizolide but these are not very common.
    - Tedizolide has very good oral bioavailability (nearly 90%).
    - It is mainly metabolised in the liver.

106. Ans (a) Erythromycin (Ref: Katzung 13th/e p884)

    Antimicrobials of choice for prophylaxis

Cholera	Tetracycline
Rheumatic fever:	Benzathine penicillin
Tuberculosis:	Isoniazid alone or with rifampicin
Meningococcal meningitis:	Ciprofloxacin
Malaria:	Mefloquine/Doxycycline
Influenza A and B	*Osetamivir*
Surgical prophylaxis:	Cefazolin
Anthrax	Ciprofloxacin/Doxycycline
Diphtheria	Erythromycin
Endocarditis	Amoxycillin/Clindamycin
Herpes Simplex	Acyclovir
Group B streptococcal infection	Ampicillin
Hemophilus influenza type B	Rifampicin
Mycobacterium avium complex (MAC)	Azithromycin/Clarithromycin/Rifabutin
Otitis media	Amoxicillin
Pertussis	Azithromycin
Plague	Tetracycline
Pneumocystis jiroveci	Cotrimoxazole/Dapsone/Atovaquone
Toxoplasmosis	Cotrimoxazole
Urinary tract infections	Cotrimoxazole

107. Ans. (b) It does not require dose adjustment in renal failure (Ref: KDT 8th/e p789)
    - Tigecycline is a glycylcycline which has same mechanism of action like tetracyclines and is thus bacteriostatic.
    - Unlike tetracyclines, it is resistant to efflux pumps.
    - It has broad spectrum of activity against most of the gram positive and gram negative cocci as well as anaerobes.
    - However of most of the Pseudomonas and proteus are resistant.
    - It is mainly secreted in bile, thus does not require dose adjustment in renal failure.

108. Ans. (d) Inhibits binding of amino acyl t-RNA to A site (Ref: KDT's 8/e p784)

109. Ans. (b) Binds to 50S ribosome and inhibits t-RNAfMet initiation complex (Ref: KDT's 8/e p807)

110. Ans. (a) Direct hair cell toxicity (Ref: Goodman and Gilman 12/e p1513, CMDT 2012/87-88)

    Aminoglycosides can lead to ototoxicity, nephrotoxicity and neuromuscular blockade.

    - **Ototoxicity** involves progressive and irreversible damage to, and eventually **destruction of, the sensory cells in the cochlea and vestibular organ of the ear.**
    - **Nephrotoxicity** consists of damage to the **proximal tubules,** and is **reversible.**
    - A rare but serious toxic reaction is paralysis caused by **neuromuscular blockade.** This is usually seen only if the agents are given concurrently with neuromuscular-blocking agents. It results from **inhibition of the Ca^{2+} uptake necessary for the exocytotic release of acetylcholine.**

111. Ans. (c) Puromycin (Ref: Harper's 27/e p378)

    Puromycin structurally resembles aminoacyl t-RNA and inhibits protein synthesis by causing premature termination. Tetracyclines inhibits the binding of aminoacyl-tRNA to the A site.

112. Ans. (d) Streptomycin (Ref: KDT 8/e p793)

113. Ans. (a) Trichomonas (Ref: KDT 8/e p788-789)

114. Ans. (a) Erythromycin (Ref: KDT 8/e p801)

115. Ans. (a) 50S ribosome (Ref: KDT 8/e p790)

116. Ans. (d) Topical in open wound (Ref: KDT 8/e p791)

117. Ans. (d) Azithromycin (Ref: KDT 8/e p793)

118. Ans. (d) Neomycin (Ref: KDT 8/e p800)

119. Ans. (d) Amikacin (Ref: KDT 8/e p799)

120. Ans. (a) Translocation of 50S ribosome (Ref: KDT 8/e p801)

121. Ans. (c) Post-antibiotic effect (Ref: Katzung 11/e p809)

122. Ans. (b) VRSA (Ref: KDT 8/e p808)

123. Ans. (d) All of the above (Ref: KDT 8/e p788-789)
    - Doxycycline is drug of choice for rickestssial infections including Q fever and for borrelliosis.
    - It can also be used for leptospirosis for which the drug of choice is penicillin G

124. Ans. (b) Clindamycin (Ref: GG 1535-1536)

125. Ans. (c) Telithromycin (Ref: GG 1529)

126. Ans. (a) E. coli (Ref: GG 1536)

    Streptogramins are effective only against gram positve bacteria

127. Ans. (b) Gentamicin (Ref: GG 1515, KDT 8/e p797)

128. Ans. (d) Campylobacter jejuni (Ref: GG 1533, KDT 8/e p803)

129. Ans. (a) Outer hair cells and base of cochlea (Ref: GG 1512, KDT 8/e p795)

130. Ans. (b) Pefloxacin (Ref: KDT 8th/e p763)

Chemotherapy A: General Considerations and Non-specific Antimicrobial Agents

- Pefloxacin is avoided in liver disease, but is safe in renal insufficiency.
- FQs are contraindicated in renal failure except
  - P: Pefloxacin
  - M: Moxifloxacin
  - T: Trovafloxacin

131. Ans (a) Levofloxacin *(Ref: Goodman and Gilman 13th/e p1016)*
Pharmacokinetics of fluoroquinolones
- These have *good oral bioavailability* (except norfloxacin) but like tetracycline multivalent cations interfere with absorption.
- **Norfloxacin** has *minimum oral bioavailability* whereas **levofloxacin** has *maximum*.
- **Excretion** of *moxifloxacin and trovafloxacin* is by *hepatic* metabolism and biliary excretion. *Sparfloxacin* and *pefloxacin* are excreted by *both* renal and hepatic route. All *other drugs* (ciprofloxacin, gatifloxacin, levofloxacin, lomefloxacin, norfloxacin and ofloxacin) are excreted by *tubular secretion in the kidneys*. Probenecid inhibits tubular secretion of these drugs. *Dose adjustment is required in renal disease for all fluoroquinolones except pefloxacin, moxifloxacin and trovafloxacin* (remembered as PMT).
- *Sparfloxacin, moxifloxacin and trovafloxacin* have **long half-lives** and can be administered once daily. **Sparfloxacin** (followed by moxifloxacin) has *longest* half-life among fluoroquinolones.

132. Ans. (d) Moxifloxacin *(Ref: KK Sharma 2/e p709-712)*
Among the given options, the drug with longest half life is moxifloxacin (around 12 hours) but overall longest acting is sparfloxacin (20 hours)

133. Ans. (a) Ciprofloxacin inhibits theophylline metabolism *(Ref: KDT 8/e p761)*

Theophylline has a narrow margin of safety (low therapeutic index) Ciprofloxacin inhibits theophylline metabolism and increases its plasma level leading to toxicity. Thus, ciprofloxacin should not be given to an asthma*tic using theophylline.*

134. Ans. (b) Inhibits DNA gyrase *(Ref: KDT 8/e p760)*
135. Ans. (a) Sulfacetamide *(Ref: KDT 8/e p757)*
136. Ans. (d) Pefloxacin *(Ref: KDT 8/e p763)*
137. Ans. (b) Inhibiting DNA gyrase *(Ref: KDT 8/e p760)*
138. Ans. (b) Sulfadoxine *(Ref: KDT 8th/e p756)*
139. Ans. (d) More active at acidic pH *(Ref: KDT 8th/e 761)*
140. Ans. (c) Competitive inhibition *(Ref: KDT 8/e p756)*
141. Ans. (d) Sprafloxacin *(Ref: KDT 8/e p764)*
142. Ans. (a) Norfloxacin *(Ref: GG 1472, KDT 8/e p763)*
Norfloxacin has minimum whereas levofloxacin has maximum oral bioavailability

143. Ans. (a) Dicloxacillin *(Ref: Harrison 19th/e p349)*
Impetigo is caused by streptococcus.

144. Ans. (d) Moxifloxacin *(Ref: Katzung 12th/e p836)*
Sparfloxacin is longest acting followed by moxifloxacin

145. Ans. (d) Mupirocin *(Ref: Harrison 19th/e p166)*

146. Ans. (c) A is true and R is false *(Ref: Katzung 13th/e p878)*
- In patients admitted in hospital for community acquired pneumonia, combination therapy of beta lactams and azithromycin is given. Beta lactams covers the gram positive and gram negative organisms whereas azithromycin covers the atypical mycobacteria like mycoplasma and chlamydia.
- Alternative to this therapy is fluoroquinolones.
- If a patient is not admitted, then either beta lactams alone or macrolides is prescribed.

147. Ans. (a) Aminopenicillins *(Ref: KDT 8th/e p744)*
- Clostridium difficile diarrhea is a super-infection also called as Pseudomembranous colitis.
- Most common cause is 3rd generation Cephalosporins
- Other causes include Clindamycin followed by Aminopenicillins (Ampicillin and Amoxycillin), and then Fluoroquinolones.
- DOC for treatment of PMC is oral Vancomycin now.
- Stool transplant can also be done.
- MAB against toxin of C.difficile: Bezlotoxumab.

148. Ans. (a) Cotrimoxazole *(Ref: KDT 8th/e p758)*
- Cotrimoxazole is combination of sulfamethoxazole with trimethoprim.
- Sulfonamides can displace bilirubin from plasma protein binding sites and may result in unconjugated hyperbilirubinemia and *kernicterus in the new born* (if given in third trimester of pregnancy).

149. Ans. (a) Doxycycline *(Ref: KDT 8th/e p788)*
- Scrub typhus is caused by Ricketssia.
- Drug of choice for all ricketssial infections is doxycycline.

150. Ans. (c) Azithromycin *(Ref: Harrison 20th/e p913)*
Drug of choice for community acquired pneumonia in outpatient setting in previously healthy person and no antibiotics taken in past 3 months is a macrolide (clarithromycin or azithromycin) or doxycycline.

151. Ans. (a) Erythromycin *(Ref: Katzung 13th/e p884)*
Antimicrobials of choice for prophylaxis

Cholera	Tetracycline
Rheumatic fever	Benzathine penicillin
Tuberculosis	Isoniazid alone or with rifampicin
Meningococcal meningitis	Ciprofloxacin
Malaria	Mefloquine/Doxycycline
Influenza A and B	Osetamivir
Surgical prophylaxis	Cefazolin
Anthrax	Ciprofloxacin/Doxycycline
Diphtheria	Erythromycin
Endocarditis	Amoxycillin/Clindamycin
Herpes Simplex	Acyclovir
Group B streptococcal infection	Ampicillin
Haemophilus influenza type B	Rifampicin
Mycobacterium avium complex (MAC)	Azithromycin/Clarithromycin/Rifabutin
Otitis media	Amoxicillin
Pertussis	Azithromycin
Plague	Tetracycline
Pneumocystis jiroveci	Cotrimoxazole/Dapsone/Atovaquone
Toxoplasmosis	Cotrimoxazole
Urinary tract infections	Cotrimoxazole

152. **Ans (a) Cloxacillin** *(Ref: Harrison 20th/e p1074)*
    - Frequent cause of mastitis is Staphylococcus aureus which may be penicillinase producing.
    - Therefore, penicillinase resistant penicillins like cloxacillin are preferred for treatment of mastitis.

153. **Ans. (b) Polymyxin B** *(Ref: Goodman and Gilman 13th edition/1058, Harrison 19th/1048)*
    First line drugs for *Burkholderia cepacia* are cotrimoxazole, meropenem and doxycycline. Some strains are susceptible to third generation cephalosporins and fluoroquinolones too. Burkholderia species are resistant to polymyxin B.

154. **Ans. (d) Ceftriaxone 250 mg i/m single dose + Azithromycin 1g oral** *(Ref: Harrison's 19/e p1009; KDT's 8/e p781)*

155. **Ans. (c) Ofloxacin** *(Ref: KDT's 8/e p761)*

156. **Ans. (c) Doxycycline** *(Ref: Goodman and Gilman 13/e p1051)*
    Tetracyclines are drug of choice for rickettsial infections including scrub typhus.

157. **Ans. (d) Azithromycin 2 g oral single dose** *(Ref: Harrison 19/e p1171)*
    Azithromycin is effective against both gonococcal and non-gonococcal (chlamydial) urethritis. Single dose is used for treatment of urethritis.

158. **Ans (a) Cotrimoxazole** *(Ref: Harrison 19/e p1361)*

    Cotrimoxazole is drug of choice for
    - Pneumocystis jiroveci
    - Nocardia
    - Burkholderia cepacia

159. **Ans. (a) Cotrimoxazole** *(Ref: Harrison 19/e p1048)*
    Cotrimoxazole, meropenem and doxycycline are the most effective agents for B. cepacia.
    Some strains are susceptible to third-generation cephalosporins and fluoroquinolones.

160. **Ans. (a) Ceftriaxone** *(Ref: Harrison 19/e p767)*
    Drug of choice for treatment of meningococcal meningitis is Penicillin G. But for empirical treatment we need to cover other likely organisms too. So, ceftriaxone is preferred that will also cover H. influenzae. Vancomycin is usually added to cover other organisms also.

161. **Ans. (a) Oral vancomycin** *(Ref: CMDT 2019/661)*
    According to new guidelines, oral vancomycin is drug of choice for pseudomembranous colitis

162. **Ans. (c) Ceftriaxone** *(Ref: Harrison 18th/e p3414, KDT 8/e p778)*
    Erythromycin and sulfamethoxazole are bacteriostatic drugs and cannot be relied upon in serious infections like bacterial meningitis. Streptomycin is an aminoglycoside effective mainly against gram negative bacteria but is not preferred for meningitis due to following reasons:

    - It cannot kill gram positive organisms responsible for bacterial meningitis like *Streptococcus, Staphylococcus and Listeria*, etc.
    - To prevent the emergence of drug resistance; as it is first line antitubercular drug.

163. **Ans. (c) Clindamycin** *(Ref: Harrison 18/e p1013-1014)*

Important points regarding pseudomembranous colitis (PMC):
- Most common organism implicated: Clostridium difficile
- Most common antimicrobial implicated: Cephalosporins > Clindamycin
- Drug of choice for treatment: Vancomycin

164. **Ans. (d) Cefotaxime + vancomycin** *(Ref: Harrison 18/e p3414)*

Antibiotics Used in Empirical Therapy of Bacterial Meningitis and Focal CNS Infections

Indication	Antibiotic
Infants <3 months	Ampicillin + Cefotaxime
3 months to 55 years	Cefotaxime (Ceftriaxone) + Vancomycin
Adults >55 years	Ampicillin + Cefotaxime (Ceftriaxone) + Vancomycin
Hospital-acquired meningitis, post-traumatic or post-neurosurgery meningitis, neutropenic patients, or patients with impaired cell-mediated immunity	Vancomycin + Cefepime

165. **Ans. (b) Cefaclor** *(Ref: KK Sharma 2/e p727)*
    Cefaclor is a second generation cephalosporin and is not active against MRSA. Resistance in MRSA occurs due to altered PBPs (transpeptidase). As the binding site is altered, therefore, no beta lactam can bind and thus all beta-lactams (penicillins, cephalosporins, carbapenems and monobactams) are ineffective against MRSA. However, recently fifth generation cephalosporins like ceftaroline and ceftobiprol have been formed, which are effective against MRSA.

166. **Ans. (a) Penicillin** *(Ref: CMDT 2012/1433, KDT 8/e p770)*
    The only acceptable treatment for syphilis in pregnancy is penicillin in dosage schedules appropriate for the stage of the disease.

Recommended treatment of Syphilis

Stage of syphilis	Treatment
Primary, secondary, or early latent	Benzathine penicillin G 2.4 million units IM once
Late	
Late latent or uncertain duration	Benzathine penicillin G 2.4 million units IM weekly for 3 weeks
Tertiary without neurosyphilis	Benzathine penicillin G 2.4 million units IM weekly for 3 weeks
Neurosyphilis	Aqueous penicillin G 18-24 million units IV daily, given every 3-4 hours or as continuous infusion for 10-14 days

167. **Ans. (b) Metronidazole** *(Ref CMDT 2010, 574, KDT 8/e p896)*
    Metronidazole is *used for pseudomembranous colitis*. However, Vancomycin is now the drug of choice.

168. **Ans. (a) Ampicillin** *(Ref: Harrison 17/e p942)*
    - K. pneumoniae and K. oxytoca are intrinsically resistant to ampicillin and ticarcillin.

Chemotherapy A: General Considerations and Non-specific Antimicrobial Agents

- Empirical treatment of serious or health care–associated Klebsiella infections should be done with amikacin, carbapenems, or tigecycline.
- Polymyxin B can be considered for use against highly resistant strains but is an agent of last resort because of its potential toxicities.

169. **Ans. (c) Colistin** *(Ref: Katzung 10/e p1194; KDT 8/e p809)*
   - Polypeptides like colistin and polymyxin B are effective against pseudomonas.
   - Carbenicillin, ticarcillin, piperacillin, azlocillin and mezlocillin are the penicillins effective against pseudomonas whereas cefoperazone, ceftazidime, cefepime and cefpirome are cephalosporins effective against pseudomonas.

170. **Ans. (d) Glycopeptides** *(Ref: CMDT-2008, 1232; KDT 8/e p806)*
   Vancomycin is a glycopeptide and is drug of choice for MRSA. Remember, no beta lactam is effective against MRSA.

171. **Ans. (d) Carbapenem** *(Ref: CMDT-2008, p1232; KDT 8/e p768)*
   MRSA do not respond to any beta lactam antibiotic (penicillins, cephalosporins, carbapenems and monobactams) because it has altered penicillin binding sites.

172. **Ans. (b) Sulfonamide** *(Ref: Harrison 17/e p346, KDT 8/e p757)*
   Sulfonamides are frequent cause of fixed drug eruptions.

173. **Ans. (c) Vancomycin** *(Ref: KDT 8/e p806)*

174. **Ans. (d) Ethambutol** *(Ref: KDT 8/e p820)*
   Aminoglycosides, Amphotericin B, cephalosporins, vancomycin, flucytosine and ethambutol require dose reduction even in mild renal failure.

175. **Ans. (c) Ciprofloxacin** *(Ref: KDT 8/e p761)*

176. **Ans. (b) Chloramphenicol**
   (Ref: KDT 8/e p791; Satoskar Bhandarkar, 19/e p694)

177. **Ans. (c) Pentamidine**
   (Ref: Robbins 7/e p640; KDT 6/e p686,806)
   - All of the options mentioned can cause folic acid deficiency resulting in megaloblastic anemia but pentamidine rarely causes this side effect.

   > - Drugs causing macrocytic anaemia are:
   >   – Co-trimoxazole
   >   – Folate anagonists like trimethoprim, pyrimethamine, methotrexate etc.
   >   – Nitrous oxide after repeated or prolonged exposure.
   >   – Oral contraceptives
   >   – Phenobarbital, phenytoin
   >   – Primidone
   >   – Triamterene

178. **Ans. (c) Clindamycin** *(Ref: KDT 8/e p805)*
   Among the given options, the answer is clindamycin but presently, IIIrd generation cephalosporris are the most common cause of pseudomembranous colitis.

179. **Ans. (c) Ampicillin** *(Ref: KDT 8/e p772)*
   Aminoglycosides (tobramycin, gentamicin, kanamycin), vancomycin and amphotericin B are highly nephrotoxic agents.

180. **Ans. (c) Erythromycin** *(Ref: KDT 8/e p802)*
   Erythromycin is secreted in bile and does not require dose adjustment in renal failure.

181. **Ans. (b) Penicillin** *(Ref: KDT 8/e p770)*

182. **Ans. (b) Aminoglycosides** *(Ref: KDT 8/e p795)*

183. **Ans. (a) Gentamicin** *(Ref: KDT 8/e p795)*
   Gentamicin is an aminoglycoside. All aminoglycosides can cause nephrotoxicity.

184. **Ans. (c) Pyrimethamine** *(Ref: KDT 8/e p884)*
   - INH causes B_6 deficiency resulting in sideroblastic anemia
   - Chloramphenicol causes aplastic anemia.
   - Pyrimethamine causes megaloblastic anemia.
   - Methyldopa causes auto immune hemolytic anemia (warm)

185. **Ans. (d) None** *(Ref: KDT 8/e p746)*

186. **Ans. (b) Penicillins**
   (Ref: CMDT 2010/1341-1342, KDT 8/e p770)

187. **Ans. (d) Oxacillin** *(Ref: Katzung 11/e p780)*

188. **Ans. (b) Chloramphenicol**
   (Ref: Katzung 11/e p803, KDT 8/e p791)

189. **Ans. (b) Ampicillin** *(Ref: KDT 8/e p746)*

190. **Ans. (b) Inj. Benzathine Penicillin** *(Ref: KDT 8/e p770)*

191. **Ans. (b) Tetracyclines** *(Ref: KDT 8/e p788)*

192. **Ans. (b) Chloramphenicol** *(Ref: KDT 8/e p790)*

193. **Ans. (d) Rifampicin** *(Ref: KDT 8/e p819)*

194. **Ans. (b) Doxycycline** *(Ref: KDT 8th/e p784)*

195. **Ans. (c) Both** *(Ref: KDT 8/e p806-807)*

196. **Ans. (c) Erythromycin** *(Ref: KDT 8/e p803)*

197. **Ans. (b) Gentamicin** *(Ref: KDT 8/e p797)*

198. **Ans. (d) Erythromycin** *(Ref: KDT 8/e p803)*

199. **Ans. (b) Ampicillin** *(Ref: KDT 8/e p745)*

200. **Ans. (b) Benzathine penicillin** *(Ref: KDT 8/e p770)*

201. **Ans. (c) Benzathine penicillin** *(Ref: KDT 8/e p770)*

202. **Ans. (d) INH** *(Ref: Harrison 15/e p432)*

203. **Ans. (d) Primaquine** *(Ref: KDT 8/e p885)*

204. **Ans. (c) Griseofulvin** *(Ref: KDT 8/e p842)*

205. **Ans. (a) Erythromycin** *(Ref: KDT 8/e p802)*

206. **Ans. (b) Cefuroxime** *(Ref: KDT 8/e p909)*

207. **Ans. (c) Azithromycin** *(Ref: KDT 8/e p804)*

208. **Ans. (d) Crystalline penicillin (Pen. G)**
   (Ref: Katzung 11/e p798)

209. **Ans. (a) Crystalline penicillin (Pen. G)**
   (Ref: Katzung 11/e p778)

210. **Ans. (b) Polymixin B** *(Ref: KDT 8th/e p809)*

211. **Ans. (b) Penicillin G** *(Ref: KDT 6th/e p768)*

212. **Ans. (a) Vancomycin** *(Ref: KDT 8th/e p806)*

213. **Ans. (c) Azithromycin** *(Ref: KDT 8th/e p804)*

214. **Ans. (b) Amikacin** *(Ref: KDT 8th/e p799)*

215. Ans. (a) Vancomycin (Ref: KDT 8th/e p762,781,809)
216. Ans. (a) Tetracycline (Ref: KDT 8th/e p788)
217. Ans. (a) Penicillin (Ref: KDT 8th/e p813)
218. Ans. (a) Tetracycline (Ref: KDT 8/e p784)
219. Ans. (b) Erythromycin (Ref: Internet)
220. Ans. (b) Doxycycline (Ref: KDT 8/e p787)
221. Ans. (b) Benzathine Penicillin (Ref: KDT 8/e p813)
222. Ans. (a) Penicillin G (Ref: KDT 8/e p813)
223. Ans. (b) Penicillin (Ref: KDT 8/e p770)
224. Ans. (b) Vancomycin (Ref: KDT 8/e p806)
225. Ans. (c) Clindamycin (Ref: KDT 8/e p762)
226. Ans. (c) Tetracycline
 (Ref: CMDT 2014/ p1415, KDT 8/e p788)
227. Ans. (b) Azithromycin (Ref: KDT 8/e p804)
228. Ans. (c) Azithromycin
 (Ref: CMDT 2014/ p162, KDT 8/e p804)
229. Ans. (a) Vancomycin (Ref: CMDT 2014/ p467, 1257)
230. Ans. (b) Vancomycin (Ref: KDT 8/e p806)
231. Ans. (a) Ethambutol (Ref: KDT 8/e p820)
232. Ans. (a) Quinolones (Ref: KDT 8/e p746)
233. Ans. (a) Gentamicin (Ref: KDT 8/e p796)
234. Ans. (c) Benzathine penicillin (Ref: KDT 8/e p770)
235. Ans. (b) 30 minutes before incision (Ref: KDT 8/e p753)
236. Ans. (d) Doxycycline (Ref: KDT 8/e p787)
237. Ans. (b) Cotrimoxazole (Ref: KDT 8/e p759)
238. Ans. (b) Methicillin (Ref: KDT 8/e p771)
239. Ans. (c) Gentamicin (Ref: KDT 8/e p797)
240. Ans. (a) Chloramphenicol (Ref: KDT 8/e p791)
241. Ans. (c) 3 mg/mL (Ref: KDT 8/e p799)
242. Ans. (c) Tetracycline (Ref: KDT 8/e p788)
243. Ans. (d) Penicillin (Ref: Harrison 15/e p432)
244. Ans. (c) Spectinomycin
 (Ref: Katzung 11/e p813, KDT 8/e p808)

CHAPTER 13
Chemotherapy B: Antimicrobials for Specific Conditions

ANTI-MYCOBACTERIAL ANTIBIOTICS

Mycobacterium causes tuberculosis and leprosy. Several atypical mycobacteria may also cause infection in humans especially in the immunocompromised patients.

TUBERCULOSIS

It is caused by *Mycobacterium tuberculosis*. The drugs used for tuberculosis are:

First line		Second line	
Essential	**Supplementary**	Thioacetazone	
Isoniazid (H)	Streptomycin (S)	PAS	Ofloxacin
Rifampicin (R)	Rifabutin	Ethionamide	Levofloxacin
Pyrazinamide (Z)	Rifapentine	Cycloserine	Moxifloxacin
Ethambutol (E)		Kanamycin	Linezolid
		Capreomycin	Clarithromycin
		Amikacin	

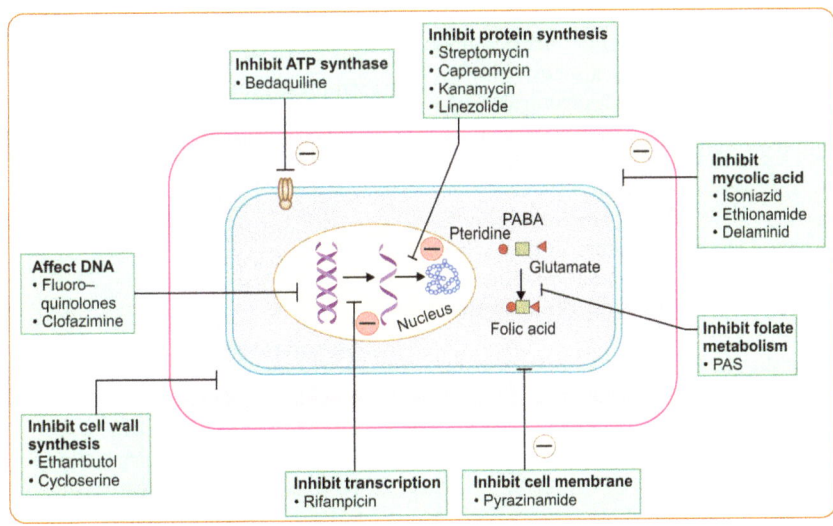

FIG. 13.1: Mechanism of action of anti-tubercular drugs

Isoniazid (H)

- It is a **prodrug** activated by **catalase-peroxidase** (coded by *KatG*). Active metabolite *inhibits* the enzyme *ketoenoylreductase* (coded by *inh A*), required for *mycolic acid synthesis*, an essential component of mycobacterial cell wall. It acts by O_2 dependent pathway such as catalase peroxidase reaction.
- It is *bacteriostatic against resting* and *bactericidal against rapidly multiplying organisms*.
- It is effective against *intra- as well as extra-cellular* mycobacteria.
- Action is most marked against rapidly multiplying bacilli (*less effective against slow multipliers*).
- It is widely distributed in the body and has **maximum CSF penetration**.
- It is effective orally and metabolized by *ACETYLATION* which is *genetically controlled*. Fast acetylators require high dose and slow acetylators are predisposed to toxicity (particularly peripheral neuritis).
- It is an essential component of multi-drug therapy of tuberculosis and is drug of choice **(used solely) for prophylaxis of tuberculosis** and for treatment of latent tuberculosis infection.
- Resistance occurs due to mutation in Kat G (gene for catalase-peroxidase) or inhA. Mutation in Kat G is responsible for high level resistance whereas mutation in inhA confers cross resistance to ethionamide.
- It causes **peripheral neuritis** that can be *prevented and treated by pyridoxine*.
- It is also **hepatotoxic** and can cause *hemolysis in G-6 PD deficient patients*. Incidence of hepatotoxicity increases with age, daily alcohol consumption and in post partum (3 months) period.
- Isoniazid also *inhibits MAO-A; thus can result in cheese reaction*.
- **Rash, fever, anemia, optic neuritis, seizures, lupus like syndrome, transient memory loss, psychosis** and **gynaecomastia** has also been reported with this drug.

Rifampicin (R)

- It is a derivative of rifamycin (other derivatives are *rifabutin and rifapentine*). It is **bactericidal** against both dividing and non-dividing mycobacterium and acts by *inhibiting DNA dependent RNA polymerase*.

- It undergoes *enterohepatic circulation* and is partly metabolized in the liver. Metabolites are coloured and can cause *orange discolouration of the urine* and secretions. It can also cause **orange staining** of **contact lens**. It is **eliminated mainly in the feces** and can be used **safely in renal dysfunction**. Food interferes with absorption, therefore it must be given *empty stomach*.

- It *penetrates all membranes* including blood brain and placental barrier.
- It is equally effective against *intra-* and *extra-*cellular bacilli.
- It is the *only bactericidal drug active against dormant bacteria* in solid caseous lesions.
- Apart from tuberculosis, it is also used in leprosy (to delay resistance to dapsone). It is the **most effective and fastest acting drug in leprosy**. It can also be used as a *prophylactic drug for meningococcal and staphylococcal carrier states*.
- It can cause light chain proteinuria and may impair antibody responses. It is also *hepatotoxic* and may cause skin rash, flu like syndrome (*more prominent with intermittent regimen*) and anemia.
- Hepatotoxicity due to rifampicin is uncommon without pre-existing liver disease. It presents as *hyperbilirubinemia without SGPT elevations*.
- Rifampicin is an *inducer of drug metabolizing enzymes* and enhances the metabolism of many drugs like anticonvulsants, oral contraceptives, oral anticoagulants, antiretroviral drugs etc. **Rifabutin has little chances of drug interactions** and is equally effective, so it is *used in* the treatment of tuberculosis in *AIDS patients* (getting antiretroviral drugs).
- The female on oral contraceptives should either increase the dose of the pill or use an alternative method of contraception, when using rifampicin as a component of antitubercular treatment.
- PAS delays absorption, therefore concomitant administration should be avoided.
- Patient *on warfarin therapy* should be shifted *to unfractionated heparin or low molecular weight heparin*, if rifampicin is being used for the treatment of tuberculosis.

Rifamycin has mechanism similar to rifampicin. It has recently been approved for oral treatment of Traveller's diarrhea.

Pyrazinamide (Z)

- This is a weakly **bactericidal** drug but is **most active against slowly replicating bacteria and in the acidic media** (intracellular sites and at the sites of inflammation). It therefore has **best sterilizing activity**.
- It is effective **only against intracellular mycobacteria**.
- Its mechanism seems to be similar to isoniazid but the exact site is not known.
- Half life of this drug is prolonged in hepatic as well as *renal impairment*.
- In 40% of the patients it causes non-gouty arthralgia.
- **Hyperuricemia** also occurs commonly but is usually asymptomatic and it *should not be stopped* if hyperuricemia develops.
- It can also cause *hepatic dysfunction, porphyria and photosensitivity*.

Ethambutol (E)

- It is a **BACTERIOSTATIC** agent for mycobacterium and acts by inhibiting the synthesis of arabinogalactan (a component of cell wall) due to **inhibition of arabinosyl transferase**.
- It is distributed throughout the body except in the CSF.

- It causes dose dependent and reversible **visual disturbances like optic neuritis** (presents as *reduced visual acuity, central scotoma and loss of ability to see green, less commonly red*). It may be due to its effect on *amacrine and bipolar* cells of retina. Because children are unable to report early visual impairment, this drug is *avoided in children*.
- It also causes *hyperuricemia and peripheral neuritis*.
- It requires dose adjustment in renal failure.

MNEMONIC

Mycobacteria	Most effective drug	
1. **Rapidly growing** (wall of cavitary lesion)		H
2. **Spurters** (within caseous material)		R
3. **Slow growing** (intracellular)		Z

Streptomycin (S)

- This is a **tuberculocidal** aminoglycoside.
- It is *not absorbed orally* and must be administered by IM injection.
- It is poorly plasma protein bound.
- Its half life is prolonged in renal failure.
- It is active **only against extra-cellular bacteria**.
- It is **NOT HEPATOTOXIC**.
- Streptomycin is *contraindicated in PREGNANCY*.

Drug	Action	Hepatotoxic	Bacteria Inhibited
H	CIDAL	Yes	Both
R	CIDAL	Yes	Both
Z	CIDAL	Yes	Intracellular
E	STATIC	No	Both
S	CIDAL	No	Extracellular

Quick Revision for First Line Drugs

- Best for rapidly growing bacteria (in wall of cavities): Isoniazid
- Maximum CSF penetration: Isoniazid
- Minimum CSF penetration: Streptomycin
- Maximum sterilizing action: Pyrazinamide
- Best for intracellular bacteria: Pyrazinamide
- Best for bacteria in casseous necrosis (spurters): Rifampicin
- Only for extracellular bacteria: Streptomycin
- Safest in renal failure: Rifampicin
- Least toxic: Rifampicin
- Associated with peripheral neuropathy: Isoniazid
- Associated with psychosis: Isoniazid
- Associated with transient memory loss: Isoniazid
- Orange discolouration of urine: Rifampicin
- Contact lens staining: Rifampicin
- Retrobulbar neuritis: Ethambutol
- Not cidal: Ethambutol
- Contraindicated in pregnancy: Streptomycin

Other Drugs

- *Thioacetazone is a tuberculostatic* drug. Major adverse effects include hepatitis, bone marrow suppression and Steven Johnson syndrome (*not used in HIV positive patients due to risk of severe hypersensitivity reactions including exfoliative dermatitis*). It is not used in intermittent regimens.
- Para amino salicylic acid (*PAS*) is related to sulfonamides, acts by similar mechanism and is *bacteriostatic*. It can cause kidney, liver and thyroid dysfunction.

- *Ethionamide* is another *tuberculostatic* drug that can cause *hepatitis, optic neuritis and hypothyroidism*. It can also be used in leprosy. It has mechanism similiar to INH and bacteria resistant to INH are *cross resistant* to ethionamide also.
- *Cycloserine* is a cell wall synthesis inhibiting drug and can cause *neuropsychiatric adverse effects*.
- *Kanamycin and amikacin* are injectable aminoglycosides, which can be used in the treatment of MDR tuberculosis.
- *Capreomycin is an injectable polypeptide. It can cause ototoxicity, nephrotoxicity, hypokalemia and hypomagnesemia*.
- *Fluoroquinolones* used for this indication include *ofloxacin, moxifloxacin and levofloxacin*. These are also effective against mycobacterium avium complex in AIDS patients.
- Newer macrolides like *azithromycin and clarithromycin* are effective against non-tubercular *atypical mycobacteria*.
- *Rifabutin is more effective than rifampicin against MAC*. It has a longer $t_{1/2}$ (45 hrs) as compared ro rifampicin (3-5 hours). Clarithromycin and fluconazole inhibit its hepatic metabolism and increase $t_{1/2}$. It has *less potential than rifampicin to induce microsomal enzymes* and thus preferred in patients on anti-HIV drugs (protease inhibitors or NNRTIs mainly nevirapine). It commonly causes gastrointestinal adverse effects. Rarely, it can cause *anterior uveitis, clostridium difficile-associated diarrhea, diffuse polymyalgia syndrome, yellow skin discoloration* **(Pseudo-jaundice)** and pancytopenia. Unlike rifampicin, it *does not require dose adjustment in liver disease*.

- **Rifabutin (as compared to rifampicin) is**
    - Less effective against TB
    - More effective against MAC
    - Longer acting
    - Less potential to induce microsomal enzymes
    - Do not require dose adjustment in liver disease

- **Rifapentine** is similar to rifampicin but is *more lipophilic and longer acting*. It is not approved for administration to patients with HIV disease because of higher rates of relapse. Its *absorption increases with meals*.

New Antitubercular Drugs

- **Bedaquiline** is an inhibitor of **mycobacterial ATP synthase**. It is indicated as a part of MDT in adults with pulmonary MDR-TB. It can cause **QT prolongation**
- **Delamanid** is a nitroimidazole (similar to metronidazole) that act by **inhibiting mycolic acid synthesis**. It can be used in XDR-tuberculosis. Major adverse effect is **QT prolongation**.
- **Pretomanid** is another nitroimidazole that **acts by inhibiting mycolic acid synthesis**. It is approved in combination with **bedaquiline** and **linezolide** (BPaL therapy; Bedaquiline, Pretomanid and Linezolide) for treatment of pulmonary MDR and XDR tuberculosis. Major adverse effects include **QT prolongation, hepatotoxicity** and **bone marrow suppression.**

Quick Revision for Second-line Drugs	
Avoided in HIV patients:	Thioacetazone
Causing hypothyroidism:	Ethionamide and PAS
Cross-resistance to isoniazid:	Ethionamide
Neuropsychiatric adverse effects:	Cycloserine
Causing pseudojaundice:	Rifabutin
Associated with uveitis:	Rifabutin
Associated with polyarthralgia:	Rifabutin

Treatment of Tuberculosis

Revised National Tuberculosis Control Programme (RNTCP) is now renamed as **National Tuberculosis Elimination Program** (NTEP). Under RNTCP, patients of TB were divided into category 1 (New patients), category 2 (old cases) and category 4 (drug resistant cases). But, NTEP guidelines do not use these categories.

Drug-sensitive Tuberculosis

All patients of drug-sensitive tuberculosis (Both category 1, new and category 2; old, patients) are now treated with six months therapy. Initial 2 months of intensive phase include 4 drugs, i.e. H, R, Z and E, whereas next 4 months of continuation phase is done with 3 drugs i.e. H, R and E.

Treatment of drug-sensitive TB
2 HRZE + 4 HRE

Drug-resistant Tuberculosis (WHO 2021 guidelines)

- **Isoniazid-resistant TB**: According to latest WHO guidelines, H-resistant TB is treated with **6 months** course of 4 drugs i.e. **R, Z, E and Levofloxacin** (Lf). Addition of streptomycin or injectable drugs is no longer recommended
- **Multi-drug resistance (MDR) or Rifampic resistance (RR):**
    When mycobacterium is resistant to both H and R, it is called MDR TB.

Three types of regimens are recommended for MDR or RR tuberculosis.

Shorter Regimen Containing Bedaquiline

The patients of MDR or RR tuberculosis possessing following criteria are candidates for this regimen:
- Resistance to FQ is excluded
- They are not exposed (or exposed for < 1 month) to second line drugs
- No extensive TB disease
- No severe extrapulmonary disease
- No pregnancy
- Age more than 6 years

    Under this **All Oral Shorter Regimen**, patients are treated for 9–11 months. Intensive phase (IP) consists of 4 months (extended to 6 months, if culture positive at the end of 4 months) and continuation phase (CP) is of 5 months. The drugs used in IP are high dose isoniazide (Hh), Z, E, levofloxacin (or moxifloxacin), clofazimine and ethionamide. All drugs are continued in CP except high dose isoniazid and ethionamide. Apart from this IP and CP, bedaquiline is given for first 6 months.
- **Injectable drugs** like amikacin (used in previous guidelines) are **no longer recommended**
- **Levofloxacin is preferred** over moxifloxacin due to risk of cardiotoxicity by later. Other FQs like gatifloxacin are not used.

SHORTER ALL ORAL MDR/RR REGIMEN
6 Bedaquiline + 4-6 Hh–Z–E–Lf–Clf–Eto + 5 Z–E–Lf– Clf

Longer Regimen for MDR/RR Tuberculosis

Patients who are not the candidates for shorter all oral regimen, can be treated with this regimen. For this regimen, antitubercular drugs are divided into three groups as follows:

BPal Regimen

It is recommend for MDR–TB patients with
- Resistance to FQ
- Not exposed to (or < 2 week exposure) bedaquine and linezolide

Under this regimen, 3 drugs are given (Bedaquiline, pretomanid and linezolide) for 6-9 months.

> BPaL Regimen
> 6–9 Bedaquiline – pretomanid – Linezolide

TB Prevention

- The close contacts of patients of active drug-sensitive tuberculosis can be given one of following regimens:
  - Isoniazid prophylaxis (6H) can be given for 6 months daily. It is given empty stomach. It has higher risk of hepatotoxicity but is safer is patient of anti HIV drugs (PL HIV)
  - 3 HP: It consists of weekly administration of 2 drugs (Isoniazide and rifapentine). It has better compliance and lesser hepatotoxicity but not suitable for PLHIV due to drug interaction potential.
- Close contacts of drug resistant TB should be given
  - 6H prophylaxis if in contact with patient with H-sensitive TB
  - Rifampicin for 4 months daily (4R) if patient is R-sensitive
  - Levofloxacin for 6 months (6L) if patient has MDR-TB but FQ sensitivity.

Group A:	Levofloxacin (or Moxifloxacin)
	Bedaquiline
	Linezolide
Group B:	Clofazimine
	Cycloserine (or Terizidone)
Group C:	Ethambutol
	Pyrazinamide
	Delamanid
	Imipenem-cilastatin (or Meropenem)
	Amikacin (or streptomycin)
	Ethionamide (or Protionamide)
	PAS

The treatment duration is **18–20 months** and may be extended. Treatment is usually continued for 15-17 months after culture conversion. Intensive phase (IP) usually consists of 6-7 months and must contain minimum 4 drugs (if sensitive; All 3 drugs from group A and 1 drug from group B). Drugs should be used from these groups in hierarchy. Continuation phase (CP) should consist of minimum 3 drugs after stopping bedaquiline.

- Injectable drugs are avoided. If required amikacin is preferred. Capreomycin and kanamycin are not recommended
- Ethionamide or PAS should be included only if bedaquiline, linezolide, clofazimine or delaminid are not used

> **LONGER MDR/RR REGIMEN**
> 6–7 Bed-Lzd-Lf-Clof + 12-Lzd-Lf-Clof

ATYPICAL MYCOBACTERIAL INFECTIONS

Clarithromycin or azithromycin is recommended for *prophylaxis of Mycobacterium avium complex* (MAC) in patients with CD_4 count less than 50 μl. **Treatment of MAC requires REC regimen** (*rifabutin + ethambutol + clarithromycin/azithromycin*). Due to its long $t_{1/2}$, *azithromycin can be used as once weekly* dose in place of once daily dose of clarithromycin for prophylaxis of MAC. Other drugs effective against atypical mycobacteria are *quinolones* (ciprofloxacin, levofloxacin, moxifloxacin and gatifloxacin) and *amikacin*.

LEPROSY

The drugs used for treatment of leprosy include rifampicin, dapsone, clofazimine, ethionamide, ofloxacin, minocycline and clarithromycin.

Dapsone

It is a **leprostatic** drug related to sulfonamides with similar mechanism of action. It is metabolized by **ACETYLATION** and *undergoes enterohepatic circulation*. It can cause gastrointestinal irritation, fever, skin rash, methemoglobinemia and hemolysis *in G-6-PD deficient* patients. Hemolytic anemia is the most common adverse effect of dapsone. It can also cause sulfone (DDS) syndrome that is also called infectious mononucleosis like syndrome. **Acedapsone** is a *repository form* of dapsone whose single intramuscular injection maintains inhibitory levels of dapsone in tissues for up to 3 months. Dapsone is also an *alternative drug for the treatment of Pneumocystis jiroveci* infection in AIDS patients. It is the **drug of choice for treatment of dermatitis herpetiformis**.

Clofazimine

It is a dye with **leprostatic and anti-inflammatory** activity. It interferes with the template function of DNA. It can cause *gastrointestinal irritation, icthyosis of skin and discolouration* of skin and secretions. Due to its anti-inflammatory action it can be *used for lepra reaction*.

Rifampicin

It is the **bactericidal** and **most effective** drug used in leprosy. It *prevents development of resistance to dapsone*.

Other Drugs

Ethionamide has antileprotic activity but causes hepatotoxicity in 10% patients. *Ofloxacin, pefloxacin and sparfloxacin* are effective drugs for leprosy **but ciprofloxacin is not active** against *Mycobacterium leprae. Minocycline and clarithromycin* can also be used in leprosy.

Types of Leprosy

Pauci-bacillary leprosy: It is the form of leprosy in which *five or less skin lesions* are present and includes TT, BT and indeterminate leprosy.

Multi-bacillary leprosy: It includes leprosy with *more than five skin lesions or smear positive cases even if the lesions are less* than five. BB, BL and LL leprosy are multi bacillary.

WHO 2018 Guidelines for Treatment of Leprosy

- **Both multibacillary** (MB) as well as **pauci-bacillary** leprosy are **treated with 3 drugs**. Treatment for adults is 600 mg rifampicin + 300 mg clofazimine (once monthly, supervised) and 100 mg dapsone + 50 mg clofazimine (once daily, at home). These drugs are given for 12 months in MB and for 6 months in PB.

- **Drug resistant leprosy is treated for 2 years.** For first 6 months, 3 drugs are used (one drug is clofazimine 50 mg and 2 drugs out of ofloxacin, minocycline and clarithromycin). For next 18 months, 2 drugs are used.

Leprosy	Drugs	Duration
MB	R-600 mg + Clof-300 mg monthly Clof-50 mg + D-100 mg daily	12 months
PB	Same as MB	6 months
R-resistance	Clof-50 mg + O-400 mg + M-100 mg[a] Clof-50 mg + O-400 mg[b]	6 months 18 months
[R + O] resistance	Clof-50 mg + M-100 mg + C-500 mg Clof-50 mg + M-100 mg[a]	6 months 18 months

(R: Rifampicin; Clof: Clofazimine; D: Dapsone; O: Ofloxacin; M: Minocycline; C: Clarithromycin)

[a] Clarithromycin 500 mg may be used in place of minocycline
[b] Minocycline 100 mg may be used as an alternative to ofloxacin

> Previously, PB leprosy was treated with 2 drugs only, i.e. clofazimine was not used. In new guidelines, PB leprosy is treated with same 3 drugs as MB leprosy.

ANTI-FUNGAL AGENTS

According to the mechanism of action these can be classified as:

Mechanism of Action of Anti-fungal Drugs

Drug class	Examples	Site of action	Mechanism
1. Polyene	Amphotericin B Nystatin Hamycin	Membrane	Binds to ergosterol and forms pores in membrane
2. Antimetabolite	5-Flucytosine	Nucleus	Inhibit nucleic acid synthesis
3. Heterocyclic benzofuran	Griseofulvin	Nucleus	Disrupts microtubule function by binding to spindle
4. Azoles a. Triazoles	Fluconazole Itraconazole Voriconazole Posaconazole Terconazole	Membrane	Inhibit lanosterol-14-α-demethylase
b. Imidazoles	Ketoconazole Clotrimazole Miconazole Econazole		
5. Allylamines	Terbinafine Butenafine Naftifine	Membrane	Inhibit squalene epoxidase
6. Echinocandins	Caspofungin Micafungin Anidulafungin	Cell wall	Inhibit β-1, 3-glycan

DRUGS USED FOR THE TREATMENT OF SYSTEMIC FUNGAL INFECTIONS

These include amphotericin B, flucytosine, triazoles, ketoconazole and echinocandins.

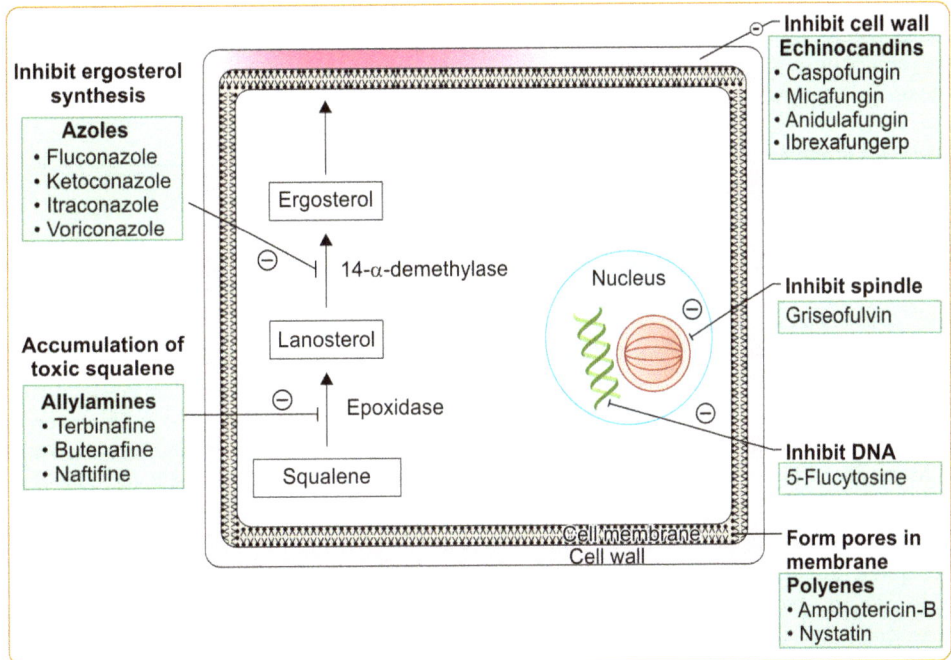

FIG. 13.2: Mechanism of action of anti-fungal drugs

Amphotericin B

- It is a **polyene** antibiotic similar to nystatin. It is *not absorbed orally* so administered by slow i.v. infusion. It is *widely distributed except in the CNS*.
- It binds to ergosterol and causes the *formation of artificial pores in fungal cell membrane*.
- Amphotericin B has the *widest antifungal spectrum [except Pseudoallescheria boydii (also called Scedosporium apiospermum) and Fusarium] and is the drug of choice or co-drug of choice for most systemic fungal infections*. It is **drug of choice for cryptococcal meningitis**, **mucormycosis** and **disseminated infections by sporothrix**. It can be used intrathecally in fungal meningitis and locally for corneal ulcers and keratitis.
- **Infusion related reactions** are seen frequently with this drug and require premedication with antihistaminics or glucocorticoids.
- **Dose limiting toxicity is nephrotoxicity** manifested by *renal tubular acidosis, hypokalemia* and *hypomagnesemia*. Infusion of normal saline before giving AMB decreases nephrotoxicity but solution of AMB should not be made in normal saline (It is made in dextrose.) Saline loading (IL of normal saline infusion before therapy) may decrease nephrotoxicity.
- It may also result in **anemia** (due to decreased erythropoietin).
- Intrathecal administration may cause seizures and neurological damage.

> *Liposomal AMB, colloidal dispersion (ABCD) and lipid complex (ABLC)* are **lipid preparations** of amphotericin B (*costlier* than conventional preparations). These formulations result in *decreased accumulation* of the drug in tissues like kidney, thus *nephrotoxicity is decreased*. Some formulations also show decreased incidence of infusion related reactions. However, these new preparations have *similar efficacy and antifungal spectrum as possessed by conventional preparations*.

Flucytosine

This is a pyrimidine analogue and is administered orally. It is converted by cytosine deaminase to 5-FU, an inhibitor of thymidylate synthase. It has *synergistic activity with amphotericin B*. Spectrum of 5-flucytosine is narrow and includes cryptococcus and candida. Major toxicities include bone marrow suppression, alopecia and liver dysfunction.

Azoles

Ketoconazole, fluconazole, voriconazole, itraconazole, posaconazole and rabuconazole are the azoles used for *systemic* fungal infections. These drugs *act by inhibiting 14 α demethylase*, which is responsible for the conversion of lanosterol to ergosterol. Due to opposite mechanism of action of AMB and azoles, the combination of these drugs is antagonistic [azoles inhibit formation of ergosterol where AMB binds to produce action].

- **Ketoconazole** has *narrow antifungal spectrum* and due to severe and frequent adverse reactions, is now *rarely used*. Ketoconazole *inhibits cytochrome P450 enzymes* (also inhibited by *fluconazole, itraconazole and voriconazole*) and increases plasma concentrations of cyclosporine, warfarin and theophylline etc. Inhibition of CYP enzymes result in decreased formation of adrenal and gonadal steroids and may lead to *gynaecomastia*, menstrual irregularities and infertility.

- **Fluconazole** has *maximum oral bioavailability and CNS penetration* among this group of drugs. It is excreted by kidney as compared to other azoles which are mainly metabolized by liver. It is the **drug of choice for candidiasis, coccidioides and cryptococcus. In cryptococcal meningitis, fluconazole is used for maintenance therapy after induction with AMB and flucytosine.**

> **MNEMONIC**
>
> Fluconazole is the drug of choice for
> - Candidiasis
> - Cryptococcus (not meningitis)
> - Coccidiodomycosis

- **Itraconazole** is the *drug of choice for blastomycosis (non-meningeal), histoplasmosis, coccidioidomycosis, paracoccidioidomycosis and sporotrichosis* (previously KI was used for sporotrichosis) infections. Its entry in the CNS is limited, therefore *not used for CNS* fungal *infections*. Fluconezole is antifungal DOC for prophylaxis of febrile neutropenia whereas voriconazole is DOC for treatment.
- **Voriconazole** has the *widest spectrum among azoles (except Mucor and Sporotrichosis)* and is the *drug of choice for invasive aspergillosis, Fusarium* and *Scedosporium*. Adverse reactions of azoles include diarrhea, rash and hepatotoxicity in preexisting liver dysfunction. It is also implicated in *prolonging QT interval*. Voriconazole causes *visual disturbances* like blurred vision, altered colour perception and photophobia. Long-term use is associated with multistep phototoxic process followed by actinic keratosis, then **squamous cell carcinoma.**
- **Posaconazole** is the only azole active against *mucormycosis*.
- **Isavuconazole** is an orphan drug for treatment of aspergillosis and mucormycosis.

Echinocandins

This is a new group of antifungal drugs that include **caspofungin, micafungin** and **anidulafungin**. These are used *intravenously* and act by *inhibiting the synthesis of $β_{1}, 3$ glycan*, a component of fungal cell wall. Caspofungin is *approved for invasive aspergillosis not responding to AMB or voriconazole*. It is quite nontoxic and causes only mild infusion related reactions.

> **MNEMONIC**
>
> **CASP** ofungin
> **A**spergillosis
> **C**andida

Ibrexafungerp

This is a new drug similar in mechanism to echinocandins i.e. **inhibits β-1,3 glycan synthesis**. However, unlike echinocandins, it is effective orally. It is used for vulvovaginal candidiasis. It is also effective against aspergillosis. This drug is effective against fungal strains which are resistant to echinocandins.

SYSTEMIC DRUGS FOR SUPERFICIAL FUNGAL INFECTIONS

1. Griseofulvin

It is used orally and its oral *absorption is increased by fatty meal*. It gets distributed to stratum corneum and *acts by interfering with microtubule function* in dematophytes. It may also inhibit synthesis and polymerization of nucleic acids. It is used for dematophytoses of skin and hair (tinea infections) because it **gets concentrated in keratin**. It causes gastrointestinal disturbances, photosensitivity and liver dysfunction. It can also cause *disulfiram like reaction* with alcohol. Its metabolism is induced by phenobarbitone.

2. Allylamines

The drugs in this group include **terbinafine, naftifine and butenafine**. These are **fungicidal** agents that act by *inhibiting squalene epoxidase* resulting in the decreased ergosterol synthesis. Inhibition of this enzyme can lead to accumulation of squalene that is toxic to the fungus. Main adverse effect of terbinafine is rash and gastrointestinal upset. Allylamines like terbinafine are oral fungicidal drugs.

3. Azoles

Ketoconazole, fluconazole and itraconazole can be used orally for superficial fungal infections but **voriconazole is not used for this purpose.**

TOPICAL DRUGS FOR SUPERFICIAL FUNGAL INFECTIONS

These include:
- **Polyenes** e.g. *nystatin* (used topically for local candida infections and orally for gastrointestinal fungi)
- **Imidazoles** e.g. *miconazole, econazole, clotrimazole, luliconazole, efinaconazole, ketoconazole, terconazole, butaconazole, tioconazole, oxiconazole, sertaconazole.*
- **Allylamines** e.g. *terbinafine, butenafine, naftifine*
- **Oxaboroles** e.g. *tavaborole*
- **Ciclopirox olamine**
- **Benzoic acid with salicylic acid** (Whitfield's ointment)
- **Tolnaftate**
- **Undecylenic acid**
- **Haloprogin.**

ANTI-VIRAL AGENTS

Antiviral drugs can act at any step of viral replication. Viral replication involves fusion of the virus to host cell membrane and penetration inside the cell. Then uncoating occurs and early proteins (like DNA polymerase) are synthesized. The nucleic acids (DNA or RNA) are then synthesized and after that late proteins (final functional proteins) are synthesized and processed. After packaging and assembly, viral particles are released (with the help of neuraminidase) and cause infection of other cells. Drugs can act at any of these steps to inhibit viral replication.

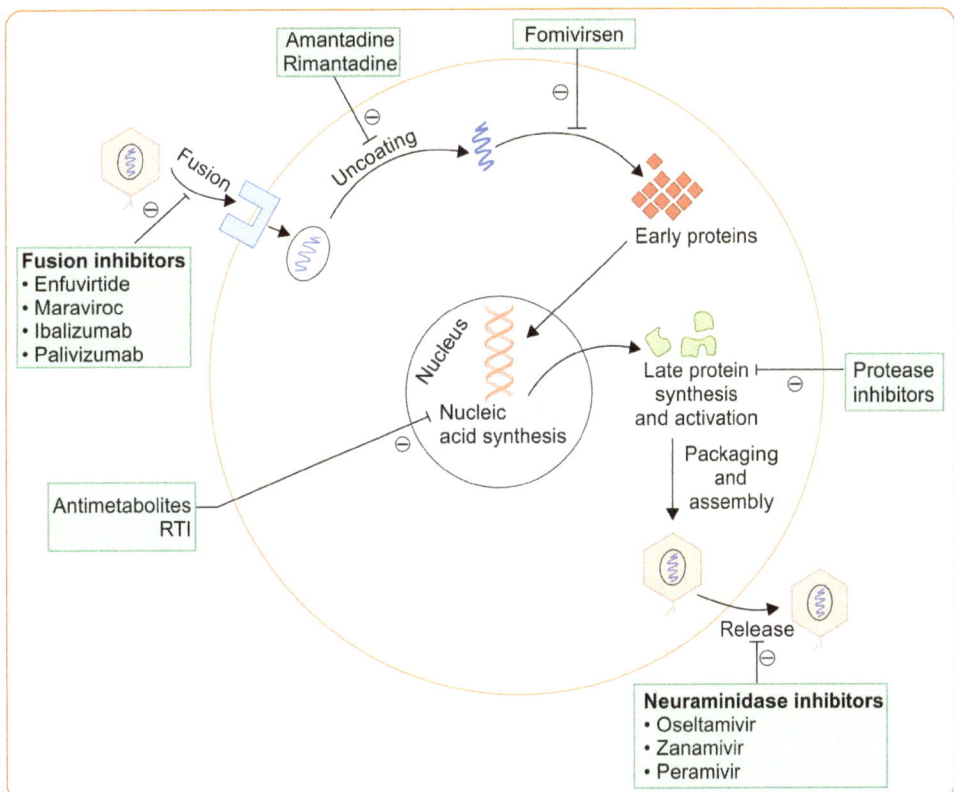

FIG. 13.3: Mechanism of action of anti-viral drugs

ANTI-HERPES DRUGS

- Most of these drugs are antimetabolites and inhibit viral DNA polymerase after bioactivation by kinases.

Acyclovir and its Congeners

- Acyclovir is a *guanosine analogue* active **against herpes simplex virus (HSV-1 and 2) and varicella zoster virus (VZV).**
- Acyclovir *is not active against CMV* infections.
- It is *activated first by a virus specific kinase (thymidine kinase) to form acyclovir monophosphate* (virus develops resistance due to mutation of this kinase) and then by host kinases to form acyclovir triphosphate. This product *competitively inhibits the action of DNA polymerase* (by competing with GTP) and also gets incorporated into the DNA and causes chain termination.
- It can be used *topically, orally or intravenously*.
- It has **very short $t_{1/2}$** and requires multiple daily dosing.
- It is primarily excreted by kidneys.

- It is used for the treatment of *mucocutaneous and genital herpes* and also for the prophylaxis of herpes infections in AIDS and immunocompromised patients.
- **Parenteral** administration for serious herpes infections cause *nephrotoxicity and neurotoxicity* (altered sensorium, tremor, myoclonus, delirium, seizures etc.) as principal dose limiting toxicities but *it does not cause bone marrow suppression*.
- *Mycophenolate* (immunosuppressant) potentiates antiherpes activity of acyclovir and related drugs by depleting intracellular GTP.
- It is essential to maintain hydration while the patient is on acyclovir therapy because *dehydration increases its nephrotoxic potential*.
- **Valacyclovir has a long half life** and gets converted to acyclovir by hepatic metabolism.
- **Famciclovir is a prodrug** that gets converted to *penciclovir* (also *developed as a separate drug*) and acts via similar mechanism.

Ganciclovir

- It is active against *CMV and HSV* and acts by inhibiting DNA polymerase. First phosphorylation step in this case also is virus specific.
- **Ganciclovir** *is used only intravenously* whereas **valganciclovir** *has good oral absorption*.
- Ganciclovir is the **drug of choice for CMV** infections including retinitis.
- Dose limiting adverse effect is **myelosuppression**. Its bone marrow suppressive action is additive to other myelosuppressive drugs like zidovudine.
- CNS side effects (headache to convulsions) also occur quite commonly.

Cidofovir

It is *activated exclusively by host cell kinases* and is active against HSV, CMV, adenovirus and papilloma virus. Its diphosphate product has prolonged $t_{1/2}$. Dose limiting toxicity is **nephrotoxicity**. Probenecid and i.v. saline can decrease nephrotoxicity. Ocular toxicity including **uveitis and iritis** is another complication. It is considered as a potential human carcinogen.

Foscarnet

It is not an antimetabolite and **does not require intracellular activation by viral or cellular kinases**. It is *used i.v for CMV infections*. Nephrotoxicity (30% incidence), *symptomatic hypomagnesemia and hypocalcemia* (increased by concomitant pentamidine) and *CNS problems* are the major adverse effects.

Other Drugs

- *Vidarabine, idoxuridine, trifluridine, fomivirsen and docosanol* (alcohol exclusively found in breast milk) are other drugs that can be used for herpes infections.
- **Fomivirsen is the first antisense oligonucleotide** and is active against *CMV retinitis (by intravitreal route)* resistant to other drugs. It can cause iritis, vitreitis and changes in intraocular pressure.
- *Idoxuridine is used only topically* for keratoconjunctivitis by HSV.
- *Docosanol is a long chain saturated alcohol* that can be used topically (as a cream) for herpes labialis. It prevents the entry of the virus in cell by inhibiting the fusion of the virus envelope with the host cell membrane.
- **Letermovir** is a CMV DNA terminase complex inhibitor. It interferes with virion maturation and is used for prophylaxis of CMV infection.

DRUG FOR SMALLPOX

Although smallpox has been eradicated but there may be risk of **bioterror attack** with this orthopox virus. **Tecovirimat** is a new drug that has activity against orthopox viruses such as smallpox and monkeypox. It inhibits the function of a major envelope protein required for production of extracellular virus. Thus, the virus is prevented from leaving an infected cell and spread of the virus within the body is prevented. Many doses of tecovirimat are stockpiled in USA for countering such bioterror attacks.

DRUGS FOR EBOLA VIRUS

The primary treatment of Ebola virus include maintaining hydration by fluids and electrolytes. Recently, monoclonal antibodies have been developed that target viral surface glycoproteins and prevent entry of virus in human cells. All these drugs are approved for Zaire Ebola virus disease. Combination of three monoclonal antibodies **Atoltivimab**, **Maftivimab** and **Odesivimab** was approved as first therapy of Zaire Ebola virus. Recently, **Ansuvimab** has also been approved for this indication.

ANTI-INFLUENZA DRUGS

These include amantadine, rimantadine, oseltamivir and zanamavir.

Amantadine and Rimantadine

These drugs *prevent uncoating* of influenza A virus (not influenza B). These drugs decrease the duration of symptoms of influenza if used prophylactically. **Rimantadine is longer acting** than amantadine. Most common adverse effects of these drugs are gastrointestinal complaints and minor CNS effects. Amantadine is also effective for the treatment *of Parkinsonism*.

Oseltamivir and Zanamavir

- These drugs act as **neuraminidase inhibitors** and prevent the virion release by causing clumping of mature virions.
- These drugs are effective against **both influenza A and influenza B**.
- **Oseltamivir is an oral prodrug** (can cause nausea and vomiting) whereas **zanamivir is administered by inhalational route** (*bronchospasm* is an important adverse effect).
- **Neuropsychiatric disorders** including suicidal tendancy have been associated with oseltamivir and zanamivir.
- These can be used prophylactically to prevent influenza during epidemics. **Oseltamivir is drug of choice for bird flu** (currently strain causing pandemic is **H5N1**) as well as swine flu (by H1N1).
- **Peramivir** is a newer drug in this category that can be administsitered *intravenously*.
- **Laninamivir** is a long-acting inhaled neuraminidase inhibitor effective even against oseltamivir resistant virus.

Baloxavir marboxil is a new drug approved for single dose oral treatment of **acute uncomplicated influenza**. It interferes with cap-dependent endonuclease activity of the influenza virus polymerase enzyme and thus inhibits viral replication.

ANTI-HEPATITIS DRUGS

Drugs active against hepatitis B (HBV) and hepatitis C virus (HCV) are interferon α (IFN-α), lamivudine, ribavirin, entecavir, adefovir and telbivudine. **Goal of therapy in chronic HBV is to** sustain suppression of HBV replication whereas in HCV, it is viral eradication.

IFN-α

It acts by JAK-STAT pathway to increase antiviral proteins and also promotes formation of natural killer (NK) cells. It is *used in chronic HBV* infections. It can also be used *with ribavirin in acute HCV* infections and prevent its progression to chronic disease. **Pegylated IFN-α 2a and 2b are superior to conventional IFN α 2a and 2b.** *Intralesional* IFNs are useful for verruca vulgaris and condyloma acuminata (imiquimod; an immunomodlator is also effective).

Lamivudine

It is a nucleoside reverse transcriptase inhibitor used in the treatment *of HIV* infections. Low dose of this drug can be used *alone or in combination with IFN-α for chronic HBV infections* (because it has longer intracellular $t_{1/2}$ in HBV than in HIV).

Ribavirin

It has a **wide antiviral spectrum** and can be given **orally**. It is used with *IFN-α in chronic HCV infection*. Although it affords no benefit in respiratory syncytial virus (RSV) infections, however, some authorities still recommend its use in immunocompromised children for this purpose. It can cause **dose dependent hemolytic anemia** and is a known human **teratogen**. DOC for chronic HBV is entecavir whereas for HCV (both acute and chronic), DOC is Peg-IFN-α plus riibavirin.

Entecavir

It is the newer HBV viral DNA polymerase inhibitor. It is effective *against HBV resistant to lamivudine* and has become first line drug for chronic HBV infection. It should be given in empty stomach.

Adefovir

It acts as an antimetabolite for HBV but nephrotoxicity is dose limiting adverse effect. It can also cause lactic acidosis with hepatomegaly and steatosis.

New Drugs for Hepatitis C Virus

Three group of new drugs have been approved for HCV. All of these are **effective orally**. These groups include HCV **protease (NS3A/4) inhibitors**, **NS5A inhibitors** and **RNA polymerase NS5B inhibitors**. These drugs are now used as first line drugs for hepatitis C in different combinations.

Protease inhibitors	NS5A inhibitors	NS5B inhibitors
Telaprevir	Elbasvir	Sofosbuvir
Boceprevir	Ledipasvir	Dasabuvir
Simprevir	Ombitasvir	
Grazoprevir	Daclatasvir	
Paritaprevir	Velpatasvir	
Glecaprevir	Pibrentasvir	
Voxilaprevir		

MNEMONIC

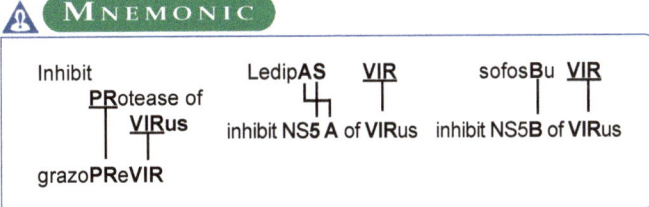

COVID-19

The pandemic of novel corona virus started in **December 2019** in **Wuhan city** of **China**. It is assumed that the virus originated from bats. It is a beta corona virus that belongs to a family containing SARS and MERS corona virus also. The full name of novel corona virus is SARS CoV2 and the disease caused by this virus is called **CO**rona **VI**rus **D**isease of 2019 (COVID-19).

Pathogenesis and Drug Targets

Entry of SARS-CoV2 virus in the lung cells is mediated by interaction between S2 protein (Spike protein) on the virus and ACE2 receptors on the lung cells. For this interaction, S2 protein is proteolysed and ACE2 receptor is glycosylated (by TMPRSS2). The virus then enters inside cells by forming endosomes. Acidification of endosomes is required for entry of virus. After entry inside the cells, an enzyme RNA dependent RNA polymerase (RdRP) forms mRNA (via replication). This RNA helps in formation of various structural and non-structural proteins. Further, this mRNA also enters the nucleus of host cells via importins. After entry in the nucleus, mRNA inhibits host cell division and also evades immune invasion (prevents release of substances required for activation of immune system). When all proteins are assembled, the new virus leaves the host cell by exocytosis and affects other cells.

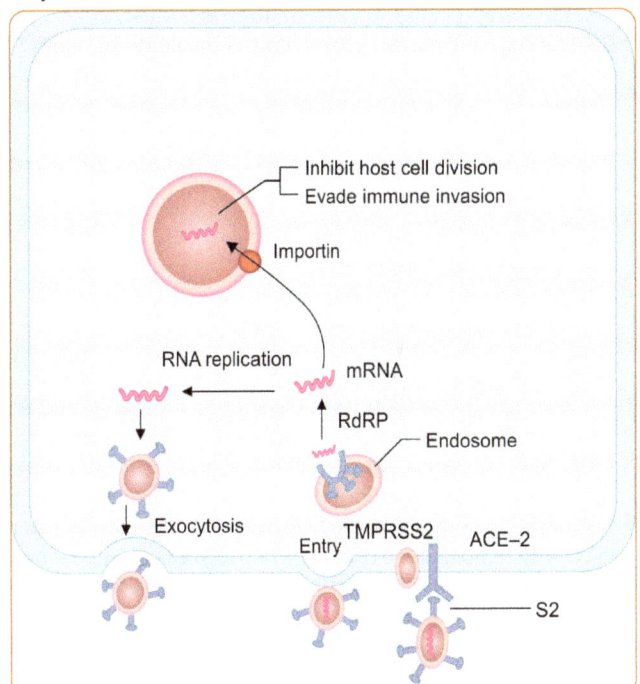

Further, in many patients, the body's immune response goes out of control resulting in cytokine storm which can result in multi-organ failure and ARDS.

Various targets of drug therapy can be:
1. Virus entry inhibitors
2. RdRP inhibitors
3. Importin inhibitors
4. Immunomodulators

1. **Virus entry inhibitors:** The drugs proposed to act by inhibiting entry of virus include:
   a. Chloroquine and Hydroxychloroquine
   b. Umifenovir (Arbidol)

c. Camostat and Nafamostat
d. Monoclonal Antibodies

- **Chloroquine and hydroxychloroquine** inhibits entry by preventing glycosylation of ACE-2, inhibiting proteolytic processing of S2 and preventing acidification of endosomal pH. Apart from this, these drugs can also decrease cytokine production and inhibit lysosomal activity. These drugs can cause **QT prolongation, retinopathy, hypoglycemia** and neuropsychiatric symptoms, chloroquine and hydroxychloroquine were tried in prophylaxis and treatment of COVID-19, however, these were soon discontinued due to lack of efficacy.
- **Umifenovir** (Arbidol) inhibits endocytosis. It is approved for influenza virus infections in Russia and China.
- **Camostat** and **Nafamostat** act by inhibiting TMPRSS-2. These are approved in Japan for Pancreatitis.
- Several **monoclonal antibodies** against spike proteins recently were approved by US-FDA for emergency use authorization (EUA). These are given in early stages to prevent hospitalization of patients with risk factors. All these drugs are **given intravenously in OPD setting**. The approved drugs are:

  - Bamlanivimab + Etesevimab
  - Casirivimab + Imdevimab
  - Sotrovimab

2. **RNA dependent RNA polymerase inhibitors**: Remdesivir and Favipiravir act as RdRP inhibitors of SARS CoV-2.
- **Favipiravir** is a purine analog and is available in Japan for influenza virus. Its use was discontinued in COVID-19.
- **Remdesivir** is an adenosine analog. It is administered IV and is the **only FDA approved drug for treatment of COVID-19. Its use is not recommended by WHO. Remdesivir is indicated in:**

  - Moderate to severe COVID-19 patients
  - Hospitalized patients
  - Patients on oxygen therapy
  - Within 10 days of disease onset.

While using remdesivir, **monitoring of KFT, LFT and PT is** required. The use of remdesivir should be **avoided if eGFR is less than 30 mL/min or ALT is more than 5 times** the upper limit. Major adverse effects include allergy, infusion related reactions and nausea, chloroquine reduces its antiviral activity. Remdesivir is commonly **used with steroids. Baricitinib can be used** with remdesivir in patients **when steroids cannot be used**.

3. **Importin inhibitors**: Ivermectin is proposed to act by inhibiting the importin protein. By this mechanism, ivermectin can prevent hijacking of cellular machinery by the virus. Ivermectin is already used for treatment of various helminthic infections and scabies. Its use for COVID-19 was discontinued due to lack of efficacy.
4. **Immunomodulators**: Several drugs can be used to inhibit the overactive immune system in COVID-19.
   a. **Steroids**: These are the **only drugs** which have been shown to **DECREASE MORTALITY** in patients with COVID-19 pneumonia. However, the use of steroids is **contraindicated in asymptomatic patients and** in those with **mild disease**. These should be started after 7 days of disease onset. The recommended dose of steroids are:

      - 6 mg dexamethasone once a day OR
      - 32 mg methylprednisolone once a day OR
      - 40 mg prednisolone once a day OR
      - 50 mg hydrocortisone thrice a day.

   Adverse effects of steroids needs to be addressed. Most important being **risk of infections including mucormycosis**. These can also result in hyperglycemia.
   b. **Tocilizumab**: It is a **monoclonal antibody against IL-6**. It is used intravenously at a dose of 8 mg/kg (max. 800 mg) to prevent cytokine storm. It is indicated in patients with:

   - Severe to critically ill COVID-19 pneumonia.
   - No improvement of oxygen requirement after 24-48 hours of steroids
   - Raised CRP (>75 mg/L)
   - No bacterial, fungal or TB infection

   However, tocilizumab should be avoided in:
   - Immunosuppressed patients
   - ALT > 5 times the upper limit
   - High risk of GI perforation
   - Uncontrolled infections
   - Absolute neutrophil count <500 cells/μL
   - Platelet count <50,000 cells/μL

   c. **Baricitinib**: It is a Janus Kinase (JAK) inhibitor being used for treatment of Rheumatoid Arthritis. It can be used for treatment of COVID-19 **in combination with remdesivir, in patients where steroids cannot be used**. It needs dose adjustment in renal and hepatic disease. Major adverse effect is increases **risk of thromboembolism**.

DGHS guidelines for treatment of COVID-19

Category	Clinical features	(June 2021) Mainstay treatment
Asymptomatic		No medication
Mild	No shortness of breath/(SOB) Respiratory rate (RR) < 24 SpO$_2$ > 94%	Anti-pyretics (acetaminophen or NSAIDs) Anti-tussives Inhalational budesonide 800 μg BD for 5 days
Moderate	No SOB RR = 24–30 SpO$_2$ = 90–93%	O$_2$ (to maintain SpO$_2$ > 92%) Steroids (if SpO$_2$ < 92%) Prophylactic anticoagulants Other therapies depending upon investigations
Severe	SOB RR > 30 SpO$_2$ < 90%	O$_2$ (to maintain SPO$_2$ >90%) Steroids Prophylactic anticoagulant Other therapies depending upon investigations

ANTI-HIV DRUGS

Human Immunodeficiency Virus (HIV) enters the CD4 cells after fusion of viral Gp41 with CCR5 or CXCR4 receptors on human cells. After entry, viral RNA is converted to DNA with the help of reverse transcriptase (RNA dependent DNA polymerase). This viral DNA integrates with human DNA to form provirus with the help of enzyme, integrase. This proviral DNA can replicate and transcript to form RNA which forms proteins via translation. The proteins formed initially are inactive and require protease enzyme for activation. Complete virus is generated from these components, which leaves the CD4 cells to infect other cells. Various drugs can target these steps and are described ahead.

Reverse Transcriptase Inhibitors

HIV is a retrovirus that forms its DNA from RNA with the help of the enzyme RNA dependent DNA polymerase (reverse transcriptase). Drugs may inhibit this enzyme either competitively (anti-metabolites) or non-competitively. The competitive inhibi-

Chemotherapy B: Antimicrobials for Specific Conditions

tors may be nucleoside reverse transcriptase inhibitors (NRTIs) or nucleotide reverse transcriptase inhibitors (e.g. tenofovir). The non-competitive inhibitors are also known as non-nucleoside/non-nucleotide reverse transcriptase inhibitors (NNRTIs).

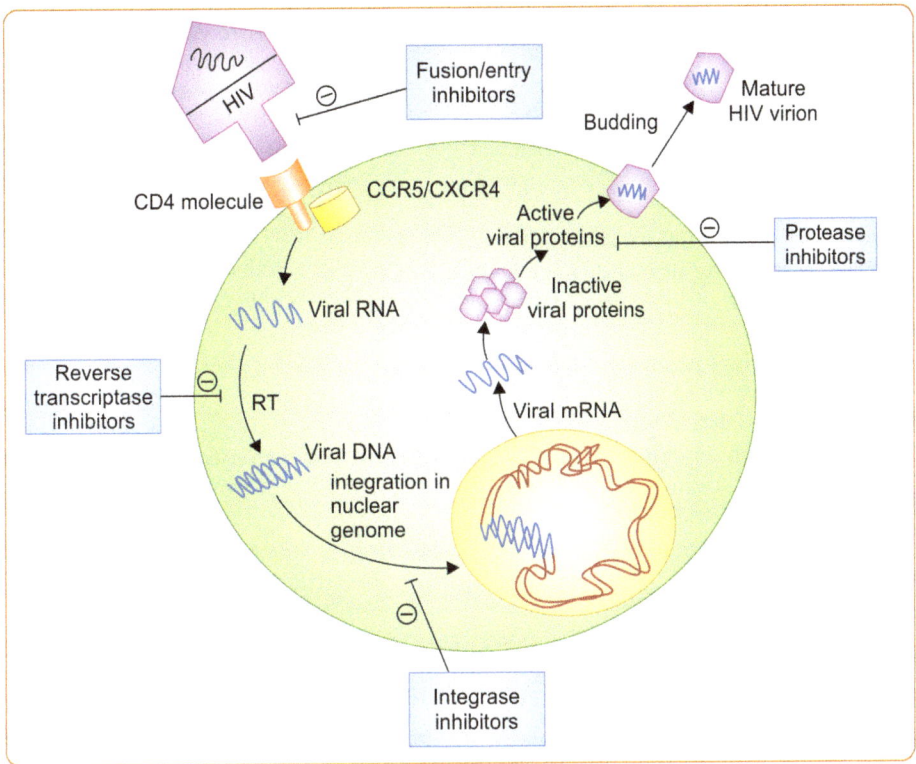

FIG. 13.4: Pathogenesis of HIV and target of various drugs

a. NRTIs

These are *prodrugs* and are activated by host cell kinases to *form triphosphates*. These drugs *competitively inhibit reverse transcriptase* and also act as chain terminators by incorporation into the DNA chain (because these lack 3′ hydroxyl group on ribose ring, attachment of next nucleotide is not possible). Resistance to these drugs emerges rapidly if used alone.

- **Zidovudine** is frequently used NRTI in the treatment of HIV infections. It *can also be used for the prophylaxis of* needle stick injury patients and for the *prevention of vertical transmission of HIV* from mother to fetus. Major adverse effect of zidovudine is **bone marrow suppression** leading to megaloblastic anemia, neutropenia and thrombocytopenia (*ganciclovir should not be combined*). It is contraindicated in patient with Hb < 8g%. It can also cause *myopathy*. Rifampicin increases the clearance of this drug. Chronic administration is associated with *lipodystrophy syndrome, nail hyperpigmentation and lipoatrophy.*

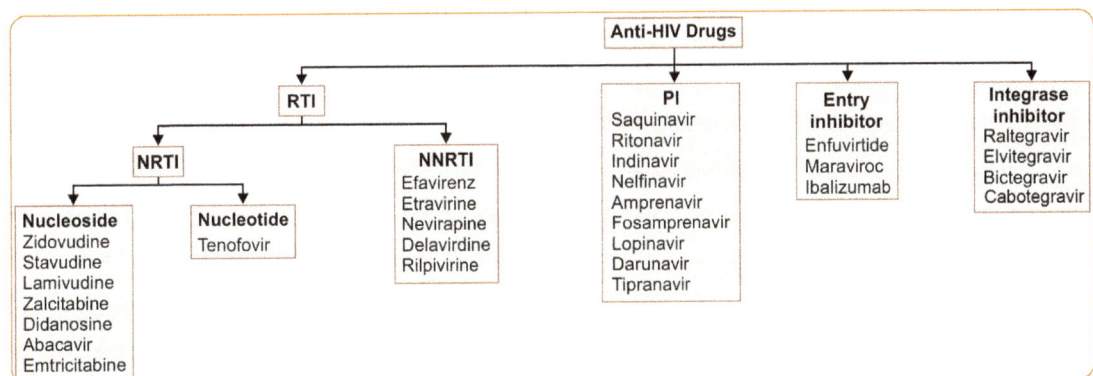

- **Didanosine** is another NRTI. Its *oral bioavailability is reduced by food*. It can lead to dose limiting *pancreatitis (maximum chances), hyperuricemia, optic neuritis* and also painful sensory peripheral neuropathy. Diarrhea is more common than with other NRTIs. It may cause *neutropenia (not anemia)* and fulminant hepatic failure and electrolyte abnormalities
- **Stavudine** causes dose limiting *peripheral neuropathy*. It has maximum chances of causing *lactic acidosis* (mitochondrial toxicity). It can also result in *pancreatitis*. It is *most strongly associated with lipodystrophy syndrome among all NRTIs and protease inhibitors.*
- **Lamivudine and emtricitabine** are *best tolerated NRTIs*. These are **not** associated with *peripheral neuropathy or pancreatitis*. Both are effective against hepatitis B. Emtricitabine is once a day alternative to lamivudine.

> **MNEMONIC**
>
> **Drugs having activity against both HIV and HBV**
> L – Lamivudine
> E – Emtricitabine
> T – Tenofovir

- **Zalcitabine** has unique toxicity to cause *oral ulceration and stomatitis* It is least effective NRTI. It also result in *peripheral neuropathy and pancreatitis.*
- **Abacavir** increases the **risk of myocardial infarction**. It may cause severe hypersensitivity reaction particularly in patients having HLA B*5701 allele. Testing of this allcle should be done before starting abacavir.
- **All NRTIs are excreted by the kidney** (require dose adjustment in renal failure) *except abacavir* which gets metabolized by alcohol dehydrogenase. *Hypersensitivity* is the major adverse reaction of abavacir (should not be restarted).
- All NRTIs may cause *lactic acidosis, hepatomegaly and steatosis* by inhibiting mammalian mitochondrial DNA polymerase. Risk factors are obesity and pre-existing liver dysfunction.
- Maximum risk of:

– Pancreatitis:	Didanosine
– Peripheral neuropathy:	Stavudine
– Lipodystrophy syndrome:	Stavudine

b. Nucleotide RTI

Tenofovir is a nucleotide and does not require bioactivation by kinases. It is excreted mainly by the kidney and renal impairment including a Fanconi like syndrome with hypophosphatemia may occur. *Oral bioavailability* of tenofovir *increases with meals* (decreased for other NRTIs). It is well tolerated and flatulence is only significant side effect. *It is also effective against hepatitis B.*

> **Note**
>
> - Lamivudine, emtricitabine and tenofovir have activity against hepatitis B virus.
> - Thymidine analog NRTIs (zidovudine and stavudine) and protease inhibitors are associated with lipodystrophy syndrome characterized by hyperlipidemia, hypercholesterolemia, glucose intolerance and fat re-distribution.
> - Strains of HIV resistant to lamivudine (due to MI84V substitution) appear to have enhanced sensitivity to other NRTIs.
> - Zidovudine is most likely to cause anemia whereas zidovudine and didanosine are most likely to cause neutropenia
> - Stavudine (followed by zidovudine) are most likely to cause lipoatrophy
> - Zidovudine and didanosine are most likely to cause peripheral neuropathy.
> - Didanosine has maximum risk of causing pancreatitis

c. NNRTIs

These drugs inhibit reverse transcriptase by acting at a site (**allosteric site**) different from that of NRTIs. These are **selective for HIV-1** and have no activity against HIV-2. *Resistance to these drugs develops very rapidly.* Drugs in this group are **efavirenz, nevirapine, etravirine and delavirdine**.

- *Skin rash* is an adverse effect of all of these drugs and *nevirapine can cause Steven Johnson syndrome* and toxic epidermal necrolysis.
- **Nevirapine is used in pregnancy to prevent vertical transmission** (*single oral dose of 200 mg* to mother during labour and single 2 mg/kg oral dose to neonate **within 3 days after birth**). *It decreases transmission to 13% as compared to 21.5% by zidovudine. However because of hepatotoxicity and less effectiveness of nivaprine, it is not preferred* for this indication.
- **Efavirenz** is *neurotoxic* and side effects may range from lack of concentration to vivid dreams to delusions and mania.
- **Etravirine** is a recently approved NNRTI. This **second generation NNRTI** is *effective against HIV resistant to first generation* NNRTI (Efavirenz, nevirapine and delavirdine). Another recently approved second generation NNRT1 is *rilpivirine.*

Doravirine is a 3rd generation NNRTI. It is approved as once daily treatment with lamivudine and tenofovir for treatment of HIV.

> **Note**
>
> - NNRTI do not cause lipodystrophy
> - Nevirapine and efavirenz are CYP 450 enzyme inducers whereas delavirdine is enzyme inhibitor.

Protease Inhibitors

Protease *helps in the maturation of infectious virions* and inhibitors of this enzyme can be used in the treatment of HIV infections (by *inhibiting the post-translational modification of viral proteins*).

- Oral bioavailability of **indinavir** is decreased by food. It *can cause crystalluria* and *kidney stones*. To prevent renal damage, good hydration must be maintained. It can also cause **asymptomatic hyperbilirubinemia.**
- This group of drugs inhibits the metabolism of several drugs by inhibiting CYP3A4. *Ritonavir in low doses can be used with other protease inhibitors to increase their plasma concentration.* **Current guidelines recommend that all protease-inhibitor containing regimens use ritonavir boosting if possible.** *Only Nelfinavir and Atazanavir can be used safely without ritonavir boosting.* **Nelfinavir** is *the only protease inhibitor for which ritonavir boosting is not recommended.*
- Concentration of **amprenavir and fosamprenavir (a long-acting prodrug of amprenavir) decrease** when co-administered **with ethinyl estradiol.**
- **Tipranavir** is the **only nonpeptidic protease inhibitor**. It is effective against HIV resistant to other protease inhibitors. It can cause *hepatotoxicity and intracranial hemorrhage.*
- **Atazanavir** frequently cause *asymptomatic unconjugated hyperbilirubinemia* (like indinavir) and *increase in PR interval in ECG*. It requires acidic pH to remain in solution, therefore should not be given with proton pump inhibitors. *Both tenofovir and efavirenz lower the serum concentration of atazanavir, therefore when used with these drugs, it must be boosted by ritonavir.*
- Amprenavir can cause Steven Johnson syndrome.
- **All** protease inhibitors are metabolized by liver and all can cause **metabolic abnormalities** including *hypercholesterolemia, diabetes mellitus, hyperlipidemia, insulin resistance and altered fat distribution* (collectively called lipodystrophy syndrome). **Atazanavir** is *devoid of this adverse effect.* **Tesamorelin** is a *synthetic analogue of growth hormone releasing factor* indicated to

Chemotherapy B: Antimicrobials for Specific Conditions

reduce excess abdominal fat in HIV-infected patients with lipodystrophy.

ENTRY Inhibitors

For entry of HIV in CD4 cells, there is interaction between virus envelope glycoproteins and proteins present on CD4 cells. GP41 and GP120 are glycoproteins present on viral envelope that binds to CD-4 receptors on cells. The entry of virus inside the cells is facilitated by co-receptors (CCR-5 or CXCR-4) present on CD-4 cells. Drugs can bind to these proteins to inhibit entry of HIV in CD-4 cells.

Binding Target	Drug
GP-41	Enfuvirtide
GP-120	Fostemsavir
CD-4	Ibalizumab
CCR-5	Maraviroc

- **Ibalizumab** is a monoclonal antibody against CD4 receptors. When given intravenously, it can inhibit the fusion of HIV with CD4 cells.
- **Enfuvirtide** is a drug that **binds to Gp 41 subunit of HIV** envelope protein *and inhibits the fusion* of viral and host cell membranes. This prevents the entry of the virus in the host cells. It is *used subcutaneously* and can cause *injection site reactions*, hypersensitivity and pneumonia. It is not effective against HIV-2
- **Fostemsavir** is an oral prodrug of temsavir. It inhibits entry of HIV in CD-4 cells by **binding to GP120**. Major adverse effects include **QT prolongation**, increase in hepatic transaminases and immune reconstitution syndrome.
- **Maraviroc** is the *first CCR5 co-receptor antagonist* to be approved for use. It is only active against "CCR-5-tropic virus" and thus, a co-receptor tropism assay should be performed before starting maraviroc. This type of HIV-1 virus tends to predominate *early in infection*. It can be *given orally*.

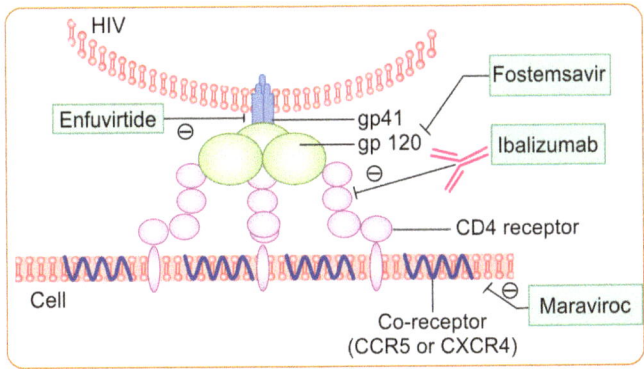

FIG. 13.5: Site of action of HIV fusion inhibitors

Integrase Inhibitors

Raltegravir, elvitegravir, dolutegravir and bictegravir are the *oral drugs* approved by FDA that act by inhibiting the integrase enzyme. **Cobicistat** is used to boost the effect of elvitegravir. Recently, cobicistat has been approved to boost the effect of darunavir and atazanavir also.

Cabotegravir + Rilpivirine has been recently approved as once monthly intramuscular injections for HIV.

Cobicistat is a new drug that inhibits the metabolism of elvitegravir. It is approved as a booster for this drug.

MNEMONIC

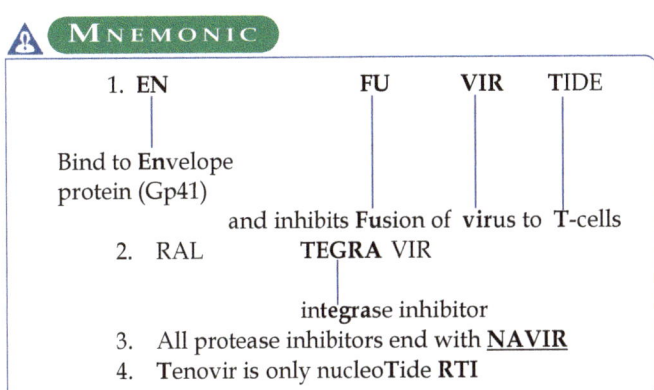

1. **EN** **FU** **VIR** **TIDE**
   Bind to **En**velope protein (Gp41)
   and inhibits **Fu**sion of **vir**us to **T**-cells
2. RAL **TEGRA** VIR
   inte**gra**se inhibitor
3. All protease inhibitors end with **NAVIR**
4. Tenovir is only nucleo**Tide** RTI

Elapegademase is a recombinant adenosine deaminase (ADA) enzyme. It is indicated by intramuscular injection **for severe combined immunodeficiency** due to ADA deficiency.

Note

Anti-HIV drug combinations that should NOT be used are:

- Zidovudine + Stavudine : Pharmacological antagonism (compete for intracellular phosphorylation)
- Atazanavir + Indinavir : Additive unconjugated hyperbilirubinemia.
- Didanosine/stavudine + Zalcitabine : Additive peripheral neuropathy.
- Lamivudine + Zalcitabine : In vitro antagonism.

ANTI-RETROVIRAL THERAPY (ART)

Highly active anti-retroviral therapy (HAART) also known as combination ART (cART) is recommended with the primary goal of complete suppression of viral replication (viral load <50 copies/mL).

WHO Guidelines for ART (2016)

A. **When to start**
- ART should be started in all HIV positive patients **regardless of WHO clinical stage and at any CD4 cell**
- For patients with TB and HIV, treatment of TB should be started first, followed by ART as soon as possible within first 8 weeks of treatment.

B. What to start

	Preferred First Line ART	Second Line ART
1. Adults	T + L (or Em) + E (2 NRTI + 1 NNRTI/II)	2 NRTI + Boosted PI
2. Adolescents	T + L (or Em) + E T + L (or Em) + D (2NRTI + 1 NNRTI/II)	2 NRTI + Boosted PI
3. Children (3–10 years)	A + L + E (2 NRTI + 1 NNRTI)	2 NRTI + Boosted PI (or RAL)
4. Children (<3 years)	A + L + LPV (2 NRTI + 1 PI/II)	2 NRTI + RAL

T: Tenofovir, L: Lamivudine, Em: Emtricitabine, E: Efavirenz, NRTI: Nucleoside/tide reverse transcriptase inhibitor, II: Integrase inhibitor, PI: Protease inhibitor, D: Dolutegravir, A: Abacavir, RAL: Raltegravir, LPV: Lopinavir + Ritonavir

C. Infant Prophylaxis: Z + N for 6 weeks
D. Post-exposure Prophylaxis: (For 28 days; start within 72 hours)

	Preferred	Alternative
Adults and adolescents	T + L + PI	RAL/DRV/E are alternative to PI
Children < 10 years	Z + L + LPV	A can be used for Z

ANTIMALARIAL DRUGS

Malarial parasite (plasmodium) undergoes a primary developmental stage in liver (pre erythrocytic stage; responsible for the cause of malaria) and then it enters the RBCs (erythrocytic stage; responsible for symptoms). Symptoms of malaria (fever, chills and rigors) correspond to the erythrocytic stage. Plasmodium may give rise to gametes in the blood which can be taken up by the female anopheles (responsible for transmission of malaria). Some schizonts remain dormant in liver and this dormant hepatic stage (exo-erythrocytic) is responsible for relapse of malaria. Exo-erythrocytic stage is absent in P. falciparum, so relapses do not occur. The drugs used for the treatment or prevention of malaria may be classified (on the basis of the stage in the life cycle of the parasite at which these act) as:

- **Primary tissue schizonticides:** These are the drugs that kill schizonts in the liver (pre-erythrocytic stage) e.g. *proguanil, primaquine* and *pyrimethamine*. These drugs are used for **causal prophylaxis.**
- **Erythrocytic schizonticides:** These drugs kill schizonts in the blood and can be used for the **treatment of acute attacks as well as suppressive prophylaxis** of malaria. All of these drugs are used for treatment of malaria but not for prophylaxis. Artemisinin derivatives are very short acting whereas quinine and sulfadoxine are toxic on long term administration, therefore are not suitable for prophylaxis. Erythrocytic schizonticides may be fast acting or slow acting:
  - **Fast acting:** *Chloroquine, mepacrine, quinine, mefloquine, halofantrine, atovaquone* and *artemisinin derivatives*
  - **Slow acting:** *Proguanil, pyrimethamine, sulfonamides, tetracyclines*

> **MNEMONIC**
>
> Fast acting Erythrocytic schizonticidal drugs
> M – Mefloquine
> A – Atovaquone
> C – Chloroquine (and amiodiaquine and piperaquine)
> H – Halofantrine (and lumefantrine)
> A – Artemisinins
> R – Res-Q (Quinine)

- **Exo-erythrocytic schizonticides:** These drugs kill the exo-erythrocytic forms and are thus used for **radical cure**, e.g. *primaquine*.

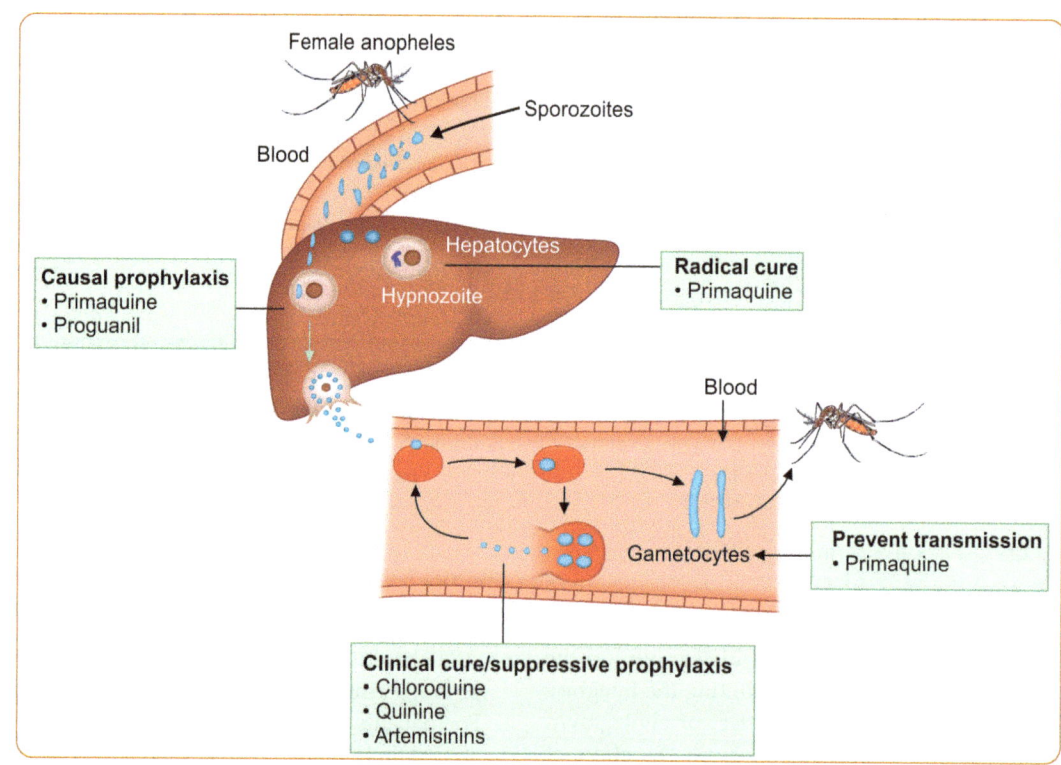

FIG. 13.6: Life cycle of malarial parasite with target of drugs

- **Sporonticides or gametocides:** These drugs kill the gametes and thus **prevent transmission** of malaria. Chloroquine, mepacrine and quinine kill the gametes of *P. vivax* only whereas *proguanil, pyrimethamine, primaquine and artemisinin* kill gametes of both P. vivax as well as *P. falciparum*.

Stage	Clinical Use
Pre-Erythrocytic	Causal prophylaxis
Erythrocytic	Clinical cure
	Suppressive prophylaxis
Exo-Erythrocytic	Radical cure
Gametocytic	Prevention of transmission

Chloroquine

It is the drug possessing **largest volume of distribution** (>1300 L). It accumulates in the food vacuole of the plasmodium. Thus, it is selectively concentrated in the parasitized erythrocytes. It *prevents polymerization of heme to hemozoin* resulting in accumulation of heme that is toxic for the parasite. It is the *drug of choice for treatment and prophylaxis of non-falciparum malaria and chloroquine sensitive P. falciparum malaria*. It is an erythrocytic schizonticide and has no effect on exo-erythrocytic stages. It is also used for other indications that are

- Rheumatoid arthritis
- Extraintestinal amoebiasis
- Discoid lupus erythematosis
- Lepra reaction
- Infectious mononucleosis
- Photogenic reactions
- Malaria
- Giardiasis

> **Note**
> This can be remembered from the mnemonic: **RED LIP M**ahatma **G**andhi

Adverse effects of chloroquine include skin rashes (lichenoid eruptions), peripheral neuropathy, hypotension, myocardial depression (T wave changes in ECG), auditory impairment and toxic psychosis. **Prolonged use of high doses can result in blindness due to retinal damage** (Bull's eye maculopathy). It can also precipitate porphyria and cause discolouration of nails and mucous membranes. Chloroquine is the drug of choice for treatment of malaria in pregnant women.

Quinine

Its mechanism of action is not clear and may be similar to chloroquine. Its major use is treatment of *P. falciparum* infections resistant to chloroquine (drug of choice). It is often used with doxycycline or clindamycin to decrease the duration of therapy and limit toxicity. To delay emergence of resistance, it is not advocated for chemoprophylaxis. It is 70% bound to plasma proteins especially α1 acid glycoprotein, such binding increases in acute attacks of malaria, so that patients of malaria can tolerate much higher doses of quinine than other subjects. Its d-isomer, quinidine can be used i.v. for severe P. falciparum infections. It can cause hypoglycemia manifested by palpitations, sweating and tachycardia. To prevent hypoglycemia, i.v. infusion of quinine should always be given in 5% dextrose solution (instead of normal saline). At toxic doses, cinchonism can occur which manifests as symptoms of gastrointestinal distress, vertigo, blurred vision, headache and tinnitus. It can also cause cardiac conduction abnormalities and hemolysis in G-6-PD deficient patients. According to WHO guidelines, quinine is safe in pregnancy and can be used for severe or chloroquine resistant malaria.

Mefloquine

It **can be used for chloroquine resistant *P. falciparum* infections, both for treatment as well as prophylaxis**. It can cause **cardiac conduction disturbances, psychosis and seizures**. Administration with *halofantrine or quinine is contraindicated* because it can cause prolongation of QT interval. It is effective as a **single dose treatment** of malaria.

Primaquine

It acts by forming redox compounds that act as cellular antioxidants. It is a tissue (pre- as well as exo-erythrocytic) schizonticide and gametocide. **It can kill the gametes of all species of plasmodium** unlike chloroquine and quinine which are effective against gametes of *P. vivax* only. It is always used along with blood schizonticides for **radical cure** of malaria. It can cause *methemoglobinemia and hemolysis in G-6-PD deficient patients*. It is **contraindicated in pregnancy**. It has **no role (for radical cure) in P. falciparum malaria** because this organism has no exo-erythrocytic stage.

> **Tafenoquine** is a new oral drug similar to primaquine. It is approved as single oral dose for radical cure of *P. vivax* malaria.

Antifolate Drugs

These include *pyrimethamine, proguanil, sulfadoxine and dapsone*. **Proguanil** is a prodrug and is activated to *form cycloguanil*. **Pyrimethamine and cycloguanil act by inhibiting DHFRase**. Pyrimethamine plus sulfadoxine act through sequential blockade. These are *slow acting blood schizonticides* that are active against chloroquine resistant *P. falciparum* infections. Proguanil plus atovaquone can be used for treatment as well as chemoprophylaxis of chloroquine resistant malaria.

Atovaquone

It is a rapidly acting blood schizonticide that acts by collapsing the parasite's membrane. Proguanil potentiates its antimalarial action. It can also be used for *Pneumocystis jiroveci* pneumonia and *Toxoplasma gondii* infections.

Artemisinin Derivatives

Artemisinin, dihydroartemisinin, artesunate, artemether and arteether are the compounds obtained from a Chinese herb Artemisia annua. Artemisinin is a prodrug and is activated in the body to dihydroartemisinin. These drugs generate highly active free radicals that damage parasite membranes. These drugs are the fastest acting drugs against malaria. Artesunate has a very short half life and can be given i.v. These can be used for the treatment of multidrug resistant malaria as well as serious forms like cerebral malaria. Artemisinin derivatives are not indicated for chemoprophylaxis of malaria. It can rarely cause QT prolongation.

Halofantrine and Lumefantrine

Halofantrine has erratic oral bioavailability and can cause potentially serious cardiotoxicity (even more if combined with mefloquine). Due to these reasons, it is not recommended for chemoprophylaxis of malaria. Use of this drug is reserved for treatment of multidrug resistant malaria. Lumefantrine is a new drug similar to halofantrine and is always used along with artemether. *Its absorption markedly increases with fatty food.*

Other Drugs

Other antimalarial drugs include *doxycycline, amodiaquine, mepacrine and pyronaridine* etc. **Mepacrine is most concentrated in collagen.**

TREATMENT AND PROPHYLAXIS OF MALARIA (NATIONAL GUIDELINES ACCORDING TO NBVDCP)

Treatment of uncomplicated malaria

Parasite	Males and Non-pregnant females	Pregnancy (1st trimester)	Pregnancy (2nd and 3rd trimester)
P. vivax (or P. ovale)	Chloroquine + Primaquine[a,b]	Chloroquine	Chloroquine
P. falciparum (or P. malariae)	ACT[c] + Primaquine[d]	Quinine	ACT[c]
Mixed	ACT[c] + Primaquine[d]	Quinine	ACT[c]

Treatment of severe/complicated malaria

P. falciparum	Artesunate[e] followed by oral ACT	Artesunate[e] followed by oral ACT	Artesunate[e] followed by oral ACT

[a] Primaquine is contraindicated in pregnancy, infants and G-6-PD deficiency
[b] For *P. vivax*, primaquine is given for 14 days to kill hypnozooites
[c] ACT is artemisinin-based combination therapy. Preferred ACT is
 – North-Eastern states: Artemether + Lumefantrine
 – Rest of India: Artesunate + Sulfadoxine/Pyrimethamine

Contd...

Contd...

[d] For *P. falciparum*, Primaquine is given as a single dose to kill gametes
[e] Artesunate is given by IV or IM route. It is continued for minimum 48 hours.

The WHO Recommended ACTs include

- Artemether-Lumefantrine
- Artesunate-Mefloquine
- Dihydroartemisinin-Piperaquine
- Artesunate-Amodiaquine
- Artesunate-Sulfadoxine-Pyrimethamine

CHEMOPROPHYLAXIS OF MALARIA

| Short-term (< 6 weeks): | Doxycycline[a,b] |
| Long-term (> 6 weeks): | Mefloquine[c,d] |

[a] Doxycycline is started 2 days before travel and continued for 4 weeks after leaving the endemic area
[b] Doxycycline is contraindicated in pregnancy and children < 8 years.
[c] Mefloquine is started 2 weeks before travel and continued for 4 weeks after leaving the endemic area
[d] Mefloquine is contraindicated in patients with history of convulsions or neuropsychiatric conditions.

DRUGS FOR AMOEBIASIS

The drugs effective against infections of *Entamoeba histolytica* can be classified as:
- Tissue (extra-intestinal) amoebicides only e.g. Chloroquine.
- Both intestinal (luminal) and extra-intestinal amoebicides e.g. nitroimidazoles (metronidazole, tinidazole secnidazole, ornidazole), emetine and dehydroemetine.
- Luminal amoebicides only e.g. diloxanide furoate, paromomycin, iodoquinol, quiniodochlor and tetracyclines.

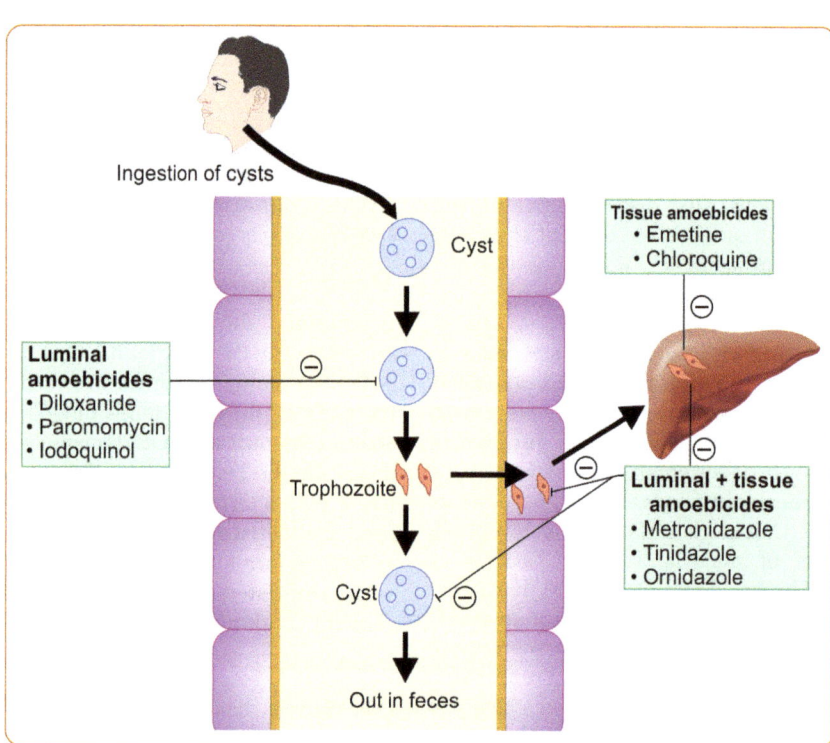

FIG. 13.7: Site of action of anti-amoebic drugs

Chemotherapy B: Antimicrobials for Specific Conditions

Nitroimidazoles

This group includes metronidazole and related drugs. These are effective orally as well as i.v. and eliminated by hepatic metabolism. Nitro group of these drugs gets bioactivated (by reduction) to form reactive cytotoxic products that damage DNA.

- **Metronidazole is the drug of choice for intestinal wall disease and amoebic liver abscess**. It is usually combined with a luminal amoebicide for these indications. It is **not a very good drug for luminal amoebiasis** *because it is almost completely absorbed* in the proximal intestine and very little amount reaches the colon.
- Metronidazole is also the **drug of choice for the treatment of trichomoniasis, giardiasis, bacterial vaginosis and pseudomembranous colitis by *C. difficile*.**
- It is also used for the treatment of infections caused by **anaerobic bacteria** like bacteroides and clostridium, and in combination therapy *H. pylori*.

Nausea, metallic taste and abdominal cramps are the most common adverse effects. It can also cause discolouration of urine, leucopenia and dizziness. Seizures can occur with the use of high dose. Opportunistic fungal infections can occur in a patient on metronidazole. It can cause **disulfiram like reaction** if used in patients taking alcohol. Metronidazole can potentiate the anticoagulant effect of coumarins. **Tinidazole, secnidazole, ornidazole and satranidazole** have similar potency and efficacy as metronidazole but are **long acting (secnidazole has longest half life)**. Satranidazole is devoid of metallic taste, neurological adverse effects as well as disulfiram like reaction.

> ⚠️ **MNEMONIC**
>
> **Metronidazole is the drug of choice for**
> **G** – Giardiasis
>   Gardernella vaginalis (Bacterial vaginosis)
>   **U** – Ulcer (Peptic ulcer) (In combination therapy for H. pylori)
>   **P** – Pseudomembranous colitis by C. difficile
>   **T** – Trichomoniasis (Strawberry vagina)
>   **A** – Ameobiasis
>   Anaerobic bacteria like Bacteroides and Clostridium

Diloxanide Furoate

It is the **drug of choice for asymptomatic intestinal amoebiasis** and is used with tissue amoebicides for extra-intestinal infections. It is also the **drug of choice for carriers**. It can cause flatulence as adverse effect.

Emetine

Emetine and dehydroemetine act by *inhibiting protein synthesis* and can be used parenterally in severe hepatic amoebiasis. Toxicity of these drugs includes **emesis, muscle weakness and cardiotoxicity** (arrhythmias and congestive heart failure). It is rarely used now.

Iodoquinol and Quinidochlor

Iodoquinol is a *luminal amoebicide* and in large doses can lead to thyroid enlargement and peripheral neuropathy. **Quinidochlor and other 8-hydroxyiodoquinolines** in high dose can cause eye defects (Subacute Myelo Optic Neuropathy or **SMON**).

Paromomycin

It is an **aminoglycoside** that can be used as luminal amoebicide. It has some activity against cryptosporidiosis in AIDS patients. **Recently** it has been **approved for the treatment of kala-azar**.

Nitazoxanide

It is a **prodrug** and is converted to tizoxanide. Latter *inhibits* the enzyme **pyruvate ferrodoxin oxidoreductase** (PFOR) which is essential for energy metabolism in anaerobic organisms. It has good activity against *cryptosporidium parvum*. It has some activity against *Entamoeba histolytica, T. Vaginalis, Ascaris, H. Nana* and metronidazole resistant *Giardia* but is approved only for the treatment of giardiasis and cryptosporidiosis.

DRUGS FOR TRYPANOSOMIASIS

Trypanosomiasis may be African or South American. African trypanosomiasis (sleeping sickness) is caused by *T. gambiense* and *T. rhodesiense*. It has an early haemolymphatic stage and in later stage CNS is involved. South American trypanosomiasis (Chagas' disease) is caused by *T. cruzi*.

Pentamidine

Its mechanism of action is not clear but it may act by interference with nucleic acid metabolism. It is *effective against early haemolymphatic stage of sleeping sickness*. It does not cross blood brain barrier, therefore is not effective against late CNS stages. It is **also used for the prophylaxis (aerosol) and treatment (i.v) of *Pneumocystis jiroveci* pneumonia and in the treatment of kala-azar**. It can cause *respiratory abnormalities, hypotension, hyperglycemia* (as well as hypoglycemia) *neutropenia and pancreatitis*.

Melarsoprol

It is an *organic arsenical* and is the **drug of choice for late stages of African trypanosomiasis**.

Other Drugs

Benznidazole is the **drug of choice for Chagas disease**.
Suramin is the drug of choice for early haemolymphatic stages of African trypanosomiasis. It is also used as an *alternative to ivermectin in onchocerciasis*.

Eflornithine is also effective in some cases of trypanosomiasis. It is also used *topically in women to dealy regrowth of facial hair following depilation*.

Trypanosomiasis	Drug of Choice
East African sleeping sickness	
Early haemo lymphatic stage	Suramin
Late CNS stage	Melarsoprol
South-American (Chagas disease)	Benznidazole (alternative is nifurtimox)

DRUGS FOR LEISHMANIASIS

- **Leishmaniasis** can be visceral (kala-azar), mucocutaneous or cutaneous. Kala azar can be diagnosed by **positive rK 39 dipstick test. Liposomal amphotericin B is the treatment of choice for visceral leishmaniasis**. Sodium stibogluconate

(pentavalent antimonial compound) is the most commonly used treatment for all forms of the disease. But it must be administered parenterally and is a cardiotoxic (cause QT prolongation) drug. The alternative agents for visceral leishmaniasis are pentamidine, miltefosine and sitamaquine. Last two drugs can be administered orally. Paromomycin has recently been approved for the treatment of kala-azar. **Miltefosine** is drug of choice for post kala-azar dermal leishmaniasis.
- Fluconazole or metronidazole can be used for cutaneous lesions and amphotericin B can be used for mucocutaneous lesions. However, sodium stibogluconate remains the first line therapy.
- Other drugs effective against leishmaniasis are ketoconazole, mepacrine and allopurinol.

DRUG OF CHOICE FOR SOME PROTOZOAL INFECTIONS

Organism	Drug of choice
Babesia	Clindamycin + Quinine
Balantidium coli	Tetracyclines
Cryptosporidium	Nitazoxanide/Paromomycin
Cyclospora	Cotrimoxazole
Isospora	Cotrimoxazole
Pneumocystis jiroveci	Cotrimoxazole
Leishmania donovani	Liposomal amphotericin B
Giardia lamblia	Metronidazole
Trichomonas vaginalis	Metronidazole
Toxoplasma gondii	Pyrimethamine + Sulfadiazine + Folinic acid
T. gondii in pregnancy	Spiramycin
Early African trypanosomiasis	Suramin
Late (CNS) African trypanosomiasis	Melasoprol
Chagas disease	Benznidazole

> **Note**
> DOC for Kala-azar – Liposomal amphotericin-B
> DOC for dermal Leishmaniasis – Miltefosine
> Most commonly used drug for Leishmania – Sodium stibogluconate

ANTI-HELMINTHIC DRUGS

Various helminthes causing human infestation are:

1. Nematodes
- Round worm (*Ascaris lumbricoides*)
- Hook worm (*Necator americanus* and *Ancylostoma duodenale*)
- Pinworm (*Enterobius vermicularis*)
- Threadworm (*Strongyloides stercoralis*)
- Filarial worm (*Wuchereria bancrofti* and *Brugia malayi, Onchocerca volvulus*)
- Whip worm (*Trichuris trichiura*)
- Trichinea worm (*Trichinella spiralis*)
- Guinea worm (*Dracunculus medinensis*)

2. Trematodes
- Blood fluke (*Schistosoma haematobium, mansoni* and *japonicum*)
- Lung fluke (*Paragonimus westermani*)
- Liver fluke (*Fasciola hepatica*)

3. Cestodes
- Pork tapeworm (*Taenia solium*)
- Beef tapeworm (*Taenia saginata*)
- Fish tapeworm (*Diphyllobothrium latum*)
- Dog tapeworm (*Echinococcus granulosus*)
- Dwarf tapeworm (*Hymenolepis nana*)

CLASSIFICATION

Based on mechanism of action, these drugs may be classified as:
- Drugs inhibiting polymerization of beta tubulin: Albendazole, mebendazole, thiabendazole, triclabendazole
- Drugs causing spastic paralysis (NN receptor agonist): Pyrantel pamoate, levamisole
- Drugs causing flaccid paralysis (GABAA agonist): Piperazine, ivermectin
- Drugs altering microfilarial membrane and increasing phagocytosis: Diethylcarbamazine (DEC)
- Drugs causing uncoupling of oxidative phosphorylation: Bithionol, niclosamide
- Drugs causing influx of calcium: Praziquantal.

IMPORTANT POINTS

- Albendazole, mebendazole and pyrantel pamoate have wide antihelminthic spectrum.
- Albendazole is the drug of choice for the treatment of all nematode infestations including cutaneous larva migrans (creeping eruption), visceral larva migrans (toxocariasis) and neurocysticercosis except enterobius (mebendazole), wuchereria and brugia (DEC), onchocerca and strongyloides (ivermectin) and dracunculus (Metronidazole).
- Praziquantal is the drug of choice for all trematode and cestode infestations except Fasciola hepatica (triclabendazole) and hydatid disease (albendazole).
- High dose albendazole if used for greater than 3 months (as for hydatid disease) may cause hepatotoxicity.
- DEC acts on both microfilaria and adult whereas ivermectin acts only on microfilaria.
- Onchocerciasis is also known as river blindness and is treated by ivermectin.
- Ivermectin should be avoided in children below 5 years old.
- Niclosamide is used for most cestodes. However it has been superseded by praziquantal for this indication.
- Ivermectin has recently been approved for topical treatment of inflammatory lesions of rosacea.

Moxidectin is a new **oral** drug for treatment of onchocerciasis. It acts by binding to glutamate and GABA chloride channels.

Golden Points

1. Isoniazid is metabolized by ACETYLATION which is genetically controlled. Slow acetylators are predisposed to peripheral neuritis.
2. Rifampicin is secreted in bile, so does not require dose adjustment in renal failure.
3. While penicillin is DOC for treatment of meningococcal meningitis, it is not indicated for prophylaxis where rifampicin (or ceftriaxone) is DOC because only rifampicin and 3rd generation cephalosporins can eliminate nasal carriers.
4. Rifampicin is the least toxic anti-tubercular drug and is also the safest drug in pregnancy.
5. Ethambutol is bacteriostatic.
6. Pyrazinamide acts only on intra-cellular mycobacteria
7. Ethambutol and streptomycin are NOT hepatotoxic.
8. Rifaximin is a rifampicin derivative indicated for Traveller's diarrhea (E. coli) and hepatic encephalopathy
9. H and Z have maximum CNS penetration whereas E and S do not cross BBB. R has moderate CNS entry.
10. MDR tuberculosis is defined as resistance to minimum H and R whereas XDR tuberculosis is defined as resistance to H and R, all fluoroquinolones and atleast one injectable agent.
11. Dapsone is the drug of choice for treatment of dermatitis herpetiformis.
12. Drug of choice for Type 1 as well as Type 2 lepra reaction is corticosteroids.
13. MC adverse effect of AMB is infusion-related reactions whereas MC dose-dependent adverse effect of AMB is nephrotoxicity.
14. Dose limiting toxicity of AMB is nephrotoxicity manifested by renal tubular acidosis, hypokalemia and hypomagnesemia.
15. Infusion of normal saline before giving AMB decreases nephrotoxicity but solution of AMB should not be made in normal saline (It is made in dextrose).
16. Fluconazole is antifungal DOC for prophylaxis whereas voriconazole is DOC for treatment of febrile neutropenia
17. Voriconazole has very wide spectrum anti-fungal action but not effective against mucormycosis.
18. Allylamines like terbinafine are oral fungicidal drugs.
19. Drug of choice for cryptococcal meningitis is amphotericin B whereas for other cryptococcal infections, it is fluconazole.
20. Oseltamivir is drug of choice for bird flu (H5N1) as well as swine flu (H1N1).
21. Abacavir increases the risk of myocardial infarction and a hypersensitivity reaction particularly in patients having HLA B*5701 allele. Testing of this allele should be done before starting abacavir.
22. Nelfinavir is the only protease inhibitor for which ritonavir boosting is not recommended.
23. All protease inhibitors can cause lipodystrophy syndrome. Atazanavir is devoid of this adverse effect.
24. Tesamorelin is a synthetic analogue of growth hormone releasing factor indicated to reduce excess abdominal fat in HIV-infected patients with lipodystrophy.
25. Exo-erythrocytic stage is absent in P. falciparum, so relapses do not occur.
26. P. falciparum do not form hypnozooites (exo-erythrocytic stage). Therefore, it does not show relapse.
27. Prolonged use of high doses of chloroquine can result in blindness due to retinal damage (Bull's eye maculopathy).
28. Primaquine is contraindicated in G-6-PD deficiency.
29. Mefloquine is effective as a single dose treatment of malaria.
30. DOC for radical cure of P. vivax malaria is primaquine
31. Proguanil potentiates the action of atovaquone
32. Artemisinins are the fastest acting drugs against malaria.
33. Diloxanide furoate is the drug of choice for asymptomatic intestinal amoebiasis
34. Satranidazole does not cause disulfiram-like reaction
35. Liposomal amphotericin B is the treatment of choice for visceral leishmaniasis.
36. Miltefosine can be administered orally for kala-azar.
37. 8-hydroxyquinolines like quiniodochlor can cause SMON
38. Albendazole is the drug of choice for the treatment of all nematode infestations including cutaneous larva migrans (creeping eruption), visceral larva migrans (toxocariasis) and neurocysticercosis except enterobius (mebendazole), wuchereria and brugia (DEC), onchocerca and strongyloides (ivermectin) and dracunculus (Metronidazole).
39. Praziquantal is the drug of choice for all trematode and cestode infestations except Fasciola hepatica (triclabendazole) and hydatid disease (albendazole).

Drug of Choice

Conditions	Drug of choice
Mycobacterial diseases	
Tuberculosis	See text
Leprosy	See text
Type 1 Lepra reaction	Corticosteroids
Type 2 Lepra reaction	Corticosteroids
M. avium intracellulare	Azithromycin + Ethambutol ± Rifabutin
M. kansasii	Isoniazid + Rifampicin ± Ethambutol
M. fortuitum chelonei	Cefoxitin + clarithromycin
Fungal diseases	
Candida albicans	Fluconazole
Candida glabrata	Caspofungin
Candida krusei	Caspofungin
Candida endocarditis	Amphotericin B (AMB)
Histoplasmosis	
Meningeal	AMB
Non-meningeal	Itraconazole
Coccidioidomycosis	AMB
Para-coccidioidomycosis	Itraconazole[1]
Sporotrichosis	Itraconazole
Blastomycosis	
Mild and Non-CNS	Itraconazole
Severe or CNS	AMB
Penicillium marneffei	Itraconazole[1]
Chromoblastomycosis	Itraconazole
Mycetoma	
Eumycetoma	Itraconazole
Actinomycetoma	Itraconazole
Cryptococcal meningitis	
Induction	AMB (for 2 weeks)
Maintenance	Fluconazole (for further 8 weeks)
Aspergillosis	
Invasive	Voriconazole
Allergic broncho-pulmonary (AMBA)	Prednisolone + Itraconazole/ Voriconazole
Mucormycosis	AMB[2]
Pseudoallescheria boydii	Voriconazole
Fusarium	Voriconazole
Exserohilum	AMB
Febrile neutropenia	
Treatment	Voriconazole
– Prophylaxis	Fluconazole

Contd...

Contd...

Viral diseases	
• Herpes simplex	
– Keratitis	Topical vidarabine/Trifluridine
– Neonatal	Acyclovir
– Encephalitis	Acyclovir
– Dissemnated	Acyclovir
– Esophagitis	Acyclovir
– Genital	Acyclovir
– Bell's Palsy	Prednisolone
• Varicella	Acyclovir
• Herpes zoster	
– Acute	Valacyclovir
– Post herpetic neuralgia	Gabapentin
• Epstein Barr virus	Symptomatic (no antiviral)
• Cytomegalo virus	
– Retinitis	Ganciclovir
– Post-transplant	
* Mild	Valganciclovir
* Severe	Ganciclovir
• Measels	Ribavirin[3]
• Prion disease	Flupirtine[4]
• Viral hemorrhagic fever	
– Lassa virus	Ribavirin
– Rift Valley fever	Ribavirin
– Congo crimean hemorrhage fever	Ribavirin
– Hantaan virus	Ribavirin
• Respiratory syncytial virus	
– High risk patient, acute	Ribavirin (aerosolized)
– Prophylaxis (infants)	Palivizumab
• Influenza virus	
– Seasonal influenza	Oseltamivir
– Avian influenza (including bird flu)	Oseltamivir
Oseltamivir-resistant influenza	Zanamivir
• Human immunodeficiency virus (HIV)	
– Treatment	Zidovudine + Lamivudine + Nevirapine
– Post-exposure prophylaxis	Zidovudine + Lamivudine ± Atazanavir
Protozoal diseases[5]	
• Ameobiasis	
– Asymptomatic intestinal	Diloxanide furoate

Contd...

Contd...

- Mild, moderate and severe intestinal — Metronidazole + diloxanide
- Extra-intestinal (hepatic abcess) — Metronidazole + diloxanide
- Primary ameobic meningo-encephalitis (*Naegleria fowleri*) — AMB
- Acanthameoba keratitis — Topical propamidine isethionate

- Coccidiosis
  - Cryptosporidiosis — Nitazoxanide/Paromomycin
  - Isoporiasis — Cotrimoxazole
  - Cyclosporiasis — Cotrimoxazole
  - Microsporidiosis — Albendazole[6]
  - Sacrocytosis — No treatment[7]

Helminthic diseases

- Flukes
  - Schistosoma — Praziquantal
  - Clonorchis — Praziquantal
  - Opisthorchis — Praziquantal
  - Paragonimus — Praziquantal
  - Fasciolopsis — Praziquantal
  - Fasciola — Triclabendazole
- Tapeworms
  - Taenia solium — Praziquantal
  - T. saginata — Praziquantal
  - D. latum — Praziquantal
  - H. nana — Praziquantal
  - Echinococcus — Albendazole

Contd...

Contd...

- Neurocysticercosis — Albendazole
- Nematodes
  - Ascaris — Albendazole
  - Trichuris — Albendazole
  - Ancylostoma — Albendazole
  - Necator — Albendazole
  - Enterobius — Albendazole
  - Trichinella — Albendazole
  - Cutaneous larva migrans — Albendazole
  - Visceral lara migrans — Albendazole
  - Dracunculus (Guinea worm) — Metronidazole
- Filarial worm
  - W. bancrofti — Di Ethyl Carbamezine (DEC)
  - B. malayi — DEC
  - B. timori — DEC
  - Loa loa — DEC
  - Onchocerca volvulus — Ivermectin
- Strongyloides stercoralis — Ivermectin

> **Note**
> 1. For severe cases, AMB is drug of choice
> 2. Posaconazole should be given after disease has stabilized
> 3. Indicated only when severe pneumonitis is present
> 4. Decreases cognitive decline but does not stop mortality
> 5. For other protozoa, see text
> 6. Fumagillin topically should be added for ocular disease
> 7. Sulfadiazine may clear cysts

Image Based Questions

1. According to mechanism of action of different anti-viral drugs (shown in the figure), which of the following is likely to be baloxavir marboxil?

   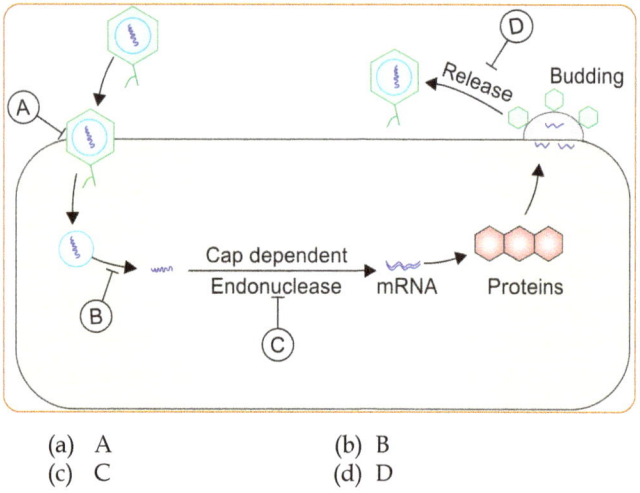

   (a) A
   (b) B
   (c) C
   (d) D

2. A patient of rheumatoid arthritis was on DMARDs since 7 years. The fundus examination revealed the features shown in the image. Which of the following is the likely drug responsible for these features?

   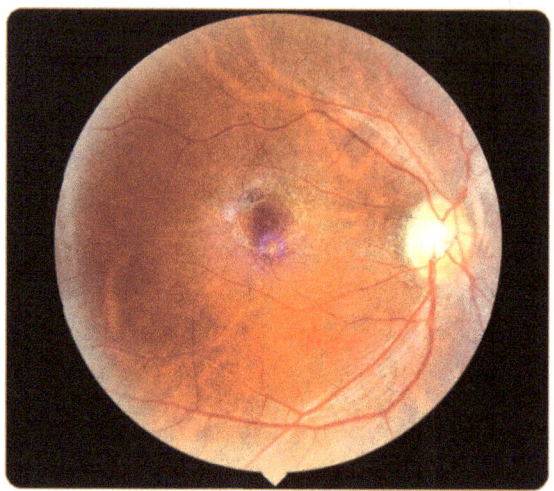

   (a) Methotrexate
   (b) Hydroxychloroquine
   (c) Leflunomide
   (d) Sulfasalazine

3. A patient of HIV developed visual problems. The fundus examination revealed the features shown in the figure. Drug of choice for treatment of this condition is:

   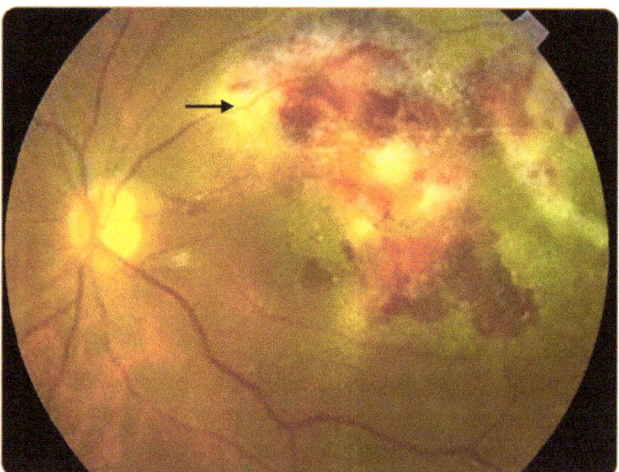

   (a) Cotrimoxazole
   (b) Ganciclovir
   (c) Acyclovir
   (d) Ceftriaxone

Explanations

1. **Ans. (c) C**
   Baloxavir marboxil is a new drug that acts by inhibiting cap-dependent endonuclease of the influenza virus.

2. **Ans. (b) Hydroxychloroquine**
   The image shows the characteristic Bull's Eye maculopathy. It is caused by chloroquine group of drugs.

3. **Ans. (b) Ganciclovir**
   The fundus shows the characteristic features of CMV retinitis. Drug of choice for this condition is ganciclovir.

Multiple Choice Questions

ANTI-MYCOBACTERIAL DRUGS

1. Which of the following is used for the treatment of paucibacillary leprosy? *(NEET Pattern 2020)*
   - (a) 2 drugs for 6 months
   - (b) 2 drugs for 12 months
   - (c) 3 drugs for 6 months
   - (d) 3 drugs for 12 months

2. Which of the following anti-tubercular drug can cause ophthalmological toxicity? *(AIIMS Nov. 2018)*
   - (a) Isoniazid
   - (b) Rifampicin
   - (c) Ethambutol
   - (d) Pyrazinamide

3. Dapsone is used for treatment of bacterial and fungal infections as well as for immunomodulatory actions. What is mechanism of dapsone for these indications? *(AIIMS Nov. 2018)*
   - (a) Inhibition of cell wall synthesis
   - (b) Inhibition of ergosterol in cell membranes
   - (c) Inhibition of protein synthesis
   - (d) Competition with PABA in folic acid synthesis

4. Which anti-tubercular drug can result in peripheral neuropathy due to deficiency of pyridoxine? *(Recent Question 2017-2018)*
   - (a) Isoniazid
   - (b) Rifampicin
   - (c) Ethambutol
   - (d) Pyrazinamide

5. In MDR TB, mycobacterium tuberculosis is resistant to: *(Recent Question 2016-17)*
   - (a) Isoniazid and Rifampicin
   - (b) Isoniazid and ethambutol
   - (c) Only Rifampcin
   - (d) Pyrazinamide and Ethambutol

6. Which of the following antitubercular drug is responsible for red green colour blindness? *(Recent Question 2016-17)*
   - (a) Rifampicin
   - (b) Isoniazid
   - (c) Pyrizinamide
   - (d) Ethambutol

7. Which of the following anti tubercular drug causes optic neuritis? *(Recent Question 2016-17)*
   - (a) Ethambutol
   - (b) Rifampicin
   - (c) Isoniazid
   - (d) Pyrazinamide

8. Ethambutol is safer in patient of: *(Recent Question 2016-17)*
   - (a) Liver disease
   - (b) Kidney disease
   - (c) Both liver and kidney diseases
   - (d) Gout

9. Antitubercular drug causing sideroblastic anemia: *(Recent Question 2016-17)*
   - (a) Ethambutol
   - (b) Rifampicin
   - (c) Isoniazid
   - (d) Pyrazinamide

10. Mutation in which of the following genes is responsible for rifampicin resistance? *(Recent Question 2016-17)*
    - (a) EpoA
    - (b) EpoRf
    - (c) RpoA
    - (d) RpoB

11. Which of the following antitubercular drug can cause hyperuricemia? *(Recent Question 2016-17)*
    - (a) Rifampicin
    - (b) Pyrazinamide
    - (c) Isoniazid
    - (d) Ethambutol

12. Which of the following is a bactericidal drug for Mycobacterium leprae? *(AIIMS May, 2017)*
    - (a) Ofloxacin
    - (b) Ciprofloxacin
    - (c) Amoxicillin
    - (d) Erythromycin

13. A 12-year-old child presents with 4 lesions of leprosy on back and four lesions on left arm. What should be the treatment of this child? *(AIIMS May, 2017)*
    - (a) [Rifampicin 600 mg + Clofazimine 300 mg] once monthly and [Dapsone 100 mg + Clofazamine 50 mg] daily
    - (b) Rifampicin 600 mg once monthly + Dapsone 100 mg daily
    - (c) [Rifampicin 450 mg + Clofazimine 150 mg] once monthly + Dapsone 50 mg daily + Clofazimine 50 mg alternate day
    - (d) Rifampicin 450 mg once monthly + Dapsone 50 mg daily

14. Which of the following statements is not true about rifabutin as compared to rifampicin? *(AIIMS Nov, 2016)*
    - (a) It has longer half-life than rifampicin
    - (b) It is more effective for newly diagnosed TB as compared to rifampicin
    - (c) It has lesser incidence of drug interactions as compared to rifampicin
    - (d) It is more effective against MAC as compared to rifampicin

15. Which of the following is the new drug for the treatment of multi drug resistant tuberculosis? *(AIIMS Nov, 2015)*
    - (a) Bedaquiline
    - (b) Linezolide
    - (c) Levofloxacin
    - (d) Cefepime

16. Which of the following antitubercular drugs is associated with hypothyroidism? *(AIIMS May, 2014)*
    - (a) Rifampicin
    - (b) Pyrazinamide
    - (c) Ethionamide
    - (d) Streptomycin

17. Pseudojaundice is an adverse effect of: *(Recent NEET Pattern Question)*
    - (a) Phenytoin
    - (b) Rifabutin
    - (c) Omeprazole
    - (d) Chlorpromazine

Chemotherapy B: Antimicrobials for Specific Conditions

18. Commonest side effect of Dapsone is:
    (a) Hemolytic anemia   *(Recent NEET Pattern Question)*
    (b) Thrombocytopenia
    (c) Cyanosis
    (d) Bone marrow depression

19. Ethambutol causes: *(Recent NEET Pattern Question)*
    (a) Retrobulbar neuritis   (b) Deafness
    (c) Red urine   (d) Peripheral neuritis

20. Which of the following antitubercular drugs is safe in hepatitis?   *(Recent NEET Pattern Question)*
    (a) Isoniazid   (b) Rifampicin
    (c) Pyrazinamide   (d) Ethambutol

21. Most effective drug against extracellular mycobacteria is:
       (Recent NEET Pattern Question)
    (a) Isoniazid   (b) Rifampicin
    (c) Pyrazinamide   (d) Ethambutol

22. Hypothyroidism is caused by which of the following anti-tubercular drug?   *(Recent NEET Pattern Question)*
    (a) Streptomycin   (b) Ethionamide
    (c) Thioacetazone   (d) Ethambutol

23. ATT causing orange coloured urine is:
       (Recent NEET Pattern Question)
    (a) Rifampicin
    (b) Isoniazid
    (c) Streptomycin
    (d) Pyrazinamide

24. Which of the following antitubercular drug is not hepatotoxic?   *(Recent NEET Pattern Question)*
    (a) Isoniazid   (b) Rifampicin
    (c) Ethionamide   (d) Streptomycin

25. Which of the following is active against atypical mycobacteria?   *(Recent NEET Pattern Question)*
    (a) Clarithromycin   (b) Rifabutin
    (c) Ciprofloxacin   (d) All of the above

26. ATT most commonly implicated in causing peripheral neuropathy is: *(Recent NEET Pattern Question)*
    (a) Rifampicin   (b) Pyrazinamide
    (c) INH   (d) Ethambutol

27. Arthralgia is commonly caused by which ATT drug?
       (Recent NEET Pattern Question)
    (a) INH   (b) Rifampicin
    (c) Pyrazinamide   (d) Ethambutol

28. Which of the following antitubercular drugs can be safely used in severe renal failure?   *(Recent NEET Pattern Question)*
    (a) Streptomycin   (b) Ethambutol
    (c) Capreomycin   (d) Rifampicin

29. A patient of multidrug resistant tuberculosis is on antitubercular drugs. After a few months he develops an inability to distinguish between red and green color. Most likely drug causing these symptoms is: *(Recent NEET Pattern Question)*
    (a) Rifampicin
    (b) Ethambutol
    (c) Cycloserine
    (d) Ethionamide

30. Which of the following drugs is useful in the treatment of infection by Mycobacterium avium complex?
       (Recent NEET Pattern Question)
    (a) Isoniazid   (b) Clarithromycin
    (c) Cycloserine   (d) Rifampicin

31. Which of the following antitubercular drugs can cause psychosis?   *(Recent NEET Pattern Question)*
    (a) Ofloxacin   (b) Cycloserine
    (c) Capreomycin   (d) Rifampicin

32. INH induced peripheral neuropathy results from deficiency of vitamin: *(Recent NEET Pattern Question)*
    (a) B_1 (b) B_2
    (c) B_6 (d) B_{12}

33. Antitubercular drug which DOES NOT cross blood brain barrier is: *(Recent NEET Pattern Question)*
    (a) Streptomycin   (b) INH
    (c) Rifampicin   (d) Pyrazinamide

34. Which of the following antitubercular drugs can be used in patients with hepatic dysfunction?
       (Recent NEET Pattern Question)
    (a) Streptomycin   (b) INH
    (c) Pyrazinamide   (d) Rifampicin

35. INH can be used safely in the presence of:
       (Recent NEET Pattern Question)
    (a) Jaundice   (b) Chronic renal failure
    (c) Epilepsy   (d) Coronary artery disease

36. Which of the following antitubercular drug is preferred in severe liver disease?   *(Recent NEET Pattern Question)*
    (a) Streptomycin + Isoniazid
    (b) Streptomycin + Ethambutol
    (c) Isoniazid + Rifampicin
    (d) Rifamicin + Ethambutol

37. Which of the following ATT has maximum CSF penetration?   *(Recent NEET Pattern Question)*
    (a) Streptomycin   (b) INH
    (c) Rifampicin   (d) Ethambutol

38. Common dose dependent side effects of ethambutol is:
       (Recent NEET Pattern Question)
    (a) Red-urine   (b) Optic neuritis
    (c) Nephropathy   (d) Peripheral neuropathy

39. Most common drug used in Leprosy is:
       (Recent NEET Pattern Question)
    (a) Dapsone   (b) Clofazimine
    (c) Ethionamide   (d) Ofloxacin

40. The bacterial drug resistance in tuberculosis results from:
       (Recent NEET Pattern Question)
    (a) Transduction   (b) Transformation
    (c) Plasmid mediated   (d) Mutation

41. INH and pyridoxine are given together in antituberculous chemotherapy: *(Recent NEET Pattern Question)*
    (a) To prevent peripheral neuritis
    (b) To prevent emergence of INH resistance
    (c) As a nutrient supplement
    (d) As a synergistic combination

42. Bacteriostatic antitubercular drug among the following is: *(Recent NEET Pattern Question)*
    (a) Isoniazid (b) Rifampin
    (c) Streptomycin (d) Ethambutol

43. Dapsone is used in all *except*: *(Recent NEET Pattern Question)*
    (a) Dermatitis herpetiformis
    (b) Leprosy
    (c) Pneumocystis jiroveci pneumonia
    (d) Tuberculosis

44. In Lepra reaction, the drug useful is: *(Recent NEET Pattern Question)*
    (a) Pencillins (b) Clofazimine
    (c) Dapsone (d) Rifampicin

45. Antitubercular drug that can cause hyperuricemia is: *(Recent NEET Pattern Question)*
    (a) Rifampicin (b) INH
    (c) Pyrazinamide (d) Streptomycin

46. Treatment of lepromatous leprosy is: *(Recent NEET Pattern Question)*
    (a) Rifampicin + Dapsone
    (b) Rifampicin + Clofazimine
    (c) Rifampicin + Dapsone + Clofazimine
    (d) Rifampicin + Ofloxacin + Minocycline

47. Ethambutol should be used very cautiously in childhood tuberculosis due to which of its side effect? *(Recent NEET Pattern Question)*
    (a) Ocular toxicity (b) Renal damage
    (c) Hepatotoxicity (d) Neurotoxicity

48. Which of the following drugs can produce dramatic improvement in patients with Type II lepra reaction? *(Recent NEET Pattern Question)*
    (a) Thalidomide (b) Steroids
    (c) Dapsone (d) Clofazamine

49. Mechanism of action of rifampicin is: *(Recent NEET Pattern Question)*
    (a) Inhibition of mycolic acid synthesis
    (b) DNA dependent RNA polymerase inhibition
    (c) Protein synthesis inhibition
    (d) Inhitits synthesis of arabinogalactone

50. Drug that crosses placenta is: *(Recent NEET Pattern Question)*
    (a) Isoniazid (b) Rifampicin
    (c) Pyrazinamide (d) All

51. Treatment of Mycobacteria avium complex include all *except*: *(Recent NEET Pattern Question)*
    (a) Ciprofloxacin (b) Clarithromycin
    (c) Rifabutin (d) Pyrazinamide

52. Which one of the following drugs is not used in the treatment of mycobacterium avium intercellulare infection? *(Recent NEET Pattern Question)*
    (a) Clarithromycin (b) Eflornithine
    (c) Ethambutol (d) Rifabutin

53. Most important side effect of ethambutol is: *(Recent NEET Pattern Question)*
    (a) Hepatotoxicity (b) Renal toxicity
    (c) Peripheral neuropathy (d) Retrobulbar neuritis

54. The following drugs are useful in the treatment of isoniazid poisoning: *(Recent NEET Pattern Question)*
    (a) Pyridoxine (b) Diazepam
    (c) Bicarbonate (d) All of the above

55. Treatment of lepra reaction includes: *(Recent NEET Pattern Question)*
    (a) Chloroquine (b) Corticosteroids
    (c) Stoppage of drug (d) All of above

56. Leprosy treatment includes following drugs *except*: *(Recent NEET Pattern Question)*
    (a) Dapsone (b) Rifampicin
    (c) Penicillin (d) Clofazimine

57. Which fluoroquinolone is highly active against Mycobacterium leprae and is being used in alternative multidrug therapy regimens? *(Recent NEET Pattern Question)*
    (a) Norfloxacin (b) Ofloxacin
    (c) Ciprofloxacin (d) Lomefloxacin

58. The tetracycline with highest antileprotic activity is: *(Recent NEET Pattern Question)*
    (a) Minocycline (b) Doxycycline
    (c) Demeclocycline (d) Oxytetracycline

59. Which of the following drugs was initially developed as an antitubercular drug, but later found to have mood elevating properties? *(Recent NEET Pattern Question)*
    (a) Isoniazid (b) Selegeline
    (c) Fluoxetine (d) Lithium

60. Drug used in prophylaxis of H. influenzae is: *(Recent NEET Pattern Question)*
    (a) Doxycycline (b) Rifampicin
    (c) Erythromycin (d) None

61. Which anti-tubercular drug cause pneumonia like syndrome? *(Recent NEET Pattern Question)*
    (a) INH (b) Rifampicin
    (c) Ethambutol (d) Pyrazinamide

62. Maximum sterilising action is shown by which anti TB drug? *(Recent NEET Pattern Question)*
    (a) Rifampicin (b) INH
    (c) Pyrazinamide (d) Streptomycin

63. Slow acetylators of isoniazid are more prone to develop: *(Recent NEET Pattern Question)*
    (a) Failure of therapy (b) Peripheral neuropathy
    (c) Hepatotoxicity (d) Allergic reactions

64. The adverse reaction that absolutely contraindicates further use of rifampicin in the treatment of tuberculosis: *(Recent NEET Pattern Question)*
    (a) Respiratory syndrome
    (b) Cutaneous syndrome
    (c) Flu like syndrome
    (d) Abdominal syndrome

65. ATT drug causing contact lens staining is: *(Recent NEET Pattern Question)*
    (a) INH (b) Rifampicin
    (c) Pyrazinamide (d) Thioacetazone

Chemotherapy B: Antimicrobials for Specific Conditions

66. Anti-tubercular drug associated with psychosis is:
    (Recent NEET Pattern Question)
    (a) INH (b) Rifampicin
    (c) Ethambutol (d) Streptomycin

67. Oral contraceptive (OCP) failure by rifampicin is due to:
    (Recent NEET Pattern Question)
    (a) Decreased absorption of OCPs
    (b) Increased binding of OCPs by rifampicin and reduced free drug concentration
    (c) Increased metabolism of OCPs
    (d) Increased chances of ovulation due to rifampicin

68. Dapsone is used in: *(Recent NEET Pattern Question)*
    (a) Dermatitis herpetiformis
    (b) Pityriasis rosacea
    (c) Contact dermatitis
    (d) Oculocutaneous albinism

69. Drug causing icthyosis and hyperpigmentation, when used in leprosy is: *(Recent NEET Pattern Question)*
    (a) Rifampicin (b) Dapsone
    (c) Clofazimine (d) Ethionamide

70. Antitubercular drug which reaches inside the caseous material is? *(Recent NEET Pattern Question)*
    (a) Isoniazid (b) Rifampicin
    (c) Pyrazinamide (d) Ethambutol

71. Side effects of isoniazid are all *except*:
    (Recent NEET Pattern Question)
    (a) Hepatitis (b) Optic neuritis
    (c) Peripheral neuropathy (d) Thrombocytopenia

72. Which of the following is a bacteriostatic antitubercular drug? *(Recent NEET Pattern Question)*
    (a) Streptomycin (b) Ethambutol
    (c) Isoniazid (d) Rifampicin

73. All are true about rifampicin *except*:
    (Recent NEET Pattern Question)
    (a) Microsomal enzyme inducer
    (b) Used in treatment of meningiococcal meningitis
    (c) May cause OCP failure
    (d) Bactericidal in nature

74. Rifampicin acts by inhibiting:
    (Recent NEET Pattern Question)
    (a) DNA dependent RNA polymerase
    (b) RNA dependent DNA polymerase
    (c) Mycolic acid inhibition
    (d) Mycolic acid incorporation defects

75. The most effective antitubercular drug against slow multiplying intracellular mycobacteria is:
    (Recent NEET Pattern Question)
    (a) Rifampicin (b) Isoniazid
    (c) Pyrazinamide (d) Ethambutol

76. Which vitamin is most likely to be deficient in patients on treatment with isoniazid?
    (Recent NEET Pattern Question)
    (a) Vitamin B_1 (b) Vitamin B_2
    (c) Vitamin B_6 (d) Vitamin B_{12}

77. MDR tuberculosis is defined by:
    (Recent NEET Pattern Question)
    (a) Resistance to all first and second line anti-tubercular agents
    (b) Resistance to any three first line anti-tubercular agents
    (c) Resistance to all first line and any three classes of second line anti-tubercular agents
    (d) Resistance to isoniazid and rifampicin

78. Isoniazid induced peripheral neuropathy responds to administrations of: *(Recent NEET Pattern Question)*
    (a) Pyridoxine (b) Riboflavin
    (c) Thiamine (d) Cobalamin

79. Which of the following anti-tubercular agent does not cause hepato-toxicity? *(Recent NEET Pattern Question)*
    (a) Isoniazid (b) Rifampicin
    (c) Ethambutol (d) Pyrazinamide

80. All of the following can cause visual adverse effects *except*: *(Recent NEET Pattern Question)*
    (a) Ethambutol (b) Rifampicin
    (c) Chloroquine (d) Digoxin

81. Drug resistance in Mycobacterium tuberculosis is due to:
    (Recent NEET Pattern Question)
    (a) Conjugation (b) Transduction
    (c) Mutation (d) None of the above

82. Which one of the anti-tubercular drug may precipitate gout? *(Recent NEET Pattern Question)*
    (a) Pyrazinamide (b) Rifampicin
    (c) Streptomycin (d) Isoniazid

83. Which one of the following therapies would be safe in a patient with pulmonary tuberculosis having markedly abnormal liver function? *(Recent NEET Pattern Question)*
    (a) Streptomycin + isoniazid
    (b) Ethambutol + isoniazid
    (c) Rifampicin + isoniazid
    (d) Streptomycin + ethambutol

84. Antitubercular drug which should not be given to a patient having both tuberculosis as well as AIDS is:
    (Recent NEET Pattern Question)
    (a) INH (b) Pyrazinamide
    (c) Ethambutol (d) Thiacetazone

85. Which of the following drugs is not used in the treatment of leprosy? *(Recent NEET Pattern Question)*
    (a) Rifampicin (b) Dapsone
    (c) Kanamycin (d) Clofazimine

86. Fastest acting drug on the lepra bacilli is:
    (Recent NEET Pattern Question)
    (a) Rifampicin (b) Dapsone
    (c) Kanamycin (d) Clofazimine

87. Dapsone is used in the treatment of:
    (Recent NEET Pattern Question)
    (a) Malaria (b) Dermatitis herpetiformis
    (c) TB (d) Kala-azar

88. Which of the following is the major side effect of rifampicin? *(Recent NEET Pattern Question)*
    (a) Renal failure
    (b) Hepatotoxicity
    (c) Bone marrow suppression
    (d) Blood dyscrasias

89. Which of the following anti TB drugs can be safely given in a patient with renal failure?
    (Recent NEET Pattern Question)
    (a) INH   (b) Rifampicin
    (c) Streptomycin   (d) Kanamycin

90. ATT safe in hepatic failure are:
    (Recent NEET Pattern Question)
    (a) Pyrazinamide and ethambutol
    (b) INH and Rifampicin
    (c) Streptomycin and Ethambutol
    (d) Rifampicin and Streptomycin

91. Optic neuritis is caused by:
    (a) Ethambutol   (b) INH
    (c) Rifampicin   (d) Chlormycetin

92. The following anti T.B. drug should not be given to AIDS patient: *(Recent NEET Pattern Question)*
    (a) Rifampicin   (b) Ethambutol
    (c) Streptomycin   (d) Pyrazinamide

93. Which of the following drugs results in the production of orange coloured urine? *(Recent NEET Pattern Question)*
    (a) Rifampicin   (b) Isoniazid
    (c) Pyrazinamide   (d) Ethambutol

94. Least hepatotoxic anti TB drug is:
    (Recent NEET Pattern Question)
    (a) Ethambutol   (b) Rifampicin
    (c) Pyrazinamide   (d) Isoniazid

ANTI-FUNGAL AND ANTIVIRAL (EXCEPT HIV) DRUGS

95. Which of the following drugs is used as nail lacquer for fungal infections? *(NEET Pattern 2020)*
    (a) Fluconazole   (b) Nystatin
    (c) Itraconazole   (d) Terbinafine

96. Drug of choice for invasive aspergillosis is:
    (NEET Pattern 2020)
    (a) Posaconazole   (b) Voriconazole
    (c) Liposomal AMB   (d) Caspofungin

97. Which of the following is True or False regarding drugs used for viral infections? *(AIIMS Nov. 2020)*
    (a) Treatment of HCV with ribavirin is considered better than sofosbuvir
    (b) Ombitasvir is inhibitor of proteins synthesis
    (c) Imiquimod is used for Condyloma acuminata
    (d) Simprevir inhibits protease of hepatitis C
    (e) Oseltamivir is used for swine flu

98. Which of the following statements regarding foscarnet are True or False? *(AIIMS Nov. 2019)*
    (a) It is used for resistant CMV infections
    (b) Renal toxicity is seen
    (c) It is activated by viral thymidine kinase
    (d) Regular monitoring of serum electrolytes is required
    (e) It can cause genital ulceration

99. Which of the following is wrongly matched regarding mechanism of action of anti-fungal drugs?
    (AIIMS May 2018)
    (a) Azoles: Inhibit lanosterol alpha demethylase thereby preventing ergosterol synthesis
    (b) Flucytosine: Inhibits microtubule thereby preventing mitosis
    (c) Echinocandins: Inhibit glycan synthesis by inhibiting beta 1,3 glycan synthase
    (d) Amphotericin B: Impair barrier mechanism in cell membrane

100. Mechanism of action of oseltamivir is:
     (NEET Pattern 2019)
     (a) Neuraminidase inhibition
     (b) Inhibit thymidylate synthase
     (c) Inhibit RNA transcription
     (d) Inhibit uncoating of the virus

101. Mechanism of action of triazoles is:
     (NEET Pattern 2019)
     (a) Inhibit ergosterol synthesis
     (b) Inhibit mitotic spindle
     (c) Create pores in the membrane
     (d) Inhibit beta 1,3 glycan

102. Amphotericin B produce antifungal action by acting on:
     (Recent Question 2017-2018)
     (a) Cell membrane   (b) Cell wall
     (c) Ribosome   (d) Nucleic acid

103. Mechanism of action of oseltamivir is:
     (a) Neuraminidase inhibitor *(AIIMS May 2017)*
     (b) Blocks M2 protein
     (c) Apoptosis of respiratory epithelial cells
     (d) Block DNA dependent RNA polymerase

104. A diabetic patient presents with fungal infection of sinuses and peri-orbital region with significant visual impairment. The best drug for treatment of this patient is:
     (a) Amphotericin B   *(AIIMS May 2014)*
     (b) Itraconazole
     (c) Ketoconazole
     (d) Broad spectrum antibiotics

105. Griseofulvin is not useful in one of the following:
     (Recent NEET Pattern Question)
     (a) Tinea capitis   (b) Tinea cruris
     (c) Tinea versicolor (d) Tinea pedis

106. Avian influenza is treated by:
     (Recent NEET Pattern Question)
     (a) Amantadine   (b) Ribavarin
     (c) Cidofovir   (d) Oseltamivir

107. Amphotericin-B is obtained from:
     (Recent NEET Pattern Question)
     (a) Streptomyces nodosus   (b) Streptomyces pimprina
     (c) Streptomyces nousseri (d) Streptomyces fragilis

108. Which of the following is NOT true about anti-fungal drugs? *(Recent NEET Pattern Question)*
     (a) Amphotericin B is given only parenterally
     (b) Griseofulvin is effective orally
     (c) Ciclopirox olamine is effective in systemic mycoses
     (d) Fluconazole is effective orally as well as i.v.

Chemotherapy B: Antimicrobials for Specific Conditions

109. **Topically used antifungal agent is:**
     (Recent NEET Pattern Question)
     (a) Ketoconazole (b) Clotrimazole
     (c) Amphotericin B (d) Physostigmine

110. **Which of the following is a broad spectrum systemic antifungal agent?** *(Recent NEET Pattern Question)*
     (a) Econazole (b) Miconazole
     (c) Ketoconazole (d) Clotrimazole

111. **Which of the following anti-metabolites act as an antifungal agent?** *(Recent NEET Pattern Question)*
     (a) Paclitaxel (b) 5-Flucytosine (5 FC)
     (c) Chlorambucil (d) Decarbazine

112. **Drug of choice for herpes simplex virus infection is:**
     (Recent NEET Pattern Question)
     (a) Acyclovir (b) Zidovudine
     (c) Indinavir (d) Ribavarin

113. **All can be used for systematic fungal infections *except*:**
     (Recent NEET Pattern Question)
     (a) Ketoconazole (b) Fluconazole
     (c) Amphotericin B (d) Griseofulvin

114. **Drug of choice for chronic hepatitis B is:**
     (Recent NEET Pattern Question)
     (a) Lamivudine (b) IFN-alpha
     (c) Ribavirin (d) Zidovudine

115. **All are effective against Tinea versicolor *except*:**
     (All India 2002)
     (a) Fluconaozole (b) Clotrimazole
     (c) Ketoconazole (d) Griseofulvin

116. **Drugs that can be used to treat candida infection are all *except*:** *(Recent NEET Pattern Question)*
     (a) Ketoconazole (b) Nystatin
     (c) Amphotericin (d) Griseofulvin

117. **Which of the following anti-fungal drugs has only topical action?** *(Recent NEET Pattern Question)*
     (a) Fluconazole (b) Ketoconazole
     (c) Itraconazole (d) Clotrimazole

118. **Drug that can cause complete histopathological resolution in patients with hepatitis B is:**
     (Recent NEET Pattern Question)
     (a) Cyclosporine (b) Ribavarin
     (c) Entecavir (d) None of the above

119. **Mechanism of action of terbinafine is:**
     (a) Binds to ergosterol *(Recent NEET Pattern Question)*
     (b) Prevents formation of purine
     (c) Inhition of microtubule formation
     (d) Inhibition of ergosterol synthesis

120. **In dermatophytosis, which antifungal drug is not indicated:** *(Recent NEET Pattern Question)*
     (a) Fluconazole (b) Terbinafine
     (c) Griseofulvin (d) Amphotericin B

121. **Treatment of choice for coccidiodomycosis is:**
     (Recent NEET Pattern Question)
     (a) Amphotericin (b) Fluconazole
     (c) Flucytosine (d) Griseofulvin

122. **Most serious adverse effect of ketoconazole is:**
     (a) Adrenal insufficiency *(Recent NEET Pattern Question)*
     (b) Pellagra like skin lesion
     (c) Liver injury
     (d) Prostate cancer

123. **Induction of treatment in serious fungal infections is mostly done by:** *(Recent NEET Pattern Question)*
     (a) IV amphotericin B (b) Ketoconazole
     (c) 5 – Flucytosine (d) Fluconazole

124. **Which one of the statements is false regarding adefovir dipivoxil?** *(Recent NEET Pattern Question)*
     (a) Acyclic nucleotide analogue
     (b) Well tolerated orally
     (c) Used in chronic hepatitis B infection
     (d) Used in anti-retroviral therapy

125. **Drug of choice for Herpes simplex encephalitis is:**
     (a) 5-Hydroxy deoxyuridine (5-HU)
     (b) Acyclovir *(Recent NEET Pattern Question)*
     (c) Gancyclovir
     (d) None of the above

126. **Which of the following is oral drug for treatment of hepatitis C?** *(AIIMS Nov 2015)*
     (a) Ledipasvir (b) Peg-interferon
     (c) Lamivudine (d) Ribamivir

127. **All of the following drugs are useful in swine flu *except*:** *(AIIMS Nov 2015)*
     (a) Oseltamivir (b) Peramivir
     (c) Zanamivir (d) Abacavir

128. **Which of the following has poorest oral bioavailability?**
     (Recent NEET Pattern Question)
     (a) Oseltamivir (b) Zanamivir
     (c) Rimantidine (d) Amantadine

129. **Drug of choice for acyclovir resistant herpes is:**
     (Recent NEET Pattern Question)
     (a) Cidofovir (b) Gancyclovir
     (c) Valacyclovir (d) Foscarnet

130. **Cidofovir can be used for:** *(Recent NEET Pattern Question)*
     (a) Respiratory papillomatosis
     (b) Herpes simplex
     (c) CMV
     (d) All of the above

131. **Antifungal used as cancer chemotherapeutic agent is:**
     (Recent NEET Pattern Question)
     (a) Flucytosine (b) Nystatin
     (c) Voriconazole (d) Terbinafine

132. **The drug used to treat acyclovir resistant Herpes Simplex Virus (HSV) and Varicella Zoster Virus (VZV) infection is:** *(Recent NEET Pattern Question)*
     (a) Foscarnet (b) Valacyclovir
     (c) Abacavir (d) Ganciclovir

133. **Oseltamivir dose is** *(Recent NEET Pattern Question)*
     (a) 75 mg BD x 5 days orally
     (b) 75 mg BD x 5 days IV
     (c) 200 mg BD x 5 days orally
     (d) 200 mg BD x 5 days IV

134. Acyclovir is used in: *(Recent NEET Pattern Question)*
    (a) Herpes keratitis (b) CMV retinitis
    (c) Hepatitis C (c) Hepatitis B

135. The antifungal which has a bactericidal mode of action against dermatophyte infections in therapeutic doses is:
    (Recent NEET Pattern Question)
    (a) Fluconazole (b) Terbinafine
    (c) Itraconazole (d) Ketoconazole

136. Drug of choice in herpes simplex encephalitis is:
    (Recent NEET Pattern Question)
    (a) Acyclovir (b) Vidarabine
    (c) Interferon (d) Amantadine

137. Antifungal drug used for systemic fungal infection is:
    (Recent NEET Pattern Question)
    (a) Griseofulvin (b) Clotrimazole
    (c) Amphotericin B (d) Econazole

138. Acyclovir is used for the following viral infection:
    (a) Rabies virus *(Recent NEET Pattern Question)*
    (b) Cytomegalovirus
    (c) Herpes simplex virus
    (d) Human immunodeficiency virus

139. Acyclovir is given in: *(Recent NEET Pattern Question)*
    (a) Enteric fever (b) Malaria
    (c) Herpes infection (d) Bacillary dysentery

140. Drug of choice for herpes simplex keratitis is:
    (Recent NEET Pattern Question)
    (a) Acyclovir (b) Ganciclovir
    (c) Amantadine (d) Interferon

ANTI-HIV DRUGS

141. A nurse got accidental prick from the HIV infected needle. Which of the following statements is false regarding the management of this nurse? *(AIIMS Nov. 2019)*
    (a) Zidovudine is used as monotherapy for post-exposure prophylaxis
    (b) Washing hands with soap and water is advised
    (c) Baseline viral markers of healthcare personnel should be done at the time of prick
    (d) Follow up viral markers of healthcare personnel should be measured at 6 weeks

142. A patient of HIV is on treatment with indinavir, zidovudine, lamivudine and ketoconazole. He developed nephrolithiasis, hyperlipidemia, central obesity, hyperglycemia and insulin resistance. *(AIIMS Nov. 2018)*
    (a) Lamivudine (b) Indinavir
    (c) Zidovudine (d) Ketoconazole

143. Which of the following is most appropriate treatment of a patient of tuberculosis in which mycobacterium is resistant to both isoniazid and rifampicin?
    (AIIMS Nov. 2018)
    (a) 6 drugs for 4 months and 4 drugs for 12 months
    (b) 6 drugs for 6 months and 4 drugs for 18 months
    (c) 6 drugs for 6 months and 4 drugs for 4 months
    (d) 5 drugs for 2 months, 4 drugs for one month and 3 drugs for 5 months

144. Which of the following statements regarding mechanism of action of anti-HIV drugs is correct? *(AIIMS May 2018)*
    (a) Enfuvirtide binds to Gp 120 and CCR5
    (b) Raltegravir inhibits integrase enzyme
    (c) Ritonavir inhibits HIV reverse transcriptase
    (d) Tenofovir is the protease inhibitor of HIV

145. Which of the following drug has dual action on HIV and hepatitis B virus? *(Recent Question 2017-2018)*
    (a) Enfuvirtide (b) Emtricitabine
    (c) Abacavir (d) Acyclovir

146. Mechanism of action of protease inhibitors is:
    (AIIMS May 2017)
    (a) Prevents maturation of new viral particles
    (b) Prevents translation of viral RNA
    (c) Causes apoptosis of the affected cells
    (d) Inhibits proviral RNA synthesis

147. Which of the following drug acts by inhibiting the protease enzyme of HIV? *(AIIMS May 2015)*
    (a) Saquinavir (b) Nevirapine
    (c) Abacavir (d) Enfuvirtide

148. Non-nucleoside reverse transcriptase inhibitors (NNRTIs) include all of the following *except:* *(AIIMS May 2014)*
    (a) Nevirapine (b) Delavirdine
    (c) Etravirine (d) Lamivudine

149. All of the following drugs have activity against hepatitis B virus *except:* *(AIIMS Nov 2014)*
    (a) Lamivudine (b) Zidovudine
    (c) Emtricitabine (d) Telbivudine

150. All of the following are common adverse effects of HAART therapy *except:* *(AI 2012)*
    (a) Steatosis (b) Lipodytrophy
    (c) Optic neuritis (d) Increased cholesterol

151. A person is being treated for Human Immunodeficiency Virus-1. He developed hypertriglyceridemia and hypercholesterolemia. Most likely drug implicated for these adverse effects is: *(AI 2012)*
    (a) Ritonavir (b) Raltegravir
    (c) Didanosine (d) Efavirenz

152. Which of the following drug is a reverse transcriptase inhibitor? *(Recent NEET Pattern Question)*
    (a) Indinavir (b) Ritonavir
    (c) Nelfinavir (d) Abacavir

153. The basis of combining ritonavir with lopinavir:
    (Recent NEET Pattern Question)
    (a) Pharmaceutical compatibility
    (b) CYP3A4 inhibition by ritonavir
    (c) Long elimination half life of ritonavir
    (d) Ability to counteract side-effects of lopinavir

154. Zidovudine and didanosine used in HAART act by:
    (Recent NEET Pattern Question)
    (a) Inhibitory effects on viral DNA
    (b) Nucleoside reverse transcriptase inhibition
    (c) Inhibit the synthesis of gp41
    (d) Protease inhibition

155. Zidovudine causes: *(Recent NEET Pattern Question)*
    (a) Neurotoxicity (b) Nephrotoxicity
    (c) Neutropenia (d) Ototoxicity

Chemotherapy B: Antimicrobials for Specific Conditions

156. Antiviral drug having dual antiviral activity against HIV and HBV is: *(Recent NEET Pattern Question)*
    (a) Enfuvirtide (b) Emtricitabine
    (c) Abacavir (d) Entecavir

157. Which of the following statements about lamivudine is FALSE? *(Recent NEET Pattern Question)*
    (a) Possess Anti–HIV and anti-HBV activity
    (b) Dose lower for blocking HIV replication than HBV replication
    (c) Should not be used as monotherapy in HBV/HIV infected patients
    (d) Anti-HBe seroconversion occurs in minority of patients

158. Which of the following is most common side effect of zidovudine? *(Recent NEET Pattern Question)*
    (a) Anemia (b) Peripheral neuropathy
    (c) Lactic acidosis (d) All

159. A laboratory technician was accidentally exposed to a HIV serum positive sample, which of the following shall be the role of zidovudine in treatment of this patient? *(Recent NEET Pattern Question)*
    (a) Protects against acquiring the HIV infection
    (b) Makes the patient seronegative
    (c) Delays the progression of disease
    (d) None

160. Prophylactic therapy should be started against Pneumocystis carinii pneumonia in AIDS patients with CD4 counts below: *(Recent NEET Pattern Question)*
    (a) < 50/microL (b) < 150/microL
    (c) < 200/microL (d) < 400/microL

161. Which of the following anti-HIV drug should never be given as rechallange once history of producing allergic reaction with drug is known? *(Recent NEET Pattern Question)*
    (a) Lamivudine (b) Abacavir
    (c) Zidovudine (d) Nelfinavir

162. All are protease inhibitor *except*: *(Recent NEET Pattern Question)*
    (a) Ritonavir (b) Amprenavir
    (c) Tenofovir (d) Nelfinavir

163. Which protease inhibtor has boosting effect? *(Recent NEET Pattern Question)*
    (a) Amprenavir (b) Tenovir
    (c) Nelfinavir (d) Ritonavir

164. Which of the following is a protease inhibitor? *(Recent NEET Pattern Question)*
    (a) Lamivudine (b) Saquinavir
    (c) Delavirdine (d) Zidovudine

165. Following drugs act against HIV-2 *except*: *(Recent NEET Pattern Question)*
    (a) Ritonavir (b) Tenofovir
    (c) Efavirenz (d) Zalcitabine

166. Enfuvirtide belongs to the class of: *(Recent NEET Pattern Question)*
    (a) Fusion inhibitors
    (b) Protease inhibitors
    (c) Gp 120 inhibitors
    (d) Nucleotide reverse transcriptase inhibitors

167. Drug which produces Steven Johnson's syndrome in HIV infected individuals is: *(Recent NEET Pattern Question)*
    (a) Paraaminosalicylate (b) Cycloserine
    (c) Thioacetazone (d) Rifampicin

168. In anti retroviral therapy, Zidovudine should not be combined with: *(Recent NEET Pattern Question)*
    (a) Lamivudine (b) Nevirapine
    (c) Didanosine (d) Stavudine

169. The HIV fusion inhibitor, enfuvirtide, acts at the site of: *(Recent NEET Pattern Question)*
    (a) Gp 120 (b) Gp 41
    (c) P24 (d) CXCR4

170. Viral HIV integrase inhibitor is: *(Recent NEET Pattern Question)*
    (a) Zidovudine (b) Maroviroc
    (c) Raltegravir (d) Enfuvirtide

171. All the following antiretroviral drugs produce dyslipidemia *except*: *(Recent NEET Pattern Question)*
    (a) Atazanavir (b) Saquinavir
    (c) Amprenavir (d) Nelfinavir

172. Peripheral neuropathy not caused by which anti-retroviral drug? *(Recent NEET Pattern Question)*
    (a) Lamivudine
    (b) Didanosine
    (c) Zidovudine
    (d) Zalcitabine

173. Which of the following is a reverse transcriptase inhibitor? *(Recent NEET Pattern Question)*
    (a) Ritonavir (b) Saquanavir
    (c) Amprenavir (d) Tenofovir

174. Pancreatitis is a common complication of which one of the following: *(Recent NEET Pattern Question)*
    (a) Zidovudine (b) Didanosine
    (c) Zalcitabine (d) Stavudine

175. All of the following are anti HIV agents *except*: *(Recent NEET Pattern Question)*
    (a) Ritonavir (b) Acyclovir
    (c) Didanosine (d) Zidovudine

176. All of the following are HIV protease inhibitors *except*: *(Recent NEET Pattern Question)*
    (a) Saquinavir (b) Atazanavir
    (c) Abacavir (d) Amprenavir

177. The other name for reverse transcriptase is: *(Recent NEET Pattern Question)*
    (a) DNA dependent DNA polymerase
    (b) RNA dependent RNA polymerase
    (c) DNA dependent RNA polymerase
    (d) RNA dependent DNA polymerase

178. The minimum period required for post-exposure chemoprophylaxis for HIV is: *(Recent NEET Pattern Question)*
    (a) 4 weeks (b) 6 weeks
    (c) 8 weeks (d) 12 weeks

ANTI-MALARIAL DRUGS

179. Which of the following is clinical use of tafenoquine?
     (AIIMS Nov. 2019)
     (a) Radical cure of Plasmodium vivax malaria
     (b) Prophylaxis of malaria in pregnancy
     (c) Treatment of severe falciparum malaria
     (d) Treatment of endemic malaria in children < 2 years

180. Mention the true/false statements about drug resistant malaria: *(AIIMS Nov. 2019)*
     (a) Not present in India
     (b) Quinine with clindamycin or doxycycline is still effective treatment
     (c) Chloroquine with sulfadoxine-pyrimethamine is effective
     (d) Artemether with lumefantrine is useful
     (e) Monotherapy with artemisinin derivatives is not useful due to high risk of recrudescence

181. Which of the following drug has gametocidal action against all species of Plasmodium? *(AIIMS Nov. 2018)*
     (a) Primaquine
     (b) Chloroquine
     (c) Quinine
     (d) None of these

182. A patient from north-eastern states was diagnosed to have infection with P. falciparum malaria. What is the most appropriate drug for this patient? *(AIIMS May 2018)*
     (a) Artemether plus lumefantrine
     (b) Sulfadoxine plus pyrimethamine
     (c) Chloroquine
     (d) Mefloquine

183. Dose of Mefloquine in adults for Malaria prophylaxis:
     (Recent Question 2016-17)
     (a) 150 mg   (b) 250 mg
     (c) 300 mg   (d) 500 mg

184. All of the following are adverse effects of quinine *except*:
     (Recent Question 2016-17)
     (a) Hypotension   (b) Hypoglycemia
     (c) Bull's eye retinopathy (d) Arrhythmias

185. Fastest acting erythrocytic schizontocidal drug for malaria is:
     (a) Primaquine   (b) Pyrimethamine
     (c) Artemisinin   (d) Proguanil

186. According to the new WHO 2013 malaria treatment guidelines, which of the following statements is true?
     (AIIMS Nov 2015)
     (a) ACT should not be used in falciparum malaria
     (b) Presumptive treatment with chloroquine should be given
     (c) Primaquine is contraindicated in infants and pregnant women
     (d) Primaquine is to be given for 7 days in falciparum malaria

187. Most effective treatement for severe malaria is:
     (AIIMS Nov. 2014)
     (a) Artesunate   (b) Chloroquine
     (c) Quinine   (d) Primaquine

188. The development of resistance to conventional treatment has led WHO to recommend the use of combination therapies containing artemisinin derivative (artemisinin-based combination therapies also known as ACTs). All of the following combination therapies are recommended if such resistance is suspected, *except*:
     (Recent NEET Pattern Question)
     (a) Artemether plus lumefantrine
     (b) Artesunate plus quinine
     (c) Artesunate plus pyrimethamine-sulfadoxine
     (d) Artesunate plus mefloquine

189. Chloroquine is used in the treatment of:
     (Recent NEET Pattern Question)
     (a) DLE   (b) Pemphigus
     (c) Psoriasis   (d) Nummular eczema

190. Chloroquine is useful in: *(Recent NEET Pattern Question)*
     (a) Discoid lupus erythematosis
     (b) Rheumatoid arthritis
     (c) Infectious mononucleosis
     (d) All of the above

191. Drug of choice for treatment of chloroquine resistant falciparum malaria is: *(Recent NEET Pattern Question)*
     (a) Quinine   (b) Chloroquine
     (c) Pyrimethamine (d) Primaquine

192. Tissue schizontocide which prevents relapse of vivax malaria is: *(Recent NEET Pattern Question)*
     (a) Quinine   (b) Primaquine
     (c) Pyrimethamine (d) Chloroquine

193. Chloroquine is given in high loading dose because of:
     (Recent NEET Pattern Question)
     (a) High volume of distribution
     (b) Poor GIT absorption
     (c) High first pass metabolism
     (d) All

194. Which of the following can cause hypoglycemia in a patient of severe cerebral malaria on treatment?
     (Recent NEET Pattern Question)
     (a) Quinine   (b) Chloroquine
     (c) Halofantrine (d) Mefloquine

195. Radical cure is required for malaria caused by:
     (Recent NEET Pattern Question)
     (a) *P. falciparum* and *P. vivax*
     (b) *P. falciparum* and *P. malariae*
     (c) *P. vivax* and *P. malariae*
     (d) *P. vivax* and *P. ovale*

196. Which antimalarial drug is known to cause neuropsychiatric adverse reaction? *(Recent NEET Pattern Question)*
     (a) Artesunate   (b) Artimisnin
     (c) Quinine   (d) Mefloquine

197. Drawback of artesunate is: *(Recent NEET Pattern Question)*
     (a) Poor bioavailability
     (b) Rapid recrudescence of malaria
     (c) Hypoglycemia
     (d) Hemolysis

Chemotherapy B: Antimicrobials for Specific Conditions 411

198. Absorption of which of the following anti-malarial drug increases with food intake? *(Recent NEET Pattern Question)*
    (a) Mefloquine
    (b) Lumefantrine
    (c) Chloroquine
    (d) Amodiaquine

199. Patient is being admininstered i.v. quinine following which he developed restlessness and sweating, the most likely cause is: *(Recent NEET Pattern Question)*
    (a) Hypoglycaemia
    (b) Cinchonism
    (c) Arrhythmias
    (d) Sweating

200. Which one of the following antimalarial drugs is safe for use in pregnancy? *(Recent NEET Pattern Question)*
    (a) Atovaquone
    (b) Tetracycline
    (c) Proguanil
    (d) Primaquine

201. Chloroquine is given as 600 mg loading dose because: *(Recent NEET Pattern Question)*
    (a) It is rapidly absorbed
    (b) It is rapidly metabolized
    (c) It has increased tissue binding
    (d) It is rapidly eliminated

202. Drug of choice for chloroquine resistant malaria in pregnancy is: *(Recent NEET Pattern Question)*
    (a) Quinine
    (b) Mefloquine
    (c) Artemisinin
    (d) Sulphadoxine+ pyrimethamine

203. Radical cure of Plasmodium vivax is by: *(Recent NEET Pattern Question)*
    (a) Chloroquine
    (b) Tetracycline
    (c) Primaquine
    (d) Artesunate

204. Volume of distribution for chloroquine is: *(Recent NEET Pattern Question)*
    (a) 5–8 L
    (b) 9–15 L
    (c) 100–650 L
    (d) Above 1300 L

205. Which of the following antimalarial is a slow acting schizonticide ? *(Recent NEET Pattern Question)*
    (a) Artemether
    (b) Mefloquine
    (c) Pyrimethamine
    (d) Quinine

206. Chemoprophylaxis in an Englishman visiting chloroquine and mefloquine resistant malaria region is done with: *(Recent NEET Pattern Question)*
    (a) Primaquine
    (b) Doxycycline
    (c) Amodiaquine
    (d) Hydroxychloroquine

207. Drug of choice for exo-erythrocystic stage of malaria is: *(Recent NEET Pattern Question)*
    (a) Chloroquine
    (b) Primaquine
    (c) Proguanil
    (d) Mefloquine

208. Drug not given for malaria prophylaxis is: *(Recent NEET Pattern Question)*
    (a) Chloroquine
    (b) Proguanil
    (c) Doxycycline
    (d) Artesunate

209. Antimalarial agent safe for use in pregnancy is: *(Recent NEET Pattern Question)*
    (a) Atovaquone
    (b) Pyrimethamine
    (c) Primaquine
    (d) Proguanil

210. Which one of the following drug may be used for prevention of relapse of *P. vivax* infection? *(Recent NEET Pattern Question)*
    (a) Chloroquine
    (b) Primaquine
    (c) Atovaquone
    (d) Tetracycline

211. The infective form of malarial parasite is: *(Recent NEET Pattern Question)*
    (a) Trophozoites
    (b) Sporozoites
    (c) Hypnozoites
    (d) Merozoites

212. First line drug for falciparum malaria in pregnancy is: *(Recent NEET Pattern Question)*
    (a) Chloroquine
    (b) Quinine
    (c) Primaquine
    (d) Tetracycline

213. Which antimalarial drug is implicated in causing hypoglycemia? *(Recent NEET Pattern Question)*
    (a) Chloroquine
    (b) Pyrimethamine
    (c) Quinine
    (d) Primaquine

214. Drug of choice for the treatment of a pregnant woman with P vivax malaria is: *(Recent NEET Pattern Question)*
    (a) Quinine
    (b) Chloroquine
    (c) Artemether
    (d) Paracetamol

215. Drug not used in chloroquine resistant malaria is: *(Recent NEET Pattern Question)*
    (a) Sulfadoxine-pyrimethamine
    (b) Fluoroquinolones
    (c) Quinine
    (d) Artemisinins

ANTI-PROTOZOAL, ANTI-HELMINTHIC AND MISCELLANEOUS DRUGS

216. Drug of choice for treatment of bacterial vaginosis in pregnancy is: *(AIIMS Nov. 2019)*
    (a) Clindamycin
    (b) Metronidazole
    (c) Erythromycin
    (d) Rovamycin

217. Match the following drugs with the organism they are used for: *(AIIMS Nov. 2019)*

Drug	Organism
1. Praziquantal	A. Filaria
2. Diethylcarbamezine	B. Giardia
3. Nitazoxanide	C. Strongyloides
4. Mebendazole	D. Tapeworms
	E. Leishmania
	F. Ascaris lumbricoides

218. A 50-year-old male had fever for 1 week, abdominal distention and loss of appetite. It is not responding to antibiotics and antimalarials. Widal test is negative but RK39 dipstick test was positive. Which drug can be used? *(AIIMS Nov. 2018)*
    (a) Bedaquiline
    (b) Linezolid
    (c) Fluconazole
    (d) Amphotericin B

219. Ivermectin is used for the treatment of: *(Recent Question 2016-17)*
    (a) Scabies
    (b) Fungal infection
    (c) Cholera
    (d) Ascaris

220. True about uses of benzyl benzoate is:
    (Recent Question 2016-17)
    (a) It is topically used for the treatment of scabies
    (b) It is present in cough or asthma preparations
    (c) It is used for the treatment of hypogonadism
    (d) All are true

221. Drug of choice for the treatment of tapeworms is:
    (Recent Question 2016-17)
    (a) Prolozone   (b) Piperazine
    (c) Pyrantel palmoate (d) Praziquantel

222. A female presented with frothy, greenish vaginal discharge with a musty smell. On examination 'strawberry vagina' was noted. A diagnosis of trichomonas vaginalis was made. Drug of choice is: (AIIMS May, 2017)
    (a) Metronidazole (b) Tetracycline
    (c) Erythromycin   (d) Fluconazole

223. A patient was being treated with a drug that interferes with the activity of enzyme pyruvate ferredoxin oxidoreductase. Which of the following is the most likely organism causing infection in this patient? (AI 2012)
    (a) Beef tapeworm
    (b) Whipworm
    (c) Cryptosporidium
    (d) Trypanosoma

224. Potassium iodide is useful in the treatment of:
    (Recent NEET Pattern Question)
    (a) Sporotrichosis (b) Impetigo
    (c) Viral warts   (d) Dermatitis herpetiformis

225. Bull's eye retinopathy is seen in:
    (Recent NEET Pattern Question)
    (a) Chloroquine (b) Methanol
    (c) Ethambutol   (d) Steroids

226. The drug of choice for schistosomiasis is:
    (Recent NEET Pattern Question)
    (a) Albendazole   (b) Metronidazole
    (c) Praziquantel (d) Triclabendazole

227. Hepatotoxic drugs are all *except*:
    (Recent NEET Pattern Question)
    (a) Methotrexate (b) Isoniazid
    (c) Cycloserine   (d) Ethionamide

228. Drug of choice for neurocysticercosis is:
    (Recent NEET Pattern Question)
    (a) Praziquantel (b) Albendazole
    (c) Levamisole   (d) Piperazine

229. Which of the following drug causes flaccid paralysis of ascaris? (Recent NEET Pattern Question)
    (a) Albendazole   (b) Pyrantel pamoate
    (c) Piperazine   (d) Ivermectin

230. Which of the following is TRUE about drugs useful in amoebiasis? (Recent NEET Pattern Question)
    (a) Diloxanide furoate is useful in intestinal and extra-intestinal amoebiasis
    (b) Emetine is well tolerated orally
    (c) Chloroquine is effective only in hepatic amoebiasis
    (d) Mepacrine is useful in chronic cyst passers

231. DEC (Di-ethyl-carbamazine) is used for the treatment of:
    (Recent NEET Pattern Question)
    (a) Filariasis   (b) Dracunculiasis
    (c) Schistosomiasis (d) Taeniasis

232. Which of the following drug is deposited in the retina?
    (a) Isoniazid   (Recent NEET Pattern Question)
    (b) Chloroquine
    (c) Rifampicin
    (d) Pyrizinamide

233. Round worm infection is best treated with:
    (Recent NEET Pattern Question)
    (a) Metronidazole (b) Mebendazole
    (c) Albendazol   (d) Pyrantel pamoate

234. Drug of choice for bacterial vaginosis is:
    (a) Metronidazole   (Recent NEET Pattern Question)
    (b) Ampicillin
    (c) Ciprofloxacin
    (d) Fluconazole

235. Mebendazole cannot be used for:
    (Recent NEET Pattern Question)
    (a) Ascariasis
    (b) Entrobius vermicularis
    (c) Onchocercosis
    (d) Hydatid cyst disease

236. Drug of choice for medical treatment of hydatid cyst of liver is: (Recent NEET Pattern Question)
    (a) Praziquantel (b) Thiabendazole
    (c) Ivermectin   (d) Albendazole

237. What is the dose of niclosamide used in treatment of Taenia saginata infection in children?
    (Recent NEET Pattern Question)
    (a) 40 mg/kg single dose
    (b) 40 mg/kg/day for 3 days
    (c) 40 mg/kg/day for 7 days
    (d) 40 mg/kg/day for 21 days

238. Drug commonly used in the treatment of echinococosis is:
    (Recent NEET Pattern Question)
    (a) Albendazole   (b) Ivermectin
    (c) Pyrental prermeated (d) Metronidazole

239. Ivermectin is used for the treatment of:
    (a) Filariasis   (Recent NEET Pattern Question)
    (b) Ascariasis
    (c) Teniasis
    (d) Hookworm infestation

240. Drug amphotericin B is used for treatment of:
    (Recent NEET Pattern Question)
    (a) Sleeping sickness (b) Kala azar
    (c) Malaria   (d) Filaria

241. Drug that is not used in renal failure is:
    (Recent NEET Pattern Question)
    (a) Ethambutol (b) Rifampicin
    (c) Isoniazid   (d) Streptomycin

242. The antiretroviral drug which is also effective in chronic active hepatitis-B infection is: (Recent NEET Pattern Question)
    (a) Zidovudine (b) Nelfinavir
    (c) Efavirenz   (d) Lamivudine

Chemotherapy B: Antimicrobials for Specific Conditions

243. **Drug of choice for hookworm infestation is:**
     (Recent NEET Pattern Question)
     (a) Piperazine citrate
     (b) Bephenium hydroxynaphthoate
     (c) Mebendazole
     (d) Albendazole

244. **Drug of choice for ascariasis is:**
     (Recent NEET Pattern Question)
     (a) Piperazine citrate
     (b) Bephenium hydroxynaphthoate
     (c) Mebendazole
     (d) Albendazole

245. **Drugs of choice for the treatment of neurocysticercosis are:** *(Recent NEET Pattern Question)*
     (a) Hydroquinone and metronidazole
     (b) Metronidazole and pyrental palmoate
     (c) Albendazole and praziquantel
     (d) Cyclophosphamide

246. **Which of the following is not used as treatment for lymphatic filariasis?** *(Recent NEET Pattern Question)*
     (a) Ivermectin
     (b) Diethyl carbamazine
     (c) Praziquantel
     (d) Albendazole

247. **Metrifonate is effective against:**
     (Recent NEET Pattern Question)
     (a) Amoebiasis
     (b) Leishmaniosis
     (c) Schistosomiasis
     (d) Giardiasis

248. **Disulfiram like interaction with alcohol is seen with all of the following drugs except:** *(Recent NEET Pattern Question)*
     (a) Metronidazole   (b) Cefoperazone
     (c) Griseofulvin   (d) Satranidazole

249. **Scabies can be effectively treated systemically by:**
     (Recent NEET Pattern Question)
     (a) Psoralens   (b) Ivermectin
     (c) Permethrin   (d) Contrimoxazole

250. **The treatment of choice for bacterial vaginosis is:**
     (a) Clindamycin   *(Recent NEET Pattern Question)*
     (b) Erythromycin
     (c) Ampicillin
     (d) Metronidazole

251. **Drug of choice for kala-azar is:**
     (Recent NEET Pattern Question)
     (a) Sodium stibogluconate
     (b) Amphotericin B
     (c) Pentamidine
     (d) None of the above

252. **Metronidazole is effective in all of the following conditions except:** *(Recent NEET Pattern Question)*
     (a) Pseudomembranous colitis
     (b) Neurocysticercosis
     (c) Giardiasis
     (d) Amebic liver abscess

253. **Albendazole is effective against all of the following except:** *(Recent NEET Pattern Question)*
     (a) Roundworm   (b) Hookworm
     (c) Tapeworm   (d) Pinworm

254. **All of the following drugs can be used for intestinal ameobiasis except:** *(Recent NEET Pattern Question)*
     (a) Metronidazole
     (b) Chloroquine
     (c) Diloxanide furoate
     (d) Tinidazole

255. **Dosage of albendazole in ascariasis is:**
     (Recent NEET Pattern Question)
     (a) 400 mg once
     (b) 400 mg bd for one day
     (c) 400 mg tds for one day
     (d) 400 mg bd for 5 days

256. **Poly drug Resistance in tuberculosis is:**
     (Recent Question 2016-17)
     (a) Resistance to two or more first-line drugs but not to both isoniazid and rifampicin
     (b) Resistance to two or more first-line drugs including isoniazid and rifampicin
     (c) Resistance to one first-line drugs and atleast one of three injectable second-line drugs
     (d) Resistant to isoniazid and rifampin, plus any fluoroquinolone and at least one of three injectable second-line drugs

Explanations

1. **Ans. (c) 3 drugs for 6 months** *(Ref: NLEP guidelines 2019)*
   According to the latest guidelines treatment of multibacillary and paucibacillary leprosy is same except for duration of treatment.

	Multibacillary	Paucibacillary
Rifampin	600 mg once a month supervised	600 mg once a month supervised
Clofazimine	300 mg once a month supervised + 50 mg daily self administered	300 mg once a month supervised + 50 mg daily self administered
Dapsone	100 mg daily self administered	100 mg daily self administered
Duration	12 months	6 months

2. **Ans. (c) Ethambutol** *(Ref: KDT 8th/e p820)*
   Ethambutol (E)
   - It is a **BACTERIOSTATIC** agent for mycobacterium and acts by inhibiting the synthesis of arabinogalactan (a component of cell wall) due to **inhibition of arabinosyl transferase**.
   - It is distributed throughout the body except in the CSF.
   - It causes dose dependent and reversible **visual disturbances like optic neuritis** (presents as *reduced visual acuity, central scotoma and loss of ability to see green, less commonly red*). It may be due to its effect on *amacrine and bipolar* cells of retina. Because children are unable to report early visual impairment, this drug is *avoided in children*.
   - It also causes *hyperuricemia and peripheral neuritis*.
   - It requires dose adjustment in renal failure.

3. **Ans. (d) Competition with PABA in folic acid synthesis** *(Ref. KDT 8th/e p831)*
   - Folic acid synthase (dihydropteroate synthase) results in the formation of folic acid by incorporation of PABA.
   - *Sulfonamides, dapsone and paraaminosalicylic acid (PAS)* are structural analogues of paraaminobenzoic acid (PABA).
   - These drugs act as competitive inhibitors of folic acid synthase.

4. **Ans. (a) Isoniazid** *(Ref: KDT 8th/e p817)*
5. **Ans. (a) Isoniazid and Rifampicin** *(Ref: KDT 8th/e p826)*
6. **Ans. (d) Ethambutol** *(Ref: KDT 8th/e p820)*
7. **Ans. (a) Ethambutol** *(Ref: KDT 8th/e p820)*
8. **Ans. (a) Liver disease** *(Ref: KDT 8th/e p820)*
9. **Ans. (c) Isoniazid** *(Ref: KDT 8th/e p817)*
   Isoniazid causes deficiency of pyridoxine which is associated with sideroblastic anemia.
10. **Ans. (d) RpoB** *(Ref: KDT 8th/e p817)*
11. **Ans. (b) Pyrazinamide** *(Ref: KDT 8th/e p819)*
12. **Ans. (a) Ofloxacin** *(Ref: KDT 7th/e p782)*
    Ofloxacin, pefloxacin, moxifloxacin and sparfloxacin are fluoroquinolones effective against leprosy and fluoroquinolone are bactericidal drugs.

13. **Ans. (c) (Rifampicin 450 mg + Clofazimine 150 mg) once monthly + Dapsone 50 mg daily + Clofazimine 50 mg alternate day** *(Ref: National Leprosy Eradication programme)*
    This is a case of multibacillary leprosy. The multi drug therapy for in adults (15 years or above) is
    Rifampicin 600 mg plus clofazimine 300 mg once monthly and Dapsone 100 mg plus Clofazimine 50 mg daily for 12 months
    As the patient is child, the doses used are less, rest of the treatment is similar
    Rifampicin 450 mg and Clofazimine 150 mg monthly and dapsone 50 mg daily. As clofazimine less than 50 mg tablet is not available, so 50 mg is given on alternate day.

14. **Ans. (b) It is more effective for newly diagnosed TB as compared to rifampicin** *(Katzung 13th/e p817,820)*

	Rifampicin	Rifabutin
Half life	Shorter	Longer
CYP inhibition (drug interactions)	Marked	Weak
Efficacy against Mycobacterium tuberculosis	More	Less
Efficacy against MAC	Less	More
Hepatotoxic potential	Present	Absent

15. **Ans. (a) Bedaquiline** *(Ref: Harrison 19th/e p1115, KDT 8th/e p823)*
    Ref: Bedaquiline is a new drug approved for MDT tuberculosis. It acts by inhibiting ATP synthase in mycobacteria. Major adverse effect of this drug is QT prolongation.

16. **Ans. (c) Ethionamide** *(Ref: KDT 8th/e p821)*
    Ethionamide and PAS are two antitubercular drugs associated with hypothyroidism and goiter.

17. **Ans. (b) Rifabutin** *(Ref: Goodman and Gilman 12th/e p1553)*

18. **Ans. (a) Hemolytic anemia** *(Ref: Goodman and Gilman 12th/e p1564, KDT 8th/e p832)*
    Hemolysis develops in almost every individual treated with 200-300 mg dapsone per day. Doses of less than 100 mg in healthy persons and less than 50 mg per day in persons with G-6PD deficiency do not cause hemolysis. Methemoglobinemia is also very common.

19. **Ans. (a) Retrobulbar neuritis** *(Ref: Katzung 10/e p774; KDT 8th/e p820)*
    Ethambutol causes retrobulbar neuritis and can result in red green colour blindness.

20. **Ans. (d) Ethambutol** *(Ref: Katzung 10/e p774; KDT 8th/e p820)*
    Isoniazid, rifampicin and pyrazinamide can cause hepatotoxicity whereas ethambutol and streptomycin do not cause hepatotoxicity.

21. **Ans. (b) Rifampicin** *(Ref: Goodman & Gilman 11th/e p1205, 1208, 1211; KDT 8th/e p818)*

Chemotherapy B: Antimicrobials for Specific Conditions

- Ethambutol is bacteriostatic drug.
- INH and rifampicin are equally effective against intra as well as extracellular mycobacteria. INH require a concentration of 0.025 µg/mL whereas rifampicin inhibits the growth of bacteria at a concentration of 0.005 µg/mL.
- Pyrazinamide acts more in acidic pH and it requires a concentration of 12.5 µg/mL.
- Thus, most active drug for extra-cellular bacteria is rifampicin.

22. **Ans. (b) Ethionamide** *(Ref: KDT 8th/e p821)*
PAS and ethionamide can lead to hypothyroidism.

23. **Ans. (a) Rifampicin**
(Ref: Goodman & Gilman 11th/e p1209; KDT 8th/e p819)

24. **Ans. (d) Streptomycin** *(Ref: KDT 8th/e p820)*
Streptomycin and ethambutol are not hepatotoxic. Read carefully, option (c) is ethionamide not ethambutol.

25. **Ans. (d) All of the above** *(Ref: KDT 8th/e p829)*
- Most atypical Mycobacteria are resistatnt to the usual antitubercular drugs, though pulmonary disease caused by M. avium complex or M. kansasii may respond to prolonged treatment with Rifampicin, Isoniazid and Ethambutol.

- Drugs that are used are:
    - **Rifabutin**
    - Clofazimine
    - **Quinolones e.g. ciprofloxacin**
    - Newer macrolides like clarithromycin and azithromycin.

26. **Ans. (c) INH** *(Ref: KDT 8th/e p818)*
- Peripheral neuritis and a variety of neurological manifestations (paraesthesias, numbness, mental disturbances, rarely convulsions) are the most important dose dependent toxic effects of INH.
- These are due to interference with utilization of pyridoxine and its increased excretion in urine.

27. **Ans. (c) Pyrazinamide** *(Ref: KDT 8th/e p819)*
- Arthralgia is caused by pyrazinamide, which may be non-gouty or due to hyperuricemia secondary to inhibition of uric acid secretion in the kidney.
- Ethambutol also produces hyperuricemia due to interferance with urate excretion.

28. **Ans. (d) Rifampicin** *(Ref: KDT 8th/e p818)*
Streptomycin and capreomycin are nephrotoxic whereas ethambutol accumulates in renal failure and thus should be avoided in presence of severe renal failure.

29. **Ans. (b) Ethambutol** *(Ref: KDT 8th/e p820)*

30. **Ans. (b) Clarithromycin** *(Ref: KDT 8th/e p829)*
- Treatment of MAC infection is REC (Rifabutin + Ethambutol + Clarithromycin)
- Clarithromycin alone can be used for the prophylaxis of MAC infections in HIV positive patients.
- Azithromycin can also be used in place of clarithromycin.

31. **Ans. (b) Cycloserine** *(Ref: KDT 8th/e p821)*

32. **Ans. (c) B_6** *(Ref: KDT 8th/e p817-818)*
Pyridoxine (vitamin B_6) is administered for the prevention as well as treatment of isoniazid induced peripheral neuropathy.

33. **Ans. (a) Streptomycin** *(Ref: KDT 8th/e p820)*
Streptomycin and ethambutol do not cross blood brain barrier whereas INH and pyrazinamide have maximum CNS penetration.

34. **Ans. (a) Streptomycin** *(Ref: KDT 8th/e p820)*
Ethambutol and streptomycin are first line anti-tubercular drugs that are NOT hepatotoxic.

35. **Ans. (d) Coronary artery disease** *(Ref: KDT 8th/e p818)*
INH causes hepatitis, peripheral neuritis and neurological manifestations (paresthesias, numbness, mental disturbance rarely convulsion). Its toxic metabolitre accumulates in the presence of renal failure.
So we are left with last option; coronary artery disease, which is our answer of exclusion.

36. **Ans. (b) Streptomycin + Ethambutol** *(Ref: KDT 8th/e p820)*

37. **Ans. (b) INH** *(Ref: Katzung 11/e p825)*

38. **Ans. (b) Optic neuritis** *(Ref: Katzung 11/e p827)*

39. **Ans. (a) Dapsone** *(Ref: Katzung 11/e p831)*

40. **Ans. (d) Mutation** *(Ref: Katzung 11/e p824,826,827)*

- Resistance to INH occurs due to point mutation in inhA or katG genes.
- Resistance to rifampicin occurs due to point mutation in rpoB genes.
- Resistance to ethambutol is due to mutations resulting in overexpression of embB gene.

41. **Ans. (a) To prevent peripheral neuritis** *(Ref: KDT 8th/e p818)*

42. **Ans. (d) Ethambutol** *(Ref: KDT 8th/e p819)*

43. **Ans. (d) Tuberculosis** *(Ref: KDT 8th/e p832)*

44. **Ans. (b) Clofazimine** *(Ref: KDT 8th/e p833)*
Anti-inflammatory drugs are used in lepra reaction. Steroids, clofazimine and thalidomide can be used.

45. **Ans. (c) Pyrazinamide** *(Ref: KDT 8th/e p819)*

46. **Ans. (c) Rifampicin + Dapsone + Clofazimine**
(Ref: KDT 8th/e p836)

47. **Ans. (a) Ocular toxicity** *(Ref: KDT 8th/e p820)*

48. **Ans. (a) Thalidomide** *(Ref: KDT 8th/e p837)*
Steroids are drug of choice for both type 1 as well as type 2 lepra reaction. Thalidomide is used in steroid resistant type 2 lepra reaction.

49. **Ans. (b) DNA dependent RNA polymerase inhibition**
(Ref: KDT 8th/e p818)

50. **Ans. (d) All** *(Ref: KDT 8th/e p818-819)*
All first line antitubercular drugs can cross placenta. Streptomycin is contraindicated in pregnancy whereas other drugs are found to be safe.

51. **Ans. (d) Pyrazinamide** *(Ref: KDT 8th/e p819)*

52. **Ans. (b) Eflornithine** *(Ref: KDT 8th/e p829)*
Eflornithine is used for the treatment of some cases of trypanosomiasis. It is also used topically in women to delay regrowth of facial hair following depilation.

53. **Ans. (d) Retrobulbar neuritis** *(Ref: KDT 8th/e p820)*

54. Ans. (d) All of the above
(Ref: Harrison 17th ed/Table e35.4; American academy of family physicians, http://www.aafp.org/afp/980215ap/romero.html)

> **Management of isoniazid toxicity**
> - Five gram of IV pyridoxine given over 5 to 10 minutes is sufficient to counteract the neurotoxic effects of isoniazid in most cases.
> - Diazepam, 5 to 10 mg administered intravenously, is the initial approach to seizure control, with the dose repeated as necessary.
> - The acidosis associated with isoniazid toxicity appears to be lactic acidosis secondary to the seizure activity. Therefore, as the seizures are controlled, the acidosis usually decreases in severity. Since sodium bicarbonate may assist in correcting severe cases of acidosis, its administration should be considered if the pH is less than 7.1.

55. Ans. (d) All of above (Ref: Katzung 11/e p831, KDT 8th/e p837)

56. Ans. (c) Penicillin (Ref: KDT 8th/e p836)

57. Ans. (b) Ofloxacin (Ref: Harrison 19th/e p1127)

58. Ans. (a) Minocycline (Ref: Harrison 19th/e p1127)

59. Ans. (a) Isoniazid (Ref: Goodman Gilman 12th/e p1558)
Isoniazid caused euphoria as an adverse effect. This lead to development of structurally similar drugs (MAO inhibitors) as antidepressants.

60. Ans. (b) Rifampicin
(Ref: Harrison 19th/e p205, KDT 8th/e p819)
Rifampicin is drug of choice for prophylaxis of meningococcal and H. influenzae meningitis

61. Ans. (b) Rifampicin
(Ref: Harrison 19th/e p205, KDT 8th/e p819)

62. Ans. (c) Pyrazinamide (Ref: Katzung 13th/e p819)
Pyrazinamide is most active against slow growing bacteria inside macrophages. Thus, it possesses strong sterilizing activity.

63. Ans. (b) Peripheral neuropathy
(Ref: Goodman Gilman 12th/e p1556, KDT 8th/e p817-818)

64. Ans. (a) Respiratory syndrome
(Ref: Williams Chemtherapy Vol 3 Pg 10)

65. Ans. (b) Rifampicin (Ref: Goodman Gilman 12th/e p1553)
Rifampicin cause discoloration (orange) of secretions leading to contact lens staining.

66. Ans. (a) INH (Ref: Goodman Gilman 12th/e p1556)
Isoniazid can cause neuropsychiatric adverse effects like seizures, transient loss of memory and psychosis.

67. Ans. (c) Increased metabolism of OCPs
(Ref. KDT 8th/e p818)

68. Ans. (a) Dermatitis herpetiformis
(Ref. Goodman Gilman 12/e p1219)

69. Ans. (c) Clofazimine (Ref: KDT 8th/e p833)

70. Ans. (b) Rifampicin (Ref: KDT 8th/e p823)

71. Ans. (d) Thrombocytopenia (Ref: KDT 8th/e p817-818)

72. Ans. (b) Ethambutol (Ref: KDT 8th/e p820)

73. Ans. (b) Used in treatment of meningiococcal meningitis
(Ref: KDT 8th/e p819)
- Rifampicin is drug of choice for prophylaxis of meningococcal meningitis.
- Penicillins are used for treatment of meningococcal meningitis.

74. Ans. (a) DNA dependent RNA polymerase
(Ref: KDT 8th/e p818)

75. Ans. (c) Pyrazinamide (Ref: KDT 8th/e p819)

76. Ans. (c) Vitamine B_6 (Ref: KDT 8th/e p817-818)

77. Ans. (d) Resistance to isoniazid and rifampicin
(Ref: KDT 8th/e p776)

78. Ans. (a) Pyridoxine (Ref: KDT 8th/e p818)

79. Ans. (c) Ethambutol (Ref: KDT 8th/e p820)

80. Ans. (b) Rifampicin (Ref: KDT 8th/e p818-819)

81. Ans. (c) Mutation (Ref: KDT 8th/e p817)

82. Ans. (a) Pyrazinamide (Ref: KDT 8th/e p819)

83. Ans. (d) Streptomycin + ethambutol (Ref: KDT 8th/e p827)

84. Ans. (d) Thiacetazone (Ref: KDT 8th/e p818)

85. Ans. (c) Kanamycin (Ref: KDT 8th/e p831)

86. Ans. (a) Rifampicin (Ref: KDT 8th/e p833)

87. Ans. (b) Dermatitis herpetiformis
(Ref: Goodman Gilman 12/e p1823)

88. Ans. (b) Hepatotoxicity (Ref: KDT 8th/e p818)

89. Ans. (b) Rifampicin (Ref: KDT 8th/e p818)

90. Ans. (c) Streptomycin and Ethambutol
(Ref: KDT 8th/e p820)

91. Ans. (a) Ethambutol (Ref: KDT 8th/e p820)

92. Ans. (a) Rifampicin (Ref: KDT 8th/e p818)

93. Ans. (a) Rifampicin (Ref: KDT 8th/e p819)

94. Ans. (a) Ethambutol (Ref: KDT 8th/e p820)

95. Ans. (d) Terbinafine (Ref: KDT 8th/e p874)
- Ciclopirox olamine is most commonly used drug as nail lacquer for onychomycosis. Terbinafine is also available as nail lacquer.
- Azoles like fluconazole and itraconazole are available only by oral route for dermatophytosis.
- Terbinafine
  - Fungicidal
  - Has high affinity for keratin
  - DOC for dermatophytoses
  - Available as topical (nail lacquer) as well as for systemic administration

96. Ans. (b) Voriconazole (Ref: KDT 8th/e p846)
- Voriconazole is the drug of choice for invasive aspergillosis
- Posaconazole is the only azole active against mucormycosis. However, drug of choice for mucormycosis is liposomal amphotericin B

Chemotherapy B: Antimicrobials for Specific Conditions

- Caspofungin is approved for invasive aspergillosis not responding to AMB or voriconazole. It is quite nontoxic and causes only infusion related reactions.
- Liposomal AMB is the drug of choice or co-drug of choice for most systemic fungal infections. It can be used intrathecally in fungal meningitis and locally for corneal ulcers and keratitis.

97. **Ans. (a) F, (b) F, (c) T, (d) T, (e) T**
    (Ref: KDT 8th/e p853,856,858)
    - For hepatitis C virus infections, along with ribavirin, injectable interferons needs to be administered (which has lot of adverse effects). Sofosbuvir is a new oral drug that acts by inhibiting NS5B. It is preferred over ribavirin because of better efficacy.
    - Ombiasvir acts as RNA polymerase (NS5A) inhibitor of HCV. Therefore, it acts via inhibition of transcription (not protein synthesis)
    - Simprevir is a protease inhibitor of HCV.
    - Oseltamivir (as well as zanamivir) is the most effective drug for influenza A, including H5N1 and HIN1 (swine flu) strains.
    - Imiquimod is an immunomodulator used for viral warts like condyloma accuminata.

Protease Inhibitors	NS5A inhibitors	NS5B inhibitors
Telaprevir	Elbasvir	Sofosbuvir
Boceprevir	Ledipasvir	Dasabuvir
Simprevir	Ombitasvir	
Grazoprevir	Daclatasvir	
Paritaprevir	Velpatasvir	

98. **Ans. (a) T, (b) T, (c) F, (d) T, (e) T** *(Ref: KDT 8th/e p852,853)*
    - Drug of choice for herpes simplex virus and varicella zoster virus infection is acyclovir.
    - Drug of choice for cytomegalovirus is ganciclovir.
    - Both acyclovir and ganciclovir are pro-drugs and require activation by kinases.

    Foscarnet
    - It is a simple straight chain phosphonate.
    - It does not require activation by kinases.
    - It is active against H. simplex (including strains resistant to acyclovir), CMV (including ganciclovir-resistant ones) and other herpes group viruses.
    - Oral absorption is poor. Its t½ is 4–8 hours, and it is not metabolized by liver.
    - Toxicity of foscarnet is high. It damages kidney and produces a **renal** diabetes like condition; acute **renal failure** can also occur. Anemia, phlebitis, tremors, convulsions, **genital ulceration** and other neurological as well as constitutional symptoms due to **hypocalcemia** are frequent.
    - It is administered by iv infusion

99. **Ans. (b) Flucytosine: Inhibits microtubule thereby preventing mitosis**
    (Ref: KDT 8th/e p842-843)
    Flucytosine acts as an antimetabolite whereas griseofulvin inhibits mitotic spindle.

Group	Example	Mechanism
Polyene	Amphotericin B	Create artificial pores in membrane by binding to ergosterol
Azoles	Fluconazole Itraconazole	Inhibit Lanosterol-14-alpha-demethylase
Allylamines	Terbinafine Butenafine	Inhibit squalene epoxidase
Anti-metabolite	5-Flucytosine	Inhibit DNA formation
Benzofuran	Griseofulvin	Binds to tubulin and inhibit mitosis
Echinocandins	Caspofungin Micafungin	Inhibit beta 1,3 glycan in fungal cell wall

100. **Ans. (a) Neuraminidase inhibition**
     (Ref: Goodman and Gilman 13th/e p1114)
     Neuraminidase inhibitors like oseltamivir, zanamivir and peramivir are used for the treatment of bird flu and swine flu.

101. **Ans. (a) Inhibit ergosterol synthesis**
     (Ref: Goodman and Gilman 13th/e p1091)

Anti-fungal drug group	Example	Mechanism
Polyene	Amphotericin B	Create artificial pores in membrane by binding to ergosterol
Azoles (Imidazole and triazoles)	Fluconazole Itraconazole	Inhibit Lanosterol-14-alpha-demethylase
Allylamines	Terbinafine Butenafine	Inhibit squalene epoxidase
Anti-metabolite	5-Flucytosine	Inhibit DNA formation
Benzofuran	Griseofulvin	Binds to tubulin and inhibit mitosis
Echinocandins	Caspofungin Micafungin	Inhibit beta 1,3 glycan in fungal cell wall

102. **Ans. (a) Cell membrane** *(Ref: KDT 8th/e p839)*
     Amphotericin B binds to ergosterol which is an important component of fungal cell wall.

103. **Ans. (a) Neuraminidase inhibitor** *(Ref: CMDT 2017/1412)*
     Oseltamivir acts as a **neuraminidase inhibitor** and prevents the virion release by causing clumping of mature virions. Another drugs in this group are zanamivir and peramivir.

     > - These drugs are effective against both **influenza A** and **influenza B**.
     > - **Oseltamivir is an oral prodrug** (can cause nausea and vomiting) whereas **zanamivir is administered by inhalational route** (bronchospasm is an important adverse effect).
     > - **Neuropsychiatric disorders** including suicidal tendancy have been associated with oseltamivir and zanamivir.

104. **Ans. (a) Amphotericin B** *(Ref: Harrison 18th/e p1663)*
     The diagnosis is **rhinocerebral mucormycosis.**
     - Mucormycosis typically occurs in patients with diabetes mellitus, solid organ or hematopoietic stem

cell transplantation (HSCT), prolonged neutropenia, or malignancy
- Amphotericin B deoxycholate remains the only licensed antifungal agent for the treatment of mucormycosis. However, lipid formulations of AmB are significantly less nephrotoxic, can be administered at higher doses, and may be more efficacious than AMB deoxycholate for this purpose.

105. **Ans. (c) Tinea versicolor** *(Ref: CMDT-2010/110)*
    - Griseofulvin is used for dermatophytoses including Tinea capitis, Tinea cruris, Tinea pedis, Tinea unguum and Tinea corporis etc.
    - Tinea versicolor is caused by a yeast *Malassezia furfur*. It is treated by **selenium sulfide and ketoconazole shampoo**.

106. **Ans. (d) Oseltamivir** *(Ref: KDT 8th/e p853)*
    Oseltamivir and zanamavir are used for avian influenza (bird flu).

107. **Ans. (a) Streptomyces nodosus** *(Ref: KDT 8th/e p839)*

Organism	Antibiotic obtained
S. pimprina	Hamycin
S. venezuelac	Chloramphenicil
S. erythrens	Erythromycin
S. grisens	Aminoglycosides
S. mediterranei	Rifampicin
S. nodosus	Amphotericin B

108. **Ans. (c) Ciclopirox olamine is effective in systemic mycoses** *(Ref: KDT 8th/e p848)*
    - Amphotericin B is the drug of choice for most serious systemic infections but it has to be administered parenterally.
    - Griseofulvin is the drug that is used for the treatment of dermatophytosis by oral route.
    - Fluconazole can be used orally as well as parenterally.
    - Cyclopirox olamine is used only topically for mild fungal infections.

109. **Ans. (b) Clotrimazole** *(Ref: KDT 8th/e p843)*
110. **Ans. (c) Ketoconazole** *(Ref: KDT 8th/e p844)*
111. **Ans. (b) 5-Flucytosine (5 FC)**
    (Ref: Katzung 11/e p838, KDT 8th/e p843)
112. **Ans. (a) Acyclovir** *(Ref: KDT 8th/e p850)*
113. **Ans. (d) Griseofulvin** *(Ref: KDT 8th/e p842)*
114. **Ans. (a) Lamivudine**
    (Ref: KDT 8th/e p862, Katzung 11th/e p870)
    Now, the drug of choice for hepatitis B is entecavir.

115. **Ans. (d) Griseofulvin** *(Ref: KDT 8th/e p842)*
116. **Ans. (d) Griseofulvin** *(Ref: KDT 8th/e p842)*
117. **Ans. (d) Clotrimazole** *(Ref: KDT 8th/e p843)*
118. **Ans. (c) Entecavir** *(Ref: KDT 8th/e p854)*
119. **Ans. (d) Inhibition of ergosterol synthesis**
    (Ref: KDT 8th/e p847)

120. **Ans. (d) Amphotericin B** *(Ref: KDT 8th/e p840-841)*
121. **Ans. (b) Fluconazole** *(Ref: CMDT 2014, KDT 8th/e p845)*
122. **Ans. (a) Adrenal insufficiency** *(Ref: Katzung 11th/e p839, KK Sharma 2nd/e p768)*
123. **Ans. (a) IV amphotericin B** *(Ref: KDT 8th/e p840)*
124. **Ans. (d) Used in anti-retroviral therapy**
    (Ref: KDT 8th/e p855)
    Adefovir is approved, at lower and less toxic doses, only for treatment of HBV infection.

125. **Ans. (b) Acyclovir** *(Ref: KDT 8th/e p851)*
126. **Ans. (a) Ledipasvir**
    (Ref: Harrison 19th/e p2049, KDT 8th/e p859)
    Ledipasvir is a new NS5A polymerase inhibitor for oral treatment of hepatitis C viral infections.

    New drugs for Hepatitis C virus
    Three group of new drugs have been approved for HCV. All of these are effective orally. These groups include HCV protease (NS3A/4) inhibitors, RNA polymerase NS5A inhibitors and RNA polymerase NS5B inhibitors.
    Protease Inhibitors

Protease inhibitors	NS5A inhibitors	NS5B inhibitors
Telaprevir	Elbasvir	Sofosbuvir
Boceprevir	Ledipasvir	Dasabuvir
Simprevir	Ombitasvir	
Grazoprevir	Daclatasvir	
Paritaprevir		

127. **Ans. (d) Abacavir** *(Ref: Harrison 19th/e p1214; Goodman Gilman 12th/e p1609, 1615; Katzung 12th/e p886, 887; KDT 8th/e p861)*
    Abacavir is a NRTI used for HIV whereas all other drugs are given in the options are drugs used for bird flu and swine flu.

128. **Ans. (b) Zanamivir** *(Ref: KDT 8th/e p854)*
129. **Ans. (d) Foscarnet** *(Ref: CMDT 2014 p1308, KDT 8th/e p852)*
130. **Ans. (d) All of the above** *(Ref: Goodman Gilman 12/e p1601)*
    - **Cidofovir** can be used for
        - Acyclovir resistant Herpes simplex
        - CMV retinitis
        - Molluscum contagiosum
        - Anogenital warts
        - Respiratory papillomatosin

131. **Ans. (a) Flucytosine** *(Ref: KDT 8th/e p843)*
132. **Ans. (a) Foscarnet** *(Ref: KDT 8th/e p853)*
133. **Ans. (a) 75 mg BD x 5 days orally** *(Ref: KDT 8th/e p853)*
134. **Ans. (a) Herpes keratitis** *(Ref: KDT 8th/e p851)*
135. **Ans. (b) Terbinafine** *(Ref: KDT 8th/e p847)*
136. **Ans. (a) Acyclovir** *(Ref: KDT 8th/e p851)*
137. **Ans. (c) Amphotericin B** *(Ref: KDT 8th/e p840)*
138. **Ans. (c) Herpes simplex virus** *(Ref: KDT 8th/e p850)*
139. **Ans. (c) Herpes infection** *(Ref: KDT 8th/e p850)*
140. **Ans. (a) Acyclovir** *(Ref: KDT 8th/e p851)*
141. **Ans. (a) Zidovudine is used as monotherapy for post-exposure prophylaxis** *(Ref: KDT 8th/e p872)*

Chemotherapy B: Antimicrobials for Specific Conditions

Post-exposure prophylaxis:
- Treatment should be started within 72 hours of exposure, preferably as early as possible
- At first the wound is washed with soap and water.
- Secondly before initiating drug therapy blood samples are taken to measure the baseline viral markers
- Then, triple drug therapy is given which includes Tenofovir, Lamivudine and a boosted protease inhibitor for 28 days.
- After 6 weeks again viral markers are measured to check for the infection.

142. Ans. (b) Indinavir *(Ref: KDT 8th/e p865)*

HIV protease inhibitors
- Protease *helps in the maturation of infectious virions* and inhibitors of this enzyme can be used in the treatment of HIV infections (by *inhibiting the post-translational modification of viral proteins*).
- This group of drugs inhibits the metabolism of several drugs by inhibiting CYP3A4. *Ritonavir in low doses can be used with other protease inhibitors to increase their plasma concentration.* **Current guidelines recommend that all protease-inhibitor containing regimens use ritonavir boosting if possible.** Only Nelfinavir and Atazanavir can be used *safely without ritonavir* boosting. **Nelfinavir is *the only protease inhibitor for which ritonavir boosting is not recommended.***
- **All protease inhibitors are metabolized by liver and all can cause metabolic abnormalities** including *hypercholesterolemia, diabetes mellitus, hyperlipidemia, insulin resistance and altered fat distribution* (collectively called lipodystrophy syndrome). **Atazanavir** is *devoid of this adverse effect.* **Tesamorelin** is a *synthetic analogue of growth hormone releasing factor* indicated to **reduce excess abdominal fat in HIV-infected patients with lipodystrophy.**
- **Atazanavir** frequently cause *asymptomatic unconjugated hyperbilirubinemia* (like indinavir) and *increase in PR interval in ECG.* It require acidic pH to remain in solution, therefore should not be given with proton pump inhibitors. *Both tenofovir and efavirenz lower the serum concentration of atazanavir, therefore when used with these drugs, it must be boosted by ritonavir.*
- Amprenavir can cause Steven Johnson syndrome.
- Oral bioavailability of **indinavir** is decreased by food. It can cause crystalluria and kidney stones. To prevent renal damage, good hydration must be maintained. It can also cause **asymptomatic hyperbilirubinemia.**

143. Ans. (b) 6 drugs for 6 months and 4 drugs for 18 months *(Ref: RNTCP 2016 guidelines)*
- When *Mycobacterium* is resistant to **both isoniazid and rifampicin**, tuberculosis is called MDR. Isolated rifampicin resistance is treated like MDR cases (except H is added).
- Treatment of MDR tuberculosis includes minimum 6 drugs for 6 months in intensive phase and minimum 4 drugs for 18 months in continuation phase. The drugs are chosen based on drug sensitivity testing.
- Usually pyrazinamide, Ethambutol, Levofloxacin, Kanamycin, Ethionamide and Cycloserine are given in intensive phase and pyrazinamide and kanamycin are stopped after intensive phase and rest 4 drugs are continued in continuation phase.

144. Ans. (b) Raltegravir inhibits integrase enzyme *(Ref: KDT 8th/e p861)*
- Enfuvirtide binds to Gp 41 and inhibit fusion of virus with CD4 cells
- Raltegravir is an integrase inhibitor
- Ritonavir is a protease inhibitor
- Tenofovir is an NRTI.

145. Ans. (b) Emtricitabine *(Ref: CMDT 2018/1369)*

146. Ans. (a) Prevents maturation of new viral particles *(Ref: KDT 7/e p809)*

Function of protease enzyme in HIV is to break inactive polyproteins to functional components. This post-translational modification is required for maturation of new viral particles. Protease inhibitors like atazanavir inhibit this step.

147. Ans. (a) Saquinavir *(Ref: Goodman Gillman 12th/e p1648; Katzung 12th/e p870; KDT 8th/e p866)*
- Drugs whose name end with 'NAVIR' are HIV protease inhibitors. Thus among the given options, saquinavir is a protease inhibitor.
- Enfuvirtide is HIV fusion inhibitor.
- Nevirapine is NNRTI whereas Abacavir is NRTI

148. Ans. (d) Lamivudine *(Ref: Katzung 12th/e p870, KDT 8th/e p861)*
Lamivudine is nucleoside reverse transcriptase inhibitor (NRTI), not the non-nucleoside reverse transcriptase inhibitor (NNRTI).

149. Ans. (b) Zidovudine *(Ref: KDT 8th/e 861-864)*
Anti-HIV drugs effective against HBV are

- **L:** Lamivudine
- **E:** Emtricitabine
- **T:** Tenofovir

Apart from these, other drugs for HBV are

- Interferons
- Telbivudine
- Entecavir
- Adefovir

150. Ans. (c) Optic neuritis *(Ref: Goodman and Gilman 12th/e p1659)*

HAART therapy is highly active anti-retroviral therapy for treatment of HIV infection and AIDS.
- All NRTIs commonly cause lactic acidosis, hepatomegaly and steatosis.
- All protease inhibitors are associated with lipodystrophy syndrome characterized by hypercholesterolemia, weight gain, insulin resistance and hyperglycemia.

Thus, steatosis, lipodystrophy and hypercholesterolemia can be observed commonly in patients taking HAART whereas optic neuritis is not a common adverse effect of antiretroviral drugs.

151. Ans. (a) Ritonavir *(Ref: KK Sharma 2/e p793, KDT 8th/e p866)*

Ritonavir is a protease inhibitor and can cause hypertriglyceridemia and hypercholesterolemia.

- All protease inhibitors are metabolized by liver and all can cause metabolic abnormalities including hypercholesterolemia, diabetes mellitus, hyperlipidemia, insulin resistance and altered fat distribution (lipodystrophy).
- Atazanavir is devoid of this adverse effect.
- Tesamorelin is a synthetic analogue of growth hormone releasing factor indicated to reduce excess abdominal fat in HIV-infected patients with lipodystrophy.

152. Ans. (d) Abacavir *(Ref: KDT 8th/e p861)*
All drugs ending with navir are protease inhibitors. Abacavir is an NRTI.

153. Ans. (b) CYP3A4 inhibition by ritonavir
(Ref: Katzung 10th/e p810; KDT 8th/e p866)
Ritonavir is a microsomal enzyme inhibitor particularly of CYP3A4. It decreases the metabolism of other drugs and thus lower dose of lopinavir can be used in treatment of HIV when combined with ritonavir.

154. Ans. (b) Nucleoside reverse transcriptase inhibition
(Ref: KDT 8th/e p861, 862)

155. Ans. (c) Neutropenia
(Ref: Katzung 11th/e p856, KDT 8th/e p862)

156. Ans. (b) Emtricitabine *(Ref: KDT 8th/e p863)*

157. Ans. (b) Dose lower for blocking HIV replication than HBV replication *(Ref: CMDT 2014/654-655)*
- Lamivudine can be used for both HIV as well as HBV. The dose for HIV is 150 mg twice a day whereas a lower dose of 100 mg daily is used in HBV.
- It should not be used alone as resistance develops quickly.
- Seroconversion from HBeAg positive to anti HBe occurs in only 20% of patients.

158. Ans. (a) Anemia *(Ref: KDT 8th/e p862)*

159. Ans. (a) Protects against acquiring the HIV infection
(Ref: KDT 8th/e p861)

160. Ans. (c) < 200/microL *(Ref: KDT 8th/e p860)*

161. Ans. (b) Abacavir
(Ref: Katzung 11th/e p857, CMDT 2014/1294, KDT 8th/e p863)

162. Ans. (c) Tenofovir
(Ref: Katzung 11th/e p859, KDT 8th/e p861)

163. Ans. (d) Ritonavir
(Ref: Katzung 11th/e p863, KDT 8th/e p866)

164. Ans. (b) Saquinavir *(Ref: KDT 8th/e p866)*

165. Ans. (c) Efavirenz *(Ref: KDT 8th/e p863)*

166. Ans. (a) Fusion inhibitor *(Ref: KDT 8th/e p867)*

167. Ans. (c) Thioacetazone
(Ref: KDT 8th/e p743, Harrison's 17th/e p1181, 346)

168. Ans. (d) Stavudine *(Ref: KDT 8th/e p862)*

169. Ans. (b) Gp 41 *(Ref: KDT 8th/e p867)*

170. Ans. (c) Raltegravir
(Ref: Harrison 17th/e p1191; Katzung 11//866, KDT 8th/e p866)

171. Ans. (a) Atazanavir *(Ref: Katzung 11/e p863)*

Unlike other protease inhibitors, atazanavir does not appear to be associated with dyslipidemia, fat redistribution or metabolic syndrome'.

172. Ans. (a) Lamivudine *(Ref: KDT 8th/e p862)*
173. Ans. (d) Tenofovir *(Ref: KDT 8th/e p863)*
174. Ans. (b) Didanosine *(Ref: KDT 8th/e p862)*
175. Ans. (b) Acyclovir *(Ref: KDT 8th/e p861)*
176. Ans. (c) Abacavir *(Ref: KDT 8th/e p861)*
177. Ans. (d) RNA dependent DNA polymerase
(Ref: KDT 8th/e p860-861)
178. Ans. (a) 4 weeks *(Ref: KDT 8th/e p871)*
179. Ans. (a) Radical cure of Plasmodium vivax malaria
(Ref: KDT 8th/e p878)

Radical cure: Several patients of P. vivax malaria relapse due to persistence of exo-erythrocytic stage. Drugs which attack this stage (hypnozoites) given together with a clinical curative achieve total eradication of the parasite from the patient's body.

Drug of choice for radical cure of vivax and ovale malaria is:
- Primaquine 15 mg daily for 14 days
- Tafenoquine is a new long-acting exo-erythrocytic schizontocidal drug. It has been developed as a single dose radical cure for vivax malaria.

180. Ans. (a) F, (b) T, (c) F, (d) T, (e) T *(Ref: KDT 8th/e p876-877)*
- Plasmodium falciparum is now the most common cause of malaria as well as most common cause of drug resistant malaria in India (Option a is false)
- DOC for multiple drug resistant P falciparum is artemisinin compounds, but they are short acting. The short action is responsible for recrudescences when used as monotherapy in malaria. So they are combined with long acting drugs (known as ACT; Artemisinin based Combination Therapy) like
  - Artemether + Lumefantrine: DOC in North-Eastern states.
  - Artesunate + Sulfadoxine/Pyrimethamine: DOC all over India except NE states.
- Artemisinins are contraindicated in first trimester of pregnancy; but can be given in second and third trimester.
- So, if drug resistant malaria occurs in 1st trimester of pregnancy, DOC is Quinine. To reduce its toxicity, we commonly add clindamycin (in pregnancy and children) or doxycycline (in other patients).
- Chloroquine is not effective in drug resistant malaria. So artesunate (not Chloroquine) is combined with sulfadoxine-pyrimethamine (Option c)

181. Ans. (a) Primaquine *(Ref: KDT 8th/e p878)*
- Primaquine has gametocidal action against all species of Plasmodium.
- Artemisinins have weak gametocidal action against early stages but not against mature gametes
- Proguanil does not kill gametes, however, it inhibit their development in the mosquito.

182. Ans. (a) Artemether plus lumefantrine *(Ref: KDT 8th/e p889)*

Chemotherapy B: Antimicrobials for Specific Conditions

Malaria	Drug of choice
P. vivax	Chloroquine
P. falciparum in North Eastern states	Artemether + Lumefantrine
P. falciparum in rest of India	Artesunate + Sulfadoxine/Pyrimethamine

183. Ans. (b) 250 mg *(Ref: KDT 8th/e p881)*
184. Ans. (c) Bull's eye retinopathy *(Ref: KDT 8th/e p882, 883)*
185. Ans. (c) Artemisinin *(Ref: KDT 8th/e p887)*
186. Ans. (c) Primaquine is contraindicated in infants and pregnant women *(Ref: Harrison 19th/e p1383; http://nvbdcp.gov.in/Doc/Diagnosis-Treatment-Malaria-2013.pdf)*

    According to WHO 2013 malaria guidelines
    - Primaquine is used to prevent relapse but is contraindicated in pregnant women, infants and individuals with G6PD deficiency.
    - *P. falciparum* cases should be treated with ACT (Artesunate 3 days + Sulfadoxine Pyrimethamine 1 day). This is to be accompanied by single dose primaquine preferably on day 2. The role of primaquine here is to prevent transmission due to its gameticidal action.
    - Primaquine is given for 14 days in treatment of P.vivax malaria. The role of primaquine here is to prevent relapse (by killing exo-erythrocytic stage). This is also known as radical cure.
    - In cases where parasitological diagnosis is not possible due to non-availability of either timely microscopy or RDT, suspected malaria cases will be treated with full course of chloroquine, till the results of microscopy are received. Once the parasitological diagnosis is available, appropriate treatment as per the species, is to be administered. Presumptive treatment with chloroquine is no more recommended.

187. Ans. (a) Artesunate
     (Ref: Harrison 19th/e p1699-1701, KDT 8th/e p 887)
     Drug of choice for severe or complicated malaria is artesunate. For more details, see text.

188. Ans. (b) Artesunate plus quinine *(Ref: CMDT 2010/1356)*

     The WHO recommended ACTs include:
     - Artemether-lumefantrine
     - Artesunate-amodiaquine
     - Artesunate-mefloquine
     - Artesunate-sulfadoxine-pyrimethamine
     - Dihydroartemisinin-piperaquine

189. Ans. (a) DLE *(Ref: Katzung 10th/e p849; KDT 8th/e p880)*
190. Ans. (d) All of the above *(Ref: KDT 8th/e p880)*
191. Ans. (a) Quinine *(Ref: KDT 8th/e p883)*
     Among the given options, quinine is the best answer. DOC for uncomplicated chloroquine resistant P. falciparum malaria is ACT [artemisinin-based combination therapy.]
192. Ans. (b) Primaquine *(Ref: KDT 8th/e p885)*
193. Ans. (a) High volume of distribution *(Ref: KDT 8th/e p880)*
194. Ans. (a) Quinine *(Ref: KDT 8th/e p883)*
195. Ans. (d) *P. vivax* and *P. ovale* *(Ref: KDT 8th/e p878)*
196. Ans. (d) Mefloquine *(Ref: KDT 8th/e p881)*
197. Ans. (b) Rapid recrudescence of malaria *(Ref: KDT 8th/e p887)*
198. Ans. (b) Lumefantrine *(Ref: KDT 8th/e p889)*
199. Ans. (a) Hypoglycemia *(Ref: KDT 8th/e p883)*
200. Ans. (c) Proguanil *(Ref: KDT 8th/e p883)*
201. Ans. (c) It has increased tissue binding *(Ref: KDT 8th/e p880)*
202. Ans. (a) Quinine *(Ref: CMDT 2010, 1358, KDT 8th/e p883)*
203. Ans. (c) Primaquine *(Ref: KDT 8th/e p878)*
204. Ans. (d) Above 1300 L *(Ref: Katzung 11th/e p39)*
205. Ans. (c) Pyrimethamine *(Ref: KDT 8th/e p884)*
206. Ans. (b) Doxycycline *(Ref: KDT 8th/e p875)*
207. Ans. (b) Primaquine *(Ref: KDT 8th/e p885)*
208. Ans. (d) Artesunate *(Ref: KDT 8th/e p887)*
209. Ans. (d) Proguanil *(Ref: KDT 8th/e p883)*
210. Ans. (b) Primaquine *(Ref: KDT 8th/e p885)*
211. Ans. (b) Sporozoites *(Ref: Goodman Gilman 12/e p1384)*
212. Ans. (b) Quinine *(Ref: KDT 8th/e p883)*
213. Ans. (c) Quinine *(Ref: KDT 8th/e p883)*
214. Ans. (b) Chloroquine *(Ref: KDT 8th/e p880)*
215. Ans. (b) Fluoroquinolones *(Ref: KDT 8th/e p877)*
216. Ans. (b) Metronidazole *(Ref: KDT 8th/e p894-896)*
     - Metronidazole is drug of choice for bacterial vaginosis (with or without pregnancy).
     - Alternative to metronidazole is clindamycin.
     - Rovamycin i.e. spiramycin (which is a macrolide) is drug of choice for toxoplasmosis in pregnancy.

217. Ans. 1. D, 2. A, 3. B, 4. F *(Ref: KDT 8th/e p907)*
     - Drug of choice for treatment of flukes (except liver fluke) and tapeworms (except dog tapeworm) is Praziquantal.
       - Drug of choice for treatment of liver fluke is triclabendazole.
       - Drug of choice for dog tapeworm (Echinococcus) is albendazole
     - Drug of choice for all nematodes (see exceptions below) is albendazole (or Mebendazole)
       - Drug of choice for treatment of filariasis is Diethylcarbamezine.
       - Drug of choice for treatment of Onchocerca and Strongyloides is ivermectin.
     - Nitazoxanide: DOC for Cryptosporidium and also used for Giardia (DOC is metronidazole and tinidazole)

218. Ans. (d) Amphotericin B *(Ref: KDT 8th/e p902)*
     RK 39 dipstick test is positive in infection with Leishmania. So, it is a case of visceral Leishmaniasis or Kala azar. The drug of choice is amphotericin B.

219. Ans. (a) Scabies *(Ref: KDT 8th/e p911)*
220. Ans. (a) It is topically used for the treatment of scabies *(Ref: KDT 8th/e p962)*
221. Ans. (d) Praziquantel *(Ref: KDT 8th/e p913)*
222. Ans. (a) Metronidazole *(Ref: CMDT 2017/e p1531)*
     The diagnosis is trichomonas vaginitis. The drug of choice is metronidazole or tinidazole

223. **Ans. (c) Cryptosporidium** *(Ref: Goodman Gilman 12th/e p1433)*
Pyruvate ferredoxin oxidoreductase (PFOR) enzyme dependent electron transfer is essential for anaerobic metabolism in many protozoa and bacterial species. The drug that acts by interfering with this reaction is **nitazoxanide**. It is the only drug available for cryptosporidiosis. It is also **approved for** treatment of **Giardiasis**.

224. **Ans. (a) Sporotrichosis** *(Ref: Harrison 17th/e p1265)*
Previously oral saturated solution of KI was used for sporotrichosis but now oral itraconazole is the drug of choice for cutaneous and lymphocutaneous sporotrichosis.

225. **Ans. (a) Chloroquine** *(Ref: Kanski Clinical Ophthalmology 6th/e p842-843)*
Chloroquine can cause Bull's eye maculopathy. The risk of retinotoxicity increases significantly with cumulative dose of more than 300 g (i.e. 250 mg daily for 3 years). It is rare if duration is less than one year.

226. **Ans. (c) Praziquantel** *(Ref: KDT 8th/e p913)*
Praziquantel is the drug of choice for all trematode and cestode infestations except Fasciola hepatica (triclabendazol) and hydatid disease (albendazole).

227. **Ans. (c) Cycloserine** *(Ref: KDT 8th/e p818, 821)*
- Rifampicin, INH and pyrazinamide are first line drugs for TB that are hepatotoxic.
- Ethionamide is also hepatotoxic. Remember, ethambutol is not hepatotoxic.
- Cycloserine does not cause hepatotoxicity. Its major adverse effect is neuropsychiatric reactions.

228. **Ans. (b) Albendazole** *(Ref: KDT 8th/e p909)*

229. **Ans. (c) Piperazine** *(Ref: KDT 8th/e p910)*

Drug	Mechanism of action
Albendazole	Blocks glucose uptake
Pyrantel Pamoate	Spastic Paralysis
Piperazine	Flaccid Paralysis
Ivermectin	Tonic Paralysis

230. **Ans. (c) Chloroquine is effective only in hepatic amoebiasis** *(Ref: KDT 8th/e p897)*

- **Drugs used for the treatment of amoebiasis are:**
  - Luminal ameobicide only *e.g.*, Diloxanide furoate, paromomycin and quiniodochlor.
  - Tissue ameobicide only *e.g.*, Chloroquine.
  - Both tissue as well as luminal ameobicides *e.g.*, Metronidazole, emetine etc.

- Metronidazole is the drug of choice for all forms of amoebiasis except very mild intestinal disease and carrier state.
- Diloxanide furoate is the agent of choice for mild intestinal amoebiasis and carriers.
- Emetine and dehydroemetine are rarely used now due to their emetic and cardiotoxic potential.

231. **Ans. (a) Filariasis** *(Ref: KDT 8th/e p910)*
- DEC kills microfilaria (Mf) of W. bacrofti and B. malayi from peripheral blood in 7 days, but microfilaria present in nodules and transudate are not killed.
- DEC is active against Mf of both Loa-loa and Onchocerca (but not against adult worms of onchocerca).

232. **Ans. (b) Chloroquine** *(Ref: KDT 8th/e p880)*

233. **Ans. (c) Albendazole** *(Ref: KDT 8th/e p909)*

234. **Ans. (a) Metronidazole** *(Ref: KDT 8th/e p895)*

235. **Ans. (c) Onchocercosis** *(Ref: KDT 8th/e p908)*

236. **Ans. (d) Albendazole** *(Ref: KDT 8th/e p909)*

237. **Ans. (a) 40 mg/kg single dose** *(Ref: KDT 8th/e p912)*
The dose in children (2-6 years) is 1g single dose. So, the best answer is option "A".

238. **Ans. (a) Albendazole** *(Ref: KDT 8th/e p909)*

239. **Ans. (a) Filariasis** *(Ref: KDT 8th/e p911)*

240. **Ans. (b) Kala azar** *(Ref: KDT 8th/e p903)*

241. **Ans. (d) Streptomycin** *(Ref: KDT 8th/e p798)*

242. **Ans. (d) Lamivudine** *(Ref: KDT 8th/e p862)*
Lamivudine is a nucleoside reverse transcriptase inhibitor used in the treatment *of HIV* infections. Low dose of this drug can be used *alone or in combination with IFN-α for chronic HBV infections* (because it has longer intracellular $t_{1/2}$ in HBV than in HIV).

243. **Ans. (d) Albendazole** *(Ref: Katzung 11th/e p924, KDT 8th/e p909)*

244. **Ans. (d) Albendazole** *(Ref: Katzung 11th/e p924, KDT 8th/e p 909)*

245. **Ans. (c) Albendazole and praziquantel** *(Ref: KDT 8th/e p909, 913)*

246. **Ans. (c) Praziquantel** *(Ref: KDT 8th/e p906)*

247. **Ans. (c) Schistosomiasis** *(Ref: KDT 8th/e)*

248. **Ans. (d) Satranidazole** *(Ref: KDT 8th/e p895, 897)*

249. **Ans. (b) Ivermectin** *(Ref: KDT 8th/e p911)*

250. **Ans. (d) Metronidazole** *(Ref: KDT 8th/e p895)*

251. **Ans. (b) Amphotericin B** *(Ref: KDT 8th/e p902)*

252. **Ans. (b) Neurocysticercosis** *(Ref: KDT 8th/e p895-896)*

253. **Ans. (c) Tapeworm** *(Ref: KDT 8th/e p909)*

254. **Ans. (b) Chloroquine** *(Ref: KDT 8th/e p894)*

255. **Ans. (a) 400 mg once** *(Ref: KDT 8th/e p909)*

256. **Ans. (a) Resistance to two or more first-line drugs but not to both isoniazid and rifampicin** *(Ref: Park 24th)*

Chapter 14: Chemotherapy C: Antineoplastic Drugs

Neoplastic cells are quite similar to normal cells, therefore the drugs targeted to kill these cells can also kill normal cells. As most of these drugs are acting on rapidly dividing cells, the normal cells having quick turnover are most susceptible to toxicity. *Bone marrow suppression, alopecia and mucositis* are thus commonly caused by anti-cancer drugs. New drugs targeting specific steps in the cells are devoid of these adverse effects.

Anticancer drugs may be divided (on the basis of stage of cell cycle at which these act) into two groups – cell cycle specific (CCS) and cell cycle non-specific (CCNS). CCS drugs are effective when the cells are proliferating whereas CCNS drugs are effective whether the cells are dividing or are in the resting phase.

TABLE 14.1: Cell cycle effects of anticancer drugs

Phase	CCS drugs	CCNS drugs
G_1	Etoposide	**Alkylating agents**
S	**Antimetabolites**	• Melphalan
	• Methotrexate	• Cyclophosphamide
	• 6-MP	• Nitrosourea
	• Cladribine	**Platinum compounds**
	• 5–FU	• Cisplatin
	• Capecitabine	• Carboplatin
G_2	**Topoisomerase inhibitors**	• Oxaliplatin
	• Irinotecan	**Anthracyclines**
	• Topotecan	• Doxorubicin
	• Etoposide	• Daunorubicin
	Bleomycin	• Epirubicin
M	**Vinca alkaloids**	• Mitoxantrone
	• Vincristine	**Antitumor antibiotics**
	• Vinblastine	• Dactinomycin
	• Vinorelbine	• Mitomycin–C
	Taxanes	
	• Paclitaxel	
	• Docetaxel	
	• Cabazitaxel	
	Erbulin	
	Estramustine	
	Ixabepilone	

Anticancer drugs can be discussed broadly under these groups:

1. Cytotoxic drugs
2. Targeted anticancer drugs
3. Hormones and related drugs
4. Other anticancer drugs

CYTOTOXIC DRUGS

Alkylating Agents

i. *Nitrogen mustards*: Mechlorethamine, cyclophosphamide, ifosfamide, melphalan, chlorambucil
ii. *Ethylenimines*: Thio-TEPA, hexamethylmelamine (altretamine)
iii. *Alkyl sulfonates*: Busulfan
iv. *Nitrosoureas*: Carmustine, lomustine, streptozocin
v. *Triazines* : Procarbazine, dacarbazine, temozolomide

Platinum Compounds

Cisplatin, carboplatin, oxaliplatin.

Antimetabolites

i. *Pyrimidine analogs* : 5-FU, cytarabine, gemcitabine
ii. *Purine analogs*: 6-MP, 6-thiogunanine, pentostatin, cladribine
iii. *Folic acid analogs*: Methotrexate, pemetrexed

Natural Products

i. *Vinca alkaloids*: Vincristine, vinblastine, vinorelbine
ii. *Taxanes*: Paclitaxel, docetaxel
iii. *Epipodophyllotoxins*: Etoposide, teniposide
iv. *Camptothecins*: Topotecan, irinotecan
v. *Antitumor antibiotics*: Anthracyclines (daunorubicin, doxorubicin, epirubicin, idarubicin, mitoxantrone), bleomycin, dactinomycin, mitomycin-C
vi. *Enzymes*: L-asparaginase

Alkylating Agents (Fig. 14.1)

All alkylating agents and related drugs (procarbazine, dacarbazine and platinum compounds) **are CCNS drugs** and thus act on both resting as well as dividing cells. These drugs alkylate nucleophilic groups on DNA bases **(N7 of guanine is most susceptible)** and may lead to cross-linking of bases, abnormal base-pairing and DNA strand breakage. **Gastrointestinal distress, bone marrow suppression, alopecia, secondary leukemias and sterility are common adverse effects of all the alkylating agents.**

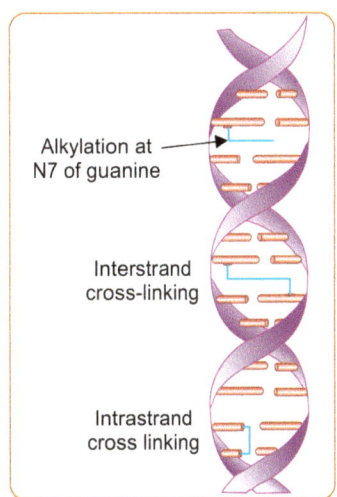

FIG. 14.1: Site of action of alkylating agents

Nitrogen Mustards

- **Cyclophosphamide** is a **prodrug** and is activated by hepatic biotransformation to aldophosphamide. One of its degradation products is **acrolein** that is responsible for **hemorrhagic cystitis** (its characteristic adverse effect). This adverse effect can be decreased by vigorous hydration and by the use of mercapto ethane sulfonic acid (**mesna**). Cyclophosphamide may also result in **cardiac dysfunction, pulmonary toxicity and syndrome of inappropriate ADH secretion**. Ifosfamide produces *chloracetaldehyde* (nephrotoxic) and *acrolein* as metabolites. Ifosfamide has same toxicity profile as cyclophosphamide, however it has HIGHER risk of neurotoxicity and hemorrhagic cystitis. Cyclophosphamide is the **drug of choice for Wegener's granulomatosis**. It is a powerful vesicant

> **Key Points**
>
> **HEMORRHAGIC CYSTITIS**
> Drugs causing:
> - *Ifosfamide*
> - *Cyclophosphamide*
>
> Metabolite responsible:
> - *Acrolein*
>
> Treatment:
> - *Mesna*

- **Mechlorethamine** is best known for its use in **Hodgkin's disease**. It is a **powerful vesicant**.
- **Melphalan** is the drug of choice for **multiple myeloma**.

Nitrosoureas

Drugs like **carmustine** (BCNU), **lomustine** (CCNU) and **semustine** (methyl CCNU) etc. are highly lipid soluble and can cross blood brain barrier. Thus, these are used for the treatment of **brain tumors like gliomas**. These can cause **delayed neutropenia**.

- Dacarbazine primarily affects RNA and protein synthesis unlike alkylating agent.
- **Streptozocin** can destroy beta cells of pancreas, and is thus used for *islet cell tumors*. It has minimum bone marrow toxicity.

Other Alkylating Agents

- **Busulfan** causes adrenal insufficiency, *pulmonary fibrosis*, skin hyperpigmentation and hyperuricemia.
- **Procarbazine is most leukemiogenic** and causes **disulfiram like reaction** with alcohol. It also causes CNS effects like hypnosis and vivid dreams.
- **Chlorambucil** spares myelocytes, used for CLL.
- **Lurbinectedin** is an alkylating agent with additional mechanism of inhibiting RNA polymerase II and macrophage infiltration into tumor tissue. It is approved for treatment of small cell carcinoma of lung. Major distinctive adverse effect of lurbinectedin is hepatotoxicity.

Distinctive Toxicities of Alkylating Agents

Drug	Toxicity
Cyclophosphamide	Alopecia, Hemorrhagic cystitis, SIADH
Ifosfamide	Hemorrhagic cystitis, SIADH
Busulfan	Pulmonary fibrosis, Hyperpigmentation, Adrenal insufficiency
Procarbazine	Secondary leukemias, Disulfiram like reaction, Behavioral changes, CNS depression
Cisplatin	Emesis, Nephrotoxicity, Peripheral sensory neuropathy, Ototoxicity
Lurbinectedin	Hepatotoxicity

Platinum Compounds

These include **cisplatin, carboplatin and oxalplatin**. These are *not alkylating agents* in true sense but are discussed here because of similar mechanism of action. Only difference is that these use platinum instead of alkyl group to form dimers of DNA. Most common adverse effect of these agents is **nausea and vomiting (maximum among all anti-cancer drugs)**. These drugs are mild bone marrow suppressants and are **nephrotoxic, ototoxic as well as neurotoxic**. *Cisplatin* is most *nephrotoxic* whereas *carboplatin* is more *hematotoxic* (bone marrow suppressant). Carboplatin has less nephrotoxic, ototoxic and neurotoxic potential than cisplatin. **Oxaliplatin is effective against the cells showing resistance to cisplatin or carboplatin. Its dose limiting toxicity is neurotoxicity** (peripheral neuropathy).

- It is important to establish chloride diuresis prior to cisplatin therapy in order to *prevent renal toxicity*. Chloride diuresis has *no effect on ototoxicity*.
- Cisplatin is always given as **slow IV infusion** (never bolus) to prevent intense nausea and acute rise in serum creatinine.
- *Aluminium inactivates cisplatin*, therefore aluminium containing equipments or needles should not be used with cisplatin.
- **Amifostine** is labelled for *reduction* of cisplatin induced *nephrotoxicity*.
- **Amifostine** is also used to *reduce xerostomia* in patients undergoing irradiation of head and neck involving parotid.
- Cisplatin has less chances of causing bone marrow suppression.
- **Cisplatin** *reduces all ions in serum* i.e. causes hypomagnesemia, hypokalemia, hypocalcemia and hypophosphatemia. (Remember, *cyclosporine*, an immunosuppressive drug *cause hyperkalemia*).
- Cisplatin has been *associated with development of AML*, usually 4 years or more after treatment.

> **Note**
> - Nitrosoureas and ifosfamide may lead to renal failure.
> - All alkylating agents are myelosuppressive.
> - Nitrosoureas and mechlorethamine have strong vesicant properties (cause local irritation and damage).
> - Alkylating agents also can cause sterility and secondary leukemias (less common with cyclophosphamide).
> - All alkylating agents have caused pulmonary fibrosis.
> - In high dose, all alkylating agents can cause veno-occlusive disease of liver which can be reversed by defibrotide.

Antimetabolites

These drugs act in the **S-phase** of cell cycle (CCS drugs), thus only dividing cells are responsive. These drugs possess immunosuppressive properties apart from their antineoplastic effects.

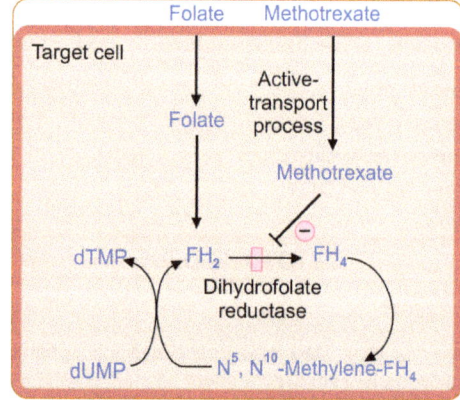

FIG. 14.2: Mechanism of action of methotrexate

Folic Acid Analogs

- **Methotrexate, pemetrexed** and **pralatrexate** are the **inhibitors of** dihydrofolate reductase **(DHFRase)**. These drugs also inhibit **thymidylate synthase (TS)** and the enzymes involved in early purine synthesis **(Fig. 14.2)**.
- Methotrexate forms polyglutamates inside the cell that helps to trap it within the cells and thus is important for cytotoxicity to neoplastic cells.

> - **Methotrexate resistance** can occur due to:
>   - *Impaired transport* of methotrexate into cells,
>   - Production of *altered forms of DHFRase* that have decreased affinity for the inhibitor,
>   - *Increased* concentrations of *intracellular DHFRase* through gene amplification or altered gene regulation, *decreased* ability to synthesize *methotrexate polyglutamates*
>   - Increased expression of a drug *efflux transporter*, of the MRP (multidrug resistance protein) class.

- Methotrexate can be **sequestered in third-space collections** and leech back into general circulation, causing prolonged immunosuppresion.
- Clearance of methotrexate depends on renal function and **vigorous hydration is required to prevent its crystallization in renal tubules**.
- It is the **drug of choice** for the treatment of **choriocarcinoma**. It is also useful for acute leukemias, non-Hodgkin lymphoma, cutaneous T-cell lymphoma and breast cancer. It can be used by intrathecal route for *meningeal leukemias*.
- Methotrexate is **also indicated in the management of rheumatoid arthritis, psoriasis and ectopic pregnancy**.

> **MNEMONIC**
>
> Uses of Methotrexate
> Inhibit –Immunosuppressant
> C –Crohn's disease
> A –Abortion
> N –Non Hodgkin Lymphoma
> C –Choriocarcinoma
> E –Ectopic pregnancy
> R –Rheumatoid arthritis

- Adverse effects of methotrexate are **bone marrow suppression and mucositis**. The toxicity of methotrexate to normal cells can be **reduced by** administration of N_{10} **formyl- tetrahydrofolic acid (folinic acid, citrovorum factor or leucovorin)**. This strategy is known as *leucovorin rescue. Leucovorin do not prevent neurotoxicity.* Alkalinization of urine can also reduce methotrexate toxicity. In extreme cases, toxicity can be treated by dialysis or administration of **GLUCARPIDASE**, a methotrexate cleaving enzyme. Long term use of methotrexate may also lead to **hepatotoxicity**, pulmonary infiltrates and fibrosis. NSAIDs like aspirin, penicillins and cephalosporins may decrease the renal excretion of methotrexate and result in toxicity.
- Pemetrexed is approved for treatment of *mesothelioma. Folic acid and vitamin* B_{12} *supplementation decreases the toxicity of pemetrexed without interfering with its clinical efficacy.*
- **Pralatrexate** is a similiar drug indicated for peripheral T-cell lymphoma.

Purine Analogs

- **6-mercaptopurine** (6-MP) and **6-thioguanine** (6-TG) are the purine antimetabolites that are activated by hypoxanthine-guanine phosphoribosyl transferase (HGPRTase). The resulting nucleotides inhibit several enzymes in purine biosynthesis and metabolism. 6-MP is metabolized by xanthine oxidase.
- When administered along **with allopurinol** (*xanthine oxidase inhibitor), the* **dose of 6-MP (and also azathioprine) should be reduced** to 1/4th of the original dose.
- Purine antimetabolites are used mainly for the treatment of leukemias (both acute leukemias and CML).
- Dose limiting toxicity is bone marrow suppression but hepatotoxicity can also result.
- Other important purine analogs are fludarabine phosphate and cladribine (adenine analogs).
- Because **cladribine** is resistant to degradation by adenosine deaminase, it is **drug of choice** for the treatment of **hairy cell leukemia.**
- **Fludarabine** is *drug of choice* for chronic lymphocytic leukemia **(CLL)**. *Use of pentostatin with fludarabine may result in severe pulmonary toxicity.*
- All purine analogs may cause immunosuppression on long-term use and patients should be given cotrimoxazole for prophylaxis of *Pneumocystis*.

Pyrimidine Analogs

- Drugs in this group include **cytarabine** (cytosine arabinoside), **5-fluorouracil** (5-FU), **capecitabine, gemcitabine, 5-azacytidine and decitabine.**
- **Cytarabine** is the single *most effective agent for induction of remission in AML.*
- Cytarabine is activated by kinases to form arabinoside CTP that is an inhibitor of DNA polymerase.
- High dose of **cytarabine** can lead to neurotoxicity (**ataxia and peripheral neuropathy**).
- 5-FU is converted to 5'-dUMP that inhibits TS. Its major route of metabolism is by conversion to CO_2 and elimination by respiratory pathway.
- **Capecitabine** is an **oral pro-drug of 5-FU**. It can cause hyperbilirubinemia.
- Thiopurines (6-MP and 6-TG) are metabolized by the thiopurine methyl transferase (TPMT) whereas 5-FU is catabolized by dihydropyrimidine dehydrogenase (DPD). Both TPMT and DPD have pharmaco-genetic deficiencies in some persons.
- **Capecitabine and 5-FU** can cause **hand and foot syndrome** (a form of erythromelalgia manifested as tingling, numbness, pain, erythema, swelling and increased pigmentation). Uridine triacetate is recently approved for oral treatment of 5-FU and capecitabine toxicity
- *Leucovorin augments the action of 5-FU.*
- 5 FU cause single strand breaks and thus affects both DNA & RNA.
- **Gemcitabine** is a *very potent radiosensitizer.*
- **Gemcitabine** is the **drug of choice** for **pancreatic cancer.**
- **5'-Azacytidine** acts by **DNA hypomethylation** and is approved for treatment of **myelodysplasia**. Decitabine is another drug acting by same mechanism.
- **Cedazuridine** is a cytidine deaminase inhibitor. It is given in combination with decitabine for myelodysplastic syndrome and chronic myelomonocytic leukemia.

Distinctive Toxicities of Antimetabolites

6-MP and 6 TG	Hepatotoxicity
Methotrexate	Mucositis, hepatotoxicity
5-FU	Hand and foot syndrome, neurotoxicity
Capecitabine	Hand and foot syndrome, Hyperbilirubinemia
Cytarabine	Cerebellar ataxia
Fludarabine	Arthralgia
Gemcitabine	Diarrhea

> **Note**
> - All antineoplastic antimetabolites can cause bone marrow suppression.
> - Alkylating agents are used for chronic leukemias whereas antimetabolites are commonly used for acute leukemias.

Mitotic Spindle Inhibitors (Fig. 14.3)

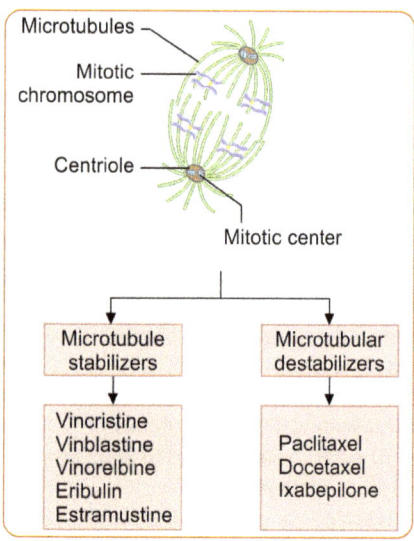

FIG. 14.3: Mitotic spindle inhibitors

Vinca Alkaloids

Vincristine, vinblastine and vinorelbine are the vinca alkaloids that act by **inhibiting polymerization of microtubules** (thus inhibiting formation of mitotic spindle). Therefore, these are effective in M-phase of cell cycle. Vinblastine causes bone marrow suppression whereas **vincristine is 'marrow sparing'** but is neurotoxic (peripheral neuropathy). Vinca alkaloids can also result in **SIADH**.

- **Vinblastine's** most important clinical use is the curative therapy of *metastatic testicular tumors*.
- **Vincristine with glucocorticoids** is the *treatment of choice* for inducing remission in *childhood leukemias*. It can *also* be used for *pediatric solid tumors* (Wilm's tumor, neuroblastoma and rhabdomyosarcoma) and *lymphomas*.

Taxanes

Paclitaxel and docetaxel interfere with mitotic spindle formation by **preventing disassembly of microtubules**. Paclitaxel causes hypersensitivity reactions (due to Cremophor-containing vehicle) whereas docetaxel is devoid of this adverse effect. **Protein bound paclitaxel (nab-paclitaxel)** has *decreased risk of hypersensitivity reactions*. Both of these drugs can cause *bone marrow suppression* and *neurotoxicity*. Cisplatin decreases paclitaxel clearance and paclitaxel can decrease doxorubicin clearance. **Cabazitaxel** is a microtubule inhibitor indicated in combination with prednisone for hormone refractory metastatic prostate cancer.

Ixabepilone

It is a new drug approved for treatment of *advanced breast carcinoma* resistant to anthracyclines and taxanes. It is given in combination with capecitabine. It acts by *binding to tubulin and promoting microtubule stabilization*, thereby arresting cells in the G_2-M phase of cell cycle.

Erbulin Mesylate

It is a microtubule inhibitor recently approved for treatment of patients with metastatic **breast cancer**. It has also been approved for **liposarcoma.**

Estramustine

It is a **combination of estrogen and mechlorethamine** (nitrogen mustard) and is used for the treatment of **prostatic carcinoma**. It acts as *anti-mitotic drug* by binding to tubulin. It can produce estrogenic side effects (gynaecomastia and impotence).

Topoisomerase Inhibitors

Camptothecins

Irinotecan and **topotecan** are obtained from *Camptotheca acuminata* tree and act by **inhibiting topoisomerase I** (this enzyme nicks, introduces negative supercoils and reseals the DNA strand). Topotecan is used in advanced ovarian carcinoma and is excreted by renal route. **Irinotecan is a prodrug** that is converted in the liver to an active metabolite, SN-38. It is eliminated in bile and feces and thus its **dose should be reduced in hepatic failure. Irinotecan is now the treatment of choice for advanced colorectal carcinoma** *in combination with 5-FU.*

- Dose limiting toxicity of *topotecan is neutropenia* whereas it is *diarrhea for irinotecan.*
- Irinotecan can also lead to myelosuppression.
- *Irinotecan can also result in a cholinergic syndrome* (manifested as diarrhea, sweating, hypersalivation, lacrimation, rhinorrhea, abdominal cramps and bradycardia) due to inhibition of acetylcholine esterase. It occurs within 24 hours.

Epipodophyllotoxins

Podophyllotoxin was used for its emetic, cathartic and antihelminthic effects. It acts by binding to tubulin but its derivatives; **etoposide** and **teniposide** act by **inhibiting topoisomerase II** resulting in DNA damage through strand breakage. These drugs act at the junction of late S and early G_2 phase of cell cycle. These drugs can cause *gastrointestinal distress and myelosuppression.*

- Etoposide is indicated for testicular, prostatic and oat cell carcinoma [of lung].
- **Etoposide therapy can result in acute non-lymphocytic** (acute monocytic or monomyelocytic) **leukemia.** This leukemia develops at a *short time interval* (1 to 3 years) after the end of therapy as compared to alkylating agents induced leukemia (require 4-5 years). Another distinguishing feature of this leukemia is *absence of myelodysplastic period preceeding leukemia.*
- At high doses, *etoposide is hepatotoxic.*

Antitumor Antibiotics

This group includes **anthracycline antibiotics** (*doxorubicin* also known as *adriamycin, daunorubicin, epirubicin and idarubicin*), mitoxantrone, bleomycin, dactinomycin and mitomycin. **Except bleomycin (acts in G_2 phase), all other drugs are CCNS drugs.** *All antitumor antibiotics are obtained from Streptomyces.*

- Anthracycline antibiotics act by inhibiting topoisomerase II. Doxorubicin and daunorubicin are primarily used in acute leukemias whereas idarubicin and epirubicin display broader activity against solid tumors (breast carcinoma, Osteosarcoma, Ewing's sarcoma and soft tissue sarcoma). These agents also generate semiquinone free radicals that are responsible for cardiotoxicity (manifested in the form of dilated cardiomyopathy and congestive heart failure). This adverse effect can be reduced by using α-tocopherol and dexrazoxane (a free radical scavenger). Liposomal forms of these drugs have decreased cardiac toxicity. Dilated cardiomyopathy is cumulative, dose-dependent and may present even after discontinuation of the anthracyclines. Earliest morphological feature is swelling of endoplasmic reticulum. It is followed by loss of cardiomyocytes (myofibrillar dropout). Symptoms are similar to CHF including exertional dysponea, orthopnea and peripheral edema. These drugs also can cause red coloured urine (not hematuria). Another important feature of these drugs is that these can cause "radiation recall reaction" (erythema and desquamation of skin seen at the sites of prior radiation exposure). Mitoxantrone seems to be less cardiotoxic than the other drugs of this group. Mitoxantrone has been approved for AML, advanced hormone resistant prostate cancer and treatment of late stage, secondary progressive multiple sclerosis. It is less cardiotoxic but can result in acute promyelocytic leukemia. Valrubicin is approved for intravesical therapy of BCG-refractory urinary bladder carcinoma in situ.
- **Dactinomycin** (Actinomycin-D) acts by inhibiting DNA dependent RNA synthesis. It is indicated for solid tumors in children (rhabdomyosarcoma and Wilm's tumor) and choriocarcinoma. It is a radiosensitizer (like metronidazole and 5-FU).
- **Bleomycin** is a CCS *glycopeptide* drug that acts in the G_2 phase by causing DNA strand breakage and free radical formation. It can result in *cutaneous toxicity* (hyperpigmentation, hyperkeratosis, erythema and ulcers), pneumonitis, **pulmonary fibrosis,** hypersensitivity and mucocutaneous reactions (particularly flagellated pigmentation of skin). **Earliest indicator of an adverse effect is decreased in DLco**. It causes necrosis of type I pneumocytes that results in compensatory hyperplasia of type II pneumocytes. Bleomycin is *metabolized by bleomycin hydrolase*, whose concentration is less in skin and lungs (thus major organs involved in toxicity). Bleomycin toxicity may *become apparent after exposure to transient very high PIO_2* because bleomycin dependent electron transport is dependent on O_2.
- **Mitomycin** acts as an **alkylating agent**. It may be used as **intravesical therapy** to treat **superficial bladder cancers** and **anal carcinoma** (with radiation therapy). Rarely, it *can cause hemolytic uremic syndrome*. It is **best available** drug for use as an adjuvant to X-ray radiation **to attack hypoxic tumor cells.** (because, it is converted to active alkylating agent by reduction). It can cause **delayed bronchospasm.** It is also used in patients with **treacheal or laryngeal stenosis.**

Distinctive Toxicities of Natural Anticancer Drugs

Bleomycin	Pulmonary fibrosis (Marrow sparing)
Anthracyclines	Cardiotoxicity
Paclitaxel	Peripheral neuropathy, Hypersensitivity
Docetaxel	Peripheral neuropathy, Fluid retention
Irinotecan	Diarrhea
Vincristine	Peripheral neuropathy (**Marrow sparing**), SIADH

> **Note**
> All natural anticancer products can cause bone marrow suppression except bleomycin and vincristine.

TARGETED ANTICANCER THERAPIES

Unlike cytotoxic drugs, these drugs are specifically targeted against some molecules present on cancer cells. These can be divided into:
- Monoclonal antibodies
- Small molecule inhibitors

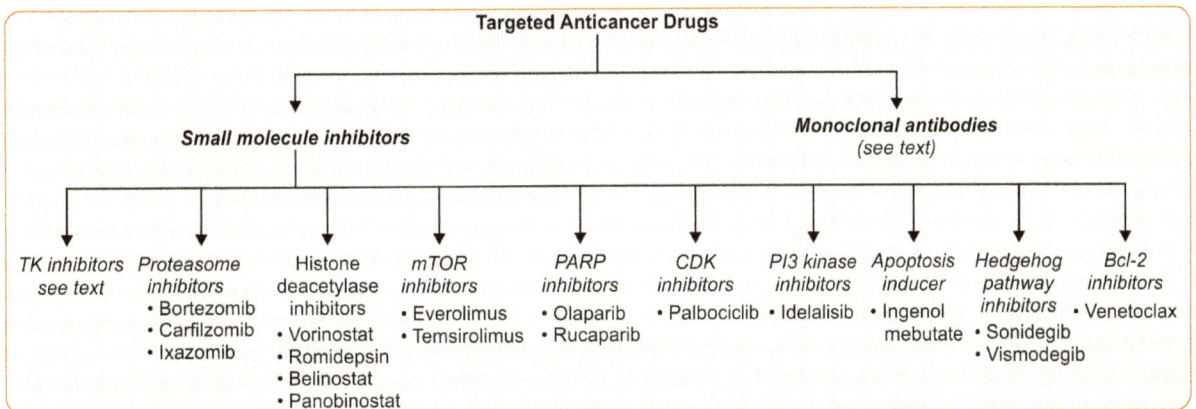

Monoclonal Antibodies

Monoclonal antibodies are produced from hybridomas (monoclonal antibody producing cells). Later are formed by fusion of antibody producing spleen cells (obtained from mice) with myeloma cells. Monoclonal antibiodies may be developed against many targets to kill cancer cells. The important types are:

1. **Disinhibition of T-cells brakes:** (Immune check point inhibitors): *James P. Allison and Tasuku Honjo* received **Noble**

prize in physiology or medicine for their discovery of cancer therapy by inhibition of negative immune regulation. Normally, there are certain checkpoints, so that immune cells (like T-cells) do not attack self antigens. Certain receptors like PD-1 (programmed death receptors) or CTLA-4 (cytotoxic T-lymphocyte associated protein) are present on T-cells. When ligands on other cells (PDL-1 or CD-80/86 respectively) bind to these receptors, T-cells are inhibited. Same method is utilized by some cancer cells to evade destruction from T-cells. These tumor cells overexpress the ligands like PDL-1 and inhibit T-cells. Monoclonal antibodies targeting these interactions result in disinhibition of these brakes and thus, T-cells can destroy cancer cells.

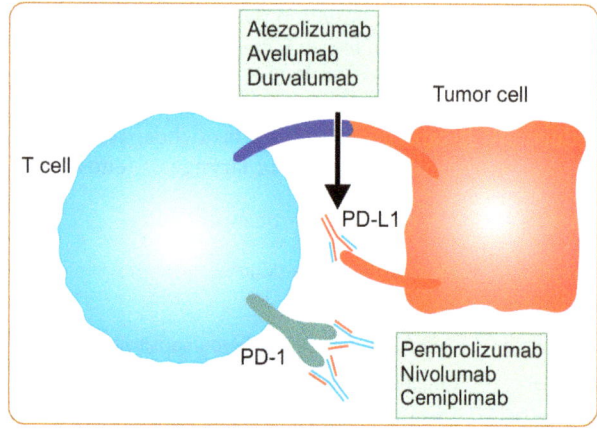

(a) *PD-1 and PDL-1 inhibitors*
- **Nivolumab**, **Pembrolizumab** and **Cemiplimab** are monoclonal antibodies against PD-1 receptors on T-cells.
- **Atezolizumab**, **Avelumab** and **Durvalumab** are monoclonal antibodies against PDL-1 present on cancer cells.

(b) *CTLA-4 Inhibitor:*
Normally CD-80 or CD-86 present on antigen presenting cells bind to CD-28 present on T-cells. Cytotoxic T-lymphocyte Antigen-4 (CTLA-4) is a CD-28 homologue expressed on T-cells. Binding of this with CD-80/86 molecules inhibit the T-cells. **Ipilimumab** acts as CTLA-4 inhibitor resulting in T-cell activation and destruction of cancer cells. It is approved for treatment of **malignant melanoma**.

	Drug	Targete	Use
1.	Nivolumab	PD-1	Hodgkin's lymphoma Non-small cell lung cancer Metastatic melanoma
2.	Pembrolizumab	PD-1	Metastatic melanoma Non-small cell lung cancer Endometrial cancer Esophageal cancer Small cell lung cancer Renal cell carcinoma Head and Neck cancer
3.	Cemiplimab	PD-1	Squamous cell carcinoma of skin
4.	Dostarlimab	PD-1	Endometrial cancer
5.	Avelumab	PDL-1	Merkel cell carcinoma Renal cell carcinoma
6.	Durvalumab	PDL-1	Urothelial carcinoma
7.	Atezolizumab	PDL-1	Urothelial carcinoma Non-small cell lung carcinoma
8.	Ipilimumab	CTLA-4	Malignant melanoma

2. **Monoclonal antibodies against CD-antigens**
Several monoclonal antibodies have been developed against CD-antigens present on immune cells. Their targets and uses are given in table below

	Drug	Target	Indications
1.	Blinatumomab	CD-3 and CD-19	Philadelphia negative ALL
2.	Tafasitamab	CD-19	DLBCL
3.	Loncastuximab	CD-19	DLBCL
4.	Rituximab	CD-20	Non-Hodgkin lymphoma CLL
5.	Ofatumumab	CD-20	CLL
6.	Tositumomab	CD-20	B-cell lymphoma
7.	Ibritumomab	CD-20	B-cell lymphoma
8.	Obintuzumab	CD-20	B-cell Non-Hodgkin lymphoma, CLL, SLL
9.	Inotuzumab	CD-22	B-cell, ALL
10.	Moxetumomab	CD-22	Hairy cell leukemia
11.	Brentuximab	CD-30	Hodgkin lymphoma T-cell lymphoma
12.	Gemtuzumab	CD-33	CD-33 positive AML
13.	Daratumumab	CD-38	Multiple myeloma
14.	Isatuximab	CD-38	Multiple myeloma
15.	Alemtuzumab	CD-52	CLL Low grade lymphoma
16.	Polatuzumab	CD79B	DLBCL
17.	Emapalumab	IFN-γ	Hemophagocytic lymphohistiocytosis

> **MNEMONIC**
>
> Rituximab is a monoclonal antibody against CD20. It is used for treatment of:
> R – **R**h. arthritis
> e
> L – **L**upus (SLE)
> I – **I**TP
> A – **A**utoimmune hemolytic anemia
> N – **N**on-Hodgkin Lymphoma
> C – **C**LL
> e

3 **Monoclonal antibodies against growth factor receptors**
Activation of receptors of various growth factors (like EGF, VEGF, HER-2, PDGF, etc.) is associated with development of certain cancers.
- **Cetuximab**, **Panitumumab** and **Necitumumab** are monoclonal antibodies against Epidermal Growth Factor Receptor (EGFR). It is also called as Human Epidermal growth factor Receptor-1 (HER-1).
  – **Cetuximab** is a monoclonal antibody *against EGFR*. It is approved for *colon cancer* [with irinotecan] and *head and neck cancer* [with radiation therapy]. Its main adverse effects are skin rash, hypomagnesemia and hypersensitivity reactions.
  – **Panitumumab** is a fully human monoclonal antibody **against EGFR**. It is similar to cetuximab but do not cause hypersensitivity reactions [because it is fully human]. It is approved for **colo-rectal cancer**.
  – **Trastuzumab** and **Pertuzumab** are monoclonal antibodies against Human Epidermal growth factor Receptor-2 (Her-2/neu).

Chemotherapy C: Antineoplastic Drugs

- Trastuzumab is useful for the treatment of **breast carcinoma** but **cardiotoxicity** limits its use. Recently, It has also been approved for cancer of stomach or gastroesophageal junction.
- **Ado-trastuzumab mertansine** is a **conjugate** of trastuzumab (monoclonal antibody against her-2) and mertansine (microtubule inhibitor). It is approved for treatment of her-2 positive metastatic breast cancer.
- **Pertuzumab** is a monoclonal antibody against her-2/neu. It is used in combination with trastuzumab (bind to different region of her-2 receptor) for metastatic breast carcinoma.

- **Bevacizumab** is monoclonal antibody against vascular Endothelial Growth Factor (VEGF) whereas **Ramucirumab** is targeted against VEGF Receptor (VEGFR-2)
  - **Bevacizumab** is a monoclonal antibody against vascular endothelial growth factor (VEGF). Latter is an essential requirement for angiogenesis. It is approved for *colorectal, breast, glioblastoma, metastatic renal cell carcinoma and non-small cell lung cancer*. Its main safety concerns are hypertension, thromboembolism, wound healing complications and gastrointestinal perforations.
  - **Ramucirumab** is approved for non-small cell lung carcinoma and gastro-esophageal junction cancer.
- **Olaratumab** is monoclonal antibody against Platelet Derived Growth Factor Receptor-α (PDGFR-α). It is approved for soft tissue sarcoma

	Drug	Targete	Indications
1.	Amivantamab	EGFR, MET	Non-small cell lung cancer
2.	Cetuximab	EGFR	Colo-rectal carcinoma Head and Neck Cancer
3.	Panitumumab	EGFR	Colo-rectal carcinoma
4.	Necitumumab	EGFR	Non-small cell lung cancer
5.	Trastuzumab	HER-2/neu	Breast cancer Adenocarcinoma of gastro-esophageal junction
6.	Enfortumab	HER-2	Breast cancer
7.	Pertuzumab	HER-2/neu	Breast cancer
8.	Margetuximab	HER-2	Breast cancer
9.	Ramucirumab	VEGFR-2	Non-small cell lung cancer Hepatocellular carcinoma Gastro-esophageal junction cancer
10.	Bevacizumab	VEGF	Colo-rectal carcinoma Renal cell carcinoma Brain tumors Ovarian carcinoma Non-small cell lung cancer
11.	Olaratumab	PDGFR-α	Soft tissue sarcoma
12.	Naxitamab	GD-2	Neuroblastoma

4. **Other Targets**
- **Denosumab** is a monoclonal antibody against RANK-ligand. It is approved for treatment of **Giant cell tumor** of bone apart from osteoporosis.
- **Dinutuximab** is targeted against glycolipid GD-2. It is approved for **neuroblastoma**.
- **Elotuzumab** is monoclonal antibody against SLAM-F7 and is used for **multiple myeloma**.
- **Mogamulizumab** is recently developed monoclonal antibody against CCR-4. It is approved for treatment of mycosis fungoides and Sezary syndrome.

	Drug	Targete	Indications
1.	Denosumab	RANK-L	Giant cell tumor of bone
2.	Dinutuximab	Glycolipid-GD2	Neuroblastoma
3.	Elotuzumab	SLAM-F7	Multiple myeloma
4.	Mogamulizumab	CCR-4	Mylosis fungoides Sezary syndrome
5.	Belantamab	BCMA	Multiple myeloma
6.	Sacituzumab	Trop-2	Breast cancer

Small Molecule Inhibitors

These may act by inhibiting enzymes like tyrosine kinase, PI3 kinase, mTOR, etc. Unlike monoclonal antibodies, these are smaller in size.

(a) Tyrosine Kinase Inhibitors

- All tyrosine kinase inhibitors are metabolized by CYP 3A4 enzymes. Thus, these have the potential of drug interactions.
- All tyrosine kinase inhibitors can be administered orally.
- **Imitinab** is an oral drug used for chronic phase of CML. It acts by inhibiting tyrosine kinase activated due to *abl-bcr fusion* (t 9, 22; Philadelphia chromosome). It is a **competitive inhibitor of ATP-binding of the abl** kinase in the inactive conformation. **Dasatinib** and **Nilotinib** are similar drugs used in case of imatinib resistance. **Imatinib is the drug of choice for CML and gastro-intestinal stromal tumor (GIST)**.

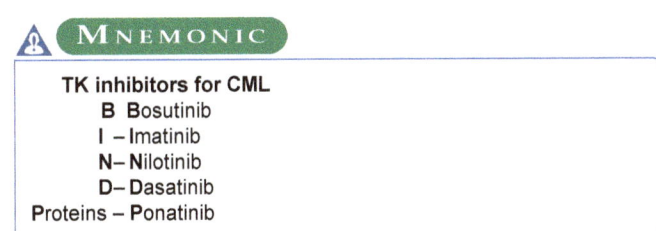

TK inhibitors for CML
  B Bosutinib
  I – Imatinib
  N – Nilotinib
  D – Dasatinib
Proteins – Ponatinib

- **Geftinib and Erlotinib** are inhibitors of tyrosine kinase associated with **epidermal growth factor receptor (EGFR)**. These are indicated for *non-small cell lung cancer*. **Erlotinib** is especially effective in cases affecting *women, nonsmokers,* and persons of *Asian* ethnicity as well as cases involving *adenocarcinoma and bronchioalveolar carcinoma* histology. Erlotinib is also indicated for **pancreatic carcinoma** with gemcitabine. **Food increases the absorption** of Erlotinib to 100%. It is metabolized by **CYP3A4** enzyme system. Acneiform **skin rash, diarrhea, anorexia and fatigue** are the most common adverse effects of this drug. Molecular studies have shown that patients with EGFR mutations respond to **Erlotinib** at significantly high rates, but patients with Kras mutations do not respond and should not be offered this drug.

TK inhibitors for NSCLC
Operate Osimertinib
After – Afatinib
           Alectinib
    E – Erlotinib
    C – Crizotinib
       – Ceritinib
    G – Geftinib

- **Sorafenib** and **Sunitinib** are small molecules that **inhibit multiple tyrosine kinases**. Both can be used for *renal cell cancer*. In addition *sorafenib* is indicated for *hepatocellular cancer* and *sunitinib* for *GIST*. These can cause hypertension as an adverse effect.

> **MNEMONIC**
>
> TK inhibitors for GIST
> S – Sunitinib
> I – Imatinib
> R – Regorafenib

- **Lapatinib** is indicated for breast carcinoma. It inhibits tyrosine kinase associated with EGFR and HER-2/neu receptors.
- **Midostaurin** is a multi-kinase inhibitor. It can inhibit FLT3 and PDGF signalling among others. It is approved for **FLT3 positive AML, systemic mastocytosis** and **mast cell leukemia**.
- **Pazopanib** is a multi targeted tyrosine kinase inhibitor against VEGF receptors, PDGF receptor and c-kit. It is approved for treatment of **advanced renal cell carcinoma**.
- **Larotectinib** is an inhibitor of tropomyosin kinases (like Trk A, Trk B). It is the **first drug** to be specifically developed and approved to treat any cancer containing certain mutation. It is approved *for solid tumors with NTRK mutation*.

> **MNEMONIC**
>
> TK inhibitors for RCC
> P – Pazopanib
> A – Axitinib
> S – Sorafenib
> S – Sunitinib

> **MNEMONIC**
>
> TK inhibitors for malignant melanoma
> **Cause** Cobemetinib
> D – Dabrafenib
> V – Vemurafenib
> T – Trameltinib

Drug	Inhibit TK activated by	Indication
Acalabrutinib	Bruton TK (BTK)	Mantle cell lymphoma
Afatinib	EGFR, HER-2, HER-4	Non-small cell lung carcinoma (NSCLC)
Alectinib	ALK, RET	NSCLC
Axitinib	VEGFR-1, 2, 3	Advanced renal cell carcinoma (RCC)
Binimetinib	MEK	Malignant melanoma
Bosutinib	abl-bcr, src	CML
Brigatinib	ALK, ROS-1, IGF-1R, FLT-3	NSCLC
Cabozantinib	c-MET, VEGFR-2	Medullary carcinoma thyroid RCC
Capmatinib	C-MET	NSCLC
Ceritinib	ALK	NSCLC
Cobimetinib	MEK, MAPK	Metastatic melanoma
Crizotinib	c-MET, ALK	Non-small cell lung carcinoma
Dabrafenib	BRAF	Metastatic melanoma

Drug	Inhibit TK activated by	Indication
Dacomitinib	EGFR	Non-small cell lung cancer
Dasatinib	abl-bcr	CML
Encorafenib	BRAF	Malignant melanoma
Entrectinib	TRK, ROS-1, ALK	NSC LC, NTRK + Solid tumors
Erlotinib	EGFR	Non-small cell lung carcinoma, Pancreatic carcinoma
Erdafitinib	FGFR	Bladder cancer
Geftinib	EGFR	Non-small cell lung carcinoma
Fedratinib	JAK-2	Myelofibrosis
Gilteritinib	FLT-3	FLT-3 positive AML
Ibrutinib	Btk	CLL
Imatinib	abl-bcr, c-KIT, PDGF	CML, GIST
Infigratinib	FGFR	Cholangiocarcinoma
Larotrectinib	Trk A, Trk B, Trk C	Solid tumors with NTRK mutation
Lapatinib	her-2/neu, erb-B2	Breast carcinoma
Lenvatinib	VEGF	I[131] refractory differentiated thyroid cancer, HCC, RCC
Lonafarnib	Farnesyl Transferase	Hutchinson Gilford Progeria syndrome
Lorlatinib	ALK	ALK positive NSCLC
Nilotinib	abl-bcr	CML
Nintedanib	PDGFR, FGFR, VEGFR	Idiopathic pulmonary fibrosis, NSCLC
Osimertinib	EGFR	NSCLC
Pazopanib	VEGFR-1,2,3 PDGFR α, β c-KIT	Advanced renal cell carcinoma
Pemigatinib	FGFR-2	Cholangiocarcinoma
Pexidartinib	KIT, CSF-1R, FLT 3	Tenosynovial giant cell tumor
Ponatinib	abl-bcr	CML, Philadelphia positive ALL
Pralsetinib	RET	NSCLC
Regorafenib	VDGFR2, TIE2	Colorectal carcinoma GIST
Ripretinib	KIT, PDGFR	GIST
Ruxolitinib	JAK 1, 2	Myelofibrosis
Selpercatinib	RET	NSCLC, medullary carcinoma of thyroid
Sorafenib	VEGFR, PDGFR RAF	Renal cell carcinoma, Hepatocellular carcinoma
Selumetinib	MEK	Neurofibromatosis-1
Sunitinib	VEGFR, PDGFR c-KIT, FLT-3 RET	Renal cell carcinoma, Pancreatic neuroendocrine tumors, GIST
Sotorasib	RAS	NSCLC
Tepotinib	C-MET	NSCLC
Tofacitinib	JAK	Rheumatoid arthritis
Tivozanib	VEGF	RCC
Trametinib	MEK	Metastatic melanoma
Tucatinib	HER-2	Breast cancer
Vandetanib	VEGFR, EGFR	Medullary carcinoma thyroid
Vemurafenib	BRAF	Malignant melanoma
Zanubrutinib	BTK	Mantle cell lymphoma

Chemotherapy C: Antineoplastic Drugs

(b) Proteasome Inhibitors

Bortezomib, carfilzomib and **ixazomib** act by *inhibiting proteasome* resulting in down regulation of NF-κB (involved in cell survival). These have been approved for treatment of *resistant multiple myeloma*.

(c) Histone Deacetylase Inhibitors

Vorinostat and Romidepsin *are histone deacetylase inhibitors* approved *for cutaneous T-cell lymphoma*. **Panobinostat** is a new drug in this category that is approved for *multiple myeloma*. **Belinostat** is another drug in this group appoved for relapsed or refractory *peripheral T-cell lymphoma*.

Tazametostat is a histone methyltransferase EZH2 inhibitor. It is approved as oral therapy of **epithelioid sarcoma**. It is given with venetoclax.

(d) mTOR Inhibitors

This group include **everolimus** and **Temsirolimus** (a prodrug that is converted to sirolimus). These act as specific inhibitors of mTOR. **Temsirolimus** is approved for **advanced renal cell carcinoma** whereas **everolimus** *is used for breast, pancreatic, brain and renal cell carcinoma*. These are associated with interstitial lung disease.

(e) PARP Inhibitors

Olaparib and **rucaparib** are poly ADP-ribose polymerase (PARP) inhibitors and are used for oral treatment of **ovarian cancer**. **Niraparib** is new drug in this group that is indicated for ovarian, fallopian tube or primary peritoneal cancer. **Talazoparib** has been recently approved for advanced breast carcinoma with BRCA mutations.

(f) CDK Inhibitors

Palbociclib, abemaciclib and **ribociclib** are orally effective cyclin dependent kinase (cdk) 4 and 6 inhibitors. These are approved for post-menopausal women with ER + ve and HER-2 negative **breast cancer**. **Trilaciclib** is a new cdk-4 and cdk-6 inhibitor. It is used **to prevent bone marrow suppression** caused by chemotherapy of small cell lung carcinoma.

(g) PI 3 Kinase Inhibitors

Idelalisib is a small molecular inhibitor of PI3 kinase delta. It is approved for oral treatment of **relapsed CLL, follicular B-cell NHL and SLL. Copanlisib** is a new PI3 kinase inhibitor indicated in follicular lymphoma. **Duvelisib** is a dual inhibitor of PI3Kδ as well as PI3Kγ. It is approved for treatment of **CLL** and **follicular lymphoma**. **Umbralisib** is PI3 kinase inhibitor approved for marginal zone lymphoma and follicular lymphoma whereas **alpelisib** is approved for breast cancer.

(h) Apoptosis Inducers

Ingenol mebutate is an inducer of apoptosis specifically indicated for topical treatment of **actinic keratosis** of face, scalp, trunk and extremities.

(i) Protein Synthesis Inhibitors

Omacetaxine is a protein synthesis inhibitor approved for **chronic phase of CML**. It binds to A-site and prevents elogation step in protein synthesis.

(j) Hedgehog Pathway Inhibitors

Abnormalities in hedgehog pathway is associated with basal cell carcinoma. **Sonidegib** and **vismodegib** are new anticancer drugs that inhibit this pathway and used for **basal cell carcinoma**. **Glasdegib** is the only hedgehog pathway inhibitor approved for **AML**.

(k) Bcl-2 Inhibitors

Bcl-2 is an antiapoptotic protein. **Venetoclax** induces apoptosis by inhibiting this protein and is indicated in **CLL**.

(l) Isocitrate Dehydrogenase 2 (IDH2) Inhibitor

IDH2 mutation may result in AML. **Enasidenib** and **Ivosidenib** are inhibitors of IDH2 enzyme and are approved for IDH2 mutation positive AML.

(m) Selinexor

It is a selective inhibitor of nuclear export (SINE). Exportin-1 (XPO-1) helps in nuclear export of several proteins like oncogenes, tumor suppressor genes etc. from nucleus to cytoplasm. It is overexpressed in certain cancers. By inhibiting XPO-1, selinexor results in accumulation of tumor suppressor genes in nucleus of malignant cells and also reduces the level of oncogene products which drive cell proliferation. This leads to cell death by apoptosis. It is approved for oral treatment of multiple myeloma and diffuse large B-cell lymphoma. Major adverse effects include thrombocytopenia and hyponatremia.

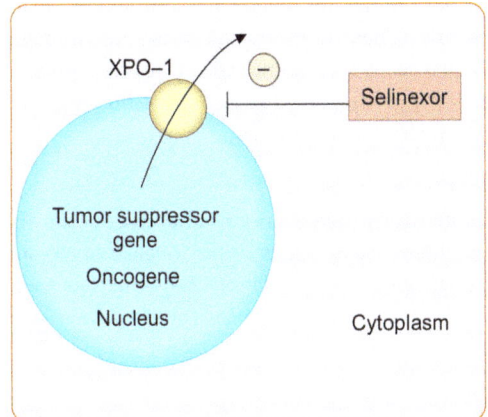

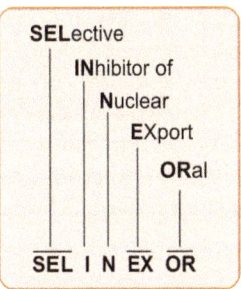

HORMONES AND RELATED AGENTS

Glucocorticoids

Prednisolone is the most commonly used glucocorticoid in cancer chemotherapy. It is used for the combination chemotherapy in leukemia and lymphomas. It is **also combined with ondansetron** for the management of chemotherapy induced **vomiting**.

Estrogens

Previously **high dose estrogen** therapy was used for the treatment of **breast carcinoma** but now it has been replaced with antiestrogen therapy. Estrogen is also effective in **prostate cancer** because it suppresses androgen production.

Progestins

These include **medroxyprogesterone acetate, hydoxyprogesterone caproate and megestrol**. These are useful as second line hormonal therapy for metastatic hormone dependent **breast cancer and endometrial cancer**. In addition, progestins stimulate appetite and restore a sense of well being.

Androgen Inhibitors (Antiandrogens)

Flutamide, nilutamide, enzalutamide, bicalutamide and **darolutamide** bind to androgen receptor and inhibit the actions of androgens. These are thus effective for the treatment of **prostatic carcinoma**. These are used **along with gonadotropin releasing hormone agonists**. This strategy is known as **complete androgen blockade**. *Flutamide can cause hot flushes, hepatic dysfunction and gynaecomastia.*

Gonadotropin Releasing Hormone (GnRH) Agonists

Goserelin, nafarelin, and leuprolide act as agonists of LHRH. Continuous administration of these agents lead to transient release of LH and FSH (and thus **flaring up** of symptoms in prostatic carcinoma) followed by inhibition of release of gonadotropins. These are indicated in the management of advanced **prostatic carcinoma**. Main adverse effects include transient flaring up of disease, hot flushes, impotence, gynaecomastia and osteoporosis.

GnRH Antagonists

Cetrorelix, ganirelix, degarelix and abarelix are the antagonists of LHRH. These drugs decrease the release of gonadotropins without causing initial stimulation. *Degarelix has been approved for the treatment of prostatic carcinoma without the risk of flare up reaction.*

Antiestrogens

Tamoxifen and **toremifen** are selective estrogen receptor modulators (SERMs) that are useful for chemoprevention as well as treatment of both early stage and metastatic **breast carcinoma**. These can lead to transient flare up reaction, menopausal symptoms and other estrogenic adverse effects. **Fulvestrant** is *pure ER antagonist* (selective estrogen receptor down regulator; SERD) having improved safety profile, faster onset and long duration. It is indicated for metastatic breast cancer.

Key Points

Fulvestrant
- Is a SERD
- Indicated in tamoxifen-resistant breast cancer
- Safer than SERMs
- Faster onset
- Long duration

Aromatase is an enzyme responsible for the conversion of androstenedione (an androgen precursor) to estrone (estrogenic hormone). Drugs inhibiting aromatase include aminoglutethimide, anastrozole, exemestane and letrozole. These are classified into first generation (aminoglutethimide), second generation (formestane, fadrozole, rogletimide) and third generation (exemestane, anastrozole, letrozole and vorozole) drugs. Aromatase inhibitors are useful in advanced breast carcinoma. Adverse effects include hot flushes, arthralgia and fatigue. Aminoglutethimide also causes adrenal insufficiency and myelosuppression.

Selected Toxicities of Hormonal Agents

• Flutamide	Hot flushes, liver dysfunction
• SERMs	Menopausal symptoms, fluid retention, thromboembolism, increased incidence of endometrial cancer
• Progestins	Fluid retention
• Corticosteroids	Fluid retention, hypertension, diabetes, increased susceptibility to infections
• GnRH agonists	Transient flare up reaction, hot flushes, impotence, gynecomastia, osteoporosis
• Aminoglutethimide	Adrenal insufficiency, myelosuppression, rash
• Aromatase inhibitors	Fatigue, hot flushes, arthralgia

OTHER ANTICANCER DRUGS

Asparaginase Specific Enzymes

L-Asparaginase is an enzyme used for the treatment of **acute lymphoid leukemia (ALL)**. These tumors require exogenous asparagine for growth. L-asparaginase acts by depleting this amino acid in the serum. It is administered by i.v. route and may cause **severe hypersensitivity reactions, acute pancreatitis and cortical vein thrombosis.**

Calaspargase pegol is a long acting asparagine specific enzyme recently approved for treatment of ALL in children and young adults (1 month to 21 years).

Pentostatin

This drug is used for the treatment of **hairy cell leukemia** (*DOC is cladribine*). It acts by **inhibiting the enzyme adenosine deaminase** (although the name is statin but it has no HMG CoA reductase inhibiting action).

Lutelium 177 Dotatate

Dotatate is a compound containing tyrosine octreotate. It acts a **somatostatin receptor (SSR) antagonist**. There is massive overexpression of SSR receptors in several neuroendocrine tumors. When a radioactive substance Lutetium 177 is added to dotatate, it selectively enters tumor cells containing SSR. Lutetium 177 dotatate is selectively approved for treatment of SSR positive gastropancreatic **neuroendocrine tumors** including foregut, hindgut and midgut neuroendocrine tumors in adults.

Chemotherapy C: Antineoplastic Drugs

Tagraxofusp
It consists of **truncated diphtheria toxin conjugated with IL-3**. Blastic Plasmacytoid Dendritic Cell Neoplasm (BPDCN) is a rare hematological malignancy. Key feature of malignant cells in this cancer is the overexpression of CD123, also known as IL-3 receptors. Malignant cells in BPDCN require constant presence of IL-3 for survival. Tagraxofusp binds to cells expressing IL-3 receptors and delivers in them the diphtheria toxin after binding. Diphtheria toxin inhibit protein synthesis in these malignant cells and the cells undergo apoptosis. Tagraxofusp is indicated **for the treatment of BPDCN** in adults and pediatric patients over 2 years.

Octreotide
It is a **long acting somatostatin analog** and is useful in the treatment of **islet cell carcinoma** (decreases both insulin and glucagon secretion). Other uses of octreotide include secretory diarrheas, **esophageal varices and acromegaly**.

Plicamycin
It is used for **hypercalcemia of malignancy** and **metastatic testicular carcinoma** because it decreases serum calcium levels.

Hydroxyurea
It is the drug used for **sickle cell anemia, essential thrombocytosis and polycythemia vera**. It can also be used in **CML**. It acts by inhibiting ribonucleoside reductase (rate limiting step in synthesis of DNA). In sickel cell anemia, it increases the solubility of hemoglobin by *inducing the synthesis of fetal hemoglobin* (reduces vaso-occlusive events). In essential thrombocytosis, it is the drug of choice **(if not responding, anagrelide may be added)**. It can be used orally for all these purposes.

Tretinoin (ATRA)
All-trans retinoic acid (ATRA) induces *70% or more* rate of complete remission in *acute promyelocytic leukemia*. It can cause various toxicities:

Vitamin A toxicity	Headache, fever, dryness, skin rash, pruritis, conjunctivitis
Retinoic acid syndrome	Fever, leucocytosis, dyspnea, weight gain, pulmonary infiltrates, pleural or pericardial effusion.
CNS toxicity	Dizziness, anxiety, depression, confusion, agitation
Hypercholesterolemia	
Hypertriglyceridemia	
Abdominal pain and diarrhea	

AS₂O₃
It is used for the treatment of **acute promyelocytic leukemia** (APML). It may causes *hyperglycemia* and *prolonged QT interval*. Like tretinoin, it also acts as a differentiating agent.

Sipuleucel-T
It is a cell-based cancer immunotherapy for **prostate cancer**. Patient's antigen presenting cells are extracted by leukapheresis and are incubated with a fusion protein (consising of prostatic acid phosphatase and GM-CSF). This is then re-infused into the patient to cause an immune response against the tumor cells carrying prostatic acid phosphatase antigen. It is approved for hormone refractory prostate cancer.

Thalidomide

- Its major actions are:
  - Inhibition of angiogenesis
  - Inhibition of TNF-α
  - Increased production of IL-10
  - Reduces phagocytosis
  - Alteration of adhesion molecule expression
  - Enhances cell-mediated immunity via interactions with T-cells.
- Currently, it is indicated for
  - Multiple myeloma at initial diagnosis
  - Relapsed-refractory cases of multiple myeloma
  - Erythema nodosum leprosum (Provides dramatic relief; drug of choice for steroid resistant cases)
  - Skin manifestations of SLE
- Its major adverse effects are:
  - Teratogenicity
  - Peripheral neuropathy
  - Constipation
  - Rash
  - Hypothyroidism
  - Increased risk of DVT
- Immunomodulatory derivatives of thalidomide are called IMiDs. One of these is Lenalidomide, which is approved as a first line therapy for multiple myeloma with dexamethasone and bortezomib.
- Another group of thalidomide analogs are called SelCIDs (Selective cytokine Inhibiotry Drugs).

This drug was used in 1960s as a sedative and anti-emetic drug (for morning sickness) but was banned because of teratogenic effects (phocomelia). Now it has come again in the market for use as an anticancer drug in **multiple myeloma and melanoma**. **Lenalidomide** is its more potent and non-teratogenic derivative. It has recently been **approved for mantle cell lymphoma** also *Thalidomide* most commonly *causes sedation and constipation* in cancer patients. It can also cause *peripheral sensory neuropathy*. Two enantiomers of thalidomide (R and S) are present but these are interconvertible in body, therefore racemic mixture is used. **Pomalidomide** is a newer thalidomide analogue.

New Therapies for Cancer Arranged Alphabetically According to Cancer

Cancer	TK inhibitor	Monoclonal antibody	Other new drugs
Acute Myeloid Leukemia	Gilteritinib	Gemtuzumab ozogamicin	Enasidenib Ivosidenib Glasdegib
Acute Lymphocytic Leukemia	Imatinib Dasatinib Ponatinib	Blintatumomab Inotuzumab	
Anaplastic T Cell Lymphoma		Brentuximab	
Basal Cell Carcinoma			Sonidegib Vismodegib
Brain Tumor		Bevacizumab	Everolimus
Breast Carcinoma	Lapatinib Tucatinib	Trastuzumab Azo-trastuzumab emtansine Pertuzumab Enfortumab Margetuximab Sacituzumab	Everolimus Palbociclib Ribociclib Abemaciclib Talazoparib Alpelisib

Contd...

Contd...

Cancer	TK inhibitor	Monoclonal antibody	Other new drugs
B Cell Lymphoma		Loncastuximab Tafasitamab Polatuzumab Obinutuzumab Ibrutumomab tiuxetan Tositumomab Rituximab	Idelalisib Copanlisib
Chronic Myeloid Leukemia	Bosutinib Imatinib Nilotinib Dasatinib Ponatinib		Omacetaxine
Colorectal Carcinoma	Regorafenib	Cetuximab Panitumumab Bevacizumab	Ziv-Aflibercept Trifluridine + Tipiracil
Cholangiocarcinoma	Infigratinib Pemigatinib		
Chronic Lymphoid Leukemia	Ibrutinib	Alemtuzumab Ofatumumab Obinutuzumab Rituximab	Idelalisib venetoclax Duvelisib
Cutaneous T Cell Lymphoma			Denileukin diftitox Vorinostat Romidepsin Bexarotene
Dermatofibrosarcoma Protuberans	Imatinib		
Endometrial cancer		Dostarlimab Pembrolizumab	
Giant Cell Tumor of Bone		Denosumab	
Gastrointestinal Stromal Tumor	Sunitinib Imatinib Regorafenib Ripretinib		
Hairy cell leukemia		Moxetumomab	
Gastroesophageal Junction adenocarcinoma		Trastuzumab Ramucirumab	
Head and Neck Cancer		Cetuximab	
Hepatocellular Carcinoma	Sorafenib Lenvatinib	Ramucirumab	
Merkel cell carcinoma		Avelumab	
Hodgkin Lymphoma		Brentuximab Nivolumab	
Kaposi Sarcoma			Alitretinoin
Liposarcoma			Trabectedin
Medullary Carcinoma of Thyroid	Cabozantinib Vandetanib Selpercatinib		

Contd...

Contd...

Cancer	TK inhibitor	Monoclonal antibody	Other new drugs
Malignant melanoma	Dabrafenib Vemurafenib Trametinib Cobimetinib Encoratenib Binimetinib	Ipilimumab Nivolumab Pembrolizumab	Aldesleukin
Multiple Myeloma		Daratumumab Elotuzumab Isatuximab Belantamab	Ixazomib Bortezomib Carfilzomib Panobinostat Selinexor
Myelofibrosis	Ruxolitinib Imatinib		
Mantle Cell Lymphoma	Ibrutinib Zanubrutinib Acalabrutinib		Bortezomib
Non-Small Cell Lung Carcinoma	Dacomitinib Lorlatinib Afatinib Brigatinib Ceritinib Crizotinib Erlotinib Geftinib Osimertinib Alectinib Dacomitinib Lorlatinib Capmatinib Entrectinib Nintedanib Pralsetinib Selpercatinib Sotorasib Tepotinib	Ramucirumab Nivolumab Necitumumab Pembrolizumab Bevacizumab Atezolizumab Amivantamab	
Neuroblastoma		Dinutuximab Naxitamab	
Non Hodgkin Lymphoma			
Ovarian Carcinoma		Bevacizumab	Olaparib Rucaparib Niraparib
Pancreatic carcinoma	Erlotinib Sunitinib		Everolimus
Pancreatic neuroendocrine tumors	Sunitinib		
Prostate Carcinoma			Cabazitaxel Abiraterone Enzalutamide Radium 223 Sipuleucel-T
Peripheral T Cell Lymphoma			Belinostat Pralatrexate
Renal Cell Carcinoma	Axitinib Pazopanib Sorafenib Sunitinib Lenvatinib Tivozanib	Bevacizumab Avelumab Pembrolizumab	Aldesleukin Temsirolimus Everolimus

Contd...

Chemotherapy C: Antineoplastic Drugs

Contd...

Cancer	TK inhibitor	Monoclonal antibody	Other new drugs
Soft Tissue Sarcoma	Pazopanib	Olaratumab	
Squamous cell carcinoma of skin		Cemiplimab	
Systemic Mastocytosis	Imatinib		
Thyroid Carcinoma	Lenvatinib Sorafenib		
Urothelial carcinoma	Erdafitinib	Atezolizumab Durvalumab	

Zolendronic Acid

It is a *bisphosphonate* indicated for the treatment of bony metastases and multiple myeloma.

Mitotane

It is indicated for the palliation of *inoperable adrenocortical carcinoma*. Concomitant spironolactone interferes with adrenal suppression produced by mitotane.

Aldesleukin

It is **recombinant IL-2** and can be used for the management of **renal cell carcinoma** and **malignant melanoma**.

Denileukin Deftitox

It is a **combination of IL-2 with diphtheria toxin** and is used for **cutaneous T cell lymphoma**.

Adjuvant chemotherapy is administered after surgery or radiotherapy while *neoadjuvant* chemotherapy means administration of anti-cancer drugs before surgery or radiotherapy.

Neoadjuvant chemotherapy is used for cancers of:
- Bladder
- Breast
- Colorectal
- Esophagus
- Stomach
- Lung (non-small cell)

Therapy of Choice for Various Cancers   (Ref: CMDT 2019)

	Diagnosis	Treatment of Choice
1.	ALL	Induction: Vincristine + Prednisolone + Daunorubicin + Asparaginase + Intrathecal Methotrexate
		Consolidation: Hyper-CVAD alternated with Cytarabine + Methotrexate Philadelpnia + ve → Add imatinib or other TK inhibitor
2.	AML	Cytarabine + Daunorubicin/Idarubicin
3.	CML	Imatinib (or Nilotinib or Dasatinib)
4.	CLL	< 70 years → FCR > 70 years → Chlorambucil Refractory → Ibrutinib
5.	Hairy-cell leukemia	Cladribine

Contd...

Contd...

	Diagnosis	Treatment of Choice
6.	Hodgkin disease	ABVD
7.	Non-Hodgkin Lymphoma	CHOP-R
8.	Multiple Myeloma	Bortezomib + Dexamethasone + Lenalidomide
9.	Waldenstrom macroglobulinemia	Plasmapheresis ± Bortezomib (With or without rituximab)
10.	Polycythemia vera	Hydroxyurea
11.	Non-small cell lung cancer	Cisplatin + Vinorelbine ± Bevacizumab
12.	Small cell lung cancer	Cisplatin + Etoposide
13.	Mesothelioma	Cisplatin + Pemetrexed
14.	Head and Neck cancer	Cisplatin + 5-FU
15.	Esophageal cancer	Cisplatin + 5-FU
16.	Uterine cancer	Progestins/Tamoxifen/Aromatase inhibitors OR Cisplatin + Doxorubicin
17.	Ovarian cancer	Paclitaxel + Carboplatin ± Bevacizumab
18.	Cervical cancer	Cisplatin + Paclitaxel (or cisplatin with radiation)
19.	Breast cancer	**Endocrine :** Tamoxifen (Pre-menopausal) Aromatase inhibitor (Post-menopausal) **Adjuvant chemotherapy**: Doxorubicin + Cyclophosphamide + Paclitaxel ± Trastuzumab
20.	Choriocarcinoma	Methotrexate/Dactinomycin
21.	Testicular cancer	BEP
22.	Kidney cancer	Sunitinib or sorafenib
23.	Bladder cancer	Gemcitabine + Cisplatin
24.	Prostate cancer	GnRH agonist ± Antiandrogen
25.	Astrocytoma/Glioblastoma multiforme	Temozolomide + Radiation
26.	Neuroblastoma	Cyclophosphamide + Doxorubicin + Cisplatin + Etoposide
27.	Thyroid cancer	I^{131} / Sorafenib (Vandetanib for medullary carcinoma)
28.	Stomach cancer	Epirubicin + Cisplatin + 5-FU
29.	Pancreatic cancer	Gemcitabine
30.	Colon cancer	FOLFOX-6 ± Bevacizumab FOLFIRI ± Bevacizumab (for more advanced disease)
31.	Rectal cancer	Radiotherapy + 5- FU
32.	Anal cancer	Radiation + 5-FU + Mitomycin C
33.	Insulinoma	Interferon/Streptozocin
34.	Osteosarcoma	Doxorubicin + Cisplatin
35.	Soft tissue sarcoma	MAID
36.	Gastrointestinal stromal tumors (GIST)	Imatinib or sunitinib

Contd...

Contd...

	Diagnosis	Treatment of Choice
37.	Melanoma (non-BRAF mutation)	Pembrolizumab or Nivolumab
38.	Melanoma (BRAF mutation)	Vemurafenib or Dabrefenib
39.	Hepatocellular carcinoma	Sorafenib
40.	Kaposi sarcoma	Liposomal doxorubicin/daunorubicin
41.	Adrenal cancer	Mitotane
42.	Carcinoid	Octreotide

Abbreviations:

Hyper - CVAD	Cyclophosphamide + Vincristine + Adriamycin (Doxorubicin) + Dexamethasone
ABVD	Adriamycin + Bleomycin + Vinblastine + Dacarbazine
CHOP - R	Cyclophosphamide + Hydroxydaunorubicin (Doxorubicin) + Oncovin (Vincristine) + Prednisone + Rituximab
FCR	Fludarabine + Cyclophosphamide + Rituximab
BEP	Bleomycin + Etoposide + Cisplatin
FOLFOX - 6	FOLinic acid (Leucovorin) + 5- FU + Oxaliplatin
FOLFIRI	FOLinic acid + 5-FU + IRInotecan
MAID	Mesna + Adriamycin + Ifosfamide + Dacarbazine

DRUGS USED TO PREVENT TOXICITY OF ANTI-CANCER DRUGS

Drug	Mechanism	Indications
Allopurinol	Inhibit xanthine oxidase	Prevent hyperuricemia from tumor lysis syndrome
Rasburicase	Recombinant urate oxidase	Prevent hyperuricemia from tumor lysis
Mesna	Neutralizing agent	Prevent hemorrhagic cystitis due to ifosfamide and high dose cyclophosphamide
Leucovorin	Replete Tetrahydrofolic acid	Rescue after high dose methotrexate
Amifostine	Prevent radiation-induced xerostomia and	Prevent radiation-induced xerostomia and cisplatin-induced nephrotoxicity
Dexrazoxane	Iron-chelator	Prevent cardiotoxicity due to anthracyclines
Palifermin	Keratinocyte growth factor	Prevent mucositis following chemotherapy
Pilocarpine	Cholinergic agonist	Radiation-induced xerostomia
Pamidronte and Zolendronate	Bisphosphonates	Hypercalcemia of malignancy
Epoetin-alpha and Darbopoetin-alpha	Erythropoietin	Anemia
Filgrastim, Peg-Filgrastim	G-CSF and	Febrile neutropenia prophylaxis
Sargramostim	GM-CSF	
Oprelvekin	IL-11	Thrombocytopenia
Trilaciclib	CdK-4,6 inhibitor	Prevent bone marrow suppression
Ondansetron	5-HT$_3$ antagonist	Nausea and vomiting
Granisetron		
Palonosetron		
Aprepitant	NK-1 antagonist	Cisplatin-induced delayed vomiting

Golden Points

1. N7 of guanine is most susceptible position for alkylation
2. Cyclophosphamide is the drug of choice for Wegener's granulomatosis.
3. Nitrosoureas can cause delayed neutropenia.
4. **Amifostine is indicated for**:
   - Reduction of cisplatin induced nephrotoxicity.
   - To reduce xerostomia in patients undergoing irradiation
5. Methotrexate is the drug of choice for the treatment of choriocarcinoma.
6. The toxicity of methotrexate to normal cells can be reduced by administration of N_{10} formyl- tetrahydrofolic acid (folinic acid, citrovorum factor or leucovorin).
7. In extreme cases, methotrexate toxicity can be treated by dialysis or administration of GLUCARPIDASE, a methotrexate cleaving enzyme.
8. When administered along with allopurinol the dose of 6-MP (and also azathioprine) should be reduced to 1/4th of the original dose.
9. Fludarabine is drug of choice for chronic lymphocytic leukemia (CLL).
10. **Hand and Foot Syndrome** is caused by:
    - 5 - FU
    - Capecitabine
    - Doxorubicin
11. Capecitabine and 5-FU can cause hand and foot syndrome
12. Gemcitabine is the drug of choice for pancreatic cancer.
13. **Radiosensitizers**
    - Gemcitabine
    - Metronidazole
    - Mitomycin–C
    - Fludarabine
    - Irinotecan
    - Dactinomycin
    - 5–FU
    - Hydroxyurea
    - Paclitaxel
14. **Uridine Triacetate** is indicated for
    - Hereditary orotic aciduria
    - 5-FU and capecitabine toxicity
15. **Marrow sparing cytotoxic drugs**
    - Vincristine
    - Bleomycin
    - L-asparaginase
16. Irinotecan is now the treatment of choice for advanced colorectal carcinoma in combination with 5-FU.
17. **Etoposide induced secondary leukemia**
    - Develops at short time interval
    - Lacks preceeding myelodysplastic stage.
18. Anthracycline induced cardiotoxicity can be reduced by using α-tocopherol and dexrazoxane (a free radical scavenger).
19. Anthracyclines can cause "radiation recall reaction"
20. Earliest indicator of bleomycin induced pulmonary fibrosis is decrease in DLco.
21. Mitomycin C is used in patients with treacheal or laryngeal stenosis
22. Imatinib is the drug of choice for CML and gastro-intestinal stromal tumor (GIST).
23. **Vorinostat and Romidepsin** are histone deacetylase inhibitors approved for cutaneous T-cell lymphoma.
24. **Abiraterone** acts by inhibiting 17-α hydroxylase and is indicated in refractory prostate cancer
25. **Ziv-aflibercept** is a fusion protein against VEGF and placental growth factor. It is a approved for **metastatic colorectal carcinoma** in combination with FOLFIRI
26. Tretinon and AS_2O_3 are used for treatent of acute Promyelocytic leukemia [M_3-AML]
27. **Lenalidomide** is approved for treatment of **mantle cell lymphoma** and multiple myeloma
28. Adjuvant chemotherapy is administered after surgery or radiotherapy while neoadjuvant chemotherapy means administration of anti-cancer drugs before surgery or radiotherapy.

Image Based Questions

1. Cell cycle is shown in the figure below. Which of the following drug act specifically at the stage marked with arrow?

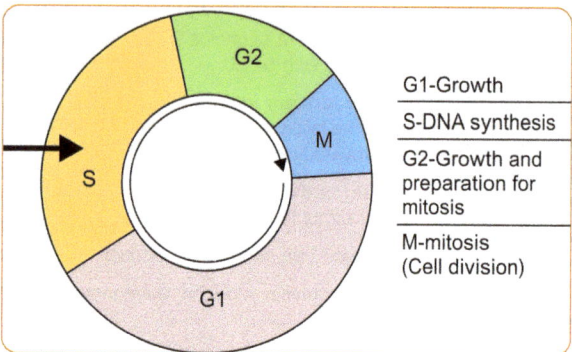

   (a) Mechlorethamine (b) Methotrexate
   (c) Vincristine (d) Paclitaxel

2. Figure shows the mechanism of action of:

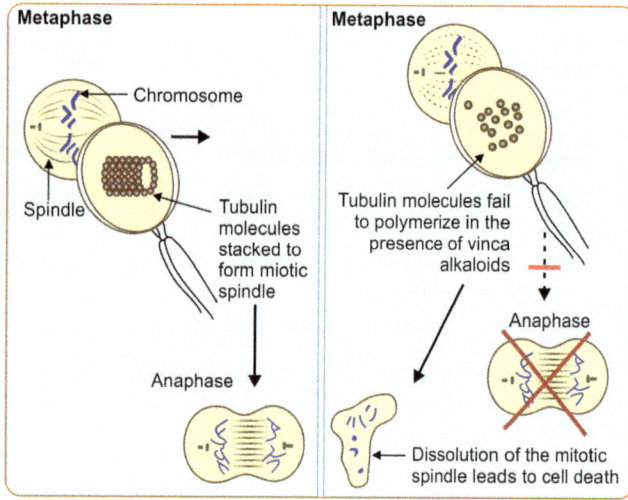

   (a) Vinblastine (b) Cisplatin
   (c) Imatinib (d) Trastuzumab

3. A patient present with the features shown in the figure below after treatment with an anticancer drug. The likely drug is:

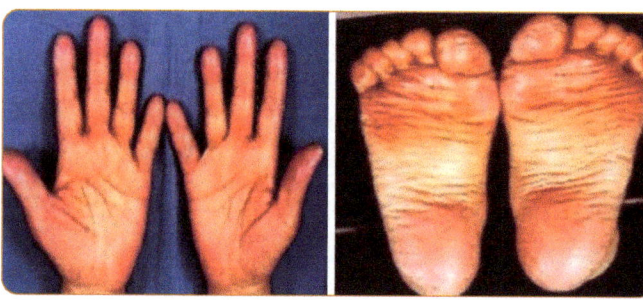

   (a) Cisplatin
   (b) 5-Fluorouracil
   (c) Methotrexate
   (d) Imatinib

4. A patient was given radiotherapy for head and neck cancer. After 6 months chemotherapy was started. The patient presented with the features shown in Figure after start of chemotherapy. It is likely due to which drug?

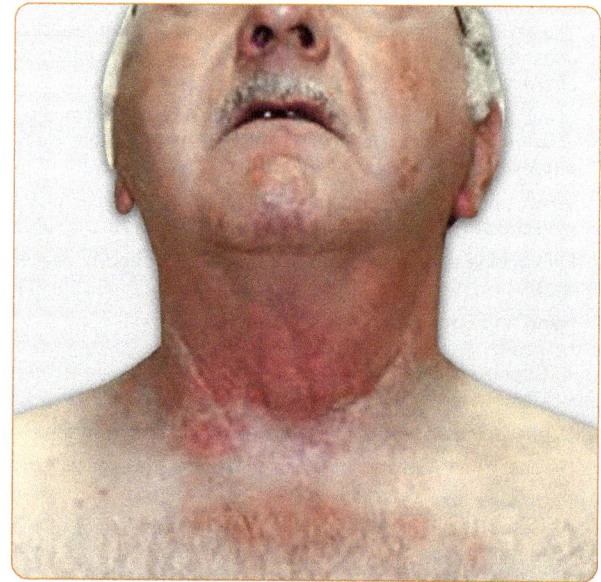

   (a) Doxorubicin (b) Cisplatin
   (c) Imatinib (d) Methotrexate

5. Figure shows the mechanism of action of which of the following drug?

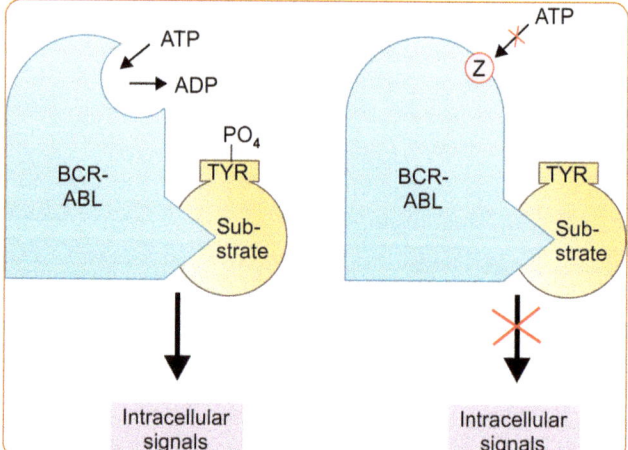

   (a) Nilotinib
   (b) Methotrexate
   (c) Pertuzumab
   (d) Cisplatin

Chemotherapy C: Antineoplastic Drugs

Explanations

1. **Ans. (b) Methotrexate**
   Anticancer drugs that act by inhibiting the metabolism (antimetabolites) specifically act on S phase of cell cycle. Antimetabolites include methotrexate, purine analogs (like 6-mercaptopurine, 6-thioguanine) and pyrimidine analogs (like 5-fluorouracil, capecitabine etc.)

2. **Ans. (a) Vinblastine**
   The mechanism shows the inhibition of polymerization of tubulin means the drug inhibit the spindle formation. This mechanism is shown by vinca alkaloids like vincristine and vinblastine.

Mechanism on spindle	Drugs
Inhibit polymerization of tubulin	Vincristine, Vinblastine
Inhibit depolymerization of tubulin	Paclitaxel, Docetaxel

3. **Ans. (b) 5-Fluorouracil**
   The figure shows Hand and Foot syndrome which is characteristic adverse effect of 5-fluorouracil and capecitabine.

4. **Ans. (a) Doxorubicin**
   The history and the figure shows the characteristic 'Radiation recall syndrome'. It is caused by doxorubicin.

5. **Ans. (a) Nilotinib**
   Tyrosine kinase activated by abl-bcr fusion result in CML. This enzyme can be inhibited by
   B: Bosutinib
   I: Imatinib
   N: Nilotinib
   D: Dasatinib
   Proteins: Ponatinib

Multiple Choice Questions

CYTOTOXIC DRUGS

1. Match the following: *(AIIMS Nov. 2019)*

Drug	Mechanism of action
1. Omalizumab	A. Anti-CD 6
2. Itolizumab	B. Anti-CD 25
3. Daclizumab	C. Anti-IgE
4. Belimumab	D. Anti-IgG 1
	E. Anti-B lymphocyte stimulator

2. Which drug is likely to cause flagellated pigmentation of skin? *(AIIMS May 2018)*
   - (a) Bleomycin
   - (b) Minocycline
   - (c) Vincristine
   - (d) Daunorubicin

3. Which anti-neoplastic drug is cell cycle specific and acts on S-phase? *(NEET Pattern Question 2016-17)*
   - (a) Vincristine
   - (b) Cyclophosphamide
   - (c) Cytarabine
   - (d) Vinblastine

4. Cerebellar ataxia is caused by which anticancer drug? *(NEET Pattern Question 2016-17)*
   - (a) Cyclophosphamide
   - (b) Chloramphenicol
   - (c) Cytarabine
   - (d) Irinotecan

5. Hand and foot syndrome is caused by which anticancer drug? *(NEET Pattern Question 2016-17)*
   - (a) Cyclophosphamide
   - (b) Chloramphenicol
   - (c) Capecitabine
   - (d) Mitomycin-C

6. Treatment for cisplatin induced delayed nausea and vomiting is: *(NEET Pattern Question 2016-17)*
   - (a) Aprepitant
   - (b) Mesna
   - (c) Ondansetron
   - (d) Metoclopramide

7. All of the following anticancer drugs act on G2 phase except: *(AIIMS May 2016)*
   - (a) Paclitaxel
   - (b) Etoposide
   - (c) Irinotecan
   - (d) Bleomycin

8. L-asparaginase is used for the treatment of: *(AIIMS May 2016)*
   - (a) Acute lymphocytic leukemia
   - (b) Acute myelocytic leukemia
   - (c) Chronic myelocytic leukemia
   - (d) Chronic lymphocytic leukemia

9. All of the following statements about paclitaxel are true except: *(AIIMS Nov 2014)*
   - (a) It is obtained from *E. coli*
   - (b) It acts by enhancing the polymerization of β-tubulin
   - (c) It can cause bone marrow suppression
   - (d) It is used in ovarian and breast cancer

10. The most common side effect of cancer chemotherapy is nausea with or without vomiting. The anticancer drugs vary in their ability to cause nausea and vomiting. Which of the following anti-cancer drugs is least likely to cause nausea and vomiting? *(AIIMS May 2014)*
    - (a) Chlorambucil
    - (b) Cisplatin
    - (c) Doxorubicin
    - (d) Daunorubicin

11. Which of the following medications is essential for ameliorating the toxicity of pemetrexed? *(AIIMS May 2014)*
    - (a) Folinic acid and vitamin B_6
    - (b) Folic acid and vitamin B_{12}
    - (c) Vitamin B_6 and Vitamin B_{12}
    - (d) Folic acid and dexamethasone

12. Topical mitomycin-C is used in: *(AI 2012)*
    - (a) Sturge-Weber syndrome
    - (b) Laryngotracheal stenosis
    - (c) Endoscopic angiofibroma
    - (d) Skull base osteomyelitis

13. Which group of anticancer drugs temozolomide belong to? *(AI 2012)*
    - (a) Oral alkylating agent
    - (b) Antitumor Antibiotic
    - (c) Antimetabolite
    - (d) Mitotic Spindle Inhibitor

14. Which of the following parameters is not monitored in a patient on methotrexate therapy? *(Recent NEET Pattern Question)*
    - (a) Liver function tests
    - (b) Lung function test
    - (c) Eye examination
    - (d) Hemogramz

15. Which of the following anticancer drugs can cross blood brain barrier? *(Recent NEET Pattern Question)*
    - (a) Cisplatin
    - (b) Nitrosourea
    - (c) Vincristine
    - (d) Vinblastine

16. Which of the following drugs produce significant nephrotoxicity? *(Recent NEET Pattern Question)*
    - (a) Cisplatin
    - (b) Carboplatin
    - (c) Vinblastine
    - (d) Vincristine

17. Folinic acid counteracts the toxicity of: *(Recent NEET Pattern Question)*
    - (a) Doxorubicin
    - (b) Methotrexate
    - (c) Cyclophosphamide
    - (d) Fluorouracil

18. Toxicity of nitrogen mustards can be decreased by: *(Recent NEET Pattern Question)*
    - (a) Amifostine
    - (b) Folinic acid
    - (c) GM-CSF
    - (d) MESNA

19. Which one of the following alkaloids is used as anti-cancer agent? *(Recent NEET Pattern Question)*
    - (a) Vincristine
    - (b) Papaverine
    - (c) Ephedrine
    - (d) Atropine

20. The antimalignancy drug which is potentially cardiotoxic is: *(Recent NEET Pattern Question)*
    (a) Doxorubicin (b) Bleomycin
    (c) Fluorouracil (d) Dacarbazine

21. "Stocking and glove" neuropathy is seen in: *(Recent NEET Pattern Question)*
    (a) Vinblastine (b) Paclitaxel
    (c) Etoposide (d) Mitoxantrone

22. Which of the following anti-cancer drug is NOT 'S'-phase specific? *(Recent NEET Pattern Question)*
    (a) Methotrexate (b) Mercaptopurine
    (c) Ifosfamide (d) Thioguanine

23. All are alkylating agents *except*: *(Recent NEET Pattern Question)*
    (a) Cyclophosphamide (b) Lomustine
    (c) Busulfan (d) Zalcitabine

24. Cisplatin does not cause: *(Recent NEET Pattern Question)*
    (a) Cardiomyopathy (b) Nephrotoxicity
    (c) Neuropathy (d) Tinnitus

25. Cyclophosphamide can cause: *(Recent NEET Pattern Question)*
    (a) Hemorrhagic cystitis (b) Cardiomyopathy
    (c) Neuropathy (d) Convulsions

26. Which of the following is not an early adverse effect of methotrexate? *(Recent NEET Pattern Question)*
    (a) Hepatic fibrosis (b) Myelosupression
    (c) Nausea (d) Stomatitis

27. Which of the following is not an antineoplastic antibiotic? *(Recent NEET Pattern Question)*
    (a) Actinomycin D (b) Doxorubicin
    (c) Bleomycin (d) Spiramycin

28. Leucovorin rescue is related to:
    (a) Methotrexate toxicity *(Recent NEET Pattern Question)*
    (b) Cyclophosphamide toxicity
    (c) Oncovin toxicity
    (d) Cisplatin toxicity

29. Which of the following causes peripheral neuritis? *(Recent NEET Pattern Question)*
    (a) Methotrexete (b) Vincristine
    (c) Busulfan (d) Cyclophosphamide

30. Which of the following is an Alkylating agent? *(Recent NEET Pattern Question)*
    (a) Doxorubicin (b) Chlorambucil
    (c) Vinblastine (d) Methotrexate

31. Which of the following statement about rituximab is FALSE? *(Recent NEET Pattern Question)*
    (a) It is a chimeric monoclonal antibody against CD-20
    (b) It has dose-dependent kinetics
    (c) It is used for treatment of non-Hodgkin lymphoma
    (d) Its most common adverse effect is infusion related reactions

32. Histopathology of cardiac muscle from a patient treated with overdose of doxorubicin shows: *(Recent NEET Pattern Question)*
    (a) Vacuolar degeneration of myofibrils
    (b) Muscle spindle whorls
    (c) Hyalinization of the bundle of muscles
    (d) Apoptosis of muscles

33. Ramesh, a young male with AML was started on doxorubicin based chemotherapy. Two months later, he presented with swelling of feet and breathlessness on exertion. Which of the following adverse effect of doxorubicin could lead to these symptoms? *(Recent NEET Pattern Question)*
    (a) Restrictive cardiomyopathy
    (b) Hypertrophic cardiomyopathy
    (c) Dilated cardiomyopathy
    (d) Pericardial fibrosis

34. Most widely used anticancer drug is: *(Recent NEET Pattern Question)*
    (a) 5-FU (b) Methotrexate
    (c) Cisplatin (d) Rituximab

35. Hemolytic uremic syndrome is adverse effect of: *(Recent NEET Pattern Question)*
    (a) Vincristine (b) Vinblastine
    (c) Cisplatin (d) Mitomycin C

36. An anti-leukemic drug acts by inhibiting DNA polymerase. Apart from myelosuppression, it can cause cerebellar ataxia. The likely drug is: *(Recent NEET Pattern Question)*
    (a) Bleomycin (b) Cytarabine
    (c) Mercaptopurine (d) Methotrexate

37. Mechanism of action of 5-FU is: *(Recent NEET Pattern Question)*
    (a) Antimetabolite
    (b) Anti-mitotic
    (c) Topoisomerase inhibitor
    (d) Direct DNA chelating agent

38. A person with mediastinal tumor was treated with chemotherapy. Now he developed high frequency hearing loss. Most probable drug implicated is: *(Recent NEET Pattern Question)*
    (a) Cisplatin (b) Etoposide
    (c) Doxorubicin (d) Methotrexate

39. Which of the following anticancer drugs is not derived from plants? *(Recent NEET Pattern Question)*
    (a) Irinotecan (b) Doxorubicin
    (c) Paclitaxel (d) Etoposide

40. Resistance to methotrexate develops due to: *(Recent NEET Pattern Question)*
    (a) Rapid cancer cell multiplication
    (b) Deficiency of thymidylate kinase
    (c) Deficiency of thymidylate synthetase
    (d) Increased production of dihydrofolate reductase

41. About vinca alkaloids, true is: *(Recent NEET Pattern Question)*
    (a) Inhibits mitotic spindle
    (b) Enhances polymerization of tubulin
    (c) Inhibits topoisomerase I
    (d) Inhibits topoisomerase II

42. **Mesna is used in:** *(Recent NEET Pattern Question)*
    (a) Hemorrhagic cystitis
    (b) Acute promyelocytic leukemia
    (c) Serous otitis media
    (d) Polycythemia vera

43. **Which of the following anti-neoplastic drugs SHOULD NOT be given by rapid IV infusion?**
    (Recent NEET Pattern Question)
    (a) Cyclophosphamide   (b) Cisplatin
    (b) Bleomycin   (d) Cytosine arabinoside

44. **Mechanism of a action of vincristine is:**
    (a) Tubulin inhibitor *(Recent NEET Pattern Question)*
    (b) Antimetabolite
    (c) Adenylate cyclase inhibitor
    (d) Anti folate

45. **Which of the following antineoplastic and immunosuppressant drugs is a dihydrofolate reductase inhibitor?**
    (Recent NEET Pattern Question)
    (a) Methotrexate   (b) Adriamycin
    (c) Vincristine   (d) Cyclophosphamide

46. **The drug of choice in choriocarcinoma is:**
    (Recent NEET Pattern Question)
    (a) Methotrexate   (b) Actinomycin-D
    (c) Vincristine   (d) 6-Thioguanine

47. **Microtubule formation is inhibited by:**
    (Recent NEET Pattern Question)
    (a) Paclitaxel   (b) Vincristine
    (c) Etoposide   (d) Irinotectan

48. **Drug not acting on tubulin is:**
    (Recent NEET Pattern Question)
    (a) Bleomycin   (b) Colchicine
    (c) Paclitaxel   (d) Vincristine

49. **Which antineoplastic drug has a very high cardiac toxicity?** *(Recent NEET Pattern Question)*
    (a) Bleomycin   (b) Actinomycin-D
    (c) Doxorubicin   (d) Mitomycin-C

50. **Methotrexate resistance is due to:**
    (Recent NEET Pattern Question)
    (a) Increased concentrations of intracellular DHFR through gene amplification
    (b) Failure of efflux pumps
    (c) Bacterial modification
    (d) Increased synthesis of poly glutamates

51. **Which of the following is not an antimetabolite?**
    (Recent NEET Pattern Question)
    (a) Methotrexate   (b) 5 Fluorouracil
    (c) Gemcitabine   (d) Vincristine

52. **Cyclophosphamide is:** *(Recent NEET Pattern Question)*
    (a) Alkylating agent   (b) Antitumor antibiotic
    (c) Monoclonal antibody   (d) Antimetabolites

53. **Most characteristic side effect of adriamycin is:**
    (Recent NEET Pattern Question)
    (a) Nephrotoxicity   (b) Neurotoxicity
    (c) Cardiotoxicity   (d) Hemorrhagic cystitis

54. **Mechanism of action of 5-FU is:**
    (Recent NEET Pattern Question)
    (a) Antimetabolite
    (b) Direct DNA chelating agent
    (c) Anti-Mitotic
    (d) Topoisomerase inhibitor

55. **Anticancer drug that causes lung fibrosis is:**
    (Recent NEET Pattern Question)
    (a) Bleomycin   (b) Cisplatin
    (c) Fulvestrant   (d) Tamoxifen

56. **Which of the following is not an alkylating agent?**
    (Recent NEET Pattern Question)
    (a) Chlorambucil   (b) Ifosfamide
    (c) Nitrosourea   (d) Cladribine

57. **Ifosfamide belong to which class?**
    (Recent NEET Pattern Question)
    (a) Alkylating agent   (b) Antimetabolite
    (c) Taxanes   (d) Antibiotics

58. **Which of the following is not an alkylating agent?**
    (Recent NEET Pattern Question)
    (a) 5-FU   (b) Busulfan
    (c) Cyclophosphamide   (d) Melphalan

59. **Pulmonary fibrosis is caused by:**
    (Recent NEET Pattern Question)
    (a) Methotrexate   (b) Cyclophosphamide
    (c) Mercaptopurine   (d) Busulfan

60. **Which of the following is a highly emetogenic chemotherapy drug?** *(Recent NEET Pattern Question)*
    (a) 5-Fluorouracil   (b) Paclitaxel
    (c) Vincristine   (d) Cisplatin

61. **Pulmonary fibrosis is side effect associated with the use of:** *(Recent NEET Pattern Question)*
    (a) Actinomycin   (b) Bleomycin
    (c) Doxorubicin   (d) Mithramycin

62. **Bleomycin toxicity primarily involves:**
    (Recent NEET Pattern Question)
    (a) Liver   (b) Bone marrow
    (c) Skin   (d) Lungs

63. **Which of the following is used to treat methotrexate toxicity?** *(Recent NEET Pattern Question)*
    (a) Folic acid   (b) Folinic acid
    (c) Riboflavin   (d) Cyanocobalamine

64. **Peripheral neuropathy as a side effect is caused by which of the following anti cancer drugs?**
    (Recent NEET Pattern Question)
    (a) Vincristine   (b) Cyclophosphamide
    (c) Etoposide   (d) Irinotecan

65. **Which of the following is an inhibitor of dihydrofolate reductase?** *(Recent NEET Pattern Question)*
    (a) Phenytoin   (b) Alcohol
    (c) Methotrexate   (d) Yeast

66. **The following are alkylating agents *except*:**
    (a) Cyclophosphamide   *(Recent NEET Pattern Question)*
    (b) Methotrexate
    (c) Mechlorethamine
    (d) Busulfan

Chemotherapy C: Antineoplastic Drugs

67. Which of the following drug causes hemorrhagic cystitis?
 (Recent NEET Pattern Question)
 (a) Cyclophosphamide (b) Cycloserine
 (c) Ciprofloxacin (d) Cyclosporine

68. Anticancer drug causing nephrotoxicity:
 (Recent NEET Pattern Question)
 (a) Cyclophosphamide (b) Busulfan
 (c) Cisplatin (d) Procarbazine

NEW DRUGS AND MISCELLANEOUS

69. Which of the following is used to treat hormone-responsive breast cancer? *(AIIMS May, 2012)*
 (a) Adriamycin (b) Clomiphene citrate
 (c) Diethylstibestrol (d) Tamoxifen

70. Which of the following is a radioprotector? *(AI 2012)*
 (a) Colony stimulating factor
 (b) Amifostine
 (c) Cisplatin
 (d) Methotrexate

71. Use of tamoxifen in carcinoma of breast patients does not lead to the following side effects: *(AIIMS May 2011)*
 (a) Thromboembolic events
 (b) Endometrial carcinoma
 (c) Cataract
 (d) Cancer in opposite breast

72. Thalidomide, used for multiple myeloma, is:
 (Recent NEET Pattern Question)
 (a) Associated with diarrhea
 (b) Characterized by enantiomeric interconversions
 (c) Metabolized extensively by hepatic CYP system
 (d) Safe for use in pregnant females

73. Phocomelia is due to teratogenic effect of:
 (Recent NEET Pattern Question)
 (a) Thalidomide (b) Chlorpromazine
 (c) Methotrexate (d) Carbamazepine

74. Drug that is radioprotective is:
 (Recent NEET Pattern Question)
 (a) Paclitaxel (b) Vincristine
 (c) Etoposide (d) Amifostine

75. Rituximab is used in: *(Recent NEET Pattern Question)*
 (a) Hodgkin's disease
 (b) Acute myeloid leukemia
 (c) Non-Hodgkin lymphoma
 (d) Multiple myeloma

76. Hydroxyurea acts by inhibiting:
 (a) DNA gyrase *(Recent NEET Pattern Question)*
 (b) DNA synthetase
 (c) Ribonucleotide diphosphate reductase
 (d) Ribonucleotide oxidase

77. Bevacizumab is: *(Recent NEET Pattern Question)*
 (a) Anti-VEGF antibody
 (b) Histone deacetylase inhibitor
 (c) Proteasome inhibitor
 (d) Her-2/neu inhibitor

78. Competitive inhibitor of tyrosine kinase is:
 (Recent NEET Pattern Question)
 (a) Imatinib (b) Letrozole
 (c) Bicalutamide (d) Fulvestrant

79. Monoclonal antibody causing cardiomyopathy is:
 (Recent NEET Pattern Question)
 (a) Trastuzumab (b) Infliximab
 (c) Adalimumab (d) Rituximab

80. Rituximab is a monoclonal antibody against:
 (Recent NEET Pattern Question)
 (a) CD-20 (b) VEGF
 (c) EGFR (d) IL-2

81. All are true regarding sunitinib except:
 (Recent NEET Pattern Question)
 (a) It inhibits tyrosine kinase
 (b) It is used for renal cell carcinoma
 (c) It is used for the treatment of GIST
 (d) It is excreted primarily in urine

82. Finasteride is a: *(Recent NEET Pattern Question)*
 (a) 5-α reductase inhibitor
 (b) Phosphodiesterase inhibitor
 (c) Alpha blocker
 (d) Androgen receptor blocker

83. Imatinib primarily acts by inhibiting:
 (Recent NEET Pattern Question)
 (a) BCR-ABL (b) Tyrosine kinase
 (c) PGDFR (d) None

84. True about Bicalutamide is: *(Recent NEET Pattern Question)*
 (a) Binds to androgen receptor
 (b) Causes gynaecomastia
 (c) It can be given as monotherapy in prostatic carcinoma
 (d) All are true

85. All drugs are used in treatment of breast carcinoma except: *(Recent NEET Pattern Question)*
 (a) Tamoxifen (b) Flutamide
 (c) Cyclophosphamide (d) Letrozole

86. Regarding trastuzumab, all of the following are true except: *(Recent NEET Pattern Question)*
 (a) Shows better response in combination with paclitaxel
 (b) Used in non-metastatic breast cancer
 (c) Causes upregulation of HER2/neu
 (d) Do not cause bone marrow toxicity

87. Thalidomide acts through: *(Recent NEET Pattern Question)*
 (a) Inhibiting angiogenesis
 (b) Inhibiting thymidylate synthase
 (c) Inhibition of Topo-isomerase I
 (d) Inhibition of Topo-isomerase II

CANCER CHEMOTHERAPY

88. Which of the following statements is not true?
 (NEET Pattern 2019)
 (a) Tamoxifen is drug of choice for postmenopausal breast cancer and aromatase inhibitors are preferred for premenopausal breast cancer
 (b) Hormonal therapy is effective in estrogen receptor positive breast cancers
 (c) Tamoxifen is given as 20 mg once a day for 5 years
 (d) Tamoxifen increases the risk of endometrial carcinoma

89. Which of the following can cause agranulocytosis?
 (NEET Pattern Question 2017-2018)
 (a) Alkylating agents (b) Corticosteroids
 (c) Paracetamol (d) Endotoxemia

90. Most common long term side effect of tamoxifen is: *(NEET Pattern Question 2016-17)*
    (a) Weight gain
    (b) Osteoporosis
    (c) Venous thrombosis
    (d) Hot flushes and sweating

91. A girl with acute promyelocytic leukemia was admitted for management. While on treatment she developed tachypnea, fever and pulmonary infiltrates. What should be done for the treatment of this problem? *(AIIMS May 2017)*
    (a) Dexamethasone
    (b) Cytarabine
    (c) Doxorubicin
    (d) Methotrexate

92. Which of the following drugs is useful for the treatment of advanced prostate cancer? *(AIIMS May 2014)*
    (a) Ganirelix
    (b) Cetrorelix
    (c) Abarelix
    (d) Goserelin

93. Which of the following drugs has been recently approved for treatment of prostate cancer? *(AIIMS Nov 2014)*
    (a) Leuprolide
    (b) Goserelin
    (c) Abarelix
    (d) Degarelix

94. A patient on treatment for leukemia, develops chest pain, pulmonary infiltrates and pleural effusion. The likely cause is: *(NEET)*
    (a) Daunorubicin
    (b) Hydroxyurea
    (c) Cytarabine
    (d) Tretinoin

95. Neoadjuvant chemotherapy is used in all *except*: *(Recent NEET Pattern Question)*
    (a) Esophageal carcinoma
    (b) Breast carcinoma
    (c) Thyroid carcinoma
    (d) Non-small cell carcinoma of lung

96. Chemotherapy is not useful in: *(Recent NEET Pattern Question)*
    (a) Chondrosarcoma
    (b) Wilm's tumor
    (c) Choriocarcinoma
    (d) All

97. All cause myelosuppression *except*: *(Recent NEET Pattern Question)*
    (a) Docetaxel
    (b) Vincristine
    (c) Methotrexate
    (d) Irinotecan

98. Proliferation independent agents include all the following *except*: *(Recent NEET Pattern Question)*
    (a) Vincristine
    (b) Carmustine
    (c) Melphalan
    (d) Cyclophosphamide

99. People with high risk for development of breast cancer should be treated by prophylactic administration of: *(Recent NEET Pattern Question)*
    (a) Tamoxifen
    (b) Aminoglutethimide
    (c) Diethylstibesterol
    (d) Flutamide

100. Which of the following is widely used in the management of carcinoma breast? *(Recent NEET Pattern Question)*
     (a) Actinomycin-D
     (b) Bleomycin
     (c) Doxorubicin
     (d) Dacarbazine

101. Allopurinol potentiates action of: *(Recent NEET Pattern Question)*
     (a) Azathioprine
     (b) Busulfan
     (c) Actinomycin
     (d) Procarbazine

102. Dronabinol is orally active cannabinoid used in the management of chemotherapy induced vomiting. Which of the following parameters should be monitored in this patient? *(Recent NEET Pattern Question)*
     (a) Blood pressure
     (b) Respiratory rate
     (c) Urine output
     (d) Temperature

103. Drug of choice for CML is: *(Recent NEET Pattern Question)*
     (a) Rituximab
     (b) Imatinib
     (c) Vincristine
     (d) Cisplatin

104. Which of the following drug is not used for multiple myeloma? *(Recent NEET Pattern Question)*
     (a) Melphalan
     (b) Thalidomide
     (c) Bortezomib
     (d) Methotrexate

105. Drug of choice for neutropenia due to cancer chemotherapy is: *(Recent NEET Pattern Question)*
     (a) Vitamin B-12
     (b) IL-11
     (c) Filgrastim
     (d) Erythropoietin

106. Treatment of chronic phase of CML is: *(Recent NEET Pattern Question)*
     (a) Imatinib
     (b) Hydroxyurea
     (c) Interferon
     (d) Cytarabine

107. The chemotherapeutic agent of choice for concurrent chemoradiation in carcinoma cervix is: *(Recent NEET Pattern Question)*
     (a) Paclitaxel
     (b) Hydroxyurea
     (c) 5 FU (fluorouracil)
     (d) Cisplatin

108. Medical adrenalectomy is seen with: *(Recent NEET Pattern Question)*
     (a) Vincristine
     (b) Vinblastine
     (c) Mitotane
     (d) Methotrexate

109. Regimen used in non-Hodgkin's Lymphoma is: *(Recent NEET Pattern Question)*
     (a) CHOP
     (b) COPP
     (c) MOPP
     (d) ABVD

110. The combination chemotherapy used in Hodgkin's Lymphoma: *(Recent NEET Pattern Question)*
     (a) Adriamycin, Bleomycin, Vincristine, Dacarbazine
     (b) Adriamycin, Bleomycin, Vinblastine, Dacarbazine
     (c) Actinomycin, BCNU, Vincristine, DTIC
     (d) Actinomycin, Bleomycin, Vinblastine, Dacarbazine

111. Drug useful in breast cancer is: *(Recent NEET Pattern Question)*
     (a) Tamoxifen
     (b) Cyproterone
     (c) Testosterone
     (d) Chlorambucil

Explanations

1. Ans. 1. C, 2. A, 3. B, 4. E *(Ref: KDT 8TH/e p251-52, 943)*

Drug	Mechanism of action	Indication
1. Omalizumab	Anti-IgE	Bronchial Asthma
2. Itolizumab	Anti-CD-6	New drug for Psoriasis
3. Daclizumab	Anti CD 25 (IL-2R antagonist)	Immunosuppressant
4. Belimumab	Anti-B lymphocyte stimulator(BlyS)	New drug for SLE

2. Ans. (a) Bleomycin *(Ref: KDT 8th/e p927)*

Bleomycin is metabolized by bleomycin hydrolase which is deficient in skin and lungs. It thus leads to characteristics adverse effects on these organs. These are:
- Flagellated pigmentation of skin
- Pulmonary fibrosis.

3. Ans. (c) Cytarabine *(Ref: KDT's 8th/e p923)*

4. Ans. (c) Cytarabine *(Ref: KDT 8th/e p923-924)*

5. Ans. (c) Capecitabine
(Ref: KDT 8th/e p923; From ROAMS 13th/e p325)

6. Ans. (a) Aprepitant *(Ref: KDT's 8th/e p718)*

7. Ans. (a) Paclitaxel *(Ref: Katzung 13th/e p921)*

Paclitaxel is a taxane that act on mitotic spindle. Drugs acting on mitotic spindle act on M phase of cell cycle.

Phase of cell cycle	Drugs acting
G1	Etoposide
S	Antimetabolites
G2	Bleomycin Etoposide Irinoctecan Topotecan
M	Vinca alkaloids Taxanes

8. Ans. (a) Acute lymphocytic leukemia
(Ref: Katzung 13th/e p938; KDT 8th/e p928)

L-Asparaginase is used for treatment of ALL. It can cause hypersensitivity and acute pancreatitis.

9. Ans. (a) It is obtained from E. coli *(Ref: KDT 8th/e p924)*
- Paclitaxel is obtained from bark of western yew tree (not from E. coli).
- Vinca alkaloids (like vincristine and vinblastine) inhibit polymerization whereas paclitaxel and docetaxel enhance polymerization of β-tubulin.
- Like most anticancer drugs, paclitaxel can also result in bone marrow suppression.
- Major indications of taxanes like paclitaxel are:

- Ovarian cancer
- Breast carcinoma
- Head and neck cancer
- Small cell carcinoma of lung
- Esophageal adenocarcinoma
- Prostate cancer

10. Ans. (a) Chlorambucil
(Ref: KDT 8th/e p918; Harrison 18th/e p708)

Cisplatin and cyclophosphamide have very high emetogenic potential whereas chlorambucil and busulfan have the least.

11. Ans. (b) Folic acid and vitamin B_{12} *(Ref: Goodman and Gilman 12th/e p1694; Harrison 18th/e p703)*

Folic acid and vitamin B_{12} are essential for ameliorating the toxicity of pemetrexed.

Pemetrexed Toxicity
- Pemetrexed toxicity mirrors that of methotrexate, with the additional feature of a prominent erythematous and pruritic rash in 40% of patients.
- Severe myelosuppression with pemetrexed, seen especially in patients with pre-existing homocystinemia and possibly reflecting folate deficiency, is largely eliminated by concurrent administration of low dosages of folic acid beginning 1–2 weeks prior to pemetrexed and continuing while the drug is administered.
- Patients should receive intramuscular vitamin B_{12} with the first dose of pemetrexed to correct possible B_{12} deficiency.
- These small doses of folate and B_{12} do not compromise the therapeutic effect.

12. Ans. (b) Laryngotracheal stenosis
(Ref: American College of Chest Physicians, 2008, KDT 8th/e p927)
- Application of topical mitomycin C after endoscopic dilation of laryngotracheal stenosis reduces the rate of restenosis.
- It is also useful for anal carcinoma and superficial bladder cancer.

13. Ans. (a) Oral alkylating agent
(Ref: Goodman Gilman 12th/e p1687, KDT 8th/e p920)

Temozolomide is an alkylating agent that can be given orally.

14. Ans. (c) Eye examination *(Ref: CMDT 2010, 1501)*

Methotrexate toxicities include:
- Myelosuppression
- Nephrotoxicity
- Hepatotoxicity
- Neurotoxicity (with intrathecal administration and high-dose therapy)
- Photosensitivity
- Pulmonary toxicity
- Multiple drug interactions which may enhance toxicities (avoid aspirin, penicillins, NSAIDs, omeprazole, TMP-SMZ)

15. Ans. (b) Nitrosourea *(Ref: KDT 8th/e p919)*

Nitrosoureas like carmustine, lomustine and semustine can cross blood brain barrier and thus are used for treatment of gliomas.

16. **Ans. (a) Cisplatin** *(Ref: KDT 8th/e p920)*
    Cisplatin is most emetogenic and highly nephrotoxic anti-cancer drug.
17. **Ans. (b) Methotrexate** *(Ref: KDT 8th/e p657)*
18. **Ans. (c) GM-CSF** *(Ref: Katzung 10th/e p538)*
    Nitrogen mustards like mechlorethamine cause bone marrow suppression as major adverse effect. Leucopenia can be reversed by sargramostim (recombinant GM-CSF). All nitrogen mustards do not cause hemorrhagic cystitis, therefore mesna is not the answer.
19. **Ans. (a) Vincristine** *(Ref: KDT 8th/e p924)*
20. **Ans. (a) Doxorubicin** *(Ref: KDT 8th/e p926)*
21. **Ans. (b) Paclitaxel** *(Ref: Katzung 11th/e p950, KDT 8th/e p925)*
22. **Ans. (c) Ifosfamide** *(Ref: Katzung 11th/e p938, KDT 8th/e p919)*
23. **Ans. (d) Zalcitabine** *(Ref: KDT 8th/e p918-919)*
24. **Ans. (a) Cardiomyopathy** *(Ref: KDT 8th/e p920)*
25. **Ans. (a) Hemorrhagic cystitis** *(Ref: KDT 8th/e p919)*
26. **Ans. (a) Hepatic fibrosis** *(Ref: Katzung 11/945, KDT 8th/e p921)*
27. **Ans. (d) Spiramycin** *(Ref: KDT 8th/e p916)*
28. **Ans. (a) Methotrexate toxicity** *(Ref: KDT/8th/e p657)*
29. **Ans. (b) Vincristine** *(Ref: KDT 8th/e p924)*
30. **Ans. (b) Chlorambucil** *(Ref: KDT 8th/e p919)*
31. **Ans. (b) It has dose-dependent kinetics** *(Ref: Goodman Gilman 12th/1746-1747, KDT 8th/e p931-932)*
    - Rituximab is a chimeric **monoclonal antibody against CD-20 B-cell antigen.** It acts by depleting B-cells.
    - Rituximab **follows first order kinetics.** Its clearance remains constant irrespective of plasma concentration. Dose-dependent kinetics means zero-order kinetics i.e. clearance and $t_{1/2}$ change with dose (plasma concentration). Drugs following zero-order kinetics are warfarin, alcohol, high dose aspirin, tolbutamide, theophylline and phenytoin.
    - **Infusion-related reactions** are seen in approximately 50% of patients receiving first infusion. The incidence decreases with subsequent infusions. Starting with low doses and pre-treatment with steroids or antihistaminics are the methods to reduce infusion-related reactions.
    - Rituximab **may cause reactivation of hepatitis B.** Patients should be screened for hepatitis B before initiation of therapy. It rarely causes reactivation of JC virus leading to progressive multifocal leukoencephalopathy.
    - Rituximab can be used for treatment of:

      - Non Hodgkin lymphoma
      - Mantle cell lymphoma
      - Chronic lymphocytic leukemia
      - Auto-immune hemolytic anemia
      - Diffuse large B cell lymphoma
      - Thrombotic thrombocytopenic purpura (TTP)
      - Gastric lymphoma
      - Rheumatoid arthritis
      - Immune thrombocytopenic purpura (ITP)
      - Pemphigus vulgaris
      - Sjogren syndrome
      - SLE

32. **Ans. (a) Vacoular degeneration of myofibrils** *(Ref: GG-1714)*
33. **Ans. (c) Dilated cardiomyopathy** *(Ref: GG-1714)*
34. **Ans. (c) Cisplatin** *(Ref: GG-1689)*
35. **Ans. (d) Mitomycin C** *(Ref: GG-1718, KDT 8th/e p927)*
    Mitomycin C and gemcitabine can cause hemolytic uremic syndrome.
36. **Ans. (b) Cytarabine** *(Ref: GG-1700)*
37. **Ans. (a) Antimetabolite** *(Ref: GG-1695, KDT 8th/e p916)*
38. **Ans. (a) Cisplatin**
39. **Ans. (b) Doxorubicin** *(Ref: KDT 8th/e p916)*
40. **Ans. (d) Increased production of dihydrofolate reductase** *(Ref: CMDT 2015/p1638)*
41. **Ans. (a) Inhibits mitotic spindle** *(Ref: KDT 7th/e p924)*
42. **Ans. (a) Hemorrhagic cystitis** *(Ref: KDT 8th/e p919)*
43. **Ans. (b) Cisplatin** *(Ref: KDT 8th/e p920)*
44. **Ans. (a) Tubulin inhibitor** *(Ref: KDT 8th/e p924)*
45. **Ans. (a) Methotrexate** *(Ref: KDT 8th/e p921)*
46. **Ans. (a) Methotrexate** *(Ref: KDT 8th/e p921)*
47. **Ans. (b) Vincristine** *(Ref: KDT 8th/e p 924)*
48. **Ans. (a) Bleomycin** *(Ref: KDT 8th/e p927)*
49. **Ans. (c) Doxorubicin** *(Ref: KDT 8th/e p926)*
50. **Ans. (a) Increased concentrations of intracellular DHFR through gene amplification** *(Ref: Goodman Gilman 12th/e p1820)*
51. **Ans. (d) Vincristine** *(Ref: KDT 8th/e p916)*
52. **Ans. (a) Alkylating agent** *(Ref: KDT 8th/e p918)*
53. **Ans. (c) Cardiotoxicity** *(Ref: KDT 8th/e p926)*
54. **Ans. (a) Antimetabolite** *(Ref: KDT 8th/e p923)*
55. **Ans. (a) Bleomycin** *(Ref: KDT 8th/e p927)*
56. **Ans. (d) Cladribine** *(Ref: KDT 8th/e p918,919)*
57. **Ans. (a) Alkylating agent** *(Ref: KDT 8th/e p919)*
58. **Ans. (a) 5-FU** *(Ref: KDT 8th/e p923)*
59. **Ans. (d) Busulfan** *(Ref: KDT 8th/e p919)*
60. **Ans. (d) Cisplatin** *(Ref: KDT 8th/e p920)*
61. **Ans. (b) Bleomycin** *(Ref: KDT 8th/e p927)*
62. **Ans. (d) Lungs** *(Ref: KDT 8th/e p927)*
63. **Ans. (b) Folinic acid** *(Ref: KDT 8th/e p921)*
64. **Ans. (a) Vincristine** *(Ref: KDT 8th/e p924)*
65. **Ans. (c) Methotrexate** *(Ref: KDT 8th/e p921)*
66. **Ans. (b) Methotrexate** *(Ref: KDT 8th/e p918-919)*
67. **Ans. (a) Cyclophosphamide** *(Ref: KDT 8th/e p919)*
68. **Ans. (c) Cisplatin** *(Ref: KDT 8th/e p920)*
69. **Ans. (d) Tamoxifen** *(Ref: KDT 8th/e p932)*

Estrogen receptor positive breast cancers are amenable to treatment with anti-estrogen drugs like
- **SERMs:** Tamoxifen, Doloxifen and Toremifene
- **SERDs:** Fulvestrant
- **Aromatase inhibitors:** Letrozole, Anastrozole, Exemestane

70. **Ans. (b) Amifostine**
    (Ref: KK Sharma 2nd/e p858, KDT 8th/e p936)
    Amifostine is used for reducing the toxicities of anticancer drugs. It is indicated for:
    1. Cisplatin induced nephrotoxicity.
    2. Radiation induced xerostomia

    Amifostine is used to prevent radiation induced toxicity whereas colony stimulating factors are used for management of chemotherapy induced leucopenia.
    - Amifostine scavenges free radicals produced by radiation and inactivates active species through formation of thioether conjugates. Amifostine has been approved by the USA FDA as a radioprotector. It is also known as "Ethyol".
    - Since amifostine acts by scavenging the free radicals, it must be given before the radiation. It is of no use in radiation protection after the event.

71. **Ans. (d) Cancer in opposite breast** *(Ref: Goodman and Gilman 12th/e p1179, CMDT 2010, 1505, KDT 8th/e p338)*
    - Tamoxifen is a SERM that acts as antagonist at estrogen receptors in the breast. It decreases the risk of contralateral breast cancer and is approved for primary prevention of breast cancer in women at high risk.

Adverse effects of Tamoxifen include:	
• Hot flushes	• Vaginal discharge or bleeding
• Menstrual irregularities	• Thromboembolic events (rare)
• Endometrial hyperplasia	• Cataracts
• Hepatotoxicity	• Tumor flare

72. **Ans. (b) Characterized by enantiomeric interconversions**
    (Ref: Goodman & Gilman 11th/e p1370, 1371, Katzung 10th/e p919)
    - Thalidomide was used for morning sickness but later withdrawn due to severe teratogenic effects (phocomelia).
    - It is not extensively metabolized by microsomal enzymes.
    - Two isomers of thalidomide; S (teratogenic) and R (sedative) are present. But giving R isomer do not protect against teratogenic potential due to enantiomeric interconversions in the body.
    - It is now being used for multiple myeloma and has dose limiting adverse effect of peripheral neuropathy. It can also result in constipation.

73. **Ans. (a) Thalidomide** *(Ref: KDT 8th/e p100)*

74. **Ans. (d) Amifostine** *(Ref: internet, KDT 8th/e p936)*

75. **Ans. (c) Non-Hodgkin lymphoma**
    (Ref: Katzung 10th/e p589, KDT 8th/e p932)
    Rituximab is a monoclonal antibody used for the treatment of non-Hodgkin lymphoma.

76. **Ans. (c) Ribonucleotide diphosphate reductase**
    (Ref: GG–1721, KDT 8th/e p927)

77. **Ans. (a) Anti-VEGF antibody**
    (Ref: GG–1732, KDT 8th/e p930-931)

78. **Ans. (a) Imatinib** *(Ref: GG–1732, KDT 8th/e p929)*
79. **Ans. (a) Trastuzumab** *(Ref: GG–1737)*
80. **Ans. (a) CD-20** *(Ref: GG–1745, KDT 8th/e p931)*
81. **Ans. (d) It is excreted primarily in urine**
    (Ref: CMDT 2015 /1607, KDT 8th/e p931)
82. **Ans. (a) 5-α reductase inhibitor** *(Ref: KDT 8th/e p932)*
83. **Ans. (b) Tyrosine kinase** *(Ref: KDT 8th/e p929)*
    - Imatinib inhibits tyrosine kinase linked with
      - abl-bcr fusion
      - PDGF receptor
      - c-kit receptor
84. **Ans. (d) All are true** *(Ref: Goodman Gilman 7th/e p1766)*
85. **Ans. (b) Flutamide** *(Ref: CMDT 2014 p715-717)*
86. **Ans. (c) Causes upregulation of HER2/neu**
    (Ref: CMDT 2014, p716)
87. **Ans. (a) Inhibiting angiogenesis** *(Ref: Goodman Gilman 12th/e p1741, KDT 8th/e p936)*
88. **Ans. (a) Tamoxifen is drug of choice for postmenopausal breast cancer and aromatase inhibitors are preferred for premenopausal breast cancer**
    (Ref: Goodman and Gilman 13th/e p1239)
    Hormonal therapy for breast cancer
    - Three type of drugs are used for hormonal therapy of breast cancer. These are
      - SERMs like tamoxifen
      - Aromatase inhibitors like letrozole
      - SERDs like fulvestrant
    - These are effective only in estrogen receptor positive breast cancer
    - Aromatase inhibitors are the preferred first line therapy in postmenopausal females whereas SERMs like tamoxifen is preferred in premenopausal female.
    - Taxomifen can increase the risk of endometrial carcinoma due to estrogen agonistic action at endometrium
    - Dose of tamoxifen is 20-40 mg per day for 5-10 years.

89. **Ans. (a) Alkylating agents** *(Ref: KDT 8th/e p917)*
90. **Ans. (c) Venous thrombosis** *(Ref: KDT's 8th/e p338)*
91. **Ans. (a) Dexamethasone** *(Ref: Harrison 19/e p1686-87)*
    The features given are known as APL differentiation syndrome which can occur while treatment with tretinoin. The treatment is with steroids.
92. **Ans. (d) Goserelin** *(Ref: Katzung12th/e p972; Goodman and Gilman 12th/e p1763-1764, KDT 8th/e p264)*
    Gonadotropin releasing hormone agonists like leuprolide and goserelin are useful for the treatment of advanced prostate cancer. Among GnRH antagonists, only degarelix is approved for the treatment of advanced prostate cancer.
93. **Ans. (d) Degarelix** *(Ref: CMDT 2015/1624)*
    - **Degarelix** is a GnRH antagonist, that has recently been approved for advanced prostate cancer.
    - GnRH agonists like **leuprolide** and **goserelin** are being used in prostate cancer since many years.
    - **Docetaxel** is first cytotoxic agent that **improve survival** in patients with hormone-refractory prostate cancer.
    - **Sipulecel-T** is an immunotherapy recently approved for prostate cancer.

- Other drugs for prostate cancer are:
    - Cabazitaxel
    - Abiraterone
    - Enzalutamide
    - Radium-223 dichloride

94. **Ans. (d) Tretinoin** *(Ref: Katzung 10th/e p899; KDT 8th/e p928)*
    Tretinoin causes chest pain, pleuritis, pulmonary infiltrates and pleural effusion. It is a known human teratogen. Daunorubicin and doxorubicin cause cardiotoxicity manifested as arrhythmias and CHF.

95. **Ans. (c) Thyroid carcinoma**
    (Ref: CMDT-2010/667,1456, 1469,1625)
    - *"Thyroid carcinomas are extra-ordinarily resistant to chemotherapy"*
    - Neoadjuvant chemotherapy is administration of chemotherapy before surgery or radiation therapy whereas adjuvant chemotherapy is used after surgery/radiation.

    - **Neoadjuvant chemotherapy is used in:**
        - Bladder cancer
        - Breast cancer
        - Colorectal cancer
        - Esophageal cancer
        - Gastric adenocarcinoma
        - Non-small cell lung cancer

96. **Ans. (a) Chondrosarcoma** *(Ref: KDT 8th/e p915)*

97. **Ans. (b) Vincristine** *(Ref: KDT 8th/e p924)*

98. **Ans. (a) Vincristine** *(Ref: KDT 8th/e p919, 924)*
    Proliferation independent means cell cycle nonspecific agents.

99. **Ans. (a) Tamoxifen** *(Ref: KDT 8th/e p338)*

100. **Ans. (c) Doxorubicin**
    (Ref: CMDT 2010, 1466-1468, KDT 8th/e p926)

101. **Ans. (a) Azathioprine** *(Ref: KDT 8th/e p922)*
    Allopurinol *inhibits degradation* of azathioprine and 6-mercaptopurine and thus potentiates their action.

102. **Ans. (a) Blood pressure** *(Ref: GG–1345)*

103. **Ans. (b) Imatinib** *(Ref: GG–1732, KDT 8th/e p929)*

104. **Ans. (d) Methotrexate** *(Ref: Harrison 19th/e p716)*

105. **Ans. (c) Filgrastim** *(Ref: KDT 8th/e p936)*

106. **Ans. (a) Imatinib** *(Ref: KDT 8th/e p929)*

107. **Ans. (d) Cisplatin** *(Ref: CMDT 2014/ p736, KDT 8th/e p920)*

108. **Ans. (c) Mitotane** *(Ref: Goodman and Gilman 12th/e p1719)*

109. **Ans. (a) CHOP** *(Ref: KDT 8th/e p935)*

110. **Ans. (a) Adriamycin, Bleomycin, Vincristine, Dacarbazine**
    (Ref: KDT 8th/e p935)

111. **Ans. (a) Tamoxifen** *(Ref: KDT 8th/e p338, 932)*

Immunomodulators

CHAPTER 15

IMMUNOSUPPRESSANTS

1. Glucocorticoids

These are most commonly used immunosuppressant drugs and act by inhibiting the production of prostaglandins, leukotrienes, histamine, bradykinin and PAF.

- These drugs also *diminish chemotactic activity* of neutrophils and monocytes.
- Glucocorticoids cause *sequestration of lymphocytes* in lymphoid tissue resulting in lymphopenia.
- By *inhibiting IL-1 production*, these drugs cause a decrease in IL-2 and IFN γ production.
- Continuous administration of glucocorticoids can *increase the catabolism of IgG*. These are used as first line immunosuppressive drugs for solid organ as well as hematological stem cell transplant recipients. These are also used for the treatment of graft rejection and graft versus host disease (GVHD), treatment of ITP, rheumatoid arthritis and bronchial asthma.

2. Calcineurin Inhibitors

Calcineurin is required for the activation of NFAT (nuclear factor of activated T cells) which in turn increases the transcription of IL-2 by activated T cells. Cyclosporine and tacrolimus (FK 506) inhibits the activation of NFAT by binding to immunophilins (cyclosporine binds to cyclophilin and tacrolimus binds to FKBP). Net result of administration of **cyclosporine and tacrolimus** is **inhibition of gene transcription of IL-2**. These are used as immunosuppressive agents for organ transplantation, GVHD and some autoimmune diseases like rheumatoid arthritis and psoriasis.

- Cyclosporine can cause *nephrotoxicity, hepatotoxicity, hypertension, hyperkalemia, hyperlipidemia, hyperuricemia, hyperglycemia, hirsutism, gum hyperplasia and neurotoxicity* (tremor, headache, motor disturbance and seizures).
- Incidence of *hyperglycemia and neurotoxicity are more with tacrolimus* than cyclosporine. Whereas **hirsutism, gum hyperplasia, hyperuricemia and hyperlipidemia are not caused by tacrolimus.**

> **Key Points**
>
> Hirsutism, gum hyperplasia, hyperuricemia and hyperlipidemia are adverse effects of cyclosporine which are not caused by tacrolimus.

> **Note**
>
> - *Tacrolimus is more potent* than *cyclosporine*.
> - Tacrolimus is a *macrolide antibiotic*.
> - Nephrotoxicity is the major indication for cessation or modification of cyclosporine therapy. Hypertension occurs in 50% of renal transplant and almost all cardiac transplant recepients.
> - Sirolimus aggravates cyclosporine induced renal dysfunction whereas cyclosporine increases sirolimus induced hyperlipidemia and myelosuppression.

3. Proliferation Signal Inhibitors

IL-2 stimulates immune system by activation of several T cells via activation of mammalian target of rapamycin (mTOR). **Sirolimus (rapamycin) binds to mTOR and inhibits the action of IL-2 without affecting its transcription.** It is used as immunosuppressive agent in organ transplantation and GVHD. It is **also incorporated in cardiac stents to decrease the chances of reocclusion**. Its major adverse effect is **thrombocytopenia** due to bone marrow suppression and hyperlipidemia. Sirolimus per se is not nephrotoxic. Lymphocele is increased in a dose dependent fashion by sirolimus. **Everolimus** is a new drug in this category having **shorter half life** (43 hours as compared to 60 hours with sirolimus) and is **useful in cardiac transplantation**. These drugs increase the risk of *hemolytic uremic syndrome*. Everolimus has recently been approved for treatment of patients with subependymal giant cell astrocytoma (SEGA) associated with tuberous sclerosis.

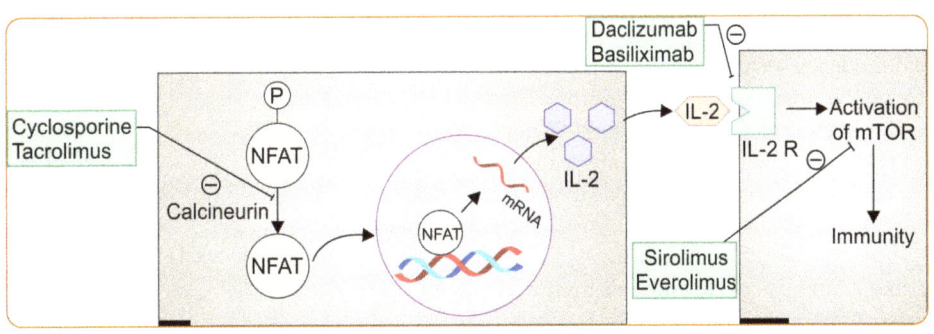

FIG. 15.1: Calcineurin pathway and its inhibitors

4. Purine Synthesis Inhibitor

Mycophenolate mofetil *inhibits inosine monophosphate dehydrogenase* after conversion to its active metabolite mycophenolic acid. This enzyme is necessary for de novo synthesis of purines. It is used as immunosuppressant in patients *who are refractory to steroids*. GI disturbances and myelosuppression are major adverse effects of this drug.

> **Key Points**
>
> Mycophenolate does not cause nephrotoxicity.

5. Antimetabolites

Azathioprine is the only antimetabolite that is used as *immunosuppressant* **but not as an anticancer drug.** It is a **prodrug** and is activated in the body to 6-mercaptopurine (anticancer drug). It lacks anticancer properties because conversion to active metabolite occurs only in lymphoid cells. Major toxic effect is bone marrow suppression. Its **dose should be reduced if allopurinol is used** concurrently because 6-MP is also metabolized by xanthine oxidase.

6. Other Cytotoxic Agents

Cyclophosphamide, chlorambucil and methotrexate are other anticancer drugs that can be used as immunosuppressants. Cyclophosphamide and chlorambucil are used in treating *childhood nephrotic syndrome*. Cyclophosphamide is also used for treatment of *SLE and Wegner's granulomatosis*.

7. Leflunomide

Active metabolite of this prodrug **inhibits dihydro-orotate dehydrogenase** resulting in inhibition of pyrimidine synthesis. It is an **orally active** drug with **long half life** of several weeks. Liver and kidney damage are major toxicities. *Cholestyramine increases its excretion*. It is increasingly being used for *polyoma virus nephropathy*.

8. Thalidomide

- It is a sedative drug that was withdrawn due to teratogenic (phocomelia) effects. It has come into market again due to its anti-angiogenic, immunomodulatory and anti-inflammatory effects.
- **Currently, it is being used for multiple myeloma, erythema nodosum leprosum and skin manifestations of SLE.**
- Important **adverse effects** of thalidomide include *tetratogenicity, peripheral neuropathy, constipation, hypothyroidism and increased risk of thrombosis particularly DVT*. Immunomodulatory derivatives of thalidomide are termed IMiDs. **Lenalidomide** is an **IMiD** approved for myelodysplastic syndrome and multiple myeloma. Anothert group of thalodomide analogs, **SelCIDs** (SELective Cytokine Inhibitory Drugs) are phosphodiesterase-4 (PDE 4) inhibitors with potent anti-TNFα activity.

9. Antibodies

Polyclonal antibodies like anti-lymphocyte and anti-thymocyte antibodies, hyperimmune immunoglobulins and Rho (D) immunoglobulin are useful as immunosuppressive drugs. Recently, several **monoclonal antibodies** have been synthesized to produce this effect.

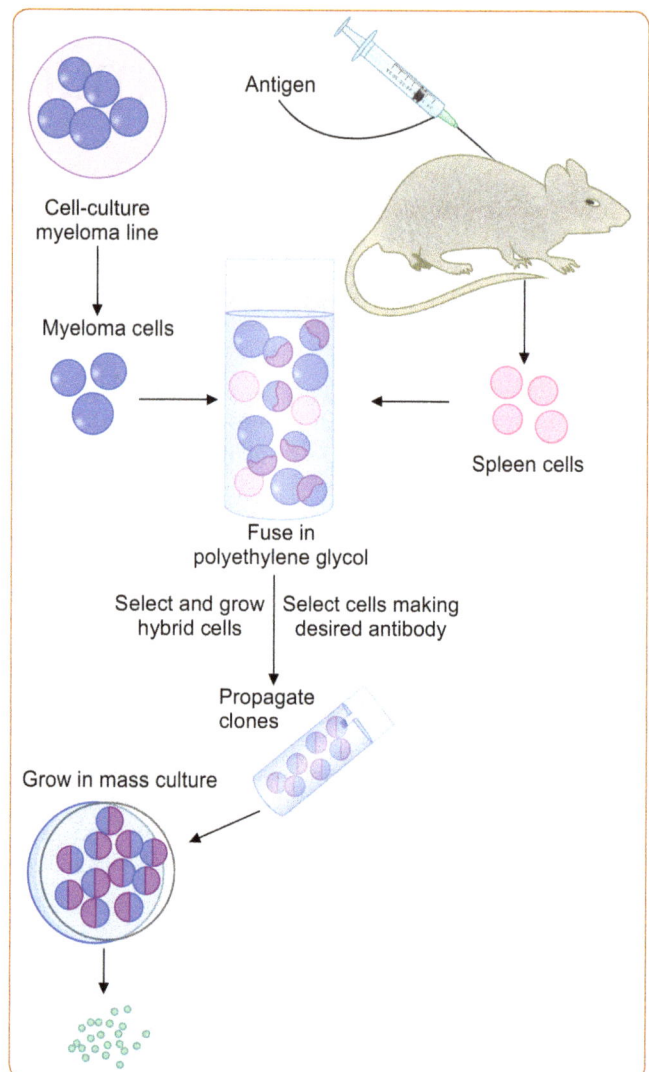

FIG. 15.2: Formation of monoclonal antibodies

Monoclonal antibody	Target	Indication
Abciximab	Gp II/IIIa	Antiplatelet
Adalimumab	TNF-α	RA Non-infectious uveitis
Alefacept	LFA-3	Plaque psoriasis
Alemtuzumab	CD 52	B cell CLL Multiple sclerosis
Amivantamab	EGFR and MET	Non small cell lung cancer
Abatacept	CD-80, 86	RA
Aflibercept	VEGFR1,2	Neovascular Age related macular degeneration
Avelumab	PD-L1	Merkel cell carcinoma, Renal cell carcinoma
Basiliximab	IL-2R (CD-25)	Immunosuppressant
Belantamab	B-cell maturation antigen	Multiple myeloma
Belimumab	BLyS	SLE

Contd...

Immunomodulators

Contd...

Monoclonal antibody	Target	Indication
Bevacizumab	VEGF	Colorectal carcinoma, Glioblastoma, Renal cell carcinoma
Belatacept	CD 80, 86	Transplantation
Bezlotoxumab	Clostridium toxin B	*Clostridium difficile* infection
Brentuximab	CD 30	Hodgkin lymphoma, Anaplastic large cell lympoma
Brodalumab	IL-17RA	Plaque psoriasis
Brolucizumab	VEGF	Neovascular age-related macular degeneration
Canakinumab	IL-1β	Cryopyrin associated periodic syndrome (CAPS)
Caplacizumab	vwF	Thrombotic thrombocytopenic purpura
Cemiplimab	PD-I	Squamous cell carcinoma of skin
Cetuximab	EFGR	Colorectal carcinoma
Certolizumab	TNFα	Crohn's disease
Crizanlizumab	P-selectin	Veno-occlusive disease in sickle cell anemia
Daclizumab	IL-2R (CD-25)	Immunosuppressant
Denosumab	RANK ligand	Osteoporosis
Dostarlimab	PD-1	Endometrial cancer
Dupilumab	IL-4R	Atopic dermatitis, Nasal polyps
Durvalumab	PD-L-1	Urothelial carcinoma
Eculizumab	C5 complement component	Paroxysomal nocturnal hemoglobinuria, Atypical hemolytic uremic syndrome
Efalizumab	CD 11a chain of LFA	Psoriasis
Emapalumab	IFN-γ	Hemophagocytic lymphohistiocytosis
Emicizumab	Factor IXa, X	Hemophilia A
Enfortumab	Nectin-4	Urothelial carcinoma
Epratuzumab	CD 22	SLE
Etanercept	TNF α	RA (rheumatoid arthritis)
Fam-trastuzumab	Her-2	Breast cancer
Gemtuzumab	CD 33	AML
Golimumab	TNFα	RA, Psoriasis, Ankylosing Spondylosis
Guselkumab	IL-23	Plaque psoriasis
Ibritumomab	CD 20	B-cell NHL
Inebilizumab	CD19	Neuromyelitis optica spectrum disorders
Infliximab	TNFα	RA, Crohn's disease, Psoriatic arthritis, Wegener's disease, Sarcoidosis
Inotuzumab	CD-22	B-cell precursor ALL
Ipilimumab	CTLA-4	Metastatic melanoma
Isatuximab	CD-38	Multiple myeloma
Ixekizumab	IL-17A	Plaque psoriasis, Ankylosing spondylosis
Loncastuximab	CD19	Large B-cell lymphoma
Margetuximab	Her-2	Breast cancer
Mogamulizumab	CCR-4	Mycosis fungoides, Sezary syndrome
Moxetumomab Pasudotox	CD-22	Hairy cell leukemia
Natalizumab	Integrin-α4	Multiple sclerosis
Naxitamab	GD-2	Neuroblastoma
Nimotuzumab	EGFR	Squamous cell carcinoma, Glioma
Nivolumab	PD-1	Non-small cell lung cancer
Obiltoxaximab	PA of bacillus anthracis	Inhalational anthrax
Obinutuzumab	CD-20	CLL, SLL
Ocrelizumab	CD-20	Breast cancer, Multiple sclerosis
Ofatumumab	CD 20	SLE
Omalizumab	Ig E	Bronchial asthma
Palivizumab	Fusion protein	RSV
Panitumumab	EGFR	Colorectal carcinoma
Pembrolizumab	PD-1	Endometrial cancer, esophageal cancer, small cell and non-small cell lung cancer, renal cell carcinoma
Pertuzumab	HER-2	Breast cancer, Multiple sclerosis
Polatuzumab	BCR	DLBCL
Ramucirumab	VEGFR-2	Non-small cell Lung cancer and cancer of gastroesophageal junction, hepatocellular carcinoma
Ranibizumab	VEGF	Neovascular Macular degeneration, Macular edema following retinal vein occlusion
Reslizumab	IL-5	Severe Asthma
Risankizumab	IL-23	Plaque psoriasis
Rituximab	CD 20	B-cell NHL
Rilonacept	IL-1	CAPS
Sacituzumab	Trop 2	Triple negative breast cancer
Sarilumab	IL-6	RA
Satralizumab	IL-6R	Neuromyelitis optica spectrum disorder
Secukinumab	IL-17a	Plaque psoriasis
Siltuximab	IL-6	Castleman's disease
Tafasitamab	CD-19	Diffuse large B-cell lymphoma (DLBCL)
Teprotumumab	IGF-1	Thyroid eye disease
Tocilizumab	IL-6R	SLE, RA, Cytokine release syndrome
Trastuzumab	her-2/neu	Breast cancer, Stomach and gastro-esophageal junction carcinoma
Ustekinumab	IL-12, IL-23	Plaque psoriasis
Vedolizumab	α₄β₇	Ulcerative colitis, Crohn's disease

NOMENCLATURE OF MONOCLONAL ANTIBODIES

Name of the monoclonal antibody can be devided into four parts.

Prefix + Target subsystem + Origin subsystem + Suffix
- **Suffix** for all monoclonal antibodies is **mab**
- Depending on the source of origin, various names are given, e.g. u stands for human, xi for chimeric etc.
- Target is identified by specific letters, e.g. vi for virus, ci for circulation.
- *Previously, target consisted of three letters (first consonant, second vowel and third consonant) but third consonant can be deleted for ease of pronounciation. In 2009, new and shorter target subsystems were introduced.*
- Prefix is different for each monoclonal antibody.

Prefix	Target subsystem			Source subsystem		Suffix
	Old	New	Meaning		Meaning	
	vi (r)	v (i)	Viral	u	Human	
	ba (c)	b (a)	Bacterial	o	Mouse	
	li (m)	l (i)	Lower immunity	a	Rat	
	fu (ng)	f (u)	Fungal	i	Primate	Mab
	ne (r)	n (e)	Nervous system	xi	Chimeric	
Variable	ki (n)	k (i)	Interleukin as target	zuaxo	Humanizedrat mouse hybrid	
	mu (l)	-	Musculoskeletal	xizu	Chimeric humanized hybrid	
	o (s)	s (o)	Bone			
	co (l)		Colonic tumor			
	me (l)		Melanoma			
	ma (r)	- t(u)	Mammary tumor			
	go (t)		Testicular tumor			
	go (v)		Ovarian tumor			
	pr (o)		Prostate tumor			
	tu (m)		Miscellaneous tumor			

Examples of each target subsystem

	Monoclonal antibody	Target subsystem	Indication
1.	Abagovomab	gov	Ovarian cancer
2.	Abciximab	ci	Antiplatelet
3.	Adalimumab	lim	Rheumatoid Arthritis
4.	Basiliximab	li	Transplantation
5.	Canakinumab	kin (IL-1β)	Rheumatoid Arthritis
6.	Capromab	pro	Prostatic cancer
7.	Cetuximab	tu	Colorectal cancer
8.	Donesumab	s	Osteoporosis
9.	Ecromeximab	me	Malignant melanoma
10.	Edrocolomab	col	Colonic cancer
11.	Efungumab	fung	Invasive candida infection
12.	Ertumaxomab	ma	Mammary tumor (Breast cancer)
13.	Infliximab	li	Rheumatoid arthritis
14.	Nacolomab	col	Colonic cancer
15.	Palivizumab	vi	Respiratory Syncytial Virus
16.	Panobacumab	bac	Pseudomonas aeruginosa infection
17.	Rituximab	tu	Non-Hodgkin lymphoma
18.	Solanezumab	ne	Alzheimer's disease
19.	Stamulumab	mul	Muscular dystrophy
20.	Trastuzumab	tu	Breast cancer
21.	Ustekinumab	kin (IL-12, IL-23)	Multiple sclerosis

10. Co-stimulation Inhibitor

Certain costimulatory molecules are present on the surface of T cells as well as antigen presenting cells (APCs). Interaction of these molecules is necessary for the activation of T cells. **Abatacept** and **belatacept** act by inhibiting CD 80 and CD 86 costimulatory molecules present on APC. Abatacept is *used for the treatment of severe rheumatoid arthritis resistant to DMARDs*. **Belatacept** is used for preventing rejection of *kidney transplants*.

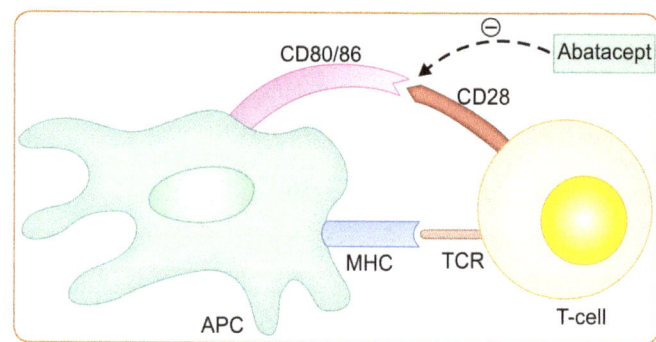

FIG. 15.3: Mechanism of action of abatacept

11. IL-1 Inhibitor

Anakinra is an *inhibitor of IL-1* being investigated for use in *septic shock and RA*.

12. Other Drugs

Nintedanib is a small molecule kinase inhibitor that blocks multiple pathways involved in scarring of lung tissue. It is approved for oral treatment of **idiopathic pulmonary fibrosis**.

Apremilast is phosphodiesterase-4 inhibitor indicated for **severe plaque psoriasis** and **psoriatic arthritis**.

IMMUNOSTIMULANTS

1. Levamisole

It is used along *with 5-FU* for treatment of *colorectal carcinoma* after surgery. **Agranulocytosis** is major adverse effect. It is **also used for the treatment of pediculosis**. It was also used as an antihelminthic drug via stimulation of ganglionic nicotinic receptors.

2. BCG

Bacillus Calmette Guerin is a viable stain of *Mycobacterium bovis* and is useful as **intravesical therapy of superficial bladder cancer**.

3. Cytokines

These include **interferons**, colony stimulating factors **(CSF) and various interleukins**.
- Recombinant form of IL-2 is **Aldesleukin** and is **useful in malignant melanoma** and **renal cell carcinoma**
- **Filgrastim** (recombinant G-CSF) and **sargramostim** (recombinant GM-CSF) are **useful for chemotherapy induced myelosuppression**.

4. Thalidomide

It was used as a sedative drug but was withdrawn from the market in 1960s due to its teratogenic effects (Phocomelia). Recently, it has been re-introduced due to its immunomodulatory properties. **Its major actions are:**
- Inhibition of angiogenesis
- Inhibition of TNF-α
- Increased production of IL-10
- Reduces phagocytosis
- Alteration of adhesion molecule expression
- Enhances cell-mediated immunity via interactions with T-cells.
- **Currently, it is indicated for**
  - Multiple myeloma at initial diagnosis
  - Relapsed-refractory cases of multiple myeloma
  - Erythema nodosum leprosum
  - Skin manifestations of SLE

 Key Points

Immunomodulatory derivatives of thalidomide are called IMiDs. One of these is Lenalidomide, which is approved as a first line therapy for multiple myeloma with dexamethasone and bortezomib.

- Its major adverse effects are:
  - Teratogenicity
  - Peripheral neuropathy
  - Constipation
  - Rash
  - Hypothyroidism
  - Increased risk of DVT
- Immunomodulatory derivatives of thalidomide are called IMiDs. One of these is Lenalidomide, which is approved as a first line therapy for multiple myeloma with dexamethasone and bortezomib.

- Another group of thalidomide analogs are called SelCIDs (Selective Cytokine Inhibitory Drugs).

 Key Points

Another group of thalidomide analogs are called SelCIDs (Selective Cytokine Inhibitory Drugs).

5. Imiquimod

It is an immune response modifier shown to be effective against external genital and peri-anal warts (i.e., condyloma acuminata) by topical route. It act by releasing IFN-α and cytokines like IL-1, IL-6 and TNF α etc. It has also been approved for basal cell carcinoma and actinic keratosis of the face and scalp.

PSORIASIS

Psoriasis is a chronic skin condition caused by an overactive immune system. There is excessive epidermal proliferation with dermal inflammation. All patients are instructed to avoid dryness and irritation of skin. The drugs used for treatment of psoriasis are:

Topical Drugs

- *Topical corticosteroids* are primary drugs for treatment of psoriasis. Most cases of localized, plaque type psoriasis can be managed with mid-potency glucocorticoids. However, long-term use can result in *tachyphylaxis* and *atrophy of skin*.
- Topical vitamin D analog is *calcipotriol*. It suppresses proliferation and enhances differentiation of keratinocytes. Because of rapid metabolism of percutaneously absorbed calcipotriol, hypercalcemia does not develop.
- *Tazarotene* is topical retinoid. It also exerts antiproliferative and anti-inflammatory effects.

Photochemotherapy

- Immunosuppressive effects of **ultraviolet (UV) light** can be used for therapeutic activity in psoriasis. Narrow band UV-B and PUVA (UV-A with psoralen) are used clinically. UV therapy is associated with *increased risk of melanoma and non-melanoma skin cancers*.

Oral Drugs

- **Oral glucocorticoids should not be used** in psoriasis due to potential for development of life-threatening pustular psoriasis when discontinued.
- **Methotrexate** (weekly) or **cyclosporine** (twice daily) can be used as immunosuppressants.
- **Acitretin** is a synthetic oral retinoid. It can be used when immunosuppression should be avoided. However, it is *highly teratogenic*.
- **Apremilast** is a new oral *phosphodiesterase inhibitor*. It is approved for both psoriasis as well as psoriatic arthritis. It can cause **depression** and should be avoided in *renal failure*.

Biological Agents

Unknown stimulus activates dermal dendritic cells and cutaneous T-cells to secrete cytokines. TNF-α, IL-12, IL-23 and IL-17 play the major role in pathogenesis of psoriasis.
- *Adalimumab, certolizumab, etanercept, infliximab and golimumab* are **TNF-α inhibitors** for psoriasis. Except infliximab

(given IV), all other drugs in this category are given subcutaneously. All these drugs *increase the risk* of infections including **TB, HIV, Hep-B and Hep-C**. TNF-α inhibitors may also *worsen CHF*.

A –	Adalimumab
C –	Certolizumab
E –	Etanercept
INhibitors –	INfliximab
GOLI –	GOLImumab
maro	

- **Ustekinumab** is monoclonal antibody against IL-12/IL-23. It is also approved for psoriasis.
- **Guselkumab and Tildrakizumab** are monoclonal antibodies against IL-23. These have recently been approved for psoriasis
- **Secukinumab and Ixekixumab** are IL-17 antagonists. These can increase the risk of exacerbation of inflammatory bowel disease
- **Brodalumab** is monoclonal antibody against IL-17 receptors. Apart from exacerbation of IBD, it can result in suicidal ideation.
- Leucocyte function antigens (LFA-1 and LFA-3) are also involved in pathogenesis of psoriasis. **Efalizumab** is a monoclonal antibody against LFA-1 whereas **Alefacept** is a fusion protein against LFA-3. Both of these drugs are used for psoriasis.

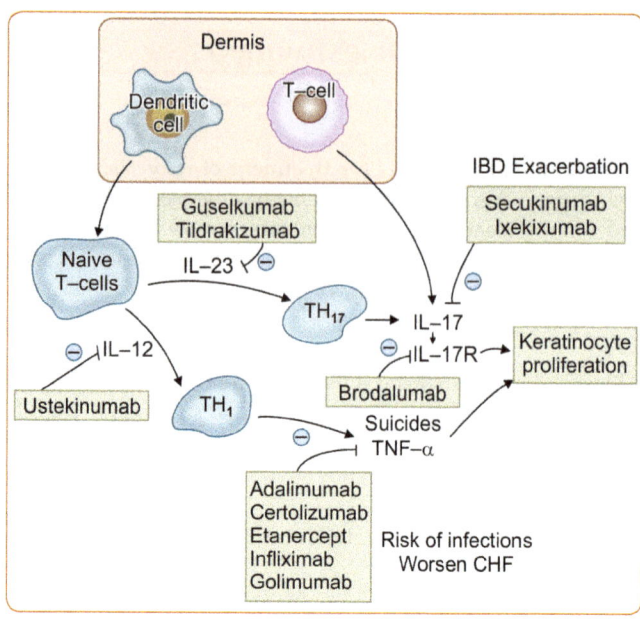

FIG. 15.4: Pathogenesis of psoriasis and drug targets

Drug of Choice

Clinical Diagnosis	Drug of Choice
• Rheumatoid arthritis	
– Pain relief	NSAIDs
– Bridge therapy	Corticosteroids
– DMARD	Methotrexate
• Psoriasis	
– Limited disease (<10% body surface area (BSA) involvement)	Topical steroid + Topical vitamin D analog (calcipotriene/calcitriol)
– Moderate (10–30% BSA)	UV phototherapy
– Severe (>30% BSA)	Narrow band UV-B (NB-UVB) Phototherapy
– Resistant to NB-UVB	PUVA
– Severe pustular	Methotrexate[1]
• Neovascular Age Related Macular Degeneration	Bevacizumab[2]
• Crohn's disease	Corticosteroids
• Paroxysmal Nocturnal Hemoglobinuria	
– Mild	No treatment
– Severe hemolysis	Eculizumab
– Wegener's granulomatosis	Cyclophosphamide + corticosteroids
– Sarcoidosis	Corticosteroids
– Multiple sclerosis	Beta-interferons
– Antiphospholipid syndrome	Warfarin

1. Cyclosporine or infliximab may also be used
2. Ranivizumab or pegaptanib or aflibercept may also be used

Image Based Question

1. A baby was born with the congenital malformations shown in the figure. The likely teratogenic drug received by the mother is:

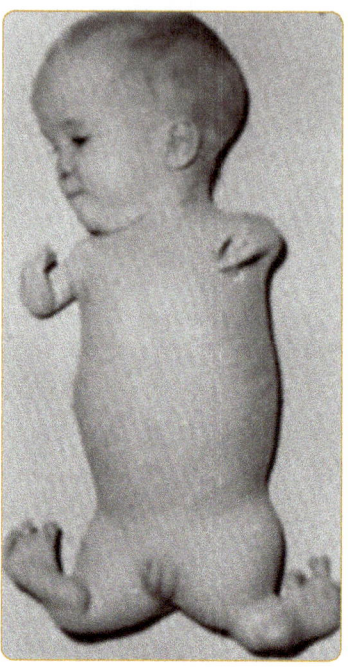

   (a) Thalidomide   (b) Alcohol
   (c) Carbimazole   (d) Heparin

Explanation

1. **Ans. (a) Thalidomide**
   The figure shows the baby with phocomelia. This is characteristic teratogenic effect of thalidomide.

Multiple Choice Questions

1. Match the following drugs poisoning with the antidotes:
   (AIIMS Nov. 2019)

Drugs overdose	Antidote
1. HCN	A. Trimethaphan
2. Paracetamol	B. Nalorphine
3. Morphine	C. Bupropion
4. Nicotine	D. Diazepam
	E. N-acetylcysteine
	F. Amyl nitrite

2. Palivizumab, a monoclonal antibody is used for the prophylaxis of: *(AIIMS Nov 2016)*
   (a) Human metapneumovirus
   (b) Para-influenza virus type 2 and 4
   (c) Influenza virus
   (d) Respiratory syncytial virus

3. Basiliximab is a monoclonal antibody against:
   (Recent Question 2017-2018)
   (a) IL-2 receptor (b) CD 20
   (c) TNF alpha (d) IL-6

4. Best time to give Rh anti-D prophylaxis is:
   (AIIMS Nov 2015)
   (a) 12 weeks of pregnancy
   (b) 28 weeks of pregnancy
   (c) 36 weeks of pregnancy
   (d) After delivery

5. Which of the following is a calcineurin inhibitor?
   (AIIMS Nov 2015)
   (a) Cyclosporine
   (b) Methotrexate
   (c) Azathioprine
   (d) Mycophenolate mofetil

6. Abatacept is a new drug approved for: *(AIIMS Nov 2014)*
   (a) SLE
   (b) Rheumatoid arthritis
   (c) Sjogren syndrome
   (d) Scleroderma

7. All of the following are adverse effects of thalidomide *except*: *(AI 2012)*
   (a) Myocarditis
   (b) Constipation
   (c) Peripheral neuropathy
   (d) Sedation

8. A 5-year-old child of severe nephrotic syndrome on treatment with tacrolimus, frusemide and prednisolone developed seizures. The investigations revealed: *(AI 2012)*
   - Serum Na+ = 136 mEq/L
   - Blood urea = 78 mg/dL
   - Serum creatinine = 0.5 mg/dL
   - Serum albumin = 1.5 g/dL
   - Serum total Ca = 7.5 mg/dL
   - Urine albumin = 2 g

   What is the likely cause of symptoms in this baby?
   (a) Hypocalcemia
   (b) Tacrolimus toxicity
   (c) Uremia
   (d) Hyponatremia

9. Cyclosporine acts by decreasing the production of:
   (Recent NEET Pattern Question)
   (a) IL-1 (b) IL-2
   (c) IL-6 (d) IL-8

10. Not true about thalidomide:
    (Recent NEET Pattern Question)
    (a) Causes phocomelia
    (b) Not tested in pregnant animals before introduction
    (c) Still has restricted clinical use
    (d) Has no antiangiogenesis action against tumour

11. Side effects of cyclosporine are all, *except*:
    (Recent NEET Pattern Question)
    (a) Nephrotoxicity
    (b) Bone marrow suppression
    (c) Hypertension
    (d) Hirsutism

12. Which of the following antineoplastic and immunosuppressant drugs is a dihydrofolate reductase inhibitor?
    (Recent NEET Pattern Question)
    (a) Methotrexate
    (b) Adriamycin
    (c) Vincristine
    (d) Cyclophosphamide

13. Which of the following act through helper T cells?
    (Recent NEET Pattern Question)
    (a) Cyclosporine (b) Azathioprine
    (c) Cytarabine (d) Cycloserine

14. All are true about cyclosporine-A *except*:
    (Recent NEET Pattern Question)
    (a) Given orally as too toxic by intravenous route
    (b) Given in renal transplant
    (c) Selectively inhibit T-lymphocytes proliferation
    (d) It causes renal toxicity

15. All of the following are side effects of cyclosporine *except*: *(Recent NEET Pattern Question)*
    (a) Post-transplant lymphoproliferative disorders (PTLDs)
    (b) Hypotension
    (c) Nephrotoxicity
    (d) Tremors

16. Infliximab is: *(Recent NEET Pattern Question)*
    (a) IgG1 chimeric monoclonal antibody against TNF-α
    (b) IgG1 fully human monoclonal antibody against TNF-α
    (c) IgG4 chimeric monoclonal antibody against TNF-α
    (d) P75 TNF receptor fusion protein

17. Monoclonal antibody to IL-5 is:
    (Recent NEET Pattern Question)
    (a) Mepolizumb
    (b) Omalizumb
    (c) Keliximab
    (d) Altrakincept

18. Anti IgE monoclonal antibody used in bronchial asthma is: *(Recent NEET Pattern Question)*
    (a) Mepolizumab
    (b) Omalizumab
    (c) Keliximab
    (d) Altrakincept

19. Etanercept used in rheumatoid arthritis act by the inhibition of: *(Recent NEET Pattern Question)*
    (a) TNF alpha
    (b) TFG beta
    (c) IL-2
    (d) IL-6

20. Tacrolimus acts by inhibiting:
    (Recent NEET Pattern Question)
    (a) DNA and RNA synthesis
    (b) Anti-lymphocyte antibody formation
    (c) T-Cell proliferation
    (d) All of the above

21. Fully humanized antibodies used in treatment of rheumatoid arthritis: *(Recent NEET Pattern Question)*
    (a) Anakira
    (b) Adalimumab
    (c) Infliximab
    (d) Leflunomide

22. The only FDA approved radioactive antibody that can be used for treatment of lymphoma:
    (Recent NEET Pattern Question)
    (a) Trastuzumab
    (b) Ibritumomab
    (c) Rituximab
    (d) Imatinib

23. All are TNF-α antagonists used in rheumatoid arthritis except: *(Recent NEET Pattern Question)*
    (a) Ifosfamide
    (b) Infliximab
    (c) Etanercept
    (d) Adalimumab

24. Tacrolimus level is increased by all except:
    (Recent NEET Pattern Question)
    (a) Erythromycin
    (b) Itraconazole
    (c) Danazole
    (d) Rifampicin

25. Bevacizumab is used in: *(Recent NEET Pattern Question)*
    (a) Diabetic retinopathy
    (b) Glaucoma
    (c) Diabetic nephropathy
    (d) Neuropathy

26. All of the following is true about "Imiquimod" except:
    (Recent NEET Pattern Question)
    (a) Direct antiviral activity
    (b) Indirect antiviral activity
    (c) Antitumor activity
    (d) It release cytokines

27. Which of the following immuno-suppressive agents acts selectively by inhibiting helper T-cells?
    (Recent NEET Pattern Question)
    (a) Cyclophosphamide
    (b) Azathioprine
    (c) Cyclosporine
    (d) Cystosine arabinoside

28. Which of the following drug does not cause renal toxicity?
    (Recent NEET Pattern Question)
    (a) Cisplatin
    (b) Tacrolimus
    (c) Mycophenolate mofetil
    (d) Naproxen

29. Anti IgE monoclonal antibody is:
    (Recent NEET Pattern Question)
    (a) Certolizumab
    (b) Rifampicin
    (c) Omalizumab
    (d) Canakinumab

30. Mechanism of action of bevacizumab is:
    (Recent NEET Pattern Question)
    (a) Acts on VEGF
    (b) EGFR antagonist
    (c) PDGF monoclonal antibody
    (d) Tyrosine kinase inhibitor

31. Which of the following is a calcineurin inhibitor?
    (Recent NEET Pattern Question)
    (a) Cyclophosphamide
    (b) Cyclosporine
    (c) Etanercept
    (d) Sirolimus

32. Basiliximab acts by antagonism against:
    (Recent NEET Pattern Question)
    (a) CD 25
    (b) CD 11a
    (c) TNF
    (d) IL-2

33. Bevacizumab is: *(Recent NEET Pattern Question)*
    (a) Monoclonal antibody against VEGF
    (b) Anti-IL-2 monoclonal antibody
    (c) Monoclonal antibody against FGFR
    (d) Monoclonal antibody against EGFR

34. Rituximab is antibody against:
    (Recent NEET Pattern Question)
    (a) CD 20
    (b) VEGF
    (c) EGER
    (d) IL-2

35. True about azathioprine is:
    (Recent NEET Pattern Question)
    (a) It has more anti tumor effect than immunosuppressant effect
    (b) It is not a prodrug
    (c) It selectively affects differentiation of T cells
    (d) It is a pyrimidine antimetabolite

36. Thalidomide is not used in:
    (Recent NEET Pattern Question)
    (a) HIV related neuropathy
    (b) Erythema nodosum leprosum
    (c) HIV related oral ulcer
    (d) Behcet's disease

37. All of the following are tumor necrosis factor blocking agents, *except*:
    (Recent NEET Pattern Question)
    (a) Adalimumab
    (b) Eternacept
    (c) Infliximab
    (d) Abciximab

38. Which of the following immunosuppressive agent requires monitoring of renal function on regular basis?
    (Recent NEET Pattern Question)
    (a) Azathioprine
    (b) Mycophenolate mofetil
    (c) Methotrexate
    (d) Cyclosporine A

39. A topical retinoid recently introduced for the treatment of psoriasis is: *(Recent NEET Pattern Question)*
    (a) Adapalene   (b) Tazarotene
    (c) Alitretinoin   (d) Bexarotine

40. Immunostimulant agent among the following is:
    (Recent NEET Pattern Question)
    (a) Pirenzepine   (b) Levamisol
    (c) Albendazole   (d) Methotrexate

41. Antihelminthic also acting as immunomodulator is:
    (Recent NEET Pattern Question)
    (a) Albendazole   (b) Levamisole
    (c) Mebendazole   (d) Piperazine

42. Cyclosporin-A acts on: *(Recent NEET Pattern Question)*
    (a) CD4 cells
    (b) CD3 cells
    (c) CD8 cells
    (d) B lymphocytes

Explanations

1. **Ans. 1. F, 2. E, 3. B, 4. A** *(Ref: KDT 8th/e p590, 223, 509, 134)*
   - **HCN poisoning:** It is cyanide poisoning. DOC is Hydroxocobalamine. Amyl nitrite (inhalational) with sodium thiosulphate (IV) can also be used.
   - Paracetamol poisoning (causes hepatoxicity) : N-acetyl-cysteine is used.
   - **Morphine poisoning:** DOC is Naloxone. Nalorphine can also be used.
   - Nicotine poisoning: Trimethaphan and Hexamethonium – Nn receptor blockers (ganglionic blockers) are used.

   Bupropion is an anti-smoking drug. It inhibits the reuptake of Noradrenaline and Dopamine (NDRI).

2. **Ans. (d) Respiratory syncytial virus** *(Katzung 13th/e p863)*
   Palivizumab is a monoclonal antibody produced by recombinant DNA technology. It is used in the prevention of respiratory syncytial virus (RSV) infections.

3. **Ans. (a) IL-2 receptor** *(Ref: KDT 8/e p943)*
   Basiliximab and daclizumab are monoclonal antibodies against CD 25 (IL-2 receptor)

4. **Ans. (b) 28 weeks of pregnancy**
   (Ref: Williams Obstetrics 24th/e p312)
   - Anti-D immune globulin is given prophylactically to all Rh D-negative, unsensitized women at approximately 28 weeks, and a second dose is given after delivery if the infant is Rh D-positive Following delivery, anti-D immune globulin should be given within 72 hours.
   - If immune globulin is inadvertently not administered following delivery, it should be given as soon as the omission is recognized, because there may be some protection up to 28 days postpartum.
   - Anti-D immune globulin is also administered after pregnancy-related events that could result in fetomaternal hemorrhage.

5. **Ans. (a) Cyclosporine**
   (Ref: Goodman Gilman 12th/e p1008; Katzung 12th/e p986; KDT 8/e p937)
   - Cyclosporine and tacrolimus act as immunosuppresants by their inhibitory action on calcineurin.

6. **Ans. (b) Rheumatoid arthritis** *(Ref: Harrison 18th/e p2748)*
   Abatacept is a co-stimulation inhibitor. Two signals are required for activation of T-cells:

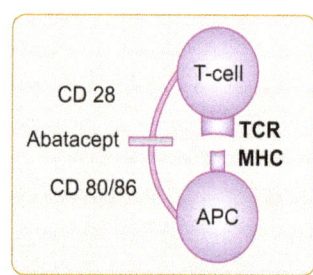

1. **Main signal:** Interaction of T-cell receptor (TCR) with MHC of antigen presenting cells (APC)
2. **Co-stimulatory signal:** Interaction of CD 28 of T-cells with CD-80/86 of APC.

When both signals are present, T-cell gets activated. Abatacept acts by blocking the co-stimulatory signal and prevents activation of T-cells. It is approved for treatment of Rheumatoid arthritis.

7. **Ans. (a) Myocarditis** *(Ref: Goodman Gilman 12/e p1742)*
   - Thalidomide was banned because of teratogenic effects (phocomelia). Now it has come again in the market for use as an anticancer drug in **multiple myeloma and melanoma.**
   - **Lenalidomide** is its more potent and non-teratogenic derivative.
   - *Thalidomide most commonly causes sedation and constipation* in cancer patients. It can also cause *peripheral sensory neuropathy.*
   - Two enantiomers of thalidomide (R and S) are present but these are interconvertible in body, therefore racemic mixture is used.

8. **Ans. (b) Tacrolimus toxicity**
   (Ref: Harrison 18/e p2272, 361, 347, 2308)
   To get to the answer, we will look at the options one by one.
   Hypocalcemia: Serum calcium in this boy is 7.5 mg/dL. Hypocalcemia can result in seizures but the level should be very low. Further, if we correct calcium with serum albumin, it will come in normal range. Corrected calcium level in the serum can be calculated by adding 0.8 mg/dL With every 1.0 g/dL decrease in serum albumin below the normal value of 4.0 g/dL. Hence, in this patient, corrected serum calcium level will be:
   $7.5 + 0.8 \times (4.0 - 1.5) = 9.5$ mg/dL
   It is in normal range (8.5-10.5 mg/dL) and thus cannot be the cause of seizures in this person.
   Uremia: Although blood urea is elevated (78 mg/dL as compared to normal value of 15-40 mg/dL) but serum creatinine is normal (0.5 mg/dL). For diagnosis of uremia, serum creatinine must be 3 times the normal value. Thus, uremia cannot be the answer.
   Hyponatremia: Serum sodium is at lower normal value (136-152 mEq/L). For causing seizures, serum sodium should be less than 125 mEq/L. Therefore, this option can also be ruled out.
   Tacrolimus toxicity: This child is on tacrolimus therapy. It is a known neurotoxin and can cause seizures. It also can cause renal failure. Further by ruling out other options, the most likely cause seem to be tacrolimus toxicity.

9. **Ans. (b) IL-2** *(Ref: KDT 8/e p936)*

Immunomodulators

10. **Ans. (d) Has no antiangiogenesis action against tumour**
    (Ref: KDT 6/e p84, 834)
    - Thalidomide was banned in 1960 because of its teratogenic effect of phocomelia (seal like limbs). It has anxiolytic, adjuvant analgesic/antipyretic properties and has been found to counteract cancer associated cachexia.
    - Its mechanism of action is by suppressing TNF and or by modulating IL-2.
    - Recently it has been reintroduced as antineoplastic drug due to its anti-angiogenesis action.

11. Ans. (b) Bone marrow suppression *(Ref: KDT 8/e p940)*
12. Ans. (a) Methotrexate *(Ref: KDT 8/e p942)*
13. Ans. (a) Cyclosporine *(Ref: KDT 8/e p939)*

Mechanism of action of:

(a)	Cyclosporine –	Through T helper cells (by inhibiting calcineurin)
(b)	Azathioprine –	Inhibits de novo purine synthesis and damges DNA. It selectively affects cytolytic T lymphocytes.
(c)	Cytarabine –	Inhibits DNA synthesis in S-phase.
(d)	Cycloserine –	Inhibits bacterial cell wall synthesis.

14. Ans. (a) Given orally as too toxic by intravenous route *(Ref: KDT 8/e p937-938)*
15. Ans. (b) Hypotension *(Ref: KDT 8/e p937-938)*
16. Ans. (a) IgG1 chimeric monoclonal antibody against TNF-α *(Ref: KDT 8/e p230)*
17. Ans. (a) Mepolizumb *(Ref: www.wikipedia.org)*
18. Ans. (b) Omalizumab *(Ref: KDT 8/e p251)*
19. Ans. (a) TNF alpha *(Ref: KDT 8/e p937)*
20. Ans. (c) T-Cell proliferation *(Ref: KDT 8/e p938)*
21. Ans. (b) Adalimumab *(Ref: Katzung 11/e p633)*
22. Ans. (b) Ibritumomab *(Ref: Katzung 11/e p978)*
23. Ans. (a) Ifosfamide *(Ref: KDT 8/e p919)*

24. **Ans. (d) Rifampicin**
    (Ref KDT 8/e p940, www.medscape.com/druginfo)
    Erythromycin, itraconazol and danazol inhibit the metabolism of tacrolimus and thus increase the plasma concentration whereas rifampicin is an enzyme inducer and decrease its plasma level.

25. **Ans. (a) Diabetic retinopathy**
    (Ref: Katzung 11//977; Harrison 17/e p512)
    Bevacizumab is a monoclonal antibody against VEGF and is used as an anti-angiogenic drug. It is mainly used for colorectal carcinoma and is used off-label by intravitreal injection to slow progression of neovascular macular degeneration.

26. Ans. (a) Direct antiviral activity *(Ref Katzung 11/e p1053)*
27. **Ans. (c) Cyclosporine** *(Ref: KDT 8/e p937)*
    Cyclosporine inhibits helper T cells (CD4) cells by inhibiting the transcription of IL-2 (via calcineurin inihibition).
28. Ans. (c) Mycophenolate mofetil *(Ref: KDT 8/e p942)*
29. Ans. (c) Omalizumab *(Ref: KDT 8/e p251)*
30. Ans. (a) Acts on VEGF *(Ref. KDT 8/e p930-931)*
31. Ans. (b) Cyclosporine *(Ref: KDT 8/e p937)*
32. Ans. (a) CD 25 *(Ref: KDT 8/e p943)*
33. Ans. (a) Monoclonal antibody against VEGF *(Ref: KDT 8/e p871)*
34. Ans. (a) CD 20 *(Ref: KDT 8/e p931)*
35. Ans. (c) It selectively affects differentiation of T cells *(Ref: KDT 8/e p942)*
36. Ans. (a) HIV related neuropathy *(Ref: KDT 8/e p837)*
37. Ans. (d) Abciximab *(Ref: KDT 8/e p937)*
38. Ans. (d) Cyclosporine A *(Ref: KDT 8/e p940)*
39. Ans. (b) Tazarotene *(Ref: KDT 8/e p954)*
40. Ans. (b) Levamisol *(Ref: KDT 8/e p910)*
41. Ans. (b) Levamisole *(Ref: KDT 8/e p910)*
42. Ans. (a) CD4 cells *(Ref: KDT 8/e p939)*

Miscellaneous Topics

CHAPTER 16

DRUGS USED IN DERMATOLOGY

1. Glucocorticoids

Potency of these agents is traditionally measured using vasoconstrictor assay (area of skin blanching). *Betamethasone, clobetasol, diflorasone, halobetasol, amcinonide, desoximetasone, fluocinonide, halcinonide, triamcinolone,* flurandrenolide, hydrocortisone, mometasone, aclometasone, dexamethasone and desonide formulations can be used topically. **Betamethasone diproprionate is most potent and hydrocortisone is least potent topically steroid.** Skin atrophy (cigarette paper skin), striae, telangictasia, purpura and acneiform eruptions are the side effects occuring by chronic use.

> **Key Points**
>
> Betamethasone diproprionate is most potent and hydrocortisone is least potent topically steroid.

> **Key Points**
>
> Skin atrophy (cigarette paper skin), striae, telangictasia, purpura and acneiform eruptions are the side effects occuring by chronic use of topical steroids.

2. Retinoids

These may be **first generation** *(retinol, tretinoin, isotretinoin and alitretinoin)*, **second generation** *(acitretin),* **third generation** *(tazarotene and bexarotene)* and **retinoid-like** *(adaplene)* compounds. These are potent **teratogens** (contraindicated in pregnancy) and may cause dry skin, nose bleeds, conjuctivitis, alopecia, muscular pain, pseudotumor cerebri and mood alterations.

- Tretinoin is used for acne vulgaris and as an adjunctive agent for treating photoaging.
- Tazarotene is approved for psoriasis and acne vulgaris.
- Alitretinoin is approved only for treatment of skin manifestations of Kaposi's sarcoma.
- Isotretinoin is indicated for the treatment of severe nodulocystic acne vulgaris. It may result in hyperlipidemia, myalgia and arthralgia.
- Acitretin (major metabolite of etretinate) was used for psoriasis but was withdrawn due to very long half life (2-3 days).
- Bexarotene is used for cutaneous T-cell lymphoma. It may cause lipid abnormalities, hypothyroidism and gastrointestinal symptoms.

3. Photochemotherapy

Ultraviolet radiations may be classified into UV-A (320-400 nm), UV-B (290-320 nm) and UV-C (100-290 nm) according to wavelength. *UV-B is most erythrogenic and melanogenic radiation.*

  PUVA: 8-Methoxypsoralen (oral) followed by UV-A is approved for treatment of *vitiligo, psoriasis and cutaneous T-cell lymphoma.* Major side effects include nausea, blistering and painful erythema. It increases the risk of melanoma and squamous cell carcinoma.

Photopheresis: After oral methoxypsoralen, leucocytes are seperated from whole blood using extracorporeal pheresis (ECP) device and then exposed to UV-A radiation. Irradiated cells are then returned to the patient. ECP is effective for *cutaneous T-cell lymphoma.*

  Photodynamic therapy: It combines photosensitizing drugs (mostly porphyrins) with visible light for the treatment of *non-melanoma skin cancers and actinic keratosis.*

4. Antimetabolites

- **Methotrexate** is used for moderate to *severe psoriasis, pemphigus vulgaris, pityriasis rubra, SLE, dermatomyositis and cutaneous T-cell lymphoma.* Pregnancy and lactation are absolute contraindications.
- **Azathioprine** is steroid sparing agent for pemphigus vulgaris, bullous pemphigoid, dermatomyositis, atopic dermatitis, SLE, psoriasis and Behcet's disease.
- **5-FU** is used for actinic keratoses and superficial basal cell carcinoma.

5. Calcineurin Inhibitors

Cyclosporine is used for atopic dermatitis, psoriasis, alopecia areata, pemphigus vulgaris, bullous pemphigoid, lichen planus and pyoderma gangrenosum. **Tacrolimus and pimecrolimus** are other agents in this group.

> **Key Points**
>
> Sun protection factor (SPF) defines a ratio of minimal dose of sunlight that produce erythema on skin with sunscreens to that without sunscreen.

6. Biological Agents

- **Alefacept and efalizumab** are aproved for moderate to severe *psoriasis.*
- **Etanercept** is approved for psoriasis, rheumatoid arthritis and ankylosing spondylitis.
- **Infliximab** is approved for Crohn's disease and rheumatoid arthritis and is in phase III trials for treatment of psoriasis.
- **Denileukin diftitox** is indicated for advanced cutaneous T cell lymphoma.

7. Sunscreens

These may protect from UV-A (avobenzone, oxybenzone, titanium oxide and zinc oxide) or UV-B (cinnamates, salicylates etc). **Sun protection factor** *(SPF)* defines a ratio of minimal dose of sunlight that produce erythema on skin with sunscreens to that without sunscreen. It provides valuable information regarding UVB protection but is *useless for UVA efficacy*.

8. Other Agents

- *Cholestasis associated pruritis* may respond to *cholestyramine, ursodeoxycholic acid, ondansetron, rifampicin and nalmefene* (opioid antagonist).
- *Pruritis of uremia* is most effectively treated with *UVB radiation*. It may also respond to *naltrexone and omeprazole*.
- *Capsaicin* is approved for the treatment of *post herpetic neuralgia and painful diabetic neuropathy*.
- **Masoprocol** is a potent 5-LOX inhibitor with antitumor activity effective for topical treatment of actinic keratosis.

AGE-RELATED MACULAR DEGENERATION

- It is of two types Dry and wet. Dry form is most common but untreatable. Vitamin supplements with zinc, lutein and zeaxanthin may delay its progression. Wet form or neovascular ARMD is amenable to therapy.
- Photodynamic therapy with verteporfin (a radiosensitizer) is the approved therapy of neovascular ARMD.
- New strategies include intravitreal administration of anti-VEGF compounds. These include pegaptanib, ranbizumab, aflibercept and bevacizumab.
- Anecorvate is an angiogenesis inhibitor indicated for ARMD.

TREATMENT OF POISONINGS

	Poisoning	Treatment
1.	Ergot Alkaloids	Nitroprusside
2.	β-blockers	Glucagon and Calcium
3.	Organophosphates	Atropine
4.	Carbamates	Atropine
5.	Benzodiazepines	Flumazenil
6.	Zolpidem	Flumazenil
7.	Cyanide	O_2 + Amyl nitrite + Sodium Thiosulphate
8.	Hydrogen Sulfide	Amyl nitrite
9.	Carbon Monoxide	Hyperbaric Oxygen
10.	Methemoglobinemia	High Dose O_2 + Methylene Blue
11.	Ethylene Glycol	Fomepizole
12.	Iron	Desferrioxamine
13.	Methanol	Fomepizole or ethanol
14.	Salicylates	Alkaline diuresis with sodium bicarbonate
15.	Isoniazid	Pyridoxine
16.	Lithium	Hemodialysis

Contd...

Contd...

17.	Serotonin syndrome	Cyproheptadine or chlorpromazine
18.	Opioids	Naloxone
19.	Scorpion sting	Prazosin
20.	Acetaminophen	N-acetylcysteine
21.	Atropine	Physostigmine
22.	Calcium channel blockers	Calcium
23.	Theophylline/caffeine	Esmolol

CHELATING AGENTS

	Drug	Uses in poisoning of
1.	Dimercaprol (BAL)	As, Pb, Hg, Au (contraindicated in Fe and Cd poisoning)
2.	Succimer	Pb, As, Cd, Hg
3.	Unithiol	Hg, As, Pb
4.	Calcium disodium EDTA	Pb, Zn, Cd, Mn, Hg, Fe
5.	DTPA	Uranium, plutonium
6.	Dicobalt EDTA	Cyanide
7.	D-penicillamine	Cu, Wilson disease, Pb, Hg, cystinuria, scleroderma
8.	Trientine	Cu
9.	Desferrioxamine	Fe
10.	Deferipirone (oral)	Fe
11.	Deferasirox (oral)	Fe

STREET NAMES OF SOME DRUGS OF ABUSE

Drug of Abuse	Street Name
Gamma Hydroxy butyrate (GHB)	Liquid ecstasy
	Grievous bodily harm
Phencyclidine and Ketamine	Angel dust
	Hog
	Special K
Cocaine	Crack (vapour to be smoked)
	Rush
	Coke
	Snow
	Blow
	Peruvian marching Powder
Methylene dioxymethamphetamine (MDMA)	Ecstasy
	Rave drug
Lysergic acid diethylamide (LSD)	Windowpane
	Twenty-five

ANTIOBESITY DRUGS

Obesity is a complex metabolic disorder resulting from the abnormality between energy intake and energy expenditure. Generally this imbalance is because of life style and behavioral origin. It is also associated with insulin resistance, dyslipidemia and cardiovascular disease.

PATHOGENESIS

Glucose forms a dependable source of energy for short-term basis whereas lipids are utilized on the long-term basis. The

arcuate nucleus in the mediobasal hypothalamus forms the main integrating centre for feeding and regulation of body weight. The following compounds/peptides play an important role in the regulation of food intake:

 Key Points

Drug treatment of obesity started if:
- BMI > 30 kg/m²
  or
- BMI > 27 with obesity related risk-factors.

Orexins and Ghrelin

- *Orexin* is a 33 amino acid peptide, which acts on the orexin receptor (oxR) to *stimulate food intake* in a dose dependent manner.
- *Ghrelin* is an acetylated peptide secreted by gastric mucosal cells that causes release of growth hormone from the pituitary. It also acts directly on the arcuate nucleus to *stimulate food intake*. The plasma level of ghrelin increases before meals and falls following intake of food.

Neuropeptide Y (NPY) and Agouti-related Peptide (AgRP)

These **two peptides; NPY and AgRP, stimulate food intake**, reduce energy expenditure and promote weight gain.

 Key Points

Bariatric surgery for obesity recommended if:
- BMI > 40 kg/m²
  or
- BMI > 35 with obesity related comorbidities

Melanocyte Stimulating Hormone (MSH) and CART (Cocaine and Amphetamine-related Transcript)

Both MSH and CART reduce food intake by eventually causing *activation of 5-HT$_2$C (serotonin) receptors.*

Insulin and Leptin

These signals are increased in obesity. These are *inhibitory to NPY and AgRP neurons and facilitatory to MSH and CART neurons.*

Cannabinoids

The endocannabinoids act on their receptor CB_1 and CB_2 to stimulate the anabolic pathway (*NPY and AgRP*). They also *inhibit the catabolic pathways (CART and MSH)* eventually *resulting in excessive food intake and obesity.*

 Key Points

FDA-approved antiobesity drugs are:
- Lorcaserin
- Phentermine + Topiramate
- Orlistat
- Liraglutide

THERAPIES FOR THE MANAGEMENT OF OBESITY

1. Diet

Which diet plan is best at promoting sustained weight loss remains a controversial issue. Four types of diets are recommended for weight loss. These are
- **Atkins** (*very low carbohydrate*)
- **Traditional** (*lifestyle, exercise, attitudes, relationships, nutrition*) [LEARN]
- **Ornish** (*very high carbohydrate*)
- **Zone** (*low carbohydrate*)

> **Note**
> These can be *remembered as* **A TO Z**

2. Drugs

5-HT$_2$ receptor activation leads to weight loss. Therefore, drugs increasing the level of serotonin (reuptake inhibitors) can be used to treat obesity.

a. **Liraglutide:** It is a **GLP-1 analog** and is primarily used in diabetes mellitus. It decreases appetite by decreasing gastric emptying as well as by its central action. It is recently approved for obesity

b. **Lorcaserin:** It is a **selective 5HT$_{2C}$ agonist**. It decreases appetite. Most common adverse effect is headache. Studies focus *concerns of breast tumors in animals, increased valvular heart disease and psychiatric adverse effects.*

c. **Phentermine + Topiramate:** This combination has been approved for obesity. Common side effects include mood changes, fatigue, insomnia and tachycardia. The combination is teratogenic and is contraindicated in pregnancy.

d. **Orlistat:** It is an *inhibitor of gastrointestinal lipases*, which are necessary for absorption of fat from the diet. This drug decreases fat absorption by up to 30%, resulting in weight loss. Adverse effects include loose stools, increased defecation and oily discharge. Most of these can be managed by the simultaneous use of natural fibre.

e. **Amphetamines, fenfluramine and dexfenfluramine:** These were used previously for the treatment of obesity but are not used now. *Fenfluramine and dexfenfluramine* are banned due to the risk of *cardiotoxicity.*

f. **Sibutramine:** It blocks the presynaptic uptake of *both norepinephrine and serotonin* resulting in the potentiation of anorexic effects of both of these neurotransmitters in the CNS. Side effects include mild elevation in BP, headache, insomnia, dry mouth and constipation.

g. **Rimonabant:** It is a *cannabinoid receptor antagonist* which acts on CB_1 receptor resulting in the increased levels of serotonin and dopamine. It blocks the orexigenic action of ghrelin and causes reduction in appetite. It also causes lipolysis and increases basal metabolic rate. Adverse effects include nausea, vomiting, depression (leading to suicidal tendencies) and anxiety. **It can decrease blood pressure.**

 Key Points

Rimonabant is an anti-obesity drug that can lower blood pressure.

h. **Naltrexone plus bupropion:** This combination has been recently approved for chronic weight management. It has the potential to cause suicidal thoughts and neuropsychiatric reactions.

Though all of the above drugs may result in weight loss but tolerance develops to the anorexic effect, when these are used for a long duration of time.

New Targets
- NPY and AgRP antagonists
- MSH and CART agonists

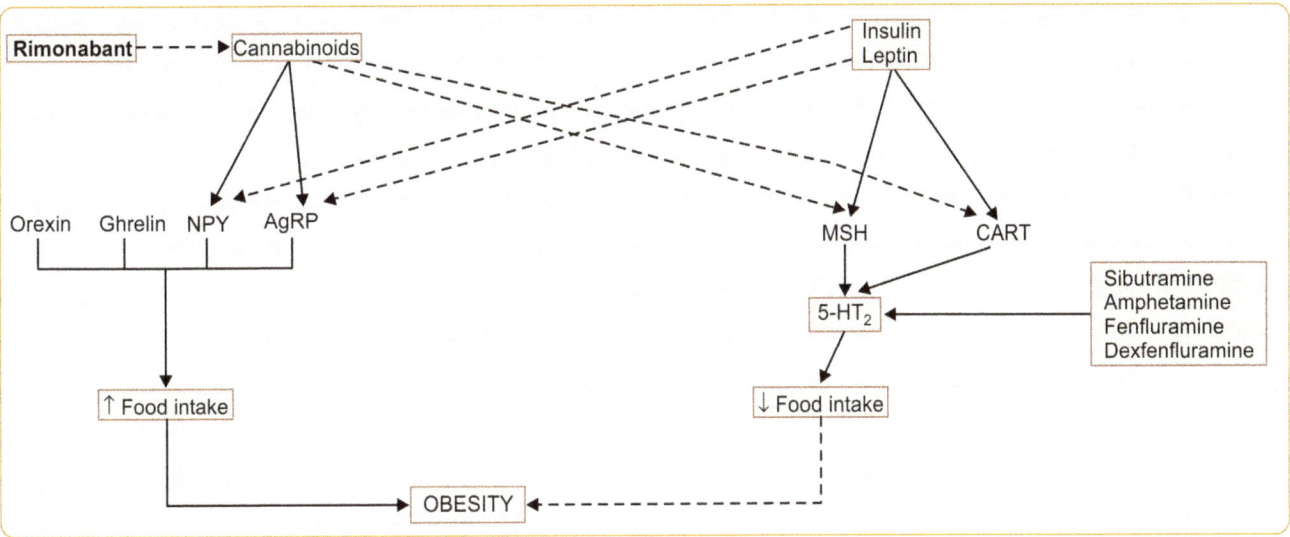

FIG. 16.1: Physiological and pharmacological regulation of food intake (Bold arrow indicates stimulation whereas dotted arrow indicates inhibition)

ERECTILE DYSFUNCTION

Inability of the male to attain and maintain penile erection for a duration sufficient to permit satisfactory intercourse is called as erectile dysfunction (ED).

Physiology of Penile Erection

Both the parasympathetic system (S2-4) and NO synthesis and release process should be intact for the normal erection of penis. NO increases the level of cGMP leading to relaxation of smooth muscles of corpora cavernosa. This leads to penile erection.

Etiology

The causes of erectile dysfunction can be psychological (most common), vascular, neurological and hormonal. Arteriosclerosis, hypertension, diabetes, smoking, alcohol consumption and drugs (like beta blockers) are the secondary causes of erectile dysfunction.

DRUGS USEFUL IN THE MANAGEMENT OF ERECTILE DYSFUNCTION

- *Phosphodiesterase inhibitors*: Normally cGMP formed by the action of NO is metabolized by phosphodiesterase. Sildenafil selectively inhibits PDE-V leading to increased cGMP levels and so is useful in erectile dysfunction. It can be administered orally. Adverse effects include headache, nasal congestion, flushing, visual disturbances (blue vision) etc. Colour vision defect is due to inhibition of PDE-VI present in the retina. Apart from their use in ED, sildenafil can also be used in the management of pulmonary hypertension. Other drugs of this group are *vardenafil, udenafil, avanafil and tadalafil*.

Key Points

Tadalafil is the longest acting phosphodiesterase inhibitor.

- **Tadalafil** is the **longest acting** phosphodiesterase inhibitor.
- These drugs should not be prescribed to a patient on nitrates due to the risk of severe hypotension.

Key Points

Phosphodiesterase inhibitors should not be prescribed to a patient on nitrates due to the risk of severe hypotension.

- Other *orally effective drugs*: Apomorphine, a dopamine agonist can also be used. Its main adverse effect is nausea. Trazodone (an antidepressant) and phentolamine (non-selective α blocker) have also shown promise for the management of ED.
- *Alprostadil*: It is a PGE_1 analogue administered directly in the cavernosal tissue (more useful in patients not responding to oral sildenafil therapy). Phentolamine is another drug which can be used intracavernosally.

Avanafil is a new PDE-5 inhibitor similar to sildenafil

- *Aviptadil*: It is the analogue of vasoactive intestinal peptide that causes smooth muscle relaxation. It can be used along with phentolamine for ED.
- *Ketanserin*: It is a $5-HT_2$ and α receptor antagonist used in combination with alprostadil for ED.
- *Thymoxamine*: It is an α blocker used as intracavernosal injection for ED.
- Recently, *naltrexone* has been tried for the restoration of erectile function.
- *Herbal drugs* (like Ginseng, kava, gingko etc.) have been claimed to be useful for erectile dysfunction but efficacy has not been established clinically.

ANTI-SMOKING DRUGS

The **first line** medications for smoking cessation are **nicotine replacement therapy (NRT)** and sustained release (SR) **Bupropion**. Other medications used as **second line** treatment are **clonidine, nortriptyline and varenicline**.

Among these, **US-FDA** approved medications for smoking-cessation include:
- Nicotine Replacement Therapy (NRT)
- Bupropion
- Varenicline.

NICOTINE REPLACEMENT THERAPY

- Nicotine acts by stimulation of neural nicotinic acetylcholine receptors (NAChRs) in the ventral tegmental area of the brain. This causes release of dopamine in the nucleus accumbens which lead to reduction in nicotine withdrawal symptoms in regular smokers who abstain from smoking.
- It does not completely eliminate the symptoms of withdrawal because none of the available nicotine delivery systems reproduce the rapid and high levels of *arterial nicotine* achieved when cigarette smoke is inhaled.
- All the available medicinal nicotine products rely on *systemic venous absorption*.
- Weight gain, is a significant problem in smoking-cessation. It can be reduced by nicotine replacement therapy (NRT).

NRT may be in the form of **slow sustained release** (transdermal patches) or **acute NRT formulations** (gums, lozenges, sub-lingual tablet, oral inhaler and nasal spray).

Transdermal Patch

Nicotine patches are applied to the skin and deliver nicotine through the skin at a relatively steady rate. It comes in the form of 24 hour patch (to be applied whole day) and 16 hour patch (to be removed before sleeping).
- The main advantage of nicotine patches over acute NRT formulations is that it is easy to administer, requires less frequent dosing, with fewer adverse effects and better compliance. It delivers nicotine more slowly than acute NRT formulations.
- The disadvantage of the patch is the lack of acute (rescue) dosing for craving episodes, which can be provided with other NRTs. In fact, the nicotine patch may be combined with other NRTs to increase its efficacy.
- The most frequently reported side effects are local skin reactions. Changing the site of patch application daily can reduce this problem. Sleep disturbances have also been commonly reported with 24-hour patches.

Acute Dosing Nicotine Products

Acute-dosing products have the benefit that both the amount and timing of doses can be titrated by the user. Control over the timing of self-dosing enables smokers to use NRT medications as "rescue medication" when they encounter particularly strong cravings or threats to abstinence. Acute dosing nicotine products include gum, lozenge, sublingual tablet, oral inhaler, and nasal spray.

Nicotine Gum

- It is not chewed like ordinary gum, but is intermittently chewed and held in the mouth over about 30 minutes, as needed, to release its nicotine.
- It is available in 2 mg and 4 mg dosage forms.
- Acidic beverages like coffee and juices should be avoided before and after the use of nicotine gum, because they decrease the absorption of nicotine. Nicotine gum also provides substitute oral activity during tobacco abstinence.

Nicotine Lozenge

- It is also available in 2 mg and 4 mg formulations.
- Lozenge is not chewed, it dissolves in the mouth over approximately 30 minutes
- As with nicotine gum, nicotine from the lozenge is absorbed slowly through the buccal mucosa and delivered into systemic circulation.
- The nicotine lozenge delivers 25% more nicotine than nicotine gum, because some nicotine is retained in the gum whereas nicotine is dissolved completely in lozenge.
- The lozenge may have better patient acceptability, especially in those who cannot use the gum because of dentures temporomandibular joint pain or for those who do not prefer chewing gum.

Nicotine Sublingual Tablet

- This product is designed to be held under the tongue where the nicotine in the tablet is absorbed sublingually.
- Like the lozenge, the tablet has the advantage of not requiring chewing.
- The levels of nicotine obtained by use of the lozenge and sublingual tablet are similar.

Nicotine Oral Inhaler

- The inhaler was designed to satisfy behavioral aspects of smoking, namely, the *hand-to-mouth ritual*.
- Although termed an "inhaler" the majority of nicotine is delivered into the oral cavity and in the GIT. Very little nicotine is delivered to the lung. Because absorption is primarily through the buccal mucosa, the rate of absorption is similar to that of nicotine gum.
- It produces peak levels of nicotine in 15 minutes (as compared to 30 minute with gum and lozenges)

Nicotine Nasal Spray

- It achieves peak venous nicotine levels within 4-15 min, faster than any other NRT.
- Due to the fast nicotine delivery, nicotine spray may have some abuse liability.
- The main disadvantage of a nasal spray is the initial local irritation.

NON-NICOTINIC DRUGS FOR SMOKING CESSATION

Varenicline

- It is an analogue of cytisine.
- It is a highly selective and partial agonist at α_4-β_2 receptor producing lesser response than that of nicotine. Thus, varenicline maintains a moderate level of dopamine release, which reduces craving and withdrawal symptoms during

abstinence. It also blocks the reinforcing effects of nicotine obtained from cigarette smoke in the case of relapse.
- Varenicline is the non-nicotine containing medication.
- The main adverse effects such as nausea, headache, vomiting, flatulence, insomnia and abnormal dreams, generally mild in nature are observed which diminish over time.
- Varenicline was also found to be safe for treating smokeless tobacco dependence.

Bupropion
- It is an anti-depressant that acts as a neuronal reuptake inhibitor of dopamine and noradrenaline.
- It is used in sustained release formulation.
- It is an oral non-nicotine therapy.
- Dopaminergic activity of bupropion affects the area implicated in the reinforcing properties of the addictive drug and the development of dependence—the reward pathway, or mesolimbic system—while its noradrenergic activity in the locus ceruleus plays a role in withdrawal from nicotine.
- Bupropion lowers the seizure threshold and should not be used in those with history of seizure disorder, serious head trauma, eating disorders (bulimia or anorexia nervosa) and in those who receive other medications that may lower seizure threshold.

Nortriptyline
- Nortriptyline is a tricyclic anti-depressant.
- It is recommended as a second-line medication for tobacco cessation.

Clonidine
- It acts on the central nervous system and may reduce withdrawal symptoms associated with smoking cessation.
- Its clinical use is limited by significant adverse effects, such as sedation, dizziness and dry mouth.
- Abrupt cessation of clonidine can led to severe hypertension.
- It is a second-line option for smoking cessation pharmacotherapy.

Nicotine Blockade Therapy
- The goal of blockade therapy is to reduce or eliminate any rewarding pharmacological effects, should the person attempt to resume the drug use.
- Mecamylamine can be used as an antagonist to block the nicotine-mediated reinforcing consequences of cigarette smoking.

Naltrexone
- It is a long acting form of opioid antagonist.
- The rationale for using naltrexone for smoking cessation is that the performance enhancing and other positive effects of nicotine may be opioid mediated.

HYPERKALEMIA

Emergency treatment of hyperkalemia is indicated when cardiac toxicity or muscular paralysis or severe hyperkalemia (> 6.5 mEq/L) is present, even in the absence of ECG changes.

Treatment of Hyperkalemia

Modality	Indication	Mechanism
1. Glucose + Insulin	Emergency	Distribution of K^+ into cells
2. β-agonists like salbutamol	Emergency	Distribution of K^+ into cells
3. Bicarbonate	Emergency	Distribution of K^+ into cells
4. Calcium gluconate	Emergency	Antagonize cardiac conduction abnormalities due to K^+
5. Loop Diuretics	Non-Emergency	Renal K^+ excretion
6. Resins [Sodium polystyrene sulfate]	Non-Emergency	Binds K^+
7. Hemodialysis	Both Emergency as well as non-emergency	Extracorporeal K^+ removal
8. Peritoneal dialysis	Non-emergency	Peritoneal K^+

SEROTONIN SYNDROME

Serotonin syndrome is a condition associated with skeletal muscle contractions, hyperthermia, hyperreflexia, diarrhea, mydriasis, agitation, myoclonus and coma. It results from excessive serotonin in the synapse. It can be caused by:

 Key Points

Myoclonus is present in serotonin syndrome but absent in neurolept malignant syndrome (NMS) whereas rigidity is present in NMS but absent in serotonin syndrome.

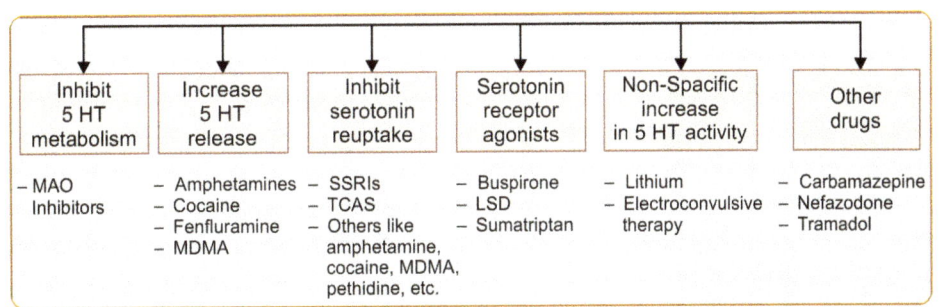

Multiple Choice Questions

1. Which of the following antihypertensive drug is avoided in patients with high serum uric acid levels?
    (NEET Pattern 2019)
    (a) Hydrochlorthiazide
    (b) Enalapril
    (c) Prazosin
    (d) Atenolol

2. Most commonly implicated drug for acute liver failure is:
    (a) Paracetamol   (NEET Pattern 2019)
    (b) Valproate
    (c) Warfarin
    (d) Tetracycline

3. Match the following drugs with their ocular adverse effects: (AIIMS Nov. 2019)

Drug	Adverse effect
1. Amiodarone	A. Blepharoconjunctivitis
2. Hydroxychloroquine	B. Angle closure glaucoma
3. Systemic steroids	C. Retinopathy
4. Digoxin	D. Optic neuritis
	E. Yellow vision
	F. Cataract

4. Drug used for smoking cessation is: (NEET Pattern 2019)
    (a) Vareniciline   (b) Acamprosate
    (c) Naloxone   (d) Sildenafil

5. All of the following drugs are used in emergency management of acute hyperkalemia except:
    (a) Calcium gluconate   (AIIMS Nov 2017)
    (b) Salbutamol
    (c) Glucose-Insulin
    (d) Intravenous magnesium sulphate

6. Which of the following drug can result in teratogenic effect shown in the diagram if given during pregnancy?
    (AIIMS May 2016)

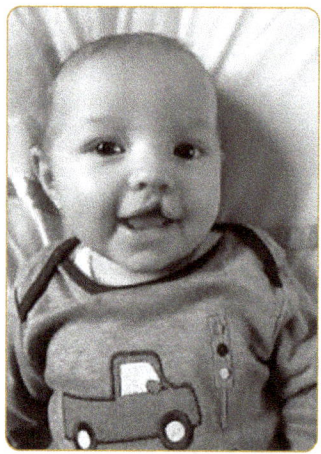

    (a) Niacin   (b) Retinoic acid
    (c) Thiamine   (d) Folic acid

7. Pigmentation of nail can be caused by all of the following drugs except: (AIIMS May 2016)
    (a) Cyclophosphamide   (b) Chlorpropamazine
    (c) Chloroquine   (d) Amiodarone

8. QT prolongation can be caused by:
    (NEET Pattern Question 2017-2018)
    (a) Lithium   (b) Quinidine
    (c) Adenosine   (d) Magnesium

9. All of the following drugs can cause hearing loss except:
    (AIIMS May 2015)
    (a) Metronidazole   (b) Kanamycin
    (c) Quinine   (d) Vancomycin

10. All of the following drugs can result in amorphous whorl like corneal opacities except: (AIIMS May 2015)
    (a) Amiodarone   (b) Chloroquine
    (c) Indomethacin   (d) Chlorpromazine

11. Ocreoplasmin is the newer drug used in which of the following conditions? (AIIMS May 2014)
    (a) Retinal break   (b) Vitreomacular adhesion
    (c) Submacular bleed   (d) Diabetic macular bleed

12. Which of the following drug is implicated in the causation of osteomalacia of the bone? (AI 2012)
    (a) Phenytoin   (b) Steroids
    (c) Heparin   (d) Estrogen

13. All of the following drugs cause tachychardia except:
    (a) Amphetamine   (b) Nifedipine   (AI 2012)
    (c) Theophylline   (d) Clonidine

14. Which of the following drugs can result in cyanide poisoning? (AI 2012)
    (a) Sodium nitroprusside (b) Amyl nitrite
    (c) Hydroxycobalamin   (d) Sodium thiosulphate

15. Treatment of choice in solar keratosis is:
    (Recent NEET Pattern Question)
    (a) Methotrexate
    (b) Topical 5 FU
    (c) Topical mechlorethamine
    (d) Topical steroids

16. All drugs cause interstitial lung disease, except:
    (Recent NEET Pattern Question)
    (a) Phenytoin sodium   (b) Sulphonamides
    (c) Busulphan   (d) Alpha methyl dopa

17. Constipation is caused by all of the following drugs except: (Recent NEET Pattern Question)
    (a) Neostigmine   (b) Atropine
    (c) Morphine   (d) Fentanyl

18. Hirsutism is caused by which drug?
    (Recent NEET Pattern Question)
    (a) Minoxidil   (b) Dactinomycin
    (c) Cycloserine   (d) Valsartan

Miscellaneous Topics

19. **Which of the following drugs can cause lipodystrophy?**
    (Recent NEET Pattern Question)
    (a) Atorvastatin (b) Probucol
    (c) Saquinavir (d) Gentamicin

20. **Which of the following drugs is not used for the treatment of hyperkalemia?** *(Recent NEET Pattern Question)*
    (a) Salbutamol (b) Calcium gluconate
    (c) Sodium bicarbonate (d) Magnesium sulphate

21. **Gastric lavage is contraindicated in:**
    (Recent NEET Pattern Question)
    (a) Salicylate poisoning
    (b) Kerosene poisoning
    (c) Morphine poisoning
    (d) Organophosphate poisoning

22. **Astringents are substances that:**
    (Recent NEET Pattern Question)
    (a) Irritate sensory nerve endings
    (b) Precipitate proteins
    (c) Penetrate target cell nucleus for their action
    (d) All of the above

23. **All of the following drugs can cause cholestatic jaundice *except*:** *(Recent NEET Pattern Question)*
    (a) Erythromycin estolate (b) INH
    (c) OC pills (d) Chlorpromazine

24. **All of the following drugs cause hirsutism *except*:**
    (Recent NEET Pattern Question)
    (a) Phenytoin (b) Minoxidil
    (c) Corticosteroids (d) Heparin

25. **Correctly matched pair of heavy metals and their chelating agents is:** *(Recent NEET Pattern Question)*
    (a) Iron-BAL
    (b) Mercury-Calcium disodium edetate
    (c) Copper-d-penicillamine
    (d) Aresenic-Desferrioxamine

26. **All are true about nitric oxide *except*:** *(AIIMS Nov., 2007)*
    (a) Vasodilation
    (b) Smooth muscle relaxation
    (c) Beneficial in ARDS
    (d) cAMP mediated

27. **Which of the following drugs are used for smoking cessation?** *(Recent NEET Pattern Question)*
    (a) Bupropion (b) Buspirone
    (c) Venlafaxine (d) Fluoxetine

28. **Which one of the following is a cholestatic drug?**
    (Recent NEET Pattern Question)
    (a) Erythromycin
    (b) Phenothiazines
    (c) Oral contraceptives
    (d) All of the above

29. **Which one of the following is not a cause for hyperkalemia?** *(Recent NEET Pattern Question)*
    (a) Digoxin
    (b) Potassium sparing diuretic
    (c) Renin angiotensin system blockers
    (d) Cyclosporine

30. **Vitamin, which acts as a hormone is:**
    (Recent NEET Pattern Question)
    (a) A (b) C
    (c) D (d) E

31. **Which of the following drug has disulfide groups?**
    (Recent NEET Pattern Question)
    (a) BAL (b) EDTA
    (c) Penicillin (d) Penicillamine

32. **In nodulocystic acne treatment is:**
    (Recent NEET Pattern Question)
    (a) Steroids (b) Antibiotics
    (c) Isotretinoin (d) Antifungal

33. **Iron poisoning in 4 year child is treated by:**
    (Recent NEET Pattern Question)
    (a) Stomach lavage
    (b) Desferrioxamine IV 100 mg
    (c) X-ray abdomen
    (d) Blood transfusion

34. **Drug therapy used in treatment of Wernicke's encephalopathy:** *(Recent NEET Pattern Question)*
    (a) Diazepam (b) Disulfiram
    (c) Thiamine (d) Cynocobalamine

35. **Which of the following chelating agent is the degradation product of Penicillin?**
    (Recent NEET Pattern Question)
    (a) EDTA (b) Dimercaprol
    (c) Penicillamine (d) Desferrioxamine

36. **Pulmonary fibrosis occurs most commonly by:**
    (Recent NEET Pattern Question)
    (a) Clindamycin (b) Amiodarone
    (c) Nikkomycin (d) Kanamycin

37. **Scleromatous skin changes are seen in all *except*:**
    (Recent NEET Pattern Question)
    (a) Adriamycin (b) Bleomycin
    (c) Steroid (d) Busulphan

38. **Pulmonary fibrosis is noted with all *except*:**
    (Recent NEET Pattern Question)
    (a) Busulfan (b) Bleomycin
    (c) Nitrofurantoin (d) Bumetanide

39. **Vitamin-B_6 deficiency is seen with the use of all of the following drugs *except*:** *(Recent NEET Pattern Question)*
    (a) Cycloserine (b) Cyclosporine
    (c) INH (d) d-Penicillamine

40. **Severe myopathy commonly is a side effect of:**
    (Recent NEET Pattern Question)
    (a) Rosuvastatin (b) Nicotinic acid
    (c) Ezetimibe (d) Colesevelam

41. **The following drugs can produce ototoxicity *except*:**
    (Recent NEET Pattern Question)
    (a) Ethacrynic acid (b) Aztreonam
    (c) Gentamicin (d) Frusemide

42. **Gynaecomastia is an adverse effect of all of the following drugs *except*:** *(Recent NEET Pattern Question)*
    (a) Spironolactone (b) Finasteride
    (c) Cortisol (d) Cimetidine

43. Drug not causing hyperuricemia:
    (Recent NEET Pattern Question)
    (a) Probenecid (b) Thiazide
    (c) Pyrazinamide (d) Ethambutol

44. Drugs which produce gynaecomastia are all *except*:
    (Recent NEET Pattern Question)
    (a) Cimetidine (b) Digoxin
    (c) Cortisol (d) Spironolactone

45. The appearance of markedly vacuolated, nucleated red cells in the marrow, anemia and reticulocytopenia are characteristic dose-dependent side effects of:
    (Recent NEET Pattern Question)
    (a) Azithromycin (b) Chloramphenicol
    (c) Clindamycin (d) Doxycycline

46. The following drugs cause methemoglobinemia:
    (Recent NEET Pattern Question)
    (a) Aniline (b) Dapsone
    (c) Nitrates (d) All of the above

47. Iodophores are mixtures of the following:
    (Recent NEET Pattern Question)
    (a) Iodine and alcohol
    (b) Iodine and aldehyde
    (c) Iodine and surface active agents
    (d) Iodine and phenol

48. Flushing with alcohol is seen in all *except*:
    (Recent NEET Pattern Question)
    (a) Amoxicillin (b) Co-trimoxazole
    (c) Furazolidone (d) Chlorpropamide

49. Which of the following drug causes hemolytic anemia in glucose-6-phosphate dehydrogenase deficient individual?
    (Recent NEET Pattern Question)
    (a) Chloramphenicol (b) Acetaminophin
    (c) Prednisolone (d) Griseofulvin

50. Pleural fibrosis is caused by: *(PGI June, 2002)*
    (a) Phenytoin *(Recent NEET Pattern Question)*
    (b) Methysergide
    (c) Amiodarone
    (d) Ergotamine
    (e) Ranitidine

51. Which of the following drug causes hirsutism?
    (Recent NEET Pattern Question)
    (a) Phenytoin (b) Valproate
    (c) Carbamazepine (d) Phenobarbitone

52. Sildenafil acts by inhibiting:
    (Recent NEET Pattern Question)
    (a) Phosphodiesterase-2 (b) Phosphodiesterase-5
    (c) Adenyl cyclase (d) Guanyl cyclase

53. Drug contraindicated in a diabetic patient is:
    (Recent NEET Pattern Question)
    (a) Mannitol (b) Steroids
    (c) Enalapril (d) Glycerol

54. Drugs used in the treatment of obesity is/are:
    (Recent NEET Pattern Question)
    (a) Orlistat (b) Sibutramine
    (c) Rimonabant (d) All of the above

55. Nicotine replacement therapy is available in all forms *except*:
    (Recent NEET Pattern Question)
    (a) Chewing gum (b) Lozenges
    (c) Patch (d) Tablets

56. A person on anti-tubercular drugs complained of deafness and tinnitus in one ear. Drug implicated is:
    (Recent NEET Pattern Question)
    (a) Streptomycin (b) Isoniazid
    (c) Ethambutol (d) Rifampicin

57. Drug of choice for malaria in pregnancy is:
    (Recent NEET Pattern Question)
    (a) Proguanil (b) Chloroquine
    (c) Arteminsin (d) Halofantirine

58. Regarding sildenafil, all of the following statements are correct *except*: *(Recent NEET Pattern Question)*
    (a) Should not be used with nitrates
    (b) Inhibitor of phospho-di-esterase V
    (c) Increases libido and prolongs orgasm
    (d) Its side effects are potentiated by inhibition of CYP 3A4

59. Warm antibody haemolytic anemia is seen in:
    (Recent NEET Pattern Question)
    (a) Methyldopa (b) Penicillin
    (c) Quinine (d) Stibophen

60. Which drug does not cause thyroid dysfunction?
    (Recent NEET Pattern Question)
    (a) Amiodarone (b) Lithium
    (c) PAS (d) Paracetamol

61. Highly vestibulotoxic drug is:
    (Recent NEET Pattern Question)
    (a) Cisplatin
    (b) Streptomycin
    (c) Dihydrostreptomycin
    (d) Quinine

62. Which of the following drug can cause thyroid dysfunction? *(Recent NEET Pattern Question)*
    (a) Amiodarone (b) Ampicillin
    (c) Ibutilide (d) Acyclovir

63. Drug causing peripheral neuropathy is:
    (Recent NEET Pattern Question)
    (a) Zalcitabine
    (b) Isoniazid
    (c) Nitrofurantoin
    (d) All of the above

64. Which of the following drugs does not cause gynecomastia? *(Recent NEET Pattern Question)*
    (a) Ketoconazole (b) Cimetidine
    (c) Digitalis (d) Pyrazinamide

Explanations

1. **Ans. (a) Hydrochlorthiazide** *(Ref: KDT 8th/e p633)*
   Adverse effect of Hydrochlorthiazide is hyperuricemia. Therefore, it is contraindicated in patients with gout.
   - Enalapril, Prazosin and Atenolol have no effect on serum uric acid levels.

2. **Ans. (a) Paracetamol** *(Ref: KDT 8th/e p223)*
   - All the four drugs given Paracetamol, Valproate, Warfarin and Tetracyclines can cause hepatotoxicity.
   - Paracetamol among these is the most common cause particularly in patients with liver disease and in alcoholics.

3. **Ans. 1. D, 2. C, 3. F, 4. E**
   (Ref: KDT 8th/e p880, 318, 560, Goodman Gilman 13th/e p564)
   Ocular adverse-effects of drugs:
   - Amiodarone:
     - Corneal deposits (cornea verticallata)
     - **Optic neuritis**
   - Hydroxychloroquine:
     - Bull's eye maculopathy **(retinopathy).**
   - Systemic steroids:
     - Given topically — cause open angle glaucoma
     - Given systemically — cause posterior subcapsular **cataract**.
   - Digoxin:
     - Yellow vision

4. **Ans. (a) Vareniciline**
   (Ref: Goodman and Gilman 13th/e p437-438)
   Anti-Smoking drugs
   - **Vareniciline:** It is a **direct acting nicotinic agonist** having selectivity for **α4β2 isoform of NN receptors**. It can be used orally and has a half life of 14-20 hours. Its adverse effects include headache, nausea and sleep disturbances.
   - **Nicotine:** A transdermal patch containing nicotine is applied to the patient's body. The dose of nicotine is then slowly decreased and finally withdrawn. It is effective in only 18-20% of the patients. It is also available in the form of lozenges.
   - **Bupropion:** It is an anti-depressant drug that can be used for cessation of smoking. It acts by **inhibition of neuronal reuptake of 5-HT**, NE and DA. The duration of treatment is for 8-10 weeks. It can result in CNS stimulation leading to seizures.
   - **Clonidine:** It is a very effective drug for reducing the **withdrawal effects of nicotine.** It is better than nicotine chewing gum as it can be used in patients with cardiac diseases also. It decreases the craving as well as is useful for insomnia.
   - **Rimonabant:** It is a cannabinoid receptor antagonist that results in the increased 5-HT and dopamine levels. The adverse effects include nausea, vomiting, suicidal tendencies (depression) and anxiety.

5. **Ans. (d) Intravenous magnesium sulphate**
   (Ref: Harrison 19/e p312)
   - Magnesium sulphate has no role in acute hyperkalemia.
   - Calcium gluconate, salbutamol and glucose-insulin are all used in acute hyperkalemia.

6. **Ans. (b) Retinoic acid**
   (Ref: Katzung 13thth/e p1042; KDT 8th/e p154)
   Retinoic acid and isotretinoin are well known teratogens. These can result in cleft lip and other congenital anomalies.

7. **Ans. (d) Amiodarone**
   (Ref: Nail and its disorders by S. Sachidanand pg 80)
   Pigmentation of nail is called **chromonychia**. It can be caused by several factors.

Drugs causing nail pigmentation
• Anticancer drugs
– Melphalan
– Hydroxyurea
– Doxorubicin
– Busulfan
– 5-FU
– Methotrexate
– **Cyclophosphamide**
– Bleomycin
• Tetracyclines
• 8-Methoxypsoralen
• **Chloroquine**
• Sulfonamides
• Phenothiazines
– **Chlorpromazine**
– Thioridazine
• Phenytoin
• Timolol
• Mercury
• Gold

8. **Ans. (b) Quinidine** *(Ref: KDT 8th/e p574)*

9. **Ans. (a) Metronidazole**
   (Ref: Goodman Gillman 12th/e p1512, 1542, 1407; Katzung 12th/e p824)
   Metronidazole does not cause hearing loss

Important drugs causing ototoxicity are:
• Aminoglycosides
• Vancomycin
• Cisplatin
• Loop diuretics (Ethacrynic acid, Furosemide)
• Quinine
• Salicylates

10. **Ans. (d) Chlorpromazine**
    (12th/e p1793; Khurana 5th/e p69; Parsons21stth/e p214, Clinical ocular Pharmacology/803)
    - **Amorphous whorl like corneal deposit suggests a case of cornea verticillata (or vortex keratopathy). It is seen in Fabry's disease and it may be drug induced.**
    - The whorl-like pattern shows the direction of migration of corneal epithelial cells
      - Phenothiazines like chlorpromazine and thioridazine are mainly associated with pigmentation of endothelium and descment's membrane.

> **Drugs associated with whorl like corneal opacities are:**
> - Amiodarone
> - Chloroquine
> - Hydroxychloroquine
> - Indomethacin
> - Atovaquone
> - Tamoxifen

11. **Ans. (b) Vitreomacular adhesion**

    (Ref: http://www.revophth.com/content/d/retinal_sider/c/40601/)

    Ocriplasmin is a recombinant protease with activity against fibronectin and laminin, components of the vitreoretinal interface. It is approved by FDA for treatment of symptomatic vitreomacular adhesion (VMA). It works by dissolving the proteins that link the vitreous to the macula, resulting in posterior detachment of the vitreous from the retina.

    There are two primary indications for ocriplasmin. The first is for patients who have mild to moderate symptomatic VMA, and also have good visual acuity. Vitrectomy surgery would not be a viable option for this group, because their vision is too good to risk the complications associated with surgery. The FDA approval of ocriplasmin provided surgeons with a minimally invasive means of treating these patients who previously had no viable option.

    The second set of patients are those with more moderate VMA whose visual acuity has deteriorated to 20/80 or worse, sufficient to justify surgery. Ocriplasmin is the ideal first choice in these patients.

12. **Ans. (a) Phenytoin** *(Ref: CMDT 2012/1120; KDT 8th/e p441)*

    Phenytoin inhibits the hepatic production of 25 hydroxy vitamin D and also directly inhibit bone mineralization and thus may result in osteomalacia. Steroids and heparin result in osteoporosis not osteomalacia.

> **Important drugs causing osteomalacia are:**
> - Phenytoin
> - Carbamazepine
> - Valproate
> - Phenobarbitone
> - Bisphosphonates

13. **Ans. (d) Clonidine**

    (Ref: KK Sharma 2th/e p174; KDT 8th/e p140)
    - Clonidine is α_2 agonist and decreases the central sympathetic outflow. It decreases blood pressure as well as heart rate.

14. **Ans. (a) Sodium Nitroprusside**

    (Ref: CMDT 2012/1533; KDT 8th/e p614)

15. **Ans. (b) Topical 5 FU** *(Ref: CMDT-2010/113)*

    Solar (actinic) keratosis is treated by application of liquid nitrogen. Alternative treatment is 5-FU. Imiquimod cream can also be used.

16. **Ans. (d) Alpha methyl dopa**

    (Ref: CMDT-2010/262, Katzung 11th/e p943)

> **Drugs causing interstitial lung disease are:**
> - Amiodarone
> - Nitrofurantoin
> - Sulfonamides
> - Busulfan
> - Bleomycin
> - Cyclophosphamide
> - Methotrexate
> - Nitrosoureas
> - Gold salts
> - Penicillamine
> - Phenytoin

17. **Ans. (a) Neostigmine** *(Ref: KDT 6th/e p101, 455)*
    - Neostigmine is an inhibitor of acetylcholinesterase and thus acts like a cholinergic drug. Therefore, it can produce diarrhea (not constipation).
    - Atropine is an anti-cholinergic drug, thus can cause constipation.
    - Morphine and fentanyl are opioids. These can also result in constipation.

18. **Ans. (a) Minoxidil** *(Ref: KDT 6th/e p548)*
    - Minoxidil is a potassium channel opener, useful as antihypertensive drug. It can cause hirsutism in females and is used for the treatment of alopecia in males.

19. **Ans. (c) Saquinavir** *(Ref: Goodman & Gilman 11th/e p1301)*
    - All protease inhibitors are associated with HIV-lipodystrophy. Saquinavir is a protease inhibitor.
    - All NRTIs are associated with lactic acidosis. Stavudine can also cause lipoatrophy (maximum among NRTIs).
    - Insulin can also result in lipodystrophy.

20. **Ans. (d) Magnesium sulphate**

    (Ref: Harrison 16th/e p262-263)
    - Calcium gluconate decreases membrane excitability and reverses ECG changes of severe hyperkalemia.
    - Insulin and bicarbonate can shift pottassium inside the cells. Glucose is added to prevent hypoglycemia due to insulin.
    - β_2 agonists like salbutamol can also move pottassium inside the cells.

21. **Ans. (b) Kerosene poisoning** *(Ref: KDT 8th/e p81)*

    Gastric lavage is contraindicated in kerosene and acid or alkali i.e. corrosive poisonings.

22. **Ans. (b) Precipitate proteins** *(Ref: KDT 8th/e p947)*
    - Astringents are substances that precipitate proteins, but do not penetrate cells, thus affect the superficial layer only.

23. **Ans. (b) INH** *(Ref: Harrison 17th/e p765)*
    - Drugs causing cholestatic hepatitis:
        - Acetohexamide
        - Anabolic steroids
        - Androgens
        - Chlorpropamide
        - Clavulanic acid/amoxicllin
        - Cyclosporine
        - Erythromycin estolate
        - Flucloxacillin
        - Gold salts
        - Methimazole
        - Nitrofurantoin
        - Oral contraceptives
        - Phenothiazines

Miscellaneous Topics

- INH doesnot produces cholestatic jaundice, rather it causes diffuse hepatocellular damage.

24. **Ans. (d) Heparin** *(Ref: Harrison 17th/e p01)*
    - Drugs causing hirsutism:
        - Androgens
        - Oral contraceptives containing androgenic progestins
        - Minoxidil
        - Phenytoin
        - Diazoxide
        - Cyclosporine (Not tacrolimus)
    - Heparin produces transient and reversible alopecia.

25. **Ans. (c) Copper-d penicillamine** *(Ref: KDT 8th/e p807)*

26. **Ans. (d) cAMP mediated** *(Ref: Katzung 10th/e p309, 310)*
    - NO acts through cGMP and not through cAMP
    - Nitric oxide (NO) is a signaling molecule having important role in various pathophysiological conditions. It is also known as endothelium derive relaxing factor (EDRF).
    - NO formed from the action of NOS binds to iron in heme and causes an increase in the concentration of cGMP by stimulating guanylyl cyclase. This cGMP is responsible for its vasodilatory actions.
    - It is beneficial in ARDS and pulmonary artery hypertension.

27. **Ans. (a) Bupropion**
    (Ref: Harrison 16th/e p2575; Katzung 11th/e p521,1110)
    Drugs used for smoking cessation are:

    - Nicotine (gum, patch, nasal inhaler, oral inhaler)
    - Bupropion
    - Clonidine (oral, patch)
    - Nortriptyline
    - Rimonabant
    - Varenicilline
    - Amfebutamone
    - Mecamylamine

28. **Ans. (d) All of the above** *(Ref: Harrison 16th/e p434)*
29. **Ans. (a) Digoxin** *(Ref: Harrison 15th/e p432)*
30. **Ans. (c) D** *(Ref: KDT 8th/e p336)*
31. **Ans. (a) BAL** *(Ref: KDT 8th/e p964)*
32. **Ans. (c) Isotretinoin** *(Ref: KDT 8th/e p954)*
33. **Ans. (b) Desferrioxamine IV 100 mg** *(Ref: KDT 8th/e p652)*
34. **Ans. (c) Thiamine** *(Ref: KDT 8th/e p973)*
35. **Ans. (c) Penicillamine** *(Ref: KDT 8th/e p966)*
36. **Ans. (b) Amiodarone** *(Ref: KDT 8th/e p578)*
37. **Ans. (c) Steroid** *(Ref: KDT 8th/e p317)*
38. **Ans. (d) Bumetanide** *(Ref: Harrison 15th/e p430-432)*
39. **Ans. (b) Cyclosporine** *(Ref: KDT 8th/e p940)*
40. **Ans. (a) Rosuvastatin** *(Ref: KDT 8th/e p686)*
41. **Ans. (b) Aztreonam** *(Ref: Dhingra's Ent 4th/e p34)*
42. **Ans. (c) Cortisol** *(Ref: CMDT 2010/1064)*
43. **Ans. (a) Probenecid** *(Ref: KDT 8th/e p232–233)*

44. **Ans. (c) Cortisol** *(Ref: KDT 8th/e p560,635,698)*
    Drugs causing gynaecomastia are:

D	Digitalis
I	Isoniazid
S	Spironolactone
C	Cimetidine and Ketoconazole
O	Oestrogens

45. **Ans. (b) Chlormaphenicol** *(Ref: KDT 8th/e p791)*
    The features given are of bone marrow suppression which a very significant adverse effect of chlormaphenicol.

46. **Ans. (d) All of the above**
    (Ref: KDT 8th/e p587,832, Harrison 17th/e p35.4)
    Drugs causing Methemoglobinemia are:

    - Aniline derivatives
    - Dapsone
    - Prilocaine
    - Nitrates
    - Nitrites
    - Nitrogen oxides
    - Nitro- and nitrosohydrocarbons
    - Phenazopyridine
    - Primaquine
    - Sulfonamides

47. **Ans. (c) Iodine and surface active agents**
    (Ref: Katzung 11th/e p880)

48. **Ans. (a) Amoxicillin** *(Ref: KDT 8th/e p383; Niraj Ahuja 5th/e p43)*
    DRUGS CAUSING DISULFIRAM LIKE REACTION
    - Metronidazole
    - Cefoperazone
    - Cefamandole
    - Cefotetan
    - Moxalactam
    - Chlorpropamide
    - Procarbazine
    - Griseofulvin

49. **Ans. (a) Chloramphenicol** *(Ref: Harrsion 15th/e p433)*

50. **Ans. (b) Methysergide; (c) Amiodarone**
    (Ref: KDT 8th/e p190,578)
    - Methylsergide and amidarone causes pleural fibrosis
    - Others drugs mentioned here, donot cause pleural fibrosis.

51. **Ans (a) Phenytoin** *(Ref: KDT 7th/e p414)*
52. **Ans (b) Phosphodiesterase – 5** *(Ref: KDT 7th/e p303)*
53. **Ans (b) Steroids** *(Ref: KDT 7th/e p294)*
54. **Ans. (d) All of the above** *(Ref: KDT 7th/e p139)*
55. **Ans. (d) Tablets** *(Ref: CMDT 2014 p8)*
    Nicotine replacement is available as:

    - Patch
    - Gum
    - Lozenges
    - Nasal sprays
    - Inhalers

56. **Ans. (a) Streptomycin** *(Ref: KDT 8th/e p794)*
57. **Ans. (b) Chloroquine** *(Ref: KDT 7th/e p823)*

58. **Ans. (c) Increases libido and prolongs orgasm**
    (Ref: KDT 7th/e p303-304)
    - Sildenafil inhibits PDE-5 and result in erection. It is not an aphrodisiac, do not increase libido.
59. **Ans. (a) Methyldopa** *Ref: KDT 8th/e p618)*

60. **Ans. (d) Paracetamol** *(Ref: KDT 8th/e p223)*
61. **Ans. (b) Streptomycin** *(Ref: KDT 8th/e p794-795)*
62. **Ans. (a) Amiodarone** *(Ref: KDT 8th/e p578)*
63. **Ans. (d) All of the above** *(Ref: KDT 7th/e p760, 767, 808)*
64. **Ans. (d) Pyrazinamide** *(Ref: KDT 7th/e p793, 650, 516, 769)*

CHAPTER 17

New Drugs with Mnemonics

FDA-APPROVED DRUGS IN 2020-2021

Drug	Mechanism	Route	Indication
Abametapir	Metalloproteinase inhibitor	Topical	Pediculosis
Aducanumab	Mab against β-amyloid	Intravenous	Alzheimer's disease
Amisulpiride	D2 antagonist	Intravenous	Postoperative nausea and vomiting
Amivantamab-vmjw	Mab against EGFR and MET	Intravenous	Non-small cell lung carcinoma
Anifrolumab-fnia	Mab against type 1 interferon	Intravenous	Systemic lupus erythematosis
Ansuvimab-zykl	Zaire ebolavirus (EBOV) glycoprotein 1 (GP1)-directed recombinant, human IgG 1 monoclonal antibody	Intravenous	Zaire EBOLA virus disease
Atoltivimab, maftivimab, and odesivimab-ebgn	Mab against Gp of zaire Ebola virus • Maftivimab is a neutralizing antibody that blocks entry of the virus into susceptible cells. • Odesivimab is a non-neutralizing antibody that induces antibody-dependent effector function through FcyRIIIa signaling when bound to its target. • Atoltivimab combines both neutralization and FcyRIIIa signaling activities.	Intravenous	Zaire Ebola virus
Avalglucosidase alfa-ngpt	Enzyme replacement therapy	Intravenous	Pompe's disease
Avapritinib	PDGF kinase inhibitor	Oral	GIST
Belantamab mafodotin	B-cell maturation antigen (BCMA)-directed antibody and microtubule inhibitor conjugate	Intravenous	Multiple myeloma
Belumosudil	Rho kinase inhibitor	Oral	Chronic graft versus host disease
Belzutifan	HIF-2α inhibitor	Oral	Von Hippel-Lindau disease
Bempedoic acid	Adenosine triphosphate-citrate lyase (ACL) inhibitor	Oral	Heterozygous familial hypercholesterolemia
Berotralstat	Plasma kallikrein inhibitor	Oral	Prophylaxis of hereditary angioneurotic edema
Cabotegravir and rilpivirine	Cabotegravir: Integrase inhibitor Rilpivirine: NNRTI	Intramuscular	HIV
Capmatinib	MET kinase inhibitor	Oral	Non-small cell lung carcinoma
Casimersen	Anti-sense oligonucleotide that binds to exon 45 of dystrophin pre-MRNA resulting in its exclusion	Intravenous	Duchenne's muscular dystrophy
Clascoterone	Androgen receptor inhibitor	Topical	Acne vulgaris
Dasiglucagon	Recombinant glucagon	Subcutaneous	Severe hypoglycemia
Difelikefalin	K opioid agonist	Intravenous	Pruritus associated with chronic kidney disease
Dostarlimab-gxly	Mab against PD-1	Intravenous	Endometrial carcinoma
Drospirenone and estetrol tablets	Inhibit ovulation	Oral	Contraceptive
Eptinezumab	CGRP antagonist	Intravenous	Prophylaxis of migraine
Evinacumab-dgnb	Mab against Angiopoietin like 3 receptor	Intravenous	Homozygous familial hypercholesterolemia

Contd...

Contd...

Drug	Mechanism	Route	Indication
Fexinidazole	Generate cytotoxic products that damage DNA, lipid and proteins	Oral	African trypanosomiasis
Finerenone	Non-steroidal mineralocorticoid receptor antagonist	Oral	To reduce the risk of kidney and heart complications in chronic kidney disease associated with type 2 diabetes
Fosdenopterin	Replace the missing cyclic pyranopterin monophosphate	Intravenous	Molybdenum cofactor deficiency Type A
Fostemsavir	Fusion inhibitor by binding to Gp120	Oral	HIV-1
Ibrexafungerp	Inhibit beta 1,3 glycan in fungal cell wall	Oral	Vulvovaginal candidiasis
Inebilizumab	CD19-directed cytolytic antibody	Intravenous	Neuromyelitis optica spectrum disorder
Infigratinib	FGFR kinase inhibitor	Oral	Cholangiocarcinoma
Isatuximab	CD-38 directed cytolytic antibody	Intravenous	Multiple myeloma
Lacticol	Osmotic laxative	Oral	Chronic idiopathic constipation
Lonafarnib	Farnesyl transferase inhibitor	Oral	• To reduce risk of mortality in Hutchinson-Gilford Progeria Syndrome • For treatment of processing-deficient Progeroid Laminopathies
Lonapegsomatropin-tcgd	Human growth hormone	Subcutaneous	To treat short stature due to inadequate secretion of endogenous growth hormone
Loncastuximab tesirine-lpyl	Mab against CD-19	Intravenous	Large B cell lymphoma
Lumasiran	Small interfering RNA against hydroxy acid oxidase 1	Subcutaneous	Primary hyperoxaluria type 1
Lurbinectidin	Oncogenic transcription inhibitor	Intravenous	Small cell lung carcinoma
Margetuximab	Anti-HER2 mab	Intravenous	HER-2 positive breast cancer
Melphalan flufenamide	Alkylating agent	Intravenous	Multiple myeloma
Mobocertinib	Kinase inhibitor of EGFR	Oral	On-small cell lung cancer with EGFR exon 20 insertion mutations
Naxitamab-gqgk	A GD2-binding monoclonal antibody	Intravenous	Neuroblastoma
Odevixibat	Ileal bile acid transport inhibitor	Oral	Pruritis
Olanzapine/samidorphan	Samidorphan is opioid mu receptor antagonist	Oral	Schizophrenia and bipolar disorder
Oliceridine	Opioid agonist	Intravenous	Acute severe pain
Opicapone	COMT inhibitor	Oral	Off episodes of Parkinsonism
Osilodrostat	Cortisol synthesis inhibitor	Oral	Cushing syndrome
Ozanimod	Sphingosine 1-phosphate receptor modulator	Oral	Multiple sclerosis
Pegcetacoplan	Complement C3 inhibitor	Subcutaneous	Paroxysmal Nocturnal Hemoglobinuria
Pemigatinib	FGFR inhibitor	Oral	Cholangiocarcinoma
Ponesimod	Sphinosine-1 phosphate receptor modulator	Oral	Multiple sclerosis
Pralsetinib	RET Tyrosine kinase inhibitor	Oral	Non-small cell carcinoma lung
Relugolix	GnRH antagonist	Oral	Prostate cancer
Remdesivir	RNA dependent RNA polymerase inhibitor	Intravenous	Severe COVID-19
Remimazolam	Short acting benzodiazepine	Intravenous	For producing sedation during procedures
Rimegepant	CGRP receptor antagonist	Oral	Acute treatment of migraine
Ripretinib	KIT and PDGFR alpha TK inhibitor	Oral	Gastrointestinal stromal tumor
Risdiplam	SMN2 splicing modifier	Oral	Spinal muscular atrophy
Sacituzumab govitecan	Trop-2 directed mab with topoisomerase inhibitor	Intravenous	Triple negative breast cancer
Satralizumab	Mab against IL-6 receptor	Subcutaneous	Neuromyelitis optica spectrum disorder
Selpercatinib	RET kinase inhibitor	Oral	Non-small cell lung cancer, Medullary carcinoma thyroid
Selumetinib	MEK kinase inhibitor	Oral	Neurofibromatosis-1

Contd...

Contd...

Drug	Mechanism	Route	Indication
Serdexmethylphenidate and dexmethylphenidate	Dopamine Noradrenaline reuptake inhibitor	Oral	ADHD
Setmelanotide	A melanocortin 4 (MC4) receptor agonist	Subcutaneous	Chronic weight management in obesity due to proopiomelanocortin (POMC), proprotein convertase subtilisin/kexin type 1 (PCSK1), or leptin receptor (LEPR) deficiency
Somapacitan-beco	Human Growth hormone analog	Subcutaneous	Growth hormone deficiency
Sotorasib	RAS kinase inhibitor	Oral	Non-small cell lung carcinoma
Tafasitamab	CD19-directed cytolytic antibody	Intravenous	Diffuse large B cell lymphoma
Tazemetostat	EZH2 Histone methyltransferase inhibitor	Oral	Epithelioid sarcoma
Tepotinib	C-MET kinase inhibitor	Oral	Non-small cell lung cancer
Teprotumumab	Mab against IGF-1	IV	Thyroid eye disease
Tirbanibulin	Microtubule inhibitor	Topical	Actinic keratosis of face and scalp
Tivozanib	VEGF kinase inhibitor	Oral	Renal cell carcinoma
Triheptanoin	Medium chain triglyceride	Oral	Long-chain fatty acid oxidation disorders (LC-FAOD)
Trilacicilib	Cdk-4 and cdk-6 inhibitor	Intravenous	Chemotherapy induced myelosuppression
Tucatinib	Her-2 tyrosine kinase inhibitor	Oral	Breast cancer
Umbralisib	PI3 kinase inhibitor	Oral	Marginal zone lymphoma Follicular lymphoma
Vericiguat	Soluble guanylate cyclase agonist	Oral	Congestive heart failure
Vibegron	Selective beta-3 adrenergic receptor agonist	Oral	Overactive bladder
Viloxazine	Norepinephrine reuptake inhibitor	Oral	Attention deficit hyperkinetic disorder
Viltolarsen	Antisense nucleotide	Intravenous	Duchenne muscular dystrophy
Voclosporin	Calcineurin inhibitor	Oral	Lupus nephritis

FDA-APPROVED DRUGS IN 2019-2020

Drug	Mechanism	Route	Indication
Afamelanotide	Melanocortin 1 receptor agonist	Subcutaneous	Phototoxicity in patients with erythropoietic protoporphyria
Alpelisib	PI3 kinase inhibitor	Oral	Breast cancer
Apremilast	PDE-4 inhibitor	Oral	Oral ulcers associated with Behcet disease
Atezolizumab	MAb against PDL-1	IV	Extensive stage-Small Cell Lung Cancer
Avelumab + Axitinib	Avelumab: Anti-PDL-1 Axitinib: anti-VEGF kinase	Avelumab: IV Axitinib: Oral	Renal cell carcinoma
Bremelanotide	Melanocortin receptor agonist	subcutaneous	Hypoactive sexual desire disorder in females
Brexanolone	GABA-A modulator	Intravenous	Postpartum depression
Brolucizumab	VEGF inhibitor	Intravitreal	Neovascular Age-related Macular Degeneration
Cedazuridine	Cytidine deaminase inhibitor	Oral	Myelodysplastic syndrome
Cefiderocol	Cell wall synthesis inhibitor	IV	UTI due to gram negative bacteria
Cenobamate	Voltage gated Na channel blocker	Oral	Focal seizures
Clascoterone	Androgen receptor blocker	Topical	Acne vulgaris
Crizanlizumab	MAb against P-selectin	IV	Veno-occlusive disease in sickle cell anemia
Darolutamide	Androgen receptor antagonist	Oral	Prostate carcinoma
Diroximel fumarate	Forms monomethyl fumarate	Oral	Multiple sclerosis
Dupilumab	MAb against IL-4R alpha. It stops signaling of IL-4 and IL-13	SC	Chronic rhinosinusitis with nasal polyposis

Contd...

Contd...

Drug	Mechanism	Route	Indication
Elexacaftor/Ivacaftor/Tezacaftor	CFTR corrector and potentiator	Oral	Cystic fibrosis
Enfortumab vedotin	Nectin-4-directed antibody and microtubule inhibitor conjugate	IV	Urothelial carcinoma
Entrectinib	Tyrosine kinase inhibitor of ROS-1 and NTRK	Oral	ROS-1 positive Non-small cell lung cancer and NTRK positive solid tumors
Erdafitinib	FGFR Tyrosine kinase inhibitor	Oral	Urothelial carcinoma
Esketamine	Non-competitive NMDA antagonist	Intranasal	Treatment resistant depression
Fam-Trastuzumab Deruxtecan	HER2-directed antibody and topoisomerase inhibitor conjugate	IV	Breast cancer
Fedratinib	JAK-2 Inhibitor	Oral	Myelofibrosis
Givosiran	Small interfering RNA against ALS synthase	SC	Acute hepatic porphyria
Golodirsen	Antisense oligonucleotide that causes exon 53 skipping in dystrophin gene	IV	Duchenne's muscular dystrophy
Istradefylline	Adenosine A2 receptor antagonist	Oral	Off episode in Parkinsonism
Ixekizumab	MAb against IL-17a	Subcutaneous	Ankylosing Spondylitis
Lasmiditan	5HT1F agonist	Oral	Acute severe migraine
Lefamulin	Inhibit protein synthesis in bacteria	IV and oral	Community acquired bacterial pneumonia
Lemborexant	Dual orexin receptor (OX-1 and OX-2) antagonist (DORA)	Oral	Insomnia
Lenvatinib	VEGFR tyrosine kinase inhibitor	Oral	Endometrial carcinoma (with pembrolizumab)
Lumateperone tosylate	5HT-2A antagonist and partial agonist at D1 and D2 receptors	Oral	Schizophrenia
Luspatercept	Binds TGF-beta and decreases SMAD signalling	Subcutaneous	Anemia in patients with beta thalassemia
Netarsudil + Latanoprost	Netarsudil: Rho kinase inhibitor Latanoprost: PGF2 apha	Topical	Open angle glaucoma
Nintedanib	Tyrosine kinase inhibitor of PDGFR, VEGFR, FGF, FLT-3	Oral	To slow decline in pulmonary function in systemic sclerosis associated with interstitial lung disease
Onasemnogene abeparvovec	AAV vector based gene therapy to transfer SMN gene	Intravenous	Spinal muscular atrophy
Pembrolizumab	MAb against PD-1	IV	• Endometrial carcinoma (with lenvatinib) • Esophageal cancer • Small cell lung cancer • Non-small cell lung cancer • Renal cell carcinoma
Pexidartinib	TK inhibitor of Colony Stimulating Factor 1 Receptor	Oral	Tenosynovial Giant Cell Tumor
Pitolisant	H3 antagonist/inverse agonist	Oral	Narcolepsy
Polatuzumab vedotin	MAb against C79b component of B cell receptor	Intravenous	Diffuse large B cell lymphoma
Pralsetinib	RET Tyrosine kinase inhibitor	Oral	Non-small cell lung cancer
Pretomanid	Inhibit mycolic acid synthesis	Oral	For XDR and MDR TB (in combination with bedaquiline and linezolide)
Ramucirumab	VEGF antagonist	Intravenous	Hepatocellular carcinoma
Relebactam	Beta lactamase inhibitor	Intravenous	In combination with imipenem and cilastatin for intraabdominal infections and UTI
Rimabotulinumtoxin B	Inhibits release of acetylcholine	Injected in salivary glands	Chronic siallorhea
Risankizumab	MAb against IL-23	Subcutaneous	Plaque psoriasis
Romosozumab	MAb against sclerostin	Subcutaneous	Post-menopausal osteoporosis
Ruxolitinib	JAK-1 and JAK-2 inhibitor	Oral	Steroid resistant acute graft vs host disease

Contd...

Contd...

Drug	Mechanism	Route	Indication
Selinexor	Selective inhibitor of nuclear export	Oral	Multiple myeloma Diffuse large B cell lymphoma
Semaglutide	GLP-1 agonist	Oral	Type 2 diabetes mellitus
Siponimod	Sphingosine-1 phsophate receptor modulator	Oral	Multiple sclerosis
Solriamfetol	DA and NA reuptake inhibitor	Oral	For excessive day time sleepiness in Obstructive sleep apnea and Narcolepsy
Somapacitan	Human GH analog	Subcutaneous	GH deficiency
Tafamidis meglumine	Act as chaperone to stabilize TTR protein	Oral	To prevent cardiomyopathy in TTR amyloidosis
Tenapanor	NHE-3 inhibitor	Oral	IBS with constipation
Trifarotene	Retinoic acid receptor agonist	Topical	Acne vulgaris
Ubrogepant	CGRP antagonist	Oral	Acute attack of migraine
Upadacitinib	JAK inhibitor	Oral	Rheumatoid Arthritis
Venetoclax + Obinutuzumab	Venetoclax: BCL-2 inhibitor Obinutuzumab: Binds to CD-20 on B cells	Venetoclax: Oral Obintuzumab: IV	Chronic lymphoid leukemia Small lymphocytic leukemia
Voxelotor	HbS polymerization inhibitor	Oral	Sickle cell anemia
Zanubrutinib	Bruton tyrosine kinase inhibitor	Oral	Mantle cell lymphoma

FDA-APPROVED DRUGS IN 2018-2019

Drug	Mechanism	Route	Indication
Amifampridine	K channel blocker	Oral	Lambert Eaten myasthenic syndrome
Andexanet alpha	Bind to Factor Xa inhibitors	Intravenous	To reverse overdose of rivaroxaban and apixaban
Apalutamide	Androgen receptor antagonist	Oral	Prostate carcinoma
Avatrombopag	Thrombopoietin receptor agonist	Oral	Thrombocytopenia in patients with chronic liver disease
Baloxavir marboxil	Inhibit viral replication by inhibiting Cap-dependent endonuclease activity of viral polymerase	Oral	Single dose treatment of acute uncomplicated influenza
Baricitinib	Janus Kinase inhibitor	Oral	Rheumatoid arthritis
Bictegravir	Integrase inhibitor	Oral	HIV
Binimetinib	MET tyrosine kinase inhibitor	Oral	BRAF V600E or V600K mutation-positive malignant melanoma
Burosumab	Monoclonal antibody against FGF-23	Subcutaneous	X-linked hypophosphatemia
Calaspargase pegol	Asparagine specific enzyme	Intravenous	Acute lymphocytic leukemia
Cannabidiol	Unknown	Oral	Lennox-Gastaut syndrome Dravet syndrome
Caplacizumab	vWF-directed antibody fragment	IV/SC	Thrombotic thrombocytopenic purpura
Cemiplimab	Monoclonal antibody against Programmed Death receptor (PD-1)	Intravenous	Squamous cell carcinoma of skin
Cenegermin	Recombinant human nerve growth factor	Eye drops	Neurotrophic keratitis
Dacomitinib	EGFR tyrosine kinase inhibitor	Oral	Non-small cell lung cancer with EGFR exon 19 deletion or exon 21 L858R substitution mutations
Doravirine	Non-nucleoside Reverse Transcriptase Inhibitor	Oral	HIV
Duvelisib	Inhibitor of PI-3 kinase gamma and delta	Oral	Small lymphocytic lymphoma Follicular lymphoma Chronic lymphoid leukemia
Elagolix	GnRH antagonist	Oral	Pain associated with endometriosis
Elapegademase	Recombinant Adenosine deaminase enzyme	Intramuscular	Adenosine deaminase—severe combined immunodeficiency
Emapalumab	Monoclonal antibody against IFN-gamma	Intravenous	Primary hemophagocytic lymphohistiocytosis

Contd...

Contd...

Drug	Mechanism	Route	Indication
Encorafenib	BRAF-Kinase Inhibitor	Oral	BRAF V600E or V600K mutation-positive malignant melanoma
Eravacycline	Inhibit protein synthesis like other tetracyclines	Intravenous	Complicated intra-abdominal infections
Erenumab	Monoclonal antibody against CGRP	Subcutaneous	Migraine prophylaxis
Fostamatinib disodium hexahydrate	Spleen tyrosine kinase inhibitor	Oral	ITP
Fremanezumab	Monoclonal antibody against CGRP	Subcutaneous	Migraine prophylaxis
Galcanezumab	Monoclonal antibody against CGRP	Subcutaneous	Migraine prophylaxis
Gilteritinib	FLT3 kinase inhibitor	Oral	Acute myeloid leukemia
Glasdegib	Hedgehog pathway inhibitor	Oral	Acute myeloid leukemia
Ibalizumab	MAb against CD4	IV	HIV
Inotersen	Antisense oligonucleotide against transthyretin mRNA	Subcutaneous	Polyneuropathy of hereditary transthyretin-mediated amyloidosis
Ivosidenib	Isocitrate dehydrogenase 2 (IDH2) inhibitor	Oral	Acute myeloid leukemia with IDH2 mutation
Lanadelumab	Monoclonal antibody against plasma kallikrein	Subcutaneous	Hereditary angioneurotic edema
Larotrectinib	NTRK kinase inhibitor	Oral	Solid tumors with NTRK mutation
Lofexidine	Alpha 2 agonist	Oral	To decrease opioid withdrawal symptoms
Lorlatinib	ALK kinase inhibitor	Oral	Non small cell carcinoma of lung
Lusutrombopag	Thrombopoietin receptor agonist	Oral	Thrombocytopenia in patients with chronic liver disease
Lutetium lu 177 dotatate	Peptide receptor radionuclide therapy	Intravenous	Gastro-entero-pancreatic neuroendocrine tumors
Megalastat	Pharmacological chaperone for Alpha galactosidase	Oral	Fabry's disease
Mogamulizumab	Monoclonal antibody against CCR-4	Intravenous	Mycosis fungoides Sezary syndrome
Moxetumomab pasudotox	Monoclonal antibody against CD22 conjugated with Pseudomonas exotoxin	Intravenous	Hairy cell leukemia
Moxidectin	Bind to Glutamate and GABA chloride channels	Oral	Onchocerciasis
Omadacycline	Inhibit protein synthesis like other tetracyclines	Oral Intravenous	Community acquired bacterial pneumonia Acute skin and skin structure infections
Patisiran	Small Interfering RNA based therapy against mutant transthyretin	Intravenous	Polyneuropathy in patients with transthyretin mediated amyloidosis
Pegvaliase	Substitute of Phenylalanine hydroxylase	Subcutaneous	Phenylketonuria
Plazomicin	Inhibit protein synthesis like other aminoglycosides	Intravenous	Complicated UTI
Prabotulinum toxin-A	Inhibit release of ACh	Intramuscular	Temporary improvement of glabellar lines
Prucalopride	5HT4 agonist	Oral	Chronic idiopathic constipation
Ravulizumab	C5 Complement inhibitor	Intravenous	Paroxysomal nocturnal hemoglobinuria
Revefenacin	Anticholinergic	Inhalational	COPD
Rifamycin	Inhibit beta subunit of RNA polymerase	Oral	Traveller's diarrhea
Sarecycline	Inhibit protein synthesis like other tetracyclines	Oral	Inflammatory lesions of non-nodular moderate to severe acne
Segesterone + ethinyl estradiol	Inhibit ovulation	Vaginal ring	Contraception (once yearly)
Sodium zirconium cyclosilicate	Binds to K and increase fecal excretion	Oral	Hyperkalemia
Stiripentol	Increases GABAergic activity	Oral	Dravet syndrome
Tafenoquine	Free radical mediated killing of hypnozoites	Oral	Single dose radical cure of *P. vivax* malaria
Tagraxofusp	Anti-CD-123	Intravenous	Blastic plasmacytoid dendritic cell neoplasm
Talazoparib	PARP inhibitor	Oral	Breast cancer with a germline BRCA mutation
Tecovirimat	Inhibit formation of extracellular viral forms	Oral	Smallpox
Tildrakizumab	MAb against IL-23	Subcutaneous	Plaque psoriasis
Tizacaftor + Ivacaftor	CFTR stimulator and potentiator	Oral	Cystic fibrosis
Tolvaptan	Vasopressin V2 receptor antagonist	Oral	To slow kidney function decline in adult polycystic kidney disease

FDA-APPROVED NEW DRUGS BEFORE 2018

Name	Mechanism	Route	Use
Adalimumab	MAb against TNF-alpha	Subcutaneous	Non-infectious uveitis
Albiglutide Tediglutide Dulaglutide Lixisenatide	GLP-1 agonists	Subcutaneous	Type 2 diabetes mellitus
Alogliptin	DPP-4 inhibitors	Oral	Type 2 diabetes mellitus
Aminolevulinic acid hydrochloride	Porphyrin precursor	Topical	Actinic keratosis
Apremilast	PDE-4 inhibitor	Oral	Psoriasis
Asfotase alfa	Tissue non-specific alkaline phosphatase	Subcutaneous	Hypophosphatemia
Avibactam	Beta lactamase inhibitor	Intravenous	In combination with ceftazidime for complicated abdominal infections
Bedaquiline	Mycobacterial ATP synthase inhibitor	Oral	MDR tuberculosis
Belatacept	Co-stimulation inhibitor	Intravenous	Renal transplant rejection
Belimumab	MAb against B lymphocyte stimulator (BLyS)	Intravenous	SLE
Bezlotoxumab	MAb against Clostridium difficile toxin B	Intravenous	Clostridium difficile infection
Boceprevir Paritaprevir Grazoprevir Simeprevir Asunaprevir	HCV protease inhibitor	Oral	Hepatitis C virus
Brexipiprazole	Atypical antipsychotic D2 partial agonist	Oral	Schizophrenia Major depressive disorder
Brivaracetam	Binds SV2A like levetiracetam, mechanism unknown	Oral	Focal seizures
Calcifediol	Vitamin D3 analog	Oral	Secondary hyperparathyroidism
Canagliflozin Dapagliflozin Empagliflozin	SGLT-2 inhibitors	Oral	Type 2 diabetes mellitus
Cangrelor	P_2Y_{12} antagonist	Intravenous	Antiplatelet
Cariprazine	Atypical antipsychotic	Oral	Schizophrenia Bipolar I disorder
Cobicistat	CYP3A4 inhibitor	Oral	To boost the effect of elvitegravir or protease inhibitors (atazanavir or darunavir) in HIV treatment
Crisaborole	PDE-4 inhibitor	Topical	Atopic dermatitis
Crofelemer	Reduce chloride secretion via CFTR	Oral	Diarrhea in HIV
Daclizumab	MAb against IL-2R	Subcutaneous	Relapsing remitting multiple sclerosis
Deflazacort	Steroid	Oral	Duchenne muscular dystrophy
Defibrotide	Mixture of oligodeoxyribonucleotides	Intravenous	Hepatic veno-occlusive disease
Dronabinol	Tetrahydrocannabinol derivative	Oral	Anorexia associated with AIDS Chemotherapy induced nausea and vomiting
Droxidopa	Prodrug of norepinephrine	Oral	Neurogenic hypotension
Eculizumab	MAb against C5 complement component	Intravenous	Paroxysmal nocturnal hemoglobinuria
Edoxaban Rivaroxaban	Xa inhibitor	Oral	Anticoagulant
Efinaconazole	Inhibit ergosterol synthesis	Topical	Onychomycosis
Eluxadoline	Mu agonist and Delta antagonist	Oral	IBS with diarrhea
Eslicarbazepine	Na channel blocker	Oral	Focal seizures
Etelcalcetide	Calcium sensing receptor agonist	Intravenous	Secondary hyperparathyroidism in CKD patients on dialysis

Contd...

Contd...

Name	Mechanism	Route	Use
Eteplirsen	Antisense oligonucleotide that excludes exon 51 of dystrophin pre mRNA	Intravenous	Duchenne muscular dystrophy
Evolocumab Alirocumab	MAb against PCSK-9	Subcutaneous	Hyperlipidemia
Ezogabine (retigabine)	K channel opener	Oral	Focal Seizures
Fidaxomicin	RNA polymerase inhibitor	Oral	Pseudomembranous colitis
Flibanserin	5HT1A agonist and 5HT2A antagonist	Oral	Hypoactive sexual desire disorder
Golimumab	MAb against TNF alpha	Subcutaneous	Ulcerative colitis
Icatibant	Bradykinin antagonist	Subcutaneous	Hereditary angioedema
Idarucizumab	MAb against dabigatran	Intravenous	Dabigatran toxicity
Isavuconazonium sulphate	Prodrug of isavuconazole that inhibit fungal ergosterol biosynthesis	Oral, Intravenous	Mucormycosis Invasive aspergillosis
Ivabradine	I_f blocker	Oral	Chronic CHF Angina
Ivacaftor	CFTR stimulator	Oral	Cystic fibrosis
Lesinurad	URAT-1 inhibitor	Oral	Gout
Lifitegrast	LFA-1/ICAM-1 inhibitor	Oral	Dry eye disease
Linaclotide	sGC stimulator	Oral	IBS with constipation
Lomatapide	MTP inhibitor	Oral	Familial homozygous hypercholesterolemia
Lubiprostone	Cl channel activator	Oral	IBS with constipation
Macitentan	Endothelin receptor antagonist	Oral	Pulmonary hypertension
Mepolizumab Reslizumab	MAb against IL-5	Subcutaneous	Asthma
Mipomersen	Antisense nucleotide against apoB	Subcutaneous	Familial homozygous hypercholesterolemia
Naloxegol	Peripheral Mu receptor antagonist	Oral	Opioid induced constipation
Nintedanib	Tyrosine kinase inhibitor for PDGFR, EGFR and VEGFR	Oral	Idiopathic pulmonary fibrosis
Nusinersen	Antisense oligonucleotide directed against survival motor neuron 2, It increases exon 7 inclusion	Intrathecal	Spinal muscular atrophy
Obeticholic acid	FXR agonist	Oral	Primary biliary cirrhosis
Olodaterol	Long acting beta 2 agonist	Inhalation	COPD
Omapatrilat	Vasopeptidase inhibitor		Chronic CHF
Ombitasvir Ledipasvir Elbasvir Daclatasvir Velpatasvir	NS5A inhibitor	Oral	Hepatitis C virus
Oritavancin	Cell wall synthesis inhibitor similar to vancomycin	Intravenous	Gram-positive infections
Ospemifene	SERM		Post menopausal dyspareunia
Paroxetine	SSRI	Oral	Vasomotor symptoms of menopause
Patiromer	K binder	Oral	Hyperkalemia
Perampanel	AMPA receptor antagonist	Oral	Focal seizures
Peramivir	Neuraminidase inhibitor	Intravenous	Influenza virus A and B
Pimavanserin	5HT2A antagonist, atypical antipsychotic	Oral	Hallucination and delusions associated with Parkinsonism
Pirfenidone	Reduce fibroblast proliferation by reducing TGF beta	Oral	Idiopathic pulmonary fibrosis
Plecanatide	Soluble guanylyl cyclase agonist	Oral	Chronic idiopathic constipation

Contd...

Contd...

Name	Mechanism	Route	Use
Prasterone	Inactive steroid converted to estrogen in the body	Oral	Dyspareunia
Raxibacumab Obiltoxaximab	MAb against PA component of toxin of Bacillus anthracis	Intravenous	Anthrax
Rifaximin	RNA polymerase inhibitor	Oral	IBS with diarrhea
Riociguat	Soluble guanylate cyclase stimulator	Oral	Pulmonary hypertension
Rolapitant	NK1 receptor antagonist	Oral	Delayed vomiting due to chemotherapy
Sacubitril	Inhibit NEP	Oral	Chronic CHF
Secukinumab Ixekizumab Brodalumab	MAb against IL-17	Subcutaneous	Psoriasis
Sebelipase alfa	Enzyme	Intravenous	Lysosomal acid lipase deficiency
Selexipag	PGI2 receptor agonist	Oral	Pulmonary hypertension
Siltuximab	MAb against IL-6	Intravenous	Castleman's disease
Sofosbuvir Dasabuvir Beclabuvir	NS5B inhibitors	Oral	Hepatitis C virus
Sugammadex	Selective muscle relaxant binding agent	Intravenous	Reversal of muscle relaxants
Suvorexant	Orexin receptor antagonist	Oral	Insomnia
Tasimelteon	Melatonin receptor agonist	Oral	Sleep wake cycle disorder in blind
Tavaborole	Inhibit leucyl tRNA synthetase	Topical	Topical drug for onychomycosis
Ticagrelor	P_2Y_{12} antagonist	Oral	Antiplatelet
Tocilizumab	MAb against IL-6	Intravenous, Subcutaneous	Rheumatoid arthritis
Umeclidinium	Long acting M3 blocker	Inhalation	COPD
Uridine triacetate	Pyrimidine analog	Oral	Hereditary orotic aciduria 5-FU or capecitabine overdose
Vedolizumab	MAb against α4β7 integrin	Intravenous	Ulcerative colitis Crohn's disease
Vorapaxar	PAR antagonist	Oral	Antiplatelet

MNEMONICS

MNEMONIC
TALAZOPARIB

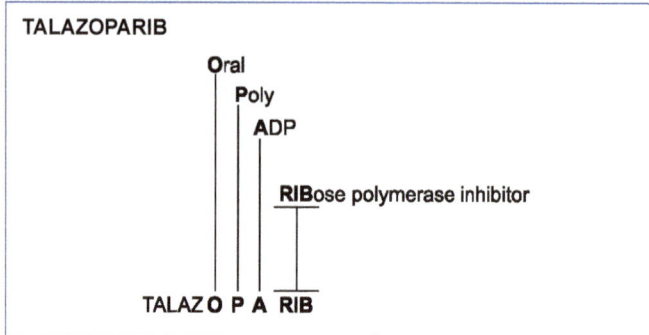

MNEMONIC
INOTERSEN

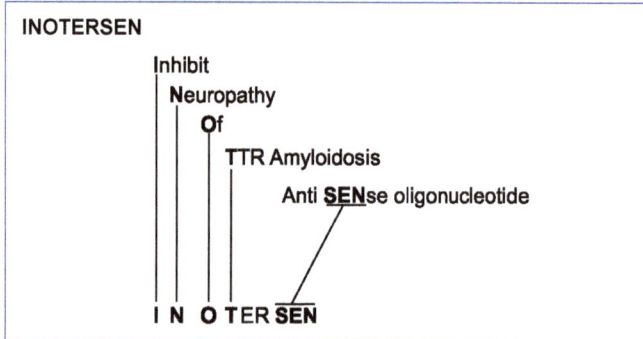

MNEMONIC
ELAPEGADEMASE—LVLR

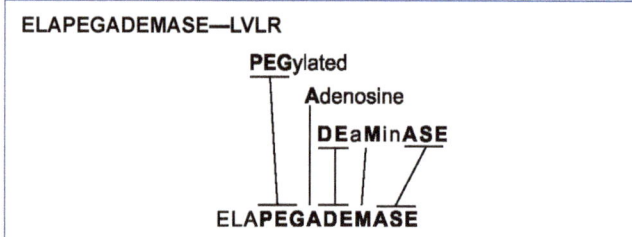

MNEMONIC
CENEGERMIN—BKBJ
- Recombinant Human Nerve Growth Factor
- Approved for neurotrophic keratitis
- Used as Eye drops

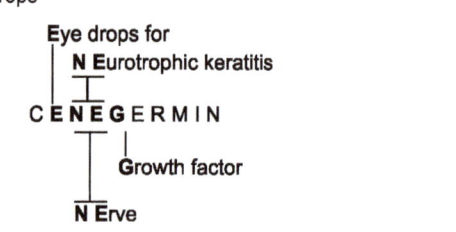

MNEMONIC
TECOVIRIMAT
- Against orthopoxviruses such as smallpox and monkeypox.
- Targets the viral p37 protein, necessary for the viral envelopment and inhibits the production of extracellular viral forms, which are responsible for the systemic spread of infection
- Does not inhibit the formation of intracellular forms of the virus
- Smallpox was declared eradicated in 1980, but variola virus (VARV), which causes smallpox, still exists
- Two million doses of tecovirimat are stockpiled in the US Strategic National Stockpile should and orthopoxvirus based bioterror attack occur.

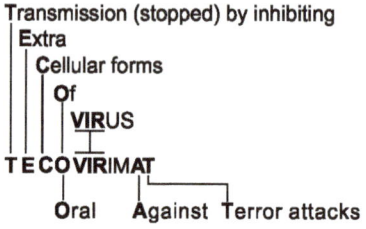

MNEMONIC
LANADELUMAB
- Monoclonal antibody against plasma kallikrein
- Plasma kallikrein is involved in conversion of HMW kininogen to bradykinin.
- Lanadelumab inhibits formation of bradykinin
- It is approved for Hereditary Angioneurotic Edema

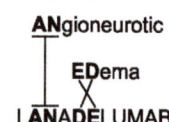

MNEMONIC
PATISIRAN
- First small interfering RNA-based drug
- It is a gene silencing drug that interferes with the production of an abnormal form of transthyretin.
- Approved for the treatment of polyneuropathy in people with hereditary transthyretin-mediated amyloidosis.

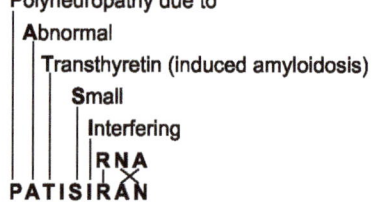

New Drugs with Mnemonics

MNEMONIC

MIGALASTAT
- Pharmacological chaperone
- Fabry disease occurs due to mutations of α-Galactosidase (GalA) on X chromosome.
- Some mutations result in misfolding of α-GalA
- This results in accumulation of Globotriaosylceramide (GL3)
- Migalastat given orally binds to α-GalA and shifts the folding behaviour towards the proper conformation, resulting in a functional enzyme.

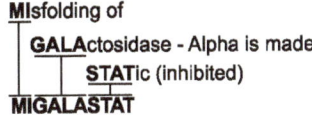

MIsfolding of
GALActosidase - Alpha is made
STATic (inhibited)
MIGALASTAT

MNEMONIC

ELAGOLIX SODIUM
- GnRH antagonist for the treatment of pain associated with endometriosis in women.
- Short-acting GnRH antagonist
- Second-generation" GnRH modulator due to its non-peptide and small molecule nature and its oral activity

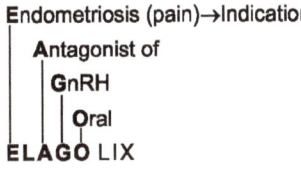

Endometriosis (pain)→Indication
Antagonist of
GnRH
Oral
ELAGO LIX

MNEMONIC

ANTI-CGRP ANTIBODIES
- Calcitonin Gene Related Peptide (CGRP) is involved in causing neurogenic inflammation and vasodilation seen in migraine
- Monoclonal antibodies against CGRP are approved for prophylaxis of migraine.
- The drugs include:
  - ERENUMAB-AOOE
  - GALCANEZUMAB-GNLM
  - FREMANEZUMAB-VFRM

How to remember

MAN CAN RAN (REN) away from **migraine headache**

fre**MAN**ezumab, gal**CAN**ezumab, e**REN**umab

MNEMONIC

BICTEGRAVIR
- Bictegravir is intergrase strand transfer inhibitor (INSTI) of HIV similar to raltegravir.

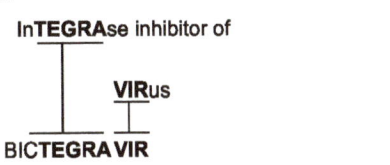

In**TEGRA**se inhibitor of
VIRus
BICTEGRAVIR

MNEMONIC

FOSTAMATINIB DISODIUM HEXAHYDRATE
- It is a tyrosine kinase inhibitor with demonstrated activity against spleen tyrosine kinase.
- The major metabolite of fostamatinib, R406, inhibits signal transduction of Fe-activating receptors and B-cell receptor and reduces antibody-mediated destruction of platelets.
- It is specifically indicated for the oral treatment of thrombocytopenia in adult patients with chronic immune thrombocytopenia (ITP) who have had an insufficient response to a previous treatment.

How to remember
- The name ends with **NIB** means it is a tyrosi**N**e kinase inhl**B**itor.
- Name contains **S** (fo**S**tamatinib) means it inhibits **S**pleen tyrosine kinase.
- Name contains **I** (fostamat**I**nib) means **I**diopathic and **T** (fos**T**amatinib) means **T**hrombocytopenia, so it can be used to remember that it is used for ITP.

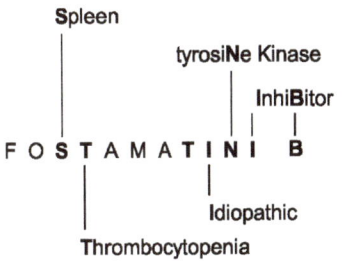

MNEMONIC

PEGVALIASE—PQPZ
- It is a phenylalanine-metabolizing enzyme.
- It is a PEGylated phenylalanine ammonia lyase (PAL) enzyme that converts phenylalanine to ammonia and trans-cinnamic acid.
- It substitutes for the deficient phenylalanine hydroxylase enzyme activity in patients with phenylketonuria and reduces blood phenylalanine concentrations.
- It is specifically indicated to reduce blood phenylalanine concentrations in adult patients with phenylketonuria who have uncontrolled blood phenylalanine concentrations greater than 600 micromol/L on existing management.
- It is supplied as a solution for subcutaneous injection.
- It comes with the boxed warning of development of anaphylaxis.

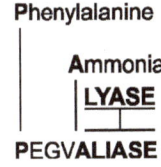

Phenylalanine
Ammonia
LYASE
PEGVALIASE

MNEMONIC

SODIUM ZIRCONIUM CYCLOSILICATE
- It is a highly-selective, oral potassium-removing agent.
- It is a non-absorbed zirconium silicate that preferentially captures potassium in exchange for hydrogen and sodium.
- It increases fecal potassium excretion through binding of potassium in the lumen of the gastrointestinal tract. Binding of potassium reduces the concentration of free potassium in the gastrointestinal lumen, thereby lowering serum potassium level.
- It is specifically indicated for the treatment of hyperkalemia in adults.
- The most common adverse reaction associated with the use of this drug is mild to moderate edema.

How to remember

Name contains **ZERO** (**ZIR**c**O**nium) potas**SIUM** (zir**C**on**IUM**), that can be used to remember that it will decrease K in the blood, so used for hyperkalemia.

```
ZER  O
         potassIUM
ZIR C O N   IUM
```

MNEMONIC

ERENUMAB AOOE
- It is a human monoclonal antibody that binds to the calcitonin gene-related peptide (CGRP) receptor and antagonizes CGRP receptor function.
- This is the receptor that is believed to transmit signals that can cause incapacitating pain.
- It is specifically indicated for the preventative treatment of migraine in adults by subcutaneous route once monthly.
- It can result in injection site reactions and constipation

How to remember

1. Name contains **REN** which can be used to remember the use as mig**RAIN**e.
2. Name ends with **MAB** that tells it is a Monocolonal AntiBody.

```
        migRAINe
                Monoclonal
                  Anti
                    Body
ERENU   M A B
```

MNEMONIC

AVATROMBOPAG AND LUSUTROMBOPAG
- These are orally bioavailable, small molecule thrombopoietin (TPO) receptor agonist that stimulates proliferation and differentiation of megakaryocytes from bone marrow progenitor cells resulting in an increased production of platelets.
- These do not compete with TPO for binding to the TPO receptor and has an additive effect with TPO on platelet production.
- These are specifically indicated for the treatment of thrombocytopenia in adult patients with chronic liver disease who are scheduled to undergo a procedure.

```
THROMBOPoietin
        AGonist
AVATROMBOPAG
```

MNEMONIC

OPRELVEKIN
- It is recombinant IL-11.
- Interleukin-11 acts as megakaryocyte growth factor.
- It is used to prevent thrombocytopenia induced by cancer chemotherapy

How to remember

The name ends with **KIN** means it is interleu**KIN**.
Remove the KI from the name and see the name, it appears to be ending with **ELeVEN**. (opr**ELVE**ki**N**)

```
     InterleuKIN
     ELEV     N
OPRELVEKIN
```

MNEMONIC

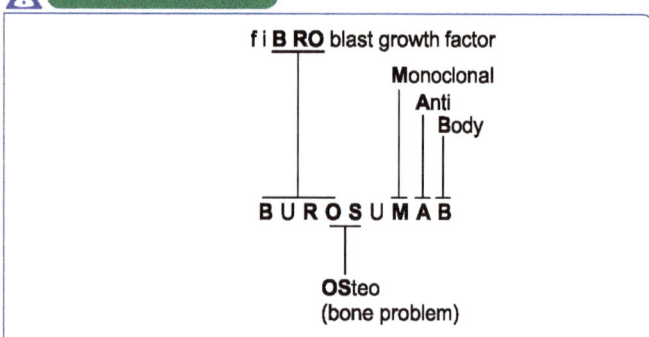

MNEMONIC

LOMITAPIDE
- It is indicated for the treatment of patients with **homozygous familial hypercholesterolemia**.
- It acts by **inhibiting** the **microsomal triglyceride transfer protein (MTP or MTTP)** which is necessary for **very low-density lipoprotein (VLDL)** assembly and secretion in the liver.

```
    MIcrosomal
      Triglyceride transport
        Protein
          Inhibitor
LOMITAPIDE
```

New Drugs with Mnemonics

MNEMONIC

ETEPLIRSEN

- **Duchenne muscular dystrophy (DMD)** may result from **mRNA** that contains out-of-frame mutations (e.g. deletions, insertions or splice site mutations), resulting in frameshift or early termination so that in most muscle fibers no functional dystrophin is produced.
- **Antisense oligonucleotides**, structural analogs of DNA, allow faulty parts of the dystrophin gene to be skipped when it is transcribed to RNA for protein production, permitting a still-truncated but more functional version of the protein to be produced.
- **Eteplirsen** is an **antisense oligonucleotide** designed to bind to **exon 51** of dystrophin **pre-mRNA**. This result in exclusion of this **exon** during **mRNA** processing in patients with genetic mutations that is amenable to **exon 51** skipping.
- It is specifically indicated for the treatment of **DMD** in patients who have a confirmed mutation of the **DMD** gene that is amenable to **exon 51** skipping.

How to remember
- All drugs ending with **RSEN** bind to RNA and are antiSENse oligonucleotides
- Name starts with E means Exon and contains LI, which in Roman means 51, so it causes skipping of EXON-51

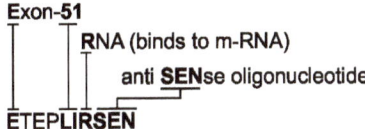

MNEMONIC

VENETOCLAX
- Overexpression of **BCL-2** has been demonstrated in **chronic lymphocytic leukemia (CLL)** cells where it mediates tumor cell survival and has been associated with resistance to chemotherapeutics.
- **Venetoclax** is a **BCL-2** inhibitor and helps to restore the process of apoptosis and is specifically indicated for the treatment of patients with **CLL** with **17p** deletion.
- It is supplied as tablets for oral administration.

How to remember
- BCL-2 contains CL-2 means CLL (L is 2 times) means it is overactive in CLL
- Name contains O means it is Oral drug
- Name contains CL means it is used for CLL

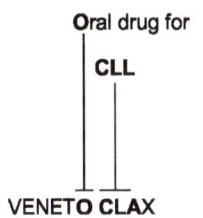

MNEMONIC

RUCONEST
- It is the commercial name of a recombinant **C1 esterase** inhibitor.
- **Hereditary angioneurotic edema** attacks stem from a deficiency of the **C1** inhibitor protein in the blood.
- It is specifically indicated for the treatment of **acute angioedema** attacks in adult and adolescent patients with hereditary angioedema.
- It is given by **intravenous route**.

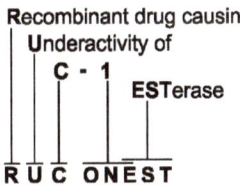

MNEMONIC

HEDGEHOG PATHWAY INHIBITORS
- VISMODEGIB
- SONIDEGIB
- GLASDEGIB

- **Hedgehog** signaling pathway is typically over-activated in **basal cell carcinoma** and **some patients of AML.**
- Vismodegib and sonidegib are approved for the treatment of adults with metastatic **basal cell carcinoma**, whereas glasdegib is approved for AML.

How to remember
- Name contains DEG, which on rearranging becomes DGE, the last 3 letters of heDGEhog pathway
- Name ends with IB which is for inhIBitor.

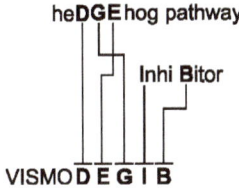

MNEMONIC

PAR-1 ANTAGONISTS
- VORAPAXAR
- ATOPAXAR

- **Thrombin** stimulates protease activated receptors-1 (**PAR-1**) on the surface of platelets to cause aggregation. These are antagonists of **PAR-1** receptor of thrombin.
- These are specifically indicated for the **reduction of thrombotic cardiovascular events** in patients with a history of myocardial infarction (MI) or with peripheral arterial disease (PAD).

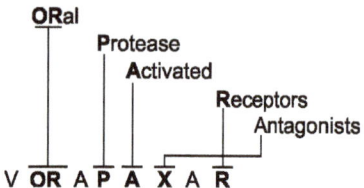

MNEMONIC

INOTUZUMAB OZOGAMICIN
- It is a **CD22**-directed antibody-drug conjugate (**ADC**) specifically indicated for the intravenous treatment of adults with relapsed or refractory **B-cell precursor acute lymphoblastic leukemia**.
- It comes with a boxed warning of risk of severe hepatotoxicity including veno-occlusive disease or sinusoidal obstruction syndrome.

How to remember
- **MAB** suggests it is a Monoclonal AntiBody.
- Name contains **TU** means it is for **TU**mor (anticancer drug)
- Name starts with **INO** which means say **NO** to I (me), think about **ALL** means used for Acute Lymphoblastic Lymphoma.

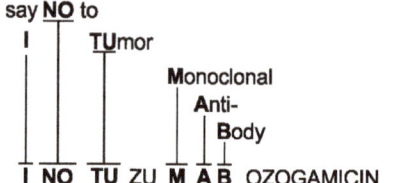

MNEMONIC

OCRELIZUMAB
- It is a **CD20**-directed **cytolytic** antibody. It is specifically indicated for the treatment of adult patients with relapsing or primary progressive forms of **multiple sclerosis** by intravenous route.

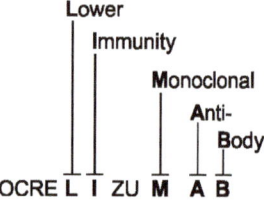

MNEMONIC

GUSELKUMAB
- It is an **interleukin-23** blocker and thus inhibits the release of pro-inflammatory cytokines and chemokines.
- It is specifically indicated for the treatment of adults with moderate-to-severe plaque psoriasis by subcutaneous administration.

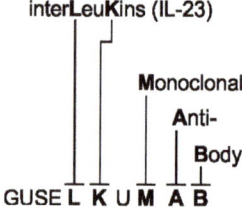

MNEMONIC

LETERMOVIR
- It is a **CMV DNA** terminase complex inhibitor which is required for viral DNA processing and packaging.
- It affects the production of proper unit length genomes and interferes with **virion** maturation.
- It is specifically indicated for **prophylaxis of cytomegalovirus (CMV) infection** and disease in adult CMV-seropositive recipients [R+] of an allogeneic hematopoietic stem cell transplant by oral route or by intravenous injection.

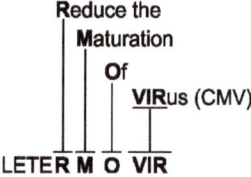

MNEMONIC

VESTRONIDASE ALFA—VJBK
- It is a recombinant **human lysosomal beta glucuronidase**. It is an enzyme replacement therapy that works by replacing the missing enzyme. It is specifically indicated for pediatric and adult patients for the treatment of **Mucopolysaccharidosis VII** by intravenous infusion.

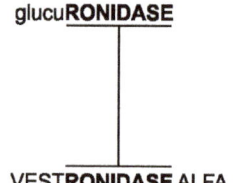

New Drugs with Mnemonics

MNEMONIC

EMICIZUMAB—KXWH
- It is a **bispecific** factor **IXa**- and factor **X-directed** antibody that brings these together **to help in clotting**.
- It is specifically indicated for routine prophylaxis to prevent or reduce the frequency of **bleeding** episodes in adult and pediatric patients with **hemophilia A** (congenital factor VIII deficiency) with factor VIII inhibitors.
- It is supplied as a **solution** for subcutaneous injection.
- It comes with the boxed warning of cases of thrombotic microangiopathy and thrombotic events.

CIrculation
Monoclonal
Anti-
Body
EMI CI ZU M A B – KXWH

MNEMONIC

CERLIPONASE ALFA
- **Ceroid lipofuscinosis type 2 (CLN-2 disease)** is a **neurodegenerative** disease caused by deficiency of the **lysosomal** enzyme **tripeptidyl peptidase-1 (TPP1)**, which catabolizes polypeptides in the **CNS**.
- Deficiency in **TPP-1** activity results in the accumulation of **lysosomal** storage materials in the central nervous system, leading to progressive decline in **motor** function.
- **Cerliponase alfa** is a hydrolytic lysosomal **N-terminal** tripeptidyl peptidase.
- It is specifically indicated to slow the loss of ambulation in symptomatic
- Pediatric patients 3 years of age and older with late infantile neuronal **CLN-2**

CERoid
LIPOfuscinosis
Neuronal
CER LIPO NASE - ALPHA

MNEMONIC

DUPILUMAB
- It is an **interleukin-4** receptor alpha antagonist and inhibits **interleukin-4** and interleukin-13 signaling by specifically binding to the **IL-4Rα** subunit shared by the **IL-4** and **IL-13** receptor complexes.
- It is specifically indicated for the subcutaneous treatment of adults with moderate-to-severe **atopic dermatitis** whose disease is not adequately controlled with topical prescription therapies or when those therapies are not advisable.

How to remember
- Name ends with **MAB** means it is Monoclonal AntiBody
- Name contains **IL** means it is against Interleukin, name starts with D (fourth letter of alphabet) means it is against IL-4.
- Name starts with **D** means it is used for Dermatitis (atopic)

IL - 4
Monoclonal
Anti-Body
DUPILUMAB
Dermatitis (atopic) is use

MNEMONIC

AMANTADINE
- It is a **weak** uncompetitive antagonist of the **NMDA** receptors.
- It has recently been approved for the treatment of **dyskinesia in patients with Parkinson's disease** receiving levodopa-based therapy, with or without concomitant dopaminergic medications. It is supplied as an extended release capsule for oral administration.

How to remember
- Name contains M, A, D and N (aMantADiNe), rearranging it forms **NMDA**, name also contains ANT (amANTadine) means it is **NMDA ANTagonist**

NMDA
ANTagonist
AMANTADINE

MNEMONIC

PI-3 KINASE INHIBITORS
– COPANLISIB
– LDELALISIB
– DUVELISIB
- These are small molecule inhibitor of **phosphatidylinositide-3 kinase (PI3K)**, an intracellular signaling component.
- These are indicated for B cell lymphomas.

phosphatidy LInoSItide kinase
InhiBitor
COPANLISIB
Used for Lymphoma

MNEMONIC

OBILTOXAXIMAB
- It is a monoclonal antibody that binds the **PA** of **B. anthracis**.
- It is indicated for use in adult and pediatric patients for the treatment of **inhalational anthrax**.

BacILLus anthracis
TOXin
Monoclonal
Anti-
Body
O B I L T O X A X I M A B

MNEMONIC

RAXIBACUMAB
- A human monoclonal antibody indicated for the prophylaxis and treatment of **inhalational anthrax**.
- It targets the protective antigen (**PA**) component of the lethal toxin of **Bacillus anthracis**.

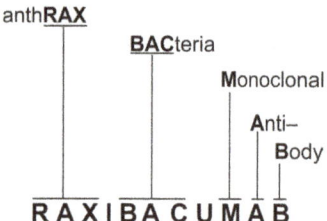

MNEMONIC

LESINURAD
- It is a **URAT-1** inhibitor indicated in combination with a **xanthine oxidase** inhibitor for the treatment of **hyperuricemia** associated with **gout** in patients who have not achieved target serum uric acid levels with a xanthine oxidase inhibitor alone.
- After secretion in the proximal tubules, uric acid comes back in the blood through **URAT-1**. Inhibition of this transporter helps in excessive secretion of uric acid, thus uricosuric effect.

How to remember
- Name starts with **LES** and contains **URA**, which can be used to remember it result in **LES**s **URA**te in the body, so can be used in gout.
- Name contains SIN, if we rearrange, it becomes **INS** which can be used to remember that it **IN**creases the Secretion of **URA**te.

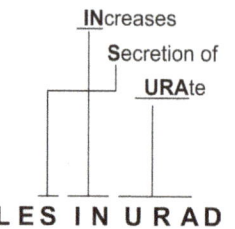

MNEMONIC

FLIBANSERIN
- It is indicated for the treatment of premenopausal women with acquired, generalized hypoactive sexual desire disorder (**HSDD**) as characterized by low sexual desire that causes marked distress or interpersonal difficulty and is NOT due to:
  – A co-existing medical or psychiatric condition,
  – Problems within the relationship, or
  – The effects of a medication or other drug substance.
- It is not indicated for the treatment of **HSDD** in postmenopausal women or in men.
- It is not indicated to enhance sexual performance.
- It has agonist activity at **5-HT1A** and antagonist activity at **5-HT2A**. It also has moderate antagonist activities at the **5-HT2B, 5-HT2C,** and dopamine **D4** receptors.

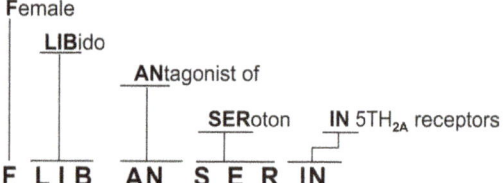

MNEMONIC

RIOCIGUAT
- It is a stimulator of soluble guanylate cyclase that increases **cGMP** resulting in vasodilation.
- It is specifically indicated for persistent/ recurrent chronic thromboembolic **pulmonary hypertension by Oral Route**.

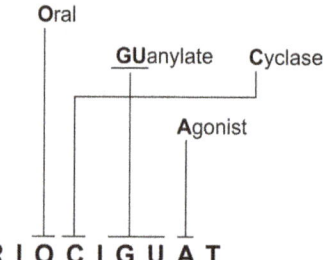

MNEMONIC

PIMAVANSERIN
- It is an atypical antipsychotic specifically indicated for the oral treatment of **hallucinations and delusions associated with Parkinson's disease**.
- The effect of pimavanserin could be mediated through a combination of inverse agonist and antagonist activity at serotonin 5-HT2A receptors and to a lesser extent at serotonin 5-HT2C receptors.

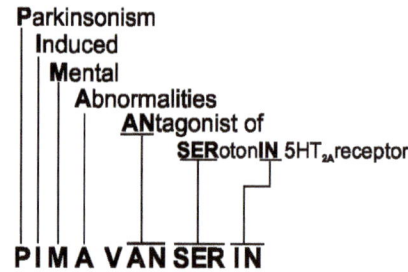

MNEMONIC

SELEXIPAG
- It is an oral prostacyclin receptor agonist indicated for the treatment of pulmonary arterial hypertension.

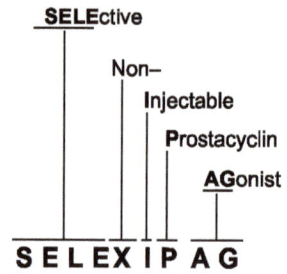

MNEMONIC

SUVOREXANT
- The orexin neuropeptide signaling system is a central promoter of wakefulness. Blocking the orexin receptor suppresses wakefulness.
- Suvorexant is an orexin receptor antagonist. It is specifically indicated for the treatment of insomnia (by oral route) characterized by difficulties with sleep onset and/or sleep maintenance.

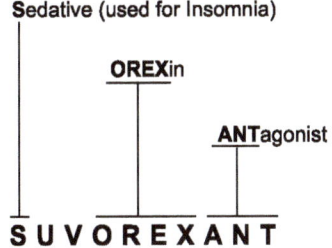

MNEMONIC

BRUTON TYROSINE KINASE INHIBITORS
- IBRUTINIB
- ACALABRUTI NIB

- Orally available selective inhibitors of Bruton's tyrosine kinase (Btk)
- BTK is a signaling molecule of the B-cell antigen receptor (BCR) and cytokine receptor pathways.
- These are approved for **mantle cell lymphoma.**

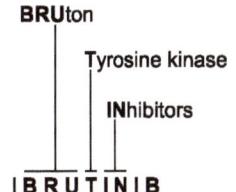

MNEMONIC

IVACAFTOR
- It is a cystic fibrosis transmembrane conductance regulator (CFTR) potentiator.
- Cystic fibrosis is caused by mutations in a gene that encodes for the CFTR protein that regulates ion (such as chloride) and water transport in the body. The defect in chloride and water transport results in the formation of thick mucus that builds up in the lungs, digestive tract and other parts of the body leading to severe respiratory and digestive problems.
- Ivacaftor is specifically approved for the treatment of **cystic fibrosis** in patients age 6 years and older who have a G55 I D mutation in the CFTR gene.

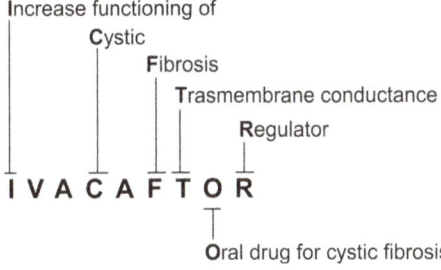

MNEMONIC

ECULIZUMAB
- It is a monoclonal antibody that specifically binds to the complement protein C5 with high affinity thereby inhibiting its cleavage to C5a and C5b and preventing the generation of the terminal complement complex C5b-9.
- It has now been approved for **atypical hemolytic uremic syndrome (aHUS)** to inhibit complement-mediated thrombotic microangiopathy.
- It is already being used for **Paroxysmal Nocturnal Hemoglobinuria (PNH)**.
- **Ravulizumab** is a new C5 inhibitor approved for PNH

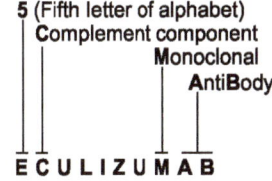

MNEMONIC

ICATIBANT
- Hereditary angioneurotic edema (HAE) is caused by an absence or dysfunction of C1-esterase-inhibitor resulting in excessive bradykinin.
- Bradykinin is a vasodilator which is thought to be responsible for the characteristic HAE symptoms of localized swelling, inflammation, and pain.
- Icatibant is a competitive antagonist selective for the bradykinin B2 receptor.
- Icatibant is specifically approved for the treatment of **acute attacks of HAE** in adults by **subcutaneous** route.

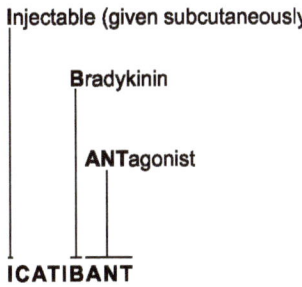

MNEMONIC

BEZLOTOXUMAB
- It is a human monoclonal antibody that binds to *C. difficile* toxin B and neutralizes its effect.
- It is specifically indicated to reduce recurrence of **Clostridium difficile infection (CDI)** in patients 18 years of age or older who are receiving antibacterial drug treatment of CDI and are at a high risk for CDI recurrence.

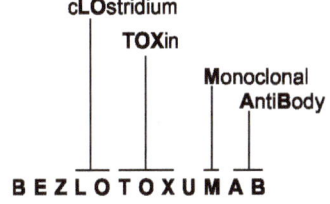

MNEMONIC

TELOTRISTAT ETHYL
- It is a **tryptophan hydroxylase inhibitor** that stops the overproduction of serotonin.
- It is specifically indicated for the oral treatment of **carcinoid syndrome** diarrhea in combination with somatostatin analog (SSA) therapy in adults inadequately controlled by SSA therapy.

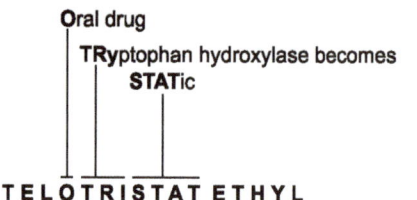

MNEMONIC

CYCLIN DEPENDENT KINASE INHIBITORS
- RIBOCICLIB
- PALBOCICLIB
- ABEMACICLIB
- Indicated for oral use for the treatment of women with hormone receptor-positive, HER2-negative advanced or metastatic **breast cancer**.

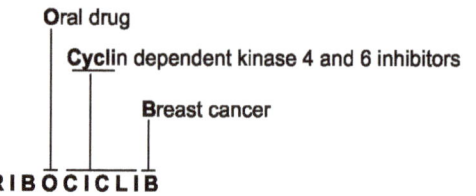

MNEMONIC

PARP INHIBITORS
- OLAPARIB
- RUCAPARIB
- NIRAPARIB

- Poly ADP Ribose Polymerase (PARP-1 and PARP-2) play a role in DNA repair.
- PARP inhibitors result in DNA damage, apoptosis and cell death.
- These are specifically indicated for the oral treatment of adults with recurrent epithelial **ovarian cancer**.

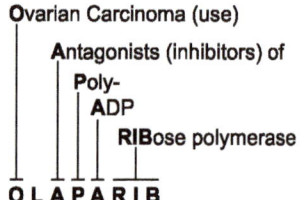

MNEMONIC

HCV PROTEASE INHIBITORS
- BOCEPREVIR
- TELAPREVIR
- SIMPREVIR
- GRAZOPREVIR
- PARITAPREVIR
- GLECAPREVIR

- These are oral drugs for **HCV** that act by inhibiting the enzyme protease of the virus.

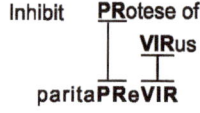

MNEMONIC

TOCILIZUMAB
- It is a monoclonal antibody against IL-6.
- It is used for Rheumatoid arthritis as DMARD.
- Recently, it has been approved for Cytokine release syndrome.
- It is given IV and increases the risk of infections.

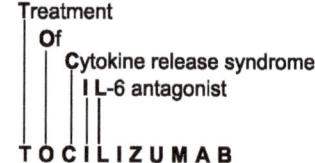

MNEMONIC

ENASIDENIB AND IVOSIDENIB
- These are oral small molecule inhibitors of the isocitrate dehydrogenase 2 (IDH2) enzyme that works by blocking several enzymes that promote cell growth.
- These are specifically indicated for the treatment of adult patients with relapsed or refractory **acute myeloid leukemia** (AML) with an isocitrate dehydrogenase-2 (IDH2) mutation as detected by an FDA-approved test.
- It comes with a Black Box Warning that an adverse reaction known as differentiation syndrome can occur and can be fatal if not treated.

How to remember
- Name contains **A** means it is used for **AML**
- After A, there is **SID** in the name, rearranging it forms **ISD**, which suggests **IS**ocitrate **D**ehydrogenase
- **EN** stands for **EN**zyme
- **IB** means **I**nhi**B**itor

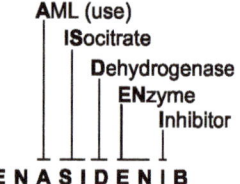

MNEMONIC

SGLT-2 INHIBITORS
- CANAGLIFLOZIN
- DAPAGLIFLOZIN
- EMPAGLIFLOZIN
- ERTUGLIFLOZIN

- These drugs inhibit the reabsorption of glucose from proximal tubule by inhibiting the **S**odium **GL**ucose **C**o**T**ransproter-2 (**SGLT-2**).
- Therefore, these drugs act by causing glucosuria. Most common adverse effect of these drugs is UTI.

How to remember

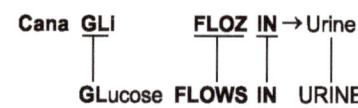

New Drugs with Mnemonics

MNEMONIC

MIDOSTAURIN
- It is a multikinase inhibitor. It is specifically indicated (by oral route) for the treatment of adult patients with newly diagnosed **acute myeloid leukemia (AML)** who are FLT3 mutation positive, as detected by an FDA approved test. It is used in combination with standard cytarabine and daunorubicin induction and cytarabine consolidation chemotherapy.

How to remember
- If you follow cricket, there is a batsman of South Africa Hashim **AML**a. When he is in **MID**dle of the crease, he is a **STAR**
- Midostaurin name contains **MID**dle and **STA**uRin (**STAR**) and used for **AML** (from **AMLA**)

MNEMONIC

SARILUMAB
- It is an interleukin-6 (IL-6) receptor antagonist treatment of adult patients with moderately to severely active **rheumatoid arthritis** who have had an inadequate response or intolerance to one or more DMARDs. It is administered subcutaneously.
- It comes with a Black Box warning of the potential for serious infections.

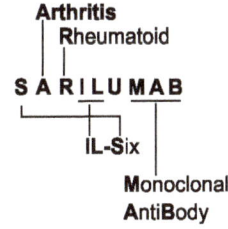

MNEMONIC

DURVALUMAB
It is a programmed death-ligand 1 (PD-L1) blocking antibody. It is specifically indicated for the intravenous treatment of patients with locally advanced or metastatic **urothelial carcinoma** who have disease progression following platinum-containing chemotherapy.

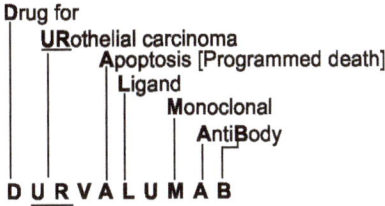

MNEMONIC

CONESTAT-ALPHA
It is recombinant C-1 inhibitor for hereditary angioneurotic edema.

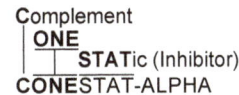

MNEMONIC

VERICIGUAT
It is soluble guanylate cyclase agonist approved for CHF.

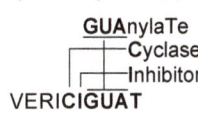

MNEMONIC

ADUCANUMAB
It is a monoclonal antibody against l AB-amyloid to target underlying cause of Alzheimer's disease.

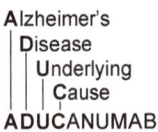

MNEMONIC

SELINEXOR
It is selecting inhibitor of nuclear export for oral treatment of multiple myeloma and diffuse large B-cell lymphoma

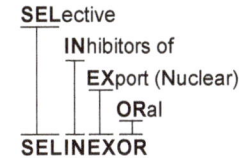

MNEMONIC

SIPONIMOD
It is sphingosine-1-phosphate modulator for multiple sclerosins

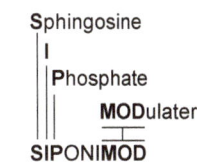

MNEMONIC

PEGCETACOPLAN
It is a pegylated C-3 antagonist for PNH.

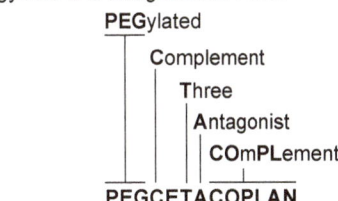

Latest Papers

INI CET MAY 2022

1. Which of the following factor in PC vs time graph is a measure of extent of drug absorption of a drug?
   (a) Area under the curve
   (b) Half life
   (c) C_{max}
   (d) T_{max}

2. Manufacturer of a drug company labels the drug contains 500 mg paracetamol. On quantitative analysis by the authorities, it was found to contain only 200 mg of drug. According to drugs and cosmetics act 1940, this type of drug is known as:
   (a) Spurious drug
   (b) Adulterant drug
   (c) Unethical drug
   (d) Misbranded drug

3. Which of the following statement is correct regarding the given graph?

   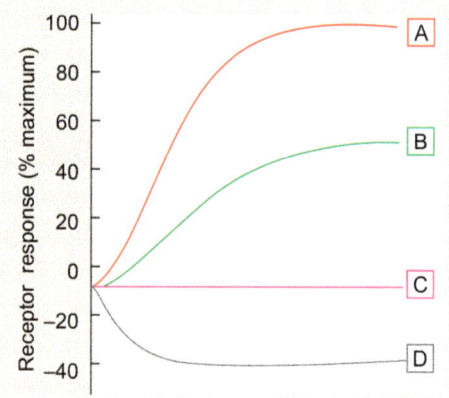

   (a) Drug A represents agonist and Drug B represents inverse agonist
   (b) Drug C represents agonist and Drug D is inverse agonist
   (c) Drug A is agonist and Drug D is inverse agonist
   (d) Drug B is partial agonist and Drug C is inverse agonist

4. Type of stimulatory G protein in PIP2-Phospholipase activation pathway is:
   (a) Gs
   (b) Gi
   (c) Gq
   (d) Go

5. Identify the type of inhibition from the given graph:

   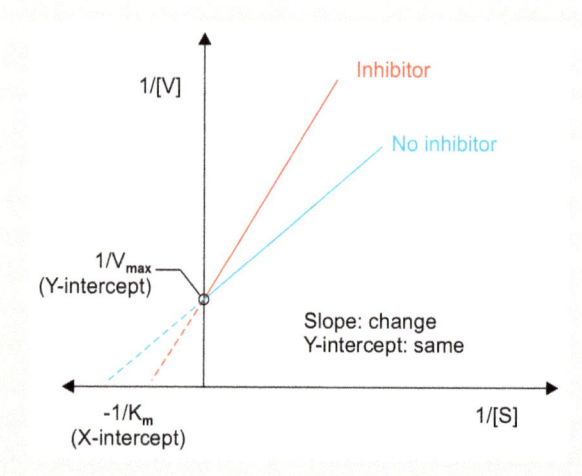

   (a) Competitive
   (b) Noncompetitive
   (c) Uncompetitive
   (d) Allosteric

6. A 20-year-old boy was brought to emergency room after consuming some unknown substance. The patient was sweating profusely, saliva was drooling from mouth and tears were present. The boy had involuntary urination and diarrhea. On examination, the heart rate was 58 beats per minute and blood pressure was 80/60 mm Hg. Which of the following is the drug of choice for treatment of this patient?
   (a) Atropine
   (b) N-acetylcysteine
   (c) Naloxone
   (d) Physostigmine

7. A patient with pre-existing liver disease consumed a drug and developed worsening of liver dysfunction. The metabolite of the drug responsible is N-acetyl-para-amino-benzo-quinone-imine. The likely implicated drug in this case is:
   (a) Paracetamol
   (b) Valproate
   (c) Amiodarone
   (d) Lorazepam

8. Which of the following is not the primary treatment agent in Rheumatoid arthritis?
   (a) Methotrexate
   (b) Hydroxychloroquine
   (c) Sulfasalazine
   (d) Azathioprine

9. Identify the correct match regarding the drug and its adverse drug reaction:
   (a) Hydralazine: Heart failure
   (b) Verapamil: Constipation
   (c) Aliskiren: Hypokalemia
   (d) Atenolol: Hemolytic anemia

10. Which of the following anti-diabetic drugs is associated with increased risk of fractures in a female with osteoporosis?
    (a) Canagliflozin
    (b) Rosiglitazone
    (c) Voglibose
    (d) Repaglinide

11. Half life of letrozole is:
    (a) 45 hours
    (b) 72 hours
    (c) 96 hours
    (d) 120 hours

12. Which of the following statement/statements regarding use of 5-alpha reductase inhibitors in BPH are correct? (multiple correct)
    (a) Decrease in serum PSA
    (b) Increase in serum PSA
    (c) Decrease in cellular testosterone
    (d) Decrease in cellular DHT

13. A 42-year-old chronic alcoholic presents to emergency department with altered sensorium and seizures. He has not consumed alcohol for last two days. On investigations, his serum ALT is 150, AST is 180 and GGT is 563 units per liter. Best drug for first line management of this patient is:
    (a) Lorazepam
    (b) Diazepam
    (c) Clonazepam
    (d) Alprazolam

14. ACTH is the treatment of:
    (a) Juvenile myoclonic epilepsy
    (b) West syndrome
    (c) Dravet syndrome
    (d) Lennox-Gastaut syndrome

15. A patient of psychosis was being treated with risperidone. He presented to emergency with upward fixed gaze. What will be the treatment of this patient?
    (a) Wait and assurance
    (b) Intramuscular promethazine
    (c) Injection diazepam
    (d) Injection lorazepam

16. A 30-year-old female presented to psychiatry OPD with symptoms of hypomania. She has a past history of mania and wants to conceive. Which of the following drug is most teratogenic?
    (a) Valproate
    (b) Lithium
    (c) Carbamazepine
    (d) Olanzapine

17. Which of the following options correctly represent the increasing order of potency of inhalational anaesthetic agents?
    (a) N_2O < Isoflurane < Halothane < Methoxyflurane
    (b) Methoxyflurane < Halothane < Isoflurane < N_2O
    (c) Halothane < Isoflurane < Methoxyflurane < N_2O
    (d) Isoflurane < N_2O < Halothane < Methoxyflurane

18. From the given diagram, identify the mechanism of action of isoniazid:
    (a) Drug A
    (b) Drug B
    (c) Drug C
    (d) Drug D

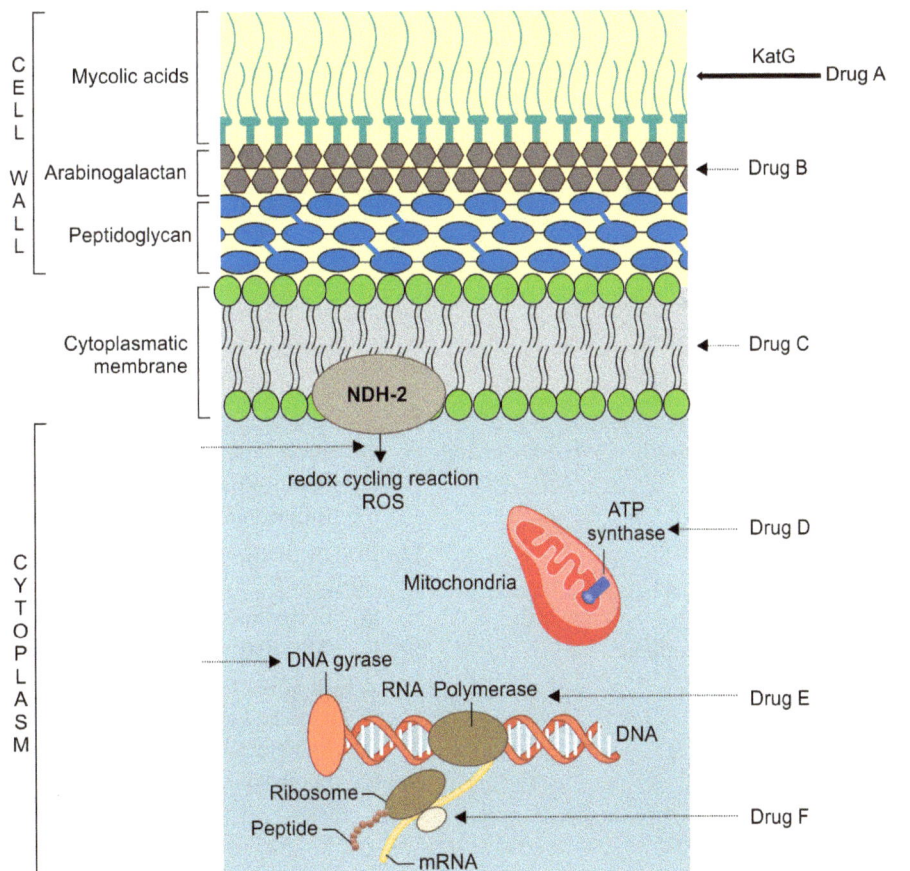

19. The given diagram shows the steps in formation of bacterial cell wall. Identify the site of action of beta lactam antimicrobials.
    (a) A
    (b) B
    (c) C
    (d) D

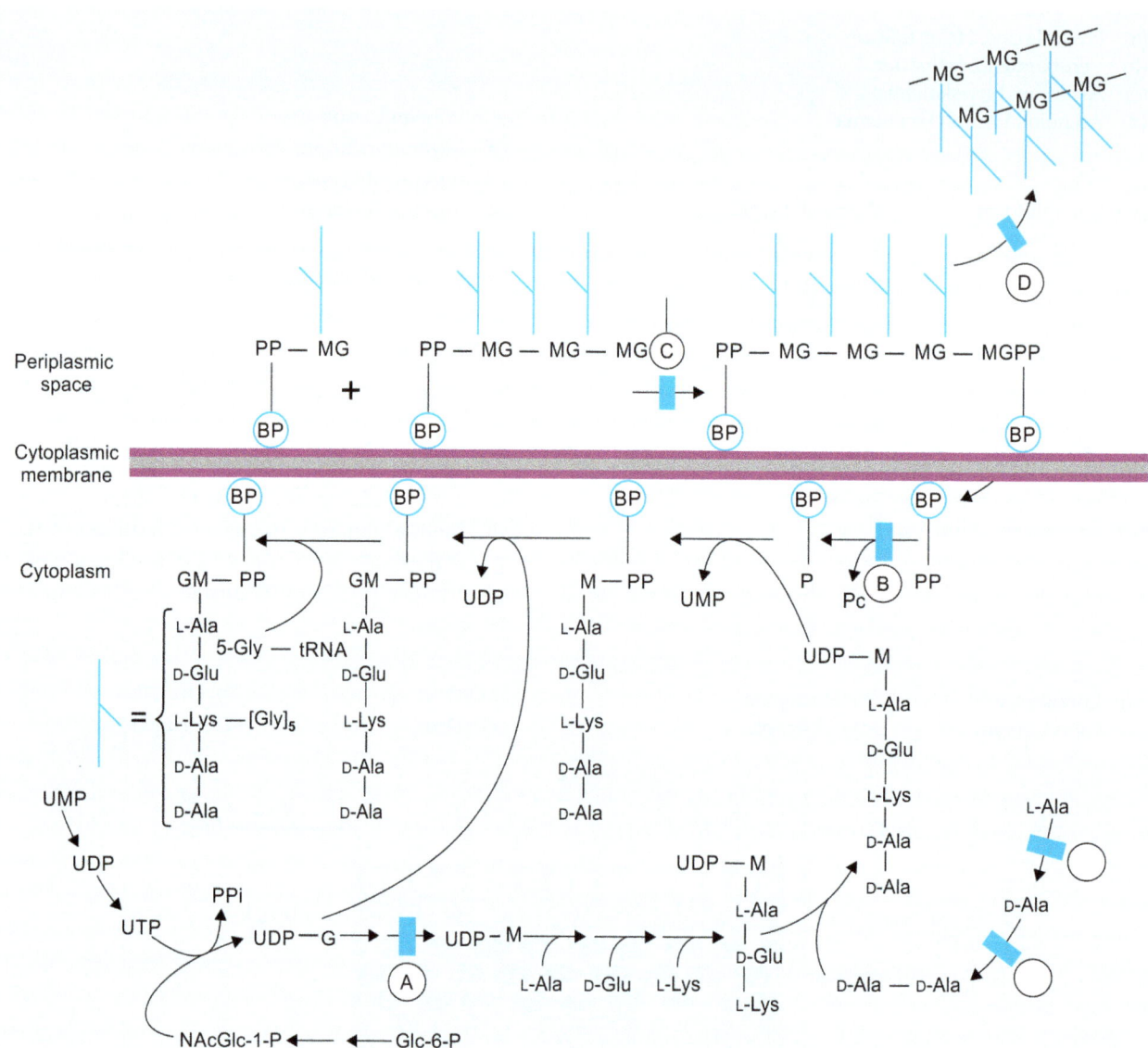

20. A pregnant female with history of lepromatous leprosy presents to OPD with type 2 lepra reaction. What should be the management?
    (a) Thalidomide
    (b) Stop MDT and start steroids
    (c) Add corticosteroids
    (d) Antibiotics

21. Active metabolite of cyclophosphamide is:
    (a) 4-ketoacyl cyclophosphamide
    (b) 4-hydroxy cyclophosphamide
    (c) N-Acetyl cyclophosphamide
    (d) N-Methylcyclophosphamide

22. Immune checkpoint inhibitor approved for treatment of advanced endometrial carcinoma is:
    (a) Pembrolizumab
    (b) Nivolumab
    (c) Ipilimumab
    (d) Trastuzumab

23. Which of the following is not an immune check point inhibitor?
    (a) Cetuximab
    (b) Pembrolizumab
    (c) Atezolizumab
    (d) Nivolumab

24. Which of the following drug is not indicated in treatment of Sickle cell anemia?
    (a) Bebtelovimab
    (b) L-glutamine
    (c) Hydroxyurea
    (d) Voxelotor

EXPLANATIONS

1. Ans. (a) Area under the curve
(Ref: Modern Pharmacology with Clinical Applications p49)

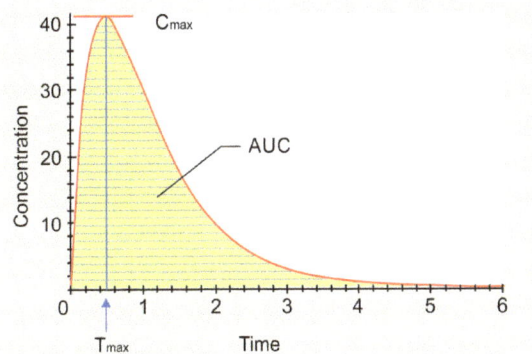

- AUC tells about the extent of absorption of the drug
- T_{max} tells about the time to reach maximum concentration, i.e. rate of absorption
- C_{max} is the maximum concentration of a drug that can be obtained

2. Ans. (d) Misbranded drug *(Ref: Drugs and Cosmetics Act)*

The Drugs and Cosmetics (amendment) Act, 2008 provides deterrent penalties for offences relating to manufacture of spurious or adulterated drugs which have serious implications on public health.

Spurious drugs: These products are manufactured concealing the true identity of the product and made to resemble another drug, especially some popular brand, to deceive the buyer and cash on the popularity of original product. The product may or may not contain the active ingredients. Spurious drugs are usually manufactured by unlicensed anti-social elements but sometimes licensed manufacturers may also be involved.

Adulterated drugs: These are those drugs which are found to contain an adulterant/substituted product or contaminated with filth rendering it injurious to health.

Misbranded drugs: A drug shall be deemed to be misbranded
(a) If it is so colored, coated, powdered or polished that damage is concealed or if it is made to appear of better or greater therapeutic value than it really is; or
(b) If it is not labeled in the prescribed manner; or
(c) If its label or container or anything accompanying the drug bears any statement, design or device which makes any false claim for the drug or which is false or Misleading in any particulars.

3. Ans. (c) Drug A is agonist and Drug D is inverse agonist
(Ref: KDT 8th/p49)

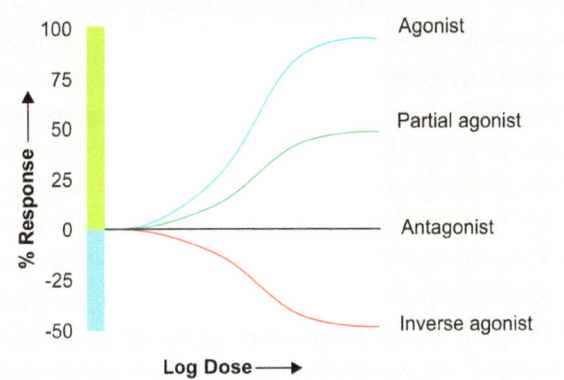

In the given graph,
- Drug A produces the maximum effect, so it is agonist
- Drug B has submaximal action, so it is partial agonist
- Drug C has no effect, so it is antagonist
- Drug D produces negative intrinsic activity, so it is inverse agonist

4. Ans. (c) Gq *(Ref: KDT 8th/p57)*

G Protein Coupled Receptors: Drugs bind to the receptor which in turn activates a G protein (GTP activated protein). This may result in one of the three actions:
1. **Activation (by Gs) or inhibition (by Gi) of enzyme adenylate cyclase:** It changes the concentration of cAMP that acts by activating protein kinases (e.g. protein kinase A). Latter produce action by phosphorylation of their substrates. Examples include beta-receptors (increase cAMP) and somatostatin (works by decreasing cAMP).
2. **Activation of phospholipase C (by Gq):** This enzyme converts PIP2 to IP3 and DAG. Final result is increase in intracellular calcium and thus action e.g. alpha-receptors, vasopressin V1 receptors.
3. Stimulation or inhibition of ion channels e.g. M2 receptors of ACh.

5. Ans. (a) Competitive *(Ref: KDT 8th/p46)*

Lineweaver-Burk plots for enzyme inhibition

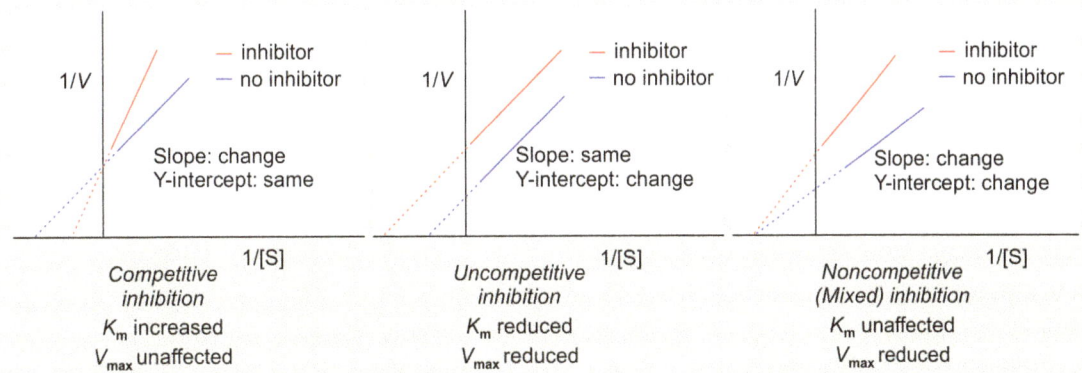

Lineweaver-Burk Plot (Double Reciprocal Plot): It is a graph between 1/V (on (y-axis) and 1/substrate (on x-axis). It was used to determine enzyme kinetics and type of enzyme inhibition. Intercept of the graph on y-axis is a measure of V_{max} (higher intercept means lower V_{max}) and intercept on x-axis is a measure of K_m (Lesser the negative lesser is K_m)

- Competitive inhibitors have same Y-intercept as uninhibited enzyme. Since V_{max} is unaffected, so $1/V_{max}$ also does not change.
- Noncompetitive inhibitors have same X-intercept as uninhibited enzyme. Since K_m is unaffected, so 1/substrates also does not change.
- Uncompetitive inhibitor will have graph shifted to left for both X- and Y-intercepts, as both V_{max} and K_m decrease.

6. Ans. (a) Atropine *(Ref: CMDT 2022/p1586)*

This is a classical case of organophosphate poisoning. Drug of choice is atropine.

- Symptoms of anticholinesterase poisoning are simply the extension of the pharmacological actions of ACh and are manifested as pin-point pupil, salivation, lacrimation, sweating, bronchoconstriction, diarrhea, urination, bradycardia, hypotension and coma. Blood pressure and heart rate may increase rarely due to stimulation of nicotinic receptors.
- Atropine is an antidote of choice for both organophosphate and carbamate poisoning.

7. Ans. (a) Paracetamol *(Ref: CMDT 2022/p1590)*

- Paracetamol is metabolized to N-acetyl para-aminobenzo quinone-imine (NAPQI) by microsomal enzymes. This metabolite has high affinity for sulfhydryl groups and can combine with the enzymes and other biomolecules resulting in hepatotoxicity.
- Normally acetaminophen is a safe drug because glutathione (contain sulfhydryl group due to presence of sulfur containing amino acid, cysteine) produced by the liver combines with NAPQ to detoxify it. However chronic alcoholics are predisposed to toxicity because:
  - Glutathione production decreases due to liver disease.
  - Alcohol is a powerful inducer of microsomal enzymes. It increases the production of NAPQ from acetaminophen resulting in toxicity.
- Acetaminophen toxicity can be decreased by providing sulfhydryl donors like N-acetylcysteine (antidote of choice). Gastric lavage (with activated charcoal) should be done to prevent further absorption but it is ineffective after 4 hours of ingestion.

8. Ans. (d) Azathioprine *(Ref: CMDT 2022/p835-837)*

- Corticosteroids are used as bridge therapy for treatment of Rheumatoid arthritis
- Methotrexate, hydroxychloroquine and sulfasalazine are synthetic disease modifying anti-Rheumatoid drugs and are used as first line drugs in treatment of Rheumatoid arthritis.
- Azathioprine is an immunosuppressant drug and is not the first line drug in treatment of rheumatoid arthritis.

9. Ans. (b) Verapamil: Constipation *(Ref: CMDT 2022/p980)*

- Calcium channel blockers like verapamil and diltiazem cause constipation as an adverse effect.
- Hydralazine is used for treatment of heart failure. It is not the adverse effect of this drug.
- Renin inhibitors like aliskiren cause hyperkalemia by decreasing the formation of aldosterone.
- Hemolytic anemia is an adverse effect of methyldopa and not of atenolol.

10. Ans. (b) Rosiglitazone *(Ref: CMDT 2022/p1225)*

Thiazolidinediones like rosiglitazone and pioglitazone are associated with a increase in risk of fractures in women (not in men).

11. Ans. (a) 45 hours *(Ref: KDT 8th/p340)*

- Letrozole is an aromatase inhibitor.
- It is used for induction of ovulation and also for treatment of post menopausal breast cancer.
- Half life of letrozole is approximately 40 hours.

12. Ans. (a) Decrease in serum PSA, (d) Decrease in cellular DHT *(Ref: CMDT 2022/p974-975)*

- 5-Alpha-reductase inhibitors like finasteride and dutasteride block the conversion of testosterone to dihydrotestosterone. This result in decrease in cellular DHT levels.
- These medications impact the epithelial component of the prostate, resulting in reduction in size of the gland and improvement in symptoms.
- Serum PSA is reduced by approximately 50% in patients receiving finasteride therapy, but the % free PSA is unchanged. Therefore, in order to compare with pre-finasteride PSA levels, the serum PSA of a patient taking finasteride should be doubled.

13. Ans. (a) Lorazepam *(Ref: CMDT 2022/p1100-1102)*

- Drug of choice for alcohol withdrawal seizures are benzodiazepines.
- Normally chlordiazepoxide or diazepam are used. However in liver disease patients, the preferred drug is lorazepam.

14. Ans. (b) West syndrome *(Ref: Nelson 20th/p2840)*

- West syndrome starts between the ages of 2 and 12 months and consists of a triad of infantile epileptic spasms that usually occur in clusters (particularly in drowsiness or upon arousal), developmental regression, and a typical EEG picture called hypsarrhythmia.
- It is best treated with ACTH.

15. Ans. (b) Intramuscular promethazine *(Ref: KDT 8th/p468,471)*

- Risperidone is an atypical antipsychotic drug with maximum D2 blockade potency.
- It can result in dystonias like upward fixed gaze.
- Drug of choice for this adverse effect is centrally acting anticholinergic drugs like benzhexol. If these are not available then first generation antihistaminics like promethazine can be used.

16. Ans. (a) Valproate *(Ref: KDT 8th/p444)*

- Most of the drugs used in treatment of mania and bipolar disorder are teratogenic.
- Least teratogenic are antipsychotic drugs like olanzapine, so these are drug of choice for treatment of bipolar disorder in pregnancy.
- Valproate is most teratogenic drug and should be avoided.

Latest Papers

17. Ans. (a) N₂O < Isoflurane < Halothane < Methoxyflurane
(Ref: KDT 8th/p405)

- Potency is inversely proportional to minimum alveolar concentration of an inhalational anesthetic agent.

Anaesthetic MAC
Nitrous oxide 104
Desflurane 6.0
Sevoflurane 2.05
Enflurane 1.68
Isoflurane 1.15
Halothane 0.74
Methoxyflurane 0.16

18. Ans. (a) Drug A *(Ref: KDT 8th/p817)*

- Isoniazid is activated by catalase peroxidase (which is encoded by bacterial gene *katG*) and it inhibits the formation of mycolic acid in mycobacteria.
- Mutation in KatG can result in resistance to isoniazid.

19. Ans. (d) D *(Ref: KDT 8th/p766-67)*

- Beta lactams like penicillins, cephalosporins, carbapenems and monobactam act by inhibiting an enzyme transpeptidase.
- This enzyme helps in cross-linking of peptidoglycan moieties in cell wall of bacteria.
- Drugs acting at different sites in the above diagram are:
  - A: Fosfomycin
  - B: Bacitracin
  - C: Vancomycin
  - D: Beta lactams

20. Ans. (c) Add corticosteroids *(Ref: KDT 8th/p837)*

- Drug of choice for both type 1 as well as type 2 lepra reaction is corticosteroids.
- Anti-leprosy treatment should not be stopped.

21. Ans. (b) 4-hydroxy cyclophosphamide
(Ref: Goodman and Gilman 13th/p862)

- Cyclophosphamide is activated by CYP2B to 4-hydroxycyclophosphamide, which is in a steady state with the acyclic tautomer aldophosphamide.
- The active cyclophosphamide metabolites (e.g., 4-hydroxycyclophosphamide and aldophosphamide) are carried in the circulation to tumor cells, where aldophosphamide cleaves spontaneously, stoichiometrically generating phosphoramide mustard and acrolein.
- Phosphoramide mustard is responsible for antitumor effects, while acrolein causes hemorrhagic cystitis often seen during therapy with cyclophosphamide.
- 4-Hydroxycyclophosphamide may be oxidized further by aldehyde oxidase, either in liver or in tumor tissue, and perhaps by other enzymes, yielding the inactive metabolites carboxyphosphamide and 4-ketocyclophosphamide.

22. Ans. (a) Pembrolizumab *(Ref: CMDT 2022/p1626)*

Pembrolizumab is an immune check point inhibitor, it binds to PD-1 and stops the inhibitory signals for T cells resulting in activation of T cells against tumor cells. It is used for wide variety of cancers including advanced endometrial carcinoma.

23. Ans. (a) Cetuximab *(Ref: CMDT 2022/p1626)*

Cetuximab is a monoclonal antibody against EGFR whereas other drugs mentioned in the options are immune check point inhibitors.

Immune checkpoint inhibition using PD-1 or PD-L1 inhibitors (nivolumab, pembrolizumab, atezolizumab, and durvalumab) has an important role in the treatment of various cancers. Checkpoint inhibitors release T cells from the inhibitory signals they receive from tumor cells via the PD-1 pathway, restoring antitumor immunity.

However, significant side effects and toxicity have been reported with checkpoint inhibitors, especially autoimmune manifestations such as hepatitis, thyroiditis, hypophysitis, colitis, pneumonitis, and type 1 diabetes mellitus.

Drugs:
New:	Nivolumab
Drugs:	Durvalumab
Act:	Avelumab
At:	Atezolizumab
Immune:	Ipilimumab
Check:	Cemiplimab
Point:	Pembrolizumab

24. Ans. (a) Bebtelovimab *(Ref: CMDT 2022/p515)*

Bebtelovimab is a monoclonal antibody used for COVID-19. Other drugs mentioned in the options are used for sickle cell anemia.

Treatment options for Sickle cell anemia:

- Allogeneic hematopoietic **stem cell transplantation**, if performed before the onset of significant end-organ damage, can cure more than 80% of children with sickle cell anemia who have suitable HLA-matched donors, with a reasonably good quality of life.
- **Hydroxyurea** increases hemoglobin F levels epigenetically. It reduces the frequency of painful crises in patients whose quality of life is disrupted by frequent vaso-occlusive pain episodes.
- **Omega-3 fatty acid** supplementation may also reduce vaso-occlusive episodes and reduce transfusion needs in patients with sickle cell anemia.
- **L-glutamine** has been shown to favorably modulate sickle pain crises and acute chest syndrome.
- **Crizanlizumab** is a monoclonal antibody against P-selectin that reduces vaso-occlusive episodes by 50%. It acts by disrupting the adverse interactions of platelets, red blood cells, and leukocytes with the endothelial wall.
- **Voxelotor** inhibits the polymerization of deoxygenated sickle red blood cells and increases the hemoglobin in SS patients age 12 years or older.

INI CET NOVEMBER 2021

1. Elimination rate constant of a drug is 0.05/hr. What is its half life?
   - (a) 6.5 hr
   - (b) 20 hr
   - (c) 13.9 hr
   - (d) 8 hr

2. Anionic and slightly acidic drugs usually bind to:
   - (a) Albumin
   - (b) Alpha acid glycoprotein
   - (c) Ceruloplasmin
   - (d) Globulin

3. The following table gives the data of area under the curve (AUC) of drug A alone and AUC of drug A when combined with drug B. p value is <0.01. Which of the following statement regarding these drugs is most correct?

Drug	Area under the curve
A alone	550 ± 150
A plus B	850 ± 150

   - (a) Drug B decreases the first pass metabolism of drug A
   - (b) Drug B increases the systemic metabolism of drug A
   - (c) Drug B decreases the intestinal absorption of drug A
   - (d) Drug B increases the renal clearance of drug A

4. Category A, B, C, D, X division of drugs is based on:
   - (a) Safety in pregnancy
   - (b) Dose adjustment in renal failure
   - (c) Therapeutic index and safety
   - (d) Over the counter use of drug

5. Which dose of dopamine act preferably on beta-1 receptors?
   - (a) Less than 2 mcg/kg/min
   - (b) 2–10 mcg/kg/min
   - (c) 10–20 mcg/kg/min
   - (d) More than 20 mcg/kg/min

6. A patient is diagnosed with cluster headache. Treatment of choice is:
   - (a) 8 L/min of oxygen for 5 min
   - (b) 6 L/min of oxygen for 10 min
   - (c) Subcutaneous sumatriptan
   - (d) Sumatriptan

7. A patient presents with grade 2 pulmonary artery hypertension. Vasoreactive stimulation test is negative. Which is the most preferred initial management of this patient?
   - (a) Epoprostenol
   - (b) Amlodipine
   - (c) Alprostadil
   - (d) Ambrisentan

8. Resistant hypertension is defined as inability to attain goal blood pressure inspite of the concurrent use of 3 antihypertensive agents of different classes prescribed at optimal doses including:
   - (a) Alpha blockers
   - (b) Diuretics
   - (c) Reserpine
   - (d) Alpha-methyldopa

9. A 65-year-old man comes to OPD with history of fall. He is hypertensive with history of atrial fibrillation and is presently on captopril, atenolol, aspirin and amiodarone. He presents with the following finding as shown in the image. What is the most probable diagnosis?

   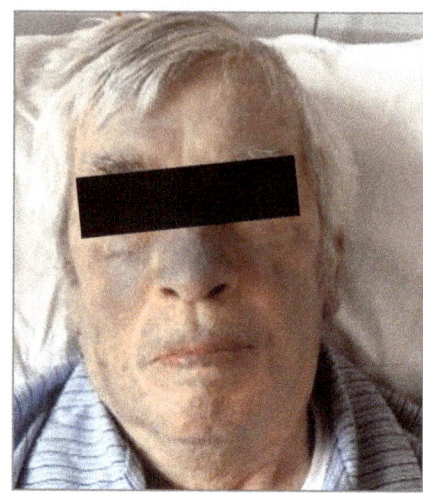

   - (a) Silver toxicity
   - (b) Lupus pernio
   - (c) Amiodarone induced skin lesion
   - (d) Captopril toxicity

10. A patient of chronic liver cirrhosis presents with ascites. Which of the following is the best diuretic to be used in this patient?
    - (a) Eplerenone
    - (b) Chlorothiazide
    - (c) Furosemide
    - (d) Triamterene

11. What is the prenatal dose of dexamethasone given for lung maturation in premature infants?
    - (a) 6 mg 2 doses 12 hours apart
    - (b) 12 mg 2 doses 24 hours apart
    - (c) 6 mg 4 doses 12 hours apart
    - (d) 6 mg 4 doses 24 hours apart

12. A 60-year-old female presents to hospital for routine check-up. She attained menopause at 52 years of age and has a past history of Colles' fracture. DEXA scan was done and T-score is -2.5. What should be the treatment given to this patient?
    - (a) Vitamin D and calcium supplementation
    - (b) Alendronate
    - (c) Repeat DEXA Scan
    - (d) Hormone replacement therapy

13. Dose of carbetocin for postpartum hemorrhage is:
    - (a) 50 mcg IV over 2 min
    - (b) 100 mcg IV over 1 min
    - (c) 150 mcg IM over 2 min
    - (d) 200 mcg IV over 1 min

14. Which of the following drug is the only medication useful in preventing disability progression in a patient with primary progressive multiple sclerosis?
    - (a) Natalizumab
    - (b) Ocrelizumab
    - (c) Siponimod
    - (d) Rituximab

15. Most effective cessation agent when used as monotherapy for smoking cessation is:
    (a) Varenicline
    (b) Nicotine gum
    (c) Sustained release bupropion
    (d) Nicotine patch

16. Which of the following is an opioid anti-tussive agent?
    (a) Diphenoxylate
    (b) Levorphanol
    (c) Ambroxol
    (d) Levopropoxyphene

17. Which of the following is a novel antidepressant drug?
    (a) Vilazodone   (b) Asenapine
    (c) Flibanserin   (d) Lurasidone

18. Which of the following antidepressant drug should be avoided in a patient of angle closure glaucoma?
    (a) Sertraline   (b) Amitriptyline
    (c) Mirtazapine   (d) Venlafaxine

19. Which of the following antiepileptic drug is used in treatment of neuropathic pain?
    (a) Gabapentin   (b) Lamotrigine
    (c) Carbamazepine   (d) Pregabalin

20. Which of the following drugs improves bioavailability and prolongs duration of action of Saquinavir?
    (a) Ritonavir   (b) Cimetidine
    (c) Vitamin C   (d) Remdesivir

21. A patient on phenytoin for seizure disorder was prescribed sucralfate 4 times a day for peptic ulcer. What should be the minimum duration between consumption of two drugs?
    (a) 30 min   (b) 60 min
    (c) 90 min   (d) 120 min

22. Mechanism of action of Remdesivir is inhibition of:
    (a) RNA dependent RNA polymerase
    (b) DNA dependent RNA polymerase
    (c) Viral protease enzyme
    (d) Cell wall synthesis

23. Which of the following cephalosporins can increase the effect of warfarin resulting in raised INR and increased risk of bleeding?
    (a) Cefoperazone   (b) Cefixime
    (c) Ceftobiprole   (d) Ceftazidime

24. A female patient presented with greenish vaginal discharge and pruritus. On colposcopy, strawberry cervix is noted. What is the drug of choice for this condition?
    (a) Ceftriaxone   (b) Metronidazole
    (c) Acyclovir   (d) Fluconazole

25. What is mechanism of action of Cyclosporine?
    (a) Calcineurin inhibitor
    (b) mTOR inhibitor
    (c) IL-2 receptor antagonist
    (d) TNF-α inhibitor

EXPLANATIONS

1. **Ans. (c) 13.9 hours** *(Ref: KDT 8th/p39)*

   $T_{1/2} = 0.693/k$
   Where k is elimination rate constant
   Thus, in this case
   $T_{1/2} = 0.693/0.05 = 13.9$ hours

2. **Ans. (a) Albumin** *(Ref: KDT 8th/p25)*
   - Acidic drugs like barbiturates, most NSAIDs, etc. mostly bind to albumin.
   - Basic drugs like atropine, morphine etc bind to alpha 1 acid glycoprotein.

3. **Ans. (a) Drug B decreases the first pass metabolism of drug A** *(Ref: KDT 8th/p22-23)*
   - Drug B increases the area under the curve (AUC) of drug A. Latter is a measure of extent of absorption (bio-availability). As drug B is increasing the bioavailability of drug A, the only relevant option becomes decrease in first pass metabolism of A.

4. **Ans. (a) Safety in pregnancy** *(Ref: KDT 8th/p1017)*

   The various categories of drug according to safety in pregnancy are:

   Category A
   Adequate and well-controlled studies have failed to demonstrate a risk to the fetus in the first trimester of pregnancy (and there is no evidence of risk in later trimesters). Examples include levothyroxine, folic acid, etc.

   Category B
   Animal reproduction studies have failed to demonstrate a risk to the fetus and there are no adequate and well-controlled studies in pregnant women. Examples are metformin, amoxicillin, etc.

   Category C
   Animal reproduction studies have shown an adverse effect on the fetus and there are no adequate and well-controlled studies in humans, but potential benefits may warrant use of the drug in pregnant women despite potential risks. Examples are gabapentin, trazodone, etc.

   Category D
   There is positive evidence of human fetal risk based on adverse reaction data from investigational or marketing experience or studies in humans, but potential benefits may warrant use of the drug in pregnant women despite potential risks. Examples include losartan.

   Category X
   Studies in animals or humans have demonstrated fetal abnormalities and/or there is positive evidence of human fetal risk based on adverse reaction data from investigational or marketing experience, and the risks involved in use of the drug in pregnant women clearly outweigh potential benefits. Examples include thalidomide, methotrexate, etc.

5. **Ans. (b) 2–10 mcg/kg/min** *(Ref: Harrison 19th/p1761)*

   Dopamine act on different receptors at different doses.
   - Less than 2 mcg/kg/min: D1 stimulation: Renal vasodilation
   - 2–10 mcg/kg/min: Beta 1 stimulation: Cardiac stimulation
   - More than 10 mcg/kg/min: Alpha 1 stimulation: Vasoconstriction

6. **Ans. (d) Sumatriptan** *(Ref: CMDT 2022/p981)*
   - Cluster headache is one of the trigeminal autonomic cephalgias.
   - Treatment of an individual attack with oral medications is generally unsatisfactory, but subcutaneous (6 mg) or intranasal (20 mg/spray) sumatriptan or inhalation of 100% oxygen (12–15 L/min for 15 minutes via a non-rebreather mask) may be effective.
   - Zolmitriptan (5- and 10-mg nasal spray) is also effective.
   - Dihydroergotamine (0.5–1 mg intramuscularly or intravenously) or viscous lidocaine (1 mg of 4–6% solution intranasally) is sometimes effective.
   - Various prophylactic agents include oral medications such as lithium carbonate, verapamil and topiramate.

7. **Ans. (d) Ambrisentan** *(Ref: CMDT 2022/p302,434)*

   Drugs used in pulmonary hypertension may act via following three main pathways:
   (1) The nitric oxide pathway: Phosphodiesterase inhibitors (sildenafil, tadalafil) and soluble guanylate cyclase stimulators (riociguat).
   (2) The endothelin pathway: Endothelin receptor antagonists (bosentan, ambrisentan, macitentan).
   (3) The prostacyclin pathway: Prostacyclin analogs (intravenous epoprostenol; intravenous, subcutaneous, inhaled, or oral treprostinil; inhaled iloprost) and prostacyclin receptor agonist (selexipag).
   - Calcium channel blockers like amlodipine are drug of choice for pulmonary hypertension in patients with positive vasoreactive testing.
   - In vasoreactive testing is negative, the drug of choice for pulmonary hypertension are endothelin antagonists.

8. **Ans. (b) Diuretics** *(Ref: CMDT 2022/p472)*
   - Resistant hypertension is defined as the failure to reach blood pressure control in patients who are adherent to full doses of an appropriate three-drug regimen (including a diuretic).
   - Usually, the patient is resistant to ACE inhibitors/ARBs, calcium channel blockers and diuretics.
   - Aldosterone antagonists like spironolactone are effective for the treatment of resistant hypertension.

9. **Ans. (c) Amiodarone induced skin lesion** *(Ref: KDT 8th/p578)*
   - This is classical presentation of blue man syndrome caused by amiodarone.
   - Blue man syndrome is thought to stem from the deposition of lysosomal membrane-bound dense bodies, similar to lipofuscin, in the dermis of patients on chronic amiodarone therapy.

10. **Ans. (a) Eplerenone** *(Ref: CMDT 2022/p456,706)*
    - Due to ascites, there is decrease in extracellular fluid. It activates renin angiotensin pathway resulting in increased level of aldosterone in patients with cirrhosis.

- Aldosterone antagonists like spironolactone and eplerenone are highly effective diuretics in patients with cirrhosis.

11. Ans. (c) 6 mg 4 doses 12 hours apart
(Ref: CMDT 2022/p810)
- Dexamethasone and betamethasone can be used antenatally for fetal lung maturation in premature delivery.
- Both the drugs are given by intramuscular route to mother.
- Total dose of both the drugs is 24 mg.
- Betamethasone is given as two doses each of 12 mg at an interval of 24 hours.
- Dexamethasone is given as 4 doses of 6 mg each at intervals of 12 hours.

12. Ans. (b) Alendronate *(Ref: CMDT 2022/p1163)*

This is a case of post-menopausal osteoporosis and bisphosphonates like alendronate are drug of choice.
- Bisphosphonates act by inhibiting the action of osteoclasts.
- Major adverse effect of these drugs is esophageal toxicity.

13. Ans. (b) 100 mcg IV over 1 min *(Ref: KDT 8th/p357)*
- Carbetocin is a long-acting analogue of oxytocin.
- It is used for treatment of PPH and prevention of uterine atony after caesarean section.
- The dose of carbetocin is 100 mcg intravenously infused over a period of 1 min.

14. Ans. (b) Ocrelizumab *(Ref: CMDT 2022/p1032)*
- Ocrelizumab is the only drug which is effective in preventing disability progression in patients with primary progressive multiple sclerosis.
- Interferons, glatiramer and dimethylfumarate are commonly used as initial therapy to reduce frequency of attacks in relapsing remitting multiple sclerosis.
- For patients with active secondary disease, cladribine, ocrelizumab, ofatumumab and Siponimod, etc. can be used

15. Ans. (a) Varenicline
(Ref: CMDT 2022/7-8, Harrison 19th/p2731)

Anti-Smoking drugs
- Varenicline: It is the single most effective drug for smoking cessation.
  It is a direct acting nicotinic agonist having selectivity for α4β2 isoform of NN receptors.
  It can be used orally and has a half-life of 14-20 hours.
  Its adverse effects include headache, nausea and sleep disturbances.
- Nicotine: A transdermal patch containing nicotine is applied to the patient's body. The dose of nicotine is then slowly decreased and finally withdrawn. It is effective in only 18-20% of the patients. It is also available in the form of lozenges.
- Bupropion: It is an anti-depressant drug that can be used for cessation of smoking. It acts by inhibition of neuronal reuptake of 5-HT, NE and DA. The duration of treatment is for 8–10 weeks. It can result in CNS stimulation leading to seizures.
- Clonidine: It is a very effective drug for reducing the withdrawal effects of nicotine. It is better than nicotine chewing gum as it can be used in patients with cardiac diseases also. It decreases the craving as well as is useful for insomnia.

16. Ans. (d) Levopropoxyphene
(Ref: Medicinal Chemistry p502)
- Levopropoxyphene was used as an opioid antitussive drug. Its dextro isomer is used as an analgesic.
- Diphenoxylate is an opioid that is used for treatment of diarrhea.
- Ambroxol is an expectorant.
- Levorphanol is an opioid used as an analgesic.

17. Ans. (a) Vilazodone *(Ref: CMDT 2022/p1081)*
- Vilazodone is an atypical antidepressant drug like nefazodone and trazodone.
- Asenapine and lurasidone are antipsychotic drugs.
- Flibanserin is indicated for treatment of hypoactive sexual desire disorder in females.

18. Ans. (b) Amitriptyline *(Ref: KDT 8th/p486)*
- Amitriptyline is a tricyclic antidepressant.
- It possesses very strong anticholinergic properties
- Due to anti-cholinergic action, TCAs can precipitate acute attack of glaucoma in patients with closure glaucoma.
- It is therefore, avoided in patients with angle closure glaucoma.

19. Ans. (a), (c), (d) *(Ref: CMDT 2022/p94)*
- Gabapentin and pregabalin, are first-line therapies for neuropathic pain. Both medications have no significant medication interactions. However, they can cause sedation, dizziness, ataxia, and gastrointestinal side effects. Both gabapentin and pregabalin require dose adjustments in patients with kidney dysfunction.
- Serotonin norepinephrine reuptake inhibitors (SNRIs) duloxetine and venlafaxine are also first-line treatments for neuropathic pain. Patients should be advised to take duloxetine on a full stomach because nausea is a common side effect. Because venlafaxine can cause hypertension and induce ECG changes, patients with cardiovascular risk factors should be carefully monitored when starting this medication. Desvenlafaxine, the active metabolite of venlafaxine, is also available and may be tolerated better than venlafaxine.
- TCAs are another class of medications for neuropathic pain that work through the norepinephrine and serotonin pathways. Among the TCAs that are effective for neuropathic pain, nortriptyline and desipramine are preferred over amitriptyline because they cause less orthostatic hypotension and have fewer anticholinergic effects.
- Carbamazepine is used in treatment of post herpetic and trigeminal neuralgia.
- Topical medications, such as lidocaine 5% patch and capsaicin 8% patches, are considered second-line therapies.
- Other medications effective for neuropathic pain include tramadol and tapentadol, both of which are opioids with norepinephrine activity. Medical cannabis strains high in cannabidiol have proven efficacy for some types of neuropathic pain.

20. Ans. (a) Ritonavir *(Ref: CMDT 2022/p1366)*
- Saquinavir is an HIV protease inhibitor and is metabolized by hepatic microsomal enzymes CYP3A4.

- Ritonavir at low doses inhibits this enzyme and thus improves the bioavailability and duration of action of other protease inhibitors like saquinavir.
- This phenomenon is known as ritonavir boosting.

21. **Ans. (d) 120 min** *(Ref: Goodman Gilman 13th/p913)*
    - Sucralfate forms a viscous layer in the stomach that may inhibit absorption of other drugs, including phenytoin, digoxin, cimetidine, ketoconazole, and fluoroquinolone antibiotics.
    - Sucralfate therefore should be taken at least 2 hours after the administration of other drugs.
    - The "sticky" nature of the viscous gel produced by sucralfate in the stomach also may lead to the formation of bezoars in some patients, particularly in those with underlying gastroparesis.

22. **Ans. (a) RNA dependent RNA polymerase** *(Ref: CMDT 2022/p1411)*
    - Remdesivir is the only FDA approved drug used for treatment of COVID-19 pneumonia.
    - It acts by inhibiting RNA dependent RNA polymerase enzyme in the virus.
    - It is indicated in hospitalized patients with moderate to severe pneumonia.
    - It should not be used beyond 10 days of illness.

23. **Ans. (a) Cefoperazone** *(Ref: KDT 8th/p670,778)*
    - Some cephalosporins like cefoperazone, cefotetan, moxalactam etc can cause hypoprothrombinemia.
    - These can increase risk of bleeding particularly when used with warfarin like drugs

24. **Ans. (b) Metronidazole** *(Ref: CMDT 2022/p790-91)*
    - Greenish vaginal discharge, pruritis and strawberry cervix points towards the diagnosis of trichomoniasis.
    - The drug of choice for treatment of trichomoniasis is metronidazole or tinidazole.

25. **Ans. (a) Calcineurin inhibitor** *(Ref: KDT 8th/p937)*
    - Calcineurin is required for the activation of NFAT (nuclear factor of activated T cells) which in turn increases the transcription of IL-2 by activated T cells.
    - Cyclosporine and tacrolimus (FK 506) inhibit the activation of NFAT by binding to immunophilins (cyclosporine binds to cyclophilin and tacrolimus binds to FKBP).
    - Net result of administration of cyclosporine and tacrolimus is inhibition of gene transcription of IL-2. These are used as immunosuppressive agents for organ transplantation, GVHD and some autoimmune diseases like rheumatoid arthritis and psoriasis.

INI CET JULY 2021

1. Which of the following is wrongly matched?
   (a) Dabigatran: Idarucizumab
   (b) Rivaroxaban: Andexanet alpha
   (c) Fondaparinux: Ciraparantag
   (d) Apixaban: Andexanet alpha

2. A patient had symptoms of redness and photophobia. On examination, cells were present in anterior chamber with keratic precipitates. Intraocular pressure was measured to be 38 mm Hg. Which of the following anti-glaucoma drug should be avoided?
   (a) PG analogues
   (b) Beta blockers
   (c) Mannitol
   (d) Carbonic anhydrase inhibitors

3. A hypertensive patient has grade 4 renal failure and GFR less than 30 mL/min. The physician wants to prescribe a thiazide diuretic. Which is the best drug for this patient?
   (a) Hydrochlorothiazide
   (b) Chlorthalidone
   (c) Metolazone
   (d) Indapamide

4. A study was conducted to see the effect of different drugs on isolated mammalian intestinal tissue in Dale's organ bath. Which of the following is the likely drug from the graph shown below?
   (a) Acetylcholine
   (b) Barium chloride
   (c) Adrenaline
   (d) KCl

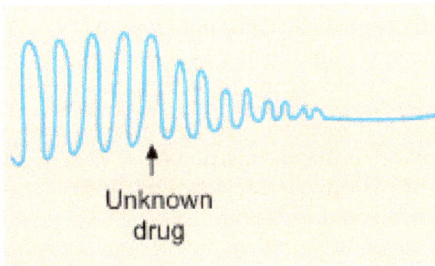

5. Inhaled NO is used for the treatment of:
   (a) Pulmonary hypertension
   (b) Migraine
   (c) Labile hypertension
   (d) Resistant epilepsy

6. Nivolumab is a monoclonal antibody used for the treatment of:
   (a) Hodgkin's lymphoma
   (b) Medulloblastoma
   (c) Retinoblastoma
   (d) Pleuropulmonary blastoma

7. A patient was taking chemotherapy cyclophosphamide, methotrexate and 5-Fluorouracil for treatment of breast cancer. She developed fever and on investigations, she had anemia and neutropenia. Which of the following antimicrobial is not indicated in this patient for treatment of this infection?
   (a) Piperacillin-tazobactam
   (b) Cefepime
   (c) Linezolid
   (d) Meropenem

8. A patient on retigabine therapy for a month for focal seizures. Phenytoin was added to therapy. What is the next step?
   (a) Change retigabine to carbamazepine
   (b) Decrease dose
   (c) Increase dose
   (d) Stop retigabine

9. Which of the following drugs can be used for the treatment of severe COVID-19 pneumonia in children?
   (a) Steroids
   (b) Remdesivir
   (c) Ivermectin
   (d) All of these

10. We administer a drug following first order kinetics. If the administered dose is doubled:
    (a) Plasma concentration and elimination half-life remains same
    (b) Plasma concentration becomes double and elimination half-life remains same
    (c) Elimination half-life becomes double and plasma concentration remains same
    (d) Elimination half-life and plasma concentration both becomes double

11. Which of the following is correctly matched regarding intrinsic resistance to antifungals?
    (a) Aspergillus niger: Voriconazole
    (b) Candida glabrata: Amphotericin B
    (c) Candida krusei: Fluconazole
    (d) Aspergillus marneffi : Micafungin

12. Identify the mechanism of action of vancomycin from the given figure:

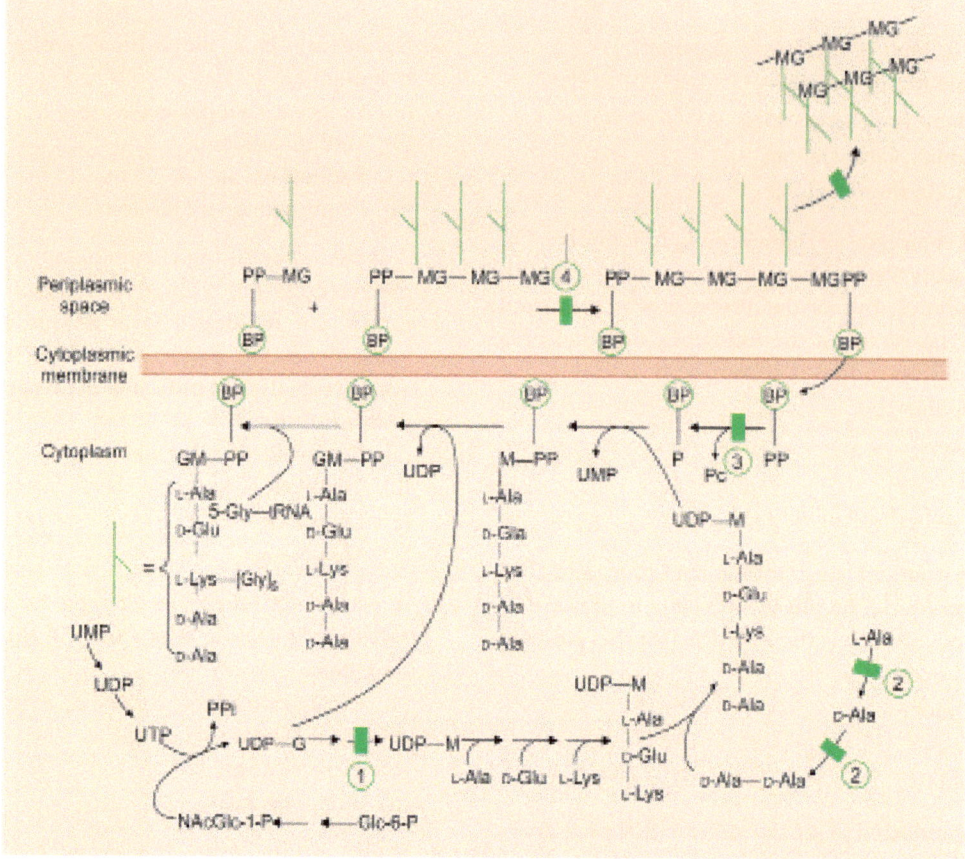

13. Topiramate is used for the treatment of:
    (a) Lennox-Gastaut syndrome
    (b) Attention deficit hyperkinetic disorder
    (c) Treatment of migraine
    (d) Prophylaxis of heat stroke

14. What is NOT the off label use of risperidone?
    (a) Post traumatic stress disorder
    (b) Obsessive compulsive disorder
    (c) Dementia
    (d) Bipolar disorder

15. Which of the following is FDA-approved drug for long term treatment of obesity?
    (a) Sibutramine   (b) Liraglutide
    (c) Metformin   (d) Fenfluramine

16. A newly diagnosed tuberculosis patients was found to be HIV positive. Which of the following statement is true about treatment of this patient?
    (a) Start ATT and ART together
    (b) ART should be started only if CD4 count is less than 50/mcL
    (c) ATT should be started first followed by ART 2 weeks later
    (d) ART should be started first followed by ATT 2 weeks later

17. A patient with stroke was started on clopidogrel. He developed another episode of stroke 6 months later. Which of the following is the likely cause?
    (a) Rapid metabolism by CYP 1A2
    (b) Poor metabolism by CYP 2C19
    (c) Poor metabolism by CYP 2D6
    (d) Poor metabolism by CYP 2E1

18. Which of the following is true about nicotine replacement therapy?
    (a) Varenicline is a form of NRT that comes with black box warning of cardiovascular adverse effects
    (b) There should be a gap of minimum 15 minutes between nicotine and coffee or acidic food
    (c) NRT is given by GI route
    (d) Nicotine gum is better because it attains 10-15 percent higher plasma concentration than lozenges

19. A patient was given ipratropium and he developed paradoxical bronchoconstriction. Which is not a likely mechanism of this bronchoconstriction?
    (a) Benzalkonium chloride
    (b) Presynaptic stimulation of M2 autoreceptors
    (c) Use of hypertonic saline in nebuliser
    (d) EDTA

20. Mechanism of action of local anaesthetics is:
    (a) Alters the resting membrane potential of the cell
    (b) Decrease transport of K across cell
    (c) Decrease transport of Na via voltage-gated channels
    (d) Binds to receptor complex and prevents activation of gates

21. For treatment of which of the following conditions, a combination of antimicrobials is usually not required?
    (a) Malaria
    (b) Gonorrhea
    (c) Intra-abdominal infection
    (d) Tuberculosis

EXPLANATIONS

1. **Ans. (c) Fondaparinux: Ciraparantag** *(Ref: CMDT 2022/p395,1593)*
   - Idarucizumab is a monoclonal antibody against dabigatran, a direct acting oral thrombin inhibitor
   - Andexanet alpha is an antidote for factor Xa inhibitors. It is FDA approved for reversing the effect of factor Xa inhibitors, rivaroxaban and apixaban. It has not been approved for reversal of anticoagulant effect of other Xa inhibitors till now.
   - Ciraparantag is an investigational drug for reversal of anticoagulant effects of a number of anticoagulants including factor Xa inhibitors (rivaroxaban, apixaban and edoxaban), dabigatran and heparins (unfractionated heparin, LMW heparin as well as fondaparinux). Although ciraparantag is antidote against fondaparinux also but it is not approved yet, so this seems to be the best answer among the given options.

2. **Ans. (a) PG analogues** *(Ref: KDT 8th/e p169)*
   - Presence of cells and Keratic precipitates in the anterior chamber suggests inflammation likely to be anterior uveitis.
   - PG analogues are contraindicated in the presence of inflammation as these are themselves mediators of inflammation.

3. **Ans. (c) Metolazone** *(Ref: CMDT 2022/p406)*
   - Thiazides are generally ineffective when the GFR falls below 30-40 mL/min.
   - Metolazone maintains its efficacy down to a GFR of approximately 20-30 mL/min.

4. **Ans. (c) Adrenaline** *(Ref: See below)*
   As the graph is showing decrease in amplitude after instillation of the drug, the drug is likely to be a smooth muscle relaxant like adrenaline.

5. **Ans. (a) Pulmonary hypertension** *(Ref: KK Sharma 3rd/e p253)*
   - Inhaled nitric oxide is the first vasodilator to produce truly selective pulmonary vasodilation.
   - It is used for treatment of pulmonary hypertension.

6. **Ans. (a) Hodgkin's lymphoma** *(Ref: CMDT 2022/p538)*
   Nivolumab is an immune checkpoint inhibitor. It is a monoclonal antibody against programmed death receptor, PD-1. It is approved for treatment of:
   - Metastatic melanoma
   - Non-small cell lung carcinoma
   - Renal cell carcinoma
   - Hodgkin's lymphoma
   - Squamous cell carcinoma of head and neck
   - Urothelial carcinoma
   - Colorectal carcinoma
   - Hepatocellular carcinoma

7. **Ans. (c) Linezolid** *(Ref: CMDT 2022/p1669)*
   - The patient is having immunosuppression due to bone marrow suppression (neutropenia).
   - Only cidal drugs should be used in immunosuppressed patients.
   - Linezolid is bacteriostatic and should be avoided in immunosuppressed conditions whereas all other options like piperacillin, cefepime and meropenem are beta lactams and bactericidal drugs.

8. **Ans. (c) Increase dose** *(Ref: Goodman Gilman 13th/e p314)*
   - Retigabine is also known as ezogabine.
   - It is a K channel opener used for focal seizures.
   - Its metabolism is induced by phenytoin and carbamazepine, so it requires increase in dosage when these drugs are given along with retigabine
   - Major adverse effect is retinal toxicity and visual problems.

9. **Ans. (a) Steroids** *(Ref: https://academic.oup.com/jpids/article/doi/10.1093/jpids/piaa045/5823622)*
   - Steroids are the only drugs which have been shown to provide mortality benefits in severe COVID-19
   - Remdesivir is indicated for management of severe COVID-19 in adults. It is however not approved in children.
   - Ivermectin can be used for mild cases of COVID-19 in adults. However it is not approved for use in adults or in children.

10. **Ans. (b) Plasma concentration becomes double and elimination half-life remains same** *(Ref: KDT 8th/e p38-42)*
    In first order kinetics
    - Half-life and clearance remains constant
    - Rate of elimination is directly proportional to plasma concentration.
    - Steady state plasma concentration is directly proportional to dosing rate

11. **Ans. (c) Candida krusei: Fluconazole** *(Ref: CMDT 2022/p1554)*
    - Candida krusei is intrinsically resistant to fluconazole. It should be treated with echinocandins or voriconazole
    - Preferred drugs for Candida glabrata are echinocandins with transition to oral fluconazole or voriconazole if isolate is susceptible. For resistant cases liposomal amphotericin B is indicated.

12. **Ans. 4.** *(Ref: KDT 8th/e p806)*
    - Vancomycin prevents chain elongation by inhibiting the transglycosylase enzyme (Option 4)
    - Fosfomycin acts by inhibiting the conversion of glucosamine to muramic acid (Option 1)
    - Cycloserine inhibits the enzyme Ala racemase and ligase (Option 2)
    - Bacitracin inhibits bactoprenol (Option 3)

13. **Ans. (a) Lennox-Gastaut syndrome** *(Ref: Goodman Gilman 13th/e p324)*
    - Topiramate is anti-epileptic drug that acts by multiple mechanisms including
      - Na channel blockade
      - K channel opening
      - Enhances GABA activity
      - Blocks AMPA glutamate receptors
      - Weak carbonic anhydrase inhibitor
    - It is particularly used for
      - Focal seizures (even for refractory seizures)
      - GTCS (even refractory)
      - Lennox-Gastaut syndrome

- Apart from epilepsy, it is also effective in
  - Anti-Craving drug of alcohol
  - Obesity
  - Migraine prophylaxis
  - Bipolar disorder

14. **Ans. (d) Bipolar disorder** *(Ref: CMDT 2019 p1082, 1065, https://psychopharmacologyinstitute.com/publication/risperidone-indications-fda-approved-and-off-label-uses-2124)*

    Bipolar disorder is approved indication of risperidone whereas all other 'off-label' uses of this drug.

    Risperidone is an atypical antipsychotic drug. It is **FDA approved** for treatment of:
    - Schizophrenia
    - Bipolar disorder
    - Autism spectrum disorders

    It is being used **off label** for treatment of:
    - Anxiety
    - Attention deficit hyperkinetic disorder
    - Obsessive compulsive disorder
    - To treat agitation in dementia (However, no antipsychotic has been shown to be reliably effective in dementia and may increase the risk of early mortality in elderly patients with dementia).
    - Post-traumatic stress disorder

15. **Ans. (b) Liraglutide** *(Ref: CMDT 2022/p1269)*

    FDA approved anti-obesity drugs include:
    - Orlistat
    - Phentermine-Topiramate
    - Naltrexone-Bupropion
    - Liraglutide
    - Semaglutide
    - Setmelanotide

16. **Ans. (c) ATT should be started first followed by ART 2 weeks later** *(Ref: CMDT 2022/p282-283)*

    Many patients with active TB have advanced HIV disease and are therefore eligible for ART. It is preferable not to initiate treatment for HIV and TB simultaneously, and when possible to delay ART till ATT is tolerated. This strategy:
    - Simplifies patient management
    - Avoids antiretroviral (ART) and TB drug interactions
    - Avoids overlapping toxicities
    - Limits risk of immune reconstitution inflammatory syndrome (IRIS)
    - Minimizes confusion about what drugs to take when, and for which disease
    - Increases adherence

17. **Ans. (b) Poor metabolism by CYP 2C19** *(Ref: CMDT 2022/p633)*
    - Clopidogrel is an anti-platelet drug.
    - It is a prodrug and is activated by CYP 2C19.
    - In people with poor metabolisers (less activity of CYP 2C19), sufficient clopidogrel is not able to get activated and thus is not able to provide anti-platelet effect.

18. **Ans. (b) There should be a gap of minimum 15 minutes between nicotine and coffee or acidic food** *(Ref: CMDT 2022/p6-7)*

    US-FDA approved medications for smoking-cessation include:
    - Nicotine Replacement Therapy (NRT)
    - Bupropion
    - Varenicline.

Nicotine Replacement Therapy

NRT may be in the form of slow sustained release (transdermal patches) or acute NRT formulations (gums, lozenges, sub-lingual tablet, oral inhaler and nasal spray).

Transdermal patch:
- The main advantage of nicotine patches over acute NRT formulations is that it is easy to administer, requires less frequent dosing, with fewer adverse effects and better compliance. It delivers nicotine more slowly than acute NRT formulations.
- The disadvantage of the patch is the lack of acute (rescue) dosing for craving episodes, which can be provided with other NRTs. In fact, the nicotine patch may be combined with other NRTs to increase its efficacy.
- The most frequently reported side effects are local skin reactions. Changing the site of patch application daily can reduce this problem. Sleep disturbances have also been commonly reported with 24-hour patches.

Acute Dosing Nicotine Products

Nicotine Gum
- It is not chewed like ordinary gum, but is intermittently chewed and held in the mouth over about 30 minutes, as needed, to release its nicotine.
- It is available in 2 mg and 4 mg dosage forms.
- Acidic beverages like coffee and juices should be avoided before and after the use of nicotine gum, because they decrease the absorption of nicotine. Nicotine gum also provides substitute oral activity during tobacco abstinence.

Nicotine Lozenge
- It is also available in 2 mg and 4 mg formulations.
- Lozenge is not chewed, it dissolves in the mouth over approximately 30 minutes
- As with nicotine gum, nicotine from the lozenge is absorbed slowly through the buccal mucosa and delivered into systemic circulation.
- The nicotine lozenge delivers 25% more nicotine than nicotine gum, because some nicotine is retained in the gum whereas nicotine is dissolved completely in lozenge.
- The lozenge may have better patient acceptability, especially in those who cannot use the gum because of dentures temporomandibular joint pain or for those who do not prefer chewing gum.

Nicotine Sublingual Tablet
- This product is designed to be held under the tongue where the nicotine in the tablet is absorbed sublingually.
- Like the lozenge, the tablet has the advantage of not requiring chewing.
- The levels of nicotine obtained by use of the lozenge and sublingual tablet are similar.

Nicotine Oral Inhaler
- The inhaler was designed to satisfy behavioral aspects of smoking, namely, the *hand-to-mouth ritual.*
- Although termed an "inhaler" the majority of nicotine is delivered into the oral cavity and in the GIT. Very little nicotine is delivered to the lung. Because absorption is primarily through the buccal mucosa, the rate of absorption is similar to that of nicotine gum.

- It produces peak levels of nicotine in 15 minutes (as compared to 30 min with gum and lozenges)

Nicotine Nasal Spray
- It achieves peak venous nicotine levels within 4-15 min, faster than any other NRT.
- Due to the fast nicotine delivery, nicotine spray may have some abuse liability.
- The main disadvantage of a nasal spray is the initial local irritation.

Non-nicotinic Drugs for Smoking Cessation

Varenicline
- It is an analogue of cytisine.
- It is a highly selective and partial agonist at α_4-β_2 receptor producing lesser response than that of nicotine. Thus, varenicline maintains a moderate level of dopamine release, which reduces craving and withdrawal symptoms during abstinence. It also blocks the reinforcing effects of nicotine obtained from cigarette smoke in the case of relapse.
- Varenicline is the non-nicotine containing medication.
- The main adverse effects such as nausea, headache, vomiting, flatulence, insomnia and abnormal dreams, generally mild in nature are observed which diminish over time.
- Varenicline was also found to be safe for treating smokeless tobacco dependence.

Bupropion
- It is an anti-depressant that acts as a neuronal reuptake inhibitor of dopamine and noradrenaline.
- It is used in sustained release formulation.
- It is an oral non-nicotine therapy.
- Dopaminergic activity of bupropion affects the area implicated in the reinforcing properties of the addictive drug and the development of dependence - the reward pathway, or mesolimbic system - while its noradrenergic activity in the locus ceruleus plays a role in withdrawal from nicotine.
- Bupropion lowers the seizure threshold and should not be used in those with history of seizure disorder, serious head trauma, eating disorders (bulimia or anorexia nervosa) and in those who receive other medications that may lower seizure threshold.

19. **Ans. (b) Presynaptic stimulation of M2 autoreceptor** *(Ref: Internet)*

    Ipratropium is an anticholinergic drug and cause bronchodilation.
    Few people may develop paradoxical bronchoconstriction with ipratropium due to:
    - Impurities like benzalkonium chloride and EDTA in preparations
    - Use of hypertonic saline in nebuliser
    - Presynaptic inhibition of M2 autoreceptors and more release of ACh

20. **Ans. (c) Decrease transport of Na via voltage-gated channels** *(Ref: KDT 8th/e p387)*

    Local anaesthetics act by blocking Na channels in the neurons. This will decrease transport of Na via voltage-gated sodium channels.

21. **Ans. (b) Gonorrhea** *(Ref: CMDT 2022/p788)*
    - Gonorrhea is usually treated by single drug, ceftriaxone.
    - Usually many drugs are given in combination for treatment of diseases like malaria, tuberculosis, leprosy, HIV and intra-abdominal infections.
        - Malaria: Combination ACT is given
        - TB: Combination of H, R, Z and E is given
        - Intra-abdominal infections: Combination antimicrobials are given

NEET PG MAY 2022

1. A patient was given intravenous botulinum toxin and the patient died. Mechanism of botulinum toxin overdose is:
   (a) Inhibits release of acetylcholine
   (b) Inhibit reuptake of nor-epinephrine
   (c) Blockade of postsynaptic nicotinic cholinergic receptors
   (d) Inhibit entry of acetylcholine in vesicle

2. Drug of choice in paracetamol overdose is:
   (a) N-acetylcysteine
   (b) Dopamine
   (c) Hydralazine
   (d) Furosemide

3. A young female presented with left sided severe throbbing headache associated with nausea, vomiting, photophobia and phonophobia. Which of the following drug can provide immediate relief to this patient?
   (a) Propranolol
   (b) Sumatriptan
   (c) Topiramate
   (d) Flunarizine

4. A patient on digoxin therapy accidently consumed 8 tablets of digoxin 0.25 mg. Two hours later, he presented to emergency with heart rate of 54 bpm and ECG evidence of third-degree AV block. What is the immediate management of this patient?
   (a) Digoxin immune Fab
   (b) Lignocaine
   (c) Phenytoin
   (d) DC cardioversion

5. An 82-year-old patient presented with acute episode of breathlessness. Chest X-ray shows pulmonary edema. History reveals that the patient has uncontrolled hypertension and is not taking the medication regularly. Which should be the management of this patient?
   (a) Intravenous nitroglycerine
   (b) Salbutamol nebulization
   (c) Intravenous salbutamol
   (d) Intravenous antibiotics plus oxygen

6. Which of the following hypolipidemic drug acts by inhibition of PCSK-9?
   (a) Atorvastatin
   (b) Evolocumab
   (c) Ezetimibe
   (d) Lomitapide

7. A patient presents with pituitary tumor that overproduces growth hormone. Surgical removal of the tumor was incomplete. What is the first line treatment of this patient?
   (a) Leuprolide
   (b) Octreotide
   (c) Nafarelin
   (d) Goserelin

8. A 40-year-old male presents with protrusion of chin, excessive sweating, impaired glucose tolerance and enlargement of hands and feet? Which of the following drugs is a growth hormone receptor antagonist used to treat this condition?
   (a) Pegvisomant
   (b) Octreotide
   (c) Cabergoline
   (d) Olcegepant

9. A 40-year-old diabetic female presented to emergency with abdominal pain, vomiting and recent onset confusion. On examination, she had irregular breathing and dehydration. Her blood sugar is 539 mg/dL and there was presence of ketone bodies in the urine. Blood pressure of the patient is 80/50 mm Hg. What is the next best step in the management of this patient?
   (a) Regular insulin
   (b) Intravenous fluids
   (c) Intravenous fluids with regular insulin
   (d) Long-acting insulin

10. A female presented with galactorrhea. Her urine pregnancy test was negative. MRI of head revealed a large pituitary tumor. Patient refused to undergo surgery for the tumor. Which of the following is the best drug for the treatment of this patient?
    (a) Octreotide
    (b) Bromocriptine
    (c) Promethazine
    (d) Clozapine

11. A patient with opioid poisoning presents with severe respiratory depression. What is the most effective drug for treatment of this patient?
    (a) Fomepizole
    (b) Naltrexone
    (c) Flumazenil
    (d) Naloxone

12. A patient on anti-depressant therapy presents with elevated body temperature, dilated pupil, palpitations and low blood pressure. ECG shows tachycardia, broad QRS complex and right axis deviation. Which of the following interventions must be done immediately?
    (a) Wait and watch
    (b) Intravenous sodium bicarbonate
    (c) Intravenous esmolol
    (d) DC cardioversion

13. A patient presents with tremors, rigidity and bradykinesia. Which of the following drugs can be used for the treatment of this patient?
    (a) Selegiline
    (b) Donepezil
    (c) Fluoxetine
    (d) Haloperidol

14. A child born by normal vaginal delivery developed repeated attacks of flexion of neck over the trunk and jerks in the hands. EEG shows the presence of hypsarrhythmia. Antiepileptic drug of choice for this patient is:
    (a) Phenobarbitone
    (b) Phenytoin
    (c) ACTH
    (d) Levetiracetam

15. An 11-year-old boy presented to emergency with vomiting. Parents gave history of consuming 10-15 tablets of ferrous sulphate a day before. What is the antidote of iron for treatment of this patient?
    (a) Dimercaprol
    (b) Desferrioxamine
    (c) d-Penicillamine
    (d) Activated charcoal

16. A deep vein thrombosis patient was started on an anticoagulant therapy. Next day, the patient presented with the features shown in the diagram below. Likely drug implicated for this adverse effect is:

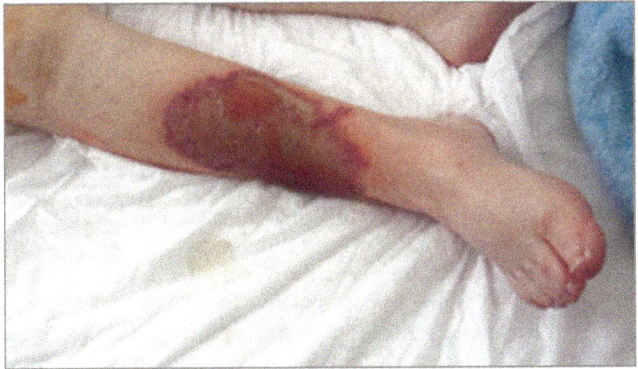

    (a) Heparin
    (b) Rivaroxaban
    (c) Warfarin
    (d) Dabigatran

17. A patient with COPD was given intravenous aminophylline therapy following which the patient developed diuresis. This is due to action on which effector?
    (a) Adenosine receptors
    (b) Beta 2 adrenergic receptors
    (c) IL-10
    (d) Histone deacetylase

18. A female with ovarian cancer was on cisplatin therapy. She presented to hospital with several episodes of vomiting. After giving an antiemetic drug, the patient developed dystonia. The antiemetic drug most likely to be responsible for these features is:
    (a) Metoclopramide   (b) Meclizine
    (c) Ondansetron   (d) Scopolamine

19. A pregnant female with urinary tract infection took antimicrobials for the same. The baby of this female developed tendon rupture and arthropathy. What is the likely mechanism of action of the antimicrobial consumed by the pregnant female?
    (a) Folic acid synthesis inhibitor
    (b) Mycolic acid synthesis inhibitor
    (c) DNA gyrase inhibitor
    (d) DNA inhibitor

20. A 48-year-old patient presented to OPD with tingling and numbness of fingers. The patient is chronic alcoholic and was recently started on antitubercular treatment. What should be the treatment of this patient?
    (a) Vitamin B_3 (b) Vitamin B_6
    (c) Vitamin B_1 (d) Vitamin B_{12}

21. In MDR tuberculosis, which of following drug combinations show resistance?
    (a) Rifampicin and Fluoroquinolones
    (b) Isoniazid and rifampicin
    (c) Isoniazid and Pyrazinamide
    (d) Rifampicin and kanamycin

22. A patient presented with hyperkalemia. Which of the following drugs can cause intracellular movement of and thus decrease in extracellular potassium levels?
    (a) Atropine   (b) Lactic acid
    (c) Epinephrine   (d) Glucagon

23. Which of the following drugs have least adverse effect on pleura?
    (a) Bromocriptine
    (b) Metformin
    (c) Nitrofurantoin
    (d) Methysergide

EXPLANATIONS

1. **Ans. (a) Inhibits release of acetylcholine**
   (Ref: KDT 8th/p110)
   - Botulinum toxin acts by inhibiting the exocytosis of acetylcholine from the vesicle.
   - Hemicholinium inhibits the uptake of choline by the neurons.
   - Vesamicol inhibits entry of acetylcholine in the vesicle.

2. **Ans. (a) N-acetylcysteine** *(Ref: CMDT 2022/p1590)*
   - Paracetamol is metabolized to N-acetyl para-aminobenzo quinone-imine (NAPQI) by microsomal enzymes. This metabolite has high affinity for sulfhydryl groups and can combine with the enzymes and other biomolecules resulting in hepatotoxicity.
   - Normally acetaminophen is a safe drug because glutathione (contain sulfhydryl group due to presence of sulfur containing amino acid, cysteine) produced by the liver combines with NAPQ to detoxify it. However chronic alcoholics are predisposed to toxicity because:
     – Glutathione production decreases due to liver disease.
     – Alcohol is a powerful inducer of microsomal enzymes. It increases the production of NAPQ from acetaminophen resulting in toxicity.
   - Acetaminophen toxicity can be decreased by providing sulfhydryl donors like N-acetylcysteine (antidote of choice). Gastric lavage (with activated charcoal) should be done to prevent further absorption but it is ineffective after 4 hours of ingestion.

3. **Ans. (b) Sumatriptan** *(Ref: CMDT 2022/p979)*

   This is a case of acute attack of migraine as suggested by headache associated with classical symptoms. Sumatriptan is used for treatment of acute attack of migraine whereas other drugs given in the options are used for prophylaxis of migraine.

4. **Ans. (a) Digoxin immune Fab** *(Ref: CMDT 2020/p1599)*

   This is a case of digoxin overdose as suggested by consumption of drug followed by symptoms like bradycardia and arrhythmias. Digoxin immune Fab (or digibind) is used for treatment of acute poisoning due to digoxin.

5. **Ans. (a) Intravenous nitroglycerine**
   (Ref: CMDT 2022/p414)
   - In full-blown pulmonary edema, the patient should be placed in a sitting position with legs dangling over the side of the bed; this facilitates respiration and reduces venous return. Oxygen is delivered by mask to obtain an arterial PO_2 greater than 60 mm Hg.
   - Morphine is highly effective in pulmonary edema and may be helpful in less severe decompensations when the patient is uncomfortable. The initial dosage is 2–8 mg intravenously (subcutaneous administration is effective in milder cases) and may be repeated after 2–4 hours. Morphine increases venous capacitance, lowering LA pressure, and relieves anxiety, which can reduce the efficiency of ventilation. However, morphine may lead to CO_2 retention by reducing the ventilatory drive. It should be avoided in patients with opioid-induced pulmonary edema, who may improve with opioid antagonists, and in those with neurogenic pulmonary edema.
   - Intravenous diuretic therapy (furosemide, 40 mg, or bumetanide, 1 mg—or higher doses if the patient has been receiving long-term diuretic therapy) is usually indicated even if the patient has not exhibited prior fluid retention. These agents produce venodilation prior to the onset of diuresis.
   - Nitrate therapy accelerates clinical improvement by reducing both BP and LV filling pressures. Sublingual nitroglycerine or isosorbide dinitrate, topical nitroglycerine, or intravenous nitrates will ameliorate dyspnea rapidly prior to the onset of diuresis, and these agents are particularly valuable in patients with accompanying hypertension.
   - Intravenous nesiritide, a recombinant form of human BNP, is a potent vasodilator that reduces ventricular filling pressures and improves cardiac output. Its hemodynamic effects resemble those of intravenous nitroglycerine with a more predictable dose–response curve and a longer duration of action. The role of nesiritide may be primarily in patients who continue to be symptomatic after initial treatment with diuretics and nitrates.
   - The role of positive inotropic agents appears to be limited to patients with refractory symptoms and signs of low cardiac output, particularly if life-threatening vital organ hypoperfusion (such as deteriorating kidney function) is present.

6. **Ans. (b) Evolocumab** *(Ref: CMDT 2022/p1679)*

   PCSK9 Inhibitors
   - Proprotein convertase subtilisin kexin type 9 (PCSK 9) is a protein that binds LDL-receptors and transport them to lysosomes where these are degraded.
   - Inhibitors of PCSK 9, therefore prevent destruction of LDL-R resulting in lowering of LDL-cholesterol.
   - Alirocumab and evolocumab are monoclonal antibodies against PCSK 9 and are approved for familial hypercholesterolemia as an adjunct to diet and maximally tolerated statin therapy.

7. **Ans. (b) Octreotide** *(Ref. CMDT 2022/p1118)*

   Acromegalic patients with an incomplete biochemical remission after pituitary surgery may benefit from medical therapy with following drugs.
   - Cabergoline is the oral dopamine agonist of choice. It is most successful for tumors that secrete both PRL and GH but can also be effective for patients with normal serum PRL levels. Cabergoline may be tried as monotherapy for patients with serum IGF-1 levels above normal but less than 2.5 times the upper limit of normal. It appears to be safe during pregnancy.
   - Octreotide LAR and lanreotide are long-acting somatostatin analogs that are given by monthly subcutaneous injection.
   - Raloxifene is a selective estrogen receptor modulator (SERM) that may be useful for persistent acromegaly in men and in women who are postmenopausal or who have had breast cancer. It does not reduce serum GH levels but normalizes serum IGF-1 levels.
   - Pegvisomant, a GH receptor antagonist, can be helpful for patients resistant to other treatments, especially when

there is associated diabetes mellitus. It blocks hepatic IGF-1 production but does not shrink GH-secreting tumors.

8. **Ans. (a) Pegvisomant** *(Ref: CMDT 2022/p1118)*
   - Pegvisomant is growth hormone receptor antagonist used for treatment of acromegaly.
   - Octreotide is a somatostatin analog indicated in treatment of acromegaly.
   - Cabergoline is a dopamine agonist used for acromegaly.
   - Olcegepant is a CGRP receptor antagonist used for migraine.

9. **Ans. (c) Intravenous fluids with regular insulin** *(Ref: CMDT 2022/p1246)*

   This is a case of diabetic ketoacidosis.
   Treatment of dehydration with IV fluids and administration of insulin are most effective treatment of diabetic ketoacidosis.

10. **Ans. (b) Bromocriptine** *(Ref: CMDT 2022/p1120)*
    - Dopamine agonists (cabergoline, bromocriptine, or quinagolide) are the initial treatment of choice for patients with giant prolactinomas and those with hyperprolactinemia desiring restoration of normal sexual function and fertility.
    - Cabergoline is the most effective and usually the best tolerated ergot-derived dopamine agonist. Bromocriptine is an alternative.
    - Women who experience nausea with oral preparations may find relief with deep vaginal insertion of cabergoline or bromocriptine tablets.
    - Patients whose tumor is resistant to one dopamine agonist may be switched to another in an effort to induce a remission.
    - Dopamine agonists are given at bedtime to minimize side effects of fatigue, nausea, dizziness, and orthostatic hypotension, which occur in up to 50% of patients.

11. **Ans. (d) Naloxone** *(Ref: KDT 8th/p511-12)*
    - Naloxone is drug of choice for treatment of acute opioid poisoning.
    - Naltrexone is used for maintenance in opioid poisoning due to its long duration of action.
    - Fomepizole is an antidote for methanol and ethylene glycol poisoning.
    - Flumazenil is used for treatment of benzodiazepine poisoning.

12. **Ans. (b) Intravenous sodium bicarbonate** *(Ref: KDT 8th/p487)*

    This is a case of TCA poisoning and most effective drug for TCA poisoning is sodium bicarbonate.

    TRICYCLIC ANTIDEPRESSANT POISONING:

    Clinical Presentation:
    The presenting signs of a TCA overdose include cardiac arrhythmias, hypotension, and anticholinergic signs (hyperthermia, flushing, dilated pupils, intestinal ileus, urinary retention, and sinus tachycardia). Central nervous system signs, such as confusion, delirium, and hallucinations, typically occur before the onset of seizures or coma. Cardiotoxic effects are responsible for the mortality in TCA overdose.

    Treatment
    - Intravenous sodium bicarbonate is the single most effective intervention for the management of TCA cardiovascular toxicity. This agent can reverse QRS prolongation, ventricular arrhythmias, and hypotension. Intravenous sodium bicarbonate is the treatment of choice for sudden-onset ventricular tachycardia, ventricular fibrillation, or cardiac arrest.
    - Lignocaine is the drug of choice for TCA-induced ventricular dysrhythmias. However, care must be taken to avoid precipitation of seizures. In comparison, many antiarrhythmic drugs should not be used with TCA overdoses. Propranolol, e.g., depresses myocardial contractility and conduction while procainamide, disopyramide, and quinidine, via membrane stabilizing effects, may enhance tricyclic toxicity
    - Intravenous fluids are the preferred therapy in hypotensive patients. Dopamine can be used if needed because it has both inotropic and vasoconstrictor activity. On the other hand, sympathomimetic vasopressor agents carry the risk of precipitating tachyarrhythmias.
    - Diazepam is the drug of choice in the management of acute-onset seizures. Phenytoin or phenobarbital may be used as second-line drugs.
    - Physostigmine, a short-acting cholinesterase inhibitor, has been referred to as the antidote for TCAs because of its ability to increase cholinergic tone and reverse anticholinergic effects. It can, however, causes severe bradycardia, seizures, and asystole by overcompensating for cholinergic tone and suppressing supraventricular and ventricular pacemakers. As a result, physostigmine should only be used in patients with coma or those with convulsion or arrhythmias resistant to standard therapy

13. **Ans. (a) Selegiline** *(Ref: KDT 8th/p458)*
    - The features of tremors, rigidity and bradykinesia points towards the diagnosis of Parkinsonism. Selegiline is a selective MAO-B inhibitor used in Parkinsonism.
    - Donepezil is used for treatment of Alzheimer's disease.
    - Fluoxetine is an anti-depressant drug of SSRI category.
    - Haloperidol is an anti-psychotic drug.

14. **Ans. (c) ACTH** *(Ref: Nelson 20th/p2840)*
    - West syndrome starts between the ages of 2 and 12 months and consists of a triad of infantile epileptic spasms that usually occur in clusters (particularly in drowsiness or upon arousal), developmental regression, and a typical EEG picture called hypsarrhythmia.
    - It is best treated with ACTH.

15. **Ans. (b) Desferrioxamine** *(Ref: KDT 8th/p652)*

    Iron Poisoning
    - Acute iron poisoning can occur in children due to accidental intake of large number of the iron tablets. The antidote of acute iron poisoning is desferrioxamine. It is given by IM injection. DTPA and calcium disodium EDTA may also be used but dimercaprol (BAL) is contraindicated because its complex with iron is itself toxic.
    - For chronic iron overload, as occurs in thalassemia patients, oral chelating agent like deferiprone is preferred.

16. **Ans. (c) Warfarin** *(Ref: KDT 8th/p668)*

    The history of anticoagulant treatment and skin necrosis points towards dermal vascular necrosis caused by warfarin.
    - Dermal vascular necrosis or purple toe syndrome is an early appearing adverse effect of warfarin.
    - It occurs within first few days of start of warfarin.
    - It occurs because warfarin inhibits the activation of clotting factors (factor 2, 7, 9 and 10) as well as anti-clotting factors (protein C and protein S). In patients with genetic deficiency of protein C, it may finish first in plasma leading to hypercoagulable state and thus dermal vascular necrosis.

17. **Ans. (a) Adenosine receptors** *(Ref: KDT 8th/p246)*

    Theophylline (and aminophylline) is a phosphodiesterase inhibitor and an antagonist of adenosine receptors. The adverse effects due to these actions include:

    Adverse effects due to phosphodiesterase inhibition:
    - GI side effects like nausea, vomiting, diarrhea
    - Arrhythmias

    Adverse effects due to adenosine receptor antagonism
    - Arrhythmias
    - Diuresis
    - Epilepsy (seizures)

18. **Ans. (a) Metoclopramide** *(Ref: KDT 8th/p714)*
    - The patient is presenting with dystonia which is an extrapyramidal symptom. It is caused by D2 antagonists like metoclopramide.
    - Drug of choice for treatment of dystonia is central anticholinergic drugs like benzhexol. Promethazine may be used as an alternative.

19. **Ans. (c) DNA gyrase inhibitor** *(Ref: KDT 8th/p759)*
    - The teratogenic effect of tendon rupture and arthropathy is caused by fluoroquinolones.
    - Fluoroquinolones act by inhibiting the enzyme DNA gyrase.

20. **Ans. (b) Vitamin B_6** *(Ref: KDT 8th/p817)*
    - Peripheral neuritis and a variety of neurological manifestations (paraesthesias, numbness, mental disturbances, rarely convulsions) are the most important dose dependent toxic effects of INH.
    - These are due to interference with utilization of pyridoxine (vitamin B_6) and its increased excretion in urine.
    - Pyridoxine is used for treatment as well as prevention of peripheral neuropathy due to isoniazid.

21. **Ans. (b) Isoniazid and rifampicin** *(Ref: KDT 8th/p824)*

    Drug resistant tuberculosis is classified as

Category	Resistance to
Mono drug resistant	Any one drug among H, Z and E
Poly drug resistance	Two or more drugs among H, Z and E
Rifampicin resistance	Resistance to R but sensitive to H
Multi drug resistance (MDR)	Both H and R
Extensive drug resistance (XDR)	H and R, Minimum one of the FQ and minimum one of the injectable drugs

22. **Ans. (c) Epinephrine** *(Ref: KDT 8th/p144)*

    Insulin and Beta 2 agonists (like salbutamol and epinephrine) result in increased movement of K towards intracellular sites. This action is utilized in treatment of hyperkalemia.

23. **Ans. (b) Metformin** *(Ref: CMDT 2022/p309)*
    - Bromocriptine and Methysergide are ergot alkaloids are associated with pleural fibrosis on long term use.
    - Nitrofurantoin can also cause pleural effusion.

NEET PG 2021

1. As an Indian medical intern, which of the following is the correct format for prescription of alprazolam?
   (a) Tablet alprazolam 0.5 mg once a day before bed time for 7 days
   (b) Tablet alprazolam 0.5 mg HS for 7 days
   (c) Tablet alprazolam 500 mcg one tablet OD for 7 days
   (d) Tablet alprazolam 0.5 mg tablet HS daily

2. Rate of administration of a drug is equal to rate of elimination. How will you calculate the dosing rate of the drug to maintain steady state concentration?
   (a) Dosing rate = Vd x target plasma concentration
   (b) Dosing rate = CL x target plasma concentration
   (c) Dosing rate = Vd/target plasma concentration
   (d) Dosing rate = CL/target plasma concentration

3. A patient with bronchial asthma presents with raised intraocular pressure. Treatment of open angle glaucoma in this patient is:
   (a) Latanoprost (b) Alprostadil
   (c) Gemeprost   (d) Carboprost

4. A patient presented with suspected cocaine overdose. Which of the following features is not seen in this patient?
   (a) Bradycardia
   (b) Agitation
   (c) Myocardial infarction
   (d) Hyperthermia

5. A child presents to hospital with agitation, photophobia and retention of urine. History reveals that he has eaten a wild fruit given by his friend. Which of the following substances is the likely cause of poisoning and its antidote respectively?
   (a) Dhatura, Physostigmine
   (b) Dhatura, Pralidoxime
   (c) Yellow Oleander, Physostigmine
   (d) Yellow Oleander, Pralidoxime

6. A 45-year-old patient being treated with low dose aspirin since 6 months presented with rectal bleeding. Inhibition of which of the following substance is likely to responsible for the bleeding?
   (a) TXA2   (b) LT
   (c) Bradykinin (d) PGI2

7. A 34 week pregnant female with polyhydramnios presents with labour pain. She was treated with indomethacin earlier. Which of the following can be likely outcome in the baby if delivery occurs at this time?
   (a) Patent ductus arteriosus
   (b) Premature closure of ductus arteriosus
   (c) Patent ductus venosus
   (d) Premature closure of ductus venosus

8. A 60-year-old female with renal disease was admitted for pyelolithotomy. Postoperative analgesic of choice in this patient is:
   (a) Diclofenac
   (b) Indomethacin
   (c) Naproxen
   (d) Acetaminophen

9. A 45-year-old patient presented with the symptoms shown in image below. Patient is a known hypertensive and was taking some antihypertensive drug. Which of the following drug is the likely cause of this condition?

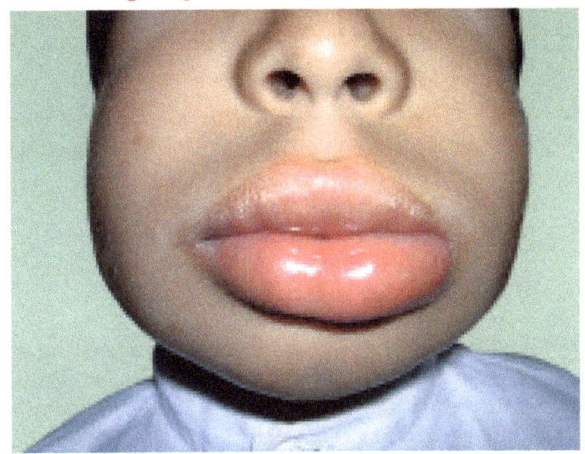

   (a) Lisinopril (b) Clonidine
   (c) Nifedipine (d) Timolol

10. Tocilizumab is an immunosuppressive drug used for Rheumatoid arthritis. It is a monoclonal antibody against:
    (a) IL-6 (b) IL-12
    (c) IL-2 (d) IL-3

11. A patient on digoxin therapy and had a level of 1 ng/mL. He was receiving several other drugs and presented 2 months later with flattening of T waves in ECG. Now the plasma level of digoxin is 3.8 ng/mL. Which of the following drug is likely to be responsible?
    (a) Triamterene   (b) Atenolol
    (c) Clarithromycin (d) KCl

12. A hypertensive patient presented with chronic renal insufficiency and pedal edema. On investigations, serum creatinine was found to be 1.9 mg/dL. Which of the following drug should be used for management of hypertension in this patient?
    (a) Prazosin   (b) Aliskiren
    (c) Chlorthalidone (d) Metoprolol

13. A 26-year-old female came to hospital for pre-conceptional counselling. Patient is a known hypertensive compliant to drug therapy. Which of the following drugs will you advise to stop?
    (a) Methyl dopa (b) Labetalol
    (c) Lisinopril (d) Nifedipine

14. Patient with a history of mitral stenosis and stroke presents with irregularly irregular heart beat. There is no clot in left atrium on TEE. Patient is already on ACE inhibitors and statins. Which of the following drug should be added for stroke prevention?
    (a) Warfarin
    (b) Dabigatran
    (c) Aspirin with clopidogrel
    (d) Aspirin

15. A 50-year-old male presents to the hospital with complaint of chest pain. Angiogram revealed left circumflex artery occlusion. Stenting is done and patient was started on aspirin 75 mg, atorvastatin 20 mg and metoprolol 50 mg. Which of the following statement is correct regarding further management of this patient?
    (a) Add a P2Y12 receptor blocker
    (b) Increase dose of aspirin
    (c) Increase dose of metoprolol to 100 mg
    (d) Add nifedipine

16. A 36 week pregnant female was taking warfarin for prosthetic heart valves and has INR value of 3. Next step in the management is:
    (a) Stop warfarin and start heparin
    (b) Stop warfarin and start heparin plus aspirin
    (c) Continue warfarin and add heparin
    (d) Switch to aspirin

17. A 60-year-old post-menopausal woman having a previous history of Colle's fracture presented with backache. Which of the following statements about anti-osteoporosis drugs is false regarding this patient?
    (a) Calcium requirement is 1200 mg per day
    (b) Oral vitamin D_3 should be given along with calcium supplements
    (c) Bisphosphonates therapy should not be given for more than one year
    (d) Teriparatide therapy should be followed by bisphosphonate therapy

18. An anesthetist injected bupivacaine in a patient for axillary nerve block. Later, the patient developed restlessness, agitation and cardiovascular collapse. Next best step in the management would be:
    (a) Cardiac resuscitation + dopamine
    (b) Cardiac resuscitation + dantrolene
    (c) Cardiac resuscitation + sodium bicarbonate
    (d) Cardiac resuscitation + 20% intralipid

19. A patient was admitted for surgery and halothane is being planned to be used as an anaesthetic agent. The patient was explained about the adverse effect of malignant hyperthermia with this drug. Which of the following drugs may also result in malignant hyperthermia?
    (a) Succinylcholine   (b) D-Tubocurarine
    (c) Dantrolene   (d) Baclofen

20. A patient presented to hospital with three bouts of vomiting and treated with anti-emetic drug. Vomiting subsided but after sometime, he developed abnormal movements. Which of the following drug is used for treatment of these motor symptoms?
    (a) Benzhexol   (b) Cyproheptadine
    (c) L-dopa   (d) Hyoscine

21. A patient having history of paronychia on finger presents with the following features as shown in image below. Drug of choice for treatment of this patient is:
    (a) CoAmoxyClav
    (b) Norfloxacin
    (c) Erythromycin
    (d) Amikacin

22. A female taking oral contraceptives acquired tuberculosis. After prescribing anti-tubercular therapy, physician advised the patient for alternative contraception. What is the probable reason of this advice?
    (a) Rifampicin causes teratogenicity
    (b) Isoniazid is teratogenic
    (c) Rifampicin increases the metabolism of oral contraceptives
    (d) Oral contraceptives decrease the efficacy of anti-tubercular therapy

23. Metronidazole is used for treatment of various anaerobic infections as well as bacterial vaginosis. Patient is instructed to avoid taking which of the following substance after metronidazole prescription to avoid possible adverse effects?
    (a) Grapefruit juice
    (b) Milk
    (c) Alcohol
    (d) Orange juice

24. A patient of borderline leprosy received multi drug therapy (MDT). He developed skin lesions as shown in the figure below. How should this patient be managed?

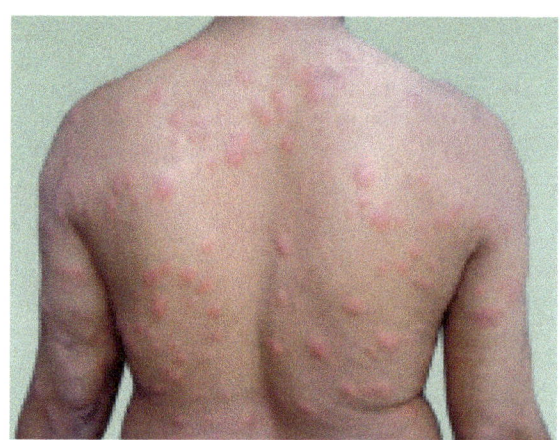

    (a) Stop MDT and give thalidomide
    (b) Continue MDT and give thalidomide
    (c) Stop MDT and give steroids
    (d) Continue MDT and give steroids

25. A 20-year-old boy presented with slow growing mass on the medial side of thigh. Investigations revealed it to be osteosarcoma and patient was started on methotrexate. Mechanism of action of methotrexate as an anticancer drug is:
    (a) Inhibition of dihydrofolate reductase
    (b) Inhibition of N5 tetrahydrofolate reductase
    (c) Inhibition of tyrosine kinase
    (d) Inhibition of purine metabolism

26. Topical application of 400 mcg/mL mitomycin C is used for:
    (a) Subglottic stenosis
    (b) Tympanoplasty
    (c) Rhinocerebral mucormycosis
    (d) Nasopharyngeal bleeding

EXPLANATIONS

1. **Ans. (a) Tablet alprazolam 0.5 mg once a day before bed time for 7 days** *(Ref: KK Sharma 3rd/e p929)*
   In the prescription, the use of abbreviations must be avoided. As the options b and d contains HS (abbreviation for bed time) and option c contains OD (abbreviation for once a day), these are not ideal prescriptions. So, the answer should be (a)

2. **Ans. (b) Dosing rate = CL x target plasma concentration** *(Ref: Katzung 13th/e p50)*
   At steady state, rate of administration is equal to rate of elimination. To maintain the steady state, the dose given is maintenance dose.
   The formula of maintenance dosing rate is CL x Target plasma concentration.

3. **Ans. (a) Latanoprost** *(Ref: Katzung 13th/e p328)*
   The drug of choice for primary open angle glaucoma is PGF2α analogs. The drugs used for this indication include latanoprost and bimatoprost.
   - Latanoprost is PGF2α used for treatment of glaucoma
   - Alprostadil is PGE1 used for keeping the ductus arteriosus patent
   - Gemeprost is PGE1 analog for cervical ripening
   - Carboprost is PGF2α for treatment of postpartum hemorrhage

4. **Ans. (a) Bradycardia** *(Ref: Katzung 13th/e p562-563)*
   Cocaine acts by inhibiting reuptake of nor-adrenaline. It thus produce sympathetic effects like tachycardia and hypertension. Bradycardia is unlikely to produce in cocaine overdose.
   - Use of cocaine causes **abnormally fast heart rhythms** and a marked elevation of blood pressure (hypertension), which can be life-threatening. This can lead to death from acute myocardial infarction, acute respiratory failure (i.e., hypoxemia, with or without hypercapnia), stroke, cerebral hemorrhage, and sudden cardiac arrest.
   - Cocaine overdose may result in **hyperthermia** as stimulation and increased muscular activity cause greater heat production. Heat loss is also inhibited by the cocaine-induced vasoconstriction. Cocaine and/or associated hyperthermia may cause muscle cell destruction (rhabdomyolysis) and myoglobinuria resulting in kidney failure.
   - Some psychological symptoms due to an overdose include **agitation**, paranoia, delirium, anxiety as well as panicked feelings.

5. **Ans. (a) Dhatura, Physostigmine** *(Ref: KDT 8th/e p132)*
   The symptoms of agitation, photophobia and retention of urine points towards anti-cholinergic drug poisoning. Dhatura is an important source of atropine and is thus likely to be the causative plant in this child. Physostigmine is an acetylcholinesterase and is used for treatment of anticholinergic poisoning like atropine, dhatura or belladonna poisoning.

6. **Ans. (a) TXA2** *(Ref: Katzung 13th/e p595)*
   Aspirin is an irreversible inhibitor of COX enzyme and results in decrease in TXA2 and PGI2. The anti-platelet action results due to decrease in TXA2 which is pro-aggregatory. This anti-platelet action is responsible for bleeding due to aspirin.

7. **Ans. (b) Premature closure of ductus arteriosus** *(Ref: Katzung 13th/e p327)*
   Indomethacin is an NSAID that decreases PG synthesis. Latter are required for keeping the ductus arteriosus patent. Decrease in PG synthesis results in premature closure of ductus areteriosus.

8. **Ans. (d) Acetaminophen** *(Ref: KDT 8th/e p224)*
   Most of the NSAIDs can result in renal toxicity due to inhibition of COX enzyme in the kidney. Acetaminophen (paracetamol) has least risk of causes nephrotoxicity.

9. **Ans. (a) Lisinopril** *(Ref: Katzung 13th/e p185)*
   The image shows the presence of angioedema which is a characteristic adverse effect of ACE inhibitors like lisinopril.

10. **Ans. (a) IL-6** *(Ref: Katzung 13th/e p629)*
    Tocilizumab is a monoclonal antibody against IL-6. It is used for:
    - Rheumatoid arthritis
    - Cytokine release syndrome
    - COVID-19 (for cytokine release syndrome)

11. **Ans. (c) Clarithromycin** *(Ref: Harrison 19th/e p34)*
    The question suggests the presence of digoxin overdose with hypokalemia (flattening of T waves). Triamterene (a K sparing diuretic), atenolol (a beta blocker that will inhibit renin secretion) and KCl are likely to cause hyperkalemia. Clarithromycin is a P-glycoprotein inhibitor and cause digoxin toxicity by inhibiting renal excretion of digoxin.

12. **Ans. (c) Chlorthalidone** *(Ref: CMDT 2022/p546)*
    The management of hypertension in chronic kidney disease includes:
    - Drug of choice are ACE inhibitors or ARBs. These are in particular preferred in patients with proteinuria. However, these should be avoided when serum creatinine is very high (> 3.5 mg/dL)
    - Diuretics like thiazides are the preferred second line drugs particularly in patients with volume overload. However, thiazides are found to be ineffective in severe renal disease (creatinine > 2.5 mg/dL or eGFR <30). Chlorthalidone is preferred agent due to its long duration of action. Metolazone is effective even in severe renal failure. Torsemide (a loop diuretic) can be used in severe renal disease
    - DHP- calcium channel blockers like amlodipine can be used as alternative second line agents in renal disease.
    - Renin inhibitors like aliskiren can be used in treatment of hypertension. However, these are not indicated in patients with renal disease.
    - Alpha blockers are preferred in treatment of hypertension when there are urinary obstructive symptoms due to benign prostatic hyperplasia
    - Beta blockers are not used as first line drugs in hypertension

    As the options does not contain ACE inhibitors or ARBs, we will prefer chlorthalidone as the answer because the patient has renal disease with volume overload (pedal edema) and serum creatinine is less than 2.5 mg/dL.

13. **Ans. (c) Lisinopril** *(Ref: KDT 8th/e p617)*
    ACE inhibitors are absolutely contraindicated in pregnancy.

Antihypertensives safe in pregnancy are:
- **B**etter: **B**eta blockers (Labetalol)
- **M**other: **M**ethyl dopa
- **C**are: **C**lonidine
- **D**uring: **D**HP calcium channel blockers like amlodipine
- **H**ypertensive: **H**ydralazine
- **P**regnancy: **P**razosin and other alpha blockers

14. **Ans. (a) Warfarin** *(Ref: CMDT 2022/337)*

    Medications to decrease risk of stroke patients with history of TIA or ischemic stroke
    - *Non-valvular atrial fibrillation (AF):*
      Direct acting oral anticoagulants (DOAC) like dabigatran, apixaban, rivaroxaban and edoxaban are preferred over warfarin. If the patient has end stage renal disease or on dialysis, then warfarin or apixaban may be used.
    - *Valvular heart disease and AF:*
      – If there is mechanical valve or moderate to severe mitral stenosis, warfarin is indicated
      – For all other valvular diseases, DOAC are preferred.
    - *Valvular disease and normal sinus rhythm:*
      – For mechanical mitral or aortic valves, warfarin is indicated
      – For all other cases (Non-rheumatic valve disease, bioprosthesis), antiplatelet (aspirin 75-100 mg) is indicated.

15. **Ans. (a) Add a P2Y12 receptor blocker** *(Ref: CMDT 2022/369)*
    - Dual anti-platelet therapy (DAPT) is indicated to prevent re-stenosis after stenting. It is also given when a patient presents with acute MI or TIA and after CABG.
    - DAPT is given for 3 months to 1 year
    - The drugs used in DAPT are aspirin (COX inhibitor) 75 mg and P2Y12 blocker (clopidogrel or prasugrel)

16. **Ans. (a) Stop warfarin and start heparin** *(Ref: KDT 8th/e p669)*

    Warfarin increase the risk of vitamin K deficiency in the baby and hemorrhagic disease of newborn. It should be replaced by warfarin in pregnancy.

17. **Ans. (c) Bisphosphonates therapy should not be given for more than one year** *(Ref: KDT 8th/e p370)*

    Management of post menopausal osteoporosis
    - Daily calcium and vitamin D must be supplemented. Calcium requirement is around 1200 mg per day. It should be supplemented with oral vitamin D_3
    - Bisphosphonates are drug of choice for post-menopausal osteoporosis. These should be continued for 5 years and then depending upon the risk of fracture, bisphosphonate holidays may be planned for 3-5 years
    - Denosuamab is another anti-resorptive therapy which can be used in females with very high-risk of fractures.
    - Teriparatide is PTH which is indicated in females with very high-risk of fractures. It is given for two years and should be followed by anti-resorptive therapy like bisphosphonates to maintain the bone mineral density.
    - Raloxifene may be used in females who are not candidates of bisphosphonate therapy, have low-risk of thromboembolic episodes or have family history of breast cancer.

18. **Ans. (d) Cardiac resuscitation + 20% intralipid** *(Ref: Katzung 13th/e p449)*

    Management of local anaesthetic toxicity:
    - Seizures should be treated with GABA agonists
    - Vasopressors may be indicated but may promote CNS toxicity
    - Total cardiovascular collapse may be treated with CPR plus 20% lipid emulsion

19. **Ans. (a) Succinylcholine** *(Ref: Katzung 13th/e p464)*

    Malignant hyperthermia may be triggered by inhaled anaesthetics (maximum with halothane) and succinylcholine.

20. **Ans. (a) Benzhexol** *(Ref: Katzung 13th/e p482)*
    - The anti-emetic leading to development of abnormal movements is likely to be metoclopramide. It can cause extrapyramidal symptoms due to its D2 receptor blocking activity in brain.
    - Treatment of drug-induced abnormal movements is central anticholinergic drugs like benzhexol. If it is not available, promethazine may be used.

21. **Ans. (a) CoAmoxyClav** *(Ref: CMDT 2019/p503)*

    The history of paronychia and given figure suggests the presence of lymphangitis. It is infection of lymphatics mostly due to infection in the proximal areas (paronychia here). Most commonly it is caused by streptococci. The treatment of lymphangitis include:
    - Cephalexin or extended spectrum penicillins like amoxicillin plus clavulanic acid are the first line drugs
    - If MRSA is the suspected agent, then cotrimoxazole should be used for treatment

22. **Ans. (c) Rifampicin increases the metabolism of oral contraceptives** *(Ref: Katzung 13th/e p712)*
    - Rifampicin is a strong enzyme inducer.
    - It induces the metabolism of estrogen and leads to failure of oral contraceptive pills

23. **Ans. (c) Alcohol** *(Ref: Katzung 13th/e p865)*

    Metronidazole can inhibit the enzyme aldehyde dehydrogenase. If a person consumes alcohol after taking metronidazole, there may be development of disulfiram like reaction.

24. **Ans. (d) Continue MDT and give steroids** *(Ref: KDT 8th/e p837)*

    History and given picture suggests the presence of type 1 lepra reaction. It should be treated with steroids but the MDT for leprosy should be continued.

25. **Ans. (a) Inhibition of dihydrofolate reductase** *(Ref: KDT 8th/e p921)*

    Methotrexate is an anticancer drug that acts by inhibiting DHFRase enzyme. It is an anti-metabolite group of anticancer drugs which are S phase selective.

26. **Ans. (a) Subglottic stenosis**

    Topical use of mitomycin C include:
    - Laryngotracheal stenosis (subglottic stenosis)
    - Intravesical treatment of bladder carcinoma

Annexures

I. History of Pharmacology

II. Drugs of Choice

III. Important Human Teratogenic Drugs

IV. Special INI-CET Pattern Questions with Explanations

Annexure I

History of Pharmacology

Scientist	Contribution
Oswald Schmiedberg	Father of Modern Pharmacology
Col. Ramnath Chopra	Father of Indian Pharmacology
Paul Ehrlich	Father of Modern Chemotherapy
David Sackett	Father of Evidence Based Medicine
Clark	Gave *Theory of drug action based on* occupation of *receptors* by specific drugs.
Otto Loewi	Direct proof of *transmission across nerve junctions* to be mediated *by neurotransmitters*.*
Ahlquist	Classified adrenergic receptors into α and β *types*.
Bergstrom, Samuelsson and Vane	Noble prize for work on *PGs and LTs*.
Banting and Best	Discovered insulin in 1921
Sanger	Worked out chemical structure of insulin in 1956
Kendall, Reichstein and Hench	Noble Prize for work on corticosteroids in Rheumatoid arthritis.
Lundy	Coined the term balanced anaesthesia
Horace Wells	Used N_2O (laughing gas) in 1844 for dental anaesthesia
Guedel	Described 4 stages of anaesthesia with Ether
Serturner	Isolated active principle of opium and named it morphine after greek God of dreams (**Morpheus**)
William Withering	Published his work on medicinal uses of Foxglove (digitalis) named 'An account of the Foxglove and some of its medicinal uses: with practical remarks on dropsy and other diseases'.
Vaughan Williams and Singh	Classification of anti-arrhythmic drugs
Ehrlich	Coined the term chemotherapy. Used the idea that if certain dyes can selectively stain microbes, they can also be toxic to these microbes. Developed arsenic compounds (Salvarsan) for treatment of syphilis.
Domagk	(a) Ushered the **Modern** era of **chemotherapy** (b) Demonstrated therapeutic effect of *prontosil* (containing sulfonamide) in pyogenic infections.
Fleming	Discovered *penicillin*
Walksman	Discovered *streptomycin*

* *Previously, it was considered to be electrical. He profused 2 frog hearts in series. Stimulation of vagus nerve of first heart caused arrest of both. Thus, a chemical must have been released by vagal stimulation of first heart (called vagusstoff now known as ACh) which passed in the perfusate and arrested the second heart.*

1. **Essential Drugs:**
   - First Model list by WHO in 1977
   - First National EDL of India in 1996
   - Current edition of India is 17th National list of Essential Medicines. It was modified in 2011. It contains 348 drugs
2. **Uppsala Monitoring Centre (Sweden)** is the international collaborating centre for Pharmacovigilance.
3. **Vasomotor reversal of Dale** was first demonstrated with **ergot alkaloids.**
4. **Centchroman** is a non-steroidal SERM **developed at CDRI India** as an oral contraceptive.
5. Synthetic toxin N-methyl-4-phenyl tetrahydropyridine (MPTP) produces nigrostrial degeneration and manifestations similar to Parkinson's disease.
6. **Blaud's pills** (for anemia) consists of FeSO4 and potassium carbonate.

7. Vitamin B$_{12}$ is also known as **Extrinsic factor of castle.**
8. Vitamin K was isolated from alfa alfa grass.
9. Rat poison contains oral anticoagulants like warfarin.
10. Name of drug warfarin is coined from **W**isconsin **A**lumni **R**esearch **F**oundation and its chemical structure being couma**RIN.**
11. New formula WHO-ORS was released in 2002. It contains low Na+ (75 mM), low glucose (75 mM) and has low osmolarity (245, mOsm/L)
12. 8-Hydroxyquinolines like quiniodochlor and iodoquinol were used in ameobic dysentry but were banned in Japan and few other countries because on long-term use these resulted in epidemics of subacute Myelo-optic Neuropathy (SMON).
13. Thalidomide caused phocomelia in Germany in 1960s when it was used for treatment of vomiting due to morning sickness.

First local anaesthetic	Cocaine (1884) for ocular anaesthesia
First i.v. anaesthetic	Thiopentone
First drug for Schizophrenia	Chlorpromazine
First ACE inhibitor	Teprotide
First oral ACE inhibitor	Captopril
First Fibrinolytic	Streptokinase
First antibiotic	Penicillin
First antitubercular drug	PAS (followed by streptomycin)

Annexure II

Drugs of Choice

	Drug of choice	Reference
Acetaminophen poisoning	ACETYLCYSTEINE	CMDT 2019/1584
Acute bronchial asthma	FORMOTEROL + INHALED CORTICOSTERIDS	CMDT 2019/259
Acute gout	NSAIDS (EXCEPT ASPIRIN)	CMDT 2019/845
Acute mania	NEUROLEPTICS (E.G. OLANZAPINE) ± LITHIUM	CMDT 2019/1097
Acute severe digitalis toxicity	DIGIBIND	CMDT 2019/1584
Acute severe migraine	SUMATRIPTAN	CMDT 2019/991
ADHD	METHYLPHENIDATE	CMDT 2019/1100
Alzheimer's disease	DONEPEZIL/RIVASTIGMINE/GALLANTAMINE	CMDT 2019/59
Ameobiasis		
– Asymptomatic intestinal	DILOXANIDE FUROATE	CMDT 2019/1530
– Symptomatic intestinal	METRONIDAZOLE + DILOXANIDE	CMDT 2019/1530
– Extraintestinal (e.g. hepatic)	METRONIDAZOLE + DILOXANIDE	CMDT 2019/1530
Anaphylactic shock	ADRENALINE (S.C./I.M.)	CMDT 2019/891
Anti thyroid in pregnancy and breast feeding	PROPYLTHIOURACIL	CMDT 2019/1144
Anticoagulant for HIT	ARGATROBAN/BIVALIRUDIN	CMDT 2019/563
Atonic seizures	VALPROATE	Harrison 19th/3262
Atropine poisoning	PHYSOSTIGMINE	CMDT 2019/1584
Atypical pneumonia	ERYTHROMYCIN	Katzung 13th/797
Babesiosis	QUININE + CLINDAMYCIN	CMDT 2019/1522
Benzodiazepine poisoning	FLUMAZENIL	CMDT 2019/1584
Beta blocker poisoning	GLUCAGON	CMDT 2019/1581
Bipolar disorder	LITHIUM	Harrison 19th/3540
Brucella	DOXYCYCLINE + RIFAMPICIN	CMDT 2019/1604
Carbamate poisoning	ATROPINE	CMDT 2019/1602
Carbon monoxide poisoning	OXYGEN	CMDT 2019/1584
Cheese reaction	PHENTOLAMINE	KDT 7th/440, 545
Chemotherapy induced vomiting (early phase)	PALONOSETRON	CMDT 2019/1678
Chloroquine resistant malaria	ARTEMISININ COMBINATION THERAPY	CMDT 2019/1520
Cholera	TETRACYCLINE	CMDT 2019/1477
Chronic lymphocytic leukemia	FLUDARABINE + RITUXIMAB ± CYCLOPHOSPHAMIDE	CMDT 2019/541
Clonidine withdrawal	PHENTOLAMINE	KDT 7th/545
Coccidiosis		
– Cryptosporidiosis	PAROMOMYCIN/NITAZOXANIDE	CMDT 2019/1532
– Isosporiasis	COTRIMOXAZOLE	CMDT 2019/1532
– Cyclosporiasis	COTRIMOXAZOLE	CMDT 2019/1532
– Microsporidiosis	ALBENDAZOLE	CMDT 2019/1532
Complicated Malaria	ARTESUNATE	CMDT 2019/1520
Cyanide toxicity	AMYL NITRITE/HYDROXOCOBALAMIN	CMDT 2019/1584
Cytomegalovirus (CMV)	GANCICLOVIR	CMDT 2019/1391

Contd...

Contd...

	Drug of choice	Reference
Depression	FLUOXETINE	Harrison 19th/3538
Diabetes insipidus		
– Central	DESMOPRESSIN	CMDT 2019/1123
– Nephrogenic	THIAZIDES	CMDT 2019/1123
– Lithium-induced	AMILORIDE	CMDT 2019/1123
Diabetes mellitus		
– Type 1	INSULIN	CMDT 2019/1244
– Type 2	METFORMIN	CMDT 2019/1246
– Ketoacidosis	REGULAR INSULIN + IV FLUIDS	CMDT 2019/1258
– Pregnancy	INSULIN	CMDT 2019/1255
DMARD	METHOTREXATE	CMDT 2019/844
Drug induced Parkinsonism	BENZHEXOL (TRIHEXYPHENYDIL)	KDT 7th/421
Echinococcosis	ALBENDAZOLE	CMDT 2019/1550
Muscle relaxant for Endotracheal intubation	SUCCINYLCHOLINE	KDT 7th/346
Enteric fever	CEFTRIAXONE	CMDT 2019/1482
Enterobiasis	ALBENDAZOLE	CMDT 2019/1553
Ethylene glycol poisoning	FOMEPIZOLE	CMDT 2019/1584
Fasciola hepatica	TRICLABENDAZOLE	CMDT 2019/1546
Febrile seizures	DIAZEPAM	KDT 7th/413
Fibrinolytics overdose	EACA	Katzung 13th/602
Filariasis	DIETHYLCARBAMAZINE	CMDT 2019/1556
Flukes (except fasciola)	PRAZIQUANTAL	Katzung 13th/924
Generalized anxiety disorder		
– Acute treatment	BENZODIAZEPINES	CMDT 2019/1063
– Sustained treatment	ANTIDEPRESSANTS (VENLAFAXINE/DULOXETINE)	CMDT 2019/1063
Giardiasis	METRONIDAZOLE/TINIDAZOLE	CMDT 2019/1543
Gonorrhoea	CEFTRIAXONE + AZITHROMYCIN/DOXYCYCLINE	CMDT 2019/1489
Grand mal epilepsy	VALPROATE	Harrison 19th/3262
Graves Opthalmopathy	I.V. METHYLPREDNISOLONE	CMDT 2019/1146
Hairy cell leukemia	CLADRIBINE	CMDT 2019/1635
Heparin overdose	PROTAMINE	Katzung 13th/593
Herpes simplex		
– Mucocutaneous	ACYCLOVIR/VALACYCLOVIR	CMDT 2019/1379
– Keratitis	VALACYCLOVIR	CMDT 2019/1379
– Neonatal	ACYCLOVIR	CMDT 2019/1379
– Encephalitis/Meningitis	ACYCLOVIR	CMDT 2019/1379
– Bell palsy	PREDNISOLONE	CMDT 2019/1379
Hookworm	ALBENDAZOLE	CMDT 2019/1551
Hypertension in pregnancy	LABETALOL	CMDT 2019/826
Hypertension with BHP	PRAZOSIN	Katzung 13th/154
Hypertensive emergencies in pregnancy	LABETALOL	CMDT 2019/476
Hypertensive emergencies	NICARDIPINE + LABETALOL	CMDT 2019/475
Hypertriglyceridemia	FIBRATES	Harrison 19th/1067
Hypothyroidism	LEVO-THYROXINE	CMDT 2019/1135
Hypovolemic shock	I.V. FLUIDS (CRYSTALLOIDS)	CMDT 2019/504
Infantile spasms	ACTH	Katzung 13th/418
Iron toxicity	DESFERRIOXAMINE	CMDT 2019/1609

Contd...

Contd...

	Drug of choice	Reference
Isoniazid poisoning	PYRIDOXINE	CMDT 2019/1584
Kala azar	LIPOSOMAL AMPHOTERICIN B	CMDT 2019/1523
Malaria (P. Vivax)	CHLOROQUINE	CMDT 2019/1520
Malaria (P. falciparum)	ARTEMISININ COMBINATION THERAPY	CMDT 2019/1520
Malignant hyperthermia	DANTROLENE	Harrison 19th/147
Methanol poisoning	FOMEPIZOLE	CMDT 2019/1584
MRSA	VANCOMYCIN	Harrison 19th/1070
Multiple myeloma	DEXAMETHASONE + LENALIDOMIDE AND/OR BORTEZOMIB	CMDT 2019/544
Mydriatic in adults	TROPICAMIDE	Katzung 13th/119
Mydriatic in children	ATROPINE	Katzung 13th/119
Myoclonic seizures	VALPROATE	Harrison 19th/3262
Neurocysticercosis	ALBENDAZOLE + CORTICOSTEROIDS	CMDT 2019/1549
Neurolept anaesthesia	FENTANYL+DROPERIDOL+NITROUS OXIDE	Katzung 13th/495
Neurolept analgesia	FENTANYL + DROPERIDOL	Katzung 13th/495
Neurolept malignant syndrome	DANTROLENE	Harrison 19th/147
Nocturnal enuresis	DESMOPRESSIN	KDT 7th/577
NSAID-induced PUD	PROTON PUMP INHIBITORS	CMDT 2019/637
OCD	FLUOXETINE	CMDT 2019/1066
OHA in obese patients	METFORMIN	CMDT 2019/1246
Onchocerciasis (river blindness)	IVERMECTIN	CMDT 2019/1557
Opioid poisoning	NALOXONE	CMDT 2019/1584
Organophosphate poisoning	ATROPINE	CMDT 2019/1584
P/O Chloroquine resistant malaria	MEFLOQUINE	CMDT 2019/1520
P/O Influenza A [H5N1 and H1N1]	OSELTAMIVIR	CMDT 2019/1432
P/O Malaria in pregnancy	CHLOROQUINE	CMDT 2019/1520
P/O Malaria	CHLOROQUINE	CMDT 2019/1529
P/O Mycobacterium avium complex	CLARITHROMYCIN/ AZITHROMYCIN	CMDT 2019/1495
P/O Plague	DOXYCYCLINE	CMDT 2019/1487
P/O Pneumocystis jiroveci pneumonia	COTRIMOXAZOLE	CMDT 2019/1565
P/O Rheumatic fever	BENZATHINE PENICILLIN	CMDT 2019/431
P/O Toxoplasmosis	COTRIMOXAZOLE	CMDT 2019/1537
P/O Whooping cough	ERYTHROMYCIN	CMDT 2019/1477
Panic attack (acute treatment)	BENZODIAZEPINES	CMDT 2019/1063
Panic disorder (sustained treatment)	SSRI (SERTRALINE)	CMDT 2019/1063
Partial seizures (temporal lobe epilepsy)	CARBAMAZEPINE	Harrison 19th/3262
Peptic ulcer disease	PPIS	CMDT 2019/637
Performance anxiety	PROPRANOLOL	Harrison 19th/2713
Petit mal epilepsy	VALPROATE	Harrison 19th/3262
Phobias	SSRI (SERTRALINE)	CMDT 2019/1065
Pneumocystis jiroveci pneumonia	COTRIMOXAZOLE	CMDT 2019/1565
POAG	LATANOPROST	CMDT 2019/187
Post menopausal osteoporosis	ALENDRONATE	Harrison 19th/2405
Post prandial hyperglycemia	NATEGLINIDE	KDT 7th/269
Post traumatic stress disorder	SSRI (SERTRALINE/PAROXETINE)	CMDT 2019/1061
Prevention of DVT	WARFARIN	Katzung 13th/600
Prophylaxis of mania	LITHIUM	Katzung 13th/502

Contd...

Contd...

	Drug of choice	Reference
Prophylaxis of MI	ASPIRIN	Katzung 13th/600
Pseudomonas	PIPERACILLIN-TAZOBACTAM/CEFTAZIDIME+ AMINOGLYCOSIDES	CMDT 2019/1322
Roundworm (Ascariasis)	ALBENDAZOLE	CMDT 2019/1550
Secondary Shock	ALPHA BLOCKERS	KDT 7th/136
Shock with oliguria	DOPAMINE	CMDT 2019/505
SMR in asthmatics	CURONIUMS LIKE VECURONIUM	Katzung 13th/460
SMR in liver and kidney disease	CIS-ATRACURIUM	Katzung 13th/453
Steroid induced osteoporosis	ALENDRONATE	CMDT 2019/1172
Status epilepticus	LORAZEPAM (I.V.)	CMDT 2019/998
Streptococcus	PENICILLIN	CMDT 2019/1321
Strongyloidiasis	IVERMECTIN	CMDT 2019/1552
Surgical prophylaxis	CEFAZOLIN	Katzung 13th/896
Syphilis		
– Primary	BENZATHINE PENICILLIN G	CMDT 2019/1505
– Secondary	BENZATHINE PENICILLIN G	CMDT 2019/1505
– Latent	BENZATHINE PENICILLIN G	CMDT 2019/1505
– Tertiary except neurosyphilis	BENZATHINE PENICILLIN G	CMDT 2019/1505
– Neurosyphlis	PENICILLIN G (AQUEOUS)	CMDT 2019/1505
– In pregnancy	PENICILLIN G (AS ABOVE)	CMDT 2019/1505
Tapeworms (except Echinococcus)	PRAZIQUANTAL	CMDT 2019/1549
Termination of acute angina	S.L. NITROGLYCERINE	CMDT 2019/366
Termination of PSVT	ADENOSINE	CMDT 2019/392
Tetanus	METRONIDAZOLE	Harrison 19th/1199
To keep ductus patent	ALPROSTADIL (PGE_1)	Katzung 13th/326
Toxoplasmosis in pregnancy	SPIRAMYCIN	CMDT 2019/1537
Toxoplasmosis	PYRIMETHAMINE + SULFADIAZINE + FOLINIC ACID	CMDT 2019/1537
Treatment of PDA	INDOMETHACIN/IBUPROFEN	Katzung 13th/326
Treatment of PPH	OXYTOCIN	Katzung 13th/289
Trichomoniasis	METRONIDAZOLE or TINIDAZOLE	CMDT 2019/1544
Trichinosis	MEBENDAZOLE/ALBENDAZOLE	CMDT 2019/1554
Trichuris	ALBENDAZOLE	CMDT 2019/1551
Trigeminal neuralgia	OXCARBAZEPINE/CARBAMAZEPINE	CMDT 2019/990
VRSA	DAPTOMYCIN	Harrison 19th/1169
Warfarin overdose	VITAMIN K_1	CMDT 2019/1601
Wegener's granulomatosis (now known as granulomatosis with polyangitis)	CYCLOPHOSPHAMIDE + STEROIDS	CMDT 2019/867

FULL FORMS OF ABBREVIATIONS

ADHD	:	Attention deficit hyperkinetic disorder
DI	:	Diabetes insipidus
DVT	:	Deep vein thrombosis
EACA	:	Epsilon amino caproic acid
HIT	:	Heparin induced thrombocytopenia
IDN	:	Isosorbide dinitrate
MRSA	:	Methicillin resistant *Staphylococcus aureus*
NTG	:	Nitroglycerine
OCD	:	Obsessive compulsive disorder
OHA	:	Oral hypoglycemic agent
P/O	:	Prophylaxis of
PDA	:	Patent ductus arteriosus
POAG	:	Primary open angle glaucoma
PPI	:	Proton pump inhibitor
PSVT	:	Paroxysmal supraventricular tachycardia
PUD	:	Peptic Ulcer Disease
VRSA	:	Vancomycin resistant *Staphylococcus aureus*

Annexure III

Important Human Teratogenic Drugs

Drug	Congenital Adomalies
Ace inhibitors	IUGR, oligohydraminos, bony malformations, PDA, hypoplasia of organs, renal anomalies
Alcohol	Fetal alcohol syndrome: IUGR, microcephaly, developmental delay, dysmorphic facies (low nasal bridge, midface hypoplasia long featureless philtrum, small palpebral fissure, thin upper lip)
Antithyroid drugs (carbimazole, methimazole, propylthiouracil)	Fetal hypothyroidism, congenital goiter, scalp defects (aplasia cutis congenita)
Androgens	Virilization; limb, esophageal and cardiac defects
Carbamazepine	Neural tube defects, defects similar to fetal hydantoin syndrome
Diethylstilbesterol	Clear cell adenocarcinoma of vagina, hypospadias
Isotretinoin	Craniofacial, heart and CNS defects
Lithium	Fetal goiter, Ebstein's anomaly
Misoprostol	Moebius syndrome
Methotrexate	Hydrocephalus, meningomyelocele, cleft palate, external ear anomalies
Phenytoin	Fetal hydantoin syndrome: Microcephaly, cleft lip, cleft palate, hypoplastic phalanges, nail hypoplasia
Progesterone	Virilization of female fetus
Tetracyclines	Discoloration of teeth, retardation of bone growth
Thalidomide	Phocomelia, polydactyly, syndactyly, external ear defects (from agenesis to pre-auricular tags), moebius syndrome, abnormalities in gut musculature
Valproate	Neural tube defects
Warfarin	Fetal warfarin syndrome (contradi syndrome): Nasal hypoplasia, calcific stippling of epiphyses, IUGR, eyes defects, hearing loss

Annexure IV

Special INI-CET Pattern Questions with Explanations

MULTIPLE TRUE FALSE TYPE QUESTIONS

1. **Following statements about pharmacokinetics of a drug are true/false?**
   (a) Most drugs are absorbed in ionized form
   (b) Basic drugs are generally bound to plasma albumin
   (c) Microsomal enzymes are located in mitochondria of hepatic cells
   (d) Blood brain barrier is deficient at CTZ
   (e) Highly plasma protein bound drugs have high volume of distribution

   Ans. False: a, b, c, e; True: d
   - Most drugs are absorbed in un-ionized form as this is the lipid soluble form
   - Acidic drugs bind to albumin and basic drugs usually bind to alpha-1 acid glycoprotein
   - Microsomal enzymes are present in smooth endoplasmic reticulum of hepatocytes.
   - Chemoreceptor trigger zone is a circumventricular organ, means it is devoid of blood brain barrier
   - If a drug has high plasma protein binding, it decreases the volume of distribution

2. **Following statements are true/false about clinical uses of atropine?**
   (a) It is used for treatment of belladonna poisoning
   (b) It is drug of choice for producing cycloplegia in children
   (c) It is preferred drug in organophosphate poisoning
   (d) It is used for treatment of bradyarrhythmias
   (e) It is first line drug in angle closure glaucoma

   Ans. True: b, c, d, False: a, e
   - Atropine is contraindicated in belladonna poisoning. Plant atropa belladonna is a source of atropine, so belladonna poisoning itself means atropine poisoning.
   - Atropine is strong cycloplegic drug and is therefore preferred in children as they have high tone of ciliary muscle.
   - Atropine is drug of choice for organophosphate and carbamate poisoning.
   - Atropine is drug of choice of Bradycardia and AV block.
   - Atropine is contraindicated in a patient with angle closure glaucoma. It may lead to precipitation of acute attack of glaucoma in such patients.

3. **The following statements are true/false about the use of drugs in Rheumatoid Arthritis?**
   (a) NSAIDs are the mainstay of therapy for slowing the disease progression
   (b) Methotrexate is most commonly used disease modifying agent
   (c) Sarilumab is a monoclonal antibody against IL-6
   (d) Abatacept is a co-stimulation inhibitor used in rheumatoid arthritis.
   (e) Etanercept should be avoided in a patient with tuberculosis.

   Ans. True: b, c, d, e False: a
   - NSAIDs are used for symptomatic treatment in Rheumatoid arthritis. These cannot slow the disease progression.
   - Methotrexate is most commonly used DMARD in rheumatoid arthritis.
   - Sarilumab is recently approved monoclonal antibody against IL-6. It is a biological DMARD.
   - Abatacept acts by inhibiting co-stimulatory signal for activation of T-cells
   - Etanercept is a fusion protein targeted to inhibit TNF-alpha. These drugs can worsen TB and hepatitis B and thus are contraindicated in such patients.

4. **Following statements are true/false about drugs affecting renin angiotensin aldosterone system?**
   (a) Aliskiren acts by inhibiting the secretion of renin
   (b) Enalapril can cause cough and angioedema
   (c) Losartan inhibits the formation of angiotensin II
   (d) Epleronone causes gynaecomastia as an adverse effect
   (e) Sampatrilat has additional inhibitory activity on neprilysin apart from inhibitory effect on ACE.

   Ans. True: b, e; False: a, c, d
   - Aliskiren is a renin inhibitor. It does not inhibit secretion of renin. Rather it inhibits the action of renin after it is secreted. Beta blockers act by inhibiting the secretion of renin.
   - ACE inhibitors like enalapril prevent the degradation of bradykinin. Excessive bradykinin can result in cough and angioedema as adverse effects.
   - Losartan is an angiotensin receptor antagonist. It does not inhibit the formation of angiotensin II.
   - Epleronone is a new aldosterone antagonist like spironolactone, however unlike spironolactone, it does not cause gynaecomastia.
   - Sampatrilat and omapatrilat are vasopeptidase inhibitors. These can inhibit two enzymes; ACE and neprilysin.

5. **Following statements are true/false about diuretics?**
   (a) Mannitol is contraindicated in pulmonary edema
   (b) Thiazides are first line drugs in hypertension
   (c) Thiazides are also used in nephrogenic diabetes insipidus
   (d) Furosemide has high ceiling diuretic effect
   (e) Acetazolamide is used for prophylaxis of mountain sickness

Ans: True: a, b, c, d, e

Explanations:
- Mannitol is contraindicated in pulmonary edema and acute renal failure.
- Thiazides are first line drugs in treatment of hypertension.
- Thiazides are also drug of choice for the treatment of nephrogenic diabetes insipidus.
- Loop diuretics like furosemide are high ceiling diuretics.
- Acetazolamide is drug of choice for prophylaxis and treatment of mountain sickness.

6. True/False statements about anti-diabetic drugs are:
   (a) Glipizide can cause hypoglycemia
   (b) Metformin causes weight gain
   (c) Sitagliptin is associated with occurrence of pancreatitis
   (d) Acarbose inhibits intestinal absorption of carbohydrates
   (e) Insulin is preferred in most patients with type 2 diabetes mellitus

Ans: True: a, c, d False: b, e
- Glipizide is a sulfonylurea. These drugs act by releasing insulin and thus can cause hypoglycemia as an adverse effect.
- Metformin is weight neutral in most patients and can also cause weight loss in few. It does not cause weight gain and is thus preferred in obese patients
- DPP-4 inhibitors like sitagliptin and GLP analogs like exenatide are associated with pancreatitis as an adverse effect.
- Acarbose inhibits the enzyme alpha glucosidase and thus decrease the absorption of carbohydrates from GIT.
- Insulin is a peptide and thus cannot be given orally. For type 2 diabetes mellitus, oral drugs are preferred first. Metformin is drug of choice. Insulin is used in patients where oral drugs are not able to control blood glucose.

7. Following statements about adverse effects of antipsychotic drugs are true/false
   (a) Clozapine can cause agranulocytosis
   (b) Haloperidol can cause tardive dyskinesia on long term use
   (c) Quetiapine can cause cataract
   (d) Sialorrhea is a common adverse effect of clozapine
   (e) Olanzapine is associated with weight gain

Ans. True: a, b, c, d, e
- Clozapine causes agranulocytosis and seizures as major adverse effects. Agranulocytosis is dose independent whereas seizures are dose dependent.
- Haloperidol is a typical antipsychotic and thus can cause all extrapyramidal symptoms including Tardive dyskinesia.
- Quetiapine is associated with cataract as an adverse effect.
- Sedation and sialorrhea are very common adverse effects of clozapine.
- Most atypical antipsychotic drugs including olanzapine and clozapine are associated with lipodystrophy syndrome characterized by weight gain, insulin resistance, hyperglycemia, hyperlipidemia etc.

8. Following statements about general anaesthetic agents is true/false?
   (a) Ketamine can produce dissociative anaesthesia
   (b) Propofol is used for day care surgery
   (c) Halothane is preferred anaesthetic for pheochromocytoma surgery
   (d) Xenon has very high blood gas partition coefficient
   (e) Etomidate can cause adrenal suppression

Ans True: a, b, e False: c, d
- Ketamine produces dissociative anaesthesia
- Propofol is most commonly used drug for day care surgery.
- Halothane is contraindicated in pheochromocytoma surgery. It sensitizes heart to arrhythmogenic actions of adrenaline.
- Xenon is fastest acting inhalational anaesthetic agent. It has lowest blood gas partition coefficient.
- Etomidate can cause adrenal suppression as an adverse effect.

9. Following statements are true/false about anticoagulants?
   (a) Rivaroxaban is an oral coagulant
   (b) Edoxaban acts as a direct factor Xa inhibitor
   (c) Andexanet is approved for overdose of apixaban like anticoagulants
   (d) Dabigatran is direct thrombin inhibitor
   (e) Idarucizumab is a monoclonal antibody for reversing the overdose of dabigatran

Ans. True: a, b, c, d, e
- Rivaroxaban is reversible oral Xa blocker. It is a new oral anti-coagulant.
- Drugs ending with xaban like rivaroxaban, edoxaban, apixaban and betrixaban are oral Xa inhibitors.
- Andexanet is recently approved for treatment of overdose of factor Xa inhibitors like apixaban.
- Dabigatran is a direct thrombin inhibitor.
- Overdose of dabigatran can be treated by a monoclonal antibody, idarucizumab.

10. Following statements are true/false about drugs used in bronchial asthma?
    (a) Salbutamol is a short acting beta 2 agonist
    (b) Formoterol can be used for acute attack as well as for prophylaxis of asthma
    (c) Beta 2 agonists can result in tremors as an adverse effect
    (d) Steroids alone are most effective drugs for acute attack of asthma
    (e) Sodium cromoglycate is ineffective in acute attack of asthma

Ans. True: a, b, c, e False: d
- Salbutamol and terbutaline are short acting beta 2 agonists. These are drug of choice for acute attack of asthma.
- Formoterol is a long and fast acting beta 2 agonist. It can be used for treatment as well as prophylaxis of asthma.
- Beta 2 agonists like salbutamol can cause tremors, tachycardia and hypokalemia as adverse effects.
- Steroids alone cannot treat acute attack of asthma. One of the bronchodilator is must for treatment of acute attack.
- Sodium cromoglycate is a mast cell stabilizer. It prevents the degranulation of mast cells and will be ineffective in acute attack of asthma where already degranulation has taken place.

MATCH THE FOLLOWING TYPE QUESTIONS

1. **Match the following regarding the mechanism of action of drugs used in treatment of peptic ulcer disease.**

A. Ranitidine	1. Proton pump inhibitor
B. Sucralfate	2. Ulcer protective
C. Lansoprazole	3. Antacid
D. Misoprostol	4. M1 antagonist
	5. PGE1 analog
	6. H2 antagonist

   Ans. A– (6), B–(2), C– (1), D– (5)
   - Ranitidine is an H_2 antagonist
   - Sucralfate is an ulcer protective
   - Lansoprazole is a proton pump inhibitor
   - Misoprostol is a PGE1 analog.

2. **Match the drug of choice with the appropriate organism**

A. MRSA	1. Penicillin G
B. Gonococci	2. Vancomycin
C. Treponema pallidum	3. Cotrimoxazole
D. Pneumocystis jiroveci	4. Ceftriaxone
	5. Doxycycline
	6. Imipenem

   Ans. A– (2), B–(4), C– (1), D– (3)
   - Drug of choice for treatment of MRSA is vancomycin.
   - Drug of choice for treatment of gonococci is ceftriaxone.
   - Drug of choice for treatment of syphilis (treponema pallidum) is penicillin G.
   - Drug of choice for treatment of Pneumocystis jiroveci is cotrimoxazole.

3. **Match the adverse effect with the anti-tubercular drug**

A. Optic neuritis	1. Rifampicin
B. Hepatotoxicity	2. Bedaquiline
C. Hearing Loss	3. Cycloserine
D. QT Prolongation	4. Ethambutol
	5. Streptomycin
	6. Linezolide

   Ans. A– (4), B–(1), C– (5), D– (2)
   - Ethambutol cause Eye problems (Optic neuritis)
   - Rifampicin, Isoniazid and pyrazinamide are hepatotoxicity
   - Streptomycin can cause nephrotoxicity and ototoxicity
   - Bedaquiline and delaminid are not anti-tubercular drugs. Both are associated with QT prolongation.

4. **Match the following monoclonal antibodies with their approved indication**

A. Durvalumab	1. Breast cancer
B. Trastuzumab	2. Osteoporosis
C. Denosumab	3. Multiple myeloma
D. Efalizumab	4. Urothelial carcinoma
	5. Psoriasis
	6. CML

   Ans. A– (4), B–(1), C– (2), D– (5)
   - Durvalumab targets the PDL-1 and is indicated in urothelial carcinoma.
   - Trastuzumab is a monoclonal antibody against her-2/neu and is used in breast cancer and gastroesophageal junction carcinoma.
   - Denosumab is a monoclonal antibody against RANK ligand and is used in osteoporosis and giant cell tumor of bone.
   - Efalizumab is targeted against LFA-1 and is used for psoriasis.

5. **Match the following immunomodulators with their mechanism**

A. Cyclosporine	1. TNF alpha inhibitor
B. Leflunomide	2. DHFRase inhibitor
C. Methotrexate	3. Calcineurin inhibitor
D. Infliximab	4. Dihydroorotate Dehydrogenase inhibitor

   Ans. A– (3), B–(4), C– (2), D– (1)
   - Cyclosporine and tacrolimus are calcineurin inhibitors used for transplantation.
   - Leflunomide is dihydro-orotate-dehydrogenase inhibitor. It is used for Rheumatoid arthritis.
   - Methotrexate acts by inhibiting dihydrofolate reductase enzyme.
   - Infliximab is a TNF-alpha blocker.

6. **Match the following drugs with their clinical indications**

A. Orlistat	1. Erectile dysfunction
B. Sildenafil	2. Smoking cessation
C. Vareniciline	3. Iron poisoning
D. Desferrioxamine	4. Hyperkalemia
	5. Obesity

   Ans. A– (5), B–(1), C– (2), D– (3)
   - Orlistat is an oral drug. It is intestinal lipase inhibitor and is approved for obesity.
   - Sildenafil is a Phosphodiesterase inhibitor and is drug of choice for erectile dysfunction.
   - Varenicline is used for smoking cessation.
   - Desferrioxamine is a chelating agent indicated in acute iron poisoning.

7. **Match these recently approved drugs with their indication**

A. Elagolix	1. X Linked hypophosphatemia
B. Baloxavir Marboxil	2. Radical cure of malaria
C. Tafenoquine	3. Influenza virus
D. Burosumab	4. Prostate carcinoma
	5. Pain due to endometriosis
	6. Rheumatoid arthritis

   Ans. A– (5), B–(3), C– (2), D– (1)
   - Elagolix is an oral GnRH antagonist. It is approved for pain due to endometriosis.
   - Baloxavir marboxil is a new drug recently approved for influenza virus.
   - Tafenoquine is a long acting drug approved for single dose radical cure of malaria.
   - Burosumab is a monoclonal antibody against FGF-23 approved for X linked Hypophosphatemia.

8. Match the drug with most important CYP involved in its metabolism

A.	Clopidogrel	1.	CYP 2C9
B.	Atorvastatin	2.	CYP 2C19
C.	Quinidine	3.	CYP 2D6
D.	Warfarin	4.	CYP 3A4

   Ans. A– (2), B–(4), C– (3), D– (1)
   - Clopidogrel is a prodrug. It is activated by CYP 2C19 to active metabolite.
   - Most of the statins including atorvastatin are metabolized by CYP 3A4.
   - Most anti-arrhythmic drugs including quinidine (except Amiodarone) are metabolized by CYP2D6.
   - Warfarin and phenytoin are primarily metabolized by CYP 2C9.

9. Match the following antiglaucoma drugs with their ocular adverse effect

A.	Adrenaline	1.	Cataract
B.	Latanoprost	2.	Conjunctival pigmentation
C.	Apraclonidine	3.	Hypertrichosis
D.	Pilocarpine	4.	Lid retraction

   Ans. A– (2), B–(3), C– (4), D– (1)
   - Adrenaline is metabolized to adrenochrome which can cause black pigmentation of conjunctiva.
   - PGF2 alpha derivatives like latanoprost are associated with hypertrichosis, heterochromia iridis and macular edema.
   - Apraclonidine can cause lid retraction.
   - Miotics like pilocarpine are associated with cataract and puntal stenosis.

10. Match the following anti-arrhythmic drugs with appropriate class

A.	Quinidine	1.	Class 1
B.	Amiodarone	2.	Class 2
C.	Propranolol	3.	Class 3
D.	Verapamil	4.	Class 4

    Ans. A– (1), B–(3), C– (2), D– (4)
    - Quinidine and procainamide are class Ia drugs
    - Amiodarone is Class 3 anti-arrhythmic agent.
    - Beta blockers like propranolol are class 2 drugs.
    - Verapamil and Diltiazem like calcium channel blockers belong to class 4.

SEQUENTIAL ARRANGEMENT TYPE QUESTIONS

1. Arrange the following drugs according to increasing volume of distribution.
   (a) Haloperidol   (b) Gentamicin
   (c) Heparin   (d) Chloroquine

   Ans. c, b, a, d
   - Chloroquine has highest volume of distribution. It is concentrated in liver and retina.
   - Heparin is high molecular weight compound and thus not able to cross most membranes. It has low Vd.
   - Gentamicin again cannot cross many membranes because of polar nature and thus has low Vd.
   - Haloperidol is a drug working in CNS. So, it must be able to cross other membranes also resulting in high Vd.
   - Thus the sequence is
     Chloroquine > Haloperidol > Gentamicin > Heparin

2. Arrange the following drugs according to their half life in increasing order
   (a) Amiodarone   (b) Adenosine
   (c) Esmolol   (d) Omeprazole

   Ans. b, c, d, a
   - Amiodarone is longest acting anti-arrhythmic drug. Its half life is more than 3 weeks.
   - Adenosine is shortest acting anti-arrhythmic drug having half life less than 10 seconds.
   - Esmolol is an ultra short acting beta blocker. It is metabolized by pseudocholinesterase and thus has half life less than 5 minutes.
   - Omeprazole has half life of 1-2 hours but works for 24 hours due to irreversible inhibition of proton pump.
   - Thus, the sequence is
     Adenosine < Esmolol < Omeprazole < Amiodarone

3. Arrange the duration of treatment of the following conditions in the increasing order
   (a) Treatment of P. vivax malaria
   (b) Treatment of multibacillary leprosy
   (c) Treatment of category 1 tuberculosis
   (d) Treatment of Hypertension

   Ans. a, c, b, d
   - Treatment of malaria is for 3 days.
   - Multibacillary leprosy is treated for 12 months.
   - Category 1 tuberculosis is treated for 6 months
   - Hypertension treatment is life long.

MULTIPLE COMPLETION TYPE QUESTIONS

1. Drugs used for the treatment of type 2 diabetes mellitus include:
   (a) Pramlintide   (b) Bromocriptine
   (c) Vildagliptin   (d) Migalastat
   1. (a), (b), (c) are correct
   2. Only (a) and (c) are correct
   3. Only (b) and (d) are correct
   4. All four options are correct

   Ans. 1. (a), (b), (c) are correct
   - Pramlintide (amylin analog), Bromocriptine (D2 agonist) and vildagliptin (DPP-4 inhibitor) are used for diabetes.
   - Migalastat is a new drug. It acts as a pharmacological chaperone for alpha galactosidase and is used for Fabry disease.

2. Adverse effects of anti-Parkinsonian drugs are given below
   (a) Levo-dopa can result in on-off phenomenon in late Parkinsonism
   (b) Amantadine can cause dyskinesia
   (c) Pramipexole is associated with impulse control disorders
   (d) Bromocriptine can result in peripheral gangrene of limbs.
   1. Options (a), (c) and (d) are correct
   2. Options (a) and (b) are correct
   3. Options (a) and (d) are correct
   4. All four options are correct

Ans. 1. (a), (c) and (d) are correct
- Levo-dopa is associated with on-off and wearing off phenomenon in late Parkinsonism.
- Amantadine has recently been approved for treatment of dyskinesia. It is assumed to be due to its NMDA receptor blocking activity.
- Pramipexole and ropinirole are associated with impulse control disorders like pathological gambling.
- Ergot derivatives like bromocriptine can cause severe vasoconstriction leading peripheral gangrene.

3. **Methotrexate is used for the treatment of the following conditions:**
   (a) Rheumatoid arthritis
   (b) Choriocarcinoma
   (c) Breast cancer
   (d) Ectopic pregnancy

   1. Options (a), (c) and (d) are correct
   2. Options (a) and (b) are correct
   3. Options (a) and (d) are correct
   4. All four options are correct

Ans. 3. Options (a) and (d) are correct

Methotrexate is used for
C: Choriocarcinoma
A: Acute leukemia
N: Non-Hodgkin lymphoma
C: Crohn's disease
E: Ectopic pregnancy
R: Rheumatoid arthritis

ASSERTION REASON TYPE QUESTIONS

1. **Assertion:** Most of the beta lactams are ineffective against MRSA.

   Reason: Resistance to MRSA occurs because of production of beta lactamases
   (a) Both Assertion and Reason are correct and Reason is correct explanation of Assertion
   (b) Both Assertion and Reason are correct and Reason is not the correct explanation of Assertion
   (c) Assertion is correct and Reason is false
   (d) Reason is correct and Assertion is false
   (e) Both Assertion and Reason are false

Ans. (c) Assertion is correct and Reason is false

- MRSA is resistant to most of the beta lactams except 5th generation cephalosporins.
- However, the reason of resistance in MRSA is altered penicillin binding proteins.

2. **Assertion:** Adrenaline is added to local anaesthetics for infiltration anaesthesia.
   Reason: By preventing systemic absorption of local anaesthetic, adrenaline make them long acting and decreases the risk of cardiotoxicity
   (a) Both Assertion and Reason are correct and Reason is correct explanation of Assertion
   (b) Both Assertion and Reason are correct and Reason is not the correct explanation of Assertion
   (c) Assertion is correct and Reason is false
   (d) Reason is correct and Assertion is false
   (e) Both Assertion and Reason are false

Ans. (a) Both Assertion and Reason are correct and Reason is correct explanation of Assertion
- Adrenaline causes vasoconstriction is prevent the absorption of local anaesthetics. This has following advantages:
- Local anaesthetic stays at the site for longer time, thus duration of action increases.
- Less systemic concentration result in decreased risk of systemic adverse effects like cardiotoxicity and neurotoxicity.
- More dose of local anaesthetic can be given safely as less will reach the systemic circulation.

3. **Assertion:** Use of atorvastatin should be avoided with microsomal enzyme inhibitors like erythromycin
   Reason: Atorvastatin is an HMG CoA reductase inhibitor
   (a) Both Assertion and Reason are correct and Reason is correct explanation of Assertion
   (b) Both Assertion and Reason are correct and Reason is not the correct explanation of Assertion
   (c) Assertion is correct and Reason is false
   (d) Reason is correct and Assertion is false
   (e) Both Assertion and Reason are false

Ans. (b) Both Assertion and Reason are correct and Reason is not the correct explanation of Assertion
- Statins like atorvastatin are HMG CoA reductase inhibitors.
- Most of the statins are metabolized by CYP3A4.
- If CYP3A4 inhibitors like erythromycin are given concomitantly with statins, there is high risk of myopathy because there metabolism is inhibited.

EU GSPR Authorised Reprsentative
Logos Europe, 9 rue Nicolas Poussin
1700, La Rochelle, France
Phone: +33 (0) 6 67 93 73 78
E-mail: contact@logoseurope.eu